AUTOIMMUNI POST-COVID19 SYNDROME AND COVID-19 VACCINATION

Volume 1

FUTURE OF AUTOIMMUNITY RESEARCH

AUTOIMMUNITY, COVID-19, POST-COVID19 SYNDROME AND COVID-19 VACCINATION

Volume 1

Edited by

YEHUDA SHOENFELD
Zabludowicz Center for Autoimmune Diseases, Sheba Medical Center, Ramat Gan, Israel; Tel Aviv University, Tel Aviv, Israel

ARAD DOTAN
Zabludowicz Center for Autoimmune Diseases, Sheba Medical Center, Ramat Gan, Israel; Sackler Faculty of Medicine, Tel Aviv University, Tel Aviv, Israel

ELSEVIER

ACADEMIC PRESS
An imprint of Elsevier

Academic Press is an imprint of Elsevier
125 London Wall, London EC2Y 5AS, United Kingdom
525 B Street, Suite 1650, San Diego, CA 92101, United States
50 Hampshire Street, 5th Floor, Cambridge, MA 02139, United States
The Boulevard, Langford Lane, Kidlington, Oxford OX5 1GB, United Kingdom

ISBN: 978-0-443-18566-3

For information on all Academic Press publications visit our website at https://www.elsevier.com/books-and-journals

Publisher: Stacy Masucci
Acquisitions Editor: Wendi Baker
Editorial Project Manager: Tim Eslava
Production Project Manager: Punithavathy Govindaradjane
Cover Designer: Mark Rogers

Typeset by TNQ Technologies

Contents

5. Laboratory characteristics of cytokine storm syndrome in COVID-19 infection

Olga Y. Tkachenko, Margarita Y. Pervakova, and Sergey V. Lapin

6. COVID-19: the impact of the cytokine storm on the immune-neuroendocrine system

Luis J. Jara, Caroline I. Gutierrez-Melgarejo, Irvin Ordoñez-González, Berenice López-Zamora, Maria F. Galaviz-Sánchez, Gabriela Medina, María Pilar Cruz-Domínguez, and Olga Vera-Lastra

7. Genetic predisposition to COVID-19 and post-COVID syndrome

Anna Malkova

8. Molecular mimicry and SARS-CoV-2

Eirini I. Rigopoulou, Arad Dotan, Georgios Efthymiou, Efthymios Dardiotis, Yehuda Shoenfeld, and Dimitrios P. Bogdanos

9. *In silico* study of molecular mimicry between SARS-CoV-2 and neutrophil extracellular traps composition in granulocyte-rich supernatants of patients with systemic lupus erythematosus and lupus nephritis

Yekbun Adiguzel and Yehuda Shoenfeld

10. COVID-19 and the hyperferritinemic syndromes

G. Zandman-Goddard and M. Tocut

11. SARS-CoV-2 and microbiome: pathology, implications and therapeutic options

Maria V. Sankova, Vladimir N. Nikolenko, Sergey V. Sankov, and Mikhail Y. Sinelnikov

12. Molecular and immunological evidence for SARS-CoV-2 being the autoimmune virus

Aristo Vojdani, Avi Rosenberg, Elroy Vojdani, and Yehuda Shoenfeld

13. Autoantibodies neutralizing antiinflammatory mediators in the context of SARS-CoV-2 infection and COVID-19

Lorenz Thurner and Christoph Kessel

14. What is common to MDA5 and COVID-19?

Daniela Noa Zohar and Yehuda Shoenfeld

15. Humoral immunity and thrombosis in COVID-19

G. Lasagni, M.O. Borghi, M. Cugno, and P.L. Meroni

16. Peripheral nervous system manifestations associated with COVID-19

Tal Davidy and Ofir Zmira

17. Central nervous system impairments in COVID-19

Polina Sobolevskaia, Andrei Kolobov, and Leonid P. Churilov

18. Neuropsychiatric side of the COVID-19

Margarita A. Mayorova, Leonid P. Churilov, Natalia N. Petrova, and Yehuda Shoenfeld

19. Myocarditis following vaccination with Pfizer-BioNTech BNT162b2 against coronavirus infection (COVID-19)

Dror Mevorach

20. Rheumatic manifestations and autoimmunity associated with COVID-19

Danielle Zemer Lev, Arad Dotan, and Michael Ehrenfeld

21. SARS-CoV-2 induction and COVID-19 manifestations related to autoimmune gastrointestinal diseases

Aaron Lerner and Carina Benzvi

22. Multisystem inflammatory syndrome in children

Nina Emeršič and Tadej Avčin

23. Anosmia in COVID-19 and post-COVID syndrome

Paula David and Anna Malkova

24. The effect of COVID-19 on patients with preexisting autoimmune diseases

Olga Vera-Lastra, Alberto Ordinola Navarro, Gabriela Medina, María Pilar Cruz-Domínguez, and Luis J. Jara

30. Maternal and fetal issues in COVID-19-mediated thromboinflammation

Victoria Bitsadze, Jamilya Khizroeva, Alexander Makatsariya, Ismail Elalamy, and Jean-Christophe Gris

31. Animal models of COVID-19 and complications

N.V. Petrova, K.K. Ganina, and S.A. Tarasov

32. Risk assessment for aerosol infection by SARS-CoV-2 and protection by respirators and surgical masks

Eitan Israeli

33. Therapeutic options in COVID-19

Ehud Horwitz, Ofer Perzon, and Dror Mevorach

34. Intravenous immunoglobulin and convalescent plasma treatment in the COVID-19 patient

MariaGiovanna Danieli, Alberto Paladini, and Eleonora Antonelli

35. Interaction between vitamin D deficiency and COVID-19

Vânia Borba and Pedro Carrera-Bastos

36. Side effects of the COVID-19 vaccines

Olga Vera-Lastra, Abihai Lucas Hernández, Alberto Ordinola Navarro, and Luis J. Jara

37. The post-COVID syndrome

Soprun Lidiia, Natalia Gavrilova, Varvara A. Ryabkova, Lukashenko Maria, and Kamaeva Evelina

38. Disease course and pathogenesis of post-COVID-19 condition

Varvara A. Ryabkova and Leonid P. Churilov

39. Long-term assessment of autoantibodies in post-COVID syndrome

Natalia Gavrilova, Anna Malkova, Soprun Lidiia, Varvara A. Ryabkova, and Kamaeva Evelina

40. Post-COVID-19 syndrome and fibromyalgia

Francesco Ursini, Piero Ruscitti, and Roberto Giacomelli

41. Treatment and prevention of the post-COVID syndrome

Natalia Gavrilova, Soprun Lidiia, Varvara A. Ryabkova, Lukashenko Maria, and Kamaeva Evelina

List of contributors

Yekbun Adiguzel Department of Medical Biology, School of Medicine, Atilim University, Kizilcasar Mah, Incek, Golbasi, Ankara, Turkey

Laura Andreoli Rheumatology and Clinical Immunology Unit, ASST Spedali Civili and Department of Clinical and Experimental Sciences, University of Brescia, Brescia, Italy

Eleonora Antonelli Postgraduate School in Internal Medicine, Dipartimento di Medicina Interna, Ospedali Riuniti di Ancona and Dipartimento di Scienze Cliniche e Molecolari, Università Politecnica delle Marche, Ancona, Italy

Lambros Athanassiou Department of Rheumatology, Asclepeion Hospital, Athens, Greece

Panagiotis Athanassiou Department of Rheumatology, St. Paul's Hospital, Thessaloniki, Greece

Tadej Avčin Department of Allergology, Rheumatology and Clinical Immunology, University Children's Hospital, University Medical Center Ljubljana, Ljubljana, Slovenia; Faculty of Medicine, University of Ljubljana, Ljubljana, Slovenia

Nina Babel Center for Translational Medicine and Immune Diagnostics Laboratory, Medical Department I, Marien Hospital Herne, University Hospital of the Ruhr-University Bochum, Herne, Germany; Charité—Universitätsmedizin Berlin, Humboldt-Universität zu Berlin, Berlin Center for Advanced Therapies, Berlin, Germany

Nicole Bechmann Institute of Clinical Chemistry and Laboratory Medicine, University Hospital Carl Gustav Carus, Technische Universität Dresden, Dresden, Germany

Carina Benzvi Chaim Sheba Medical Center, Zabludowicz Research Center for Autoimmune Diseases, Ramat Gan, Israel

Victoria Bitsadze Department of Obstetrics and Gynecology, Institute of Children's Health, I.M. Sechenov First Moscow State Medical University (Sechenov University), Moscow, Russia

Dimitrios P. Bogdanos Faculty of Medicine, School of Health Sciences, University of Thessaly, Larissa, Greece

Srinivsasa Reddy Bonam Institut National de la Santé et de la Recherche Médicale, Centre de Recherche des Cordeliers, Team Immunopathologie et Immunointervention Thérapeutique, Université de Paris, Paris, France

Vânia Borba Zabludowicz Center for Autoimmune Diseases, Sheba Medical Center, Ramat Gan, Israel; Ariel University, Ariel, Israel

M.O. Borghi Immunorheumatology Research Laboratory, IRCCS Istituto Auxologico Italiano, Milan, Italy; Department of Clinical Sciences and Community Health, University of Milan, Milan, Italy

Stefan R. Bornstein Department of Internal Medicine III, University Hospital Carl Gustav Carus, Technische Universität Dresden, Dresden, Germany

Nicola Luigi Bragazzi Laboratory for Industrial and Applied Mathematics (LIAM), Department of Mathematics and Statistics, York University, Toronto, ON, Canada; Leeds Institute of Rheumatic and Musculoskeletal Medicine (LIRMM), University of Leeds, Leeds, United Kingdom

Pedro Carrera-Bastos Centre for Primary Health Care Research, Lund University/Region Skane, Skane University Hospital, Malmö, Sweden; Faculty of Biomedical and Health Sciences, Universidad Europea de Madrid, Madrid, Spain; Centro de Estudios Avanzados en Nutrición (CEAN), Córdoba, Spain

Leonid P. Churilov Laboratory of the Mosaic of Autoimmunity, Saint Petersburg State University, Saint Petersburg, Russia; Department of Pathology, Saint Petersburg State University, Saint Petersburg, Russia; Saint Petersburg Research Institute of Phthisiopulmonology, Saint Petersburg, Russia

Francesca Crisafulli Rheumatology and Clinical Immunology Unit, ASST Spedali Civili and Department of Clinical and Experimental Sciences, University of Brescia, Brescia, Italy

María Pilar Cruz-Domínguez Division of Postgraduate Studies, Faculty of Medicine, Universidad Nacional Autónoma de México, México City, México; Direction of Education and Research, Hospital de Especialidades "Dr. Antonio Fraga Mouret" Centro Médico Nacional La Raza, Instituto Mexicano del Seguro Social, México City, México

M. Cugno Department of Pathophysiology and Transplantation, University of Milan, Milan, Italy; Fondazione IRCCS Ca' Granda Ospedale Maggiore Policlinico, Internal Medicine and Angelo Bianchi Bonomi Hemophilia and Thrombosis Center, Milan, Italy

MariaGiovanna Danieli Clinica Medica, Dipartimento di Scienze Cliniche e Molecolari and Postgraduate School in Allergology and Clinical Immunology, Università Politecnica delle Marche, Ancona, Italy

Efthymios Dardiotis Department of Neurology, Faculty of Medicine, School of Health Sciences, University of Thessaly, Larissa, Greece

Paula David Internal Medicine B, Sheba Medical Center, Ramat Gan, Israel; Zabludowicz Center for Autoimmune Diseases, Sheba Medical Center, Ramat Gan, Israel

Tal Davidy Department of Neurology, Sheba Medical Center, Ramat Gan, Tel Hashomer, Israel affiliated to Sackler Faculty of Medicine, Tel Aviv University, Tel Aviv, Israel

Silvia-Ebe-Lucia Della-Pina Rheumatology and Clinical Immunology Unit, ASST Spedali Civili and Department of Clinical and Experimental Sciences, University of Brescia, Brescia, Italy

Arad Dotan Zabludowicz Center for Autoimmune Diseases, Sheba Medical Center, Ramat Gan, Israel; Sackler Faculty of Medicine, Tel Aviv University, Tel Aviv, Israel

Marie-Agnès Dragon-Durey Laboratoire d'Immunologie, Hôpital Européen Georges Pompidou, AP-HP, Paris, France; Institut National de la Santé et de la Recherche Médicale, Centre de Recherche des Cordeliers, Team Inflammation, Complement et Cancer, Université de Paris, Paris, France

Georgios Efthymiou Faculty of Medicine, School of Health Sciences, University of Thessaly, Larissa, Greece

Michael Ehrenfeld Zabludowicz Center for Autoimmune Diseases, Sheba Medical Center, Ramat Gan, Israel; Sackler Faculty of Medicine, Tel Aviv University, Tel Aviv, Israel

Ismail Elalamy Department of Obstetrics and Gynecology, Institute of Children's Health, I.M. Sechenov First Moscow State Medical University (Sechenov University), Moscow, Russia; Medicine Sorbonne University, Hematology Department of Thrombosis Center, Tenon University Hospital, Paris, France

Nina Emeršič Department of Allergology, Rheumatology and Clinical Immunology, University Children's Hospital, University Medical Center Ljubljana, Ljubljana, Slovenia

Kamaeva Evelina Laboratory of the Mosaic of Autoimmunity, Saint Petersburg State University, Saint Petersburg, Russia

Giulia Fontana Rheumatology and Clinical Immunology Unit, ASST Spedali Civili and Department of Clinical and Experimental Sciences, University of Brescia, Brescia, Italy

Franco Franceschini Rheumatology and Clinical Immunology Unit, ASST Spedali Civili and Department of Clinical and Experimental Sciences, University of Brescia, Brescia, Italy

Véronique Fremeaux-Bacchi Laboratoire d'Immunologie, Hôpital Européen Georges Pompidou, AP-HP, Paris, France

Marvin J. Fritzler Department of Medicine, Cumming School of Medicine, University of Calgary, Calgary, AB, Canada

Maria F. Galaviz-Sánchez Centro de Investigación Clínica GRAMEL, México City, México

K.K. Ganina OOO "NPF "Materia Medica Holding", Moscow, Russia

Natalia Gavrilova Department of Faculty Therapy, Saint Petersburg State University, Saint Petersburg, Russia; Department of Pulmonology, Scientific Research Institute of Phthisiopulmonology, Saint Petersburg, Russia; Saint Petersburg State University Hospital, Saint Petersburg, Russia

Roberto Giacomelli Unit of Allergology, Department of Medicine, Campus Bio-Medico University Hospital, Roma, Italy

Jean-Christophe Gris Department of Obstetrics and Gynecology, Institute of Children's Health, I.M. Sechenov First Moscow State Medical University (Sechenov University), Moscow, Russia; Hematology Department, University of Montpellier, Nimes, France

Caroline I. Gutierrez-Melgarejo Centro de Investigación Clínica GRAMEL, México City, México

Ehud Horwitz Pharmacy Division and Department of Infectious Diseases and Clinical Microbiology, Hadassah Medical Center and the Faculty of Medicine, Hebrew University, Jerusalem, Israel

Eitan Israeli Zabludowicz Center for Autoimmune Diseases, Sheba Medical Center, Ramat Gan, Israel

Etienne Jacotot Taub Institute for Research on Alzheimer's Disease and the Aging Brain, Columbia University, New York, NY, United States; Department of Pathology and Cell Biology, Columbia University, New York, NY, United States

Luis J. Jara Rheumatology Division, Instituto Nacional de Rehabilitación "Luis Guillermo Ibarra Ibarra", México City, México

Darja Kanduc Department of Biosciences, University of Bari, Bari, Italy

Christoph Kessel Department of Pediatric Rheumatology and Immunology, Translational Inflammation Research, University Children's Hospital, Münster, Germany

Jamilya Khizroeva Department of Obstetrics and Gynecology, Institute of Children's Health, I.M. Sechenov First Moscow State Medical University (Sechenov University), Moscow, Russia

Andrei Kolobov Department of Pathology, Saint Petersburg State University, Saint Petersburg, Russia

Ifigenia Kostoglou-Athanassiou Department of Endocrinology, Asclepeion Hospital, Athens, Greece

Sergey V. Lapin Laboratory for Diagnostics of Autoimmune Diseases, Center for Molecular Medicine, Saint Petersburg Pavlov State Medical University, Saint Petersburg, Russia

G. Lasagni Department of Pathophysiology and Transplantation, University of Milan, Milan, Italy

Aaron Lerner Chaim Sheba Medical Center, Zabludowicz Research Center for Autoimmune Diseases, Ramat Gan, Israel; Ariel University, Ariel, Israel

Danielle Zemer Lev Faculty of Medicine, Ben-Gurion University of the Negev, Beersheba, Israel

Soprun Lidiia Laboratory of the Mosaic of Autoimmunity, Saint Petersburg State University, Saint Petersburg, Russia; Saint Petersburg State University Hospital, Saint Petersburg, Russia

Berenice López-Zamora Instituto Politécnico Nacional, Escuela Superior de Medicina, Campus Casco de Santo Tomás, Sección de Estudios de Posgrado e Investigación, México City, México

Jose Manuel Lozano Universidad Nacional de Colombia-Sede Bogotá, Departamento de Farmacia, Mimetismo Molecular de los Agentes Infecciosos, Bogotá, DC, Colombia

Abihai Lucas Hernández Internal Medicine Department, Hospital de Especialidades "Dr. Antonio Fraga Mouret" Centro Médico Nacional La Raza, Instituto Mexicano del Seguro Social, México City, México

Alexander Makatsariya Department of Obstetrics and Gynecology, Institute of Children's Health, I.M. Sechenov First Moscow State Medical University (Sechenov University), Moscow, Russia; Russian Academy of Sciences, Moscow, Russia

Anna Malkova Ariel University, Ariel, Israel; Saint Petersburg State University, Saint Petersburg, Russia

Lukashenko Maria Laboratory of the Mosaic of Autoimmunity, Saint Petersburg State University, Saint Petersburg, Russia

Margarita A. Mayorova Laboratory of the Mosaic of Autoimmunity, Saint Petersburg State University, Saint Petersburg, Russia

Gabriela Medina Division of Postgraduate Studies, Faculty of Medicine, Universidad Nacional Autónoma de México, México City, México; Translational Research Unit, Hospital de Especialidades "Dr. Antonio Fraga Mouret" Centro Médico Nacional La Raza, Instituto Mexicano del Seguro Social, México City, México

P.L. Meroni Immunorheumatology Research Laboratory, IRCCS Istituto Auxologico Italiano, Milan, Italy

Dror Mevorach Department of Medicine B, and Division of Rheumatology-Immunology-Allergology and the Wohl Institute for Translational Medicine, Department of Medicine, Hadassah Medical Center and the Faculty of Medicine, Hebrew University, Jerusalem, Israel

Sylviane Muller Centre National de la Recherche Scientifique-Université de Strasbourg, Unit Biotechnology and Cell Signalling, Team Neuroimmunology and Peptide Therapeutics - Strasbourg Drug Discovery and Development Institute, Strasbourg, France; Fédération Hospitalo-Universitaire OMICARE, Fédération de Médecine Translationnelle de Strasbourg, University of Strasbourg, Strasbourg, France; University of Strasbourg Institute for Advanced Study, Strasbourg, France

Natalia N. Petrova Department of Psychiatry and Addiction, Saint Petersburg State University, Saint Petersburg, Russia

Vladimir N. Nikolenko First Moscow State Medical University named after I.M. Sechenov (Sechenov University), Moscow, Russia; Lomonosov Moscow State University, Moscow, Russia

Alberto Ordinola Navarro Internal Medicine Department, Hospital de Especialidades "Dr. Antonio Fraga Mouret" Centro Médico Nacional La Raza, Instituto Mexicano del Seguro Social, México City, México; Division of Postgraduate Studies, Faculty of Medicine, Universidad Nacional Autónoma de México, México City, México; Infectious Disease Department, Instituto Nacional de Ciencias Médicas y Nutrición Salvador Zubirán, México City, México

Irvin Ordoñez-González Universidad Veracruzana, Facultad de Medicina, Veracruz, México

Alberto Paladini Postgraduate School in Internal Medicine, Dipartimento di Medicina Interna, Ospedali Riuniti di Ancona and Dipartimento di Scienze Cliniche e Molecolari, Università Politecnica delle Marche, Ancona, Italy

Margarita Y. Pervakova Laboratory for Diagnostics of Autoimmune Diseases, Center for Molecular Medicine, Saint Petersburg Pavlov State Medical University, Saint Petersburg, Russia

Ofer Perzon Department of Medicine B, Hadassah Medical Center and the Faculty of Medicine, Hebrew University, Jerusalem, Israel

N.V. Petrova FSBI Institute of General Pathology and Pathophysiology RAMS, Moscow, Russia; OOO "NPF "Materia Medica Holding", Moscow, Russia

Marko Radic Department of Microbiology, Immunology and Biochemistry, College of Medicine, University of Tennessee Health Science Center, Memphis, TN, United States

Eirini I. Rigopoulou Faculty of Medicine, School of Health Sciences, University of Thessaly, Larissa, Greece

Jorge-Manuel Rodrigues-Fernandes Internal Medicine/Autoimmune Diseases Unit, Curry Cabral Hospital, Central Lisbon University Hospital Centre, Lisbon, Portugal

Avi Rosenberg Johns Hopkins Medical Institutions, Baltimore, MD, United States

Piero Ruscitti Rheumatology Unit, Department of Biotechnological and Applied Clinical Sciences, Università degli Studi dell'Aquila, L'Aquila, Italy

Varvara A. Ryabkova Laboratory of the Mosaic of Autoimmunity, Saint Petersburg State University, Saint Petersburg, Russia; Department of Pathology, Saint Petersburg State University, Saint Petersburg, Russia; Pavlov First Saint Petersburg State Medical University, Saint Petersburg, Russia

Rafael Simone Saia Laboratory of Intestinal Pathophysiology, Department of Physiology, Ribeirão Preto Medical School, University of São Paulo, Ribeirão Preto, Brazil

Sergey V. Sankov First Moscow State Medical University named after I.M. Sechenov (Sechenov University), Moscow, Russia

Maria V. Sankova First Moscow State Medical University named after I.M. Sechenov (Sechenov University), Moscow, Russia

Yehuda Shoenfeld Zabludowicz Center for Autoimmune Diseases, Sheba Medical Center, Ramat Gan, Israel; Tel Aviv University, Tel Aviv, Israel

Mikhail Y. Sinelnikov First Moscow State Medical University named after I.M. Sechenov (Sechenov University), Moscow, Russia; Research Institute of Human Morphology, Moscow, Russia; Russian Scientific Centre of Surgery named after academician B.V. Petrovsky, Moscow, Russia

Polina Sobolevskaia Laboratory of the Mosaic of Autoimmunity, Saint Petersburg State University, Saint Petersburg, Russia

Ulrik Stervbo Center for Translational Medicine and Immune Diagnostics Laboratory, Medical Department I, Marien Hospital Herne, University Hospital of the Ruhr-University Bochum, Herne, Germany

Laura Talamini Centre National de la Recherche Scientifique-Université de Strasbourg, Unit Biotechnology and Cell Signalling, Team Neuroimmunology and Peptide Therapeutics - Strasbourg Drug Discovery and Development Institute, Strasbourg, France

S.A. Tarasov FSBI Institute of General Pathology and Pathophysiology RAMS, Moscow, Russia; OOO "NPF "Materia Medica Holding", Moscow, Russia

Lorenz Thurner Department of Internal Medicine I, Hematology/Oncology, Clinical Immunology and Rheumatology, and José Carreras Center for Immuno- and Gene Therapy, Saarland University Medical School, Homburg/Saar, Germany

Angela Tincani Rheumatology and Clinical Immunology Unit, ASST Spedali Civili and Department of Clinical and Experimental Sciences, University of Brescia, Brescia, Italy; I.M. Sechenov First Moscow State Medical University of the Ministry of Health of the Russian Federation (Sechenov University), Moscow, Russia

Olga Y. Tkachenko Laboratory for Diagnostics of Autoimmune Diseases, Center for Molecular Medicine, Saint Petersburg Pavlov State Medical University, Saint Petersburg, Russia

M. Tocut Department of Internal Medicine C, Wolfson Medical Center; Sackler Faculty of Medicine, Tel Aviv University, Tel Aviv, Israel

Francesco Ursini Medicine & Rheumatology Unit, IRCCS Istituto Ortopedico Rizzoli, Bologna, Italy; Department of Biomedical and Neuromotor Sciences (DIBINEM), University of Bologna, Bologna, Italy

Olga Vera-Lastra Division of Postgraduate Studies, Faculty of Medicine, Universidad Nacional Autónoma de México, México City, México; Internal Medicine Department, Hospital de Especialidades "Dr. Antonio Fraga Mouret" Centro Médico Nacional La Raza, Instituto Mexicano del Seguro Social, México City, México

Angelica Thomaz Vieira Centre National de la Recherche Scientifique-Université de Strasbourg, Unit Biotechnology and Cell Signalling, Team Neuroimmunology and Peptide Therapeutics - Strasbourg Drug Discovery and Development Institute, Strasbourg, France; Laboratory of Microbiota and Immunomodulation, Department of Biochemistry and Immunology, Institute of Biological Sciences, Federal University of Minas Gerais, Belo Horizonte, Brazil

Aristo Vojdani Immunosciences Lab, Inc., Los Angeles, CA, United States; Cyrex Laboratories, LLC, Phoenix, AZ, United States

Elroy Vojdani Regenera Medical, Los Angeles, CA, United States

Abdulla Watad Leeds Institute of Rheumatic and Musculoskeletal Medicine (LIRMM), University of Leeds, Leeds, United Kingdom; Sheba Medical Center, Tel Aviv, Sackler Faculty of Medicine, Tel Aviv University, Tel Aviv, Israel

G. Zandman-Goddard Department of Internal Medicine C, Wolfson Medical Center; Sackler Faculty of Medicine, Tel Aviv University, Tel Aviv, Israel

Ofir Zmira Department of Neurology, Sheba Medical Center, Ramat Gan, Tel Hashomer, Israel affiliated to Sackler Faculty of Medicine, Tel Aviv University, Tel Aviv, Israel

Daniela Noa Zohar Department of Neurology, The Chaim Sheba Medical Center, Ramat Gan, Israel

About the editors

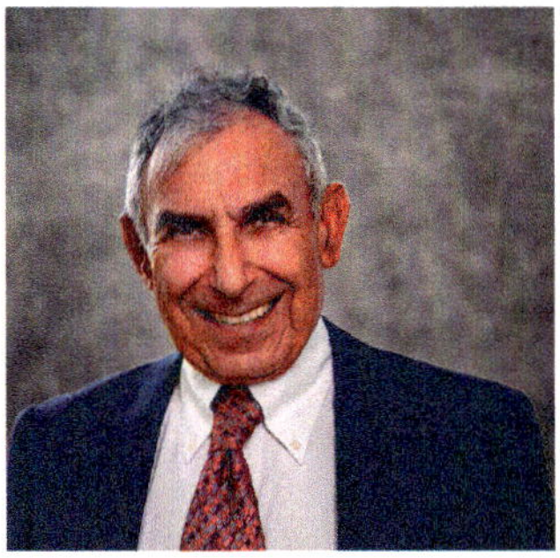

Professor Yehuda Shoenfeld, MD, FRCP, MaACR
Zabludowicz Center for Autoimmune Diseases, Sheba Medical Center, Ramat Gan, Israel; Tel Aviv University, Tel Aviv, Israel

Yehuda Shoenfeld is the Founder and Head of the Zabludowicz Center for Autoimmune Diseases, at the Sheba Medical Center, which is affiliated to the Sackler Faculty of Medicine in Tel-Aviv University, in Israel. Professor Shoenfeld was the Incumbent of the Laura Schwarz-Kipp Chair for Research of Autoimmune Diseases at the Tel-Aviv University.

Professor Shoenfeld's clinical and scientific works focus on autoimmune and rheumatic diseases, and he has published more than 2230 papers in journals such as *New Eng J Med, Nature, The Lancet, Proc Nat Acad Scie, J Clin Invest, J Immunol, Blood, FASEB, J Exp Med, Circulation, Cancer*, and others. His articles have had over 150,000 citations (H index: 130). He has written more than 350 chapters in books and has authored and edited 35 books, some of which became cornerstones in science and clinical practice, such as *The Mosaic of Autoimmunity* and *Infections and Autoimmunity* and the textbooks *Autoantibodies, Diagnostic criteria of autoimmune diseases*, and *Autoimmunity, COVID-19, Post-COVID19 Syndrome and COVID-19 Vaccination*, all of which were published by Elsevier and sold thousands of copies.

Professor Shoenfeld is on the editorial boards of 43 journals in the field of rheumatology and autoimmunity and is the Founder and the Editor of the *IMAJ* (*Israel Medical Association Journal*) the representative journal of science and medicine in the English language in Israel and also is the Founder and Editor of *Autoimmunity Reviews* (Elsevier) (Impact factor 17.3) and co-Editor of the *Journal of Autoimmunity* (Impact factor 13.3). For the past 20 years Yehuda has been the Editor of *Harefuah* – The Israel journal in medicine (Hebrew).

Professor Shoenfeld received the EULAR prize in 2005, in Vienna, Austria: "The infectious etiology of anti-phospholipid syndrome," and received a gold medal from the Slovak Society of Physicians for his contribution to Israel – Slovakia collaboration (March 2006). He is also an Honorary Member of the Hungarian Association of Rheumatology and the Royal Society of Physicians (UK). In UC Davis, USA, Professor Shoenfeld received the Nelson's Prize for Humanity and Science for 2008. In 2009 he was honored as *Doctoris Honoris Causa*, from Debrecen University (Hungary), and from 2009 he is Honorary Member of the Slovenian National Academy of Sciences. He was awarded a Life Contribution Prize in Internal Medicine in Israel, 2012, as well as the ACR Master Award in 2013. In 2019 YS was elected for the Israeli Academy of Sciences. He acted as the President of Ariel University (1920–1922). He is a member of the Israeli Academy of Sciences.

Professor Shoenfeld has educated a long list of students, more than 55 becoming Professors and Heads of departments and institutes.

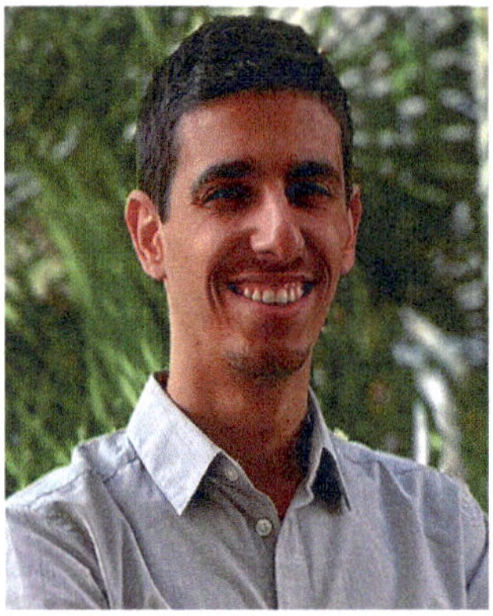

Arad Dotan
Researcher, Zabludowicz Center for Autoimmune Diseases, Sheba Medical Center, Ramat Gan, Israel; Sackler Faculty of Medicine, Tel Aviv University, Tel Aviv, Israel

Arad Dotan has a Bachelor of Medical Sciences from Ben Gurion University Medical School and Master of Public Health (MPH) from Sackler Faculty of Medicine, Tel Aviv University. Currently, he is a Researcher under the instruction of Professor Yehuda Shoenfeld at the Zabludowicz Center for Autoimmune Diseases, Sheba Medical Center, Tel-HaShomer.

Foreword

The "Severe Acute Respiratory Syndrome-related Coronavirus type 2" (SARS-CoV-2), the infectious agent responsible for the still ongoing "Coronavirus Disease 2019" (COVID-19) pandemic, represents a major environmental trigger and an important piece of the mosaic of autoimmunity and autoinflammation. Several *de novo*-onset or flares/relapses of autoimmune/autoinflammatory diseases have been reported associated either directly or indirectly with the viral agent. COVID-19 represents an - unfortunate but unique - opportunity for shedding new light and unexpected insights on virus-associated autoimmune/autoinflammatory diseases. These have, in turn, enabled the discovery of novel aspects of the COVID-19 infection, offering already approved, effective and safe drugs, as options to be repurposed in the fight against the novel coronavirus. However, there is still a dearth of information concerning the long-term impact of the virus on autoimmunity and autoinflammation—arising during post-COVID or Long COVID, which warrants further investigation.

The notion that viruses are a trigger for, and linked to the pathophysiology of, autoimmune diseases has been an accepted tenet for over half a century. Hence, it is no surprise that SARS-COV2 and COVID-19 have, from the onset of the pandemic, been implicated in a robust spectrum of autoimmune phenomena and even clinically manifested autoimmune diseases. Since it is well established that the etiology of autoimmune diseases is multifactorial (i.e., genetic, environment, sex, accelerating factors), the links of COVID-19 to autoimmune disease should include appropriate consideration of these factors and appropriate controls (e.g., age and sex-matched non-COVID acute respiratory disease).

It is widely recognized that the pathogenesis of autoimmune diseases in general, and systemic rheumatic diseases (SRD) in particular, is a multifactorial 'mosaic' that includes genetic, environmental, hormonal, and other accelerating or risk factors. Even within these 'mosaic tiles', the variables and variants are numerous, making a unified statement about how they relate to a specific SRD i.e., systemic lupus erythematosus (SLE), systemic sclerosis (SSc), autoimmune inflammatory myopathies (AIM), etc., extremely challenging.

As a matter of fact, from the onset of the SARS-COV2 pandemic in 2020, case reports, cohort studies, and meta-analyses have linked COVID-19 to autoimmunity in general and SRD in particular. The volume of SARS-CoV2 literature has increased exponentially to >2000 publications per week, resulting in a total that by far exceeds 300,000 papers. That SARS-CoV2 infection leads to an ever-widening spectrum of clinical manifestations associated with COVID-19 has been attributed to immune dysregulation evidenced as abnormalities of cytokine expression and activity, disproportionate

T-cell and B-cell levels and activities, and abnormalities of acquired and innate immunity. The pathogenic mechanisms implicating COVID-19 as a trigger of humoral and cellular autoimmune phenomena, overt SRD as well as other autoimmune diseases include increased release of self-antigens because of tissue damage, neutrophil activation and NETosis, molecular mimicry from homologous sequences of SARS-COV2 with human proteins and activation of autoreactive immune cells. A review of this literature engenders considerable debate as to whether the heightened autoinflammatory responses in COVID-19 and the immune dysregulation lead to autoimmune diseases with one consideration being that rather than triggering de novo disease, COVID-19 may only accelerate activation and progression of pre-existing sub-clinical conditions.

The timely and fast compilation of articles by outstanding experts in the field on this hot topic in this book is to be commended and will certainly attract the interest of all scientists and clinicians confronted with the multifaceted symptoms and sequelae of Covid-19.

Georg Wick, MD, Prof. emeritus
Medical University of Innsbruck, Austria

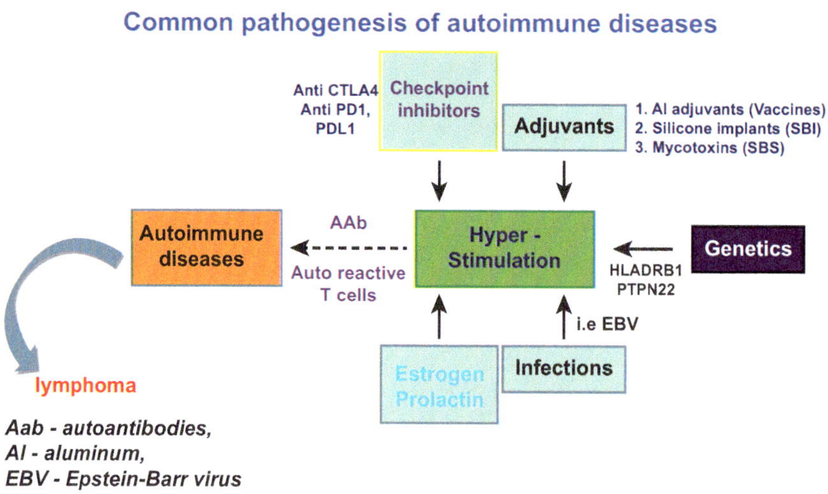

Preface

The most famous or infamous virus at the time of this writing is undoubtedly severe acute respiratory syndrome coronavirus 2 (SARS-CoV-2), the etiological agent for coronavirus disease 2019 (COVID-19). COVID-19 has become the pandemic of the new millennium, affecting hundreds of millions of people all across the globe. SARS-CoV-2 is a highly contagious disease. Unfortunately, around 20% of coronavirus-infected patients develop viral pneumonia, which may go too life-threatening. Moreover, 60% of recovered patients experience complications, such as autoimmune, endocrinal, neurological, and respiratory manifestations. This novel long-term effect of COVID-19 on recovered individuals was referred to as the "post-COVID-19 syndrome." Numerous aspects of COVID-19 raised significant concerns about the association between the virus and various autoimmune manifestations. The book aims to summarize the different links of SARS-CoV-2, COVID-19, and post-COVID-19 syndrome to autoimmunity. We hope you will enjoy the wide variety of chapters the book contains and acquire beneficial knowledge.

Yehuda Shoenfeld
Arad Dotan

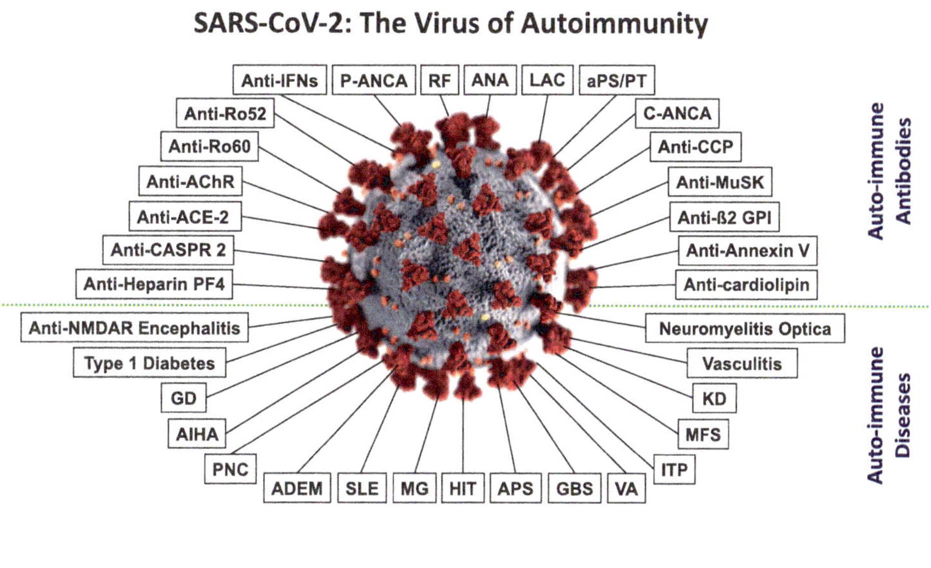

CHAPTER

1

Setting a context for autoantibodies, autoimmunity, and autoimmune diseases associated with SARS-CoV2

Marvin J. Fritzler

Department of Medicine, Cumming School of Medicine, University of Calgary, Calgary, AB, Canada

Introduction

It is widely recognized that the pathogenesis of autoimmune diseases in general, and systemic rheumatic diseases (SRD) in particular, is a multifactorial "mosaic" [1–3] that includes genetic, environmental, hormonal, and other accelerating or risk factors [4,5]. Even within these "mosaic tiles," the variables and variants are numerous making a unified statement about how they relate to a specific SRD (i.e., systemic lupus erythematous (SLE), systemic sclerosis (SSc), autoimmune inflammatory myopathies (AIM)) extremely challenging.

Virtually from the onset of the SARS-COV2 pandemic in 2020, case reports, cohort studies [2,6,7,8], and meta-analysis [9] have linked COVID-19 to autoimmunity [10–12] and SRD. The volume of SARS-CoV2 literature has increased exponentially to >2000 publications per week resulting in a total that exceeds 200,000 manuscripts [13]. SARS-CoV2 infection leading to an ever-widening spectrum of clinical manifestations associated with COVID-19 has been attributed to immune dysregulation evidenced as abnormalities of cytokine expression and activity, disproportionate T-cell and B-cell levels and activities, and abnormalities of acquired and innate immunity (reviewed in [14–17]). The pathogenic mechanisms implicating COVID-19 as a trigger of autoimmunity and SRD include increased release of self-antigens because of tissue damage, neutrophil activation and NETosis, molecular mimicry from homologous sequences of SARS-COV2 with human proteins and activation of autoreactive immune cells [14–16]. A review of this literature engenders considerable debate as to whether the heightened autoinflammatory responses in COVID-19 and the immune dysregulation leads to SRD [18–22], with one consideration being

Autoimmunity, COVID-19, Post-COVID19 syndrome and COVID-19 vaccination
https://doi.org/10.1016/B978-0-443-18566-3.00016-5

that rather than triggering de novo SRD, COVID-19 may only accelerate progression of preexisting subclinical SRD [8].

One of the puzzling issues is historical evidence that several viruses, such as Parvovirus B19, Ebstein Barr, Cytomegalovirus, Herpesvirus 6, Hepatitis A and C, and Rubella viruses, to name a few, have been identified as possible triggers of autoimmunity and SRD [12,23–27]. Even more poignantly, prior to the SARS-CoV2 pandemic, remarkable epidemics linked to other coronaviruses, such as SARS-CoV1 and Middle East Respiratory Syndrome (MERS), provide an interesting backdrop for the current coronavirus pandemic [28,29] where, by comparison to COVID-19, only a few linkages to autoimmunity were suggested [30]. Given the molecular similarity between these coronaviruses, it begs the question, "Why, then, would SARS-CoV2 have a special triggering effect"?

Early evidence suggested that concerns that SRD patients were at severe risk of COVID-19 and that SARS-CoV2 might trigger a parallel increase in SRD diagnoses currently seems misplaced since there is no convincing evidence that SLE, SSc, or other SRD had a higher infection rate, prevalence, or severe COVID-19 and, at this stage of the pandemic, no evidence that there has been a rampant increase in SRD diagnoses. Nevertheless, more recent meta-analysis and surveys of the literature tend to support the notion that COVID-19 is indeed associated with higher rates of SARS-CoV-2 infection and increased odds of mortality in SRD [9]. But, it is still unclear which factors influence SARS-CoV-2 infection in SRD such as SLE [8,31–34]. Consistent with other reports [32–34], when a local Canadian SLE cohort was compared to contemporaneous controls (individuals undergoing investigation for SRD), we found a lower rate of prepandemic seropositivity and a slightly lower to similar rate of seropositivity during the pandemic [35]. Others reported that although only 4/100 SLE patients had PCR-confirmed infection, 36% showed SARS-CoV-2 antibodies of at least one isotype, particularly IgA and IgM [31], which were also detected in prepandemic samples and had low neutralizing activity. It is likely that a number of factors influence SARS-CoV-2 infection in SLE [8,31–34], but as no prepandemic SARS-CoV2-IgG antibodies were observed in our SLE cohort [35], this seems an unlikely explanation for protection against COVID-19.

In addition to concerns that SRD patients were at higher risk of developing COVID-19, there were also concerns that the administration of SARS-CoV2 vaccines would trigger flares and worsen SRD outcomes. While long-term studies of large cohorts are yet to be completed, one study reported that <15% of SLE patients reported a "typical" flare after SARS-CoV-2 vaccination [36]. However, the majority of flares were reported as "moderate to severe" and some lasted >3 weeks. Although the low rate of flares is reassuring, potential confounders and concurrent laboratory and prospective clinical studies have yet to be reported in detail. Similarly, AIM patients receiving the Sinovac-CoronaVac vaccine at 28-day intervals had apparently normal responses irrespective of type of AIM, disease status, prescribed drugs or comorbidities [37]. In addition, vaccine-related adverse events were mild with similar frequencies in AIM patients and controls.

"Causes" of autoimmune diseases: a "mosaic" of genetic, environmental, and hormonal factors

It is well known and widely appreciated that the causes of autoimmune diseases, and SRD in particular, are multifactorial, primarily attributable to a mosaic [2] of genetic, environmental, and/or hormonal factors that in many individuals define a "risk" [4,38]. Even so-called drug-induced autoimmunity or lupus, which can be traced to a single initiating factor (procainamide, hydralazine, biologicals), require appropriate genetic and other environmental factors for progression to clinically diagnosed disease [39–41]. A thorough discussion of these factors and their implications in COVD-19-induced SRD would require a separate detailed discussion. Hence, only a broad overview and a reminder is provided here.

It is assumed that if SARS-CoV2 was a key factor in the induction of autoimmunity, it would be expected that the genes that confer high risk for SLE [42] or other SARD would also be identified in those who developed features of a SRDs. However, after numerous genetic studies, there are interesting comparisons (Table 1.1) but clear evidence showing overlaps between the "at risk" genes of developing severe COVID-19 and an autoimmune disease are lacking. Recently, robust genetic signals relating to key host antiviral defense mechanisms (i.e., antiviral restriction enzyme activators OAS1, OAS2, OAS3; in the interferon receptor

TABLE 1.1 Comparison of selected risk factors implicated in autoimmune diseases and COVID-19.

Risk factor	Autoimmune diseases	COVID-19	References
Genetics	Interferon signature; IRF-5, -7, -8; PTPN22; BLK, HLADRB1; STAT4	Interferon receptor gene IFNAR2; TYK2; ACE2; TLR7; ABO blood group locus	[42–44]
Autoantibodies capable of neutralizing type I IFN	Related to subsets of SLE, RA, SSc and SjS	Increased risk and severity	[45–48]
Selective IgA deficiency	Increased prevalence	Increased risk severe disease. More systematic studies needed	[49,50]
Age (years)	Young <45	Elderly >65	[51–55]
Sex	Primarily postpubertal females	Males	[55–57]
Hormonal status	Postpubertal/child-bearing	Postmenopausal; decreased fertility	[55,57] [58–60]
Ultraviolet/vitamin D	Decreased increased risk	Decreased increased risk	[61–63]
Air pollution	Increased risk; particulates an etiologic factor	Increased risk	[64–66]
Cigarette smoking	Increased risk	Risk of severe COVID-19 not increased	[55,67]
Obesity	Contributed to onset and progression. Role of adipokines	Increased risk. But lower BMI in MIS	[61,68–72]

Abbreviations: *AD*, autoimmune diseases; *BLK*, B lymphoid tyrosine kinase; *IFNAR2*, interferon receptor two; *IRF*, interferon regulatory factor; *MIS*, multi-inflammatory syndrome; *PTPN22*, Protein tyrosine phosphatase nonreceptor type 22; *RA*, rheumatoid arthritis; *SjS*, Sjögren syndrome; *SLE*, systemic lupus erythematosus; *SRD*, systemic rheumatic diseases; *SSc*, systemic sclerosis; *STAT4*, signal transducer and activator of transcription four; *TLR*, toll-like receptor; *TYK2*, tyrosine kinase type2.

gene IFNAR2); and mediators of inflammatory organ damage (i.e., tyrosine kinase 2 (TYK2); dipeptidyl peptidase 9 (DPP9) in COVID-19 have been reported [73]. Of note, aberrant interferon responses and "signatures" have held great interest in autoimmune diseases, particularly in SLE [74,75] and, unsurprisingly, defects in interferon, including autoantibodies to type I interferon are associated with the severity of COVID-19 [45,46,76,77]. However, as discussed later it is not clear if these "at risk" genetic signatures are unique to SARS-CoV2 or whether they are a more general feature of acute viral illnesses with particular damage to respiratory cells.

Similarly, environmental and 'lifestyle" factors, such as cigarette smoking, air pollution, ultraviolet light and vitamin D deficiency, infections, vaccinations, solvents, pesticides, and heavy metals, have a long history of being linked to autoimmunity and SRD [51,78–80] and some similarities but significant differences are noted in COVID-19 (Table 1.1). For example, the life-style demographic of "obese, elderly males" as high risk factors for developing severe COVID-19 stands in stark contrast to the hormonal and sex profiles of SRD patients who tend to be predominantly females of child-bearing age [51–54] (Table 1.1).

Moving from a comparison and contrast of COVID-19-related SRD and the prepandemic understanding of the "mosaic" of autoimmunity, it is important to appreciate key parameters that are also important in understanding SARS-Cov2 in the context of autoimmunity and SRD (Table 1.2).

Historical context

To understand the validity of claims that SARS-CoV2 virus and its severe clinical associate COVID-19 or SARS-CoV2 vaccines are responsible for triggering or "causing" autoimmune diseases or flares of SRD, it is important to evaluate these claims on the historical background of the etiology and pathogenesis of autoimmune diseases. As discussed above, one of the striking observations is the remarkable outpouring of reports of SRDs linked to SARS-CoV2 even though SARS-CoV2 is only one of several coronaviruses that infect humans. Clearly, despite having significant structural, molecular, and pathogenic features, these earlier coronaviruses did not engender the avalanche of literature linking them to autoimmunity, autoimmune disease or SRD. Further, follow-up studies of "long COVID" [15,81–83],

TABLE 1.2 Factors to consider in understanding the importance of autoimmunity in the context of the SARS-CoV2 pandemic.

- Historical Context: is SARS-CoV2 different from previous coronavirus epidemics
- The importance of controls and comparators
- Phenomenology is not pathology
- Time and timing
    - Temporarily does not equal causality
    - Studies of population-based cohorts' preinfection through infection, hospitalization and recovery
    - Sequential analysis of clinical features and biomarkers in individuals
- Role of mechanotransduction—Piezos and beyond

multiinflammatory syndrome (MIS) and "Kawasaki-like disease" in children or adults reported in SARS-CoV2 [43,84–87] was scarcely heard during other coronavirus outbreaks [30] such as SARS-CoV1 or MERs epidemics. Because of questionable links of a variety of factors including SARS-COV2 infections to autoimmune diseases, as discussed later in the section "phenomenology is not pathology," and there is a need to reconsider principles once included in Witebsky's criteria.

Controls and comparators

Controls used for any study linking an agent (e.g., SARS-CoV2) to autoimmune diseases or SRD are critical to interpretation of the results. Although observations of autoantibodies in severe COVID19 patients were reported to be associated with certain clinical features suggesting a possible causal link [19,88–90] (Table 1.3), the null hypothesis that COVID19+ individuals have the same autoimmune phenomena as similar critically ill patients was not disproven [14,17]. In many published studies, lack of proper contemporaneous controls has hindered or biased this determination. Some studies used apparently healthy controls while others stratified COVID-19 cohorts according to nominal mild, moderate, or severe

TABLE 1.3 Selected reports of autoantibodies in SARS-CoV2 and COVID-19.

Authors (reference)	COVID (N)	Controls/ Comparators	Sampling	Primary results conclusions	Comments
Lerma et al. [91]	64 27 ICU Mean age 58.3	None	CS: Single 4–37 days after Dx	30% had at least one AAB; 42% in ICU patients. AAB status not different in deceased Acute COVID-19 not associated with high prevalence SARD-AAB.	Most common ENA: anti-U1-RNP 12.5% 10.9% had previous Hx of AD. Mean age of AAB + [43] not different from AAB—[53]
Gazzarusa et al. [88]	45 hospitalized	None	CS: Single on admission	ANA 35.6%; LAC 11.1%; Anti-Ro52 4.4%; ANCA 6.6%	
Pascolini et al. [89]	33 hospitalized	25 COVID- age and sex "matched" with fever and/or pneumonia; 14 excluded because of negative PCR tests	CS: Single on admission	45.5% at least one AAB; 33% +ve ANA; 24.6% IgG ACL; 9.1% Igg or IgM anti-β2GP; 0% ANCA Patients with poor prognosis (death) had higher frequency of AAB (86% vs. 27%)	14 important comparators excluded from the study.
Sacchi et al. [90]	40 hospitalized Mean age 66.8 28M/12F	40 blood donors: no Hx of AD	"After admission"	ANA ≥1:80 57.5%; ANCA 10%; ACL 12.5%; anti-β2GP1 5%; ENA 2.5%	

(Continued)

TABLE 1.3 Selected reports of autoantibodies in SARS-CoV2 and COVID-19.—cont'd

Authors (reference)	COVID (N)	Controls/ Comparators	Sampling	Primary results conclusions	Comments
Trahtemberg et al. [14,17]	22 ICU COVID-19	20 ICU non-COVID	Longitudinal from admission to ICU	64% +ve ANA >+1:160; 38% ENA; 31% myositis-related aab; 38% anticytokine	No differences were found between COVID+ And COVID− For ANA, ENA or anticytokines
Chang et al. [19]	147 hospitalized	Healthy controls	50 samples collected longitudinally	10/73 (14%) ANA ≥1:160 1/73 (1.4%) anti-dsDNA; 1/73 (1.4%) anti-PR3; 0/73 anti-MPO; 25/51 (49%–58%) antibodies to 'traditional' CTD antigens (most common 50% antiribosomal P)	Different cohorts used for separate studies for frequency of ENA.

Abbreviations: *AAB*, autoantibodies; *AD*, autoimmune disease; *CS*, cross-sectional; *Dx*, diagnosis; *ENA*, extractable nuclear antigens; *Hx*, history; *NS*, not stated; *PCR*, primer chain reaction; *SARD*, systemic autoimmune rheumatic diseases; *RNP*, ribonucleoprotein.

disease severity. While this approach may provide comparisons of biomarkers associated with disease severity outcomes, it does not demonstrate that the biomarkers of interest are specific for SARS-CoV2 infection, nor does it provide evidence of a specific role of SARS-CoV2 as a specific inducer of autoimmunity or SRD. Confounding factors such as medications, preexisting autoimmune illnesses, and other comorbidities also need to be taken into consideration. In our published studies [14,17], we concluded that severe COVID-19 patients have similar autoantibodies and other proteomic biomarkers as compared to contemporaneous, similarly ill (e.g., ICU admission) non-COVID-19 patients. We showed that many proteomic biomarkers, particularly autoantibodies, are seen in critical illness regardless of COVID-19 status. An interpretation of the data to date should be taken to conclude that autoantibody production is a feature of immune dysfunction associated with acute systemic illness rather than a specific SARS-CoV2 driven immunopathology. This, of course, does not infer that SARS-CoV2-specific autoantibodies that associate with long-COVID and MIS will not be found.

Phenomenology is not pathology

Next, autoimmune phenomena (autoantibodies, dysregulated cytokines) should not be equated to autoimmune disease. Some attention has focused on autoantibodies such as anti-dsDNA and antiphospholipid antibodies that are thought to be "pathogenic." Historically, the Witebski criteria were developed and, up to approximately a decade ago, they were the benchmark by which claims of autoimmune disease "causes" were judged [92]. These criteria required that 1) an autoimmune reaction was identified in the form of an autoantibody or cell-mediated immune factor, 2) the corresponding antigenic target was known, and 3) an analogous response caused a similar disease in experimental animals. Hence, these three general criteria required direct evidence based on transfer of pathogenic antibody or pathogenic T cells and indirect evidence based on reproduction of the autoimmune disease in experimental animals, all in the context of circumstantial evidence from clinical observations. Today, because of scientific advancements, the Witebski criteria have largely fallen to the wayside because of logistic and even ethical challenges. For example, it is considered unethical to apply these criteria to studies of humans (e.g., transferring autoantibodies, immune activated cells, or instilling a disease "factor" (aberrant or mutated genes) into a human and studies in animals (e.g., mice) [93,94]. By no means do these claims indicate that animal models should not be considered because historically their use has been a very productive ground for investigation and breakthrough discoveries [94,95]. However, there is also the realization that what is observed in animals is often very difficult to replicate in or transfer to humans [94,96,97].

Time and timing is of the essence

Temporarily does not equal causality

The temporal appearance of an AD or SRD that developed during the pandemic in an individual should not be equated to causality. An important consideration for assessing autoimmune phenomena among critically ill patients is the need for longitudinal sampling and clinical follow-up because the development of AAB is time dependent. Therefore, a "snapshot" at arbitrary times (e.g., cross-sectional studies) is unable to capture this process.

Except for, one example, acute onset or catastrophic antiphospholipid syndrome (APS), it has been long appreciated that most autoimmune diseases and SRD take years to evolve into full-fledged disease [98,99]. Typically, SRD progress through a preclinical (perhaps asymptomatic) phase and then progress to a symptomatic phase where they may be categorized as undifferentiated autoimmune disease and then finally to full-blown disease where a patient has the key signs and symptoms and fulfills either diagnostic or classification criteria for an SRD [100–102]. It is in this context that it is important to appreciate that long-term studies will likely be required to determine the true impact of COVID-19 on human health, not to mentions SRDs. Ideally, a pre-COVD-19 cohort of uninfected individuals would be enrolled in longitudinal studies and then followed and evaluated from first symptoms SARS-COV2 infection, the development of RT-PCR confirmed COVID-19, hospital admission, discharge, and then long-term follow-up are important to truly understand if SARS-CoV2 is a key "trigger" of autoimmune disease and SRD. Our studies [14,17] provided evidence that, when observed longitudinally from admission to an intensive care unit (ICU) and then throughout hospitalization, severe COVID-19 patients had a similar autoantibody prevalence and profile as a contemporaneous comparator cohort of critically ill patients also admitted to the ICU.

Clearly, some autoimmune diseases, such as Guillain-Barré syndrome, autoimmune hemolytic anemia, and idiopathic thrombocytopenic purpura, have been convincingly attributed to SARS-CoV2 infection, but Guillain-Barré syndrome, for one, is a long-known sequelae of a number of acute viral diseases, vaccine administration, and malignancies [12,103].

Nobel 2021 PIEZO touch and temperature: COVID-19 myopathy

On October 10, 2021 it was announced that the 2021 Nobel Prize in Physiology or Medicine was jointly awarded to David Julius and Ardem Patapoutian [104]. David Julius's work focused on a novel ion channel protein which was a newly discovered capsaicin receptor named TRPV1. The discovery of TRPV1 was a major breakthrough leading to the unraveling of additional temperature-sensing receptors. Independently of one another, both David Julius and Ardem Patapoutian used the chemical substance menthol to identify TRPM8, a receptor that was shown to be activated by cold. Additional ion channels related to TRPV1 and TRPM8 were identified and found to be activated by a range of different temperatures. Ardem Patapoutian, working at the Scripps Research Institute in La Jolla, California, pursued the identity of receptors that are activated by mechanical stimuli [105]. During these studies, his laboratory discovered a novel mechanosensitive ion channel that was named Piezo1 (from Greek for pressure (í; píesi)). Eventually, a second gene named Piezo2 was discovered which was highly expressed in sensory neurons. Piezo1 and Piezo2 are ion channels directly activated on the application of pressure on cell membranes [105,106].

At first glance, it may not be apparent how these discoveries have direct relevance to SARS-COV2, COVID-19, and autoimmune diseases. Certainly, patients with severe acute respiratory distress syndrome (e.g., COVID-19) who die, usually succumb to multiorgan failure as opposed to hypoxia primarily attributed to a rampant systemic inflammatory response [107]. Even with effective use of therapeutic modalities that include extracorporeal membrane oxygenation, proning and mechanic ventilation (MV), some patients' continue on a downward spiral that is hypothetically linked to the MV used to treat the respiratory failure through a process called “"ventilator-induced lung injury" (VILI) [108], ICU-associated weakness (ICUAW) [109–111], or critical illness myopathy (CIM). Studies indicate that approximately 50% of critically ill patients on MV for more than 7 days develop CIM [112] resulting in prolonged ICU care as well as increased morbidity and mortality [110,111]. There is growing evidence that alterations of both the magnitude and the pattern of stretching the lung, results in gene expression changes accompanied by altered cellular metabolism resulting in overwhelming inflammatory and other mediator responses. This mechanism of injury has been termed “biotrauma” [107].

As discussed above, there is little evidence directly linking SARS-CoV2 and/or COVID-19 to SRD. However, a growing number of studies, including our own [14], strongly suggest that an exception may be a myopathy that bears some biomarker hallmarks (i.e., AIM-related autoantibodies) of immune-mediated necrotizing myopathy [14,113–121]. The presence of inflammatory cell infiltrates in muscle, including predominantly CD68+ macrophages and CD8+ T-cells but rare CD4+ T-cells, is compatible with an autoinflammatory process in critically ill patients [122]. In two recently reported autopsy studies, immunostaining of skeletal muscle for SARS-CoV2 markers was negative [120,121]. However, this may be explained by postmortem changes because of a prolonged (~6 days) post-mortem interval. As support for this consideration, positive RT-qPCR signals for SARS-CoV-2 were found in at least 16% (7/41) of quadriceps and 5% (2/42) of deltoid muscles [121].

ICUAW/CIM has been attributed to muscle atrophy and loss of myosin, impaired contractility, neuropathy, and molecular pathways of muscle protein degradation through the the ubiquitin proteasome system and dysregulated autophagy. Although the pathogenesis of

CIM/ICUAW is incompletely understood, there is convincing evidence that a critical mechanism involves mitochondrial dysfunction and compromised energy production related to reduced mitochondrial generation of ATP [122], which may be attributed to mitochondrial damage aggravated by inflammation, hyperglycemia, and/or free radical generation. The risk factors associated with ICUAW/CIM are described, but the impact of interventions that may alter these changes such as neuromuscular blockade, proning, and antiinflammatory drugs (i.e., corticosteroids) are not well understood. In addition, akin to studies cited above, it is unknown whether the COVID-19-associated ICUAW/CIM or biotrauma differs from other infections and sepsis that cause acute respiratory failure requiring MV [112] or whether direct viral infection of muscle is a necessary pathogenic component [123].

Turning back to the Nobel Prize work of Patapoutian and others, several interesting observations link Piezo1 to the myopathy seen in ICUAW/CIM and biotrauma. For example, interelukin-1 (IL-1), implicated in "cytokine storm" and the inflammasome of COVID-19 [124,125], increases Piezo1 expression in cells resulting in increased intracellular Ca^{++} [126]. IL-1, modulating Piezo1 expression, also lead to increased unraveling of cytoskeletal F-actin and cell deformation resulting in cell stress and death. This is further compounded by an altered alveolo-capillary barrier, a critical feature of severe COVID-19 [127].

Another interesting potential link is the relationship of Piezo1 to hyperferritinemic states such as that described in COVID-19 where overexuberant cytokine release is associated with hyperferritinemia [128]. Very high levels of ferritin occur in other diseases including hemophagocytic lymphohistiocytosis, macrophage activation syndrome, adult-onset Still's disease, catastrophic ASP, and septic shock, as discussed above all reported as part of the autoinflammatory/autoimmune spectrum of SARS-CoV2 [129–131]. High levels of free iron are known to have a deleterious effect on tissues, especially through redox damage leading to organ and tissue fibrosis.

Of interest, iron overload has been linked to Piezo1 [132] as evidenced by studies of hereditary xerocytosis, a rare disorder with gain of function mutations in PIEZO1 associated with iron overload. In addition, it was shown that mechanotransduction mediated by Piezo1 is a key regulator of macrophage phagocytic activity and erythrocyte turnover [132].

Taken together, a study of Piezo1 and other mechanotransduction molecules has potentially interesting links to COVID-19 that may be initiated and/or exacerbated by MV resulting in ICUAW/CIM or biotrauma and accompanying autoimmune and autoinflammatory features that over the long-term may progress to AIM. The potential link of MV to Piezo1 and Piezo2 (or any of the other cellular mechanotranducers) [105] to AIMs in the setting COVID-19 is worthy of study.

Summary

Numerous reports have suggested a link of SARS-CoV2 to autoimmunity, autoimmune diseases, and SRD. While the pandemic has prompted a very "fertile" field for research, with very few exceptions (e.g., Guillain Barré syndrome, autoimmune hemolytic anemia) [133] these linkages are unconvincing. However, it is important to appreciate that the evolution of SARS-CoV2 triggered autoimmunity to full blown disease will likely take years and perhaps, more than a decade. Hence, continuing attention to SARS-COV2 cohorts is warranted. One potentially important SRD is AIM where several factors, including biotrauma as result of MV may have long-term consequences and identify the leading edge of a COVID-19 AIM. Last, many studies have focused and reported on rather esoteric proteomic biomarkers and or their platforms that are not in clinical use today (e.g., not CE marked, N or 510K approved by FDA). Because of that, the "translational" aspects of determining if the repertoire of proteomic biomarkers (including autoantibodies) is worth pursuing or if some will quietly be related to the "death valley" of innovation [134].

References

[1] Shepshelovich D, Shoenfeld Y. Prediction and prevention of autoimmune diseases: additional aspects of the mosaic of autoimmunity. Lupus 2006;15:183–90.

[2] Mahroum N, Zoubi M, Lavine N, Ohayon A, Amital H, Shoenfeld Y. The mosaic of autoimmunity - a taste for more. The 12th international congress of autoimmunity 2021 (AUTO12) virtual. Autoimmun Rev September 9, 2021;20(11):102945. https://doi.org/10.1016/j.autrev.2021.102945.

[3] Gershwin ME. The mosaic of autoimmunity. Autoimmun Rev January 2008;7:161–3. https://doi.org/10.1016/j.autrev.2007.11.021.

[4] Xiao ZX, Miller JS, Zheng SG. An updated advance of autoantibodies in autoimmune diseases. Autoimmun Rev December 14, 2020;20(2):102743. https://doi.org/10.1016/j.autrev.2020.102743.

[5] Gupta S, Kaplan MJ. Bite of the wolf: innate immune responses propagate autoimmunity in lupus. J Clin Invest February 1, 2021;131:e144918. https://doi.org/10.1172/JCI144918.

[6] Bonometti R, Sacchi MC, Stobbione P, Lauritano EC, Tamiazzo S, Marchegiani A, et al. The first case of systemic lupus erythematosus (SLE) triggered by COVID-19 infection. Eur Rev Med Pharmacol Sci September 2020;24:9695–7.

[7] Galeotti C, Bayry J. Autoimmune and inflammatory diseases following COVID-19. Nat Rev Rheumatol August 2020;16:413–4. https://doi.org/10.1038/s41584-020-0448-7.

[8] Hsu TY, D'Silva KM, Patel NJ, Fu X, Wallace ZS, Sparks JA. Incident systemic rheumatic disease following COVID-19. Lancet Rheumatol June 2021;3:e402–4. https://doi.org/10.1016/S2665-9913(21)00106-5. Online.

[9] Conway R, Grimshaw AA, Konig MF, Putman M, Duarte-GarcÃa A, Tseng LY, et al. SARS-CoV-2 infection and COVID-19 outcomes in rheumatic disease: a systematic literature review and meta-analysis. Arthritis Rheumatol November 22, 2021. https://doi.org/10.1002/art.42030. Nov 22.ahead of print:.

[10] Ehrenfeld M, Tincani A, Andreoli L, Cattalini M, Greenbaum A, Kanduc D, et al. Covid-19 and autoimmunity. Autoimmun Rev August 2020;19:102597. https://doi.org/10.1016/j.autrev.2020.102597.

[11] Li J. The role of autoantibodies in arrhythmogenesis. Curr Cardiol Rep November 25, 2020;23:3–01430.

[12] Yazdanpanah N, Rezaei N. Autoimmune complications of COVID-19. J Med Virol January 2022;94:54–62. https://doi.org/10.1002/jmv.27292.

[13] National Insittues of Health, National Library of Medicine. LitCOVID. Online Source: https://www.ncbi.nlm.nih.gov/research/coronavirus. Last accessed 11/22/2021.

[14] Trahtemberg U, Fritzler MJ. On behalf of the COVID-19 chapter of the "Longitudinal Biomarkers in Lung Injury" study groupCollaborators. COVID-19-associated autoimmunity as a feature of acute respiratory failure. Intensive Care Med April 30, 2021;47(7):801–4. https://doi.org/10.1007/s00134-021-06408-z.

[15] Dotan A, Muller S, Kanduc D, David P, Halpert G, Shoenfeld Y. The SARS-CoV-2 as an instrumental trigger of autoimmunity. Autoimmun Rev February 18, 2021;20(4):102792. https://doi.org/10.1016/j.autrev.2021.102792.

[16] Berger J, Volc S. Autoantibodies in COVID-19 - a model for viral induced autoimmunity. J Eur Acad Dermatol Venereol September 2021;35:e571–3.

[17] Trahtemberg U, Rottapel R, Dos Santos CC, Slutsky AS, Baker A, Fritzler MJ. Anticardiolipin and other antiphospholipid antibodies in critically ill COVID-19 positive and negative patients. Ann Rheum Dis April 26, 2021;80(9):1236–40. https://doi.org/10.1136/annrheumdis-2021-220206.

[18] Gao ZW, Zhang HZ, Liu C, Dong K. Autoantibodies in COVID-19: frequency and function. Autoimmun Rev January 18, 2021;20(3):102754. https://doi.org/10.1016/j.autrev.2021.102754.

[19] Chang SE, Feng A, Meng W, Apostolidis SA, Mack E, Artandi M, et al. New-onset IgG autoantibodies in hospitalized patients with COVID-19. Nat Commun September 14, 2021;12:5417–25509. https://doi.org/10.1038/s41467-021-25509-3.

[20] Meroni PL, Borghi MO. Antiphospholipid antibodies and COVID-19 thrombotic vasculopathy: one swallow does not make a summer. Ann Rheum Dis August 2, 2021;80(9):1105–7. https://doi.org/10.1136/annrheumdis-2021-220520.

[21] Nikpour M, Teh B, Wicks IP, Pellegrini M. Correspondence regarding research letter to the editor by Mathian et al, 'Clinical course of coronavirus disease 2019 (COVID-19) in a series of 17 patients with systemic lupus under long-term treatment with hydroxychloroquine. Ann Rheum Dis May 29, 2020:217827. https://doi.org/10.1136/annrheumdis-2020-217827. May 29;annrheumdis. Online ahead of print.

[22] Mathian A, Amoura Z. Response to: correspondence regarding research letter to the editor by Mathian et al, 'Clinical course of coronavirus disease 2019 (COVID-19) in a series of 17 patients with systemic lupus under long-term treatment with hydroxychloroquine'' by Nikpour et al. Ann Rheum Dis May 29, 2020:217875. https://doi.org/10.1136/annrheumdis-2020-217875. May 29;annrheumdis-2020-217875. Online ahead of print.

[23] Smatti MK, Cyprian FS, Nasrallah GK, Al Thani AA, Almishal RO, Yassine HM. Viruses and autoimmunity: a review on the potential interaction and molecular mechanisms. Viruses August 2019;11(8):11080762. https://doi.org/10.3390/v11080762.

[24] Gugliesi F, Pasquero S, Griffante G, Scutera S, Albano C, Pacheco SFC, et al. Human Cytomegalovirus and autoimmune diseases: where are we? Viruses February 8, 2021;13:260.

[25] Pordeus V, Szyper-Kravitz M, Levy RA, Vaz NM, Shoenfeld Y. Infections and autoimmunity: a panorama. Clin Rev Allergy Immunol June 2008;34:283–99.

[26] de Andrade VP, De Souza FHC, Behrens Pinto GL, Shinjo SK. The relevance of anti-Jo-1 autoantibodies in patients with definite dermatomyositis. Adv Rheumatol February 2021;61:12–00171. %19.

[27] Coarelli G, Darios F, Petit E, Dorgham K, Adanyeguh I, Petit E, et al. Plasma neurofilament light chain predicts cerebellar atrophy and clinical progression in spinocerebellar ataxia. Neurobiol Dis February 23, 2021;153:105311. https://doi.org/10.1016/j.nbd.2021.105311.:105311.

[28] Huang AT, Garcia-Carreras B, Hitchings MDT, Yang B, Katzelnick LC, Rattigan SM, et al. A systematic review of antibody mediated immunity to coronaviruses: kinetics, correlates of protection, and association with severity. Nat Commun September 17, 2020;11(1):4704–18450. https://doi.org/10.1038/s41467-020-18450-4.

[29] Abdelghany TM, Ganash M, Bakri MM, Qanash H, Al-Rajhi AMH, Elhussieny NI. SARS-CoV-2, the other face to SARS-CoV and MERS-CoV: future predictions. Biomed J January 5, 2021;44(1):86–93. https://doi.org/10.1016/j.bj.2020.10.008.

[30] Esper F, Shapiro ED, Weibel C, Ferguson D, Landry ML, Kahn JS. Association between a novel human coronavirus and Kawasaki disease. J Infect Dis February 15, 2005;191(4):499–502. https://doi.org/10.1086/428291.

[31] Sjöwall J, Azharuddin M, Frodlund M, Zhang Y, Sandner L, Dahle C, et al. SARS-CoV-2 antibody isotypes in systemic lupus erythematosus patients prior to vaccination: associations with disease activity, antinuclear antibodies, and immunomodulatory drugs during the first year of the pandemic. Front Immunol August 27, 2021;12:724047. https://doi.org/10.3389/fimmu.2021.724047.

[32] Aringer M. Systemic lupus erythematosus does not prevent antibody responses to SARS-CoV-2. Lancet Rheumatol May 27, 2021;3(8):e538–40. https://doi.org/10.1016/S2665-9913(21)00153-3.

[33] Saxena A, Guttmann A, Masson M, Kim MY, Haberman RH, Castillo R, et al. Evaluation of SARS-CoV-2 IgG antibody reactivity in patients with systemic lupus erythematosus: analysis of a multi-racial and multi-ethnic cohort. Lancet Rheumatol May 27, 2021;3(8):e585–94. https://doi.org/10.1016/S2665-9913(21)00114.

[34] Ammitzbøl C, Andersen JB, Vils SR, Mistegaard CE, Mikkelsen S, Erikstrup C, et al. Isolation, behavioral changes and low seroprevalence of SARS-CoV-2 antibodies in patients with Systemic Lupus Erythematosus or Rheumatoid arthritis. Arthritis Care Res May 31, 2021. https://doi.org/10.1002/acr.24716. May 31. Online ahead of print.

[35] Mathew HR, Choi MY, Buhler K, Gukova X, Cardwell FS, Waldhauser H, et al. SARS-CoV-2 seroprevalence, seroconversion and neutralizing antibodies in a systemic lupus erythematosus cohort and comparison to controls. Lupus 2021;30(14):2318–20. https://doi.org/10.1177/09612033211063793.

[36] Barbhaiya M, Levine JM, Bykerk VP, Jannat-Khah D, Mandl LA. Systemic rheumatic disease flares after SARS-CoV-2 vaccination among rheumatology outpatients in New York City. Ann Rheum Dis June 22, 2021. https://doi.org/10.1136/annrheumdis-2021-220732. Jun 22 Online ahead of print.

[37] Shinjo SK, De Souza FHC, Borges IBP, Dos Santos AM, Miossi R, Misse RG, et al. Systemic autoimmune myopathies: a prospective phase 4 controlled trial of an inactivated virus vaccine against SARS-CoV-2. Rheumatology October 2021. https://doi.org/10.1093/rheumatology/keab773. Oct 19 Online ahead of print.

[38] Rodrigues EPS, Abreu IN, Lima CNC, da Fonseca DLM, Pereira SFG, Dos Reis LC, et al. High prevalence of anti-SARS-CoV-2 IgG antibody in the xikrin of BacajÃ¡ (KayapÃ³) indigenous population in the brazilian amazon. Int J Equity Health January 28, 2021;20:50–01392.

[39] Rubin RL. Drug-induced lupus. Expet Opin Drug Saf January 2, 2015;14:361–78.

[40] Vaglio A, Grayson PC, Fenaroli P, Gianfreda D, Boccaletti V, Ghiggeri GM, et al. Drug-induced lupus: traditional and new concepts. Autoimmun Rev July 10, 2018;17:912–8.

[41] He Y, Sawalha AH. Drug-induced lupus erythematosus: an update on drugs and mechanisms. Curr Opin Rheumatol September 2018;30:490–7.

[42] Guerra SG, Vyse TJ, Cunninghame Graham DS. The genetics of lupus: a functional perspective. Arthritis Res Ther May 29, 2012;14:211.

[43] Schulert GS, Blum SA, Cron RQ. Host genetics of pediatric SARS-CoV-2 COVID-19 and multisystem inflammatory syndrome in children. Curr Opin Pediatr September 15, 2021;33(6):549–55. https://doi.org/10.1097/MOP.0000000000001061.

[44] Shibeeb S, Khan A. ABO blood group association and COVID-19. COVID-19 susceptibility and severity: a review. Hematol Transfus Cell Ther September 2021;14:10.

[45] Bastard P, Rosen LB, Zhang Q, Michailidis E, Hoffmann HH, Zhang Y, et al. Auto-antibodies against type I IFNs in patients with life-threatening COVID-19. Science September 24, 2020;370:eabd4585. https://doi.org/10.1126/science.abd4585.

[46] Gupta S, Nakabo S, Chu J, Hasni S, Kaplan MJ. Correspondence on 'Clinical course of coronavirus disease 2019 (COVID-19) in a series of 17 patients with systemic lupus erythematosus under long-term treatment with hydroxychloroquine. Ann Rheum Dis January 15, 2021:219648. https://doi.org/10.1136/annrheumdis-2020-219648. Jan 15 Online ahead of print.

[47] Gupta S, Tatouli IP, Rosen LB, Hasni S, Alevizos I, Manna ZG, et al. Distinct functions of anti-interferon autoantibodies in systemic lupus erythematosus: a comprehensive analysis of anticytokine autoantibodies in common rheumatologic diseases. Arthritis Rheumatol January 27, 2016;68:1677–87. https://doi.org/10.1002/art.39607.

[48] Koning R, Bastard P, Casanova JL, Brouwer MC, van de Beek D. Autoantibodies against type I interferons are associated with multi-organ failure in COVID-19 patients. Intensive Care Med April 9, 2021;47(6):704–6. https://doi.org/10.1007/s00134-021-06392-4.

[49] Yel L. Selective IgA deficiency. J Clin Immunol January 1, 2010;30(1):10–6. https://doi.org/10.1007/s10875-009-9357-x.

[50] Çölkesen F, Kandemir B, Arslan, Çölkesen F, Y. ld z E., Korkmaz C, et al. Relationship between selective IgA deficiency and COVID-19 prognosis. Jpn J Infect Dis September 30, 2021. https://doi.org/10.7883/yoken.JJID.2021.281. Sept 30, Online ahead of print.

[51] Parks CG, de Souza Espindola SA, Barbhaiya M, Costenbader KH. Understanding the role of environmental factors in the development of systemic lupus erythematosus. Best Pract Res Clin Rheumatol June 2017;31:306–20.

[52] Sparks JA, Chen CY, Hiraki LT, Malspeis S, Costenbader KH, Karlson EW. Contributions of familial rheumatoid arthritis or lupus and environmental factors to risk of rheumatoid arthritis in women: a prospective cohort study. Arthritis Care Res October 2014;66:1438–46.

[53] Lahita RG. The immunoendocrinology of systemic lupus erythematosus. Clin Immunol August 2016;172:98–100. https://doi.org/10.1016/j.clim.2016.08.014.

[54] Tedeschi SK, Barbhaiya M, Malspeis S, Lu B, Sparks JA, Karlson EW, et al. Obesity and the risk of systemic lupus erythematosus among women in the Nurses' Health Studies. Semin Arthritis Rheum December 2017;47:376–83.

[55] Munipalli B, Knight D, Logvinov I, Abu Dabrh AM. Prevalence, demographics, and risk of severe acute COVID-19. Cureus October 18, 2021;13:e18851. https://doi.org/10.7759/cureus.18851.

[56] Tincani A, Nuzzo M, Motta M, Zatti S, Lojacono A, Faden D. Autoimmunity and pregnancy: autoantibodies and pregnancy in rheumatic diseases. Ann N Y Acad Sci June 2006;1069:346–52.

[57] Newson L, Manyonda I, Lewis R, Preissner R, Preissner S, Seeland U. Sensitive to infection but strong in defense-female sex and the power of oestradiol in the COVID-19 pandemic. Front Glob Womens Health May 11, 2021;2:651752. https://doi.org/10.3389/fgwh.2021.651752.

[58] Dotan A, Kanduc D, Muller S, Makatsariya A, Shoenfeld Y. Molecular mimicry between SARS-CoV-2 and the female reproductive system. Am J Reprod Immunol August 18, 2021. https://doi.org/10.1111/aji.13494. Aug 18.

[59] Bazrafkan M, Hosseini E, Nazari M, Amorim CA, Sadeghi MR. NLRP3 inflammasome: a joint, potential therapeutic target in management of COVID-19 and fertility problems. J Reprod Immunol September 21, 2021;148:103427.

[60] Zhang Y, Yang W, Li W, Zhao Y. NLRP3 inflammasome: checkpoint connecting innate and adaptive immunity in autoimmune diseases. Front Immunol October 11, 2021;12:732933. https://doi.org/10.3389/fimmu.2021.732933. eCollection@2021.:732933.

[61] Isoldi S, Mallardo S, Marcellino A, Bloise S, Dilillo A, Iorfida D, et al. Comprehensive clinic, laboratory and instrumental evaluation of children with COVID-19: a 6-months prospective study. J Med Virol February 2021;11:10.

[62] Sanchez-Flores X, Huynh T, Huang JT. Covid-19 skin manifestations: an update. Curr Opin Pediatr June 2021;14:10.

[63] Silberstein M. COVID-19 and IL-6: why Vitamin D (probably) helps but tocilizumab might not. Eur J Pharmacol March 2021;12:174031.

[64] Bernatsky S, Fournier M, Pineau CA, Clarke AE, Vinet E, Smargiassi A. Associations between ambient fine particulate levels and disease activity in patients with systemic lupus erythematosus (SLE). Environ Health Perspect January 2011;119:45–9.

[65] Zhao N, Smargiassi A, Hatzopoulou M, Colmegna I, Hudson M, Fritzler MJ, et al. Long-term exposure to a mixture of industrial SO2, NO2, and PM2.5 and anti-citrullinated protein antibody positivity. Environ Health July 29, 2020;19:86–00637.

[66] Zhang S, Chen S, Xiao G, Zhao M, Li J, Dong W, et al. The associations between air pollutant exposure and neutralizing antibody titers of an inactivated SARS-CoV-2 vaccine. Environ Sci Pollut Res Int October 2021;1:10–16786.

[67] Masso-Silva JA, Moshensky A, Shin J, Olay J, Nilaad S, Advani I, et al. Chronic E-cigarette aerosol inhalation alters the immune state of the lungs and increases ACE2 expression, raising concern for altered response and susceptibility to SARS-CoV-2. Front Physiol May 31, 2021;12:649604. https://doi.org/10.3389/fphys.2021.649604. eCollection@2021.:649604.

[68] Versini M, Jeandel PY, Rosenthal E, Shoenfeld Y. Obesity in autoimmune diseases: not a passive bystander. Autoimmun Rev August 2, 2014;13:981–1000.

[69] Tsigalou C, Vallianou N, Dalamaga M. Autoantibody production in obesity: is there evidence for a link between obesity and autoimmunity? Curr Obes Rep September 2020;9:245–54.

[70] Frasca D, Reidy L, Romero M, Diaz A, Cray C, Kahl K, et al. The majority of SARS-CoV-2-specific antibodies in COVID-19 patients with obesity are autoimmune and not neutralizing. Int J Obes November 2021;7:1–6.

[71] Strausz S, Kiiskinen T, Broberg M, Ruotsalainen S, Koskela J, Bachour A, et al. Sleep apnoea is a risk factor for severe COVID-19. BMJ Open Respir Res January 2021;8:e000845.

[72] Wood S, Harrison SE, Judd N, Bellis MA, Hughes K, Jones A. The impact of behavioural risk factors on communicable diseases: a systematic review of reviews. BMC Publ Health November 17, 2021;21:2110–12148. https://doi.org/10.1186/s12889-021-12148-y.

[73] Pairo-Castineira E, Clohisey S, Klaric L, Bretherick AD, Rawlik K, Pasko D, et al. Genetic mechanisms of critical illness in COVID-19. Nature March 2021;591:92–8.

[74] Rodero MP, Crow YJ. Type I interferon-mediated monogenic autoinflammation: the type I interferonopathies, a conceptual overview. J Exp Med November 14, 2016;213:2527–38.

[75] Crow MK, Olferiev M, Kirou KA. Type I interferons in autoimmune disease. Annu Rev Pathol January 24, 2019;14:369–93.

[76] Bastard P, Gervais A, Le VT, Rosain J, Philippot Q, Manry J, et al. Autoantibodies neutralizing type I IFNs are present in ~4% of uninfected individuals over 70 years old and account for ~20% of COVID-19 deaths. Sci Immunol August 2021;6(62):eabl4340. https://doi.org/10.1126/sciimmunol.abl434.

[77] Goncalves D, Mezidi M, Bastard P, Perret M, Saker K, Fabien N, et al. Antibodies against type I interferon: detection and association with severe clinical outcome in COVID-19 patients. Clin Transl Immunology August 17, 2021;10:e1327. https://doi.org/10.1002/cti2.1327.

[78] Choi MY, Hahn J, Malspeis S, Stevens EF, Karlson EW, Sparks JA, et al. A combination of healthy lifestyle behaviors reduces risk of incident systemic lupus erythematosus. Arthritis Rheumatol July 27, 2021. https://doi.org/10.1002/art.41935. Jul 27. Online ahead of print.

[79] Barbhaiya M, Costenbader KH. Environmental exposures and the development of systemic lupus erythematosus. Curr Opin Rheumatol September 2016;28:497–505.
[80] Barbhaiya M, Tedeschi SK, Lu B, Malspeis S, Kreps D, Sparks JA, et al. Cigarette smoking and the risk of systemic lupus erythematosus, overall and by anti-double stranded DNA antibody subtype, in the Nurses' Health Study cohorts. Ann Rheum Dis February 2018;77:196–202.
[81] Marx V. Scientists set out to connect the dots on long COVID. Nat Methods May 2021;18:449–53.
[82] Augustin M, Schommers P, Stecher M, Dewald F, Gieselmann L, Gruell H, et al. Post-COVID syndrome in non-hospitalised patients with COVID-19: a longitudinal prospective cohort study. Lancet Reg Health Eur July 2021;6:100122. https://doi.org/10.1016/j.lanepe.2021.100122.
[83] Lopez-Leon S, Wegman-Ostrosky T, Perelman C, Sepulveda R, Rebolledo P, Cuapio A, et al. More than 50 long-term effects of COVID-19: a systematic review and meta-analysis. Sci Rep March 1, 2021;1(1):16144. https://doi.org/10.1038/s41598-021-95565-8.
[84] Porritt RA, Binek A, Paschold L, Noval RM, Mc AA, Yonker LM, et al. The autoimmune signature of hyper-inflammatory multisystem inflammatory syndrome in children. J Clin Invest August 26, 2021;131(20):e151520. https://doi.org/10.1172/JCI151520.
[85] Bohn MK, Yousef P, Steele S, Sepiashvili L, Adeli K. Multi-inflammatory syndrome in children: a view into immune pathogenesis from a laboratory perspective. J Appl Lab Med August 31, 2021. https://doi.org/10.1093/jalm/jfab114. Online ahead of print:.
[86] Roe K. Explanations for 10 of the most puzzling aspects of multisystem inflammatory syndrome and other Kawasaki-like diseases. J Clin Pharm Therapeut November 2, 2021. https://doi.org/10.1111/jcpt.13560. Online ahead of print.
[87] Mercier JC, Ouldali N, Melki I, Basmaci R, Levy M, Titomanlio L, et al. Severe acute respiratory syndrome coronavirusÂ 2-related multisystem inflammatory syndrome in children mimicking Kawasaki disease. Arch Cardiovasc Dis May 2021;114:426–33. https://doi.org/10.1016/j.acvd.2021.04.005.
[88] Gazzaruso C, Carlo SN, Mariani G, Nai C, Coppola A, Naldani D, et al. High prevalence of antinuclear antibodies and lupus anticoagulant in patients hospitalized for SARS-CoV2 pneumonia. Clin Rheumatol May 27, 2020;39(7):2095–7. https://doi.org/10.1007/s10067-020-05180-7.
[89] Pascolini S, Vannini A, Deleonardi G, Ciordinik M, Sensoli A, Carletti I, et al. COVID-19 and immunological dysregulation: can autoantibodies be useful? Clin Transl Sci September 29, 2021;14:502–8. https://doi.org/10.1111/cts.12908.
[90] Sacchi MC, Tamiazzo S, Stobbione P, Agatea L, De GP, Stecca A, et al. SARS-CoV-2 Infection as a trigger of autoimmune response. Clin Transl Sci December 11, 2020;14(3):898–907. https://doi.org/10.1111/cts.12953.
[91] Lerma LA, Chaudhary A, Bryan A, Morishima C, Wener MH, Fink SL. Prevalence of autoantibody responses in acute coronavirus disease 2019 (COVID-19). J Transl Autoimmun November 27, 2020;3:100073. https://doi.org/10.1016/j.jtauto.2020.100073.
[92] Rose NR, Bona C. Defining criteria for autoimmune diseases (Witebsky's postulates revisited). Immunol Today September 1993;14:426–30.
[93] Ameratunga R, Langguth D, Hawkes D. Perspective: scientific and ethical concerns pertaining to animal models of autoimmune/autoinflammatory syndrome induced by adjuvants (ASIA). Autoimmun Rev May 2018;17:435–9.
[94] Robinson NB, Krieger K, Khan FM, Huffman W, Chang M, Naik A, et al. The current state of animal models in research: a review. Int J Surg December 2019;72:9–13. https://doi.org/10.1016/j.ijsu.2019.10.015.
[95] Leist SR, Schäfer A, Martinez DR. Cell and animal models of SARS-CoV-2 pathogenesis and immunity. Dis Model Mech September 1, 2020;13(9):046581. https://doi.org/10.1242/dmm.046581.
[96] Beyer C, Schett G, Distler O, Distler JH. Animal models of systemic sclerosis: prospects and limitations. Arthritis Rheum October 2010;62(10):2831–44. https://doi.org/10.1002/art.27647.
[97] Caspi RR. Understanding autoimmunity in the eye: from animal models to novel therapies. Discov Med March 2014;17:155–62.
[98] Choi MY, Barber MR, Barber CE, Clarke AE, Fritzler MJ. Preventing the development of SLE: identifying risk factors and proposing pathways for clinical care. Lupus July 2016;25:838–49.
[99] Choi MY, Fritzler MJ. Autoantibodies in SLE: prediction and the p value matrix. Lupus August 9, 2019;28:1285–91.
[100] Mosca M, Tani C, Talarico R, Bombardieri S. Undifferentiated connective tissue diseases (UCTD): simplified systemic autoimmune diseases. Autoimmun Rev March 2011;10:256–8.

[101] Garcia-Gonzalez M, Rodriguez-Lozano B, Bustabad S, Ferraz-Amaro I. Undifferentiated connective tissue disease: predictors of evolution into definite disease. Clin Exp Rheumatol September 2017;35:739–45.

[102] Scanzi F, Andreoli L, Martinelli M, Taraborelli M, Cavazzana I, Carabellese N, et al. Are the autoimmune/inflammatory syndrome induced by adjuvants (ASIA) and the undifferentiated connective tissue disease (UCTD) related to each other? A case-control study of environmental exposures. Immunol Res March 22, 2017;65(1):150–6. https://doi.org/10.1007/s12026-017-8912-4.

[103] Florian IA, Lupan I, Sur L, Samasca G, Timis TL. To be, or not to be? Guillain-Barré Syndrome. Autoimmun Rev October 28, 2021. https://doi.org/10.1016/j.autrev.2021.102983. Oct 28. Online ahead of print:102983.

[104] The Nobel committee for Physiology or medicine. Press release: the Nobel prize in Physiology or medicine. 2021. Online Source: https://www.nobelprize.org/prizes/medicine/2021/press-release/. Last accessed 11/22/2021.

[105] Kefauver JM, Ward AB, Patapoutian A. Discoveries in structure and physiology of mechanically activated ion channels. Nature November 2020;587:567–76. https://doi.org/10.1038/s41586-020-2933-1.

[106] Murthy SE, Dubin AE, Patapoutian A. Piezos thrive under pressure: mechanically activated ion channels in health and disease. Nat Rev Mol Cell Biol December 2017;18(12):771–83. https://doi.org/10.1038/nrm.2017.92.

[107] Dos Santos CC, Slutsky AS. The contribution of biophysical lung injury to the development of biotrauma. Annu Rev Physiol 2006;68:585–618. https://doi.org/10.1146/annurev.physiol.68.072304.113443.

[108] Curley GF, Laffey JG, Zhang H, Slutsky AS. Biotrauma and ventilator-induced lung injury: clinical implications. Chest November 2016;150:1109–17.

[109] Lad H, Saumur TM, Herridge MS, Dos Santos CC, Mathur S, Batt J, et al. Intensive care unit-acquired weakness: not just another muscle atrophying condition. Int J Mol Sci October 22, 2020;21:E7840.

[110] Latronico N, Bolton CF. Critical illness polyneuropathy and myopathy: a major cause of muscle weakness and paralysis. Lancet Neurol October 2011;10:931–41. https://doi.org/10.1016/S1474-4422(11)70178-8.

[111] Cabañes-Martínez L, Villadóniga M, González-Rodríguez L, Araque L, DÃaz-Cid A, Ruz-Caracuel I, et al. Neuromuscular involvement in COVID-19 critically ill patients. Clin Neurophysiol December 2020;131:2809–16.

[112] Tankisi H. Critical illness myopathy and polyneuropathy in Covid-19: is it a distinct entity? Clin Neurophysiol July 2021;132:1716–7. https://doi.org/10.1016/j.clinph.2021.04.001.

[113] Lazzerini PE, Laghi-Pasini F, Boutjdir M, Capecchi PL. Anti-Ro/SSA antibodies and the autoimmune long-QT syndrome. Front Med September 6, 2021;8:730161. https://doi.org/10.3389/fmed.2021.730161. eCollection;%2021.:730161.

[114] De SM, Isailovic N, Motta F, Ricordi C, Ceribelli A, Lanza E, et al. Environmental triggers for connective tissue disease: the case of COVID-19 associated with dermatomyositis-specific autoantibodies. Curr Opin Rheumatol September 9, 2021;33(6):514–21. https://doi.org/10.1097/BOR.0000000000000844.

[115] Movahedi N, Ziaee V. COVID-19 and myositis; true dermatomyositis or prolonged post viral myositis? Pediatr Rheumatol Online J June 10, 2021;19:86–00570.

[116] Veyseh M, Koyoda S, Ayesha B. COVID-19 IgG-related autoimmune inflammatory necrotizing myositis. BMJ Case Rep April 13, 2021;14. https://doi.org/10.1136/bcr-2020-239457. e239457–e239457.

[117] Zhang H, Charmchi Z, Seidman RJ, Anziska Y, Velayudhan V, Perk J. COVID-19-associated myositis with severe proximal and bulbar weakness. Muscle Nerve September 2020;62:E57–60.

[118] Mehta P, Machado PM, Gupta L. Understanding and managing anti-MDA 5 dermatomyositis, including potential COVID-19 mimicry. Rheumatol Int March 27, 2021;41(6):1021–36. https://doi.org/10.1007/s00296-021-04819-1.

[119] Rodero MP, Pelleau S, Welfringer-Morin A, Duffy D, Melki I, Bader-Meunier B. Onset and relapse of juvenile dermatomyositis following asymptomatic SARS-CoV-2 infection. J Clin Immunol August 23, 2021. https://doi.org/10.1007/s10875-021-01119-y. Aug 23. Online ahead of print:.

[120] Suh J, Mukerji SS, Collens SI, Padera Jr RF, Pinkus GS, Amato AA, et al. Skeletal muscle and peripheral nerve histopathology in COVID-19. Neurology August 24, 2021;97:e849–58. https://doi.org/10.1212/WNL.0000000000012344.

[121] Aschman T, Schneider J, Greuel S, Meinhardt J, Streit S, Goebel HH, et al. Association between SARS-CoV-2 infection and immune-mediated myopathy in patients who have died. JAMA Neurol August 1, 2021;78:948–60. https://doi.org/10.1001/jamaneurol.2021.2004.

[122] Swash M, de CM. Intensive care unit-acquired weakness: neuropathology. J Clin Neurophysiol May 2020;37:197–9.

[123] Suh J, Amato AA. Neuromuscular complications of coronavirus disease-19. Curr Opin Neurol June 21, 2021;34:669–74. https://doi.org/10.1097/WCO.0000000000000970.

[124] Ramasamy S, Subbian S. Critical determinants of cytokine storm and type I interferon response in COVID-19 pathogenesis. Clin Microbiol Rev May 12, 2021;34:e00299–20.

[125] Sghiri R, Boumiza A, Benhassine H, Elamri N, Shakoor Z, Slama F, et al. IgA rheumatoid factor is associated with bone mineral density preservation in rheumatoid arthritis. Clin Rheumatol July 2021. https://doi.org/10.1007/s10067-021-05814-4.:10-05814. %20.

[126] Lee W, Nims RJ, Savadipour A, Zhang Q, Leddy HA, Liu F, et al. Inflammatory signaling sensitizes Piezo1 mechanotransduction in articular chondrocytes as a pathogenic feed-forward mechanism in osteoarthritis. Proc Natl Acad Sci U S A March 30, 2021;118(13). https://doi.org/10.1073/pnas.2001611118. e2001611118.

[127] Kuebler WM, Jordt SE, Liedtke WB. Urgent reconsideration of lung edema as a preventable outcome in COVID-19: inhibition of TRPV4 represents a promising and feasible approach. Am J Physiol Lung Cell Mol Physiol June 1, 2020;318(6):L1239–43. https://doi.org/10.1152/ajplung.00161.2020.

[128] Perricone C, Bartoloni E, Bursi R, Cafaro G, Guidelli GM, Shoenfeld Y, et al. COVID-19 as part of the hyper-ferritinemic syndromes: the role of iron depletion therapy. Immunol Res August 2020;68:213–24.

[129] Tang KT, Hsu BC, Chen DY. Autoimmune and rheumatic manifestations associated with COVID-19 in adults: an updated systematic review. Front Immunol March 12, 2021;12:645013. https://doi.org/10.3389/fimmu.2021.645013.

[130] Widjaja G, Turki JA, Sulaiman RH, Kamal AW, Bokov DO, Suksatan W, et al. Humoral immune mechanisms involved in protective and pathological immunity during COVID-19. Hum Immunol July 1, 2021:10.

[131] Schnaubelt S, Tihanyi D, Strassl R, Schmidt R, Anders S, Laggner AN, et al. Hemophagocytic lymphohistiocytosis in COVID-19: case reports of a stepwise approach. Medicine (Baltim) March 26, 2021;100:e25170.

[132] Ma S, Dubin AE, Zhang Y, Mousavi SAR, Wang Y, Coombs AM, et al. A role of PIEZO1 in iron metabolism in mice and humans. Cell February 18, 2021;184:969–82. https://doi.org/10.1016/j.cell.2021.01.024.

[133] Freire-de-Lima L, Scovino AM, Barreto Menezes CC, Marques da FL, Santos Dos RJ, Rodrigues da Costa Santos MA, et al. Autoimmune disorders & COVID-19. Medicines (Basel) September 28, 2021;8:55.

[134] Fritzler MJ, Choi MY, Satoh M, Mahler M. Autoantibody discovery, assay development and adoption: Death valley, the sea of survival and beyond. Front Immunol 2021;12:679613. https://doi.org/10.3389/fimmu.2021.679613.

CHAPTER

2

The mosaic of autoimmunity and autoinflammation and SARS-CoV-2 as an environmental factor

Nicola Luigi Bragazzi[1,2] *and Abdulla Watad*[2,3]

[1]Laboratory for Industrial and Applied Mathematics (LIAM), Department of Mathematics and Statistics, York University, Toronto, ON, Canada; [2]Leeds Institute of Rheumatic and Musculoskeletal Medicine (LIRMM), University of Leeds, Leeds, United Kingdom; [3]Sheba Medical Center, Tel Aviv, Sackler Faculty of Medicine, Tel Aviv University, Tel Aviv, Israel

The mosaic of autoimmunity and autoinflammation

The expression "mosaic of autoimmunity" has been introduced in the scholarly literature for the first time by Shoenfeld and Isenberg in the late eighties [1] to illustrate the multifactorial, complex etiopathogenesis of autoimmunity and autoimmune disorders [2]. These exhibit a dysfunction/impairment of the immune system, which results in loss of immune tolerance against self-tissues, that are being attacked and damaged by the presence of aberrant autoreactive T and B cells [3]. The concept of autoimmunity can be further broadened to accommodate autoinflammation [4]: autoinflammatory diseases are a relatively new, emerging type of disorders characterized by self-directed inflammation, which clinically presents as periodic/recurrent fever and sometimes with episodes of acute inflammation affecting the innate immune system [5].

Autoimmune/autoinflammatory disorders can be categorized into organ-specific or systemic ones and, according to the latest classification of the "American Autoimmune Related Disease Association" (AARDA), more than 100 autoimmune/autoinflammatory diseases have been so far identified.

Autoimmunity, as well as autoinflammation, can arise from the subtle, nonlinear interplay of different variables and they can be understood as a mosaic, comprising of various cobbles and pieces, ranging from the biological make-up of the individual (the genetic and postgenetic components) [6], to behavioral (lifestyles) and environmental triggers [7,8]. The latter

Autoimmunity, COVID-19, Post-COVID19 syndrome and COVID-19 vaccination
https://doi.org/10.1016/B978-0-443-18566-3.00013-X

can include pathogens and infectious agents, like the Cytomegalovirus (CMV) and the Epstein–Barr virus (EBV), together with the influenza virus and the Human Papillomavirus (HPV) [9,10].

Environmental triggers include also occupational exposures to other agents like silica, solvents, bisphenol [11,12,13], pesticides, or ultraviolet radiation. Other environmental causes of autoimmunity can be certain drugs (allopurinol, captopril, chlorpromazine, estrogens, halothane, iodine, penicillins, rifampicins, or tetracyclines), vaccines, and other immunization practices [14], seasonality [15], behaviors and lifestyles like cigarette smoke [16,17] and physical activity [18], as well as collagen- and silicone-based implants [19,20,21].

Specifically concerning the infectious agents as potentially implicated in the genesis of autoimmunity/autoinflammation, the concepts of "infectome" and "autoinfectome" have been recently introduced, referring to the "theater" of infectious agents to which one is exposed during their lifetime and the preexisting microbiome (Fig. 2.1). Autoimmunity/

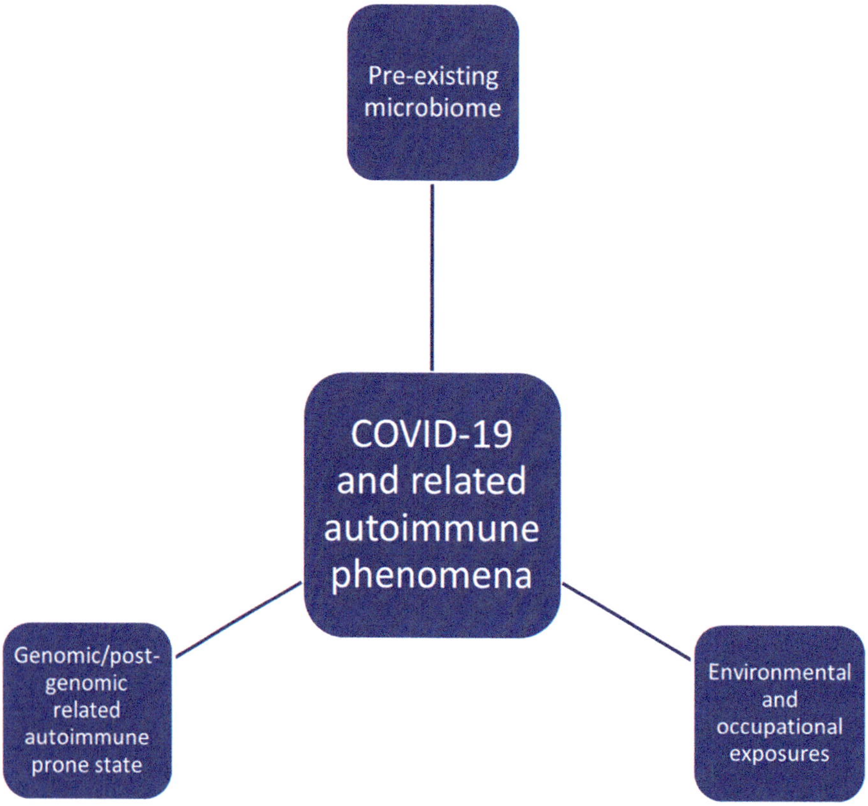

FIGURE 2.1 The subtle, complex interplay between the genetic/postgenetic predisposition to autoimmune/autoinflammatory state, the "autoinfectome"/preexisting microbiome, and environmental and occupational exposures, including the infectome, resulting in COVID-19 related autoimmune/autoinflammatory phenomena and events.

autoinflammation arises from the multi-factorial relationship between the human microbiome and exposure to the environmental infectome [22,23].

In the next paragraph, we will overview the epidemiology and the biology of a recently emerged infectious agent and, in the rest of the manuscript, we will show its interplay with autoimmune/autoinflammatory diseases (Table 2.1).

TABLE 2.1 The relationship between autoimmune/autoinflammatory diseases and COVID-19.

Autoimmune disorder	Main findings	References
Alopecia areata and *telogen effluvium*	Cases on the rise during the COVID-19 pandemic *De novo*-onset, flares and relapses after the COVID-19 infection or vaccination Unclear relationship with COVID-19	[24] [25] [26] [27] [28] [29] [30] [31] [32] [33] [34] [35] [36] [37] [38] [39] [40] [41] [42] [43] [44] [45] [46] [47] [48] [49]
Amyloidosis	*De novo*-onset after the COVID-19 infection	[50]
Ankylosing spondylitis/axial spondyloarthritis	Risk of contracting COVID-19 comparable with the general population, if not lower (potential protective role of HLA-B27) The use of drugs like DMARDs mediates favorable outcomes Subjects on NSAIDs reported poorer outcomes	[51] [52] [53]
Antiphospholipid syndrome	Less information available (from 26 cohort studies and 1 clinical case report) Some cases precipitated by the COVID-19 vaccination	[54] [55] [56] [57]
Atopic dermatitis	Higher risk of contracting the COVID-19 infection Attenuated symptoms in those on dupilumab	[58] [59] [60]

(*Continued*)

TABLE 2.1 The relationship between autoimmune/autoinflammatory diseases and COVID-19.—cont'd

Autoimmune disorder	Main findings	References
		[61] [62] [63]
Autoimmune gastritis	Potentially linked with COVID-19	[64]
Autoimmune ocular diseases	Flares/relapses of autoimmune ocular diseases, including iritis, uveitis, and Vogt-Koyanagi-Harada syndrome have been reported after the COVID-19 vaccination	[65] [66] [67] [68]
Autoimmune reproductive diseases	Scarce evidence	[69] [70]
Behçet's disease	Contrasting findings of the risk of COVID-19 (comparable with the general population for some studies, higher for other studies) Continuous antiTNF therapy may be associated with poorer clinical outcomes	[71] [72] [73] [74]
Celiac disease	Risk of COVID-19 comparable with the general population *De novo*-onset cases after the COVID-19 infection	[75] [76]
Demyelinating syndromes	After the COVID-19 vaccination	[77] [78]
Diabetes type 1	Cases of diabetes type 1 increased during the COVID-19 pandemic Higher risk of hospital admission *De novo*-onset or flares/relapses after the COVID-19 vaccination	[79] [80] [81] [82] [83]
Graves' disease	After COVID-19 vaccine administration	[83] [84]
Guillain-Barré syndrome	*De novo*-onset after the COVID-19 infection	[85]
Hashimoto's thyroiditis	*De novo*-onset after the COVID-19 infection	[86] [87] [88]
Hemolytic anemia	*De novo*-onset after the COVID-19 vaccination	[89] [90]
Immune thrombocytopenic purpura	*De novo*-onset after the COVID-19 infection	[91] [92] [93]
Inflammatory bowel disease (ulcerative colitis)	Low prevalence of COVID-19, incidence rate comparable with the general population, no increased relative risk, outcomes depending on the specific treatment received	[94] [95] [96]
Lichen planus and *lichen planopilaris*	*De novo*-onset and flares/relapses after the COVID-19 infection or vaccination	[97] [98] [99]

TABLE 2.1 The relationship between autoimmune/autoinflammatory diseases and COVID-19.—cont'd

Autoimmune disorder	Main findings	References
		[100] [101] [102] [103] [104]
Miller–Fisher syndrome	Potentially linked with COVID-19	[105]
Multiple sclerosis	Higher risk of contracting the COVID-19 infection Higher risk of severe clinical outcomes Natalizumab and ocrelizumab may be linked with worse outcomes (some studies report opposite findings), while fingolimod and siponimod may be associated with better outcomes Use of rituximab linked with poorer outcomes Use of alemtuzumab is potentially linked with a milder course of the COVID-19 infection Flares/relapses after the COVID-19 infection or vaccination	[106] [107] [108] [109] [110] [111] [112] [113] [114] [115] [116] [117] [118]
Myasthenia gravis	Worse prognosis and more severe clinical outcomes A longer length of hospital stay	[119] [120] [121] [122] [123]
Myocarditis	Unclear relationship with the virus	[124]
Myositis/polymyositis/ dermatomyositis	Potentially linked with COVID-19	[125] [126]
Pemphigus and other autoimmune blistering diseases	Higher mortality rate Relapse after the COVID-19 infection	[127] [128]
Polymyalgia rheumatica	*De novo*-onset or relapse of polymyalgia rheumatica after COVID-19 infection or vaccination	[129] [130] [131] [132] [133]
Postural orthostatic tachycardia syndrome	Positive outcomes and complete/near-complete resolution of symptoms in a few patients, with most of them exhibiting residual symptoms six-eight months after COVID-19	[134]
Primary biliary cholangitis, primary sclerosing cholangitis, and other autoimmune cholangiopathies	*De novo*-onset cases after the COVID-19 infection	[135] Ba [136] [137]
Psoriasis		

(Continued)

TABLE 2.1 The relationship between autoimmune/autoinflammatory diseases and COVID-19.—cont'd

Autoimmune disorder	Main findings	References
	The use of some drugs (like apremilast or secukinumab) may modulate good clinical outcomes Worse prognosis among those with underlying comorbidities *De novo*-onset cases, flares, and worsening of psoriasis after the COVID-19 infection or vaccination	[138] [139] [140] [141] [142] [143] [144] [145] [146]
Psoriatic arthritis	The use of some drugs (like apremilast or secukinumab) may modulate good clinical outcomes Worse prognosis among those with underlying comorbidities	[147] [148] [149] [150] [146] [151]
Rheumatoid arthritis	Inconsistent findings regarding the association between RA and COVID-19 Use of JAK inhibitors potentially protective Flares of RA after COVID-19 vaccination	[152] [153] [154]
Sarcoidosis and Löfgren's syndrome	Risk of infection comparable with the general population Higher hospitalization and mortality rates Worse symptoms in patients with underlying heart disease, on glucocorticoids and rituximab, and with moderate-to-severe lung function impairment *De novo*-onset cases after the COVID-19 infection	[155] B[156] [157] [158] [159] [160] [161] [162] [163] [164] [165] [166] [167]
Scleroderma/systemic sclerosis	Two clinical case reports – a *de novo*-onset case and flares/relapses of scleroderma after the COVID-19 infection	[168] [169]
Sjögren's syndrome	Worsening of symptoms and flares/relapses during the COVID-19 pandemic Long-term xerostomia	[170] [171] [172]
Systemic lupus erythematosus	Higher risk of contracting COVID-19 and developing severe complications Elevated ACE2 expression via oxidative stress, methylation defects, other epigenetic dysregulations, ACE2 autoantibodies, and type 1 IFN signature expression Role of extrafollicular double negative (DN2) B cell subsets Worse prognosis among patients with lupus nephritis	[173] [174] [175] [176] [177] [178] [179]

TABLE 2.1 The relationship between autoimmune/autoinflammatory diseases and COVID-19.—cont'd

Autoimmune disorder	Main findings	References
	De novo-onset or worsening after the COVID-19 infection and vaccination	[180] [181]
Vasculitis	Clinical outcomes generally positive	[182]
Vitiligo	*De novo*-onset cases or worsening after the COVID-19 vaccination	[183] [184] [185] [186] [187] [188]

SARS-CoV-2 and COVID-19

The "Severe Acute Respiratory Syndrome-Related Coronavirus Type 2" (SARS-CoV-2), initially termed as "2019 novel coronavirus" (2019-nCov), is an emerging coronavirus, which, from a morphological and molecular standpoint, is an enveloped, positive-sense, nonsegmented, single-stranded RNA virus. Viral particles resemble a crown (in Latin "*corona*"), from which the name coronavirus derives. This type of virus belongs to the *species* of Severe acute respiratory syndrome-related coronavirus, to the *subgenus* of *Sarbecovirus*, to the *genus* of *Betacoronavirus*, to the subfamily of *Orthocoronavirinae*, to the family of *Coronaviridae*, to the suborder of *Cornidovirineae*, to the order of *Nidovirales*, and to the realm of *Riboviria* [189].

In the last decades, coronaviruses have caused severe large-scale clusters of cases and outbreaks, such as those generated by the "Severe Acute Respiratory Syndrome" (SARS) virus in 2003 in mainland China, and by the "Middle East Respiratory Syndrome" (MERS) virus in 2012 in the Kingdom of Saudi Arabia (KSA, in the Middle East area) and in 2015 in South Korea [190].

The SARS-CoV-2 infects humans and other mammals, generally causing mild respiratory infections but can, occasionally, result in a severe and even lethal communicable disorder termed "Coronavirus Disease 19" (COVID-19) [189]. The SARS-CoV-2 was first identified in late December 2019, in Wuhan, province of Hubei, the People's Republic of China, where a cluster of unusual and atypical pneumonia occurred among people attending a wet market, where wild animals were slaughtered and sold in scarce hygiene conditions [190]. Since then, the virus has quickly spread out into neighboring countries and is currently circulating in more than 220 countries and territories, making the control of its diffusion a real challenge for governments, public health authorities and organisms, and scientists, as well as for all the citizens. To reflect such difficulties in counteracting and mitigating its burden, on March 11th, 2020, the World Health Organization (WHO) declared the currently ongoing outbreak as a pandemic, and on March 19th, 2020, it asked all its member states to make serious efforts to significantly curb human-to-human transmission of the virus [191].

The SARS-CoV-2 genome is approximately 30 kb in length, and is the largest among the RNA viruses, with a 5′-cap and a 3′-poly(A) tail, which are involved in the process of the viral translation. The genome consists of nine major open reading frames (ORFs) [192]. and shares high homologies with the bat coronavirus genome (in particular, with the SARSr-CoV-RaTG13 strain) [193,194]. The SARS-CoV-2 proteome comprises four major proteins, namely, the surface or spike glycoprotein (S), the membrane glycoprotein (M), the envelope (E), and the nucleocapsid phosphoprotein (N). The S protein has a molecular weight of approximately 150 kDa and plays a key role in mediating the viral binding and attachment to host receptor proteins. The M protein is characterized by a molecular weight ranging from 25 to around 30 kDa and is responsible for the curvature of the membrane, by attaching the nucleocapsid. The E protein, an integral membrane protein with a weight varying in the range 8–12 kDa, facilitates the molecular assembly and release of virions. Moreover, the protein serves also as an ion channel. All these biological activities explain the fundamental role of E in the etiopathogenesis of the infection. Finally, N is involved in the packaging of viral particles into the capsid and fosters the formation of the so-called replicase-transcriptase complex (RTC) [195,192].

Other ORFs (including ORF1a, ORF1b, ORF3a, ORF6, ORF7a, and ORF8) harbor nonstructural proteins (nsps) [192]. Specifically, the former contains nsp1, nsp2, nsp3 (known also as papain-like protease or PLpro domain), nsp4, nsp5 (known as 3C-like protease or 3CLpro), nsp6, nsp7, nsp8, nsp9, nsp10, nsp11, and nsp12 (known also as RNA-dependent RNA polymerase or RdRp). ORF1b harbors four nsps, such as nsp13 (termed as helicase or Hel, belonging to the helicase superfamily one and potentially involved in viral RNA replication through RNA-DNA duplex unwinding), nsp14 (serving as 3′-to-5′-exoribonuclease, known as ExoN), nsp15 (serving as endoribonuclease), and nsp16 (serving as mRNA cap-1 methyltransferase, 2′-O- MTase).

SARS-CoV-2 and biological mechanisms of virulence

Kumar and colleagues [192] have studied 95 SARS-CoV-2 strains, sampled from 11 countries (the USA, China, Japan, India, Taiwan, Australia, Brazil, Italy, Nepal, South Korea, and Sweden), by means of both core-genome-based and single nucleotide polymorphism (SNP)-based phylogenetic techniques, in order to dissect the molecular basis of transmission dynamics, evolutionary patterns, and divergence rates, in an effort to reveal the determinants of SARS-CoV-2 virulence. More in detail, the authors have performed a series of biogeographical genomics and postgenomics (proteomics and interactomics) analyses, studying the ORFs of the isolated specimens to identify significant unique point mutations and amino acid substitutions/additions from the comparison of various strains. Furthermore, interactomics studies showed that SARS-CoV-2 proteome significantly interacts with the human proteome, more specifically with proteins involved in events such as biochemical and biometabolic processes, viral entry (like the Notch cascade), responses to cellular stressors, protein secretion, localization, expression, assembly and composition (like the spliceosome pathway and various secretory pathways), nucleus export, ribosomal RNA (rRNA) processing, mitochondrial functioning and antiviral immune response (including the interferon signaling cascade, interleukin pathways and other inflammatory networks), among others. Finally, divergence rates were particularly high for ORF8 and ORF3a, with higher nonsynonymous substitutions with respect to synonymous ones, together with ORF1ab poly-proteins and S protein.

According to other studies, ORF7b is another ORF characterized by a significantly high rate of mutations and variants [196]. Toyoshima et al. [197] assessed 12,343 SARS-CoV-2 genome sequences sampled from six geographic territories (28 countries) and were able to identify a list of 1234 mutations. ORF1ab poly-proteins mutations (in particular, 4715L), as well as S protein mutations (specifically, 614G) were found to correlate with case fatality rates (CFR). Also, several HLA alleles, such as HLA-A*11:01, correlated with CFR.

Other scholars, like [198] have quantitatively measured the genomic variability of 48,635 SARS-CoV-2 isolates. The authors were able to observe a mean of 7.23 mutations per specimen (generally, SNPs). At least three clades emerged from the comparative phylogenomic analysis, with clade G being more common in European countries and harboring a D614G mutation at the level of the S protein [199]. Some studies have compared five SARS-CoV-2 sequences sampled from various geographical territories with those obtained from other coronaviruses (SARS, MERS, OC43, and 229E), to reveal the presence of putative miR-like sequences. Authors were able to identify seven key microRNAs (miRNAs), including miRs 8066, 5197, 3611, 3934-3p, 1307-3p, 3691-3p, and 1468-5p. Moreover, pathway and network analyses demonstrated the role of these miRNAs in events and processes related to virulence, host dynamics, and responses, thus confirming the results of Kumar and colleagues [192].

As found by these and other studies, HLA plays a key role in the etiopathogenesis of the COVID-19 infection [200]. The involvement of several immune-related pathways and cascades contributes, at least partially, to explaining the autoimmune/autoinflammatory events and phenomena observed during the disease, together with the interaction of SARS-CoV-2 with the human microbiome, which has been found to correlate with COVID-19 severity [201].

SARS-CoV-2 and COVID-19 as a further cobble of the mosaic of autoimmunity

Approximately one-third of COVID-19 patients report at least one auto-antibody against a nuclear antigen. Generally, in most cases, these autoantibodies can be detected at a low titer without high specificity [202]. Recently, the "autoantigen atlas" or "autoantigenome" of SARS-CoV-2-positive patients has been completely mapped [203]. This has enabled us to dissect at a cellular and molecular level the complex links of autoimmunity with a plethora of phenomena and events, including thrombosis, fibrosis, and smooth muscle dysfunction in COVID-19 patients [202]. As previously said, SARS-CoV-2 has been, indeed, linked with several autoimmune events [204].

SARS-CoV-2/COVID-19 and its impact on autoimmune/autoinflammatory disorders

Recently, the impact of COVID-19 on patients with autoimmune/autoinflammatory diseases has been reviewed utilizing a systematic approach [205] and, after synthesizing seven case-controlled studies, authors have found a higher risk of developing COVID-19 in patients suffering from autoimmune/autoinflammatory disorders with respect to controls (with an odds ratio, OR, of 2.19 [95% confidence interval, CI, 1.05–4.58]). Synthesizing 65 studies totaling 2766 patients, the overall rates of hospitalization and mortality were 0.35 [95%CI 0.23–0.50] and 0.066 [95%CI 0.036–0.12], respectively. Some medications, like glucocorticoids, conventional synthetic disease-modifying antirheumatic drugs (csDMARDs), and biological and targeted synthetic disease-modifying, antirheumatic drugs (b/tsDMARDs)-csDMARDs combination therapy, were associated with a worse clinical outcome, whilst b/tsDMARDs monotherapy (including antitumor necrosis factor (TNF) agents), decreased the risk of hospitalization and death.

A study conducted in Italy [206] confirmed these findings, reporting a significantly higher prevalence of COVID-19 among patients with autoimmune systemic diseases, in particular, connective tissue diseases (CTD) or suffering from autoimmune/autoinflammatory disorders not treated with DMARDs. In a study conducted in Spain [207], the population comprised 123 patients with autoimmune/autoinflammatory rheumatic diseases infected with COVID-19, 54 of which had to be hospitalized and 12 died during the hospital admission. Predictors of hospital admission were older age (OR 1.08) and autoimmune systemic condition (OR 3.55). However, exposure to DMARDs was not found to be a statistically significant covariate. In another investigation in Spain [208], 456 rheumatological (chronic inflammatory arthritis or CTDs) and matched controls were recruited. Predictors of severe COVID-19 were increasing age (OR 4.83 [95%CI 2.78–8.36]), being a male (OR 1.93 [95%CI 1.21–3.07]), and suffering from CTD (OR 1.82 [95%CI 1.00–3.30]).

In another study [209], a sample of 493,499 patients with autoimmune/autoinflammatory disorders were recruited versus 2,466,946 controls. Autoimmunity/autoinflammation was associated with a higher odds of being hospitalized for COVID-19 (matched unadjusted OR of 1.37, adjusted OR, aOR, of 1.23). The authors found a significantly higher risk of hospitalization among patients with iritis (OR 1.46), multiple sclerosis (MS, OR 1.83), psoriatic arthritis (PsA, OR 2.20), rheumatoid arthritis (RA, OR 1.42), systemic autoimmune rheumatic disorders (SARDs, with an OR of 1.47) and vasculitis (OR 2.07). Predictors of COVID-19 hospitalizations were older age, being a male, dwelling in long-term care facilities, underlying co-morbidities, and low socioeconomic status. Interestingly, the odds of complicated hospitalizations were 21% higher among all patients with autoimmune/autoinflammatory disorders, even though this association did not achieve statistical significance when correcting for confounding factors, such as socio-demographic factors and comorbidities.

Montero et al. [210] reported a rather high rate of hospitalization (67.7%) among a cohort of 62 patients with autoimmune/autoinflammatory diseases infected by COVID-19 (mean age of 60.9 years, 42% men). The mortality rate was 16%. Predictors of hospitalization were being a male (OR of 8.63), previous lung disease (OR of 27.47), and being on glucocorticoids (OR of 9.95).

Specifically focusing on rare autoimmune rheumatic diseases (RAIRDs) [211], the authors computed an age-standardized mortality rate of 3669.3 [95%CI 3500.4–3838.1] per 100,000 person-years, which was 1.44 [95%CI 1.42–1.45] times higher than the average mortality rate during the same months of the previous 5 years. In the general English population, the mortality rate during the COVID-19 pandemic was 1.38 times higher. Moreover, the mortality rate started to increase from the age of 35 upwards versus the age of 55 in the general population. When stratifying according to gender, women reported a higher increase in mortality rates.

If this data holds overall (higher COVID-19 incidence/prevalence and casualty rates among patients with autoimmunity/autoinflammation), there appear some differences among the specific autoimmune/autoinflammatory diseases. For example [212], the authors found a higher risk for RA and iritis patients and a lower risk for inflammatory bowel diseases (IBD) and MS patients [213]. They reported poorer clinical outcomes among Sjögren's syndrome (SS), vasculitis, and systemic lupus erythematosus (SLE) patients. On the other hand, some studies could not replicate these findings. For instance [214], the authors conducted an observational, cross-sectional study recruiting 1537 patients (1.49% with inflammatory articular diseases, IADs, 0.8% with RA, 0.3% with PsA, and 0.3% with ankylosing spondylitis/axial spondyloarthritis, SpA). No differences could be found between the various autoimmune/autoinflammatory diseases and comparing these patients with the general population in terms of COVID-19-related clinical outcomes, with the only predictor of fatality being older age (OR 1.1 [95%CI 1.0–1.2]).

Moreover, there are a few studies that failed to detect any statistically significant association between suffering from an autoimmune/autoinflammatory disease and contracting the COVID-19 infection, finding, on the contrary, that (at least some) autoimmune diseases could confer protection against COVID-19 [215].

These apparent discrepancies could be explained by taking into account the impact of medication [216]. Some studies found, indeed, a differential effect according to the specific drug administered. Some therapeutics, like prednisone, increased the risk of hospitalization (OR 2.05 [95%CI 1.06–3.96]), whilst other drugs, like antiTNF biologics (OR 0.40 [95%CI 0.19–0.81]) decreased such a risk [213]. Other studies confirmed these findings, with no death observed among patients with autoimmune/autoinflammatory diseases infected with COVID-19 on antiTNF therapy, whilst the use of rituximab was associated with poorer clinical outcomes. In another study [217], the use of prednisone and methotrexate were linked with hospital admission.

Finally, some de novo-onset cases or flares/relapses of autoimmune/autoinflammatory diseases have been reported after the COVID-19 infection or vaccination.

The following paragraphs will outline the major findings for each autoimmune disorder (briefly overviewed in Table 2.1), based on a comprehensive, critical appraisal of the currently available body of evidence, stressing eventual gaps in knowledge and suggesting future directions and prospects.

Alopecia areata and telogen effluvium

Alopecia areata is an autoimmune disorder characterized by an aberrant NK, T, and plasmacytoid dendritic cell (PDC) response against hair follicle self-antigens [218,219,220]. After the molecular interaction between the NKG2D receptor (NKG2DR) and the NKG2D-associated ligands (NKG2DLs, namely, major histocompatibility complex class I chain-related gene A or MICA, UL16-binding protein type 3 or ULBP3, and UL16-binding protein type 6 or ULBP6), aggregation and activation of CD8+ NKG2D + T cells is promoted, which results in the generation and release of interferon-gamma (IFN-γ) that upregulates major histocompatibility complex (MHC) class I (MHC-I) and II (MHC-II) expression via the JAK-STAT pathway. This and other cascades produce the serine protease granzyme B (GZMB) that finely modulates apoptotic cell death. Activated CD8+ NKG2D + T cells also produce γ-chain cytokines (such as interleukin (IL) type 2, IL-2, and IL-15), which contribute to creating a positive feedback loop by activating IFN-γ–producing CD8+ NKG2D + T cells. Also, other cells, including NK cells and CD4+ T cell subtypes (T helper 17, Th17, and T regulatory, T_{reg}, cells) release IFN-γ [219].

NK cells target hair follicles via the above-mentioned NKG2DL-NKG2DR pathway, but also through the expression of various CXCR3 ligands, like CXCL9, CXCL10, and CXCL11, among others. Besides this aberrant NK cell response, CD4+ T cell subtypes, fostered by upregulation of MHC-II, release a large amount of several proinflammatory cytokines and chemokines [219].

Concurrently, PDCs produce type I IFN, which, in turn, promotes and enhances the activation of CD8+, CD4+, and NK cells. However, the feedback is much more complex, in that these cells generate TNF-α, which can have a detrimental impact, by inhibiting PDCs activity and impairing keratinocytes differentiation [219].

Telogen effluvium is the abrupt interruption of *anagen* (the active phase of hair follicles growth cycle), which forces hair follicles to enter *catagen* (which is the regression phase of hair follicles growth cycle). If particularly severe, *telogen effluvium* can be accompanied by trychodinia (known also as cutaneous dysesthesia syndrome). *Telogen effluvium* can be considered an autoimmune/autoinflammatory disease [221].

Cases of *alopecia areata* and *telogen effluvium* have been on the rise during the COVID-19 outbreak [34], probably because of the increased level of stress imposed by the pandemic. Some cases of *alopecia areata* after the COVID-19 infection or vaccination have been anecdotally reported [24,25,26,27,28,30,31,32,222,35,36,37,38,39,40,42,43–45,47,48,49].

Some scholars have hypothesized different mechanisms, which could lead to hair follicle damage and subsequent loss, including the release of cytokines and chemokines inhibiting hair follicle growth, antibody-dependent enhancement (ADE), regulation of apoptotic cascades, or formation of microthrombi [223], among others. Some of these phenomena and events, as previously seen, are implicated in the multi-factorial etiopathogenesis of *alopecia areata* [219]. Furthermore, ACE2 receptors (which represent the entry of the coronavirus into human cells) are highly expressed at the level of keratinocytes and sebaceous glands, even though their precise functional role in the biology and physiopathology of hair follicles warrants further research [29]. Concerning *telogen effluvium*, besides the cytokines and chemokines released by the virus, also drugs utilized for the treatment (such as heparinoids) could play a role in its etiopathogenesis [39].

Furthermore, a cross-sectional questionnaire-based survey [41] has found that 42.5% of the participants infected by COVID-19 reported relapses of *alopecia areata*, approximately 2 months later the infection, and 74.0% of them were continuing to experience symptoms at the time of the survey. Only 12.5% of participants' relapses were not associated with the COVID-19 infection.

On the other hand, a retrospective study on 32 patients was not able to find any association between mild-to-moderate COVID-19 infection and worsening of *alopecia areata* symptoms [46]. Similarly, a national cohort study, which was conducted in Korea [33], recruited a total of 226,737 participants (7958 [3.5%] cases versus 218,779 [96.5%] controls), and confirmed the lack of relationship between COVID-19 and *alopecia areata*. The incidence rate ratio (IRR) of COVID-19 patients with a newly diagnosed *alopecia areata* compared to controls was 0.78 [95%CI 0.48–1.27] and 0.60 [95%CI 0.35–1.03], when adjusting for age and sex and for all demographic variables, respectively.

Amyloidosis

Amyloidosis is a family of autoimmune protein synthesis disorders, characterized by protein misfolding. It can affect the kidneys, heart, nervous system, gastrointestinal apparatus, glands, eyes, oral cavity, and musculoskeletal system. According to the "International Society of Amyloidosis" (ISA), there are at least 36 types of amyloidosis [224]: the most studied protein that can cause amyloidosis is the serum amyloid A (SAA), which is an important inflammatory marker of several rheumatological diseases: moreover, it plays a key role in the etiopathogenesis of several autoimmune disorders, favoring the activation of the inflammasome cascade and recruiting IL-17 producing T helper cells [225].

The potential role of SARS-CoV-2 in the pathogenesis of amyloidosis has been explored recently in a biophysical experiment based on all-atom molecular dynamic simulations [226]. The authors have found that the nine-residue segment SK9, located at the C-terminus of the envelope protein, can increase the propensity for SAA fibril formation. Three mechanisms have been hypothesized: (i) SK9 may reduce the stability of the lipid-transporting hexamer, thus shifting the equilibrium toward monomers, (ii) it may increase the frequency of aggregation-prone configurations in the resulting chains, and, finally, (iii) it may raise the stability of SAA fibrils.

A few *de novo*-onset cases after the COVID-19 infection have been described in the literature [50].

Ankylosing spondylitis

SpA is an autoimmune disease that is characterized by a progressive fusion of the *vertebrae*, leading to a hunched posture and breathing difficulties. Subjects with SpA do not appear to be at higher risk for contracting the COVID-19 infection. In a multi-center survey, recruiting 3435 individuals with SpA from 65 countries, only 41 self-reported COVID-19 like symptoms [53]. Raiker et al. [52] confirmed these results, finding that 9766 patients with axial spondyloarthritis (8842 of whom being nonradiographic) versus 691,862 controls were protected against poor COVID-19 clinical outcomes, including mortality (risk-ratio, RR, of 0.707 [95%CI 0.598–0.836]), severe COVID-19 (RR 0.791 [95%CI 0.69–0.906]), hospitalization (RR 0.872 [95%CI 0.826–0.921]), and acute kidney injury (RR 0.902 [95%CI 0.816–0.997]). Only the risk of venous thromboembolism was higher in axial spondyloarthritis patients (RR 1.219 [95%CI 1.037–1.433]). When stratifying according to gender and ethnicity, males and self-declared Black people were more likely to exhibit worse clinical outcomes. There were no substantial differences between radiographic and nonradiographic axial spondyloarthritis patients, with the only exception of hospital admission. Finally, patients on nonsteroidal anti-inflammatory drugs (NSAIDs) reported poorer outcomes.

It could be speculated that HLA-B27 may confer protection against COVID-19. It is well-known that this allele protects against the human immunodeficiency virus (HIV) [227], ensuring low viral loads, a slower decline of CD4+ T cell counts, and a slower acquired immunodeficiency syndrome (AIDS) progression. HLA-B27 protects as well against hepatitis C virus (HCV), favoring viral clearance [227]. On the other hand, the relatively mild course of COVID-19 in SpA patients could be explained by taking into account the beneficial effects of anticytokine therapy [51].

Antiphospholipid syndrome, catastrophic antiphospholipid syndrome, and HELLP syndrome

Information about the impact of COVID-19 on antiphospholipid syndrome (APS) is scarce and anecdotal, with only 26 cohort studies and one clinical case report published so far [55]. More high-quality studies are needed to draw statistically solid conclusions on the relationship between APS and the viral agent. APS is an autoimmune disorder frequently triggered by infections and characterized by multiple episodes of venous and arterial thromboses and/or recurrent fetal losses in the presence of the expression of antiphospholipid (aPL) antibodies against β_2GP1. APS is frequently accompanied by moderate thrombocytopenia and its severe form is known as catastrophic APS (CAPS) [228,229].

Two possible pathogenetic mechanisms have been hypothesized: namely, (i) a direct immune-mediated thrombotic event with dysregulation of the coagulation cascades by the viral agent – the so-called "direct hypothesis", and (ii) a belated immuno-thrombotic event, mainly caused by aPL antibodies with SARS-CoV-2 as "supporting actor" – the so-called "second hit hypothesis" [230].

In COVID-19 patients, the presence of aPL antibodies varies from 21% to 70% [230,231], with a recently published systematic literature review and meta-analysis computing a pooled percentage of 46.8% [232]. However, the precise clinical meaning of aPL antibodies in COVID-19 patients warrants further research [233].

Furthermore, some cases of APS/CAPS triggered/precipitated by the COVID-19 vaccination have been reported [54,56,57]. Interestingly, one study [234] reported that five (63%) out of eight pregnant women with symptoms of severe COVID-19 infection fulfilled the diagnostic criteria for preeclampsia/"Hemolysis, Elevated Liver enzymes, Low Platelet count" (HELLP) syndrome. Subsequent clinical case reports and case series of preeclampsia/HELLP syndrome were described by other authors [235]. An investigation synthesized these studies and performed a meta-analysis, finding that the odds of developing preeclampsia/HELLP syndrome were significantly higher among pregnant women with SARS-CoV-2 infection with respect to their counterparts without SARS-CoV-2 infection (7.0% vs. 4.8%; pooled OR 1.62 [95%CI 1.45–1.82]; pooled aOR, 1.58 [95%1.39–1.80]).

Atopic dermatitis

There are two major hypotheses explaining the etiopathogenesis of atopic dermatitis: namely, the "outside-in" and the "inside-out" hypotheses, according to which immune dysregulation would be the cause and the consequence of skin barrier impairment/breakdown, respectively. Cases of potentially COVID-19-induced atopic dermatitis have been reported, either after the infection or the vaccination [61]. Fan et al. [58] performed a case-control study and found that, in a cohort of 11,752 atopic dermatitis cases matched with 47,008 controls, atopic dermatitis patients were more likely to contract the COVID-19 infection. Atopic dermatitis remained significantly associated also after adjusting for confounding factors like sociodemographic factors and comorbidities [59]. Another study confirmed these findings, reporting that increasing age was a predictor of higher COVID-19 severity, potentially due to the higher production of IL-4 and a type-2 immune response [60]. Another study found that atopic dermatitis patients on dupilumab reported attenuated COVID-19 symptoms. This finding was confirmed by a retrospective cohort-based study by [63] and by [62]. Suffering from atopic dermatitis was associated with the COVID-19 infection (IRR 1.41 [95%CI 1.34−1.48]; adjusted IRR, aIRR, 1.18 [95%CI 1.12−1.24]) and patients on dupilumab reported better outcomes with respect to those on prednisone, cyclosporine, and/or azathioprine. A possible explanation of the increased risk of COVID-19 among atopic dermatitis patients could be that skin expresses ACE2 and that an impairment of the skin barrier may facilitate the diffusion and spread of the virus [236].

Autoimmune myopathies (myositis, dermatomyositis, and polymyositis)

De novo-onset autoimmune myopathies have been reported after the COVID-19 infection [125]. Saud et al. [126] have extracted data from 23 patient cases with COVID-19-induced acute viral myositis (generally males, with an average age from 33 to 87 years). Clinical presentation is variable, ranging from muscle weakness, and back pain to full-blown dermatomyositis with typical rashes. Levels of creatine kinase (CK) and other muscle enzymes may be also within normal ranges and have not been found to be associated with COVID-19 prognosis and clinical outcomes. Rhabdomyolysis has been reported, with a rather high mortality rate (approximately 45%). Also, dermatomyositis has been described in the extant scholarly literature, in cases positive for dermatomyositis-associated auto-antibodies, including antiMi2, antimelanoma differentiation-associated gene 5 (antiMDA5), and anti-small ubiquitin-like modifier-1 activating enzyme (antiSAE1), or antinuclear autoantibodies.

Autoimmune ocular diseases

Several cases of SARS-CoV-2 induced iritis, uveitis, and Vogt-Koyanagi-Harada syndrome-like symptoms [237] have been anecdotally reported after the COVID-19 infection or vaccination [65,66,67,68]. Potential mechanisms could be the direct viral activity or indirect inflammatory/immune-mediated trigger of the virus with accompanying thromboembolic complications [238]. ACE2 may be expressed at the eye level, even though contrasting findings have been reported in the literature [239].

Autoimmune reproductive diseases

SARS-CoV-2 may impact the human reproductive apparatus [70], inducing autoimmune reproductive diseases, including autoimmune oophoritis and, as previously mentioned, pre-eclampsia/HELLP syndrome. A biophysics/bioinformatics study [69,240] has found evidence of molecular mimicry and structural homology between SARS-CoV-2 spike glycoprotein-derived epitopes and human proteins linked to oogenesis, uterine receptivity, decidualization, and placentation.

Autoimmune thyroiditis, including Hashimoto's thyroiditis and Graves' disease

Hashimoto's thyroiditis is an autoimmune disease clinically presenting as hypothyroidism, whilst Graves' disease is an autoimmune disease that represents the most common cause of hyperthyroidism in developed countries, affecting mostly women and, in general, individuals between 30 and 60 years of age [241,242].

SARS-CoV-2 may affect the thyroid gland directly or indirectly, by modulating the hypothalamic-pituitary-thyroid hormone axis [243,244,245,246], inducing as such thyroid dysfunction. SARS-CoV-2 could be internalized into thyrocytes via interaction with integrin αvβ3, ACE2, or TMPRSS2. Internalization would lead to viral shedding with subsequent systemic spread of viral progeny, together with a massive release of thyroid hormones, including thyroxine, thyroglobulin, thyroperoxidase, and thyroid-stimulating hormone (TSH) receptor. This would result in acute or subacute thyroiditis. Another mechanism would imply the immune-processing of thyroid antigens by means of specialized antigen-presenting cells (APCs) and consequent activation in genetically predisposed individuals of autoreactive lymphocytes (clinically resulting in Hashimoto's thyroiditis or Graves' disease) [246].

Clausen and collaborators [244] explored the correlation between cytokine levels and thyroid function and the associated risk of death, recruiting 116 patients. At hospital admission, 18.1% of patients had biochemically thyroid dysfunction including subclinical thyrotoxicosis, overt thyrotoxicosis, hypothyroidism, nonthyroidal illness, and impaired thyroid hormone levels. Significant correlations could be found between thyroid hormones and cytokines/chemokines concentrations. Some cases of *de novo*-onset autoimmune thyroiditis have been anecdotally reported after the COVID-19 infection or vaccination [86,247,83,84,87,88].

Behçet's disease

(Adamantiades-)Behçet's disease is an autoimmune disease characterized by recurrent skin mucosa lesions accompanied by uveitis. It can sometimes affect the central nervous system too [73]. A study described 10 cases of Behçet's disease linked with COVID-19: one died because of respiratory failure and one developed *de novo*-onset deep venous thrombosis. A study by Enginar and Gundogdu [72] found that patients with Behçet's disease did not exhibit a higher risk compared to the general population in terms of the frequency of SARS-CoV-2 infection, length of hospital stay, lung involvement, intensive care unit (ICU) admission, and mortality. Correa-Rodríguez et al. [71] reported contrasting findings. The authors carried out a retrospective study recruiting 244 patients with Behçet's disease, 86.1% of whom were females, with a mean age of 43.95 ± 11.11 years. A prevalence rate of COVID-19 was computed at 14.75%, significantly higher with respect to the general population. Patients on continuous antiTNF therapy apparently reported poorer outcomes, whereas the use of oral glucocorticoids and colchicine did not confer protection against COVID-19. Opposite findings were reported by [74]. The authors found that the prevalence rate of COVID-19 among patients with Behçet's disease was even lower than the general population, with low-dose prednisolone and/or biologics (especially, antiTNF therapy) not conferring a higher risk. These discrepancies among studies could be reconciled by taking into account the different study settings and the methodology adopted (correcting or not correcting for confounding factors utilizing propensity score matching methods in order to reduce the risk of bias in observational studies [248]). However, this warrants further research in the field.

Celiac disease

Celiac disease, known also as sprue or gluten-sensitive enteropathy, is an autoimmune disorder mainly affecting the small intestine. *De novo*-onset cases after the COVID-19 infection have been anecdotally reported [75]. Some scholars have explored the mortality rate among celiac patients during the COVID-19 pandemic [76]. The authors found that celiac patients infected with COVID-19 did not carry a statistically significantly higher risk of hospitalization, mortality, thrombotic events, or ICU care requirement compared with COVID-19 patients without celiac disease following propensity score matching.

Demyelinating syndromes

Some cases after the COVID-19 infection or vaccination have been reported in the literature [78]. Ismail and Salama [77] have recently reviewed a total of 60 investigations, finding a potential link between SARS-CoV-2 and diverse demyelinating conditions, including autoimmune encephalitis/encephalomyelitis, and Guillain-Barré syndrome (GBS) [85].

Autoimmune hemolytic anemia

Cases of *de novo*-onset autoimmune hemolytic anemia after the COVID-19 vaccination have been anecdotally reported [89,90].

Immune thrombocytopenia

Immune thrombocytopenia, also known as immune thrombocytopenic purpura (ITP), is an autoimmune disease and a well-known complication of COVID-19. Alonso-Beato et al. [91] reviewed the literature and found that ITP flares/relapses may appear in both mild and severe COVID-19 cases, not being linked with the severity of the disease or a specific stage of the infection. In ITP patients infected with COVID-19, platelet counts were significantly lower than in their counterparts without COVID-19. The course of ITP was characterized, on the one hand, by higher bleeding rates, and, on the other hand, by better pharmacological responses. Some *de novo*-onset cases potentially induced/triggered by COVID-19 have been also occasionally reported [92,93].

Inflammatory arthritis/reactive arthritis

Inflammatory arthritis (IA) is an autoinflammatory condition affecting multiple joints [249]. An investigation recruited a sample of 103 IA patients (80 of whom with confirmed COVID-19 and 23 with high suspicion of COVID-19). 26% of the cohort required hospitalization and 4% died. Predictors of poorer clinical outcomes were increasing age, underlying comorbidities including hypertension and chronic obstructive pulmonary disease (COPD), and being on glucocorticoids. Being on biologics apparently conferred protection against COVID-19.

Inflammatory bowel diseases

IBDs include ulcerative colitis (UC) and Chron's disease (CD). According to a recently published systematic literature review and meta-analysis pooling together 23 investigations totaling a sample of 51,643 IBD patients and 1449 with COVID-19 [96], the prevalence rate of COVID-19 among IBD patients was rather low, being approximately 1.01%. Outcomes varied depending on the drug received. When compared with patients treated with corticosteroids, those on antiTNF therapy exhibited a lower risk of hospitalization (with a risk ratio or RR of 0.24 [95%CI 0.16–0.35]) and ICU admission (with an RR of 0.10 [95%CI 0.03–0.37]). However, the mortality risk was comparable among the different IBD subpopulations stratified according to the treatment received (RR 0.16 [95%CI 0.02–1.71]). With respect to patients on mesalamine, those on antiTNF therapy had a lower risk of hospitalizations (RR 0.37 [95%CI 0.25–0.54]), ICU admissions (RR 0.20 [95%CI 0.07–0.58]), and death (RR 0.21 [95%CI 0.04–1.00]). No differences could be found between patients on immunomodulators and those on mesalamine or antiTNF therapy.

According to another systematic review and meta-analysis synthesizing 24 studies [94,95], the pooled incidence rates of COVID-19 per 1000 IBD patients and the general population were comparable, being 4.02 [95%CI 1.44–11.17] and 6.59 [95%CI 3.25–13.35], respectively. In other words, no increase in relative risk (0.47 [95%CI 0.18–1.26]) could be detected. Furthermore, the relative risk of acquiring COVID-19 did not differ between UC and CD (1.03 [95%CI 0.62–1.71]). The overall proportion of COVID-19-positive IBD patients requiring hospitalization and ICU admission was 27.29% and 5.33% with a pooled mortality rate of 4.27%. On the other hand, the risk of developing adverse outcomes was higher in UC with respect to CD patients.

Lichen planus, lichen planopilaris, and lichen sclerosus

Lichen planus is an autoimmune disease characterized by an aberrant T-cell cytotoxic reaction against epithelial basal cells. It can be triggered by medications, drugs, and infectious agents, especially HCV. *De novo*-onset cases or flares/relapses of *lichen planus* have been described after the COVID-19 infection or vaccination [97,98,99,100,101,102,103,104].

Miller–Fisher syndrome

Miller–Fisher syndrome is a rare, acquired autoimmune eye disease, clinically characterized by weakness of the eye muscles, impaired limb coordination and unsteadiness, and absent tendon reflexes. Biswas et al. [105] presented a review of the extant scholarly literature on *de novo*-onset cases of Miller–Fisher syndrome that occurred after contracting the COVID-19 infection. Twelve patients were described, seven (58.3%) of whom were males, with a median age of 50 years (mean age of 50.2 ± 12.3 years, ranging from 31 to 74 years). The syndrome presented from 1 to 20 days after COVID-19 infection. Clinical outcomes were good, with a complete or near-complete resolution of symptoms within 1–2 weeks. Only in a few cases improvement was mild or limited, with one case exhibiting residual generalized hyporeflexia and one case of death due to the abrupt insurgence of ventricular arrhythmia and cardiac arrest. According to [105]; the novel coronavirus could infect the central nervous system, triggering an immune-mediated reaction and resulting in a neuronal infection by retrograde axonal transport. Possible explanations of the *de novo*-onset Miller–Fisher syndrome include ganglioside mimicry, complex-enhanced or -attenuated GQ1b-IgG and GQ1b-IgG autoantibodies, antigen expression on the myelin sheath, and autonomic dysfunction at the level of the preganglionic, ganglion and postganglionic fibers.

Multiple sclerosis

MS is a chronic, neurological autoimmune disease affecting the brain and the spinal cord [250].

SARS-CoV-2 could be internalized via sphingosine 1-phosphate (S1P), thus entering the central nervous system and replicating, shedding its progeny [251]. The role of S1P in the pathobiology of SARS-CoV-2 can have important, major implications, stressing the importance of sphingolipids as a druggable target in the fight against COVID-19 [252]. Fingolimod, an immunomodulatory drug targeting S1P receptors, could be a valuable therapeutic option: some data seems to support its clinical usefulness. Fingolimod withdrawal leads, indeed, to the clinical worsening of COVID-19-related symptoms [110]. MS patients on fingolimod and on siponimod have better outcomes, suggesting a putative mediating role of the drugs [253].

The extant scholarly literature reports contrasting findings: a study by [118] found that the incidence of COVID-19 among MS patients was 6.3%, not much higher than the general population. Nineteen (20.3%) patients needed to be hospitalized and two (2.2%) died. Predictors of poorer outcomes were increasing age, exposure to infected individuals, MS duration, and time on antiCD-20 therapy. Interestingly, lymphopenia or immunoglobulin levels were not correlated with COVID-19 and its severity. Similarly, in a Polish study [108], the hospitalization rate among MS patients did not differ from the rate among the general population.

However, according to a recent systematic review and meta-analysis synthesizing 13 studies [109], suffering from MS was associated with severe and worse COVID-19-related clinical outcomes. Other factors, such as age, being a male, overweight and obesity, diabetes, pulmonary and cardiovascular comorbidities, and hypertension were associated with a worse prognosis. Current or past smoking was not statistically associated. Received drugs impacted clinical outcomes: being on antiCD20 therapy increased the risk, whilst being on interferons significantly lowered the risk.

In a case-control study [111], a total of 779 patients with MS with COVID-19 were matched to 1558 MS patients without COVID-19, acting as controls. The authors found that underlying comorbidities, being a female, and younger age were associated with a higher risk of contracting COVID-19. Patients on natalizumab (OR 2.38 [95%CI 1.66–3.42]) and those undergoing an escalation treatment strategy (OR 1.57 [95%CI 1.16–2.13]) were at higher risk, as well as those requiring hospital access (OR 1.65 [95%CI 1.34–2.04]). However, the association between the use of natalizumab and poorer clinical outcomes was not replicated by another study [107]. The authors demonstrated, on the contrary, the safety profile of this drug. Similarly, a large, multi-center study from 28 countries [116] replicated this finding: while natalizumab is safe among MS patients with COVID-19, on the other hand, the use of rituximab and ocrelizumab may be associated with a worse prognosis, need for hospital admission, artificial ventilation, and ICU care. Moreover [112], a study found that MS patients on alemtuzumab exhibited a milder course of COVID-19, whereas another study [106] reported that MS patients on rituximab and natalizumab needed to be hospitalized. Utilizing a Big Data-based approach and mining the Biogen Global Safety Database [114], a study found that the use of interferons and glatiramer acetate was associated with a decreased COVID-19 risk, whilst being on anti-CD20 therapy was statistically associated with a significantly increased risk. Similar conclusions were reached by a study conducted by [117]; who found that the use of methylprednisolone and antiCD20 therapies was associated with severe COVID-19 infection.

In conclusion, MS-specific treatment may influence COVID-19-related clinical outcomes, but, given the uncertainty both in the direction and in the magnitude of the effect, further multi-center studies should be conducted. Based on a critical appraisal of the currently available body of evidence, some drugs like fingolimod or siponimod can be recommended, while caution is required when administering therapeutics like natalizumab, ocrelizumab, rituximab, cladribine, or alemtuzumab [254]. Some MS drugs could be considered being "reprofiled" for COVID-19 purposes, like teriflunomide, which could exert an antiviral activity by depleting the pool of cellular nucleotides that are necessary for viral replication, or dimethyl fumarate, which could protect against COVID-19 by activating the NRF-2 pathway [255] and mitigating against the burden imposed to cells by oxidative stress. Some experimental evidence has shown [256] that NRF-2 inhibitors, like 4-octyl-itaconate and dimethyl fumarate, can suppress SARS-CoV-2 replication and growth in different cell lines.

Finally, MS flares/relapses after the COVID-19 infection or vaccination have been described [113,115].

Myasthenia gravis and other autoimmune neuromuscular junction disorders

Myasthenia gravis is an autoimmune, neuromuscular disease, affecting the muscles of the eye and the face, clinically characterized by trouble swallowing, talking, and walking. From a cellular and molecular standpoint, the body develops autoantibodies against the nicotinic acetylcholine receptors (AChR) at the neuromuscular junction [257]. A large thymus or a thymoma is also another feature of the disease.

Abbas et al. [119] have synthesized 19 studies totaling 152 patients with myasthenia gravis, with an average age of 54.4 ± 12.7 years, 79 (52.0%) of whom were females. Invasive ventilation treatment was required for 25/59 (42.4%) of patients. The mean hospital length of stay was 18.2 ± 9.9 days and the mortality rate was 18/152 (11.8%). SARS-CoV-2 has been found to precipitate myasthenic crisis [120,122]. De novo-onset cases of myasthenia gravis after the COVID-19 infection [123] and vaccination have been anecdotally reported [121].

Autoimmune myocarditis

Autoimmune myocarditis is an inflammation of the myocardium [258]. Several cases of potentially immune-mediated myocarditis have been reported after the COVID-19 infection and vaccination. However [124], an investigation conducted a biophysics/bioinformatics study comparing SARS-CoV-2 spike protein-derived peptides and myocarditis-associated antigens, in terms of sequence similarity/identity. Also assessing discontinuous 3-D epitope similarities, the authors were not able to find any significant association between the virus and the disease in terms of homology.

Pemphigus vulgaris and other autoimmune blistering diseases

Autoimmune blistering diseases (AIBDs) include *epidermolysis bullosa acquisita*, IgA-mediated bullous dermatoses, *pemphigus*, and pemphigoid. These disorders are characterized by blisters at the level of the skin, mucosa, and membranes. Breglio et al. [127] reported COVID-19-related clinical outcomes in patients with *pemphigus vulgaris* and other AIBDs. The authors computed a higher mortality rate with respect to the general population (20% versus 1.6%–2%). Being on rituximab did not appear to confer a higher risk or a worse prognosis, even though more data would be necessary to draw robust conclusions, given the small sample size of the investigation. Flares/relapses after the COVID-19 infection have been reported [128].

Polymyalgia rheumatica

Polymyalgia rheumatica (PMR) is an autoimmune disease characterized by muscle pain, weakness, and stiffness, especially at the level of hips and shoulders. *De novo*-onset cases or relapses/flares of generally self-limiting PMR have been anecdotally described after the COVID-19 infection or after the COVID-19 vaccination [129,130,131,133]. Mettler and co-workers [132] have mined a global pharmacovigilance database, VigiBase, and found that COVID-19 vaccination was statistically linked with PMR (reporting odds-ratio, ROR, of 2.3 [95%CI 2.0–2.6]). Manzo and colleagues [130,131] have hypothesized that, since TLR7 and TLR9 are overexpressed in the peripheral mononuclear cells in patients genetically predisposed for PMR, immunizing against COVID-19 could result in the activation of intracellular TLRs and other endosolic and cytoplasmic nucleic acid receptors via, for instance, UNC931 [259], leading to the nuclear transcription, production and release of IL-6, IFN-α, TNF-α, and IL-27, among others.

Postural orthostatic tachycardia syndrome

Postural orthostatic tachycardia syndrome (POTS) is an autoimmune disease characterized by the presence of G-protein coupled receptor (GPCR) autoantibodies [260]. Blitshteyn and Whitelaw [134] collected data from 20 POTS patients, 70% of whom were females, with a median age of 40 years, ranging from 25 to 65 years. Six patients had reported preexisting minor autonomic symptoms, like occasional dizziness, palpitations, or syncope, and four had a remote history of concussion. Eighty-five percent of patients reported residual symptoms six-eight months after COVID-19. However, only three of them could return to work full-time with a complete or near-complete resolution of symptoms.

Primary biliary cholangitis, primary sclerosing cholangitis, and other autoimmune cholangiopathies

Very few data are available concerning these autoimmune disorders [135–137] Bartoli et al. [136] reported the case of a 44-year-old obese and hypertensive woman, with underlying Hashimoto's thyroiditis. She developed both primary biliary cholangitis and Guillain-Barré syndrome after the COVID-19 infection. Potential mechanisms may include the binding of the coronavirus on the ACE2 expressed at the level of bile duct cells [261,262], resulting in severe cholangiocyte injury and intrahepatic microangiopathy. Roth and colleagues [137] have introduced the concept of "post-COVID-19 cholangiopathy", warranting further investigation and follow-up concerning long-term liver morbidity.

Psoriasis

Psoriatic patients appear to be at higher risk for developing the COVID-19 infection [141,143]. From a molecular perspective, psoriatic patients have upregulated levels of ACE2, FURIN, and TMPPRSS2, which play a key role in the etiopathogenesis of COVID-19 [263,95,236]. However, patients on biologics do not seem to be at higher risk for COVID-19. Ciechanowicz et al. [140] analyzed 61 patients with moderate-to-severe psoriasis treated with biologics, 10 of whom presented antiCOVID-19 antibodies, and one developed symptom of mild COVID-19 infection. Similarly, in Italy [141], a study recruited 1193 PsO patients treated with biologics and small molecules, who were found to be at higher risk to test positive for COVID-19 (OR 3.43 [95%CI 2.25–5.73]), to be self-quarantined at home (OR 9.05 [95%CI 5.61–14.61]) and hospitalized (OR 3.59 [95%CI 1.49–8.63]), however, no increased risk of ICU admission or death could be found. Results concerning small molecules and biologics were replicated by other investigations [146].

Some *de novo*-onset cases or flares/relapses of psoriasis have been reported after the COVID-19 infection or vaccination [138,139,142,144,145]. However, given the dearth of high-quality information, further research is urgently warranted [264].

Psoriatic arthritis

Approximately one-third of psoriatic patients develop PsA. Some *de novo*-onset cases of PsA after the COVID-19 infection have been reported [150]. Queiro Silva et al. [146] presented seven patients with psoriasis and PsA and found that patients on apremilast and on secukinumab exhibited good clinical outcomes, different from patients on infliximab or with underlying comorbidities. These findings were replicated by other studies [149,151]. A number of studies did not observe any statistically significant surge in flares/relapses during the COVID-19 pandemic [147,148].

Rheumatoid arthritis

RA is a chronic systemic autoimmune disease that poses a dramatically high burden of disability and morbidity. If not properly treated, it can progress resulting in hyperplastic synovium, severe cartilage damage, bone erosion, and systemic consequences [265].

Contrasting findings have been reported in the scholarly literature, even though data taken altogether does not seem to suggest that COVID-19-driven biological phenomena and processes may lead to the development of arthritis [266]. On the one hand, a study [153] found a higher risk of contracting COVID-19 among patients suffering from RA, whereas other studies reported no statistically significant association. The former investigation recruited 33,886 RA and matched controls: during follow-up, 1503 patients contracted COVID-19, 388 of whom developed serious outcomes (including hospitalization or death). In the multivariate regression analysis, suffering from RA was associated with a higher risk of being infected by COVID-19 (adjusted hazard ratio, aHR, of 1.25 [95%CI 1.13−1.39]) and reporting a worse prognosis (aHR 1.35 [95%CI 1.10−1.66]). Predictors of severe COVID-19 were found to be the use of DMARDs, prednisone, Black race, Hispanic ethnicity, and underlying comorbidities. Cordtz et al. [267] found an increased risk of hospitalization among RA patients when compared to the general population (HR 1.72 [95%CI 1.29−2.30]), whilst, on the contrary [268], a study found that, among RA patients, the risk of hospitalization, and the ICU admission and death rates (all-cause mortality) were comparable with the general population.

Some scholars have suggested that SARS-CoV-2 could promote/potentiate initiation, progression, and perpetuation of RA via multiple, concurrent mechanisms, including cytokine release, activation of proinflammatory transcription pathways and cascades, and enhancement of cytokine/chemokine signaling networks [269]. Moreover, in RA patients, SARS-CoV-2 can lead to severe immune-mediated events, including thrombotic ones [270].

On the other hand, these potential risks appear to be mitigated by the use of JAK inhibitors. A recent data-mining analysis of a global pharmacovigilance database [152] found the use of JAK inhibitors to be protective against COVID-19.

Flares/relapses of RA have been anecdotally reported after the COVID-19 vaccination [154].

Sarcoidosis

From a cellular and molecular perspective, a link between COVID-19 and sarcoidosis has been hypothesized based on some common mechanistic pathways around the regulation and fine-tuning of autophagy shared by the two diseases [271,272]. A recently published review [160] has collected data from 27 patients with sarcoidosis from 14 studies. No significant differences could be found in the clinical presentation of patients with sarcoidosis infected by COVID-19 with respect to the general population. The risk of contracting the COVID-19 infection is comparable with the general population, as computed by a study recruiting 5200 sarcoidosis patients [156], with 116 of whom (2.23%) reporting infection and 18 (15.8%) requiring hospitalization. Increased hazard ratio (HR) for COVID-19 infection could be computed for those with a COVID-19 infected roommate (HR 27.44), working as a healthcare provider (HR 2.4), suffering from pulmonary sarcoidosis (HR 2.48), or neurosarcoidosis (HR 2.02), or on rituximab (HR 5.40). However, even though the risk of infection was comparable with the general population, clinical outcomes were worse [156,167].

More specifically, the rates of hospitalization and mortality were computed at 48.1% and at 7.4%, respectively, significantly higher than the average mortality rate of 2.1% among the general population [160]. This was confirmed by a population cohort-based study [155], which found an HR of 1.36 [95%CI 1.10–1.68] for hospital admission among sarcoidosis patients. In particular, the hospitalization rate was higher among sarcoidosis patients with underlying cardiovascular diseases (HR 3.19) [156]. Outcomes were worse in patients treated with glucocorticoids [161], even though another study failed to replicate such a finding [156]. Hydroxychloroquine, which has been hypothesized to be effective as COVID-19 pre or postexposure prophylaxis, does not appear to confer protection against SARS-CoV-2 [157], whilst DMARDs and antiTNF therapy appear to be effective [163], even though these preliminary findings should be replicated by high-quality, larger clinical trials. Predictors of worse prognosis were moderate-to-severe lung function impairment (aOR 7.8, 95% CI 2.4–25.8), from a cohort study of 7337 patients, 37 of whom (0.5%) with sarcoidosis [165], whereas self-declared Black race does not appear to be associated with severe outcomes [156,163] as well as old age and comorbidities other than heart disease [156]. However, another study [273] found that increasing age was associated with a worse prognosis and a greater risk of hospitalization, with an aOR of 1.18 [95%CI 1.04–1.35]. Synthesizing all available cohort studies, including the clinical case series by [159,162,167]; among sarcoidosis patients, the COVID-19 infection rate ranges from 2.1% to 8.9%. The hospitalization rate ranges from 0.8% to 50.5%, the ICU admission rate varies from 21.4% to 100% and, finally, the mortality rate ranges from 1.3% to 32.4%.

De novo-onset sarcoidosis cases have been anecdotally reported after the COVID-19 vaccination, including cases of systemic sarcoidosis or Löfgren's syndrome [164,166].

Sjögren's syndrome

Sjögren's syndrome is an autoimmune disease affecting moisture-producing glands and is characterized by systemic symptoms, including feelings of weakness and fatigue. Worsening of disease activity and flares/relapses have been described during the COVID-19 pandemic [170]. Furthermore, a new nosological entity, termed "long-term xerostomia" has been introduced [158,171]: briefly, SARS-CoV-2 may be internalized within salivary and epithelial gland cells via ACE2, leading to infection and, potentially, to long-term retention. Viral replication may give rise to immune reactions, overproduction of proinflammatory cytokines, resulting in tissue damage, expression of novel autoantigens/epitopes, B-cell activation, autoantibodies production, and release, and, finally, autoimmune sialoadenitis [274].

Of note, some cases of "phenotypic switches" along the *continuum* of autoimmunity and autoinflammation have been reported in the literature [172]: for instance, the case report of an old man who had an inactive Sjögren's syndrome and began to clinically express full-blown SLE.

Systemic lupus erythematosus

SLE is an autoimmune disease affecting a plethora of human organs and structures, from joints, and skin, to the brain, lungs, kidneys, and blood vessels. Patients with SLE may be at higher risk for contracting and developing severe COVID-19. From a cellular and molecular perspective, ACE2 expression could be upregulated in SLE patients by underlying oxidative stress and DNA methylation defects (involving genes, such as CD40LG, CD70, ITGAL/CD11A, and the KIR gene cluster) and other epigenetic dysregulations. Furthermore, type

1 IFN signature, which is typical of SLE, could increase susceptibility to COVID-19 and, more specifically, its severe complications [275,276,277]. Moreover, SLE patients may present autoantibodies to ACE2 [278] and ACE2 may elevate further if patients are on glucocorticoids [279,231]. Some recently published studies have emphasized also the role of extrafollicular double negative (DN2) B cell subsets [280], which expand in the case of severe or critical COVID-19 [281] and the levels of which correlate with inflammation markers [282,283].

Sakthiswary et al. [284] have performed a systematic literature review and meta-analysis and have pooled together 24 articles totaling 48 patients. The authors found that the median age at diagnosis of COVID-19 infection was 41 years, ranging from 11 to 66 years. The median SLE disease duration prior to the diagnosis of COVID-19 was 9 years, ranging from 0 to 30 years. Slightly less than half of SLE patients (22/48, 45.83%) had severe-to-critical COVID-19. Baseline medications did not appear to influence clinical outcomes. SLE patients with lupus nephritis were significantly more likely to develop the severe-to-critical disease (OR 5.40 [95%CI 1.120–26.045]). Predictors of contracting the virus were found to be increasing age, prednisone escalation, and having infected relatives [176]. Some cases of de novo-onset SLE have been described after the COVID-19 infection or vaccination [173,174,175,177,178,179,180,181].

Systemic sclerosis and scleroderma

Systemic sclerosis/scleroderma is an autoimmune disease clinically characterized by fibrosis and vascular abnormalities affecting the skin, joints, and internal organs (above all the esophagus, and the lower gastrointestinal tract, as well as the lungs, the heart, and the kidneys). Only two clinical case reports about the relationship between COVID-19 and systemic sclerosis/scleroderma have been published so far in the extant scholarly literature. One case report concerned a 47-year-old apparently healthy woman, without any underlying comorbidities and without a story positive for autoimmune diseases, who developed a de novo-onset scleroderma after the COVID-19 infection [168]. The other case report described a deterioration of scleroderma-associated symptoms after the COVID-19 infection [169].

Type 1 diabetes

Type 1 diabetes, known also as juvenile diabetes or insulin-dependent diabetes, is an autoimmune disease characterized by complex pathogenesis. It has been reported in 0.15%–28.98% of patients with COVID-19 [82], with the infection making the control of diabetes-associated symptoms quite challenging [80]. Clinical presentation includes symptoms such as fever, dry cough, nausea and vomiting, elevated blood glucose, and diabetic ketoacidosis, among others [79]. Diabetes type 1 has been reported on the rise during the COVID-19 pandemic [81]. Utilizing data from the multicenter "German Diabetes Prospective Follow-up Registry", in Germany, the observed incidence of diabetes type 1 in 2020/21 was significantly higher than the expected incidence (IRR, of 1.15 [1.10–1.20]), especially during June and July 2020, March, and June 2021. These findings could be confirmed by other studies [80].

Vasculitis

Vasculitis represents an inflammation of the human blood vessels. Cordtz et al. [267] found an increased risk of hospitalization for patients with vasculitides compared to the general population (HR 1.82 [95%CI 0.91–3.64]). Wong et al. [182] synthesized eight studies (7 clinical case reports and one clinical case series) discussing 9 cases of vasculitis secondary to COVID-19. The average age was 29.17 ± 28.2 years, ranging from 6 months to 83 years, with a male-to-female ratio of 4:5. Concerning the clinical presentation, maculopapular, violaceous, papular, and erythematous rashes were commonly reported. Heparin, corticosteroids (in particular, methylprednisolone), and intravenous immunoglobulin (IVIG) were prescribed for these patients. Significant clinical improvement was observed in eight out of nine patients. Only one person died during the treatment.

Finally, Gracia-Ramos and colleagues [55] reported 46 cases of de novo vasculitis after COVID-19 infection: 28 cases of small-vessel vasculitis, 13 cases of medium-vessel vasculitis, and 5 cases of large-vessel vasculitis.

Vitiligo

Vitiligo is an autoimmune disease, affecting melanocytes, causes a loss of skin color in patches. De novo-onset cases or worsening of vitiligo have been anecdotally reported after the COVID-19 infection or vaccination [183,184,185,186,187]. Some scholars have hypothesized a mediating role of increased stress during the pandemic [188], with the link between emotional factors and the disease being well-known.

Conclusions and future prospects

SARS-CoV-2 represents a major environmental trigger and an important piece of the mosaic of autoimmunity and autoinflammation [285]. Several de novo-onset or flares/relapses of autoimmune/autoinflammatory diseases have been reported associated either directly or indirectly with the viral agent. Overall, patients with autoimmune/autoinflammatory diseases, in particular CTDs, are at higher risk of COVID-19 [286,287]). However, there may be a group of diseases, including ankylosing spondylitis/axial spondyloarthropathy (SpA), PsA, and potentially also RA, that appears to be protected against COVID-19. Moreover, some studies have reported contrasting findings. These apparent discrepancies can be reconciled by taking into account the mediating effect of medications: some drugs may increase or decrease the risk of contracting the coronavirus. Not all studies have conducted subgroup analyses, stratifying by treatment, or adequately performed sensitivity analyses.

COVID-19 has represented a unique opportunity for shedding new light and unexpected insights on autoimmune/autoinflammatory diseases. These have, in turn, enabled the discovery of novel aspects of the COVID-19 infection, offering already approved, effective and safe drugs, as options to be repurposed in the fight against the novel coronavirus. However, there is still a dearth of information concerning the long-term impact of the virus on autoimmunity and autoinflammation – the so-called long-COVID or postCOVID [288,289], which warrants further investigation.

References

[1] Shoenfeld Y, Isenberg DA. The mosaic of autoimmunity. Immunol Today April 1989;10(4):123–6. https://doi.org/10.1016/0167-5699(89)90245-4. PMID: 2665774.

[2] Brickman CM, Shoenfeld Y. The mosaic of autoimmunity. Scand J Clin Lab Invest Suppl 2001;235:3–15. PMID: 11712689.

[3] Zhernakova A, Withoff S, Wijmenga C. Clinical implications of shared genetics and pathogenesis in autoimmune diseases. Nat Rev Endocrinol November 2013;9(11):646–59. https://doi.org/10.1038/nrendo.2013.161. Epub 2013 Aug 20. PMID: 23959365.

[4] Arakelyan A, Nersisyan L, Poghosyan D, Khondkaryan L, Hakobyan A, Löffler-Wirth H, Melanitou E, Binder H. Autoimmunity and autoinflammation: a systems view on signaling pathway dysregulation profiles. PLoS One November 3, 2017;12(11):e0187572. https://doi.org/10.1371/journal.pone.0187572. PMID: 29099860; PMCID: PMC5669448.

[5] Doria A, Zen M, Bettio S, Gatto M, Bassi N, Nalotto L, Ghirardello A, Iaccarino L, Punzi L. Autoinflammation and autoimmunity: bridging the divide. Autoimmun Rev November 2012;12(1):22–30. https://doi.org/10.1016/j.autrev.2012.07.018. Epub 2012 Aug 2. PMID: 22878274.

[6] Zenewicz LA, Abraham C, Flavell RA, Cho JH. Unraveling the genetics of autoimmunity. Cell March 19, 2010;140(6):791–7. https://doi.org/10.1016/j.cell.2010.03.003. PMID: 20303870; PMCID: PMC3491807.

[7] de Carvalho JF, Pereira RM, Shoenfeld Y. The mosaic of autoimmunity: the role of environmental factors. Front Biosci June 1, 2009;1:501–9. https://doi.org/10.2741/e46. PMID: 19482664.

[8] Perricone C, Agmon-Levin N, Shoenfeld Y. Novel pebbles in the mosaic of autoimmunity. BMC Med April 4, 2013;11:101. https://doi.org/10.1186/1741-7015-11-101. PMID: 23557479; PMCID: PMC3635901.

[9] Borba V, Malkova A, Basantsova N, Halpert G, Andreoli L, Tincani A, Amital H, Shoenfeld Y. Classical examples of the concept of the ASIA syndrome. Biomolecules October 12, 2020;10(10):1436. https://doi.org/10.3390/biom10101436. PMID: 33053910; PMCID: PMC7600067.

[10] Ryabkova VA, Churilov LP, Shoenfeld Y. Neuroimmunology: what role for autoimmunity, neuroinflammation, and small fiber neuropathy in fibromyalgia, chronic fatigue syndrome, and adverse events after human Papillomavirus vaccination? Int J Mol Sci October 18, 2019;20(20):5164. https://doi.org/10.3390/ijms20205164. PMID: 31635218; PMCID: PMC6834318.

[11] Aljadeff G, Longhi E, Shoenfeld Y. Bisphenol A: a notorious player in the mosaic of autoimmunity. Autoimmunity December 2018;51(8):370–7. https://doi.org/10.1080/08916934.2018.1551374. Epub 2018 Dec 28. PMID: 30590961.

[12] Lazurova Z, Lazurova I, Shoenfeld Y. Bisphenol A as a factor in the mosaic of autoimmunity. Endocr Metab Immune Disord Drug Targets May 2021;13. https://doi.org/10.2174/1871530321666210516000042. Epub ahead of print. PMID: 33992069.

[13] Sharif K, Kurnick A, Coplan L, Alexander M, Watad A, Amital H, Shoenfeld Y. The putative adverse effects of bisphenol A on autoimmune diseases. Endocr Metab Immune Disord: Drug Targets February 10, 2021. https://doi.org/10.2174/1871530321666210210154309. Epub ahead of print. PMID: 33568039.

[14] Bragazzi NL, Watad A, Amital H, Shoenfeld Y. Debate on vaccines and autoimmunity: do not attack the author, yet discuss it methodologically. Vaccine October 9, 2017;35(42):5522–6. https://doi.org/10.1016/j.vaccine.2017.08.018. Epub 2017 Sep 4. PMID: 28882443.

[15] Watad A, Azrielant S, Bragazzi NL, Sharif K, David P, Katz I, Aljadeff G, Quaresma M, Tanay G, Adawi M, Amital H, Shoenfeld Y. Seasonality and autoimmune diseases: the contribution of the four seasons to the mosaic of autoimmunity. J Autoimmun August 2017;82:13–30. https://doi.org/10.1016/j.jaut.2017.06.001. Epub 2017 Jun 16. PMID: 28624334.

[16] Gomes JP, Watad A, Shoenfeld Y. Nicotine and autoimmunity: the lotus' flower in tobacco. Pharmacol Res February 2018;128:101–9. https://doi.org/10.1016/j.phrs.2017.10.005. Epub 2017 Oct 16. PMID: 29051105.

[17] Perricone C, Versini M, Ben-Ami D, Gertel S, Watad A, Segel MJ, Ceccarelli F, Conti F, Cantarini L, Bogdanos DP, Antonelli A, Amital H, Valesini G, Shoenfeld Y. Smoke and autoimmunity: the fire behind the disease. Autoimmun Rev April 2016;15(4):354–74. https://doi.org/10.1016/j.autrev.2016.01.001. Epub 2016 Jan 7. PMID: 26772647.

[18] Sharif K, Watad A, Bragazzi NL, Lichtbroun M, Amital H, Shoenfeld Y. Physical activity and autoimmune diseases: get moving and manage the disease. Autoimmun Rev January 2018;17(1):53–72. https://doi.org/10.1016/j.autrev.2017.11.010. Epub 2017 Nov 3. PMID: 29108826.
[19] Bizjak M, Selmi C, Praprotnik S, Bruck O, Perricone C, Ehrenfeld M, Shoenfeld Y. Silicone implants and lymphoma: the role of inflammation. J Autoimmun December 2015;65:64–73. https://doi.org/10.1016/j.jaut.2015.08.009. Epub 2015 Aug 29. PMID: 26330346.
[20] Watad A, Bragazzi NL, Amital H, Shoenfeld Y. Hyperstimulation of adaptive immunity as the common pathway for silicone breast implants, autoimmunity, and lymphoma of the breast. Isr Med Assoc J August 2019;21(8):517–9. PMID: 31474010.
[21] Watad A, Rosenberg V, Tiosano S, Cohen Tervaert JW, Yavne Y, Shoenfeld Y, Shalev V, Chodick G, Amital H. Silicone breast implants and the risk of autoimmune/rheumatic disorders: a real-world analysis. Int J Epidemiol December 1, 2018;47(6):1846–54. https://doi.org/10.1093/ije/dyy217. PMID: 30329056.
[22] Bogdanos DP, Smyk DS, Invernizzi P, Rigopoulou EI, Blank M, Pouria S, Shoenfeld Y. Infectome: a platform to trace infectious triggers of autoimmunity. Autoimmun Rev May 2013;12(7):726–40. https://doi.org/10.1016/j.autrev.2012.12.005. Epub 2012 Dec 22. PMID: 23266520; PMCID: PMC7105216.
[23] Dotan A, Mahroum N, Bogdanos DP, Shoenfeld Y. COVID-19 as an infectome paradigm of autoimmunity. J Allergy Clin Immunol January 2022;149(1):63–4. https://doi.org/10.1016/j.jaci.2021.11.009. Epub 2021 Nov 24. PMID: 34826507; PMCID: PMC8610602.
[24] Abrantes TF, Artounian KA, Falsey R, Simão JCL, Vañó-Galván S, Ferreira SB, Davis TL, Ridenour W, Goren A, Tosti A, Wambier CG. Time of onset and duration of post-COVID-19 acute telogen effluvium. J Am Acad Dermatol October 2021;85(4):975–6. https://doi.org/10.1016/j.jaad.2021.07.021. Epub 2021 Jul 21. PMID: 34302903; PMCID: PMC8294706.
[25] Aksoy H, Yıldırım UM, Ergen P, Gürel MS. COVID-19 induced telogen effluvium. Dermatol Ther November 2021;34(6):e15175. https://doi.org/10.1111/dth.15175. Epub 2021 Nov 6. PMID: 34708909; PMCID: PMC8646871.
[26] Berbert Ferreira S, Gavazzoni Dias MFR, Berbert Ferreira R, Neves Neto AC, Trüeb RM, Lupi O. Rapidly progressive alopecia areata totalis in a COVID-19 patient, unresponsive to tofacitinib. J Eur Acad Dermatol Venereol July 2021;35(7):e411–2. https://doi.org/10.1111/jdv.17170. Epub 2021 Mar 20. PMID: 33587766; PMCID: PMC8013294.
[27] Capalbo A, Giordano D, Gagliostro N, Balampanos CG, Persechino F, Orrù F, Persechino S. Alopecia areata in a COVID-19 patient: a case report. Dermatol Ther March 2021;34(2):e14685. https://doi.org/10.1111/dth.14685. Epub 2021 Jan 12. PMID: 33331017; PMCID: PMC7883233.
[28] Deng J, Ngo T, Zhu TH, Halverstam C. Telogen effluvium, Beau lines, and acral peeling associated with COVID-19 infection. JAAD Case Rep July 2021;13:138–40. https://doi.org/10.1016/j.jdcr.2021.05.026. Epub 2021 Jun 6. PMID: 34124324; PMCID: PMC8180346.
[29] Di Landro A, Naldi L, Glaser E, Paus R, Tosti A. Pathobiology questions raised by telogen effluvium and trichodynia in COVID-19 patients. Exp Dermatol July 2021;30(7):999–1000. https://doi.org/10.1111/exd.14352. Epub 2021 May 4. PMID: 33838048; PMCID: PMC8250761.
[30] Domínguez-Santás M, Haya-Martínez L, Fernández-Nieto D, Jiménez-Cauhé J, Suárez-Valle A, Díaz-Guimaraens B. Acute telogen effluvium associated with SARS-CoV-2 infection. Aust J Gen Pract August 2020;26:49. https://doi.org/10.31128/AJGP-COVID-32. PMID: 33051638.
[31] Essam R, Ehab R, Al-Razzaz R, Khater MW, Moustafa EA. Alopecia areata after ChAdOx1 nCoV-19 vaccine (Oxford/AstraZeneca): a potential triggering factor? J Cosmet Dermatol December 2021;20(12):3727–9. https://doi.org/10.1111/jocd.14459. Epub 2021 Sep 24. PMID: 34559937; PMCID: PMC8661988.
[32] FIvenson D. COVID-19: association with rapidly progressive forms of alopecia areata. Int J Dermatol January 2021;60(1):127. https://doi.org/10.1111/ijd.15317. Epub 2020 Nov 23. PMID: 33226118; PMCID: PMC7753616.
[33] Kim J, Hong K, Gómez Gómez RE, Kim S, Chun BC. Lack of evidence of COVID-19 being a risk factor of alopecia areata: results of a national cohort study in South Korea. Front Med October 13, 2021;8:758069. https://doi.org/10.3389/fmed.2021.758069. PMID: 34722594; PMCID: PMC8550157.
[34] Kutlu Ö, Aktas H, İmren IG, Metin A. Short-term stress-related increasing cases of alopecia areata during the COVID-19 pandemic. J Dermatol Treat June 2020;19:1. https://doi.org/10.1080/09546634.2020.1782820. Epub ahead of print. PMID: 32538230.

[35] Lv S, Wang L, Zou X, Wang Z, Qu B, Lin W, Yang D. A case of acute telogen effluvium after SARS-CoV-2 infection. Clin Cosmet Invest Dermatol April 16, 2021;14:385–7. https://doi.org/10.2147/CCID.S307982. PMID: 33889006; PMCID: PMC8057787.
[36] May Lee M, Bertolani M, Pierobon E, Lotti T, Feliciani C, Satolli F. Alopecia areata following COVID-19 vaccination: vaccine-induced autoimmunity? Int J Dermatol February 2, 2022. https://doi.org/10.1111/ijd.16113. Epub ahead of print. PMID: 35107173.
[37] Mieczkowska K, Deutsch A, Borok J, Guzman AK, Fruchter R, Patel P, Wind O, McLellan BN, Mann RE, Halverstam CP. Telogen effluvium: a sequela of COVID-19. Int J Dermatol January 2021;60(1):122–4. https://doi.org/10.1111/ijd.15313. Epub 2020 Nov 23. PMID: 33226117; PMCID: PMC7753411.
[38] Miola AC, Florêncio LC, Bellini Ribeiro ME, Alcântara GP, Müller Ramos P, Miot HA. Early-onset effluvium secondary to COVID-19: clinical and histologic characterization. 02914-5 J Am Acad Dermatol December 2021;11(21):S0190–9622. https://doi.org/10.1016/j.jaad.2021.09.072. Epub ahead of print. PMID: 34906662; PMCID: PMC8665661.
[39] Moreno-Arrones OM, Lobato-Berezo A, Gomez-Zubiaur A, Arias-Santiago S, Saceda-Corralo D, Bernardez-Guerra C, Grimalt R, Fernandez-Crehuet P, Ferrando J, Gil R, Hermosa-Gelbard A, Rodrigues-Barata R, Fernandez-Nieto D, Merlos-Navarro S, Vañó-Galván S. SARS-CoV-2-induced telogen effluvium: a multicentric study. J Eur Acad Dermatol Venereol March 2021;35(3):e181–3. https://doi.org/10.1111/jdv.17045. Epub 2020 Dec 9. PMID: 33220124; PMCID: PMC7753386.
[40] Olds H, Liu J, Luk K, Lim HW, Ozog D, Rambhatla PV. Telogen effluvium associated with COVID-19 infection. Dermatol Ther March 2021;34(2):e14761. https://doi.org/10.1111/dth.14761. Epub 2021 Jan 14. PMID: 33405302; PMCID: PMC7883200.
[41] Rinaldi F, Trink A, Giuliani G, Pinto D. Italian survey for the evaluation of the effects of coronavirus disease 2019 (COVID-19) pandemic on alopecia areata recurrence. Dermatol Ther April 2021;11(2):339–45. https://doi.org/10.1007/s13555-021-00498-9. Epub 2021 Feb 12. PMID: 33580408; PMCID: PMC7880634.
[42] Rizzetto G, Diotallevi F, Campanati A, Radi G, Bianchelli T, Molinelli E, Mazzanti S, Offidani A. Telogen effluvium related to post severe Sars-Cov-2 infection: clinical aspects and our management experience. Dermatol Ther January 2021;34(1):e14547. https://doi.org/10.1111/dth.14547. Epub 2020 Nov 23. PMID: 33190397; PMCID: PMC7744849.
[43] Rossi A, Magri F, Michelini S, Caro G, Di Fraia M, Fortuna MC, Pellacani G, Carlesimo M. Recurrence of alopecia areata after covid-19 vaccination: a report of three cases in Italy. J Cosmet Dermatol December 2021;20(12):3753–7. https://doi.org/10.1111/jocd.14581. Epub 2021 Nov 6. PMID: 34741583.
[44] Rossi A, Magri F, Michelini S, Sernicola A, Muscianese M, Caro G, Di Fraia M, Chello C, Fortuna MC, Grieco T. New onset of alopecia areata in a patient with SARS-CoV-2 infection: possible pathogenetic correlations? J Cosmet Dermatol 2021;20(7):2004–5. https://doi.org/10.1111/jocd.14080. Epub 2021 Mar 25. PMID: 33738910; PMCID: PMC8251072.
[45] Rossi A, Magri F, Sernicola A, Michelini S, Caro G, Muscianese M, Di Fraia M, Chello C, Fortuna MC, Grieco T. Telogen effluvium after SARS-CoV-2 infection: a series of cases and possible pathogenetic mechanisms. Skin Appendage Disord 2021;21(5):1–5. https://doi.org/10.1159/000517223. PMID: 34373830; PMCID: PMC8339054.
[46] Rudnicka L, Rakowska A, Waskiel-Burnat A, Kurzeja M, Olszewska M. Mild-to-moderate COVID-19 is not associated with worsening of alopecia areata: a retrospective analysis of 32 patients. J Am Acad Dermatol September 2021;85(3):723–5. https://doi.org/10.1016/j.jaad.2021.05.020. Epub 2021 May 26. PMID: 34051315; PMCID: PMC8149466.
[47] Scollan ME, Breneman A, Kinariwalla N, Soliman Y, Youssef S, Bordone LA, Gallitano SM. Alopecia areata after SARS-CoV-2 vaccination. JAAD Case Rep February 2022;20:1–5. https://doi.org/10.1016/j.jdcr.2021.11.023. Epub 2021 Dec 15. PMID: 34931171; PMCID: PMC8673931.
[48] Sgubbi P, Savoia F, Calderoni O, Longo R, Stinchi C, Tabanelli M. Alopecia areata in a patient with SARS-Cov-2 infection. Dermatol Ther November 2020;33(6):e14295. https://doi.org/10.1111/dth.14295. Epub 2020 Sep 21. PMID: 32909635.
[49] Sharquie KE, Jabbar RI. COVID-19 infection is a major cause of acute telogen effluvium. Ir J Med Sci August 2021;31:1–5. https://doi.org/10.1007/s11845-021-02754-5. Epub ahead of print. PMID: 34467470; PMCID: PMC8407603.

[50] Crees ZD, Stockerl-Goldstein K. COVID-19 and light chain amyloidosis, adding insult to injury. 00025-0 Am J Med January 2022;23(22):S0002−9343. https://doi.org/10.1016/j.amjmed.2022.01.005. Epub ahead of print. PMID: 35081378; PMCID: PMC8783834.

[51] Ortolan A, Lorenzin M, Cosma C, Cozzi G, Padoan A, Doria A, Plebani M, Ramonda R. SARS-CoV-2 infection in spondyloarthritis patients treated with biotechnological drugs: a study on serology. Front Immunol June 11, 2021;12:682850. https://doi.org/10.3389/fimmu.2021.682850. PMID: 34177927; PMCID: PMC8226267.

[52] Raiker R, Pakhchanian H, Kavadichanda C, Gupta L, Kardes S, Ahmed S. Axial spondyloarthritis may protect against poor outcomes in COVID-19: propensity score matched analysis of 9766 patients from a nationwide multi-centric research network. Clin Rheumatol November 2021;27:1−10. https://doi.org/10.1007/s10067-021-05979-y. Epub ahead of print. PMID: 34837569; PMCID: PMC8626282.

[53] Rosenbaum JT, Hamilton H, Weisman MH, Reveille JD, Winthrop KL, Choi D. The effect of HLA-B27 on susceptibility and severity of COVID-19. J Rheumatol April 2021;48(4):621−2. https://doi.org/10.3899/jrheum.200939. Epub 2020 Oct 15. PMID: 33060311.

[54] Chidharla A, Syed SB, Chatterjee T, Tarantino MD. A case report of COVID-associated catastrophic antiphospholipid syndrome successfully treated with eculizumab. Hematol Res Rev October 30, 2021;12:929−33. https://doi.org/10.2147/JBM.S324873. PMID: 34744467; PMCID: PMC8566005.

[55] Gracia-Ramos AE, Martin-Nares E, Hernández-Molina G. New onset of autoimmune diseases following COVID-19 diagnosis. Cells December 20, 2021;10(12):3592. https://doi.org/10.3390/cells10123592. PMID: 34944099; PMCID: PMC8700122.

[56] Jinno S, Naka I, Nakazawa T. Catastrophic antiphospholipid syndrome complicated with essential thrombocythaemia after COVID-19 vaccination: in search of the underlying mechanism. Rheumatol Adv Pract December 1, 2021;5(3):rkab096. https://doi.org/10.1093/rap/rkab096. PMID: 34909568; PMCID: PMC8665448.

[57] Moreno-Torres V, Gutiérrez Á, Valdenebro M, Ortega A, Cítores MJ, Montero E. Catastrophic antiphospholipid syndrome triggered by mRNA COVID-19 vaccine. Clin Exp Rheumatol December 7, 2021;40:1054−5. Epub ahead of print. PMID: 34874824.

[58] Fan R, Leasure AC, Damsky W, Cohen JM. Association between atopic dermatitis and COVID-19 infection: a case-control study in the All of Us research program. JAAD Int March 2022;6:77−81. https://doi.org/10.1016/j.jdin.2021.12.007. Epub 2021 Dec 28. PMID: 34977817; PMCID: PMC8712258.

[59] Grieco T, Chello C, Sernicola A, Muharremi R, Michelini S, Paolino G, Carnicelli G, Pigatto PD. Impact of COVID-19 on patients with atopic dermatitis. Clin Dermatol 2021 ;39(6):1083−7. https://doi.org/10.1016/j.clindermatol.2021.07.008. Epub 2021 Jul 17. PMID: 34920828; PMCID: PMC8285243.

[60] Kridin K, Schonmann Y, Solomon A, Onn E, Bitan DT, Weinstein O, Cohen AD. Risk of COVID-19 and its complications in patients with atopic dermatitis undergoing dupilumab treatment-a population-based cohort study. Immunol Res February 2022;70(1):106−13. https://doi.org/10.1007/s12026-021-09234-z. Epub 2021 Oct 13. PMID: 34647194; PMCID: PMC8514206.

[61] Potestio L, Napolitano M, Bennardo L, Fabbrocini G, Patruno C. Atopic dermatitis exacerbation after Covid-19 vaccination in Dupilumab-treated patients. J Eur Acad Dermatol Venereol January 2022;23. https://doi.org/10.1111/jdv.17964. Epub ahead of print. PMID: 35067996.

[62] Ungar B, Glickman JW, Golant AK, Dubin C, Marushchak O, Gontzes A, Mikhaylov D, Singer GK, Baum D, Wei N, Sanin A, Gruenstein D, Lebwohl MG, Pavel AB, Guttman-Yassky E. COVID-19 symptoms are attenuated in moderate-to-severe atopic dermatitis patients treated with dupilumab. J Allergy Clin Immunol Pract January 2022;10(1):134−42. https://doi.org/10.1016/j.jaip.2021.10.050. Epub 2021 Nov 1. PMID: 34737108; PMCID: PMC8558098.

[63] Wu JJ, Martin A, Liu J, Thatiparthi A, Ge S, Egeberg A, Thyssen JP. The risk of COVID-19 infection in patients with atopic dermatitis: a retrospective cohort study. J Am Acad Dermatol January 2022;86(1):243−5. https://doi.org/10.1016/j.jaad.2021.09.061. Epub 2021 Oct 6. PMID: 34626733; PMCID: PMC8492899.

[64] Santacroce G, Lenti MV, Aronico N, Miceli E, Lovati E, Lucotti PC, Coppola L, Gentile A, Latorre MA, Di Terlizzi F, Soriano S, Frigerio C, Pellegrino I, Pasini A, Ubezio C, Mambella J, Canta R, Fusco A, Rigano G, Di Sabatino A. Impact of COVID-19 in immunosuppressive drug-naïve autoimmune disorders: autoimmune gastritis, celiac disease, type 1 diabetes, and autoimmune thyroid disease. Pediatr Allergy Immunol January 2022;33(Suppl. 27):105−7. https://doi.org/10.1111/pai.13646. PMID: 35080315.

[65] Bolletta E, Iannetta D, Mastrofilippo V, De Simone L, Gozzi F, Croci S, Bonacini M, Belloni L, Zerbini A, Adani C, Fontana L, Salvarani C, Cimino L. Uveitis and other ocular complications following COVID-19 vaccination. J Clin Med December 19, 2021;10(24):5960. https://doi.org/10.3390/jcm10245960. PMID: 34945256; PMCID: PMC8704915.

[66] Brunet de Courssou JB, Tisseyre M, Hadjadj J, Chouchana L, Broca F, Terrier B, Duraffour P, Henriquez S. De Novo Vogt-Koyanagi-Harada disease following covid-19 vaccine: a case report and literature overview. Ocul Immunol Inflamm February 2022;3:1–4. https://doi.org/10.1080/09273948.2022.2028291. Epub ahead of print. PMID: 35113742.

[67] Kim SY, Kang MS, Kwon HJ. Bilateral panuveitis mimicking Vogt-Koyanagi-Harada disease following the first dose of ChAdOx1 nCoV-19 vaccine. Ocul Immunol Inflamm February 2022;3:1–4. https://doi.org/10.1080/09273948.2022.2026410. Epub ahead of print. PMID: 35113750.

[68] Ng XL, Betzler BK, Testi I, Ho SL, Tien M, Ngo WK, Zierhut M, Chee SP, Gupta V, Pavesio CE, de Smet MD, Agrawal R. Ocular adverse events after COVID-19 vaccination. Ocul Immunol Inflamm August 18, 2021;29(6):1216–24. https://doi.org/10.1080/09273948.2021.1976221. Epub 2021 Sep 24. PMID: 34559576; PMCID: PMC8477588.

[69] Dotan A, Kanduc D, Muller S, Makatsariya A, Shoenfeld Y. Molecular mimicry between SARS-CoV-2 and the female reproductive system. Am J Reprod Immunol December 2021;86(6):e13494. https://doi.org/10.1111/aji.13494. Epub 2021 Sep 17. PMID: 34407240; PMCID: PMC8420155.

[70] Tariq J, Chatterjee T, Andreoli L, Gupta L. COVID-19 and fertility-at the crossroads of autoimmunity and thrombosis. Rheumatol Int November 2021;41(11):1885–94. https://doi.org/10.1007/s00296-021-04977-2. Epub 2021 Aug 28. PMID: 34455463; PMCID: PMC8402971.

[71] Correa-Rodríguez M, Callejas-Rubio JL, Rueda-Medina B, Ríos-Fernández R, Hera-Fernández J, Ortego-Centeno N. Clinical course of Covid-19 in a cohort of patients with Behçet disease. 00716-8 Med Clin December 2021;28(21):S0025–7753. https://doi.org/10.1016/j.medcli.2021.11.009. Epub ahead of print. PMID: 35058051; PMCID: PMC8712259.

[72] Enginar AU, Gundogdu M. The course of COVID-19 in patients with Behçet's disease. Reumatologia 2021;59(6):356–61. https://doi.org/10.5114/reum.2021.112347. Epub 2022 Jan 12. PMID: 35079178; PMCID: PMC8768042.

[73] Yurttas B, Oztas M, Tunc A, Balkan İİ, Tabak OF, Hamuryudan V, Seyahi E. Characteristics and outcomes of Behçet's syndrome patients with Coronavirus Disease 2019: a case series of 10 patients. Intern Emerg Med November 2020;15(8):1567–71. https://doi.org/10.1007/s11739-020-02427-8. Epub 2020 Jul 9. PMID: 32647946; PMCID: PMC7344029.

[74] Zouboulis CC, van Laar JAM, Schirmer M, Emmi G, Fortune F, Gül A, Kirino Y, Lee ES, Sfikakis PP, Shahram F, Wallace GR. Adamantiades-Behçet's disease (Behçet's disease) and COVID-19. J Eur Acad Dermatol Venereol September 2021;35(9):e541–3. https://doi.org/10.1111/jdv.17325. Epub 2021 May 13. PMID: 33914986; PMCID: PMC8242698.

[75] Cakir M, Guven B, Issi F, Ozkaya E. New-onset celiac disease in children during COVID-19 pandemic. Acta Paediatr February 2022;111(2):383–8. https://doi.org/10.1111/apa.16173. Epub 2021 Nov 11. PMID: 34738264; PMCID: PMC8652844.

[76] Mansoor E, Alikhan MM, Perez JA, Schlick K, Abou Saleh M, Rubio-Tapia A. Clinical characteristics, hospitalisation and mortality rates of COVID-19 among patients with coeliac disease in the USA: a multicentre network study. gutjnl-2021-325930 Gut November 2021;11. https://doi.org/10.1136/gutjnl-2021-325930. Epub ahead of print. PMID: 34764191.

[77] Ismail II, Salama S. Association of CNS demyelination and COVID-19 infection: an updated systematic review. J Neurol February 2022;269(2):541–76. https://doi.org/10.1007/s00415-021-10752-x. Epub 2021 Aug 12. PMID: 34386902; PMCID: PMC8359762.

[78] Suri V, Pandey S, Singh J, Jena A. Acute-onset chronic inflammatory demyelinating polyneuropathy afterCOVID-19 infection and subsequent ChAdOx1 nCoV-19 vaccination. BMJ Case Rep October 4, 2021;14(10):e245816. https://doi.org/10.1136/bcr-2021-245816. PMID: 34607818; PMCID: PMC8491284.

[79] Aly HH, Fouda EM, Kotby AA, Magdy SM, Rezk AR, Nasef MWA. COVID-19-Related multisystem inflammatory syndrome in children presenting with new-onset type 1 diabetes in severe ketoacidosis: a case series. Diabetes Care February 2022;3:dc211094. https://doi.org/10.2337/dc21-1094. Epub ahead of print. PMID: 35113159.

[80] Demeterco-Berggren C, Ebekozien O, Rompicherla S, Jacobsen L, Accacha S, Gallagher MP, Todd Alonso G, Seyoum B, Vendrame F, Haw JS, Basina M, Levy CJ, Maahs DM. Age and hospitalization risk in people with type 1 diabetes and COVID-19: data from the T1D exchange surveillance study. J Clin Endocrinol Metab January 18, 2022;107(2):410–8. https://doi.org/10.1210/clinem/dgab668. PMID: 34581790; PMCID: PMC8500098.

[81] Kamrath C, Rosenbauer J, Eckert AJ, Siedler K, Bartelt H, Klose D, Sindichakis M, Herrlinger S, Lahn V, Holl RW. Incidence of type 1 diabetes in children and adolescents during the COVID-19 pandemic in Germany: results from the DPV registry. Diabetes Care January 2022;17:dc210969. https://doi.org/10.2337/dc21-0969. Epub ahead of print. PMID: 35043145.

[82] Nassar M, Nso N, Baraka B, Alfishawy M, Mohamed M, Nyabera A, Sachmechi I. The association between COVID-19 and type 1 diabetes mellitus: a systematic review. Diabetes Metabol Syndr 2021 ;15(1):447–54. https://doi.org/10.1016/j.dsx.2021.02.009. Epub 2021 Feb 10. PMID: 33592371; PMCID: PMC7872855.

[83] Patrizio A, Ferrari SM, Antonelli A, Fallahi P. A case of Graves' disease and type 1 diabetes mellitus following SARS-CoV-2 vaccination. J Autoimmun December 2021;125:102738. https://doi.org/10.1016/j.jaut.2021.102738. Epub 2021 Oct 12. PMID: 34653776; PMCID: PMC8506108.

[84] Pierman G, Delgrange E, Jonas C. Recurrence of Graves' disease (a Th1-type cytokine disease) following SARS-CoV-2 mRNA vaccine administration: a simple coincidence? Eur J Case Rep Intern Med September 2, 2021;8(9):002807. https://doi.org/10.12890/2021_002807. PMID: 34671577; PMCID: PMC8523378.

[85] Khan F, Sharma P, Pandey S, Sharma D, Kumar N, Shukla S, Dandu H, Jain A, Garg RK, Malhotra HS. COVID-19-associated Guillain-Barre syndrome: postinfectious alone or neuroinvasive too? J Med Virol October 2021;93(10):6045–9. https://doi.org/10.1002/jmv.27159. Epub 2021 Jul 6. PMID: 34170552; PMCID: PMC8426929.

[86] Knack RS, Hanada T, Knack RS, Mayr K. Hashimoto's thyroiditis following SARS-CoV-2 infection. BMJ Case Rep August 9, 2021;14(8):e244909. https://doi.org/10.1136/bcr-2021-244909. PMID: 34373245; PMCID: PMC8354276.

[87] Tee LY, Harjanto S, Rosario BH. COVID-19 complicated by Hashimoto's thyroiditis. Singapore Med J May 2021;62(5):265. https://doi.org/10.11622/smedj.2020106. Epub 2020 Jul 16. PMID: 32668831; PMCID: PMC8801861.

[88] Varol AC, Hatice U, Gorgun S. COVID-19 and hashimoto's disease. Rev Assoc Med Bras June 2021;67(5):640. https://doi.org/10.1590/1806-9282.20210242. PMID: 34550248.

[89] Gadi SRV, Brunker PAR, Al-Samkari H, Sykes DB, Saff RR, Lo J, Bendapudi P, Leaf DE, Leaf RK. Severe autoimmune hemolytic anemia following receipt of SARS-CoV-2 mRNA vaccine. Transfusion November 2021;61(11):3267–71. https://doi.org/10.1111/trf.16672. Epub 2021 Oct 3. PMID: 34549821; PMCID: PMC8661722.

[90] Jaydev F, Kumar V, Khatri J, Shahani S, Beganovic S. A case of autoimmune hemolytic anemia after the first dose of COVID-19 mRNA-1273 vaccine with undetected pernicious anemia. 2022 Case Rep Hematol January 2022;29:2036460. https://doi.org/10.1155/2022/2036460. PMID: 35103106; PMCID: PMC8799952.

[91] Alonso-Beato R, Morales-Ortega A, Fernández FJH, Morón AIP, Ríos-Fernández R, Rubio JLC, Centeno NO. Immune thrombocytopenia and COVID-19: case report and review of literature. Lupus August 2021;30(9):1515–21. https://doi.org/10.1177/09612033211021161. Epub 2021 May 30. PMID: 34053365.

[92] David P, Dotan A, Mahroum N, Shoenfeld Y. Immune thrombocytopenic purpura (ITP) triggered by COVID-19 infection and vaccination. Isr Med Assoc J June 2021;23(6):378–80. PMID: 34155853.

[93] Zulfiqar AA, Lorenzo-Villalba N, Hassler P, Andrès E. Immune thrombocytopenic purpura in a patient with covid-19. N Engl J Med April 30, 2020;382(18):e43. https://doi.org/10.1056/NEJMc2010472. Epub 2020 Apr 15. PMID: 32294340; PMCID: PMC7179995.

[94] Singh AK, Jena A, Kumar MP, Jha DK, Sharma V. Clinical presentation of COVID-19 in patients with inflammatory bowel disease: a systematic review and meta-analysis. Intest Res January 2021;18. https://doi.org/10.5217/ir.2020.00108. Epub ahead of print. PMID: 33440918.

[95] Singh MK, Mobeen A, Chandra A, Joshi S, Ramachandran S. A meta-analysis of comorbidities in COVID-19: which diseases increase the susceptibility of SARS-CoV-2 infection? Comput Biol Med March 2021;130:104219. https://doi.org/10.1016/j.compbiomed.2021.104219. Epub 2021 Jan 16. PMID: 33486379; PMCID: PMC7836641.

[96] Tripathi K, Godoy Brewer G, Thu Nguyen M, Singh Y, Saleh Ismail M, Sauk JS, Parian AM, Limketkai BN. COVID-19 and outcomes in patients with inflammatory bowel disease: systematic review and meta-analysis. izab236 Inflamm Bowel Dis October 2021;27. https://doi.org/10.1093/ibd/izab236. Epub ahead of print. PMID: 34718595; PMCID: PMC8574492.

[97] Burgos-Blasco P, Fernandez-Nieto D, Selda-Enriquez G, Melian-Olivera A, De Perosanz-Lobo D, Dominguez-Santas M, Alonso-Castro L. COVID-19: a possible trigger for oral lichen planus? Int J Dermatol July 2021;60(7):882–3. https://doi.org/10.1111/ijd.15529. Epub 2021 Mar 8. PMID: 33686658; PMCID: PMC8250697.

[98] Gimeno Castillo J, de la Torre Gomar FJ, Saenz Aguirre A. Lichen planus after SARS-CoV-2 infection treated with lopinavir/ritonavir. English, Spanish Med Clin May 7, 2021;156(9):468–9. https://doi.org/10.1016/j.medcli.2020.12.014. Epub 2021 Jan 28. PMID: 33627228; PMCID: PMC7843098.

[99] Merhy R, Sarkis AS, Kaikati J, El Khoury L, Ghosn S, Stephan F. New-onset cutaneous lichen planus triggered by COVID-19 vaccination. J Eur Acad Dermatol Venereol November 2021;35(11):e729–30. https://doi.org/10.1111/jdv.17504. Epub 2021 Jul 24. PMID: 34236718; PMCID: PMC8447319.

[100] Piccolo V, Mazzatenta C, Bassi A, Argenziano G, Cutrone M, Grimalt R, Russo T. COVID vaccine-induced lichen planus on areas previously affected by vitiligo. J Eur Acad Dermatol Venereol January 2022;36(1):e28–30. https://doi.org/10.1111/jdv.17687. Epub 2021 Oct 2. PMID: 34547122; PMCID: PMC8657361.

[101] Saleh W, SHawky E, Halim GA, Ata F. Oral lichen planus after COVID-19, a case report. Ann Med Surg (Lond) December 2021;72:103051. https://doi.org/10.1016/j.amsu.2021.103051. Epub 2021 Nov 11. PMID: 34786190; PMCID: PMC8580550.

[102] Sharda P, Mohta A, Ghiya BC, Mehta RD. Development of oral lichen planus after COVID-19 vaccination—a rare case report. J Eur Acad Dermatol Venereol February 2022;36(2):e82–3. https://doi.org/10.1111/jdv.17718. Epub 2021 Oct 18. PMID: 34606669.

[103] Sood A, Raghavan S, Batra P, Sharma K, Talwar A. Rise and exacerbation of oral lichen planus in the background of SARS-CoV-2 infection. Med Hypotheses November 2021;156:110681. https://doi.org/10.1016/j.mehy.2021.110681. Epub 2021 Sep 20. PMID: 34601231; PMCID: PMC8478127.

[104] Troeltzsch M, Gogl M, Berndt R, Troeltzsch M. Oral lichen planus following the administration of vector-based COVID-19 vaccine (Ad26.COV2.S). Oral Dis September 2021;20. https://doi.org/10.1111/odi.14025. doi: 10.1111/odi.14025. Epub ahead of print. PMID: 34543493; PMCID: PMC8661663.

[105] Biswas S, Ghosh R, Mandal A, Pandit A, Roy D, Sengupta S, De K, Swaika BC, Benito-León J. COVID-19 induced Miller Fisher Syndrome presenting with autonomic dysfunction: a unique case report and review of literature. Neurohospitalist January 2022;12(1):111–6. https://doi.org/10.1177/19418744211016709. Epub 2021 May 17. PMID: 34950397; PMCID: PMC8689536.

[106] Arrambide G, Llaneza-González MÁ, Costa-Frossard França L, Meca-Lallana V, Díaz EF, Moreno-Torres I, García-Domínguez JM, Ortega-Suero G, Ayuso-Peralta L, Gómez-Moreno M, Sotoca-Fernández JJ, Caminero-Rodríguez AB, Rodríguez de Antonio LA, Corujo-Suárez M, Otano-Martínez MA, Pérez-Miralles FC, Reyes-Garrido V, Ayuso-Blanco T, Balseiro-Gómez JJ, Muñoz-Pasadas M, Pérez-Molina I, Arnal-García C, Domingo-Santos Á, Guijarro-Castro C, Íñiguez-Martínez C, Téllez Lara N, Castellanos-Pinedo F, Castillo-Triviño T, Cerdán-Santacruz DM, Pérez-Sempere Á, Torres BS, Álvarez de Arcaya A, Costa-Arpín E, Durán-Ferreras E, Fragoso-Martínez M, González-Platas M, Landete Pascual L, Millán-Pascual J, Oreja-Guevara C, Meca-Lallana JE. SARS-CoV-2 infection in multiple sclerosis: results of the Spanish neurology society registry. Neurol Neuroimmunol Neuroinflamm June 24, 2021;8(5):e1024. https://doi.org/10.1212/NXI.0000000000001024. PMID: 34168057; PMCID: PMC8225011.

[107] Chisari CG, Toscano S, Arena S, Finocchiaro C, Montineri A, Patti F. Natalizumab administration in multiple sclerosis patients during active SARS-CoV-2 infection: a case series. BMC Neurol November 29, 2021;21(1):462. https://doi.org/10.1186/s12883-021-02421-3. PMID: 34839814; PMCID: PMC8627841.

[108] Czarnowska A, Brola W, Zajkowska O, Rusek S, Adamczyk-Sowa M, Kubicka-Baczyk K, Kalinowska-Łyszczarz A, Kania K, Słowik A, Wnuk M, Marona M, Podlecka-Pietowska A, Nojszewska M, Zakrzewska-Pniewska B, Jasińska E, Gołuch K, Lech B, Noga M, Perenc A, Popiel M, Lasek-Bal A, Puz P, Maciejowska K, Kucharska-Lipowska M, Lipowski M, Kapica-Topczewska K, Chorąży M, Tarasiuk J, Kochanowicz J, Kulikowska J, Wawrzyniak S, Niezgodzińska-Maciejek A, Pokryszko-Dragan A, Gruszka E, Budrewicz S, Białek M, Kurkowska-Jastrzebska I, Kurowska K, Stepień A, Włodek A, Ptasznik V,

Pawełczyk M, Sobolewski P, Lejmel H, Strzalińska K, Maciejowski M, Tutaj A, Zwiernik J, Litwin A, Lewańczyk B, Paprocka I, Zwiernik B, Pawlos A, Borysowicz A, Narożnik A, Michałowska A, Nosek K, Fudala M, Milewska-Jedrzejczak M, Kułakowska A, Bartosik-Psujek H. Clinical course and outcome of SARS-CoV-2 infection in multiple sclerosis patients treated with disease-modifying therapies - the Polish experience. Neurol Neurochir Pol 2021;55(2):212–22. https://doi.org/10.5603/PJNNS.a2021.0031. Epub 2021 Apr 15. PMID: 33856686.

[109] Etemadifar M, Nouri H, Maracy MR, Akhavan Sigari A, Salari M, Blanco Y, Sepúlveda M, Zabalza A, Mahdavi S, Baratian M, Sedaghat N. Risk factors of severe COVID-19 in people with multiple sclerosis : a systematic review and meta-analysis. 00743-8 Rev Neurol (Paris) November 2021;4(21):S0035–3787. https://doi.org/10.1016/j.neurol.2021.10.003. Epub ahead of print. PMID: 34836608; PMCID: PMC8566345.

[110] Gomez-Mayordomo V, Montero-Escribano P, Matías-Guiu JA, González-García N, Porta-Etessam J, Matías-Guiu J. Clinical exacerbation of SARS-CoV2 infection after fingolimod withdrawal. J Med Virol January 2021;93(1):546–9. https://doi.org/10.1002/jmv.26279. Epub 2020 Jul 15. PMID: 32644205; PMCID: PMC7361541.

[111] Iaffaldano P, Lucisano G, Manni A, Paolicelli D, Patti F, Capobianco M, Brescia Morra V, Sola P, Pesci I, Lus G, De Luca G, Lugaresi A, Cavalla P, Montepietra S, Maniscalco GT, Granella F, Ragonese P, Vianello M, Brambilla L, Totaro R, Toscano S, Malucchi S, Petracca M, Moiola L, Ferraro D, Lepore V, Mosconi P, Ponzio M, Tedeschi G, Comi G, Battaglia MA, Filippi M, Amato MP, Trojano M, Italian MS Register. Risk of getting COVID-19 in people with multiple sclerosis: a case-control study. Neurol Neuroimmunol Neuroinflamm January 19, 2022;9(2):e1141. https://doi.org/10.1212/NXI.0000000000001141. PMID: 35046084; PMCID: PMC8771668.

[112] Matías-Guiu J, Montero-Escribano P, Pytel V, Porta-Etessam J, Matias-Guiu JA. Potential COVID-19 infection in patients with severe multiple sclerosis treated with alemtuzumab. Mult Scler Relat Disord September 2020;44:102297. https://doi.org/10.1016/j.msard.2020.102297. Epub 2020 Jun 11. PMID: 32554284; PMCID: PMC7286822.

[113] Pignolo A, Aprile M, Gagliardo C, Giammanco GM, D'Amelio M, Aridon P, La Tona G, Salemi G, Ragonese P. Clinical onset and multiple sclerosis relapse after SARS-CoV-2 infection. Neurol Int December6, 2021;13(4):695–700. https://doi.org/10.3390/neurolint13040066. PMID: 34940752; PMCID: PMC8707620.

[114] Reder AT, Centonze D, Naylor ML, Nagpal A, Rajbhandari R, Altincatal A, Kim M, Berdofe A, Radhakrishnan M, Jung E, Sandrock AW, Smirnakis K, Popescu C, de Moor C. COVID-19 in patients with multiple sclerosis: associations with disease-modifying therapies. CNS Drugs March 2021;35(3):317–30. https://doi.org/10.1007/s40263-021-00804-1. Epub 2021 Mar 20. PMID: 33743151; PMCID: PMC7980129.

[115] Sarwar S, Rogers S, Mohamed AS, Ogula E, Ayantayo RA, Ahmed A, Shahzadi I, Kataria S, Singh R. Multiple sclerosis following SARS-CoV-2 infection: a case report and literature review. Cureus October 25, 2021;13(10):e19036. https://doi.org/10.7759/cureus.19036. PMID: 34858736; PMCID: PMC8612412.

[116] Simpson-Yap S, De Brouwer E, Kalincik T, Rijke N, Hillert JA, Walton C, Edan G, Moreau Y, Spelman T, Geys L, Parciak T, Gautrais C, Lazovski N, Pirmani A, Ardeshirdavanai A, Forsberg L, Glaser A, McBurney R, Schmidt H, Bergmann AB, Braune S, Stahmann A, Middleton R, Salter A, Fox RJ, van der Walt A, Butzkueven H, Alroughani R, Ozakbas S, Rojas JI, van der Mei I, Nag N, Ivanov R, Sciascia do Olival G, Dias AE, Magyari M, Brum D, Mendes MF, Alonso RN, Nicholas RS, Bauer J, Chertcoff AS, Zabalza A, Arrambide G, Fidao A, Comi G, Peeters L. Associations of disease-modifying therapies with COVID-19 severity in multiple sclerosis. Neurology November 9, 2021;97(19):e1870–85. https://doi.org/10.1212/WNL.0000000000012753. Epub 2021 Oct 5. PMID: 34610987; PMCID: PMC8601210.

[117] Sormani MP, De Rossi N, Schiavetti I, Carmisciano L, Cordioli C, Moiola L, Radaelli M, Immovilli P, Capobianco M, Trojano M, Zaratin P, Tedeschi G, Comi G, Battaglia MA, Patti F, Salvetti M, Musc-19 study group. Disease-modifying therapies and coronavirus disease 2019 severity in multiple sclerosis. Ann Neurol April 2021;89(4):780–9. https://doi.org/10.1002/ana.26028. Epub 2021 Feb 9. PMID: 33480077; PMCID: PMC8013440.

[118] Zabalza A, Cárdenas-Robledo S, Tagliani P, Arrambide G, Otero-Romero S, Carbonell-Mirabent P, Rodriguez-Barranco M, Rodríguez-Acevedo B, Restrepo Vera JL, Resina-Salles M, Midaglia L, Vidal-Jordana A, Río J, Galan I, Castillo J, Cobo-Calvo Á, Comabella M, Nos C, Sastre-Garriga J, Tintore M, Montalban X. COVID-19 in multiple sclerosis patients: susceptibility, severity risk factors and serological response. Eur J Neurol October 2021;28(10):3384–95. https://doi.org/10.1111/ene.14690. Epub 2021 Jan 9. PMID: 33340215.

[119] Abbas AS, Hardy N, Ghozy S, Dibas M, Paranjape G, Evanson KW, Reierson NL, Cowie K, Kamrowski S, Schmidt S, Tang Y, Davis AR, Touchette JC, Kallmes KM, Hassan AE, Tarchand R, Mehta M, Pederson JM, Abdelmegeed M. Characteristics, treatment, and outcomes of Myasthenia Gravis in COVID-19 patients: a systematic review. Clin Neurol Neurosurg January 22, 2022;213:107140. https://doi.org/10.1016/j.clineuro.2022.107140. Epub ahead of print. PMID: 35091255; PMCID: PMC8782728.

[120] Digala LP, Prasanna S, Rao P, Qureshi AI, Govindarajan R. Impact of COVID-19 infection among myasthenia gravis patients- a Cerner Real-World DataTM study. BMC Neurol January 27, 2022;22(1):38. https://doi.org/10.1186/s12883-022-02564-x. PMID: 35086486; PMCID: PMC8792518.

[121] Galassi G, Rispoli V, Iori E, Ariatti A, Marchioni A. Coincidental onset of ocular myasthenia gravis following ChAdOx1 n-CoV-19 vaccine against severe acute respiratory syndrome coronavirus 2 (SARS-CoV-2). Isr Med Assoc J January 2022;24(1):9–10. PMID: 35077038.

[122] Murthy JMK, Gutta AK, Yerasu MR, Boorgu SK, Osman S, Jaiswal SK, Pidaparthi L, Gudavalli BP. COVID-19 in patients with myasthenia gravis: mechanisms of respiratory failure. Neurol India 2021 ;69(6):1772–6. https://doi.org/10.4103/0028-3886.333460. PMID: 34979686.

[123] Reddy Y, Osman S, Murthy JM. Temporal association between SARS-CoV-2 and new-onset myasthenia gravis: is it causal or coincidental? BMJ Case Rep July 21, 2021;14(7):e244146. https://doi.org/10.1136/bcr-2021-244146. PMID: 34290032; PMCID: PMC8296802.

[124] Marrama D, Mahita J, Sette A, Peters B. Lack of evidence of significant homology of SARS-CoV-2 spike sequences to myocarditis-associated antigens. EBioMedicine January 2022;75:103807. https://doi.org/10.1016/j.ebiom.2021.103807. Epub 2022 Jan 6. PMID: 34998242; PMCID: PMC8733122.

[125] Liquidano-Perez E, García-Romero MT, Yamazaki-Nakashimada M, Maza-Morales M, Rivas-Calderón MK, Bayardo-Gutierrez B, Pardo-Díaz E, Scheffler-Mendoza SC. Juvenile dermatomyositis triggered by SARS-CoV-2. Pediatr Neurol August 2021;121:26–7. https://doi.org/10.1016/j.pediatrneurol.2021.05.011. Epub 2021 May 20. PMID: 34126319; PMCID: PMC8136292.

[126] Saud A, Naveen R, Aggarwal R, Gupta L. COVID-19 and myositis: what we know so far. Curr Rheumatol Rep July 3, 2021;23(8):63. https://doi.org/10.1007/s11926-021-01023-9. PMID: 34216297; PMCID: PMC8254439.

[127] Breglio KF, Sarver MM, Hall 3rd RP, Marano AL. SARS-CoV-2 infections in patients with autoimmune blistering disorders: a case series and retrospective analysis. JAAD Int January 2022;24. https://doi.org/10.1016/j.jdin.2022.01.003. Epub ahead of print. PMID: 35098172; PMCID: PMC8784432.

[128] Saleh MA, Saleh NA. Pemphigus vulgaris relapse during the coronavirus disease pandemic. Dermatol Ther February 2022;2:e15354. https://doi.org/10.1111/dth.15354. Epub ahead of print. PMID: 35108427.

[129] Izuka S, Komai T, Natsumoto B, Shoda H, Fujio K. Self-limited polymyalgia rheumatica-like syndrome following mRNA-1273 SARS-CoV-2 vaccination. Intern Med December 2021;28. https://doi.org/10.2169/internalmedicine.8829-21. Epub ahead of print. PMID: 34980802.

[130] Manzo C, Castagna A, Ruotolo G. Can SARS-CoV-2 trigger relapse of polymyalgia rheumatica? Joint Bone Spine May 2021;88(3):105150. https://doi.org/10.1016/j.jbspin.2021.105150. Epub 2021 Feb 4. PMID: 33588357; PMCID: PMC7857978.

[131] Manzo C, Natale M, Castagna A. Polymyalgia rheumatica as uncommon adverse event following immunization with COVID-19 vaccine: a case report and review of literature. Aging Med (Milton) August 15, 2021;4(3):234–8. https://doi.org/10.1002/agm2.12171. Epub ahead of print. PMID: 34518809; PMCID: PMC8426911.

[132] Mettler C, Jonville-Bera AP, Grandvuillemin A, Treluyer JM, Terrier B, Chouchana L. Risk of giant cell arteritis and polymyalgia rheumatica following COVID-19 vaccination: a global pharmacovigilance study. Rheumatology October 9, 2021:865–7. https://doi.org/10.1093/rheumatology/keab756. Epub ahead of print. PMID: 34626105.

[133] Ottaviani S, Juge PA, Forien M, Ebstein E, Palazzo E, Dieudé P. Polymyalgia rheumatica following COVID-19 vaccination: a case-series of ten patients. Joint Bone Spine December 22, 2021;89(2):105334. https://doi.org/10.1016/j.jbspin.2021.105334. Epub ahead of print. PMID: 34954076; PMCID: PMC8694785.

[134] Blitshteyn S, Whitelaw S. Postural orthostatic tachycardia syndrome (POTS) and other autonomic disorders after COVID-19 infection: a case series of 20 patients. Immunol Res April 2021;69(2):205–11. https://doi.org/10.1007/s12026-021-09185-5. Epub 2021 Mar 30. Erratum in: Immunol Res. 2021 Apr 13;: PMID: 33786700; PMCID: PMC8009458.

[135] Ampuero J, Lucena A, Hernández-Guerra M, Moreno-Moraleda I, Arenas J, Conde I, Muñoz L, Canillas L, Fernandez E, Quiñones R, Simon MA, Gómez-Dominguez E, Gutierrez ML, Fernandez-Rodriguez C, Domper-Arnal MJ, Jorquera F, Garcia-Buey ML, Garcia-Retortillo M, Morillas R, Berenguer M, Casado M, Morales-Arraez D, Sousa JM, Molina E. Primary biliary cholangitis and SARS-CoV-2 infection: incidence, susceptibility and outcomes. gutjnl-2021-325700 Gut December 2021;7. https://doi.org/10.1136/gutjnl-2021-325700. Epub ahead of print. PMID: 34876479.

[136] Bartoli A, Cursaro C, Andreone P. Severe acute respiratory syndrome coronavirus-2-associated cholangiopathies. Curr Opin Gastroenterol 2022;38(22):89–97. https://doi.org/10.1097/MOG.0000000000000808. PMID: 35098930; PMCID: PMC8815639.

[137] Roth NC, Kim A, Vitkovski T, Xia J, Ramirez G, Bernstein D, Crawford JM. Post-COVID-19 cholangiopathy: a novel entity. Am J Gastroenterol May 1, 2021;116(5):1077–82. https://doi.org/10.14309/ajg.0000000000001154. PMID: 33464757.

[138] Agarwal A, Tripathy T, Kar BR. Guttate flare in a patient with chronic plaque psoriasis following COVID-19 infection: a case report. J Cosmet Dermatol October 2021;20(10):3064–5. https://doi.org/10.1111/jocd.14396. Epub 2021 Aug 20. PMID: 34416089; PMCID: PMC8662084.

[139] Bostan E, Elmas L, Yel B, Yalici-Armagan B. Exacerbation of plaque psoriasis after inactivated and BNT162b2 mRNA COVID-19 vaccines: a report of two cases. Dermatol Ther November 2021;34(6):e15110. https://doi.org/10.1111/dth.15110. Epub 2021 Aug 30. PMID: 34427024; PMCID: PMC8646432.

[140] Ciechanowicz P, Dopytalska K, Mikucka-Wituszyńska A, Dźwigała M, Wiszniewski K, Herniczek W, Szymańska E, Walecka I. The prevalence of SARS-CoV-2 infection and the severity of the course of COVID-19 in patients with psoriasis treated with biologic therapy. J Dermatol Treat December 2020;22:1–4. https://doi.org/10.1080/09546634.2020.1861177. Epub ahead of print. PMID: 33317364.

[141] Damiani G, Pacifico A, Bragazzi NL, Malagoli P. Biologics increase the risk of SARS-CoV-2 infection and hospitalization, but not ICU admission and death: real-life data from a large cohort during red-zone declaration. Dermatol Ther September 2020;33(5):e13475. https://doi.org/10.1111/dth.13475. Epub 2020 May 19. PMID: 32356577; PMCID: PMC7261990.

[142] Elamin S, Hinds F, Tolland J. De novo generalized pustular psoriasis following Oxford-AstraZeneca COVID-19 vaccine. Clin Exp Dermatol January 2022;47(1):153–5. https://doi.org/10.1111/ced.14895. Epub 2021 Sep 30. PMID: 34398977; PMCID: PMC8444761.

[143] Elmas ÖF, Demirbas A, Kutlu Ö, Bağcıer F, Metin MS, Özyurt K, Akdeniz N, Atasoy M, Türsen Ü, Lotti T. Psoriasis and COVID-19: a narrative review with treatment considerations. Dermatol Ther November 2020;33(6):e13858. https://doi.org/10.1111/dth.13858. Epub 2020 Jul 9. PMID: 32686245; PMCID: PMC7323009.

[144] Fang WC, Chiu LW, Hu SC. Psoriasis exacerbation after first dose of AstraZeneca coronavirus disease 2019 vaccine. J Dermatol November 2021;48(11):e566–7. https://doi.org/10.1111/1346-8138.16137. Epub 2021 Sep 6. PMID: 34487570; PMCID: PMC8652484.

[145] Huang YW, Tsai TF. Exacerbation of psoriasis following COVID-19 vaccination: report from a single center. Front Med December 23, 2021;8:812010. https://doi.org/10.3389/fmed.2021.812010. PMID: 35004790; PMCID: PMC8733241.

[146] Queiro Silva R, Armesto S, González Vela C, Naharro Fernández C, González-Gay MA. COVID-19 patients with psoriasis and psoriatic arthritis on biologic immunosuppressant therapy vs apremilast in North Spain. Dermatol Ther November 2020;33(6):e13961. https://doi.org/10.1111/dth.13961. Epub 2020 Jul 27. PMID: 32618402; PMCID: PMC7361149.

[147] Ciurea A, Papagiannoulis E, Bürki K, von Loga I, Micheroli R, Möller B, Rubbert-Roth A, Andor M, Bräm R, Müller A, Dan D, Kyburz D, Distler O, Scherer A, Finckh A. Impact of the COVID-19 pandemic on the disease course of patients with inflammatory rheumatic diseases: results from the Swiss Clinical Quality Management cohort. Ann Rheum Dis February 2021;80(2):238–41. https://doi.org/10.1136/annrheumdis-2020-218705. Epub 2020 Sep 22. PMID: 32963052; PMCID: PMC7509948.

[148] Costantino F, Bahier L, Tarancón LC, Leboime A, Vidal F, Bessalah L, Breban M, D'Agostino MA. COVID-19 in French patients with chronic inflammatory rheumatic diseases: clinical features, risk factors and treatment adherence. Joint Bone Spine January 2021;88(1):105095. https://doi.org/10.1016/j.jbspin.2020.105095. Epub 2020 Nov 2. PMID: 33152484; PMCID: PMC7605756.

[149] Mugheddu C, Sanna S, Atzori L, Rongioletti F. Safety of secukinumab treatment in COVID-19 affected psoriatic patients. Dermatol Ther January 2021;34(1):e14710. https://doi.org/10.1111/dth.14710. Epub 2021 Jan 3. PMID: 33368887; PMCID: PMC7883240.

[150] Novelli L, Motta F, Ceribelli A, Guidelli GM, Luciano N, Isailovic N, Vecellio M, Caprioli M, Clementi N, Clementi M, Mancini N, Selmi C, De Santis M. A case of psoriatic arthritis triggered by SARS-CoV-2 infection. Rheumatology January 5, 2021;60(1):e21–3. https://doi.org/10.1093/rheumatology/keaa691. PMID: 33206980; PMCID: PMC7717387.

[151] Tasso M, Mostacciuolo E, Ugoccioni V, Del Puente A, Peluso R, Scarpa R, Costa L, Caso F. COVID-19 clinical spectrum in psoriatic arthritis patients on biologics and tsDMARDs: results from a cohort at an Italian epicentre of the pandemic's third wave. Clin Exp Rheumatol January 27, 2022;40:1061. Epub ahead of print. PMID: 35084304.

[152] Dernoncourt A, Schmidt J, Duhaut P, Liabeuf S, Gras-Champel V, Masmoudi K, Bennis Y, Batteux B. COVID-19 in DMARD-treated patients with inflammatory rheumatic diseases: insights from an analysis of the World Health Organization pharmacovigilance database. Fundam Clin Pharmacol February 2022;36(1):199–209. https://doi.org/10.1111/fcp.12695. Epub 2021 May 25. PMID: 33973280; PMCID: PMC8239613.

[153] England BR, Roul P, Yang Y, Kalil AC, Michaud K, Thiele GM, Sauer BC, Baker JF, Mikuls TR. Risk of COVID-19 in rheumatoid arthritis: a national veterans affairs matched cohort study in at-risk individuals. Arthritis Rheumatol December 2021;73(12):2179–88. https://doi.org/10.1002/art.41800. Epub 2021 Oct 19. PMID: 33955209; PMCID: PMC8239709.

[154] Terracina KA, Tan FK. Flare of rheumatoid arthritis after COVID-19 vaccination. Lancet Rheumatol July 2021;3(7):e469–70. https://doi.org/10.1016/S2665-9913(21)00108-9. Epub 2021 Mar 30. PMID: 33817664; PMCID: PMC8009616.

[155] Aveyard P, Gao M, Lindson N, Hartmann-Boyce J, Watkinson P, Young D, Coupland CAC, Tan PS, Clift AK, Harrison D, Gould DW, Pavord ID, Hippisley-Cox J. Association between pre-existing respiratory disease and its treatment, and severe COVID-19: a population cohort study. Lancet Respir Med August 2021;9(8):909–23. https://doi.org/10.1016/S2213-2600(21)00095-3. Epub 2021 Apr 1. PMID: 33812494; PMCID: PMC8016404.

[156] Baughman RP, Lower EE. COVID-19 infections in sarcoidosis: a prospective single center study of 886 sarcoidosis patients. Sarcoidosis Vasc Diffuse Lung Dis 2021;38(2):e2021029. https://doi.org/10.36141/svdld.v38i2.11646. Epub 2021 Jun 28. PMID: 34316261; PMCID: PMC8288208.

[157] Bénézit F, Le Bot A, Jouneau S, Lemaître F, Pronier C, Lentz PA, Patrat-Delon S, Revest M, Thibault V, Tattevin P. COVID-19 in patient with sarcoidosis receiving long-term hydroxychloroquine treatment, France, 2020. Emerg Infect Dis October 2020;26(10):2513–5. https://doi.org/10.3201/eid2610.201816. Epub 2020 Jul 1. PMID: 32609083; PMCID: PMC7510728.

[158] Brito-Zerón P, Acar-Denizli N, Romão VC, Armagan B, Seror R, Carubbi F, Melchor S, Priori R, Valim V, Retamozo S, Pasoto SG, Trevisani VFM, Hofauer B, Szántó A, Inanc N, Hernández-Molina G, Sebastian A, Bartoloni E, Devauchelle-Pensec V, Akasbi M, Giardina F, Bandeira M, Sisó-Almirall A, Ramos-Casals M. Sjögren Big Data Consortium. Post-COVID-19 syndrome in patients with primary Sjögren's syndrome after acute SARS-CoV-2 infection. Clin Exp Rheumatol 2021 ;39(Suppl. 133(6)):57–65. Epub 2021 Nov 22. PMID: 34874821.

[159] Capaccione KM, McGroder C, Garcia CK, Fedyna S, Saqi A, Salvatore MM. COVID-19-induced pulmonary sarcoid: a case report and review of the literature. Clin Imag January 13, 2022;83:152–8. https://doi.org/10.1016/j.clinimag.2021.12.021. Epub ahead of print. PMID: 35051738; PMCID: PMC8755635.

[160] George LJ, Philip AM, John KJ, George AA, Nayar J, Mishra AK, Lal A. A review of the presentation and outcome of sarcoidosis in coronavirus disease 2019. J Clin Transl Res September 27, 2021;7(5):657–65. PMID: 34778596; PMCID: PMC8580525.

[161] Györfi AH, Kopp M, May M, Vetter M, Uder M, Kremer AE, Schett G, Harrer T, Distler JHW. Glucocorticoid-induced relapse of COVID-19 in a patient with sarcoidosis. annrheumdis-2020-218258 Ann Rheum Dis June 2020;30. https://doi.org/10.1136/annrheumdis-2020-218258. Epub ahead of print. PMID: 32606044.

[162] Hadi YB, Lakhani DA, Naqvi SFZ, Singh S, Kupec JT. Outcomes of SARS-CoV-2 infection in patients with pulmonary sarcoidosis: a multicenter retrospective research network study. Respir Med October 2021;187:106538. https://doi.org/10.1016/j.rmed.2021.106538. Epub 2021 Jul 22. PMID: 34325226; PMCID: PMC8297986.

[163] Manansala M, Ascoli C, Alburquerque AG, Perkins D, Mirsaedi M, Finn P, Sweiss NJ. Case series: COVID-19 in african American patients with sarcoidosis. Front Med November 4, 2020;7:588527. https://doi.org/10.3389/fmed.2020.588527. PMID: 33251236; PMCID: PMC7672207.

[164] Mihalov P, Krajčovičová E, Káčerová H, Sabaka P. Lofgren syndrome in close temporal association with mild COVID-19—case report. IDCases 2021;26:e01291. https://doi.org/10.1016/j.idcr.2021.e01291. Epub 2021 Sep 23. PMID: 34580630; PMCID: PMC8458104.

[165] Morgenthau AS, Levin MA, Freeman R, Reich DL, Klang E. Moderate or severe impairment in pulmonary function is associated with mortality in sarcoidosis patients infected with SARS-CoV-2. Lung October 2020;198(5):771—5. https://doi.org/10.1007/s00408-020-00392-9. Epub 2020 Sep 11. PMID: 32915271; PMCID: PMC7484928.

[166] Rademacher JG, Tampe B, Korsten P. First report of two cases of Löfgren's syndrome after SARS-CoV-2 vaccination-coincidence or causality? Vaccines (Basel) November 11, 2021;9(11):1313. https://doi.org/10.3390/vaccines9111313. PMID: 34835244; PMCID: PMC8619392.

[167] Southern BD. Patients with interstitial lung disease and pulmonary sarcoidosis are at high risk for severe illness related to COVID-19. Cleve Clin J Med June 2020;18. https://doi.org/10.3949/ccjm.87a.ccc026. Epub ahead of print. PMID: 32409436.

[168] Fineschi S. Case report: systemic sclerosis after covid-19 infection. Front Immunol June 28, 2021;12:686699. https://doi.org/10.3389/fimmu.2021.686699. PMID: 34262566; PMCID: PMC8273695.

[169] Jalalzadeh M, Valencia-Manrique JC, Boma N, Chaudhari A, Chaudhari S. Antineutrophil cytoplasmic antibody-associated glomerulonephritis in a case of scleroderma after recent diagnosis with COVID-19. Cureus January 4, 2021;13(1):e12485. https://doi.org/10.7759/cureus.12485. PMID: 33564500; PMCID: PMC7861062.

[170] Carubbi F, Alunno A, Ferri C, Gerli R, Bartoloni E. The impact of SARS-CoV-2 outbreak on primary sjögren's syndrome: an Italian experience. Front Med December 7, 2020;7:608728. https://doi.org/10.3389/fmed.2020.608728. PMID: 33425954; PMCID: PMC7793887.

[171] Chowdhury F, Grigoriadou S, Bombardieri M. Severity of COVID-19 infection in primary Sjögren's syndrome and the emerging evidence of COVID-19-induced xerostomia. Clin Exp Rheumatol 2021 ;39(Suppl. 133):215—22. Epub 2021 Dec 16. PMID: 34919045.

[172] Roger G, Pavot A, Bonnet I, Ferlicot S, Mariette X. Phenotypic switch from non-active primary Sjögren's syndrome to severe systemic Lupus erythematosus after COVID-19 infection in an elderly man. Joint Bone Spine December 2021;88(6):105228. https://doi.org/10.1016/j.jbspin.2021.105228. Epub 2021 May 26. PMID: 34051388; PMCID: PMC8152205.

[173] Hidaka D, Ogasawara R, Sugimura S, Fujii F, Kojima K, Nagai J, Ebata K, Okada K, Kobayashi N, Ogasawara M, Imamura M, Ota S. New-onset Evans syndrome associated with systemic lupus erythematosus after BNT162b2 mRNA COVID-19 vaccination. Int J Hematol October 2021;23:1—4. https://doi.org/10.1007/s12185-021-03243-2. Epub ahead of print. PMID: 34687421; PMCID: PMC8536917.

[174] Joseph AK, Chong BF. Subacute cutaneous lupus erythematosus flare triggered by COVID-19 vaccine. Dermatol Ther November 2021;34(6):e15114. https://doi.org/10.1111/dth.15114. Epub 2021 Sep 6. PMID: 34455671; PMCID: PMC8646373.

[175] Mashinchi B, Aryannejad A, Namazi M, Moradi S, Masoumi Z, Parsaei A, Masoumi M. A case of C-ANCA positive systematic lupus erythematous and ANCA-associated vasculitis overlap syndrome superimposed by COVID-19: a fatal trio. Mod Rheumatol Case Rep September 2021;4:rxab007. https://doi.org/10.1093/mrcr/rxab007. Epub ahead of print. PMID: 34480174; PMCID: PMC8499895.

[176] Ramirez GA, Argolini LM, Bellocchi C, Moroni L, Della-Torre E, Farina N, Caporali RF, Beretta L, Gerosa M, Bozzolo EP, Dagna L, SMILE, Milan Lupus Consortium. Impact of the COVID-19 pandemic in patients with systemic lupus erythematosus throughout one year. Clin Immunol October 2021;231:108845. https://doi.org/10.1016/j.clim.2021.108845. Epub 2021 Aug 31. PMID: 34478882; PMCID: PMC8405598.

[177] Sekar A. Lupus nephritis flare post Moderna mRNA-1273 coronavirus vaccine. QJM January 9, 2022;114(12):882—3. https://doi.org/10.1093/qjmed/hcab284. PMID: 34791449; PMCID: PMC8690008.

[178] Slimani Y, Abbassi R, El Fatoiki FZ, Barrou L, Chiheb S. Systemic lupus erythematosus and varicella-like rash following COVID-19 in a previously healthy patient. J Med Virol February 2021;93(2):1184—7. https://doi.org/10.1002/jmv.26513. Epub 2020 Sep 28. PMID: 32926434.

[179] Zamani B, Moeini Taba SM, Shayestehpour M. Systemic lupus erythematosus manifestation following COVID-19: a case report. J Med Case Rep January 25, 2021;15(1):29. https://doi.org/10.1186/s13256-020-02582-8. PMID: 33494816; PMCID: PMC7832415.

[180] Zavala-Miranda MF, González-Ibarra SG, Pérez-Arias AA, Uribe-Uribe NO, Mejia-Vilet JM. New-onset systemic lupus erythematosus beginning as class V lupus nephritis after COVID-19 vaccination. Kidney Int December 2021;100(6):1340−1. https://doi.org/10.1016/j.kint.2021.09.009. Epub 2021 Sep 22. PMID: 34560139; PMCID: PMC8455236.

[181] Zengarini C, Pileri A, Salamone FP, Piraccini BM, Vitale G, La Placa M. Subacute cutaneous lupus erythematosus induction after SARS-CoV-2 vaccine in a patient with primary biliary cholangitis. J Eur Acad Dermatol Venereol November 2021;22. https://doi.org/10.1111/jdv.17827. Epub ahead of print. PMID: 34807495.

[182] Wong K, Farooq Alam Shah MU, Khurshid M, Ullah I, Tahir MJ, Yousaf Z. COVID-19 associated vasculitis: a systematic review of case reports and case series. Ann Med Surg (Lond) February 2022;74:103249. https://doi.org/10.1016/j.amsu.2022.103249. Epub 2022 Jan 13. PMID: 35039779; PMCID: PMC8754903.

[183] Aktas H, Ertuğrul G. Vitiligo in a COVID-19-vaccinated patient with ulcerative colitis: coincidence? Clin Exp Dermatol January 2022;47(1):143−4. https://doi.org/10.1111/ced.14842. Epub 2021 Aug 3. PMID: 34236714; PMCID: PMC8444736.

[184] Ciccarese G, Drago F, Boldrin S, Pattaro M, Parodi A. Sudden onset of vitiligo after COVID-19 vaccine. Dermatol Ther January 2022;35(1):e15196. https://doi.org/10.1111/dth.15196. Epub 2021 Nov 15. PMID: 34751491; PMCID: PMC8646249.

[185] Kaminetsky J, Rudikoff D. New-onset vitiligo following mRNA-1273 (Moderna) COVID-19 vaccination. Clin Case Rep September 26, 2021;9(9):e04865. https://doi.org/10.1002/ccr3.4865. PMID: 34603727; PMCID: PMC8465924.

[186] Koç Yıldırım S. A new-onset vitiligo following the inactivated COVID-19 vaccine. J Cosmet Dermatol February 2022;21(2):429−30. https://doi.org/10.1111/jocd.14677. Epub 2021 Dec 15. PMID: 34910371.

[187] Okan G, Vural P. Worsening of the vitiligo following the second dose of the BNT162B2 mRNA COVID-19 vaccine. Dermatol Ther December 2021;21:e15280. https://doi.org/10.1111/dth.15280. Epub ahead of print. PMID: 34931408.

[188] Rokni GR, Gholami A, Kazeminejad A, Zakariaei Z, Layegh M, Patil A, Goldust M. The relationship between stress and vitiligo during COVID-19 pandemic. J Cosmet Dermatol November 2021;20(11):3387−8. https://doi.org/10.1111/jocd.14429. Epub 2021 Oct 21. PMID: 34674365; PMCID: PMC8662130.

[189] Coronaviridae Study Group of the International Committee on Taxonomy of Viruses. The species Severe acute respiratory syndrome-related coronavirus: classifying 2019-nCoV and naming it SARS-CoV-2. Nat Microbiol April 2020;5(4):536−44. https://doi.org/10.1038/s41564-020-0695-z. Epub 2020 Mar 2. PMID: 32123347; PMCID: PMC7095448.

[190] Gralinski LE, Menachery VD. Return of the coronavirus: 2019-nCoV. Viruses January 24, 2020;12(2):135. https://doi.org/10.3390/v12020135. PMID: 31991541; PMCID: PMC7077245.

[191] Phelan AL, Katz R, Gostin LO. The novel coronavirus originating in Wuhan, China: challenges for global health governance. JAMA February 25, 2020;323(8):709−10. https://doi.org/10.1001/jama.2020.1097. PMID: 31999307.

[192] Kumar R, Verma H, Singhvi N, Sood U, Gupta V, Singh M, Kumari R, Hira P, Nagar S, Talwar C, Nayyar N, Anand S, Rawat CD, Verma M, Negi RK, Singh Y, Lal R. Comparative genomic analysis of rapidly evolving SARS-CoV-2 reveals mosaic pattern of phylogeographical distribution. mSystems July 28, 2020;5(4):e00505−20. https://doi.org/10.1128/mSystems.00505-20. PMID: 32723797; PMCID: PMC7394360.

[193] Brian DA, Baric RS. Coronavirus genome structure and replication. Curr Top Microbiol Immunol 2005;287:1−30. https://doi.org/10.1007/3-540-26765-4_1. PMID: 15609507; PMCID: PMC7120446.

[194] Zhou P, Yang XL, Wang XG, Hu B, Zhang L, Zhang W, Si HR, Zhu Y, Li B, Huang CL, Chen HD, Chen J, Luo Y, Guo H, Jiang RD, Liu MQ, Chen Y, Shen XR, Wang X, Zheng XS, Zhao K, Chen QJ, Deng F, Liu LL, Yan B, Zhan FX, Wang YY, Xiao GF, Shi ZL. A pneumonia outbreak associated with a new coronavirus of probable bat origin. Nature March 2020;579(7798):270−3. https://doi.org/10.1038/s41586-020-2012-7. Epub 2020 Feb 3. PMID: 32015507; PMCID: PMC7095418.

[195] Arya R, Kumari S, Pandey B, Mistry H, Bihani SC, Das A, Prashar V, Gupta GD, Panicker L, Kumar M. Structural insights into SARS-CoV-2 proteins. J Mol Biol January 22, 2021;433(2):166725. https://doi.org/10.1016/j.jmb.2020.11.024. Epub 2020 Nov 24. PMID: 33245961; PMCID: PMC7685130.

[196] Su YCF, Anderson DE, Young BE, Linster M, Zhu F, Jayakumar J, Zhuang Y, Kalimuddin S, Low JGH, Tan CW, Chia WN, Mak TM, Octavia S, Chavatte JM, Lee RTC, Pada S, Tan SY, Sun L, Yan GZ, Maurer-Stroh S, Mendenhall IH, Leo YS, Lye DC, Wang LF, Smith GJD. Discovery and genomic characterization of a 382-nucleotide deletion in ORF7b and ORF8 during the early evolution of SARS-CoV-2. mBio July 21, 2020;11(4):e01610−20. https://doi.org/10.1128/mBio.01610-20. PMID: 32694143; PMCID: PMC7374062.

[197] Toyoshima Y, Nemoto K, Matsumoto S, Nakamura Y, Kiyotani K. SARS-CoV-2 genomic variations associated with mortality rate of COVID-19. J Hum Genet December 2020;65(12):1075−82. https://doi.org/10.1038/s10038-020-0808-9. Epub 2020 Jul 22. PMID: 32699345; PMCID: PMC7375454.

[198] Mercatelli D, Giorgi FM. Geographic and genomic distribution of SARS-CoV-2 mutations. Front Microbiol July 22, 2020;11:1800. https://doi.org/10.3389/fmicb.2020.01800. PMID: 32793182; PMCID: PMC7387429.

[199] Arisan ED, Dart A, Grant GH, Arisan S, Cuhadaroglu S, Lange S, Uysal-Onganer P. The prediction of miRNAs in SARS-CoV-2 genomes: hsa-miR databases identify 7 key miRs linked to host responses and virus pathogenicity-related KEGG pathways significant for comorbidities. Viruses June 4, 2020;12(6):614. https://doi.org/10.3390/v12060614. PMID: 32512929; PMCID: PMC7354481.

[200] Tavasolian F, Rashidi M, Hatam GR, Jeddi M, Hosseini AZ, Mosawi SH, Abdollahi E, Inman RD. HLA, immune response, and susceptibility to COVID-19. Front Immunol January 8, 2021;11:601886. https://doi.org/10.3389/fimmu.2020.601886. PMID: 33488597; PMCID: PMC7820778.

[201] Reinold J, Farahpour F, Fehring C, Dolff S, Konik M, Korth J, van Baal L, Hoffmann D, Buer J, Witzke O, Westendorf AM, Kehrmann J. A pro-inflammatory gut microbiome characterizes SARS-CoV-2 infected patients and a reduction in the connectivity of an anti-inflammatory bacterial network associates with severe COVID-19. Front Cell Infect Microbiol November 17, 2021;11:747816. https://doi.org/10.3389/fcimb.2021.747816. PMID: 34869058; PMCID: PMC8635721.

[202] Ahmed S, Zimba O, Gasparyan AY. COVID-19 and the clinical course of rheumatic manifestations. Clin Rheumatol July 2021;40(7):2611−9. https://doi.org/10.1007/s10067-021-05691-x. Epub 2021 Mar 17. PMID: 33733315; PMCID: PMC7968918.

[203] Wang JY, Zhang W, Roehrl MW, Roehrl VB, Roehrl MH. An autoantigen atlas from human lung HFL1 cells offers clues to neurological and diverse autoimmune manifestations of COVID-19. 2021.01.24.427965 bioRxiv [Preprint] January 2021;24. https://doi.org/10.1101/2021.01.24.427965. PMID: 33501444; PMCID: PMC7836114.

[204] Halpert G, Shoenfeld Y. SARS-CoV-2, the autoimmune virus. Autoimmun Rev December 2020;19(12):102695. https://doi.org/10.1016/j.autrev.2020.102695. Epub 2020 Oct 28. PMID: 33130000; PMCID: PMC7598743.

[205] Akiyama S, Hamdeh S, Micic D, Sakuraba A. Prevalence and clinical outcomes of COVID-19 in patients with autoimmune diseases: a systematic review and meta-analysis. annrheumdis-2020-218946 Ann Rheum Dis October 2020;13. https://doi.org/10.1136/annrheumdis-2020-218946. Epub ahead of print. PMID: 33051220; PMCID: PMC7554412.

[206] Ferri C, Giuggioli D, Raimondo V, L'Andolina M, Tavoni A, Cecchetti R, Guiducci S, Ursini F, Caminiti M, Varcasia G, Gigliotti P, Pellegrini R, Olivo D, Colaci M, Murdaca G, Brittelli R, Mariano GP, Spinella A, Bellando-Randone S, Aiello V, Bilia S, Giannini D, Ferrari T, Caminiti R, Brusi V, Meliconi R, Fallahi P, Antonelli A, COVID-19 & ASD Italian Study Group. COVID-19 and rheumatic autoimmune systemic diseases: report of a large Italian patients series. Clin Rheumatol November 2020;39(11):3195−204. https://doi.org/10.1007/s10067-020-05334-7. Epub 2020 Aug 27. PMID: 32852623; PMCID: PMC7450255.

[207] Freites Nuñez DD, Leon L, Mucientes A, Rodriguez-Rodriguez L, Font Urgelles J, Madrid García A, Colomer JI, Jover JA, Fernandez-Gutierrez B, Abasolo L. Risk factors for hospital admissions related to COVID-19 in patients with autoimmune inflammatory rheumatic diseases. Ann Rheum Dis November 2020;79(11):1393−9. https://doi.org/10.1136/annrheumdis-2020-217984. Epub 2020 Aug 7. PMID: 32769150; PMCID: PMC7415073.

[208] Pablos JL, Galindo M, Carmona L, Lledó A, Retuerto M, Blanco R, Gonzalez-Gay MA, Martinez-Lopez D, Castrejón I, Alvaro-Gracia JM, Fernández Fernández D, Mera-Varela A, Manrique-Arija S, Mena Vázquez N, Fernandez-Nebro A. RIER Investigators Group; RIER investigators group. Clinical outcomes of hospitalised patients with COVID-19 and chronic inflammatory and autoimmune rheumatic diseases: a multicentric

matched cohort study. Ann Rheum Dis December 2020;79(12):1544–9. https://doi.org/10.1136/annrheumdis-2020-218296. Epub 2020 Aug 12. PMID: 32796045; PMCID: PMC7430185.

[209] Eder L, Croxford R, Drucker AM, Mendel A, Kuriya B, Touma Z, Johnson SR, Cook R, Bernatsky S, Haroon N, Widdifield J. COVID-19 hospitalizations, intensive care unit stays, ventilation and death among patients with immune mediated inflammatory diseases compared to controls. jrheum.211012 J Rheumatol February 1, 2022. https://doi.org/10.3899/jrheum.211012. Epub ahead of print. PMID: 35105713.

[210] Montero F, Martínez-Barrio J, Serrano-Benavente B, González T, Rivera J, Molina Collada J, Castrejón I, Álvaro-Gracia J. Coronavirus disease 2019 (COVID-19) in autoimmune and inflammatory conditions: clinical characteristics of poor outcomes. Rheumatol Int October 2020;40(10):1593–8. https://doi.org/10.1007/s00296-020-04676-4. Epub 2020 Aug 13. PMID: 32794113; PMCID: PMC7425254.

[211] Peach E, Rutter M, Lanyon P, Grainge MJ, Hubbard R, Aston J, Bythell M, Stevens S, Pearce F. Risk of death among people with rare autoimmune diseases compared with the general population in England during the 2020 COVID-19 pandemic. Rheumatology April 6, 2021;60(4):1902–9. https://doi.org/10.1093/rheumatology/keaa855. PMID: 33271595; PMCID: PMC7798585.

[212] Eder L, Croxford R, Drucker AM, Mendel A, Kuriya B, Touma Z, Johnson SR, Cook R, Bernatsky S, Haroon N, Widdifield J. Understanding COVID-19 risk in patients with immune mediated inflammatory diseases: a population-based analysis of SARS-CoV-2 testing. Arthritis Care Res September 2021;6. https://doi.org/10.1002/acr.24781. doi: 10.1002/acr.24781. Epub ahead of print. PMID: 34486829; PMCID: PMC8653048.

[213] Bachiller-Corral J, Boteanu A, Garcia-Villanueva MJ, de la Puente C, Revenga M, Diaz-Miguel MC, Rodriguez-Garcia A, Morell-Hita JL, Valero M, Larena C, Blazquez-Cañamero M, Guillen-Astete CA, Garrote S, Sobrino C, Medina-Quiñones C, Vazquez-Diaz M. Risk of severe COVID-19 infection in patients with inflammatory rheumatic diseases. J Rheumatol July 2021;48(7):1098–102. https://doi.org/10.3899/jrheum.200755. Epub 2021 Mar 15. PMID: 33722949.

[214] Mena Vázquez N, Manrique-Arija S, Cabezudo-García P, Godoy-Navarrete FJ, Cabezas-Lucena AM, Morales-Águila M, Redondo-Rodríguez R, Sobrino B, Ureña-Garnica I, Ordoñez-Cañizares MC, Díaz Cordovés-Rego G, Fernández-Nebro A. Incidence and case fatality rate of COVID-19 in patients with inflammatory articular diseases. Int J Clin Pract April 2021;75(4):e13707. https://doi.org/10.1111/ijcp.13707. Epub 2020 Dec 14. PMID: 32931643.

[215] Murtas R, Andreano A, Gervasi F, Guido D, Consolazio D, Tunesi S, Andreoni L, Greco MT, Gattoni ME, Sandrini M, Riussi A, Russo AG. Association between autoimmune diseases and COVID-19 as assessed in both a test-negative case-control and population case-control design. Auto Immun Highlights October 6, 2020;11(1):15. https://doi.org/10.1186/s13317-020-00141-1. PMID: 33023649; PMCID: PMC7537783.

[216] Gianfrancesco M, Hyrich KL, Al-Adely S, Carmona L, Danila MI, Gossec L, Izadi Z, Jacobsohn L, Katz P, Lawson-Tovey S, Mateus EF, Rush S, Schmajuk G, Simard J, Strangfeld A, Trupin L, Wysham KD, Bhana S, Costello W, Grainger R, Hausmann JS, Liew JW, Sirotich E, Sufka P, Wallace ZS, Yazdany J, Machado PM, Robinson PC. COVID-19 Global Rheumatology Alliance. Characteristics associated with hospitalisation for COVID-19 in people with rheumatic disease: data from the COVID-19 Global Rheumatology Alliance physician-reported registry. Ann Rheum Dis July 2020;79(7):859–66. https://doi.org/10.1136/annrheumdis-2020-217871. Epub 2020 May 29. PMID: 32471903; PMCID: PMC7299648.

[217] Nuño L, Novella Navarro M, Bonilla G, Franco-Gómez K, Aguado P, Peiteado D, Monjo I, Tornero C, Villalba A, Miranda-Carus ME, De Miguel E, Bogas P, Castilla-Plaza A, Bernad-Pineda M, García-Lorenzo E, Rodríguez-Araya T, Balsa A. Clinical course, severity and mortality in a cohort of patients with COVID-19 with rheumatic diseases. Ann Rheum Dis December 2020;79(12):1659–61. https://doi.org/10.1136/annrheumdis-2020-218054. Epub 2020 Jun 30. PMID: 32606046; PMCID: PMC7677491.

[218] Rajabi F, Drake LA, Senna MM, Rezaei N. Alopecia areata: a review of disease pathogenesis. Br J Dermatol November 2018;179(5):1033–48. https://doi.org/10.1111/bjd.16808. Epub 2018 Sep 9. PMID: 29791718.

[219] Suchonwanit P, Kositkuljorn C, Pomsoong C. Alopecia areata: an autoimmune disease of multiple players. ImmunoTargets Ther July 29, 2021;10:299–312. https://doi.org/10.2147/ITT.S266409. PMID: 34350136; PMCID: PMC8328385.

[220] Thomas EA, Kadyan RS. Alopecia areata and autoimmunity: a clinical study. Indian J Dermatol 2008;53(2):70–4. https://doi.org/10.4103/0019-5154.41650. PMID: 19881991; PMCID: PMC2763714.

[221] Trüeb RM. Telogen effluvium: is there a need for a new classification? Skin Appendage Disord September 2016;2(1–2):39–44. https://doi.org/10.1159/000446119. Epub 2016 May 21. PMID: 27843921; PMCID: PMC5096239.

[222] Hussain N, Agarwala P, Iqbal K, Omar HMS, Jangid G, Patel V, Rathore SS, Kumari C, Velasquez-Botero F, López GAB, Vishwakarma Y, Nipu AP, Ahmed NK. A systematic review of acute telogen effluvium, a harrowing post-COVID-19 manifestation. J Med Virol December 2021;20. https://doi.org/10.1002/jmv.27534. Epub ahead of print. PMID: 34931698.

[223] Sattur SS, Sattur IS. COVID-19 infection: impact on hair. Indian J Plast Surg December 13, 2021;54(4):521–6. https://doi.org/10.1055/s-0041-1740289. PMID: 34984095; PMCID: PMC8719952.

[224] Benson MD, Buxbaum JN, Eisenberg DS, Merlini G, Saraiva MJM, Sekijima Y, Sipe JD, Westermark P. Amyloid nomenclature 2020: update and recommendations by the International Society of Amyloidosis (ISA) nomenclature committee. Amyloid December 2020;27(4):217–22. https://doi.org/10.1080/13506129.2020.1835263. Epub 2020 Oct 26. PMID: 33100054.

[225] Sorić Hosman I, Kos I, Lamot L. Serum amyloid A in inflammatory rheumatic diseases: a compendious review of a renowned biomarker. Front Immunol February 19, 2021;11:631299. https://doi.org/10.3389/fimmu.2020.631299. PMID: 33679725; PMCID: PMC7933664.

[226] Jana AK, Greenwood AB, Hansmann UHE. Presence of a SARS-CoV-2 protein enhances amyloid formation of serum amyloid A. J Phys Chem B August 19, 2021;125(32):9155–67. https://doi.org/10.1021/acs.jpcb.1c04871. Epub 2021 Aug 9. PMID: 34370466; PMCID: PMC8369982.

[227] Neumann-Haefelin C. Protektiver Effekt von HLA-B27 auf den Verlauf der HIV- und Hepatitis-C-Virus-Infektion [Protective role of HLA-B27 in HIV and hepatitis C virus infection]. German Dtsch Med Wochenschr February 2011;136(7):320–4. https://doi.org/10.1055/s-0031-1272531. Epub 2011 Feb 7. PMID: 21302207.

[228] Knight JS, Kanthi Y. Mechanisms of immunothrombosis and vasculopathy in antiphospholipid syndrome. Semin Immunopathol February 2022;4. https://doi.org/10.1007/s00281-022-00916-w. Epub ahead of print. PMID: 35122116.

[229] Wang X, Gkrouzman E, Andrade DCO, Andreoli L, Barbhaiya M, Belmont HM, Branch DW, de Jesús GR, Efthymiou M, Ríos-Garcés R, Gerosa M, El Hasbani G, Knight J, Meroni PL, Pazzola G, Petri M, Rand J, Salmon J, Tektonidou M, Tincani A, Uthman IW, Zuily S, Zuo Y, Lockshin M, Cohen H, Erkan D, APS ACTION. COVID-19 and antiphospholipid antibodies: a position statement and management guidance from AntiPhospholipid syndrome alliance for clinical trials and InternatiOnal networking (APS ACTION). Lupus December 2021;30(14):2276–85. https://doi.org/10.1177/09612033211062523. Epub 2021 Dec 16. PMID: 34915764.

[230] Gil-Etayo FJ, Garcinuño S, Lalueza A, Díaz-Simón R, García-Reyne A, Pleguezuelo DE, Cabrera-Marante O, Rodriguez-Frias EA, Perez-Rivilla A, Serrano M, Serrano A. Anti-phospholipid antibodies and COVID-19 thrombosis: a Co-star, not a supporting actor. Biomedicines July 27, 2021;9(8):899. https://doi.org/10.3390/biomedicines9080899. PMID: 34440103; PMCID: PMC8389622.

[231] Tang KT, Hsu BC, Chen DY. Autoimmune and rheumatic manifestations associated with COVID-19 in adults: an updated systematic review. Front Immunol March 12, 2021;12:645013. https://doi.org/10.3389/fimmu.2021.645013. PMID: 33777042; PMCID: PMC7994612.

[232] Taha M, Samavati L. Antiphospholipid antibodies in COVID-19: a meta-analysis and systematic review. RMD Open 2021;7(2):e001580. https://doi.org/10.1136/rmdopen-2021-001580. PMID: 33958439; PMCID: PMC8103564.

[233] Stelzer M, Henes J, Saur S. The role of antiphospholipid antibodies in COVID-19. Curr Rheumatol Rep July 14, 2021;23(9):72. https://doi.org/10.1007/s11926-021-01041-7. PMID: 34259944; PMCID: PMC8278370.

[234] Mendoza M, Garcia-Ruiz I, Maiz N, Rodo C, Garcia-Manau P, Serrano B, Lopez-Martinez RM, Balcells J, Fernandez-Hidalgo N, Carreras E, Suy A. Pre-eclampsia-like syndrome induced by severe COVID-19: a prospective observational study. BJOG October 2020;127(11):1374–80. https://doi.org/10.1111/1471-0528.16339. Epub 2020 Jun 21. PMID: 32479682; PMCID: PMC7300912.

[235] Conde-Agudelo A, Romero R. SARS-CoV-2 infection during pregnancy and risk of preeclampsia: a systematic review and meta-analysis. Am J Obstet Gynecol January 2022;226(1):68–89.e3. https://doi.org/10.1016/j.ajog.2021.07.009. Epub 2021 Jul 21. PMID: 34302772; PMCID: PMC8294655.

[236] Xu Q, Zhang L, Chen L, Zhao X, Wang X, Hu M, Le Y, Xue F, Li X, Zheng J. SARS-CoV-2 might transmit through the skin while the skin barrier function could be the mediator. Med Hypotheses February

2022;159:110752. https://doi.org/10.1016/j.mehy.2021.110752. Epub 2022 Jan 3. PMID: 35002019; PMCID: PMC8721925.

[237] Lavezzo MM, Sakata VM, Morita C, Rodriguez EE, Abdallah SF, da Silva FT, Hirata CE, Yamamoto JH. Vogt-Koyanagi-Harada disease: review of a rare autoimmune disease targeting antigens of melanocytes. Orphanet J Rare Dis March 24, 2016;11:29. https://doi.org/10.1186/s13023-016-0412-4. PMID: 27008848; PMCID: PMC4806431.

[238] Szcześniak M, Brydak-Godowska J. SARS-CoV-2 and the eyes: a review of the literature on transmission, detection, and ocular manifestations. Med Sci Monit September 11, 2021;27:e931863. https://doi.org/10.12659/MSM.931863. PMID: 34508064; PMCID: PMC8439119.

[239] Grajewski RS, Rokohl AC, Becker M, Dewald F, Lehmann C, Fätkenheuer G, Cursiefen C, Klein F, Heindl LM. A missing link between SARS-CoV-2 and the eye?: ACE2 expression on the ocular surface. J Med Virol January 2021;93(1):78−9. https://doi.org/10.1002/jmv.26136. Epub 2020 Jun 12. PMID: 32497334; PMCID: PMC7300893.

[240] Dotan A, Muller S, Kanduc D, David P, Halpert G, Shoenfeld Y. The SARS-CoV-2 as an instrumental trigger of autoimmunity. Autoimmun Rev April 2021;20(4):102792. https://doi.org/10.1016/j.autrev.2021.102792. Epub 2021 Feb 19. PMID: 33610751; PMCID: PMC7892316.

[241] Antonelli A, Ferrari SM, Ragusa F, Elia G, Paparo SR, Ruffilli I, Patrizio A, Giusti C, Gonnella D, Cristaudo A, Foddis R, Shoenfeld Y, Fallahi P. Graves' disease: epidemiology, genetic and environmental risk factors and viruses. Best Pract Res Clin Endocrinol Metabol January 2020;34(1):101387. https://doi.org/10.1016/j.beem.2020.101387. Epub 2020 Feb 4. PMID: 32107168.

[242] Caturegli P, De Remigis A, Rose NR. Hashimoto thyroiditis: clinical and diagnostic criteria. Autoimmun Rev 2014 ;13(4−5):391−7. https://doi.org/10.1016/j.autrev.2014.01.007. Epub 2014 Jan 13. PMID: 24434360.

[243] Anaya JM, Monsalve DM, Rojas M, Rodríguez Y, Montoya-García N, Mancera-Navarro LM, Villadiego-Santana AM, Rodríguez-Leguizamón G, Acosta-Ampudia Y, Ramírez-Santana C. Latent rheumatic, thyroid and phospholipid autoimmunity in hospitalized patients with COVID-19. J Transl Autoimmun 2021;4:100091. https://doi.org/10.1016/j.jtauto.2021.100091. Epub 2021 Mar 2. PMID: 33681751; PMCID: PMC7920824.

[244] Clausen CL, Rasmussen ÅK, Johannsen TH, Hilsted LM, Skakkebæk NE, Szecsi PB, Pedersen L, Benfield T, Juul A. Thyroid function in COVID-19 and the association with cytokine levels and mortality. Endocr Connect September 28, 2021;10(10):1234−42. https://doi.org/10.1530/EC-21-0301. PMID: 34468398; PMCID: PMC8494417.

[245] Geslot A, Chanson P, Caron P. Covid-19, the thyroid and the pituitary - the real state of play. 00001-4 Ann Endocrinol January 2022;20(22):S0003−4266. https://doi.org/10.1016/j.ando.2021.12.004. Epub ahead of print. PMID: 35065920; PMCID: PMC8772063.

[246] Lisco G, De Tullio A, Jirillo E, Giagulli VA, De Pergola G, Guastamacchia E, Triggiani V. Thyroid and COVID-19: a review on pathophysiological, clinical and organizational aspects. J Endocrinol Invest September 2021;44(9):1801−14. https://doi.org/10.1007/s40618-021-01554-z. Epub 2021 Mar 25. PMID: 33765288; PMCID: PMC7992516.

[247] Oğuz SH, Sendur SN, İremli BG, Gürlek A, Erbas T, Ünlütürk U. SARS-CoV-2 vaccine-induced thyroiditis: safety of Re-vaccinations and clinical follow-up. J Clin Endocrinol Metab February 2022;1:dgac049. https://doi.org/10.1210/clinem/dgac049. Epub ahead of print. PMID: 35100622.

[248] Austin PC. An introduction to propensity score methods for reducing the effects of confounding in observational studies. Multivariate Behav Res May 2011;46(3):399−424. https://doi.org/10.1080/00273171.2011.568786. Epub 2011 Jun 8. PMID: 21818162; PMCID: PMC3144483.

[249] Haberman RH, Castillo R, Chen A, Yan D, Ramirez D, Sekar V, Lesser R, Solomon G, Neimann AL, Blank RB, Izmirly P, Webster DE, Ogdie A, Troxel AB, Adhikari S, Scher JU, WARCOV Investigators NYU. COVID-19 in patients with inflammatory arthritis: a prospective study on the effects of comorbidities and disease-modifying antirheumatic drugs on clinical outcomes. Arthritis Rheumatol December 2020;72(12):1981−9. https://doi.org/10.1002/art.41456. Epub 2020 Oct 25. PMID: 32725762; PMCID: PMC7722024.

[250] Goldenberg MM. Multiple sclerosis review. P T March 2012;37(3):175−84. PMID: 22605909; PMCID: PMC3351877.

[251] Meacci E, Garcia-Gil M, Pierucci F. SARS-CoV-2 infection: a role for S1P/S1P receptor signaling in the nervous system? Int J Mol Sci September 15, 2020;21(18):6773. https://doi.org/10.3390/ijms21186773. PMID: 32942748; PMCID: PMC7556035.

[252] Schneider-Schaulies S, Schumacher F, Wigger D, Schöl M, Waghmare T, Schlegel J, Seibel J, Kleuser B. Sphingolipids: effectors and achilles heals in viral infections? Cells August 24, 2021;10(9):2175. https://doi.org/10.3390/cells10092175. PMID: 34571822; PMCID: PMC8466362.

[253] Sullivan R, Kilaru A, Hemmer B, Campbell Cree BA, Greenberg BM, Kundu U, Hach T, DeLasHeras V, Ward BJ, Berger J. COVID-19 infection in fingolimod- or siponimod-treated patients: case series. Neurol Neuroimmunol Neuroinflamm November 30, 2021;9(1):e1092. https://doi.org/10.1212/NXI.0000000000001092. PMID: 34848501.

[254] Alborghetti M, Bellucci G, Gentile A, Calderoni C, Nicoletti F, Capra R, Salvetti M, Centonze D. Drugs used in the treatment of multiple sclerosis during COVID-19 pandemic: a critical viewpoint. Curr Neuropharmacol 2022;20(1):107–25. https://doi.org/10.2174/1570159X19666210330094017. PMID: 33784961.

[255] Hammer A, Waschbisch A, Kuhbandner K, Bayas A, Lee DH, Duscha A, Haghikia A, Gold R, Linker RA. The NRF2 pathway as potential biomarker for dimethyl fumarate treatment in multiple sclerosis. Ann Clin Transl Neurol April 16, 2018;5(6):668–76. https://doi.org/10.1002/acn3.553. PMID: 29928650; PMCID: PMC5989754.

[256] Olagnier D, Farahani E, Thyrsted J, Blay-Cadanet J, Herengt A, Idorn M, Hait A, Hernaez B, Knudsen A, Iversen MB, Schilling M, Jørgensen SE, Thomsen M, Reinert LS, Lappe M, Hoang HD, Gilchrist VH, Hansen AL, Ottosen R, Nielsen CG, Møller C, van der Horst D, Peri S, Balachandran S, Huang J, Jakobsen M, Svenningsen EB, Poulsen TB, Bartsch L, Thielke AL, Luo Y, Alain T, Rehwinkel J, Alcamí A, Hiscott J, Mogensen TH, Paludan SR, Holm CK. SARS-CoV2-mediated suppression of NRF2-signaling reveals potent antiviral and anti-inflammatory activity of 4-octyl-itaconate and dimethyl fumarate. Nat Commun October 2, 2020;11(1):4938. https://doi.org/10.1038/s41467-020-18764-3. Erratum in: Nat Commun. 2020 Oct 21;11(1):5419. PMID: 33009401; PMCID: PMC7532469.

[257] Jayam Trouth A, Dabi A, Solieman N, Kurukumbi M, Kalyanam J. Myasthenia gravis: a review. Autoimmune Dis 2012;2012:874680. https://doi.org/10.1155/2012/874680. Epub 2012 Oct 31. PMID: 23193443; PMCID: PMC3501798.

[258] Bruestle K, Hackner K, Kreye G, Heidecker B. Autoimmunity in acute myocarditis: how immunopathogenesis steers new directions for diagnosis and treatment. Curr Cardiol Rep March 20, 2020;22(5):28. https://doi.org/10.1007/s11886-020-01278-1. PMID: 32198622; PMCID: PMC7083821.

[259] Kim YM, Brinkmann MM, Paquet ME, Ploegh HL. UNC93B1 delivers nucleotide-sensing toll-like receptors to endolysosomes. Nature March 13, 2008;452(7184):234–8. https://doi.org/10.1038/nature06726. Epub 2008 Feb 27. PMID: 18305481.

[260] Gunning 3rd WT, Kvale H, Kramer PM, Karabin BL, Grubb BP. Postural orthostatic tachycardia syndrome is associated with elevated G-protein coupled receptor autoantibodies. J Am Heart Assoc September 17, 2019;8(18):e013602. https://doi.org/10.1161/JAHA.119.013602. Epub 2019 Sep 9. PMID: 31495251; PMCID: PMC6818019.

[261] Salamanna F, Maglio M, Landini MP, Fini M. Body localization of ACE-2: on the trail of the keyhole of SARS-CoV-2. Front Med December 3, 2020;7:594495. https://doi.org/10.3389/fmed.2020.594495. PMID: 33344479; PMCID: PMC7744810.

[262] Zhao B, Ni C, Gao R, Wang Y, Yang L, Wei J, Lv T, Liang J, Zhang Q, Xu W, Xie Y, Wang X, Yuan Z, Liang J, Zhang R, Lin X. Recapitulation of SARS-CoV-2 infection and cholangiocyte damage with human liver ductal organoids. Protein Cell October 2020;11(10):771–5. https://doi.org/10.1007/s13238-020-00718-6. PMID: 32303993; PMCID: PMC7164704.

[263] Graier T, Golob-Schwarzl N, Weger W, Benezeder T, Painsi C, Salmhofer W, Wolf P. Furin expression in patients with psoriasis-A patient cohort endangered to SARS-COV2? Front Med February 10, 2021;8:624462. https://doi.org/10.3389/fmed.2021.624462. PMID: 33644099; PMCID: PMC7902756.

[264] Piaserico S, Gisondi P, Cazzaniga S, Di Leo S, Naldi L. Assessing the risk and outcome of COVID-19 in patients with psoriasis or psoriatic arthritis on biologic treatment: a critical appraisal of the quality of the published evidence. J Invest Dermatol February 2022;142(2):355–363.e7. https://doi.org/10.1016/j.jid.2021.04.036. Epub 2021 Aug 4. PMID: 34363826; PMCID: PMC8334343.

[265] Guo Q, Wang Y, Xu D, Nossent J, Pavlos NJ, Xu J. Rheumatoid arthritis: pathological mechanisms and modern pharmacologic therapies. Bone Res April 27, 2018;6:15. https://doi.org/10.1038/s41413-018-0016-9. PMID: 29736302; PMCID: PMC5920070.

[266] Schett G, Manger B, Simon D, Caporali R. COVID-19 revisiting inflammatory pathways of arthritis. Nat Rev Rheumatol August 2020;16(8):465–70. https://doi.org/10.1038/s41584-020-0451-z. Epub 2020 Jun 19. PMID: 32561873; PMCID: PMC7304381.

[267] Cordtz R, Lindhardsen J, Soussi BG, Vela J, Uhrenholt L, Westermann R, Kristensen S, Nielsen H, Torp-Pedersen C, Dreyer L. Incidence and severeness of COVID-19 hospitalization in patients with inflammatory rheumatic disease: a nationwide cohort study from Denmark. Rheumatology October 9, 2021;60(SI):SI59–67. https://doi.org/10.1093/rheumatology/keaa897. PMID: 33369663; PMCID: PMC7798558.

[268] Bower H, Frisell T, Di Giuseppe D, Delcoigne B, Ahlenius GM, Baecklund E, Chatzidionysiou K, Feltelius N, Forsblad-d'Elia H, Kastbom A, Klareskog L, Lindqvist E, Lindström U, Turesson C, Sjöwall C, Askling J, Study Group ARTIS. Impact of the COVID-19 pandemic on morbidity and mortality in patients with inflammatory joint diseases and in the general population: a nationwide Swedish cohort study. Ann Rheum Dis February 23, 2021;80(8):1086–93. https://doi.org/10.1136/annrheumdis-2021-219845. Epub ahead of print. PMID: 33622688; PMCID: PMC8206171.

[269] Tripathy A, Swain N, Gupta B. The COVID-19 pandemic: an increased risk of rheumatoid arthritis. Future Virol June 2021. https://doi.org/10.2217/fvl-2020-0393. doi: 10.2217/fvl-2020-0393. PMID: 34181704; PMCID: PMC8221023.

[270] Bobircă A, Bobircă F, Ancuța I, Florescu A, Bojincă M, Muscă A, Florescu DN, Florescu LM, Sima RM, Florescu A, Mușetescu AE. COVID-19-A trigger factor for severe immune-mediated thrombocytopenia in active rheumatoid arthritis. Life January 6, 2022;12(1):77. https://doi.org/10.3390/life12010077. PMID: 35054471; PMCID: PMC8780601.

[271] Calender A, Israel-Biet D, Valeyre D, Pacheco Y. Modeling potential autophagy pathways in COVID-19 and sarcoidosis. Trends Immunol October 2020;41(10):856–9. https://doi.org/10.1016/j.it.2020.08.001. Epub 2020 Aug 10. PMID: 32863134; PMCID: PMC7416769.

[272] Pacheco Y, Valeyre D, El Jammal T, Vallee M, Chevalier F, Lamartine J, Sigaudo-Roussel D, Verrier B, Israel-Biet D, Freymond N, Cottin V, Calender A. Autophagy and mitophagy-related pathways at the crossroads of genetic pathways involved in familial sarcoidosis and host-pathogen interactions induced by coronaviruses. Cells August 5, 2021;10(8):1995. https://doi.org/10.3390/cells10081995. PMID: 34440765; PMCID: PMC8393644.

[273] Brito-Zerón P, Gracia-Tello B, Robles A, Alguacil A, Bonet M, De-Escalante B, Noblejas-Mosso A, Gómez-de-la-Torre R, Akasbi M, Pérez-de-Lis M, Pérez-Alvarez R, Ramos-Casals M. On behalf of the SarcoGEAS-semi registry. Characterization and outcomes of SARS-CoV-2 infection in patients with sarcoidosis. Viruses May 27, 2021;13(6):1000. https://doi.org/10.3390/v13061000. PMID: 34071924; PMCID: PMC8228115.

[274] Masuko K. Will the COVID-19 pandemic trigger future occurrence of autoimmunity like Sjögren's syndrome? Int J Rheum Dis July 2021;24(7):963–5. https://doi.org/10.1111/1756-185X.14154. Epub 2021 Jun 22. PMID: 34156141; PMCID: PMC8441922.

[275] Nln I, Fernandez-Ruiz R, Muskardin TLW, Paredes JL, Blazer AD, Tuminello S, Attur M, Iturrate E, Petrilli CM, Abramson SB, Chakravarti A, Niewold TB. Interferon pathway lupus risk alleles modulate risk of death from acute COVID-19. 00020-2 Transl Res January 2022;31(22):S1931–5244. https://doi.org/10.1016/j.trsl.2022.01.007. Epub ahead of print. PMID: 35114420; PMCID: PMC8802623.

[276] Sawalha AH, Zhao M, Coit P, Lu Q. Epigenetic dysregulation of ACE2 and interferon-regulated genes might suggest increased COVID-19 susceptibility and severity in lupus patients. Clin Immunol June 2020;215:108410. https://doi.org/10.1016/j.clim.2020.108410. Epub 2020 Apr 8. PMID: 32276140; PMCID: PMC7139239.

[277] Thanou A, Sawalha AH. SARS-CoV-2 and systemic lupus erythematosus. Curr Rheumatol Rep January 28, 2021;23(2):8. https://doi.org/10.1007/s11926-020-00973-w. PMID: 33511495; PMCID: PMC7842169.

[278] Takahashi Y, Haga S, Ishizaka Y, Mimori A. Autoantibodies to angiotensin-converting enzyme 2 in patients with connective tissue diseases. Arthritis Res Ther 2010;12(3):R85. https://doi.org/10.1186/ar3012. Epub 2010 May 14. PMID: 20470389; PMCID: PMC2911869.

[279] Tang X, Geng L, Feng X, Sun L. Decreased serum ACE2 levels in patients with connective tissue diseases. Rheumatology September 1, 2021;60(9):4401–6. https://doi.org/10.1093/rheumatology/keaa898. PMID: 33369650.

[280] Bernard NJ. Double-negative B cells. Nat Rev Rheumatol December 2018;14(12):684. https://doi.org/10.1038/s41584-018-0113-6. PMID: 30367167.

[281] Woodruff MC, Ramonell RP, Nguyen DC, Cashman KS, Saini AS, Haddad NS, Ley AM, Kyu S, Howell JC, Ozturk T, Lee S, Suryadevara N, Case JB, Bugrovsky R, Chen W, Estrada J, Morrison-Porter A, Derrico A, Anam FA, Sharma M, Wu HM, Le SN, Jenks SA, Tipton CM, Staitieh B, Daiss JL, Ghosn E, Diamond MS, Carnahan RH, Crowe Jr JE, Hu WT, Lee FE, Sanz I. Extrafollicular B cell responses correlate with neutralizing antibodies and morbidity in COVID-19. Nat Immunol December 2020;21(12):1506–16. https://doi.org/10.1038/s41590-020-00814-z. Epub 2020 Oct 7. PMID: 33028979; PMCID: PMC7739702.

[282] Cervantes-Díaz R, Sosa-Hernández VA, Torres-Ruíz J, Romero-Ramírez S, Cañez-Hernández M, Pérez-Fragoso A, Páez-Franco JC, Meza-Sánchez DE, Pescador-Rojas M, Sosa-Hernández VA, Gómez-Martín D, Maravillas-Montero JL. Severity of SARS-CoV-2 infection is linked to double-negative (CD27- IgD-) B cell subset numbers. Inflamm Res January 2022;71(1):131–40. https://doi.org/10.1007/s00011-021-01525-3. Epub 2021 Nov 30. PMID: 34850243; PMCID: PMC8631699.

[283] Sachinidis A, Garyfallos A. Double Negative (DN) B cells: a connecting bridge between rheumatic diseases and COVID-19? Mediterr J Rheumatol September 30, 2021;32(3):192–9. https://doi.org/10.31138/mjr.32.3.192. PMID: 34964023; PMCID: PMC8693305.

[284] Sakthiswary R, Chuah HY, Chiang KS, Liew YS, Muhammad Aizat NA. COVID-19 in systemic lupus erythematosus: a pooled analysis and systematic review of case reports and series. Lupus October 2021;30(12):1946–54. https://doi.org/10.1177/09612033211045057. Epub 2021 Sep 27. PMID: 34565208.

[285] Freire-de-Lima L, Scovino AM, Barreto Menezes CC, Marques da Fonseca L, Santos Dos Reis J, Rodrigues da Costa Santos MA, Monteiro da Costa K, Antonio do Nascimento Santos C, Freire-de-Lima CG, Morrot A. Autoimmune disorders & COVID-19. Medicines (Basel) September 28, 2021;8(10):55. https://doi.org/10.3390/medicines8100055. PMID: 34677484; PMCID: PMC8541336.

[286] Shah S, Danda D, Kavadichanda C, Das S, Adarsh MB, Negi VS. Autoimmune and rheumatic musculoskeletal diseases as a consequence of SARS-CoV-2 infection and its treatment. Rheumatol Int October 2020;40(10):1539–54. https://doi.org/10.1007/s00296-020-04639-9. Epub 2020 Jul 14. PMID: 32666137; PMCID: PMC7360125.

[287] Dourmishev L, Guleva D, Pozharashka J, Drenovska K, Miteva L, Vassileva S. Autoimmune connective tissue diseases in the COVID-19 pandemic. Clin Dermatol 2021;39(1):56–63. https://doi.org/10.1016/j.clindermatol.2020.12.013. Epub 2020 Dec 15. PMID: 33972054; PMCID: PMC7833035.

[288] Acosta-Ampudia Y, Monsalve DM, Rojas M, Rodríguez Y, Zapata E, Ramírez-Santana C, Anaya JM. Persistent autoimmune activation and proinflammatory state in post-COVID syndrome. J Infect Dis January 2022;25. https://doi.org/10.1093/infdis/jiac017. Epub ahead of print. PMID: 35079804.

[289] Michelen M, Manoharan L, Elkheir N, Cheng V, Dagens A, Hastie C, O'Hara M, Suett J, Dahmash D, Bugaeva P, Rigby I, Munblit D, Harriss E, Burls A, Foote C, Scott J, Carson G, Olliaro P, Sigfrid L, Stavropoulou C. Characterising long COVID: a living systematic review. BMJ Glob Health September 2021;6(9):e005427. https://doi.org/10.1136/bmjgh-2021-005427. PMID: 34580069; PMCID: PMC8478580.

CHAPTER

3

Innate immune responses in COVID-19

Etienne Jacotot[1,2], *Laura Talamini*[3], *Srinivsasa Reddy Bonam*[4], *Angelica Thomaz Vieira*[3,5], *Véronique Fremeaux-Bacchi*[6], *Marko Radic*[7], *Marie-Agnès Dragon-Durey*[6,8], *Jose Manuel Lozano*[9], *Rafael Simone Saia*[10] and *Sylviane Muller*[3,11,12]

[1]Taub Institute for Research on Alzheimer's Disease and the Aging Brain, Columbia University, New York, NY, United States; [2]Department of Pathology and Cell Biology, Columbia University, New York, NY, United States; [3]Centre National de la Recherche Scientifique-Université de Strasbourg, Unit Biotechnology and Cell Signalling, Team Neuroimmunology and Peptide Therapeutics - Strasbourg Drug Discovery and Development Institute, Strasbourg, France; [4]Institut National de la Santé et de la Recherche Médicale, Centre de Recherche des Cordeliers, Team Immunopathologie et Immunointervention Thérapeutique, Université de Paris, Paris, France; [5]Laboratory of Microbiota and Immunomodulation, Department of Biochemistry and Immunology, Institute of Biological Sciences, Federal University of Minas Gerais, Belo Horizonte, Brazil; [6]Laboratoire d'Immunologie, Hôpital Européen Georges Pompidou, AP-HP, Paris, France; [7]Department of Microbiology, Immunology and Biochemistry, College of Medicine, University of Tennessee Health Science Center, Memphis, TN, United States; [8]Institut National de la Santé et de la Recherche Médicale, Centre de Recherche des Cordeliers, Team Inflammation, Complement et Cancer, Université de Paris, Paris, France; [9]Universidad Nacional de Colombia-Sede Bogotá, Departamento de Farmacia, Mimetismo Molecular de los Agentes Infecciosos, Bogotá, DC, Colombia; [10]Laboratory of Intestinal Pathophysiology, Department of Physiology, Ribeirão Preto Medical School, University of São Paulo, Ribeirão Preto, Brazil; [11]Fédération

Autoimmunity, COVID-19, Post-COVID19 syndrome and COVID-19 vaccination
https://doi.org/10.1016/B978-0-443-18566-3.00041-4

Hospitalo-Universitaire OMICARE, Fédération de Médecine Translationnelle de Strasbourg, University of Strasbourg, Strasbourg, France; [12]University of Strasbourg Institute for Advanced Study, Strasbourg, France

Introduction

At any time since our birth, our body is subject to all kinds of attacks by infectious agents and various external and internal substances. In the course of evolution, the immune system developed to protect ourselves against a large diversity of these aggressors, already known or never met, foreign or linked to the immune self (our organs and tissues). To be efficient, two types of immune responses, said innate and adaptive, protect us. These two systems work closely together but their kinetics and specialization differ. The innate immune system provides critical mechanisms for the rapid sensing and elimination of pathogens. It is a fast process, a first line of defense, characterized de facto by a spectrum of actions, which is large and not very specialized. It responds in the same way to all germs and foreign substances. In contrast, the adaptive immune system that takes place later involves antigen-specific responses which are highly adapted to specific pathogens. Both systems include humoral and cellular components that are complex and interact between them in an interlocking manner.

Immunity and its deregulation, for example in the case of autoimmunity, remains an area in which many factors and circuits have still to be discovered. By far, the numerous signaling pathways that are involved, the rules that dictate cell trafficking, the way soluble mediators agonize or antagonize cell receptors (and the existence of many of those is certainly still ignored), and diverse other cellular and molecular aspects have to be deciphered further or reconsidered. The recent emergence of severe acute respiratory syndrome coronavirus 2 (SARS-CoV-2) infection opened the way to a new field of constructive investigations in the sense that on a worldwide scale, considerable efforts were rapidly devoted and supported to understand the multiple strategies exploited by this emerging virus and its variants to influence the innate immune system and to antagonize host antiviral response.

Coronaviruses, a group of enveloped RNA virus, have long been known to present a high pandemic risk. SARS-CoV-1, the first identified strain of a coronavirus (CoV) that causes SARS, appeared in late 2002 and subsequently triggered short-lived epidemics mostly in parts of East Asia. SARS-CoV-2 is the ninth documented coronavirus that infects humans and the seventh identified in the last 20 years [1,2]. It was first identified in December 2019 in Wuhan, China. Its origin remains a matter of debate [3]. Numerous articles have been published that describe various structural aspects of SARS-CoV-2, its mode of cell recognition via targeted receptors, its attachment and intracellular behavior and cell spreading, its pathophysiological and medical effects, its long-term consequences and the possible strategies (pharmacological, vaccinal) to fight it. Considerable work has been done to rapidly develop specific diagnostic assays in human fluids as well as in waste water and air. Protective elements have been adapted to avoid the persons to become infected and to avoid infecting others, including containment measures. At this stage, however, SARS-CoV-2 is responsible for more than five million confirmed deaths around the world (December

2021). Researchers across the world are at the forefront of global efforts to understand coronavirus disease 2019 (COVID-19) induced by SARS-CoV-2 and protect communities. A large amount of information has been acquired in a short period of time and freely disseminated. However, we still suffer from large areas of ignorance, especially with regard to several aspects of immune responses and immunity to SARS-CoV-2 [4–6].

Here, we review what we acquired since two years (2020–2021) regarding the innate immune system in the context of COVID-19. Although many more studies are required to address the causality of underlying events and mechanisms, our purpose is to highlight novel concepts and ideas that may help to produce future ways of intervention to reduce infection progression or diminish its intensity. Since excellent review articles have recently been published in this area (see Ref. [7], for example), our aim was to select a few aspects of key components that we tried to present here with a different highlight.

Innate immune responses to COVID-19: cells of the innate immune system

Innate immune cells can be rapidly mobilized in case of infection by any invading pathogen to initiate a fast inflammatory response. This step does not confer immune memory to the host. Innate immune cells include monocytes, macrophages, dendritic cells (DCs), Langerhans cells, natural killer (NK) T cells, neutrophils, eosinophils, basophils and mast cells (Table 3.1). $\gamma\delta$ T cells, as other so-called unconventional T-cell subsets bearing invariant T cell receptors (TCRs) such as CD1d-restricted NK T cells, are generally placed at the border between innate and adaptive immunity.

Cells of the innate system localize in the epithelial surfaces that form physical barriers impermeable to most infectious agents. Innate immune cells are thus found in the skin, the gastrointestinal tract, the respiratory tract, the nasopharynx, cilia, eyelashes and other hairs of the body. These natural barriers constituted by the skin and mucous membranes of the nasopharynx, bronchus, and gastrointestinal tracts maintain close contact with a number of foreign microbial species that also have permanent contact with the resident microbial flora, most of these are commensal, some symbiotic and a few pathogenic. This microbiota is fundamental for the modulation of the expression of genes of important functions for the intestine, absorption of nutrients, and other mechanisms (see section Innate immune responses to COVID-19: role of microbiota). This is important as respiratory and gastrointestinal tracts are the main target for CoV.

Once lung epithelial cells (type I alveolar cells) release cytokines and chemokines, the tissue-localized immune cells, particularly lung macrophages, get activated and secrete cytokines, chemokines, growth factors, and others effectors, which will act as signals to recruit monocytes, granulocytes, and lymphocytes to increase their functions in host defense [8] (Fig. 3.1). The so-called cytokine storm that develop is thus gradual in the course of COVID-19 disease. The host may recover quickly if the patient's status prior to infection is strong enough to sustain this condition. Based on the host immune system and other associated comorbidities, the mild form of COVID-19 steps can evolve into moderate and severe. In this case, excessive production of cytokines and other soluble factors can induce lung damage, leading to cessation of air supply, followed by multi-organ damage [8].

TABLE 3.1 Fate of innate immune cells in the COVID-19.

Innate immune cells	Observations
Monocytes	The first immune cell population recruited to the infected nasopharyngeal mucosa. In mild conditions, monocytes are differentiated into type I IFN secreting inflammatory monocytes, and in severe COVID-19 conditions, they become dysfunctional [12]. In addition, nonclassical monocytes ($CD14^{+}CD16^{++}$) are disappeared in severe COVID-19 conditions.
Macrophages	Ex vivo studies have confirmed the SARS-CoV-2 infection in alveolar macrophages [13], which generally recruit monocytes and granulocytes to the inflammation site. Compared to mild COVID-19 patients, severe patients exhibited proinflammatory macrophages in BALF [14]. In vitro studies have confirmed the direct effect of SARS-CoV-2 on MDMs. Although infected MDMs were found to be refractory to IFN responses, they produced abundant proinflammatory cytokines and chemokines [15].
Dendritic cells	In blood, decreased number of pDCs, cDC1, and cDC2 were observed in both moderate and severe COVID-19 conditions [16]. Similarly, a reduced number of mDCs and pDCs were observed in the BALFs of severe COVID-19 patients [14]. Studies on DCs from patients with acute COVID-19 revealed a lack of costimulatory (CD80/CD86) molecules that mediate T cells polarization [17]. In vitro studies on MDCs shown that SARS-CoV-2 has a direct effect on MDCs, attenuation of IFN response [15]. However, MDCs are refractory to virus replication.
NK cells	In the circulation of severe COVID-19 patients, the count of these cytotoxic cells appears significantly reduced and they expressed an exhausted phenotype [18]. In the BALFs from COVID-19 patients, the presence of NK cells could be detected in moderated conditions, while decreased NK cells were observed in severe conditions [14].
Neutrophils	Increased circulating neutrophils have become a hallmark of severe COVID-19 [12,19]. Dysfunctional and increased mature neutrophil count was observed in the severe COVID-19 conditions [18,20]. PD-L1 expression on the neutrophils is one of the prime factors for dysfunctions, which activate the myeloid-derived suppressor cells [12]. This is possibly linked with lymphopenia in COVID-19 conditions.
Eosinophils	Severe COVID-19 is associated with an increased number of eosinophils and their effector responses [16].
Basophils	The COVID-19 inflammatory environment could be prominent in the recruitment of basophils. GM-CSF has been linked with severe COVID cases [21]. In addition, GM-CSF-stimulated basophils can release histamine [22]. The number of circulating basophils is decreased during the acute phase and increased in the recovery phase of the disease [23]. Interestingly, PD-L1 expression on the basophils maintained a similar trend, namely, less expression in the acute phase and increased expression in the recovery phase [24].
Mast cells	Not much work has been done on this special type of immune population. However, it has been suggested that SARS-CoV-2 activates mast cells, and induces the release of histamine, which contributes to the cytokine storm [25]. It is well established that mast cells induce a synergistic effect on macrophages, granulocytes, and T cells.

Abbreviations not described above: cDC, conventional DC; GM-CSF, granulocyte-macrophages colony-stimulating factor; IFN, interferon; MDC, monocyte-derived dendritic cell; mDC, myeloid dendritic cell; MDM, monocyte-derived macrophage; pDC, plasmacytoid dendritic cell; PD-L1, programmed death ligand-1.

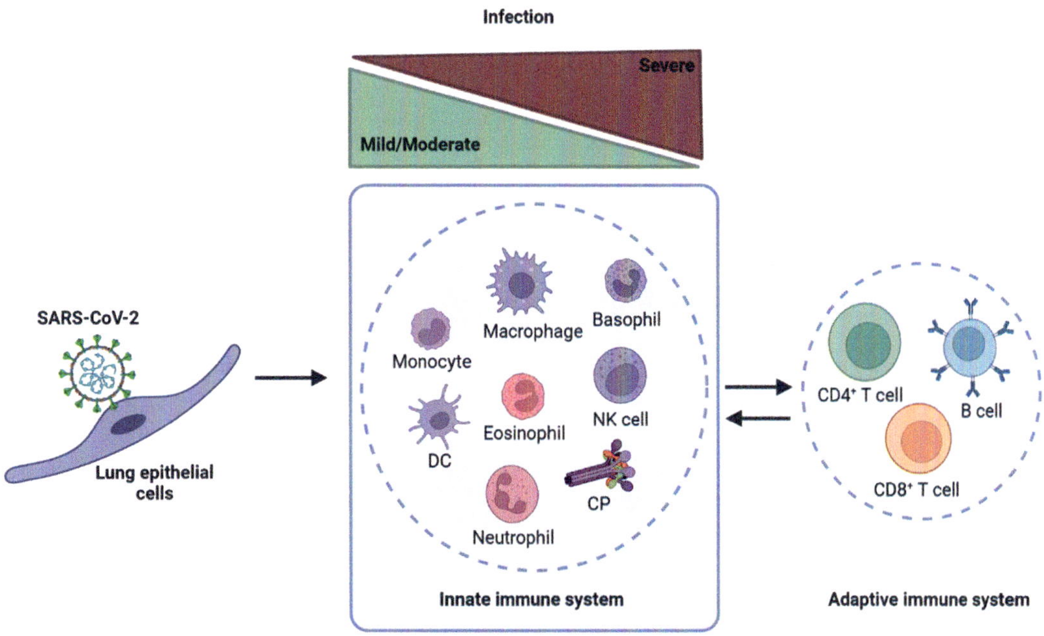

FIGURE 3.1 Innate immune system to SARS-CoV-2. Upon infection, the innate response is triggered from the signals produced by the infected epithelial cells (epithelial cells of the respiratory tract and lungs, epithelial, and nonepithelial cells of other organs that express AC2). Immune-competent hosts experience mild to moderate COVID-19, while immune-compromised or elder hosts experience severe COVID-19 conditions. Innate immune functions closely interact with the adaptive immune system. Abbreviations not described above: AC2, angiotensin I-converting enzyme two receptor; CP, complement.

Over the last two years of the pandemic, intensive efforts have been made to understand the patterns of presentation of SARS-CoV-2 infection, COVID-19 disease pathogenicity, how infected people transmit the virus, and the importance of immune responses against infection and recovery. A wide range of techniques (single-cell RNA sequencing, single-cell proteomics, mass spectrometry, multicolor flow cytometry, and others) have been used to determine changes in immune cell composition and status of their regulation in asymptomatic to mild, moderate, and severe COVID-19. To this regard, Table 3.1 highlights a few significant findings on innate immune cells responses in COVID-19 acquired, thanks to these advanced technologies.

Due to the virus incubation period, it is technically difficult to monitor the initial interactions with innate immune cells [7]. SARS-CoV-2 invades its target cells throught ACE-2, a ubiquitous receptor in human tissues and organs [9]. It appeared that innate immune cells do not directly interact with SARS-CoV-2 due to the lack of specific receptors. However, some studies describe viral RNA into macrophages. Whether the presence of viral RNA is related to a direct interaction of SARS-CoV-2 with these cells or to phagocytosis of other cells that have been infected remains to be further investigated [10]. In a similar line, human basophils are refractory to SARS-CoV-2 infection. Nevertheless, they exhibit marginal activation with SARS-CoV-2 and secrete IL-4 and IL-13 in both naïve and primed conditions (Bonam et al., personal communication). Viral RNA is detected in myeloid cells, which are derived from bronchoalveolar lavage fluid (BALF) or lungs collected from patients with severe COVID-19 [11]. At present, there is an urgent need to identify the cellular mechanisms that inhibit innate cell reprogramming in severe conditions. A clear understanding of the pathophysiology of COVID-19 in response to innate immune cells remains of prime importance in the development of therapeutics and vaccines (see section Innate immune responses to COVID-19: therapeutic developments).

Innate immune responses to COVID-19: NETosis and neutrophils

Neutrophils are the most prominent guardians of the proper functioning of healthy tissues [26]. They patrol the blood stream and exit from the vasculature to respond to altered homeostasis in any tissue that shows signs of infection or other disturbance in the normal physiologic activities occurring in tissues. Examples of perturbations that can recruit neutrophils from the vasculature to tissues include microbial infections, trauma and chronic damage, smoking, and metabolic inbalances. The common signals that guide neutrophils to respond to a wide range of altered conditions in the tissues are broadly associated with inflammation [27].

During inflammation, the local release of cytokines such as chemokine CXCL8 (also known as IL-8), tumor necrosis factor (TNF) and IL-1, induces neutrophil adhesion to receptors on luminal lining of blood vessels, their extravasation through or between endothelial cells, and the chemotaxis along and between structures comprising extracellular matrix [28]. The orchestrated motion of groups of neutrophils toward the source of a stimulus resembles the behavior of insects and is called swarming [29]. Swarms form in response to local stimuli in tissues and further orchestrate cellular movements in response to leukotriene B4. Direct cellular interactions use adhesion molecules, primarily integrins that incorporate the β2 subunit of the α/β dimers. Integrin engagement further triggers cellular interactions and activate signaling cascades that engage enzymatic activities and result in cytoplasmic movements, culminating in granule displacement [30]. Important neutrophil enzymes include neutrophil elastase (NE), myeloperoxidase (MPO), and peptidylarginine deiminase 4 (PAD4). Each of these three enzymes has a multitude of substrates, including those found in the immediate neutrophil surroundings; but it is within the neutrophil nucleus that these enzymes combine for a truly remarkable set of reactions leading to a spectacular form of cell death [31].

Like most other cells in the body, neutrophils can die by apoptosis, and apoptosis is engaged in cells that have become senescent, without having encountered an inflammatory stimulus. Because neutrophils are the most abundant white blood cell and their average life span is around 5 days, a large number of neutrophils die by apoptosis each day. However, under inflammatory conditions coupled with cellular adhesion, neutrophils are capable of dispersing nuclear chromatin in the form of "traps." Neutrophil extracellular traps (NETs), were observed using purified blood neutrophils and bacteria, yeast and viruses [32], including SARS CoV2 [33]. The NETs are produced in response to integrin engagement and depend on enzymatic activities by NE and PAD4. They incorporate MPO and NE within the chromatin meshwork that can entangle microbes, expose them to noxious enzymes and limit their infectivity. Excessive NET release, however, also may damage host tissues and the extracellular matrix [34].

Inflammation, as caused by COVID-19 in deep lung infections, causes neutrophil influx into the lung interstitium and alveolar spaces, and systemic inflammation recruits additional neutrophils from the bone marrow. This explains the high levels of circulating inflammatory cytokines and elevated numbers of blood neutrophils (neutrophilia) in severe infections [35]. Moreover, the migration of neutrophils into the lung tissue along with the release of NETs results in the edema and destruction of the fine cellular structure of airways, leading to life-threatening hypoxia and the need for assisted oxygen supporting measures. The release of neutrophil enzymes damages the extracellular matrix and leads to lung fibrosis, further aggravating the acute respiratory distress syndrome (ARDS). Initial neutrophil penetration into the lung tissues leads to the recruitment of additional neutrophils, forming neutrophil swarms that amplify the local tissue damage [36]. This set of events accounts for the major pathological findings in COVID-19 and predicts the beneficial effects of antiinflammatory and steroid therapies in severe COVID-19. Additional, more targeted approaches that may limit neutrophil migration and NET release are in clinical trials and show encouraging results (see below, section Innate immune responses to COVID-19: autophagy).

Innate immune responses to COVID-19: inflammasome

The SARS-CoV-2 infection causes severe inflammatory responses which contribute to the clinical presentation of patients with severe COVID-19 [37,38]. Early after the beginning of the pandemic, it has been proposed that hyperinflammatory response, ARDS, and multiorgan failure may be aetiologically linked through overactive inflammasome signaling [39,40]. Several studies are now accumulating that support direct (infection-induced) and indirect inflammasome activation and the critical role of inflammasomes in severe COVID-19.

Inflammasomes are (multiprotein) signaling platforms that activate inflammatory caspases to trigger several axis of defense against cellular stresses and infection, including cytokine-mediated proinflammatory cascades and immunogenic cell death [41]. The canonical inflammasomes are activation platforms of caspase-1, whereas the noncanonical inflammasomes are activation platforms of caspase-4 (also known as caspase-11 in mice) and caspase-5.

Canonical inflammasomes in COVID-19

Canonical inflammasomes are composed of three functional components: a sensor (generally a member of the so-called pattern recognition receptor/PRR family), an adaptor protein ASC (apoptosis-associated speck-like protein containing a caspase activation and recruitment domain/CARD) and the effector enzyme pro-caspase-1. Canonical inflammasomes activate when a sensor detects a molecular pattern of a pathogenic microorganism (PAMP) or an endogenous danger signal (DAMP) in the cytosol of the host cell. Five sensors capable of assembling a canonical inflammasome, each according to the type of signal received, have been well described: NLRP1 (NOD-like receptor (NLR) family, pyrin domain-containing protein 1), NLRP3, NLRC4 (NOD-, leucine-rich repeat- and CARD-containing 4), AIM2 (IFN-inducible protein also known as absent in melanoma 2), and pyrin. Activated caspase-1 converts pro-IL-1β and pro-IL-18 into functional cytokines, and cleaves gasdermin-D (GSDMD). Once cleaved, the GSDMD N-terminal fragment inserts into the plasma membrane of eukaryotic cells to form pores that are large enough to allow the release of IL-1β and IL-18, as well as various alarmins, such as ATP and high mobility group protein B1 (HMGB1) and other molecules. In several circumstances and cell types, these events culminate into a cell lysis and death process known as pyroptosis, a form of regulated necrotic cell death [42,43]. Pyroptosis is immunogenic and pro-inflammatory as it allows the massive release of PAMP and DAMP, along with IL-1β. Excessive IL-1β stimulates systemic inflammation responses by activating various signaling pathways, including nitric oxide production, the release of inflammatory arachidonic acid products such as prostaglandins and thromboxane A2, and the secretion of TNF, IL-6 and other cytokines, a pro-inflammatory complex that can lead to the so-called cytokine storm in acute inflammatory diseases (see section Innate immune responses to COVID-19: cytokines).

The NLRP3 inflammasome has important functions in RNA virus infection [44]. The idea that inflammasome sensors such as NLRP3 could serve as drivers of COVID-19 pathogenesis is reinforced by evidence in bats, which are asymptomatic reservoirs for CoV that are highly pathogenic to humans. Bats dampen host inflammation in response to both "sterile" danger signals and infections with different zoonotic RNA viruses, without affecting the viral loads in primary immune cells. Notably, bats significantly dampened activation of the NLRP3 inflammasome in bat primary immune cells compared to human or mouse counterparts [45,46].

A strong indication of inflammasome activation in COVID-19 is the fact that IL-18, the processing and secretion of which depend on inflammasome and GSDMD activation, is associated with severe COVID-19 and has emerged as a highly predictive biomarker of death [47–49]. Histological analysis of COVID-19 lung samples has shown GSDMD expression in alveolar epithelium as well as NLRP3 and caspase-1 expression in lung vascular tissue [50,51], and *post-mortem* histological sections from lung parenchyma also showed broadly elevated staining of IL-1β compared with control sections [52].

Accumulating evidences indicate that the NLRP3 inflammasome may drive COVID-19 pathology toward severe disease. The NLRP3 inflammasome is activated in response to SARS-CoV-2 infection and is active in COVID-19 patients. Studying moderate and severe COVID-19 patients, Rodrigues et al. have found active NLRP3 inflammasome in peripheral blood mononuclear cell (PBMCs) and tissues of postmortem patients upon autopsy. Direct inflammasome-derived products such as active caspase-1 (p20) and IL-18 in the sera correlated with the markers of COVID-19 severity, including IL-6 and lactate dehydrogenase (LDH). Moreover, higher levels of IL-18 and caspase-1 p20 are associated with disease severity and poor clinical outcome [47]. NLRP3 inflammasome aggregates were found in the lungs of fatal COVID-19 pneumonia thus providing an additional molecular link between viral infection and cytokine release syndrome [53]. In the lung and peripheral blood from patients with severe COVID-19, it was also observed that the pyroptosis of macrophages led to the release of the IL-1β and IL-18 by NLRP3 inflammasome activation and cleavage of caspase-1 [52]. Accordingly, high levels of endogenous DAMP molecule S100A8/A9, HMGB1 and LDH, can be detected in the serum of severe COVID-19 patients and may reflect pyroptotic cell death [54,55].

Multiple studies have shown that SARS-CoV-2 engages inflammasome and triggers pyroptosis in human monocytes, experimentally infected, and from patients under intensive care [56,57]. An important fraction of blood monocytes in COVID-19 patients is dying and infected with SARS-CoV-2. Monocyte infection activates NLRP3 and AIM2 inflammasomes, caspase-1 and GSDMD cleavage. Signs of pyroptosis (IL-1 family cytokines, LDH) in the plasma correlate with the development of severe disease [58]. SARS-CoV-2 infection of human monocyte-derived macrophages and monocyte-derived dendritic cells was found abortive, but induced the production of multiple antiviral and proinflammatory cytokines (IFN−α, IFN−β, TNF, and IL−1β, −6, and −10) and a chemokine CXCL10 [57].

Transfection or adenovirus-mediated expression of the SARS-CoV-2 nucleocapside N protein promotes NLRP3 inflammasome activation to induce hyperinflammation, and facilitates maturation of proinflammatory cytokines and induces proinflammatory responses in cultured cells and mice. This suggests one possible way to activate NLRP3 inflammasome during infection [59]. N protein interacts directly with NLRP3 protein, promotes the binding of NLRP3 with ASC, and facilitates NLRP3 inflammasome assembly. In sepsis and acute inflammation mouse models, N protein aggravates lung injury, accelerates death, and promotes IL−1β and IL−6 activation in mice. Notably, N-induced lung injury and cytokine production were suppressed in NLRP3$^{-/-}$ mice, and pharmacologically blocked by MCC950 (a specific inhibitor of NLRP3) and Ac-YVAD-cmk (an inhibitor of caspase-1).

According to another report, the SARS-CoV-2 spike (S) protein primes NLRP3 inflammasome activation and triggers IL-1β secretion in COVID-19 patient-derived macrophages but not in macrophages from healthy SARS-CoV-2 naïve individuals [60]. Most recently, it was found that the SARS-CoV-2 nonstructural protein NSP6 can impair lysosome acidification in lung epithelial cells via interacting with the vacuolar-type H^+-ATPase component ATP6AP1, thereby causing autophagic flux stagnation to instigate NLRP3 inflammasome activation and pyroptosis [61].

An unusual form of inflammasome-like activation may be related to caspase-8, which was previously viewed exclusively as an apoptotic caspase, but has now emerged as a master regulator of the three major cell death pathways, including apoptosis, pyroptosis, and necroptosis [62]. Recently, it was reported that caspase-8 can cleave GSDMD and induce the expression of pro-inflammatory cytokines and process pro-IL-1β and IL-18 in the same way as caspase-1, resulting in the release of bioactive cytokines, through either pyroptosis or necroptosis [63]. SARS-CoV-2 infection activates caspase-8 to trigger cell apoptosis and inflammatory cytokine processing in the lung epithelial cells [64]. The processed inflammatory cytokines are released through the virus-induced necroptosis pathway. Virus-induced apoptosis, necroptosis, and inflammation activation were also observed in the lung sections of SARS-CoV-2-infected HFH4-h angiotensin I-converting enzyme 2 (ACE2 transgenic mouse model). Furthermore, analysis of the *postmortem* lung sections of fatal COVID-19 patients revealed not only apoptosis and necroptosis but also massive inflammatory cell infiltration, necrotic cell debris, and pulmonary interstitial fibrosis, typical of immune pathogenesis in the lung. Thus SARS-CoV-2 infection may trigger a dual-mode of cell death pathways, and caspase-8-dependent inflammatory responses may contribute to the lung damage in COVID-19 patients. These observations may be related to the triggering of PANoptosis, a regulated and extensive inflammatory cell death mode where pyrolysis, apoptosis and necroptosis are coactivated [65].

Noncanonical inflammasomes and COVID-19

Unlike canonical inflammasomes where ligand sensing, assembly, and effector functions are carried out by multiple protein components, in the noncanonical inflammasomes, caspases −4/11 or −5 function as both sensor and effector molecules for lipopolysaccharide (LPS) from Gram-negative bacteria [66]. Once activated, caspase−4/11 can cleave GSDMD and pro-IL-18 similar to caspase-1, but it cannot cleave pro-IL-1β. On the other hand, caspase-5 also cleaves GSDMD but has only very weak activity for pro-IL-18 and pro-IL-1β [67]. The major function of noncanonical inflammasomes is therefore the induction of pyroptosis. After the occurrence of pyroptosis, the GSDMD pores release inflammatory factors, such as Il-1β and ATP, and the Ninjurin-1 pores release larger factors including HMGB1 and LDH, which collectively act as alarm signals to activate and recruit (more) immune cells and mediate the immune response.

Recent evidence also implicates the guanylate-binding protein (GBP) family as LPS cosensors and amplificators of the noncanonical inflammasome assembly through GBP hetero-oligomerization and recruitment of caspase-4 [68,69]. The arachidonic acid-derived oxidized phospholipids, oxPAPC (oxidized 1-palmitoyl-2-arachidonoyl-sn-glycero-3-phosphocholine) is a DAMP that binds caspase-4/11 and thereby trigger a pro-inflammatory response in DCs. However, while cytosolic LPS triggers caspase-11 mediated IL-1β release as well as pyroptosis, oxPAPC only induces IL-1β release, causing a hyperactivated state in the absence of cell death [70]. The noncanonic inflammasome may be important during SARS-CoV-2 infection as caspase-4/11 and caspase-5 are induced by type I and II IFNs and because plasma samples from patients with severe COVID-19 contain LPS. Alternatively, oxidized phospholipids that are known as potent inducers of ARDS, may be generated in the alveolar epithelium during SARS-CoV-2 infection and trigger caspase-4/11 activation in DCs and macrophages [71,72].

In a recent preprint, Eltobgy et al. reported that human caspase-4 is highly expressed in the lungs of COVID-19 patients, and its mouse homologue, caspase-11, is similarly induced upon SARS-CoV-2 infection of mice [73]. CASP4 expression correlates with the severity of SARS-CoV-2 infection in humans. These authors also found significantly decreased SARS-CoV-2-induced lung pathology, including blood vessel damage, in caspase-11$^{-/-}$ mice compared to wild-type (WT) and Gsdmd$^{-/-}$ mice, correlating with the preservation of caspase-11$^{-/-}$ mice body weight and their faster recovery. Furthermore, IL-1β and IL-6 were lower in the lungs of caspase-11$^{-/-}$ mice and the production of CXCL1 was dependent on caspase-11. Lungs of SARS-CoV-2-infected caspase-11$^{-/-}$ mice contained fewer neutrophils than infected WT lungs, and additionally, caspase-11$^{-/-}$ neutrophils largely failed to activate and undergo NETosis. Indeed, caspase-11$^{-/-}$ lungs accumulated less von Willebrand factor (vWF), a marker for endothelial damage, but expressed more Kruppel-like factor 2, a transcription factor that maintains vascular integrity. These results suggest that caspase-4/11, promotes detrimental SARS-CoV-2-associated inflammation and coagulopathy, largely independently of GSDMD [73–75].

Hence, both canonical and noncanonical inflammasomes participate in the pathophysiology of COVID-19 (Fig. 3.2). They may be used as markers of disease severity and could be targeted for therapeutic purposes.

Innate immune responses to COVID-19: TLRs

Toll-like receptors (TLRs) are a family of transmembrane proteins essential in activating antiviral signaling pathways. They play a crucial role in recognition of viral particles and activation of the innate immune system. The innate immune system monitors pathogens entry into the host via PRRs, such as TLR, NODs, cytosolic RIG-I-like receptors (RLRs) and lectins. CoVs are sensed by the endosomal TLRs (TLR3 and TLR7) and RLRs. Although no definitive evidence of SARS-CoV-2-induced PRRs dysregulation has been reported, the contribution of PRRs to the dismal prognosis is clear. For example, despite immunocompromised settings, the COVID-19 pandemic has a huge impact on the elderly as compared to the young, which indirectly links immunosenescence with illness severity. Poor innate immune activities, such as diminished antigen recognition, processing, efficient presentation via major histocompatibility complex (MHC) molecules, dysregulated cytokine production, are associated with age-related immunosenescence, followed by changes in the adaptive immune system development against infections [76]. These anomalies in the elderly have been increasingly recorded in response to a variety of vaccines, such as against influenza. TLR activity in human DCs has been related to a poor antibody response to influenza vaccination as people become older [77]. Furthermore, owing to inadequate PRRs activation, data demonstrate that older adults have a delayed innate immune response after vaccination, a feature that seems to also occur in the case of the various SARS-CoV-2 vaccines [78].

Interestingly, the diversified TLRs and other cytosolic sensors ended up with the induction of strong IFN responses, particularly type I and III IFNs [7,79,80]. The bystander cells recognize the secreted IFNs and produce abundant IFN responses and other proinflammatory cytokines (TNF-α, IL-1β, IL-6, and IL-18) (Fig. 3.3). In the COVID-19 conditions, IL-6 and TNF-α turned out to be predictor cytokines for disease severity and therapeutic assessment [81]. Likewise, any viral response (e.g., influenza) is abrogated by activating TLRs or other sensors of the innate immune system via producing type I/III IFN response. However, as described later, the lack of IFN-I response is observed in severe COVID-19 compared to mild and moderate conditions, which is well correlated with early IFN responses in the infected lungs [16,82]. However, the open reading frames 3b (ORF3b) protein of SARS-CoV-2 has acted as a potent antagonist to IFN-I response, which may explain the poor IFN-I response in COVID-19 patients [83], and many SARS-CoV-2 derived IFN-I antagonists have been identified [84,85]. In these proinflammatory aspects, the strategy that targets deviating or avoiding innate immune response would be a great outlook (see section Innate immune responses to COVID-19: therapeutic developments). As SARS-CoV-2 hijacks the type I IFN response (Fig. 3.3), drugs or immunomodulators that enhance the type I IFN response might play a vital role in combating COVID-19 (see section Innate immune responses to COVID-19: therapeutic developments).

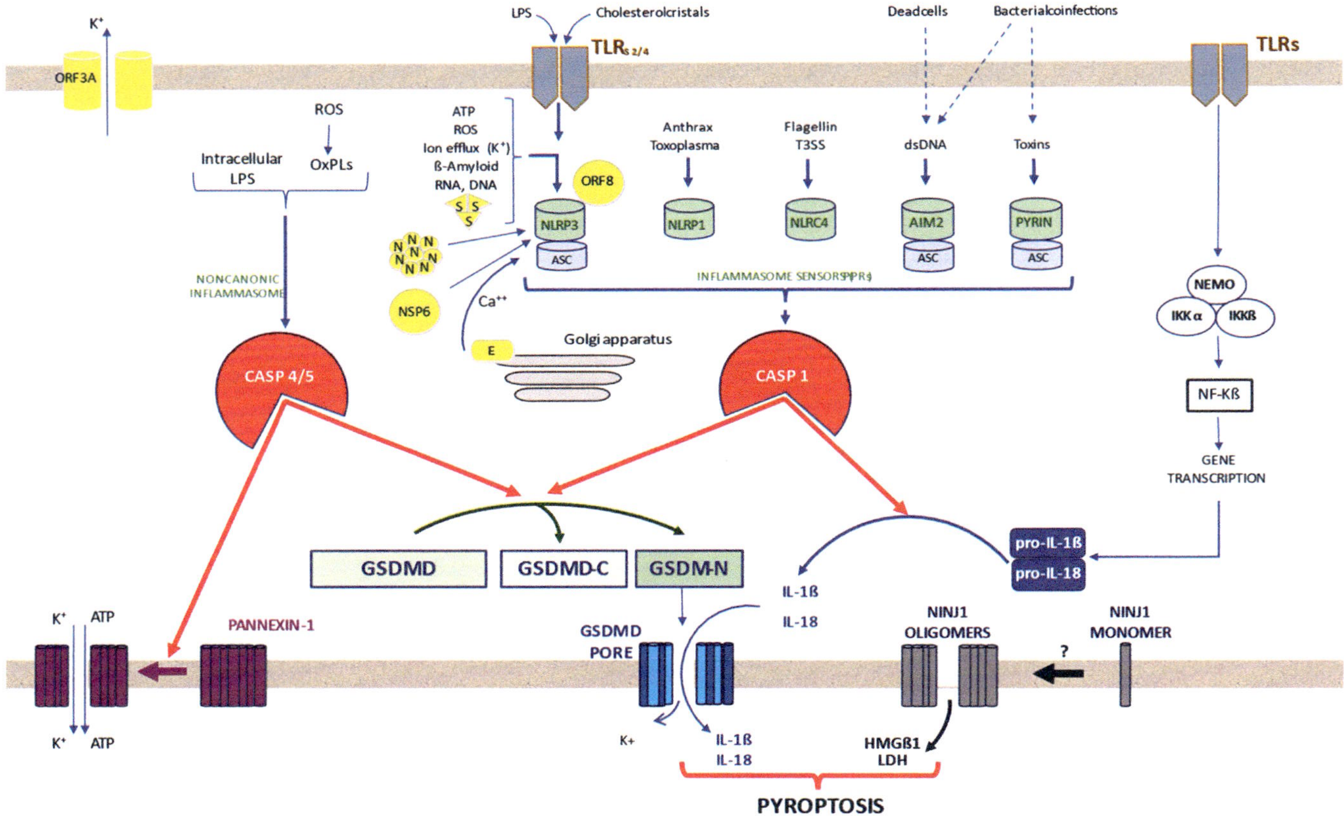

FIGURE 3.2 Both canonical and noncanonical inflammasomes participate in the pathophysiology of COVID-19. Viral proteins (yellow forms): SARS-CoV-2 virions enter epithelial cells via ACE2 and can enter monocytes by binding to anti-spike antibodies followed by FcγR-mediated internalization. Upon translation of the viral genome, the viroporins ORF3a and E can trigger K^+ efflux or Ca^{2+} influx to promote NLRP3 activation. Viral nucleocapside (N) protein can bind directly to NLRP3, resulting in its activation. The nonstructural protein NSP6 impairs lysosome acidification and triggers NLRP3-dependent pyroptosis by targeting ATP6AP1 [61]. Viral spike glycoprotein (S) also indirectly activate NLRP3-inflammasome. Host-intrinsic mechanisms: oxidation of lung surfactant phospholipids results in oxPLs, which can activate caspase-4 and/or caspase-5 to promote noncanonical inflammasome activation. LPS, often present in patients activates both TLR4 and so the NLRP3 inflammasome, and directly bind caspase-4 and -5. Complement products such as C5a can activate NLRP3 by promoting accumulation of ROS. ATP released by dead cells binds to P2X7 receptor, which causes K^+ efflux and NLRP3 activation. Dead cells, bacterial co-infection or damaged mitochondria can result in cytosolic dsDNA, which activates the AIM2 inflammasome. NLRP3 and AIM2 (and possibly other canonic inflammasome sensors activated by toxin or coinfection) inflammasome assembly activate caspase 1, which cleaves full-length GSDMD into amino-terminal (GSDMD-N) and carboxy-terminal (GSDMD-C) fragments. The GSDMD-N fragment binds to the plasma membrane, oligomerizes and inserts itself as a pore. Caspase-1 also cleaves pro-IL-1β and pro-IL-18 into their mature forms, which are released through the GSDMD pore. Caspase-4 also cleaves GSDMD to trigger GSDMD pore formation and IL-1β/IL-18 release, but doesn't mature IL-1β. IL-1β can activate macrophages to secrete additional proinflammatory cytokines such as IL-6. Pyroptosis results after further membrane damage, and under the control of Ninj-1 that oligomerize and form larger pores (than the GSDMD pore) that allow the release of HMGB1 and LDH. Ninj1 pores are essential for the final plasma membrane disruption in pyroptosis [74]. Pyropotic-mediated release of cell internal contents is associated with the formation of tissue factor-enriched extracellular vesicles which likely contributes to disseminated intravascular coagulation and thrombosis. Abbreviations not described above: dsDNA, double-stranded DNA; FcγR, Fc receptor for IgG; Ninj-1, Ninjurin-1; oxPLs, oxidized phospholipids, ROS, reactive oxygen species; TNF, tumor necrosis factor [75].

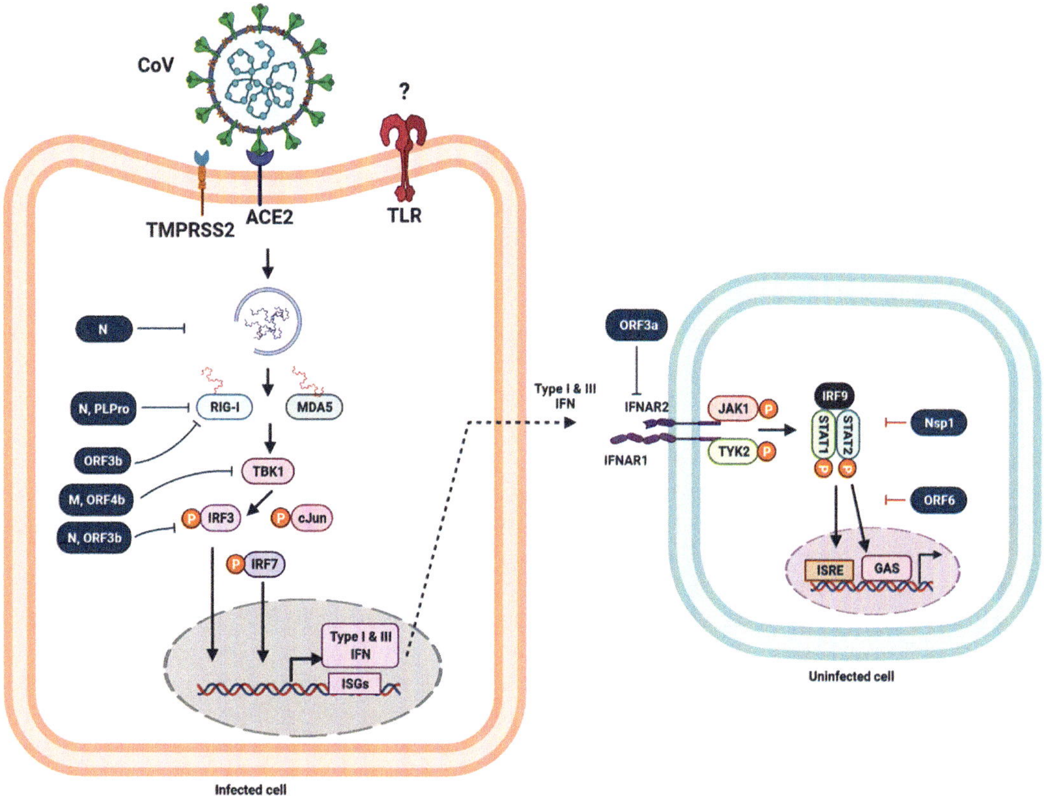

FIGURE 3.3 Innate immune evasion by CoVs. After their entry, in general, both single and dsRNA viruses are sensed by the intracellular and endosomal TLR or RLR sensors, followed by the activation of type I/III response (via IFN-regulatory factor family). As a result, the secreted IFNs binds to their receptors and activate ISGs. In parallel, signaling pathways linked to proinflammatory cytokines (such as NF-kB) are activated and show synergistic effects on the innate immune response. CoVs are known for developing innate immune evasion strategies (for more information [4,7]). Similarly, SARS-CoV-2 has changed its tropism and avoided the first-line defense. Abbreviations not described above: GAS, γ-IFN activation site; IRF, IFN regulatory factor; ISGs, IFN-stimulated genes; ISRE, interferon-sensitive response element; IFNAR, interferon-α/β receptor; JAK1, Janus kinase one; M, membrane protein; MDA5, melanoma differentiation-associated protein five; Nsp1, nonstructural protein one; PLpro, papain-like cysteine protease; RIG-1, retinoic acid-inducible gene I; STAT1/3, signal transducer and activator of transcription 1/3; TBK1, TANK Binding Kinase one; TMPRSS2, transmembrane serine protease two; TYK2, tyrosine kinase 2.

Innate immune responses to COVID-19: cytokines

The severe form of COVID-19 is known to be associated with an excessive elevation of many cytokines, a condition that was termed "cytokine storm" [86]. The immune system is a sophisticated mechanism able to counteract various pathogens, and cytokines are essential actors [87]. Cytokines are small soluble secreted proteins mainly responsible for the interaction and crosstalk between immune and nonimmune cells. They govern the action of the immune system in terms of pathogen recognition, eradication, and restoration of homeostasis equilibrium [88]. They are produced by several immune cells including macrophages, DCs, NK cells but also the T and B lymphocytes. Their half-life is usually short in order to provide a rapid response against foreign materials. However, an elevated production of cytokines can cause damage to vital organs. In response to a viral infection, MDMs are recruited from the peripheral blood to the site of infection and, using PRRs present on their cell membrane, they can recognize characteristic structures of the virus. The interaction between PAMPs and PRRs triggers phagocytosis, the phagolysosome-mediated digestion of the virus, and subsequently the activation of several signaling pathway such as the release of pro-inflammatory cytokines [89].

The SARS-CoV-2 virus enters various types of cells, in particular airway epithelial cells, via ACE2 receptors leading to tissue damage, activation of type I IFN signaling and then pro-inflammatory cytokine release. However, a failure of the negative feedback mechanism of the immune system, which usually occurs to prevent hyperinflammation and overproduction of cytokines, is observed in some COVID-19 patients [90]. This failure has as a consequence high and sustained release of diverse cytokines, such as IL-1, −2, −6, −7, −8, −10, −12, −17, −18, TNF-α, IFN-γ, granulocyte colony-stimulating factors (G-CSF), GM-CSF, as well as chemokines, as monocyte chemoattractant protein 1 (MCP-1), CXCL-10 and macrophage inflammatory protein alpha (MIP1α), what is referred under the term of cytokine "storm" [91,92]. From a clinical point of view, the massive release of soluble mediators directly correlates with lung injury, ARDS [93,94], multiorgan failure, and unfavorable prognosis of COVID-19 [89]. Cytokine storm was observed in other forms of immune malfunction, dysregulation or hyperactivation such as graft-*versus*-host disease syndrome, autoimmune conditions, hemophagocytic lymphohistiocytosis (HLH), chimeric antigen receptor (CAR) T-cell therapy, as well as other human coronavirus infections [86]. Secondary HL (sHLH), for example, is characterized by fulminant and fatal hypercytokinemia with multiorgan failure. Viral infection triggers sHLH and occurs in 3.7%−4.3% of sepsis cases in adults [95,96]. sHLH-like cytokine profile, is associated with COVID-19 disease severity, characterized by increased IL-2, IL-7, IFN-inducible protein 10, GMCSF, MIP1, MCP-1, and TNF [97]. A recent retrospective fatality predictor's multicenter study of 150 confirmed COVID-19 cases in Wuhan (China) included elevated ferritin and IL-6, suggesting that mortality might be due to virally driven hyperinflammation [98].

Compared to the latter indications, however, the cytokine storm induced by SARS-CoV-2 is different. Indeed, SARS-CoV-2 does not always induce specific cytokines like other cytokine storms and displays a specific dysregulation of IFN-I response and its downstream signature [99]. In addition, quite recently Perreau et al., analysing the sera of three cohorts of COVID-19 patients at the time of hospital admission identified, two cytokines, hepatocyte growth factor (HGF) and C-X-C motif chemokine ligand 13 (CXCL13), respectively, as the best predictors of intensive unit care (ICU) admission among 49 soluble mediators analyzed [100].

Earlier, Del Valle et al. investigated predictive biomarkers of SARS-CoV-2 inflammation and they pointed out that high serum IL-6 and TNF-α level at the time of hospitalization were strong biomarkers of disease severity and death in two cohorts of patients [81]. Other studies have also described the remarkably increased serum level of IL-6 in patients with severe COVID-19 [101−103] and it has been reported that levels of IL-6 $>$ 80 pg/mL and C-reactive protein (CRP) $>$ 97 mg/L are predictors of respiratory failure [104] (see section Innate immune responses to COVID-19: protecting or aggravating factors, biomarkers of severity). Therefore, IL-6 has attracted high interest to be targeted to quell the cytokine storm.

IL-6 is a glycoprotein produced by several cells, monocytes, macrophages, endothelial cells, B and T cells, DCs and others, and it is the key activator of Janus kinase (JAK)/STAT3 pathway during inflammation [91]. Its plasma concentration rises during septic shock and various attacks such as trauma and burns [105]. IL-6 is a pleiotropic cytokine with functions on both innate and adaptive immune responses. It is involved in immune cells differentiation, mediator in responding to pathogen invasion, in the growth and differentiation of B lymphocytes and generation of platelets [106]. It also activates the hepatocytes and induces the secretion of inflammation proteins such as CRP and fibrinogen [107]. IL-6 transcription and sustained release are observed after respiratory epithelium infections [108]. Therefore data suggested its inhibiting production or blocking could be an important therapeutic approach. In this regard, IL-6 therapy draws attention since there are already on the market biological drugs that can target the cytokine itself, and its receptor or inhibit IL-6 trans-signaling by blocking the soluble IL-6 receptor [109,110] (see section Innate immune responses to COVID-19: therapeutic developments). For instance, tocilizumab (monoclonal antibody targeting the IL-6 receptor) that was approved for the treatment of rheumatoid arthritis and recently for cytokines storm occurring after CAR-T cell therapy, is under investigation in different clinal trials for COVID-19. Although different studies showed positive clinical outcomes following the IL-6 blockade [111–113], others did not demonstrate an improved benefit in terms of survival rate or only a modest effect [114–116]. The advantage of blocking IL-6 pathway needs further investigations, and hitherto, it is still debated. It is increasingly emerging that the efficacy of IL-6 targeting depends on three key factors: the healthy status of the patient, the severity of the disease and the timing of the intervention [117]. These points must be considered in the next clinical studies (see section Innate immune responses to COVID-19: therapeutic developments).

IL-1β is another well-known cytokine involved in the process of inflammation. It is secreted by macrophages, and participates in the migration of immune cells to inflamed tissue. IL-1β is also involved in the differentiation of Th17 cells and in the production of other cytokines, adhesion and release factors as well as on the activation of NF-kB pathway [118]. Several authors reported elevated levels of IL-1β in the serum of COVID-19 patients [97,119,120]. Whereas IL-6 inhibition generated conflicting results, IL-1β inhibition showed more promising results. Drugs targeting IL-1β signaling including canakinumab (IL-1β antagonist) and anakinra (IL-1β receptor antagonist) have been tested. A clinical trial conducted in three different centers reported that early-stage COVID-19 patients treated with anakinra improved clinical outcomes and rapidly decreased fever and CRP [121]. The beneficial effect of anakinra in reducing clinical signs of hyperinflammation was also reported in other clinical studies [122,123]. In non-ICU COVID-19 patients, canakinumab therapy caused rapid and long-lasting improvement in oxygenation levels [124] (see section Innate immune responses to COVID-19: therapeutic developments).

TNF-α is the initial driver of the NF-kB pathway; it can promote the release of pro-inflammatory and antiapoptotic genes. Its role is still unclear and contradictory data are reported in the literature about TNF-α levels in COVID-19 patients. Further studies are required to define and understand the role of this cytokine, taking into account that the TNF-α/NF-kB pathway is involved in restoring cellular homeostasis and thus a nonspecific involvement may impair its protective function [125]. Previous studies for the treatment of autoimmune diseases found that administration of anti-TNF to patients led to a reduction in all inflammatory cytokines. It is therefore reasonable to predict that anti-TNF therapy could reduce inflammation-driven capillary leak in COVID-19. At the moment, very few studies are examining anti-TNF therapy (infliximab) and are still under investigation [126].

In the context of TNF, an interesting link has been established between this critical pro-inflammatory cytokine and a disintegrin metalloprotease 17 (ADAM17), also called TACE (TNF converting enzyme). ADAM17 plays a decisive role in the release of soluble TNF. TNF is initially synthesized as a transmembrane molecule, and upon activation by stimuli, transmembrane TNF is released under a soluble form by the action ADAM17. Both TNF forms (transmembrane and soluble) mediate diverse functions (beneficial in the context of the innate immune system or pathogenic in chronic diseases) through interaction with their receptors, TNFR1 and TNFR2, which also are shed by the ADAM17 proteolytic action. In addition, ADAM17 mediates the shedding of ACE2 that represent a major receptor for SARS-CoV-2 (Fig. 3.1). Although it is well documented that ADAM17 is activated during the SARS-CoV infection, which hydrolyses ACE-2 and leads to the release of its catalytic domain into the extracellular compartment, there is still some controversy related to its role in severe COVID-19. However, it becomes evident that ADAM17 may constitute a pharmacological target in SARS-CoV-2 infection. Blockade of ADAM17 could potentially have beneficial effects for COVID patients.

In this respect, the rhomboid type 2 (iRhom2) protein is necessary for ADAM17 maturation and its transport from the endoplasmic reticulum to the plasma membrane [127]. It is not known if the release of ACE depends on iRhom2 or can be compensated by the related iRhom1 protein. However, deficiency of iRhom2 leads to increased susceptibility to RNA and DNA virus infections suggesting that iRhoms might have important functions in the clearance of viral infections [128], and of COVID infection in particular. Pharmacological molecules could represent inhibitors of ADAM17. Intranasal or intraperitoneal administration of ADAM17 inhibitor TMI-1 (1, 4-[[4-(2-butynyloxy)phenyl]sulfonyl]-N-hydroxy-2,2-dimethyl-(3S)thiomorpholinecarboxamide), which potently inhibits LPS-induced TNF-α secretion in human primary monocytes, and human whole blood might represent an efficient candidate. The thiomorpholine hydroxamate compound TMI-1 has been previously designed to inhibit metalloproteinase activity for the treatment of rheumatoid arthritis. Besides, Apratastat, a reversible dual inhibitor of ADAM17 and matrix metalloproteinases significantly reduces cytokine production and decreases the recruitment of inflammatory leukocytes to the lung [129]. These types of pharmacological approaches may offer a potential strategy to prevent severe COVID-19 infections, which could, in turn, decrease the need for critical care as well as reduce the lethality of this disease.

Day-by-day, a better understanding of cytokine storm induced by the SARS-CoV-2 virus is being pictured and it appears clear that the hyperactivation of the immune system in COVID-19 presents peculiar characteristics compared to other similar situations. However, yet it is not totally clear how the virus triggers the aberrant profile of cytokines. Regarding the treatment, specific intervention strategies directly targeting diverse inflammatory cytokines have been evaluated with moderate benefits in some cases, while others did not even achieve the expected outcomes (see section Innate immune responses to COVID-19: therapeutic developments).

Innate immune responses to COVID-19: the human leukocyte antigen genotype

A normal being has the ability to defend himself against harmful agents found in his environment, thanks to a series of mechanisms present from birth, some of which do not depend on their effectiveness on previous experiences with a specific microorganism or antigen. Thus the immunity could be understood as the properties of the host thanks to which it offers resistance to harmful agents such as viruses, bacteria, fungi, protozoans, and even worms. Resistance can have varying degrees from almost complete susceptibility to complete resistance and consequently, the term immunity is relative and implies the susceptibility of a certain host to a specific agent to a greater or lesser degree.

Innate or natural immunity is a nonspecific mechanism and can be effective against a wide range of harmful agents. The main mechanisms of innate immunity are genetically controlled. For example, the natural resistance activation macrophage protein coded by the natural resistance-associated macrophage protein one gene encodes proteins responsible for iron ions sequestration within macrophages phagocytic vacuoles and prevents it from being used by phagocytosed bacteria. Innate immunity also varies widely between species and to a lesser degree between individuals of the same species. The species, race, age, gender, hormonal balance, the degree of genetic control, among other characteristics, play an important role in the characteristics of this immunity. Epithelial cells, phagocytes, and DCs have molecules in their membrane surface that recognize pathogens and in doing so activate signaling and messenger pathways that allow the modification of the cytoskeleton and thus increasing cell motility and chemotaxis, as well as the delivery of molecular elements to the cell's nucleus to provide instructions for the activation of genes that code for the production of microbicidal molecules and regulation of some defense mechanisms. Failure of these mechanisms leads to acquired immunity. In invertebrates, innate immunity is sufficient to defend against external aggressors.

Cell populations such as epithelial cells, polymorphonuclear neutrophils, phagocytes, DCs, and monocytes produce mediators in inflammatory processes and also contain TLRs responsible for nonspecifically binding to a multitude of invading microbial cells. Mast cells, eosinophils, and basophils, for their part, mediate vasodilation mechanisms in inflammatory processes, increasing capillary permeability to facilitate the arrival of defense molecules at the site of microbial invasion. Besides, NK cells express nonspecific receptors for lipid antigens present, for example, on the surface of viral capsids as could be the case of SARS-CoV-2. An additional defense mechanism is the constitutive and induced expression of an arsenal of compounds of protein known as antimicrobial peptides such as defensins, β-defensins, cryptidins, lysozyme, lactoferricins, and structural analogues of others such as magainins, mastoparans, and cecropins.

At the intersection between innate immunity and adaptative immunity the human leukocyte antigen (HLA) loci is a leading genetic candidate for infectious disease susceptibility. HLAs are classified as MHC molecules because of their important role in enabling the immune system to recognize "self" versus "non-self" antigens. The HLA gene family is located on the short arm of chromosome 6. It is known to be the most polymorphic genetic system in humans, with several thousand alleles encoding for functional polypeptides. This high level of polymorphism and heterozygosity enable the immune system with a selective advantage against the diversity of microorganisms and antigens the host encounters.

HLA/MHC class I molecules (A, B and C) are expressed on the surface of almost all nucleated cells. Proteins (both native and foreign, such as viral proteins) produced inside cells are displayed as small fragments (8–10 amino acid residues) on MHC class I at the cell surface. Foreign antigens presented by MHC class I attract cytotoxic T-cells which kill the foreign presenting cells. HLA/MHC class II molecules (DP, DM, DO, DQ and DR) are expressed only on B lymphocytes, antigen-presenting cells (monocytes, macrophages, and dendritic cells), and activated T lymphocytes. MHC class II proteins present antigens from outside of the cell to T lymphocytes. When a foreign pathogen enters the body, antigen-presenting cells (APCs) engulf the pathogen through phagocytosis. Proteins from the pathogen are digested into small peptides and loaded onto MHC class II. These class II presented antigens stimulate the multiplication of T helper $CD4^+$ cells, which in turn produce a variety of effects and cell-to-cell interactions to eliminate the pathogen, including the stimulation of antibody-producing B cells to produce antibodies to that specific antigen. HLAs corresponding to MHC class III encode components of the complement system.

The impact of COVID-19 varies not only between individuals but also between different populations. From the onset of virus infection in 2019/2020, efforts have been focused on understanding of how genetic variability across the three MHC class I genes (human leukocyte antigens HLA-A, -B, and -C) may affect susceptibility to and severity of SARS-CoV-2 [130]. Researchers of Oregon Health and Science University in Portland (OR, USA) have executed a comprehensive in silico analysis of viral peptide-MHC class I binding affinity across all known HLA-A, -B, and -C genotypes for all SARS-CoV-2 peptides. Further exploration of the potential for cross-protective immunity conferred by prior exposure to four common human coronaviruses was also conducted. To date, it is known that the SARS-CoV-2 proteome is successfully sampled and presented by a diversity of HLA alleles. However, some evidence found that HLA-B*46:01 had the fewest predicted binding peptides for SARS-CoV-2, suggesting individuals with this allele may be particularly vulnerable to COVID-19, as they were previously shown to be for SARS [131]. Conversely, this research presented evidence that HLA-B*15:03 showed the greatest capacity to present highly conserved SARS-CoV-2 peptides that are shared among common human coronaviruses, suggesting it could enable cross-protective T-cell based immunity [132].

An earlier study was conducted by researchers of the Chinese University of Hong Kong, in 90 Chinese patients by assessing the HLA types A, B, DR, and DQ alleles with serologically confirmed SARS infections. The authors identified a strong association between HLA-B*0703 and -DRB1*0301 and the development of SARS. Moreover, the frequency of B * 0703 and B60 coinheritance in the SARS group was significantly higher than that expected in the general population (0.4%). They have predicted that such genetic data would critically affect both the study of the pathogenesis of SARS and the design of future vaccination programs [133].

An effort toward cytotoxic T lymphocytes (CTLs) epitope prediction was based on the previous lessons and gained experience of the first SARS-CoV outbreak in China in November 2002. A SARS-associated CoV was identified as its etiologic agent; however, the immunopathogenesis of SARS-CoV and the role of specific CTLs in virus clearance were largely uncharacterized by that time. In a subsequent study, potential HLA-A*0201-restricted S and NP protein-derived peptides were selected from an online database and screened for potential

CTL epitopes by in vitro refolding and T2 cell-stabilization assays. The antigenicity of nine peptides, which could refold with HLA-A*0201 molecules was assessed with an IFNχ-ELISPOT assay to determine the capacity to stimulate CTLs from PBMCs of HLA-A2$^+$ SARS-recovered donors. An HLA-A*0201-restricted decameric epitope named P15 derived from the S glycoprotein was identified and found to localize within the AC2 receptor-binding region of the S1 domain. P15 could significantly enhance the expression of HLA-A*0201 molecules on the T2 cell surface, stimulate IFN-χ-producing CTLs from the PBMCs of former SARS patients, and induce specific CTLs from P15-immunized HLA-A2.1 transgenic mice in vivo. Significantly P15-specific CTLs were induced from HLA-A2.1-transgenic mice immunized by a DNA vaccine encoding the S glycoprotein suggesting that P15 was a naturally processed epitope. Thus, P15 was proposed as SARS-associated coronavirus-specific CTL epitope and a potential target for characterization of virus control mechanisms and evaluation of candidate SARS vaccines [134].

Evidence suggests that various HLA gene profiles affect susceptibility to SARS-CoV-2, however, it is poorly known how they affect individual risk from COVID-19. It was earlier described that a higher frequency of HLA-A*01:01 correlates these alleles with a number of high infections and mortality rate in different Italian populations. In particular, the presence of HLA-A*01:01 allele was associated with high risk, while HLA-A*02:01 and HLA-A*03:01 mainly contributed to low risk [135]. Besides, taking advantage of the low genetic polymorphism in the Sardinian population (Italy), genetic and immunogenetic factors, with particular attention to HLA class I and II molecules to evaluate their influence on susceptibility to SARS-CoV-2 infection and the clinical outcome, suggested that the extended haplotype HLA-A*02:05, B*58:01, C*07:01, DRB1*03:01 has a protective effect against SARS-CoV-2 infection in this population [136].

Altogether, it is clear that a better understanding of specific and precise SARS-CoV-2 interactions to the host's HLA-I and II molecules structure, binding and affinity properties could become the Rosseta stone to be deciphered toward a better design of more effective treatment strategies and potent vaccines for controlling and preventing COVID-19. This deserves studies on large and diversified patient cohorts, including asymptomatic infected individuals, patients with long-COVID, and patients with various levels of severity and forms of the disease. It is possible that distinct correlations can be found when different SARS-CoV-2 variants are examined. Such data may provide important information regarding the type of vaccines or pharmaceuticals that will be applied individually to affected patients.

Innate immune responses to COVID-19: autophagy

Autophagy is a vital self-degradative process found in all eukaryotic cells. It plays a central role in balancing sources of energy at critical times in development and in response to nutrient stress. This basal process is essential for removing misfolded or aggregated proteins and clearing damaged organelles such as mitochondria, endoplasmic reticulum, and peroxisomes. Three major types of autophagy have been described, namely, macroautophagy, microautophagy, and chaperone-mediated autophagy (CMA), which are associated with many other selective forms of canonical and noncanonical autophagy [137]. Among these main forms of autophagy, macroautophagy has been the best studied. This conserved process is achieved through the coordination of different autophagy-related (ATG) genes coding for proteins whose function is increasingly well known.

Xenophagy is a selective autophagy process described first in 1984 that is used to eliminate invading pathogens. This mechanism typically follows the same steps as macroautophagy, except that the triggering signal is the TLR-mediated cytoplasmic recognition of PAMPs. In this setting, autophagy acts as an innate immune response that restricts the growth of viruses.

LC3-associated phagocytosis (LAP) is another emerging pathway involved in pathogen elimination. LAP does not involve the formation of double-membrane autophagosome. Instead, it uses the canonical ATG genes to conjugate the family of microtubule-associated proteins 1A/1B light-chain (MAP1LC3) proteins to single-membrane phagosomes containing the pathogens. The resulting vesicles (called LAPosomes) fuse with lysosomes where the process of degradation takes place. The molecular mechanisms underlying LAP are not yet clearly understood [138].

Along with its decisive functions in the intracellular recycling degradation system that maintains cellular homeostasis, autophagy is also a key component of innate immunity that contributes to host defense against microbial infection. In fact, in cases of infection, autophagy may have dual effects [96,139]. Viruses have been extensively shown to induce autophagy to benefit viral growth in infected cells. This represents a pro-viral mechanism enhancing the survival and persistence of pathogens that exploit host autophagy. On the opposite, host cells use autophagy processes as a defense against viral infection. Autophagy initiates a first line of (innate) immune response by cooperating with PRR signaling to induce IFN production. It also selectively degrades immune components associated with viral particles. Following degradation in double-membrane vesicles called autolysosomes (autophagosomes fused with lysosomes), autophagy coordinates adaptive immunity by delivering virus-derived antigens for presentation to T lymphocytes. It is noticeable that NSP6 of SARS-CoV-2 was shown to interfere with autophagosome formation, compromising the fusion to lysosome to generate autolysosomes [140]. Autophagy dysfunction has been linked to major human diseases including cardiovascular, neurodegenerative, metabolic, pulmonary, renal, immune, and other disorders [141]. Patients with significant comorbidities associated with impaired autophagy responses might be deficient at mounting a protective innate response to SARS-CoV-2. Conversely, individuals with a fully efficient autophagy system may have increased natural resistance to COVID-19.

Numerous review articles have presented autophagy as an emerging target for possible treatment for SARS-CoV-2 infection [142–147] (see section Innate immune responses to COVID-19: therapeutic developments). Several molecules known to induce or modulate autophagy have shown some effects on the replication of CoVs (SARS-CoV, Middle East respiratory syndrome/MERS-CoV, mouse hepatitis virus) in cell cultures. They especially include (hydroxy-) chloroquine (that alters autophagy by raising the lysosomal pH), reserpine (that inhibits autophagy flux by blocking autolysosome formation), 3-methyl adenine (that blocks autophagosome formation through the inhibition of class III PI3K), wortmannin (an inhibitor of PtdIns3K and PI3Ks, as also does LY294002), nitazoxanide/Alinia (that blocks late-stage lysosome acidification), everolimus/Afinitor, niclosamide, nitazoxanide, or rapamycin/Sirolimus (all inhibitors of MTORC1, also known as mammalian target of rapamycin complex 1), and many others. Some compounds, already evaluated in several inflammatory indications, have not yet been explored in the context of infection and of COVID-19 in particular. This is the case, for example, of peptide P140 that targets CMA and also influences macroautophagy [148]. The efficacy of these various molecules in real situations has not been proven today and their perfect harmlessness has still to be demonstrated, especially in immuno-deficient patients and individuals with acute infection. Conflicting data and opposite effects of certain molecules on the autophagy process have also been published, showing for example that MTORC1 inhibition by rapamycin promotes virus growth [143]. Autophagy plays a vital role in adaptive immune response and interfering with this vital process that participated in the elimination of pathogens needs special attention. There is also a crucial requirement to develop therapeutic strategies that target specific elements of the autophagy pathway and not the whole process or other intracellular death programs such as apoptosis or necrosis (see section Innate immune responses to COVID-19: therapeutic developments).

Innate immune responses to COVID-19: the complement system

The complement system, as part of the innate immunity, works as the first line against pathogens invasion. It may be activated by three pathways based on the chemical recognition of different activators allowing the generation of active molecules. These complement bioactive molecules may act not only by their capacity to directly destroy pathogens or infected cells through the membrane attack complex (MAC) formation, but also by recruiting and activating innate and adaptive immune cells.

The SARS-CoV-2 infection induces a highly variable phenotype, from asymptomatic forms to ARDS and death. Immunological abnormalities have been reported in severe COVID-19 forms, with cytokine storm that can lead to multiorgan failure (see section Innate immune responses to COVID-19: cytokines). The mechanisms leading to this hyperinflammatory syndrome are not completely understood, and the implication of the complement system in this process is not formally established. Indeed, on the one hand, the complement system, acting as an early phase in the fight against infection may be beneficial for viral elimination, but on the other hand, due to its high capacity to activate platelets, immune and endothelial cells and to induce inflammation, it also may be highly deleterious and participate to the pathological mechanisms of the COVID-19 severe forms (Fig. 3.4). End of 2021, more than 1400 publications in less than 2 years may be retrieved in PubMed with the keywords "complement" and "COVID," illustrating the impressive research work performed in the field. Several aspects are discussed below but there is still much more to acquire to decipher the bases of this complex system in COVID-19.

Mechanisms of complement activation during the SARS-CoV-2 infection

During the SARS-CoV-2 infection, the complement system may be potentially activated by its three pathways (Fig. 3.4).

First, the lectin pathway may be activated by several pattern-recognition molecules, such as MBL (mannose-binding lectin), interacting with surface sugars of a wide series of

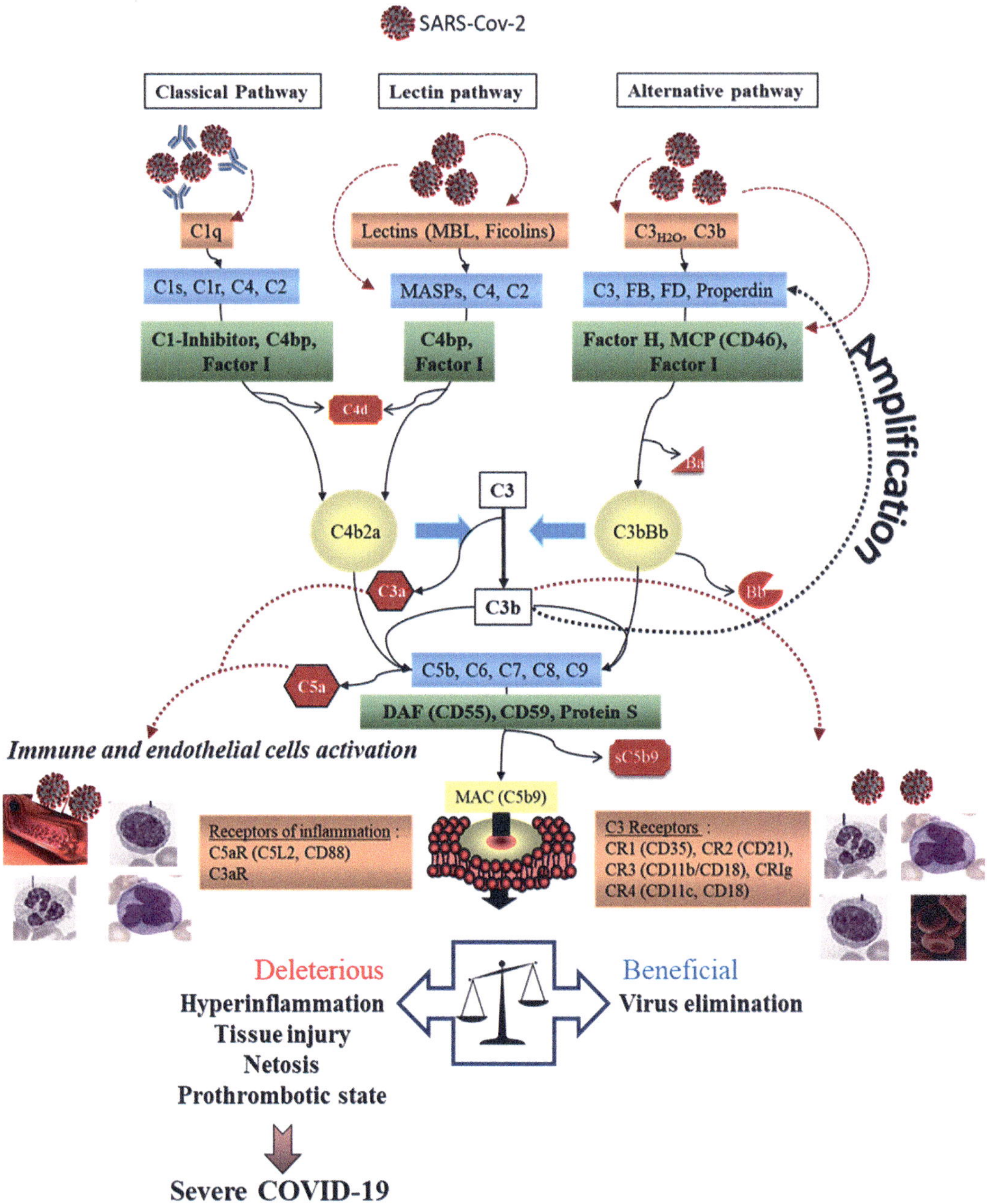

FIGURE 3.4 Representation of the complement cascade showing the pathways that may be activated by SARS-CoV-2. Complement activation induces production of activated fragments (in red) that have biological properties (C3a, C5a, C3b) after their binding to specific receptors (in orange) present on immune and nonimmune cells (platelets, endothelial cells). These fragments can be measured (C3a, C5a, C4d, Ba, Bb,sC5b9) or detected on tissues (C4d, C3b, C5b9). The regulators are shown in green. The complement system participating in the mechanisms of virus elimination may be beneficial but excessive complement activation also participates in the pathological mechanisms of the severe form of COVID-19. Abbreviations not described above: C4bp, C4-binding protein; C5aR, receptor to C5a; C3aR, receptor to C3a; CR, complement receptor; CRIg, complement receptor of immunoglobulin superfamily; DAF, decay accelerating factor; FB, facteur B; FD, facteur D; MAC, membrane attack complex; MASPS, mannose-binding lectin(MBL)-associated serine proteases; sC5b9, soluble C5b9.

microorganisms. During the previous CoV infections, notably by SARS-CoV-1, some low productive MBL polymorphisms have been identified as susceptibility factors [149]. One study demonstrates that lectin pathway (LP) recognition molecules of the complement system, such as MBL, ficolin-2 and collectin-11, bind to SARS-CoV-2 S- and N-proteins [150]. Activation of MBL pathway has also been reported in severe COVID-19 patients [151]. Of note, as MBL concentration decreases with age, this pathway may participate in disease susceptibility observed in the elderly.

Second, during the establishment of the specific anti-SARS-CoV humoral response that occurs between the 8th and 15th day after the first symptoms, the immune complexes formed between the viral proteins and specific IgA may activate the LP, while the IgM and then IgG may activate the classical pathway [152]. Both pathways lead to the formation of the classical C3 convertase (C4b2a) and the cleavage of C3 into C3a and C3b, a highly potent opsonin.

Third, the alternative pathway (AP) may be activated indirectly by the amplification loop induced by the activation of the classical pathway or the LP, leading to the alternative pathway C3 convertase (C3bBb), which allows intense C3b generation and opsonization and C3a production. But AP may also be activated directly by the binding of SARS-CoV-2 S protein on heparan sulfate on cell surfaces [153]. The formation of both (classical and alternative) C3 convertases induces C3b formation and its opsonization on pathogens and/or cell surface, and generation of the anaphylatoxin C3a implicated in the recruitment and activation of immune and nonimmune cells (notably platelets and endothelial cells), promoting phagocytosis and inflammation.

Then, the activation of the final common pathway, through the C5 convertases formation, induces the production of the anaphylatoxin C5a and the formation of MAC (C5b9) at the cell surface. C5a is a potent activator of innate immune cells, favoring phagocytosis and cytokines secretion to allow pathogens elimination, and C5b9 deposition participates in the destruction of infected cells.

In addition to these activation pathways, different studies have shown direct interaction between some viral proteins and complement components. The extracellular soluble N protein dimers may interact with the mannose-binding lectin-associated serine protease-2 (MASP-2), a lectin pathway pro-enzyme, inducing MASP-2 auto-activation and binding to MBL [150]. The structural study has found homology (48% similarity) between ORF8 protein and C-terminus serine-protease domain of human complement factor I (FI). Comparative protein-protein interaction modeling predicts ORF8 binding with overlapping FI-interacting region on C3b with higher binding energy than FI-C3b complex, potentially impairing its regulation [154].

Mechanisms of complement pathogenicity in severe forms of COVID-19

Very early at the start of the pandemic, low C3 plasma levels, in association with neutrophilia, lymphocytopenia and low $CD4^+$ T cells, have been identified as a predictor of mortality in patients with COVID-19 [155]. Overexpression of complement genes has been observed in PBMC (C2, C1 Inhibitor, C1q, CR1, CD46, complement decay-accelerating factor/DAF, also known as CD55, properdin) from COVID-19 patients according to their clinical stages [156–158], in nasopharyngeal swabs (C2, C1 inhibitor, C1q, C4, C3, complement Factor B/CFB, complement factor H/CFH) [159] or within cells present in the BALFs (mainly C1r, C1s, FB, C3, representing 14% of the genes) [160]. Factor D concentration has been demonstrated to be higher two weeks after symptom onset in patients presenting with severe as compared to mild forms [161]. In addition, properdin has been found overexpressed in PBMC but decreased in concentration in plasma from severe COVID-19 patients suggesting protein consumption or deposition [158]. Several studies have shown evidence of systemic activation of the complement system, proportional to the disease severity [151,162–164].

Numerous studies have shown that disease severity is linked to 1) occurrence of a hyper-inflammatory syndrome due to a cytokine storm, 2) tissue damage occurring mainly in the lungs but also in other organs, and 3) a hypercoagulation state due to the endothelial cells and platelets activation. Different consequences of complement overactivation have been reported to participate in the immune mechanisms of severe COVID-19.

Very recently, a study demonstrated that, in the context of severe COVID-19, C3a is able to promote differentiation of CD16 highly expressing cytotoxic T cells which do not need TCR stimulation to degranulate in the presence of immune complexes and induce endothelium injury [161]. Overall, this kinetic corresponds to the occurrence of the first symptoms of severity associated with the cytokine storm. The increasing number of these $CD16^+$ T cells with age may participate in the particular susceptibility of older people to develop severe forms of the disease [165].

C5a is one of the most potent inflammatory peptides with a broad spectrum of functions. C5a robustly boosts the production of inflammatory cytokines such as IL-8, IL-6, IL-17, TNF-α by a variety of immune (granulocytes, monocytes, macrophages, activated lymphocytes) and nonimmune cells (endothelial cells). Excessive stimulation of C5aR1 may induce cellular hyperactivation generating damaging release of oxygen radicals and activated enzymes by granulocytes, excessive release of inflammatory cytokines by macrophages and lymphocytes. This central function makes C5a a powerful weapon [166]. Different studies have shown the association between high levels of C5a and disease severity [167–170]. In addition, the induction of NETosis by C5a has been emphasized [168,171] (See section Innate immune responses to COVID-19: NETosis and neutrophils).

C5b-9 deposits have been found in the skin, lung, and kidney tissues [172] mainly localized at the vessels, on endothelial cells, the main cellular targets of the virus [173,174]. Endothelium injury has been demonstrated to have a central role in the SARS-CoV-2 induced organ damage that affects lungs and kidneys but also skin, brain and heart. This cellular type is particularly sensitive to complement activation as demonstrated by several pathological conditions, that is, in antineutrophil cytoplasmic antibodies-induced vasculitis [175], atypical hemolytic uremic syndrome [176] or antiphospholipid syndrome [177]. In addition, the C5a and C5aR axis is prone to participate in the pro-coagulation state of endothelial cells and platelets during COVID-19 [178,179].

In summary, the huge inflammatory response observed during COVID-19 infection may be the result of the complement system activation with the liberation of C3a [161], C5a [162,163,180], deposition of the C5b-9 complexes on tissues [172] (and release of sC5b-9 in the circulation [181], with major impact on immune (granulocytes, $CD16^+$ T lymphocytes) and endothelial cells.

Targeting complement for the treatment of COVID-19

During the two first outbreaks of CoV-induced infection (SARS and MERS), the complement system had been identified as a key player in the immune response [182] and a complement blockade strategy was studied as a potentially effective treatment [183]. During the current outbreak, different studies have shown the involvement of the C5a-C5aR axis, in the activation of immune cells at the systemic levels [162,180] as well as in the heart of the tissue damage that also exhibited MAC (C5b-9) deposition [172,184]. These data support the potential use of available drugs targeting this pathway such as the C5 by drugs like eculizumab (Soliris) [164], ravulizumab [185], zilucoplan (ZILU-COV trial (NCT04382755, UCB Pharma) or C5a receptor by Avacopan [186] or avdoralimab (Innate Pharma, NCT04371367) [180].

However, C5a and C5b-9 reflect the activation of the terminal pathway and the upstream events occurring in the classical, lectins of alternative pathways could be also targeted by other available drugs [187,188]. For example, the use of recombinant C1 Inhibitor (Conestat alfa, Pharming Technologies B.V.) has been tested in the context of COVID-19, hypothesizing that the treatment may regulate complement activation and collateral lung damage and by direct inhibition of the kinines/kalikrein system, may reduce capillary leakage and pulmonary edema [189]. The study is terminated and enrolling 120 patients was deemed not sufficient to show a difference in the primary outcome measure. Standard of care treatment recently changed adding further heterogeneity to trial population when including future participants (NCT04414631).

Factor D inhibition has been shown to prevent in vitro the alternative pathway activation induced by SARS-CoV-2 S proteins one and two on TF1PIGAnull cells from a myeloid progenitor cell line lacking the complement membrane regulator molecules CD55 and CD59 [153].

Altogether these data highlight the crucial role that the complement system may play in the different phases of the SARS-CoV-2 infection, from the early fight against the virus to an active role into the pathological mechanisms of the severe forms of the disease by participating in induction of the hyperinflammation syndrome, the endothelial cells activation and tissue damage. These data provide hope for the efficacy of the different molecules targeting the complement system currently tested in several clinical trials. Both clinical and basic science studies suggest that uncontrolled activity of the complement system may be a central player in the pathogenesis of COVID-19. Clinical trial evidence is now beginning to confirm this suspicion [190–192]. However, their place in the therapeutic strategy remains to be determined. A decision could benefit from identifying specific complement biomarkers measured at crucial time points of the disease.

Innate immune responses to COVID-19: protecting or aggravating factors, biomarkers of severity

The SARS-CoV-2 infection has a wide spectrum of clinical manifestations and unpredictable disease course. The heterogeneous severity ranges from 30% to 80% of asymptomatic or self-limiting recovery cases, to pneumonia, ARDS, multiorgan failure associated with hospital admission and intensive care needs [193–195]. The novel CoV shares similar features to the prior SARS-CoV-1 (2002–03) and MERS (2012-ongoing) outbreaks. These viral infections commonly present fever, dry cough, sore throat, dyspnea and myalgia, affecting the lower respiratory tract with unfavourable clinical outcomes in elderly patients, smokers and those with underlying comorbidities (e.g., diabetes, hypertension, and chronic kidney disease). In 2003, 8096 SARS-CoV cases were reported by the World Health Organization (WHO), having a total of 774 deaths across 29 countries [196]. MERS is still ongoing, with 2578 laboratory-confirmed cases and 888 deaths due to the infection or related complications, by the end of October 2021 [197,198]. The case-fatality rates are expressively higher for SARS and MERS; however, the global dissemination of the new β-coronavirus SARS-CoV-2 surpassed the absolute values of infected people and deceased, as compared to the past outbreaks.

The CoV pandemics have imposed a burden on global health and medical systems, leading efforts toward the recognition of predictors of disease course and allowing stratification of patients at high risk of adverse outcomes. Epidemiological studies have pointed out shared prognostic factors for disease severity among SARS-CoV-1, MERS, and COVID-19, including 1) demographic characteristics (advanced age, male gender, preexisting chronic diseases) [199–201]; 2) immunological (IL-6, IP-10, MCP-1, platelet factor 4 and β-thromboglobulin); 3) inflammatory and laboratory indicators (CRP, truncated forms of α1-antitrypsin, LDH, blood urea nitrogen and albumin) [199,202–204]; and 4) hematological (lymphocytopenia and neutrophilic leukocytosis) elements [201]. Nevertheless, recent studies have highlighted new biomarkers for COVID-19, which reflect our better understanding of the pathophysiology of this viral infection, and that may contribute to guide medical management of severe cases and to developing more efficient adjuvant therapies.

A molecular biomarker is defined as "a characteristic that is objectively measured and evaluated as an indicator of normal biological processes, pathogenic processes, or pharmacological responses to a therapeutic intervention" [205]. Some prognostic biomarkers of COVID-19 with the strongest scientific evidence to date are described in the following topics, based on studies with a large enrollment of patients, meta-analyses, and systematic reviews.

C-reactive protein (CRP)

CRP is a plasma protein produced by hepatocytes and normally detected at very low levels. Its production may be induced by the acute inflammatory response (mainly proinflammatory cytokines, such as IL-6, IL-1β, and TNF-α) and is suggestive of viral or bacterial infections. CRP is not only an acute indicator of inflammation, but its increased levels stimulate phagocytosis, activate the complement cascade, have antibacterial activity, and modulate the immune system [206–208]. In COVID-19, most patients showed augmented CRP levels, which have been associated with severe and critical forms of the disease, as well as nonsurvivors and positive microbiological cultures/coinfections during hospitalization [19,209,210]. In February 2020, clinical characteristics of COVID-19 patients in China were described, where the CRP levels were increased in 60.7% of them and 81.5% in severe cases [194]. About 91.1% of patients with CRP levels as ≥10 mg/L required admission to the intensive care unit, mechanical ventilation or had unfavourable outcome [194,210]. Additionally, the CRP levels at the admission were also strongly correlated with adverse outcomes and the eventual requirement of mechanical ventilation in obese patients younger than 65-year-old [211,212].

Age is one relevant factor that affects the noninfectious levels of CRP. The "inflammaging" represents the chronic activation of the innate immune system and, consequently, results in higher circulating concentrations of cytokines that occur in advanced ages. CRP has also been considered an age-related marker of poor prognosis [213]. Similar results were found in a smaller study with geriatric patients hospitalized for SARS-CoV-2 infection, whereas the cut-off CRP value was $\geq$35 mg/L [214].

There are growing evidence regarding CRP as an independent discriminator of disease severity and poor prognosis on hospital admission [215]. Thereat, the measurement of classical and accessible biomarkers, such as CRP, may help the clinicians assessing the inflammatory status and adopt immunomodulatory therapies in severe and critical cases [216].

Procalcitonin (PCT)

PCT is a precursor of calcitonin, primarily produced in thyroid parafollicular C cells and its plasma basal levels are usually very low or undetectable. The PCT mRNA expression may be induced in various extrathyroid tissues after an inflammatory challenge by LPS or other cytokines (IL-6 and TNF-α) [217]. PCT has been considered a useful predictive biomarker in clinical conditions, including sepsis and pneumonia, therefore its role as a tool for the type of microbial infection is still controversial [218,219]. Clinical investigations showed that increased PCT levels are restricted to systemic bacterial infections, whereas its levels do not change in viral infections [220]. However, patients with a severe respiratory viral infection and lethal murine influenza infection exhibited raised PCT production, a fact that is better associated with indices of severity (e.g., organ failures and mortality) than bacterial coinfections [221].

Several studies have suggested a strong correlation with elevated PCT in severe forms of SARS-CoV-2, ARDS and the existence of secondary bacterial infections, such as ventilator-associated pneumonia or tracheobronchitis [222–225]. Furthermore, meta-analysis studies showed that increased PCT levels (>0.5 ng/mL) were associated to $\approx$5-fold higher risk of severe COVID-19 and adverse outcome [216,226]. The COVID-19 survivor patients exhibited a reduction in serum PCT levels from the admission to discharge, while nonsurvivors had an opposite pattern on serial blood measurements [223,225]. PCT has also been considered a good criterion for monitoring antibiotic therapy in COVID-19 patients. Based on low PCT levels $\leq$0.25 ng/mL, withholding antibiotics did not impact the 28-day outcome and prevented risks of adverse consequences of excessive antibiotic use, especially in elderly patients [227].

Liver transaminases and albumin

SARS-CoV-2 invades the host cells through ACE2 and transmembrane serine protease 2 (TMPRSS2) as entry receptors [228]. The ACE2 mRNA and its protein are expressed in a subpopulation of cholangiocytes, but discretely in hepatocytes or other liver cell types [229–231]. Liver biopsies from nonsurvivors infected with SARS-CoV-2 were characterized by macrovesicular steatosis, mild lobular and/or portal inflammation and vascular alterations/microthrombotic disease [232,233]. Thus, these findings suggested that the virus does not promote a direct cytopathic damage and that liver dysfunction is most likely a secondary complication associated with the infectious context. Among the plausible causes for liver abnormalities, it may be mentioned the systemic inflammation, use of hepatotoxic therapies, mitochondrial dysfunction and also, altered hepatic perfusion secondary to microthrombotic disease [234].

Serum biochemical proteins have been routinely used to evaluate liver function, including hepatocyte injury [aspartate transferase (AST) and alanine transferase (ALT)], bile duct injury [γ-glutamyltransferase (GGT) and alkaline phosphatase (ALP)] and liver synthesis capacity [albumin and prothrombin time (PT)]. In COVID-19, transient AST, ALT, and GGT elevations, reaching less than 5 times the reference limit, were found between 4% and 58% of patients in Chinese and US cohorts [97,194,235–238]. Elevated liver enzymes have been associated with severe forms of SARS-CoV-2 infection, 1.5 to 3 times higher risk of poor outcome and acute-on-chronic liver failure [216,239]. The prognostic value of transaminases in CoV infections is still under debate, as well as the viral mechanisms related to these clinical findings. Not rarely, patients with increased serum ALT levels were positively correlated with other inflammatory biomarkers, such as CRP, ferritin, D-dimer and IL-6 [240–242]. Although extra-hepatic tissues also release transaminases when injured, rhabdomyolysis is uncommonly reported in COVID-19 and ALT and AST levels were not correlated with marker of muscle breakdown (creatine kinase) [243,244]. In 2002, a retrospective study in China with 182 patients also reported altered liver function in SARS-CoV-1 infection, affecting 70.3% the ALT levels and 31.3% the AST [245].

Albumin is one of the most abundant proteins found in humans, synthesized in hepatocytes, important for the maintenance of the osmotic pressure and transport of diverse molecules. Also, albumin has antioxidant properties since it provides numerous free thiols that are able to scavenge reactive oxidant species during inflammation and protect cells from oxidative stress [246]. Hypoalbuminemia was reported in ≈55% of hospitalized patients with COVID-19 (<40 g/L), while in severe and critical illnesses it increases to almost 90% [247]. Several studies considered hypoalbuminemia at admission as an independent predictor of outcome, regardless of other indicators such as lymphocyte counts, age and comorbidities [235,247–249]. Moreover, serum albumin levels were negatively correlated with CRP and AST, suggesting it as another biomarker for disease severity [250]. The mechanisms underlying hypoalbuminemia in SARS-CoV-2 have been investigated, but they may be a consequence of decreased liver protein synthesis, increased serum albumin catabolism, malnutrition, increased capillary permeability and the escape of albumin to the interstitial space [251].

Cardiac biomarkers

Preexisting diseases of the heart and blood vessels such as peripheral arterial disease, coronary heart disease and congenital heart disease, have been associated with serious clinical SARS-CoV-2 complications and worse prognosis [252,253]. Indeed, hypertension is a common global comorbidity especially in elderly, and it contributes to the risk of fatal outcomes in hospitalized COVID-19 patients when compared to those without cardiovascular diseases [254,255]. Furthermore, coronavirus infection also affects the cardiovascular system and promotes acute myocardial injury, a clinical condition that might be related to the disease severity in symptomatic cases [256]. The incidence of cardiac damage varied from 20% in hospitalized patients to more than 50% in those who required intensive care needs, being manifested by cardiac arrest, arrhythmia, myocarditis, myocardial infarction, venous thromboembolism and cardiogenic shock [67–71]. Patients with cardiac impairment showed severe illnesses, abnormal radiographic findings [257–261], higher levels of CRP and creatinine, as well as the requirement for mechanical ventilation and vasopressor agents [258].

Heart damages caused by COVID-19 are explained by multiple mechanisms, including direct viral infection and indirect imbalanced immune response [261]. ACE2 is highly expressed in the vasculature and heart, which facilitates the viral invasion in cardiomyocytes, intracellular replication and consequently, cell degeneration and necrosis [262]. Moreover, hyperactivation of the immune response releases several inflammatory mediators that lead to microcirculation disturbance, ischemia and hypoxia of the heart tissue. The ischemic injury overloads the heart functioning, maintains it at high output, low resistance state and changes the laboratory markers [261,263]. Acute cardiac injury is defined as a blood level of cardiac biomarkers (e.g., troponin) above the 99th percentile upper reference limit, regardless new abnormalities seen on electrocardiography (ECG) and echocardiography [264]. The more specific cardiac biomarkers include creatine kinase-muscle/-brain activity, cardiac troponin I (cTnI), myoglobin (Mb) and N-terminal pro-brain-type natriuretic peptide (NT-proBNP).

The cTnI is an isoform expressed only in myocardial tissue. It composes a 3-unit troponin complex (troponin I, T and C) along with tropomyosin that regulates the calcium-dependent interaction of myosin with actin, and consequently, the muscle contraction [265]. On the other hand, human cardiac muscle contains four troponin cTnT isoforms, but only one is expressed in adults and attaches the troponin complex to the actin filament [266]. The blood levels of high-sensitivity hs-cTnI and hs-cTnT were elevated in COVID-19 patients, mainly in nonsurvivors and critically ill [258–260]. A meta-analysis of 56 studies found that patients with cardiac injury had 13-fold higher mortality risk than those without this clinical complication, highlighting the prognostic predictive value of cardiac biomarkers in SARS-CoV-2 infection [257,267]. Beyond the life-threatening risk, the cTn elevation was correlated with clinical complications, such as ARDS ($\approx 58\%$), need for mechanical ventilation and malignant arrhythmia ($\approx 17\%$), when compared with those with lower cTnI levels [258,259]. The combination of raised hs-cTnI and copeptin (fragment of vasopressin precursor) upon admission may be considered an independent predictor of ICU admission or mortality in hospitalized patients with COVID-19 [268]. Elevated levels of cardiac biomarkers are related to a high rate of abnormal admission ECGs, therefore hs-cTnI was not directly associated with ventricular dysfunction, since most patients showed normal ejection fraction [268,269].

Natriuretic hormones are produced primarily within the heart and released into the circulation in response to volume wall stretch [270]. In contrast to atrial natriuretic peptide (ANP), brain natriuretic peptide (BNP) is secreted from the atria and the ventricles [271]. It has been postulated that BNP and NT-proBNP are valuable biomarkers of ventricular dysfunction and heart failure, but the half-life of NT-proBNP in the circulation is 6 times higher than BNP [272]. Similar findings have been reported for NT-proBNP in SARS-CoV-2 infection, whose serum levels were increased during hospitalization in nonsurvivors but not among survivors [241,269]. Elevated levels of NT-proBNP were also associated with more severe symptoms, disease progression and 28-day mortality of COVID-19 [273,274].

Creatine kinase-muscle/-brain is another biomarker of myocardial damage, which clinical relevance has been replaced by the high-sensitivity troponin quantification. However, meta-analysis with meta-regression of 15 studies and 11,791 patients has shown that higher creatine kinase-muscle/-brain levels at admission were significantly associated with worse prognosis and reduced survival in COVID-19 patients [275].

Moreover, Mb is a cytoplasmic protein that stores oxygen on a heme group in skeletal and cardiac muscles. As mentioned above for creatine kinase-muscle/-brain, elevated Mb levels at admission in patients with SARS-CoV-2 may serve as a predictor of adverse outcomes [276].

Coagulation markers

Coronaviruses may directly invade endothelial cells and the microcirculation impairment in vascular beds contributes to life-threatening complications of COVID-19, such as venous thrombosis, myocardial injury and multiple organ failure [277,278]. The thromboembolic events, commonly found in severe cases of the disease, have a scenario composed of endothelial injury, activation of the complement cascade, procoagulable state and thrombin production, factors that elevate the risks of deep vein thrombosis and pulmonary embolism [279]. In a Chinese cohort study, the disease severity (critical > severe > moderate) was correlated with the severity of the coagulopathy, which was characterized by thrombocytopenia, increased PT, D-dimer and fibrin degradation products, and also inflammatory markers (CRP and LDH) [280].

D-dimer is a soluble fibrin degradation product that is released when a blood clot begins to break down, it is considered as a biomarker of fibrinolysis and activation of coagulation [281]. A meta-analysis of 35 studies and 6427 patients also confirmed that higher levels of D-dimer, low platelet count and prolonged PT were parameters associated with severe cases and non-survivors patients, corroborating the risk of disseminated intravascular coagulation in the progression of COVID-19 course [282]. Similar findings were reported in a meta-analysis of 75 studies and 17,052 patients, where thromboinflammatory biomarkers, such as D-dimer, fibrinogen and CRP, were associated with increased severity and adverse outcome in SARS-CoV-2 infection [283,284]. These clinical evidence contribute to better guide the timing to start antithrombotic therapies and minimize complications during hospitalization. In fact, those coagulation parameters abnormalities remained from admission to 30 days of hospitalization in severe COVID-19 patients and also reinforced the importance of post-discharge thromboprophylaxis in high-risk cases [263].

vWF is a glycoprotein produced by endothelial cells and megakaryocytes, whose release from the Weibel-Palade bodies may be stimulated by inflammation, endothelial damage and hypoxia [285]. In accordance with other coagulation markers, COVID-19 patients have elevated vWF antigen levels, almost fivefold increase in ICU and severely ill patients, as well as nonsurvivors [178,279,286]. Patients with a peak vWF antigen $\geq$300% had a fivefold increase in risk of death, 30-fold risk of prolonged length of hospital stay and the peak D-dimer value had also the same prognostic prediction of worse prognosis [287]. Other biomarkers of endothelial dysfunction, including tissue-type plasminogen activator (t-PA), plasminogen activator inhibitor-1 antigen (PAI-1) and soluble thrombomodulin showed higher levels in SARS-CoV-2 infection. Meta-analysis of 17 studies and 1187 patients associated the increased production of the mentioned endothelial biomarkers with poor outcomes in infected patients [279].

The understanding of a COVID-19 prognostic biomarkers will be helpful in differentiating severely ill patients, guiding the appropriate treatment and preventing complications of disease course. This section detailed biomarkers of multiple tissues and organs affected in coronaviruses infections; however, results from meta-analysis need to be further confirmed by rigorous prospective studies and randomized controlled trials. Modern high-resolution methodologies such as quantitative proteomic will improve the study of host response to infectious diseases and allow the identification of new biomarkers in various samples, tissues or cells [288,289].

The current pandemic clearly showed us ideal characteristics of a prognostic predictive biomarker, which include 1) methodological simplicity to be performed in remote areas far from large urban centers and with limited access of resources; 2) low cost for the assay performance, ability to be applied in low- and middle-income countries and also on large scale; 3) produce fast results with high sensitivity, a fact that could prevent the interpersonal contamination and the viral dissemination; and also 4) high specificity and assertive results to distinguish heterogeneous population with varied preexisting diseases and lifestyle choices.

Innate immune responses to COVID-19: role of microbiota

The mammalian body harbors a huge number of microorganisms that coevolved in symbiosis with the host. This diverse and dynamic microbial ecosystem, commonly called microbiota, provides a platform that influences several physiological functions such as digestion, metabolism, mucosal barrier integrity, organ functions, and immune homeostasis of the host [290,291]. In particular, mounting evidence suggests the intricate well-balanced bidirectional interaction between the microbiota and the immune system, with the microbiota playing a fundamental role in the development of the immune system and in return, the immune system shaping the microbiota composition, establishing a balanced relationship [292–295]. Dysbiosis is a consequence of changes in the microbial community equilibrium, which paves the way for opportunistic pathogens and disturbance on the host's immunity. Recent studies have shown that patients with severe COVID-19 present with significant alterations in fecal microbiota which is characterized by enriched pathogenic bacteria and depletion of beneficial commensal bacteria [296,297]. At this stage of our knowledge, it still remains to be elucidated how gut microbiota in collaboration with host immunity can contribute to the pathogenesis of COVID-19.

The crosstalk between the intestinal microbiota and respiratory tract has been extensively explored and this bidirectional interaction is known as the gut-lung axis [298,299]. Alteration of gut microbiota due to acute respiratory viral respiratory infections has consequences on disease outcomes such as secondary bacterial infections. As such, it is reasonable to assume that dysbiosis might also affect patients with COVID-19 [300]. Although it is well known that SARS-CoV-2 affects the lung, recent evidence has shown that the gastrointestinal tract is also a target of the disease with viral titers being detected in fecal samples collected from COVID-19 patients [301,302]. Interestingly, COVID-19 patients who were respiratory negative for viral RNA and discharged from the hospital continued to show gastrointestinal manifestations, with their fecal samples remaining positive for months after discharge. These findings indicate a different kinetic profile of gastrointestinal SARS-CoV-2 with delayed viral clearance and suggest an involvement of the gastrointestinal system during COVID-19 [303,304].

A key role of commensal gut microbiota is to maintain mucosal integrity. However, during dysbiosis there are major morphological and functional changes in the gut permeability. These changes include increases in intraepithelial permeability allowing the translocation of macromolecules, microorganisms and/or their components into the bloodstream, leading to systemic inflammation [305]. Increased tight junction biomarkers correlate strongly with higher levels of systemic inflammation markers and immune activation [37,306,307]. Interestingly, recent studies have found increases in these biomarkers in the blood of COVID-19 patients as well as the translocation of bacterial and fungal products [308]. This increased permeability is thought to be caused by the reduction of commensal microbiota producers of short-chain fatty acids [309]. Short-chain fatty acids, a metabolite produced from commensal gut microbiota, induce protection against viral lung infection through activation of a G-coupled protein receptor-43 [277,310]. These microbial metabolites are largely known to promote immune regulation, stimulating resolution of inflammation by inducing apoptosis of neutrophils, increasing macrophages efferocytosis, as well as reduction in pro-inflammatory cytokines secretion by these innate immune cells [311,312].

The inflammasome pathway might also be a key player in these processes, as the inflammasome pathways are highly activated in COVID-19 patients [47]. This might be due to the dysbiosis identified in COVID-19 patients, as the microbiota is known to activate the inflammasome pathways, through sensing of bacterial structure components [313] or, through bacterial metabolites such as acetate [314,315], promoting inflammation mainly by the production of the IL-18 and IL-1β (see section Innate immune responses to COVID-19: inflammasome).

In humans, the cellular entry of the SARS-CoV-2 depends on the binding of the S protein to hACE2 and primarily targets type II pneumocytes within the lung [316]. In rodents, ACE2 is highly expressed in the lung, as well in the gut epithelium [317]. However, conventional laboratory strains of mice cannot be infected efficiently with SARS-CoV-2 because hACE2, but not mouse ACE2, supports SARS-CoV-2 binding. Nevertheless, the importance of this receptor in microbiota colonization was confirmed in a study with germ-free rats, whereby the authors elegantly demonstrated that gut microbiota regulated the colonic expression of ACE2 [318]. Thus, it is possible that ACE2 may be involved in the gastrointestinal symptoms observed in severe cases of COVID-19 [319–322].

The lung and gut microbiota of healthy individuals differ significantly in taxonomic composition, diversity, and function. In contrast to the thriving resident gut microbiota, the lung microbiota is composed of transient microorganisms mainly from the upper respiratory tract (URT). Imbalance in the diversity and function of the gut microbiota has been shown to increase host susceptibility to infections in the lungs and vice versa, highlighting the bidirectional link between these two organs [323]. Recent studies have revealed that patients infected with SARS-CoV-2 present with intestinal dysbiosis, which correlates with the susceptibility and severity of COVID-19 [303,324]. Compared to healthy individuals, where *Eubacterium, Faecalibacterium prausnitzii, Roseburia,* and *Lachnospiraceae* taxa are prevalent, the gut microbiome of patients during hospitalization with COVID-19 showed enrichment of opportunistic pathogens, such as, *Enterococcus* and *Enterobacteriaceae* and at the same time depletion of commensals [303]. These changes occurred for patients that had received antibiotics as well as those that had not received antibiotics. In nonhuman primates infected with SARS-CoV-2, 16S ribosomal RNA analysis of the microbial gut community showed changes in the taxonomic composition, with the relative abundance of *Acinetobacter* and *Ruminococcaceae* being positively correlated with the presence of SARS-CoV-2 in the URT. In addition, SARS-CoV-2 infection significantly alters metabolite composition reducing the levels of short-chain fatty acids, bile acids, and tryptophan metabolites [309]. Most importantly, gut dysbiosis persists during the COVID-19 disease course, even after clearance/recovery of SARS-CoV-2 infection [303]. The findings indicated that dysbiosis seen in COVID-19 patients might drive inflammation and fuel long-COVID-19 symptoms [303], such as fatigue, sleep disturbance, joint pain, anxiety/depression, headache, and diarrhea [325]. Although there is no current evidence to support this suggestion, there is a strong body of evidence linking the gut microbiota dysbiosis and comorbidities which increase the risk of COVID-19 severity such as in aging [326], cardiovascular diseases [327], obesity [328], and diabetes [329], thus reinforcing the hypothesis that gut microbiota might contribute or support the progression of COVID-19. It is well clear nowadays that dysbiosis in the gut microbiota can influence the immune system, lung, and brain through the gut-lung axis and gut-brain axis, and other organs. Indeed, strategies of gut microbiota modulation, such as probiotics, have already been tested on acute COVID-19 and show promising effects [330,331], with reduction in cytokine storm and inflammation [301,323,332], but more clinical research is needed to further validate these benefits (see below).

Innate immune responses to COVID-19: therapeutic developments

The therapeutic approaches against COVID-19 can be divided into four categories, which are potentially combinable: antivirals, modulators of the adaptative immune response, modulators of the innate immune response, and cytoprotectors. Antivirals aim at preventing the viral cycle by targeting either components of the virus or cellular components that SARS-CoV-2 uses to complete its cycle of multiplication. Antiviral small molecules, such as remdesivir or nirmatrelvir (authorized by the US Food and Drug Administration (FDA) late December 2021), and neutralizing antibodies will not be discussed in this chapter, as well as approaches aimed at modulating adaptative immunity, such as vaccination. Anticoagulation therapeutic tools have been evaluated [333] but will not be discussed in this section.

Early guidelines from the WHO advised against the systematic use of glucocorticoids in COVID-19, for fear of suppressing antiviral immune responses [334]. The dexamethasone RECOVERY trial was the first drug trial demonstrating a modest, but significant mortality reduction in defined subgroups of treated COVID-19 patients. In the subgroup subjected to invasive mechanical ventilation, death occurred in 29.3% of the dexamethasone-treated and 41.4% of the control patients. Then, numerous ongoing glucocorticoid trials stopped patient recruitment since it was considered unethical to randomize patients on glucocorticoids or placebo when the mortality reduction was demonstrated in a large trial. Dexamethasone treatment became rapidly part of the treatment guidelines. A meta-analysis of seven clinical trials, by the WHO, confirmed that oral or injected dexamethasone reduces death in critically ill COVID-19 patients [335]. However, methylprednisolone and hydrocortisone failed to demonstrate clinical benefit in hospitalized COVID-19 patients. Then, a recent Cochrane meta-analysis including 11 randomized, controlled trials with 8075 enrolled patients, showed that systemic glucocorticoids reduced all-cause mortality slightly. The study identified a need to determine the effective dose and the subgroup of patients who may most profit from corticosteroid application [336].

Several therapeutic attempts have been based on the blockade of pro-inflammatory cytokines that rise during the cytokine storm [86]. Indeed, most patients with severe COVID-19 exhibit substantially elevated serum levels of pro-inflammatory cytokines including IL-6, IL-1β, IL-18, GM-CSF, and TNF, as well as many other cytokines and chemokines, characterized as cytokine storm (see section Innate immune responses to COVID-19: cytokines). Elevated levels of IL-6 that being under the control of IL-1 were early found to be a stable indicator of poor outcome in patients with severe COVID-19. Markers of systemic inflammation (e.g., C-reactive protein) and of coagulopathies (e.g., D-dimer) are found to be abnormally high and also correlate with severity in COVID-19 patients. Pulmonary infiltration with large numbers of inflammatory macrophage infiltration was found in patients with severe COVID-19. Pathogenic T cells and inflammatory monocytes release GM-CSF and IL-6, which recruit more inflammatory cells into the lungs (and other organs) and further aggravate the inflammatory storm [86].

IL-6

Multiple clinical studies have examined IL-6 blockade to treat COVID-19. Studies included IL-6 receptor antagonists [tocilizumab [111,337–339] and sarilumab [340] and IL-6 inhibitors [siltuximab [341]]. The outcome of these trials is often difficult to compare owing to small sample sizes and methodological differences. When used in severe COVID-19 patients, IL-6 receptor antagonist ameliorated several clinical parameters, such as lymphocyte counts and C-reactive protein values, as well as CT opacities, while it reduced oxygen uptake [111]. In other studies, however, there was not a clear clinical benefit [342,343]. If large randomized controlled phase three trials of recombinant humanized monoclonal antibodies targeting IL-6 receptor (tocilizumab and sarilumab) have shown some improvement in ICU-hospitalized patients [338], it is difficult to conclude from the reported studies if the slight statistical improvement was related or not to combination with glucocorticoids and/or antivirals. It was hoped that IL-6 blockade would show widespread efficacy, but overall these trials do not support the widespread use of IL-6 antagonists in hospitalized patients with mild-to-moderate disease. It is also still unclear whether the dominant role of IL-6 in COVID-19 would be to promote viral containment or to contribute to local immune pathology and systemic complications [110].

GM-CSF

As a proinflammatory cytokine and myelopoietic growth factor, GM-CSF plays an essential role in mediating alveolar macrophage homeostasis and lung inflammation in COVID-19.

In the severe forms of COVID-19, increased GM-CSF levels are thought to serve as a link between T cell-mediated acute pulmonary inflammation and a self-amplifying proinflammatory cytokine loop. Several monoclonal antibodies targeting the GM-CSF pathway have been clinically evaluated. Mavrilimumab, a monoclonal antibody that binds to the α subunit of the GM-CSF receptor, did not improve clinical outcome in a small prospective cohort study of nonmechanically ventilated patients [344], but another study showed that mavrilumumab can improve outcomes in severe COVID-19 patients [345]. A third clinical trial in patients with COVID-19 requiring supplemental oxygen therapy without mechanical ventilation showed a reduced requirement of mechanical ventilation and slightly improved survival in a patient treated with mavrilimumab [346]. Otilimab, an anti-GM-CSF monoclonal antibody, has been evaluated in a double-blind, randomized, placebo-controlled study in adult patients who required high-flow oxygen, noninvasive ventilation, or invasive mechanical ventilation. In the overall population, otilimab (a single 90 mg infusion) did not confer a significant improvement in the primary outcome of proportion of patients alive and free of respiratory failure at day 28, although a post-hoc analysis suggested benefit in those aged 70 years and older [347]. In a phase-2 study, namilumab, a human monoclonal antibody against GM-CSF, reduced inflammation as measured by CRP concentration in hospitalized patients with COVID-19 pneumonia [348]. Lenzilumab, a recombinant monoclonal antibody targeting human GM-CSF, with high binding affinity in the picomolar range, was found to prevent immune hyperstimulation and is associated with faster clinical improvements and slower progression to severe disease or death in some high-risk COVID-19 patients with severe pneumonia [349]. Lenzilumab was further evaluated in a phase-3 randomised, placebo-controlled trial in hospitalised adult patients with COVID-19 pneumonia not requiring invasive mechanical ventilation [350]. This trial showed that Lenzilumab treatment of hospitalised patients with COVID-19 can slightly (6%) improve the likelihood of survival without the need for mechanical ventilation. The observed benefit was greater than that provided by standard background care including remdesivir and corticosteroids.

IL-1 and IL-1R

The IL-1 family (a group of 11 cytokines) plays a central role in the regulation of immune and inflammatory responses. IL-1α and IL-1β are the most studied members, they possess a strongly proinflammatory effect. IL-1s (IL-1α and IL-1β) are the major intrinsic pyrogenic factors (at 1–10 ng/kg) and are master cytokines of local and systemic inflammation, the blocking of which could inhibit the activation of the innate immune response. IL-1s are intensely produced by living macrophages, monocytes, fibroblasts, and dendritic cells, and higher quantities can be released when these cells die through pyroptosis. IL-1α and IL-1β bind to the same receptor molecule, which is called type I IL-1 receptor (IL-1R1). To trigger signaling IL-1s must interact with both IL-1R1 and the co-receptor IL-1R3 (IL-1RAcP). There is a third ligand of IL-1R1, the Interleukin one receptor antagonist (IL-1Ra). IL-1Ra binds to IL-1R1 but not IL-1R3, and is as an inhibitor of IL-1s signaling.

There are four agents available for targeting the IL-1 pathway: anakinra, a recombinant form of intrinsic human IL-1Ra; rilonacept, a recombinant fusion protein including the extracellular protein of human IL-1R1 and IL-1R3 fused with the Fc portion of human IgG1; and canakinumab and Bermekimab (MABp1), monoclonal antibodies against IL-1β and IL-1α, respectively.

Anakinra works as an antagonist of IL-1R1, competing with both IL-1α and IL-1β. It was the first biological drug of a selective IL-1R1 antagonist to receive approval from the FDA. Anakinra has been applied for a wide range of inflammatory diseases with no reported serious adverse effects. Anakinra use in COVID-19 has been reported in several retrospective and prospective studies, as well as in randomized controlled trials. When anakinra was used in patients with severe COVID-19, it showed a significant increase in survival without severe adverse effects [115]. Anakinra attenuated the inflammatory responses as shown by the decrease of IL-6 and of CRP circulating concentrations and by the increase of the absolute lymphocyte counts. Interestingly, anakinra showed a significant survival benefit when given without dexamethasone but not when co-administered [351]. Anakinra was also used in a study that stratified patients on the basis of high plasma suPAR levels, thus at high risk for respiratory failure, and led to decreased 28-day mortality, and shortened hospital stay [352]. On the other hand, a randomized clinical trial that addressed the therapeutic potential of anakinra in mild-to-moderate COVID-19 patients, was stopped before completion, as no significant difference was found between the groups [353]. Therefore, anakinra could be considered a safe therapeutic option for reducing mortality risk in COVID-19 patients presenting with hyperinflammation, but not in less severe cases.

Exploratory clinical trial in hospitalized adult patients with mild or severe non-ICU COVID-19, showed that canakinumab caused rapid and long-lasting improvement in oxygenation levels in the absence of any severe adverse events [124]. However, treatment of severe COVID-19 with single injection of canakinumab, in randomized, double-blind, placebo-controlled phase three trial did not significantly increase the likelihood of survival without invasive mechanical ventilation at day 29 [354]. To our knowledge (January 2022), there are no reported efficacy trials in COVID-19 patients with rilonacept, and no ongoing clinical evaluation of bermekimab in COVID-19 patients.

Interferons (IFNs)

Two major cytokine families, IFNs type I and type III (also termed IFNλs or IL-28/29), constitute the host's initial natural defense against viral infections. These cytokines are produced in response to viral infection, and induce antiviral programs both in an autocrine and paracrine manner, while at the same time they potentiate the adaptive immune response. Type I IFNs constitute a family of cytokines originally described over 60 years ago and comprise 13 IFN-α subtypes, IFN-β and IFN-ω, −κ, and −ε. They signal through the IFNαR1/IFNαR2 heterodimeric complex to up-regulate hundreds of genes collectively known as ISGs. These signaling pathways exhibit multiple antiviral functions including inhibition of viral replication, degradation of viral nucleic acids and induction of viral resistance to neighboring cells, and account for the potent antiviral activity of type I IFNs [355]. There are four type III IFNs in humans (IFN-λ1/IL-29, IFN-λ2/IL-28A, IFN-λ3/IL-28B and IFN-λ4). Type III IFNs signal through a unique heterodimeric receptor complex, IL28Rα-IL10Rβ, that induces downstream signaling similar to that of type I IFNs, and involves the phosphorylation of JAK-family kinases, and the activation of STAT and IRF transcription factors, driving the expression of ISGs and so on the induction of antiviral responses. Following respiratory influenza virus infection, IFN-λ is induced first, before and in excess levels to type I IFNs, and acts locally at the epithelial barrier to limit initial viral spread without activating inflammation. In contrast, type I IFNs come into play later on, once infection escapes IFN-λ control, to provide further antiviral resistance but at the same time induce pro-inflammatory responses essential for dealing with infection but also mediating tissue damage [356].

IFNs constitute major antiviral proteins, and their impaired production has been linked with severe cases of COVID-19. SARS-CoV-2, after entering the cells, is recognized by PRRs, like TLR3, TLR7, RIG-I and MDA5, to initiate signaling pathways that induce that production of type I and III IFNs. IFNs bind to their receptors in the same or nearby cells to activate pathways that lead to the induction of ISGs and the initiation of the antiviral response. SARS-CoV-2 viral products have been shown to inhibit various steps of these processes. Four SARS-CoV-2 nonstructural proteins (NSP16, NSP1, NSP8, and NSP9) were identified to inhibit splicing, protein translation and/or protein trafficking after infection, and thereby suppress the interferon response to infection [85,357]. Other SARS-CoV-2 proteins were shown to interfere with IFN signaling including NSP6 (that binds TBK1 to suppress IFR3 phosphorylation), NSP13 (that blocks TBK1 phosphorylation), ORF6 (that bind the importin KPNA2 to inhibit IFR3 nuclear translocation, and that also hijacks Nup98 to block STAT nuclear import), M protein (that interact with the RIG-I/MDA-5-MAVS signaling complex, N protein (that inhibits the phosphorylation of STAT1 and STAT2, and ORF9b (that target NEMO, thereby inhibiting NFkB signaling and subsequent IFN production; that interact with mitochondrial TOM70; and that also target multiple molecules of the innate immune response and impedes phosphorylation and nuclear translocation of IRF3 [358–364]. Using a reporter replicon of SARS-CoV-2 Xia et al., also reported the suppression of IFN-I signaling by multiple SARS-CoV-2 proteins: nsp1, nsp6, nsp13, ORF3a, M, and ORF7b blocked STAT1 phosphorylation; nsp6, nsp13, ORF7a, and ORF7b suppressed STAT2 phosphorylation; and ORF6 inhibited nuclear translocation of STAT1 [365].

An impaired and delayed production of type I and III IFNs has been shown in the plasma of severe COVID-19 patients [82,156,366]. COVID-19 patients have increased levels of IFN-α and IFN-λ during the first week of symptoms that are sustained also later on in patients with severe disease, while they decline in patients with moderate disease. In those COVID-19 patients where IFN-λ was detected, higher IFN-λ concentrations correlated with lower viral load in bronchial aspirates and faster viral clearance, while a higher IFN-λ to type I IFN ratio correlated with improved outcome in critically ill patients. Moreover, genetic mutations in key molecules of IFN signaling pathways have been linked to impaired immune responses in severe COVID-19 patients. Of note, autoantibodies against type I IFN family members, constitute another mechanism of impaired IFN response detected in severe cases of COVID-19.

Consequently, various IFN family members have been tested in clinical protocols. In a retrospective multicenter cohort study of COVID-19 hospitalized patients, early administration of IFN-α2b was associated with reduced in-hospital mortality in comparison with no administration of IFN-α2b, whereas late administration of IFN-α2b was associated with increased mortality, pinpointing the importance of the timing of administration and the different roles IFN may have during the progress of COVID-19 [367]. In another study, inhaled IFN-α2b treatment administered in moderate COVID-19 patients correlated with accelerated viral clearance in the upper airways, and in a reduction in serum IL-6 and CRP [368].

In a randomized phase-2 trial, administration of IFN-β1b in combination with three modestly active antivirals (lopinavir, ritonavir, and ribavirin) resulted in a reduced virus titer, a limited inflammatory response, and mild clinical disease in patients infected with SARS-CoV-2 [369]. This study did not include severe cases. Another randomized, placebo-controlled multicenter, phase-2 trial evaluating the safety and efficacy of inhaled IFNβ-1a (produced in mammalian cells), in patients admitted to hospital with COVID-19, has shown that IFNβ-1a, given as a daily inhaled dose via nebuliser for 14 days, was associated with greater odds of improvement versus placebo and more rapid recovery with a greater proportion of patients recovering during the 28-day study period [370]. A phase-3 trial with the same inhaled IFNβ-1a is ongoing to evaluate the safety and efficacy endpoints in hospitalized patients receiving oxygen with confirmed SARS-CoV-2 infection (NCT04732949). A recent phase-3 trial, however, argues against the beneficial effect of IFN-β, as subcutaneous administration of IFN-β1a in combination with remdesivir did not have any effect in nonhospitalized COVID-19 patients when compared to remdesivir alone, while it even worsened the outcome of patients who required high-flow oxygen at baseline and received corticosteroids [371].

Type III IFNs are considered promising alternatives to type I IFNs for COVID-19 treatment as they lack many of the pro-inflammatory activities types I IFNs exhibit [372]. A pegylated version of IFN-λ (peginterferon lambda) was administered in outpatients diagnosed with COVID-19, and although it was found in one study to accelerate the viral decline, increasing the proportion of patients with viral clearance by day 7 [373], but in another study, it displayed no efficacy [374]. A possible explanation is the higher viral load detected in patients in the former study.

JAKs

JAKs are a family of intracellular tyrosine kinases that play an essential role in the signaling of numerous cytokines that have been implicated in the pathogenesis of inflammatory diseases. The human JAK family comprises JAK1, JAK2, JAK3, and TYK2. There are nine clinically approved JAKs inhibitors.

Tofacitinib is an orally administered selective inhibitor of JAK1 and JAK3, which means that it interferes with the JAK-STAT signaling pathway. Tofacitinib modulates the action of various cytokines including IFNs and IL-6, decreasing the release of cytokines by type 1 and type 17 helper T cells, which are implicated in the pathogenesis of the ARDS. In a randomized, double-blind, placebo-controlled trial involving hospitalized patients with COVID-19 pneumonia, tofacitinib was found superior to placebo in reducing the incidence of death or respiratory failure. These effects were consistent regardless of sex, age, duration of symptoms, and use of glucocorticoids at baseline; they were also consistent across different levels of supplemental oxygen use at baseline [375].

Baricitinib is an oral, selective inhibitor of Janus kinases JAK1 and JAK2 with potent anti-inflammatory activity. It is clinically approved for the treatment of rheumatoid arthritis. Baricitinib inhibits the intracellular signaling pathway of cytokines, including IL-2, IL-6, IL-10, and IFN-γ. In a large double-blind, randomized, placebo-controlled trial evaluating baricitinib plus remdesivir in hospitalized adults with COVID-19, the combination was found superior to remdesivir alone in reducing recovery time and accelerating improvement in clinical status. Notably patients receiving high-flow oxygen or noninvasive ventilation at enrollment had a time to recovery of 10 days with combination treatment and 18 days without. Baricitinib/remdesivir-treated patients showed a better improvement in clinical status at day 15 than those receiving only remdesivir, but the 28-day mortality did not differ significantly [376]. In a recently published multicenter, double-blind, placebo-controlled phase-3 trial, oral baricitinib plus standard of care showed a meaningful reduction in mortality compared with placebo plus standard of care, most notably for participants receiving high-flow oxygen or non-invasive ventilation [377]. In this trial, standard of care included systemic corticosteroids, such as dexamethasone, and antivirals, including remdesivir. Glucocorticoids are likely to be most effective in severely ill COVID-19 patients. JAKs inhibition represents an additional therapeutic option for treating COVID-19 pneumonia in patients who are not yet receiving invasive mechanical ventilation.

Inflammasomes (sensors)

Based on recent knowledge, an array of therapeutic options are currently evaluated to treat COVID-19 patients by targeting directly or indirectly the diverse components of canonic and non-canonic inflammasomes. What it must be taken into account is that each inflammasome complex has many possible sensors (e.g., NLRP3, AIM2, etc; see section Innate immune responses to COVID-19: inflammasome), a small group of effectors (the inflammatory caspases), and a dominant terminal effector, the GSDMD.

There is since several years a biopharmaceutical race to either repurpose NLRP3-related inflammasome inhibitors and/or develop new direct NLRP3 inhibitors. Several small molecules were found to inhibit the NLRP3 inflammasome. This is the case of glyburide, a drug widely used in the US for the treatment of type 2 diabetes because it inhibits ATP-sensitive K^+ (KATP) channels in pancreatic β cells. However, the in vivo doses of glyburide to exert its inhibitory effect on inflammasome are quite high, which causes hypoglycemia, therefore its usage is limited to type 2 diabetes only [378].

Many other NLRP3 inhibitors are still in early development stages. In 2012, a small NLRP3 inhibitor, cytokine release inhibitory drug 3 (CRID3; renamed MCC950), was selected among a series of diarylsulfonylurea-containing compounds, as a potent and specific NLRP3 inhibitor but having no effect on AIM2, NLRC4 or NLRP1 inflammasomes, nor on TLR signaling [379]. Although MCC950 worked well in various animal models of hyperinflammation, MCC950 raised blood levels of a liver enzyme in early human trials, so it was instead used as a starting point to develop new compounds. Interestingly, MCC950 was found to inhibit caspase-1 activation and secretion of IL-1β in primary human monocytes infected with SARS-CoV-2 in vitro [47].

Recent phase-2 clinical trials have tested direct NLRP3 inhibition in patients with either mild or severe COVID-19. IFM-2427 (renamed DFV890 after buying by Novartis) is a first-in-class small molecule designed to inhibit the activity of NLRP3 outside the central nervous system by directly binding to the protein, thereby blocking its activation that leads to the maturation of the pro-inflammatory cytokines IL-1, IL-18 along with pyroptosis. A phase-2, randomized, controlled, open-label multicenter study to assess the efficacy and safety of DFV890 for the treatment of SARS-CoV-2 infected patients with COVID-19 pneumonia and impaired respiratory function, was completed in late 2021. However, there was no significant improvement with DFV890 plus standard care as compared to standard care alone (Novartis, NCT04382053). Another compound, dapansutrile (OLT1177) has been developed by Olatec Therapeutics. Dapansutrile is a novel β-sulfonyl nitrile compound, that is orally active and inhibits the NLRP3 inflammasome, but not NLRC4 and AIM2 inflammasomes. Dapansutrile prevents the assembly of the NLRP3 inflammasome and inflammatory signals such as IL-1β and IL-18 [380]. This drug also inhibits pyroptosis. However, dapansutrile also inhibits several kinases such as Src, Fyn, HcK, and STAT3 [381]. A randomized, double-blind, placebo-controlled trial phase-2 trial on the safety and efficacy of dapansutrile for people with moderate COVID-19 symptoms is ongoing (Olatec Therapeutics, NCT04540120).

Metformin, another diabetes drug, indirectly inhibits NLRP3 by regulating MTOR. Metformin was recently shown to inhibit NLRP3 activation and lung inflammation in SARS-CoV-2-infected mice and a retrospective study in patients with diabetes type 2 diagnosed with COVID-19 clearly showed that metformin use was associated with reduced mortality [382,383]. However, it remains unclear whether this protective effect is related to inflammasome or other mechanisms of action [384].

The microtubule-depolymerizing drug colchicine, an anti-inflammatory drug that is used to treat a variety of conditions, including gout, recurrent pericarditis, and familial Mediterranean fever, has also been evaluated in COVID-19 patients. Colchicine has several potential mechanisms of action, including reducing the chemotaxis of neutrophils, inhibiting indirectly (NLRP3) inflammasome signaling, and decreasing the production of cytokines, such as IL-1β [385,386]. A small randomized controlled trial in patients with moderate to severe disease demonstrated its ability to reduce oxygen requirement and hospitalization; in this study, low overall mortality precluded a determination of its effect on death [387]. A larger randomized, double-blind trial involving nonhospitalized patients with COVID-19 treated with orally administered colchicine had a slight decreased rate of hospitalization or death combined. This primary endpoint occurred in (4.7%) in the colchicine arm and (5.8%) in the placebo arm. There were no statistically significant differences in the secondary outcomes between the arms. However, the benefits of colchicine appeared to be more marked in patients with diabetes and men [388]. Other clinical trials with colchicine have shown no improvement both for the treatment of nonhospitalized patients with COVID-19 and for the treatment of hospitalized patients with COVID-19 (https://www.covid19treatmentguidelines.nih.gov/therapies/immunomodulators/colchicine/).

Gasdermins

The discovery in 2015 linking GSDMD to pyroptosis after inflammasome activation was a major breakthrough. GSDMD is indeed an attractive target as pore formation occurs downstream of all inflammasome sensors but upstream of IL-1β and DAMP release [389]. Two known small-molecule drugs have recently been described to inhibit GSDMD.

Disulfiram, a small-molecule drug approved by the FDA for alcohol dependence used for 70 years, covalently inhibits GSDMD pore formation and protects against LPS-induced sepsis and inflammatory cytokine secretion in mice [390]. Disulfiram is currently being studied in two controlled phase-2 clinical trials that are testing efficacy in symptomatic patients with mild to moderate disease (DISCO trial; NCT04485130), as well as in patients in hospitalized subjects over the age of 50 diagnosed with moderate COVID-19 (NCT04594343).

Fumarate, the Krebs cycle intermediate, and dimethyl fumarate, an FDA-approved therapeutic for multiple sclerosis (MS), were recently shown to inhibit GSDMD and pyroptosis [391]. Interestingly, a case series of several patients with MS being treated with dimethyl fumarate showed that their SARS-CoV-2 infection was self-limiting without their receiving any specific treatment [392]. Dimethyl fumarate is being tested in one arm of the RECOVERY trial (UK), a randomized phase-2/3 open-label trial for its effect in preventing death in patients with COVID-19 (NCT04381936). It should be noted that disulfiram and dimethyl fumarate may have antiviral effects. Disulfiram inhibits the SARS-CoV-2 protease in vitro (IC_{50} ~ 9 μM [393]). Dimethyl fumarate activates a nuclear factor erythroid 2-related factor 2 (NRF2)-dependent antiviral program to inhibit replication of SARS-CoV-2 in lung epithelial cells [394].

Inflammatory caspases and pan-caspase inhibition

At the frontier of inflammation and cell death, the targeting of inflammatory caspases, a strategy initially neglected, has recently entered into clinical trials. There are three inflammatory caspases in humans: caspase-1, caspase-4 and caspase-5 (see section Innate immune responses to COVID-19: inflammasome). Human caspase-4 is highly similar to mouse caspase-11 and it is considered that the human *casp-4* and *casp-5* genes originate from a duplication of the *casp-11* gene, their ortholog in mice. Caspase-1 is the central effector component of the canonic inflammasomes. Indeed, whatever the sensor used (NLPR1, NLRP3 NLRC4, AIM2, Pyrin), upon its relevant stimulation, it associates with procaspase-1 (and with ASC in the cases of NLRP3, AIM2, and Pyrin) to form a multimeric activation platform of caspase-1. Caspase-4/11 (optionally replaced by caspase-5) is the central effector component of noncanonic inflammasomes. Consequently, in humans, whatever the nature of the danger signal (DAMP or PAMP), inflammasomes require caspase-1 to cleave efficiently and mature IL-1β and IL-18 (caspase-1) and at least one of the three inflammatory caspases to cleave GSDMD (optionally gasdermin-E) and in fine trigger inflammatory cytokine release and sometimes the regulated inflammatory and immunogenic cell death termed pyroptosis (see section Innate immune responses to COVID-19: inflammasome). Of note, the discovery that caspase-4/11 (or alternatively) can act as the intracellular receptor of LPS, has been a major discovery leading to a renewed understanding of the molecular mechanisms of sepsis [66,289,395,396].

Two inhibitors of inflammatory caspases have been developed, pralnacasan (VX740) and belnacasan (VX765). Pralnacasan (VX-740, HMR-3840) is a reversible caspase-1 inhibitor developed 20 years ago by Vertex pharmaceuticals for the treatment of inflammatory diseases. Pralnacasan has been evaluated in a phase-2 clinical trial for the treatment of rhumatoid polyarthritis and found to provide clinical improvement as well as reduction of inflammatory markers. Three clinical trials have found Pralnacasan safe and well-tolerated after chronic administration. However, its development has been stopped in 2003 due to the results of a prolonged (9 months) chronic toxicology study in animals showing hepatic abnormalities.

Belnacasan (VX-765) is an acetyl pro-drug with a reversible leaving group (aldehyde). Under the action of esterases, its active metabolite is produced (VRT-043,198) [397]. Belnacasan is orally active and well-tolerated in humans; it acts as a potent inhibitor of both caspase 1 ($K_i = 0.8$ nm) and caspase-4 ($K_i < 0.6$ nM) and has a more moderate effect on caspase-8 ($K_i = 100$ nM), weak on caspase-9 ($K_i = 1$ μM), and very low on caspase-3 ($K_i = 16$ μM) and −7 ($K_i = 21.5$ μM). Belnacasan was found to be more potent than pralnacasan in cellular models of IL-1β release after LPS treatment. It has shown significant efficacy in animal models of osteoarthritis but also epilepsy, myocardial infarction (in combination with a platelet inhibitor), brain sepsis [398], and neurodegenerative diseases with an inflammatory component such as Alzheimer's disease or MS [399,400]. As Belnacasan has the advantage to inhibit caspase-1 as well as caspase-4/5 and so to block both canonic and noncanonic inflammasomes, its repurposing for the treatment of COVID-19 has been proposed [401]. Late december 2021, a proof of concept, randomized, double-blind, placebo-controlled phase-2 clinical trial has started to evaluate of orally administered belnacasan tablets for the treatment of mild to moderate COVID-19 (Medstar Health Research Institute; NCT05164120).

SARS-CoV-2 infection appears to lead to multiple forms of cell death including, apoptosis, necroptosis, pyroptosis, and a combination of them recently named PANoptosis. Although the existing evidence only comes from mouse models, inhibition of cell death is a potentially promising therapeutic idea in life-threatening infectious diseases caused by inflammatory storms including COVID-19. Consequently, the use of pan-caspase inhibition has also been suggested [402] and initiated at the clinical level. Emricasan (IDN-6556/PF-034911390) was the first pan-caspase inhibitor to be evaluated in humans [403]. It irreversibly inhibits Caspases with a very strong effect on caspase-8 ($k_3/K_I = 2{,}940{,}000\ M^{-1}s^{-1}$) and caspase-9 ($k_3/K_I = 2{,}191{,}000\ M^{-1}s^{-1}$), which gives it a potent antiapoptotic effect in numerous cell models and in mouse models of hepatic injury. Emricasan also exhibits anti-inflammatory effects (caspase-1 $k_3/K_I = 689{,}000\ M^{-1}s^{-1}$). Initially developed for the treatment of liver damage associated with chronic hepatitis C virus infection and islet transplants in patients with diabetes, Emricasan has been then evaluated in large phase 2b and 3 studies in patients with nonalchoolic steato-hepatitis (NASH). Emricasan has proven human safety and good tolerance both in acute and chronic administration but has failed to demonstrate efficacy against NASH in these large clinical trials [404,405]. A phase-1 trial is ongoing to evaluate the safety and tolerability of emricasan in symptomatic patients diagnosed with mild COVID-19 (NCT04803227).

General comments and outlook

In the last two years, COVID-19 has rapidly turned into a threat to global health and a progressive pandemic disease capable of collapsing the global healthcare infrastructure [406]. As the COVID-outbreak rapidly evolved, with successive series of waves of infection and momentary respites, the scientific community as a whole has learned a lot in many scientific and social areas, especially in immunology whether natural, innate or acquired. Giant strides have been made, in only two years, in understanding many novel molecular and cellular fundamental aspects linked to new pathophysiological pathways, leading to rapidly developing new therapeutic strategies, with innovative vaccines and repurposed drugs. If we all recognize that non-COVID—related research has been delayed over this period, it can be anticipated that in the long term, many areas will be enriched thanks to the global efforts of all members of the international community. We should recognize however that certain observations have been published rapidly to meet the societal demands. They deserve much more effort to be analyzed in full detail, compared to others and reconciled. In this chapter, some discrepancies that remain unexplained have been highlighted and interesting outlooks are proposed to attempt to sort out the "true" from the "false" in the published results. At this stage, important challenges remain to have the capacity to reduce the burden of infectious diseases that will certainly emerge at a pace that is likely to accelerate. In the context of immunology, other types of questions should be (and are currently) investigated. For example, it would be important to understand, with experimental supportive data, the natural resistance of certain individuals to COVID-19, the immunology of asymptomatic SARS-CoV-2 infection and the close relations between SARS-CoV infection (and possibly vaccination) and systemic or organ-specific autoimmunity. In this chapter, important innate immune responses are summarized, including cytokines and complement, and many immune cell subtypes that rapidly intervene to halt infection (for an overall summary, see Box 3.1).

BOX 3.1

Salient features observed during the COVID-19 pandemic

- Differences in the innate immune cell populations and their altered response favor SARS-CoV-2 infection.
- SARS-CoV-2 changes its genetic diversity and infection pattern with numerous mutations, possibly due to the innate immune system's defensive role [407].
- Although SARS-CoV-2 is potentially highly pathogenic for any human host, the environment and host individual health system are essential dynamic factors in the susceptibility to SARS-CoV-2 and maintenance (long or chronic COVID) of COVID-19 [408]. This includes numerous factors including the quality of microbiota, the activity of principal signal transduction pathways leading to cell death and other individual innate elements.
- Certain HLA alleles (e.g., HLA-A*01:01, HLA-B*46:01 and others) display a weak predicted capacity to bind SARS-CoV-2 peptides, suggesting that individuals with these alleles may be particularly vulnerable to COVID-19. Other HLA alleles could be protective.
- TLRs, NODs and RLRs may be involved both in the initial failure of viral clearance and in the subsequent development of the deadly clinical manifestations of severe COVID-19.
- SARS-CoV-2 is likely to reduce autophagy activity, leading to the assumption that compound-driven induction of autophagy could limit SARS-CoV-2 propagation.
- Older people are more prone to infections and risk of fatality due to the

Continued

BOX 3.1 *(cont'd)*

lack of spontaneous innate responses (pDCs and alveolar macrophages) along with preexisting adaptive immunity, the possible existence of autoantibodies to type I IFN, and others [409]. At the same time, youngsters and children are partly resistant to severe COVID-19 [410].

- An important aspect that should also consider is sex differences; male patients had higher innate immune responses than female patients [410].
- Vitamin D is involved in different pathophysiological processes, such as expression of ACE2, activation of innate and adaptive immune cells and clinical manifestations, such as coagulation/thrombotic disorders and ARDS. TLRs and vitamin D produce synergistic effects during infectious diseases [411].
- Overactivation of inflammasome signaling and pyroptosis are increasingly likely drivers of COVID-19 pathogenesis

It is too early to define how strong will be the long-term SARS-CoV-2 memory B- and T cell-mediated immune responses in patients recovering from infection or individuals who have been vaccinated with mRNA preparations. It will be decisive to follow different pathophysiological, immunological, and behavorial aspects that will develop in patients with long COVID. Such studies in patients of different races and environments over the world will be central. Numerous clinical trials are ongoing, exploring highly diverse clinical hypotheses, and therapeutic regimens. The huge ongoing international fundamental, biopharmaceutical, and clinical research race will provide rapid answers to decipher the multiple ideas, define the best preventive methods, improve vaccines, give each patient the right combination of antiviral and immunomodulatory drugs, and prepare at best for the next global infectious threats which humanity will be facing in the next decade(s).

Acknowledgments

Research in Strasbourg (France) was supported by the French Center National de la Recherche Scientifique (CNRS); the University of Strasbourg Institute for Advanced Study (USIAS); the Interdisciplinary Thematic Institute IMS, as part of the ITI 2021–28 program of the University of Strasbourg, CNRS and Inserm (ANR-10-IDEX-0002) and SFRI (STRAT'US project, ANR-20-SFRI-0012); the European Regional Development Fund of the European Union in the context of the INTERREG V Upper Rhine program; the FHU ARRIMAGE and the OMAGE project granted by Region Grand-Est and FEDER. SM also acknowledges the TRANSAUTOPHAGY COST Action (CA15138) and the Club francophone de l'autophagie (CFATG). EJ acknowledges support from the Fondation iXLife-iXCore-iXBlue pour la recherche and from the Schaefer Research Scholars Program Awards of the Vagelos College of Physicians and Surgeons of Columbia University. Research on SARS-CoV-2 immunoprevention conducted at the Universidad Nacional de Colombia, was supported by grants to JML from Vicerrectoría de Investigación HERMES (grant numbers 49586, 50090 and 54836). RSS acknowledges the support of the Brazilian National Council for Scientific and Technological Development (CNPq), the São Paulo Research Foundation (FAPESP) and Foundation for Support to Teaching, Research and Assistance (FAEPA) of the Clinics Hospital of the Ribeirão Preto Medical School, University of São Paulo, Brazil. SRB is grateful to Prof. Jagadeesh Bayry (INSERM, Center de Recherche des Cordeliers, Sorbonne Universités, Université de Paris, France and IIT Palakkad, Palakkad, Kerala, India) for providing a post-doctoral position. ATV acknowledges Conselho Nacional de Desenvolvimento Científico e Tecnológico (CNPq), Coordenação de Aperfeiçoamento de Pessoal de Nível Superior (CAPES), Fundação de Amparo à Pesquisa de Minas Gerais (FAPEMIG) and Instituto Serrapilheira [Serra-1912-31552]. EJ also thanks Tinoray Jacotot, for multiple inflammasome-related discussions and her helpful participation in the drawing of Fig. 3.2. The funders had no role in the preparation of this chapter.

Author contributions
All authors wrote the manuscript.

Researcher IDs
Srinivasa Reddy Bonam: 0000-0002-2888-2418.
Marie-Agnès Dragon-Durey: 0000-0002-5909-8122.
Véronique Frémeaux-Bacchi: 0000-0002-4865-8528.
Jose Manuel Lozano: 0000-0001-6039-0213.
Etienne Jacotot: 0000-0002-5301-1569.
Sylviane Muller: 0000-0002-0481-0620.
Marko Radic: 0000-0002-8004-282×
Rafael Simone Saia: 0000-0002-9771-7627.
Laura Talamini: 0000-0001-6010-2947.
Angelica T Vieira: 0000-0002-4556-7671.

References

[1] Lednicky JA, Tagliamonte MS, White SK, Elbadry MA, Alam MM, Stephenson CJ, et al. Emergence of porcine delta-coronavirus pathogenic infections among children in Haiti through independent zoonoses and convergent evolution. Preprint. medRxiv. 2021;2021.03.19:21253391. https://doi.org/10.1101/2021.03.19.21253391.

[2] Vlasova AN, Diaz A, Damtie D, Xiu L, Toh T-H, Lee JS-Y, et al. Novel canine coronavirus isolated from a hospitalized patient with pneumonia in East Malaysia. Clin Infect Dis 2021:ciab456. https://doi.org/10.1093/cid/ciab456.

[3] Holmes EC, Goldstein SA, Rasmussen AL, Robertson DL, Crits-Christoph A, Wertheim JO, et al. The origins of SARS-CoV-2: a critical review. Cell 2021;184:4848–56. https://doi.org/10.1016/j.cell.2021.08.017.

[4] Vabret N, Britton GJ, Gruber C, Hegde S, Kim J, Kuksin M, et al. Immunology of COVID-19: current state of the science. Immunity 2020;52:910–41. https://doi.org/10.1016/j.immuni.2020.05.002.

[5] Boyton RJ, Altmann DM. The immunology of asymptomatic SARS-CoV-2 infection: what are the key questions? Nat Rev Immunol 2021;21:762–8. https://doi.org/10.1038/s41577-021-00631-x.

[6] Terrier O, Si-Tahar M, Ducatez M, Chevalier C, Pizzorno A, Le Goffic R, et al. Influenza viruses and coronaviruses: knowns, unknowns, and common research challenges. PLoS Pathog 2021;17:e1010106. https://doi.org/10.1371/journal.ppat.1010106.

[7] Schultze JL, Aschenbrenner AC. COVID-19 and the human innate immune system. Cell 2021;184:1671–92. https://doi.org/10.1016/j.cell.2021.02.029.

[8] Bonam SR, Kotla NG, Bohara RA, Rochev Y, Webster TJ, Bayry J. Potential immuno-nanomedicine strategies to fight COVID-19 like pulmonary infections. Nano Today 2021;36:101051. https://doi.org/10.1016/j.nantod.2020.101051.

[9] Karlsson M, Zhang C, Méar L, Zhong W, Digre A, Katona B, et al. A single–cell type transcriptomics map of human tissues. Sci Adv 2021;7:eabh2169. https://doi.org/10.1126/sciadv.abh2169.

[10] Jiang M, Kolehmainen P, Kakkola L, Maljanen S, Melén K, Smura T, et al. SARS-CoV-2 isolates show impaired replication in human immune cells but differential ability to replicate and induce innate immunity in lung epithelial cells. Microbiol Spectr 2021;9:e0077421. https://doi.org/10.1128/Spectrum.00774-21.

[11] Xu G, Qi F, Li H, Yang Q, Wang H, Wang X, et al. The differential immune responses to COVID-19 in peripheral and lung revealed by single-cell RNA sequencing. Cell Discov 2020;6:73. https://doi.org/10.1038/s41421-020-00225-2.

[12] Schulte-Schrepping J, Reusch N, Paclik D, Baßler K, Schlickeiser S, Zhang B, et al. Severe COVID-19 is marked by a dysregulated myeloid cell compartment. Cell 2020;182:1419–1440.e23. https://doi.org/10.1016/j.cell.2020.08.001.

[13] Chu H, Chan JF-W, Wang Y, Yuen TT-T, Chai Y, Hou Y, et al. Comparative replication and immune activation profiles of SARS-CoV-2 and SARS-CoV in human lungs: an ex vivo study with implications for the pathogenesis of COVID-19. Clin Infect Dis 2020;71:1400–9. https://doi.org/10.1093/cid/ciaa410.

[14] Liao M, Liu Y, Yuan J, Wen Y, Xu G, Zhao J, et al. Single-cell landscape of bronchoalveolar immune cells in patients with COVID-19. Nat Med 2020;26:842–4. https://doi.org/10.1038/s41591-020-0901-9.

[15] Yang D, Chu H, Hou Y, Chai Y, Shuai H, Lee AC-Y, et al. Attenuated interferon and proinflammatory response in SARS-CoV-2-infected human dendritic cells is associated with viral antagonism of STAT1 phosphorylation. J Infect Dis 2020;222:734–45. https://doi.org/10.1093/infdis/jiaa356.

[16] Lucas C, Wong P, Klein J, Castro TBR, Silva J, Sundaram M, et al. Longitudinal analyses reveal immunological misfiring in severe COVID-19. Nature 2020;584:463–9. https://doi.org/10.1038/s41586-020-2588-y.

[17] Zhou R, To KK-W, Wong Y-C, Liu L, Zhou B, Li X, et al. Acute SARS-CoV-2 infection impairs dendritic cell and T cell responses. Immunity 2020;53:864–877.e5. https://doi.org/10.1016/j.immuni.2020.07.026.

[18] Zheng M, Gao Y, Wang G, Song G, Liu S, Sun D, et al. Functional exhaustion of antiviral lymphocytes in COVID-19 patients. Cell Mol Immunol 2020;17:533–5. https://doi.org/10.1038/s41423-020-0402-2.

[19] Qin C, Zhou L, Hu Z, Zhang S, Yang S, Tao Y, et al. Dysregulation of immune response in patients with coronavirus 2019 (COVID-19) in Wuhan, China. Clin Infect Dis 2020;71:762–8. https://doi.org/10.1093/cid/ciaa248.

[20] Lourda M, Dzidic M, Hertwig L, Bergsten H, Palma Medina LM, Sinha I, et al. High-dimensional profiling reveals phenotypic heterogeneity and disease-specific alterations of granulocytes in COVID-19. Proc Natl Acad Sci U S A 2021;118. https://doi.org/10.1073/pnas.2109123118. e2109123118.

[21] Thwaites RS, Sanchez Sevilla Uruchurtu A, Siggins MK, Liew F, Russell CD, Moore SC, et al. Inflammatory profiles across the spectrum of disease reveal a distinct role for GM-CSF in severe COVID-19. Sci Immunol 2021;6:eabg9873. https://doi.org/10.1126/sciimmunol.abg9873.

[22] Tedeschi A, Salmaso C, Di Donato M, Lorini M, Miadonna A. Granulocyte-macrophage colony-stimulating factor and interleukin-3 cause basophil histamine release by a common pathway: downregulation by sodium. Immunology 1999;96:164–70. https://doi.org/10.1046/j.1365-2567.1999.00697.x.

[23] Rodriguez L, Pekkarinen PT, Lakshmikanth T, Tan Z, Consiglio CR, Pou C, et al. Systems-level immunomonitoring from acute to recovery phase of severe COVID-19. Cell Rep Med 2020;1:100078. https://doi.org/10.1016/j.xcrm.2020.100078.

[24] Chen J, Vitetta L. Increased PD-L1 expression may Be associated with the cytokine storm and CD8+ T-cell exhaustion in severe COVID-19. J Infect Dis 2021;223:1659–60. https://doi.org/10.1093/infdis/jiab061.

[25] Conti P, Caraffa A, Tetè G, Gallenga CE, Ross R, Kritas SK, et al. Mast cells activated by SARS-CoV-2 release histamine which increases IL-1 levels causing cytokine storm and inflammatory reaction in COVID-19. J Biol Regul Homeost Agents 2020;34:1629–32. https://doi.org/10.23812/20-2EDIT.

[26] Nathan C. Neutrophils and immunity: challenges and opportunities. Nat Rev Immunol 2006;6:173–82. https://doi.org/10.1038/nri1785.

[27] Nourshargh S, Alon R. Leukocyte migration into inflamed tissues. Immunity 2014;41:694–707. https://doi.org/10.1016/j.immuni.2014.10.008.

[28] Friedl P, Weigelin B. Interstitial leukocyte migration and immune function. Nat Immunol 2008;9:960–9. https://doi.org/10.1038/ni.f.212.

[29] Lämmermann T, Afonso PV, Angermann BR, Wang JM, Kastenmüller W, Parent CA, et al. Neutrophil swarms require LTB4 and integrins at sites of cell death in vivo. Nature 2013;498:371–5. https://doi.org/10.1038/nature12175.

[30] Mócsai A, Walzog B, Lowell CA. Intracellular signalling during neutrophil recruitment. Cardiovasc Res 2015;107:373–85. https://doi.org/10.1093/cvr/cvv159.

[31] Sollberger G, Tilley DO, Zychlinsky A. Neutrophil extracellular traps: the biology of chromatin externalization. Dev Cell 2018;44:542–53. https://doi.org/10.1016/j.devcel.2018.01.019.

[32] Brinkmann V, Zychlinsky A. Beneficial suicide: why neutrophils die to make NETs. Nat Rev Microbiol 2007;5:577–82. https://doi.org/10.1038/nrmicro1710.

[33] Ackermann M, Anders H-J, Bilyy R, Bowlin GL, Daniel C, De Lorenzo R, et al. Patients with COVID-19: in the dark-NETs of neutrophils. Cell Death Differ 2021;28:3125–39. https://doi.org/10.1038/s41418-021-00805-z.

[34] Kaplan MJ, Radic M. Neutrophil extracellular traps: double-edged swords of innate immunity. J Immunol 2012;189:2689–95. https://doi.org/10.4049/jimmunol.1201719.

[35] Narasaraju T, Tang BM, Herrmann M, Muller S, Chow VTK, Radic M. Neutrophilia and NETopathy as key pathologic drivers of progressive lung impairment in patients with COVID-19. Front Pharmacol 2020;11:870. https://doi.org/10.3389/fphar.2020.00870.

[36] Isles HM, Loynes CA, Alasmari S, Kon FC, Henry KM, Kadochnikova A, et al. Pioneer neutrophils release chromatin within in vivo swarms. Elife 2021;10:e68755. https://doi.org/10.7554/eLife.68755.

[37] Polidoro RB, Hagan RS, de Santis Santiago R, Schmidt NW. Overview: systemic inflammatory response derived from lung injury caused by SARS-CoV-2 infection explains severe outcomes in COVID-19. Front Immunol 2020;11:1626. https://doi.org/10.3389/fimmu.2020.01626.

[38] Vardhana SA, Wolchok JD. The many faces of the anti-COVID immune response. J Exp Med 2020;217:e20200678. https://doi.org/10.1084/jem.20200678.

[39] Yap JKY, Moriyama M, Iwasaki A. Inflammasomes and pyroptosis as therapeutic targets for COVID-19. J Immunol 2020;205:307–12. https://doi.org/10.4049/jimmunol.2000513.

[40] Lee S, Channappanavar R, Kanneganti T-D. Coronaviruses: innate immunity, inflammasome activation, inflammatory cell death, and cytokines. Trends Immunol 2020;41:1083–99. https://doi.org/10.1016/j.it.2020.10.005.

[41] Man SM, Kanneganti T-D. Converging roles of caspases in inflammasome activation, cell death and innate immunity. Nat Rev Immunol 2016;16:7–21. https://doi.org/10.1038/nri.2015.7.

[42] Liu X, Zhang Z, Ruan J, Pan Y, Magupalli VG, Wu H, et al. Inflammasome-activated gasdermin D causes pyroptosis by forming membrane pores. Nature 2016;535:153–8. https://doi.org/10.1038/nature18629.

[43] Shi J, Zhao Y, Wang K, Shi X, Wang Y, Huang H, et al. Cleavage of GSDMD by inflammatory caspases determines pyroptotic cell death. Nature 2015;526:660–5. https://doi.org/10.1038/nature15514.

[44] Wang X, Jiang W, Yan Y, Gong T, Han J, Tian Z, et al. RNA viruses promote activation of the NLRP3 inflammasome through a RIP1-RIP3-DRP1 signaling pathway. Nat Immunol 2014;15:1126–33. https://doi.org/10.1038/ni.3015.

[45] Ahn M, Anderson DE, Zhang Q, Tan CW, Lim BL, Luko K, et al. Dampened NLRP3-mediated inflammation in bats and implications for a special viral reservoir host. Nat Microbiol 2019;4:789–99. https://doi.org/10.1038/s41564-019-0371-3.

[46] Goh G, Ahn M, Zhu F, Lee LB, Luo D, Irving AT, et al. Complementary regulation of caspase-1 and IL-1β reveals additional mechanisms of dampened inflammation in bats. Proc Natl Acad Sci USA 2020;117:28939–49. https://doi.org/10.1073/pnas.2003352117.

[47] Rodrigues TS, de Sá KSG, Ishimoto AY, Becerra A, Oliveira S, Almeida L, et al. Inflammasomes are activated in response to SARS-CoV-2 infection and are associated with COVID-19 severity in patients. J Exp Med 2021;218:e20201707. https://doi.org/10.1084/jem.20201707.

[48] Junqueira C, Crespo Â, Ranjbar S, Ingber J, Parry B, Ravid S, et al. SARS-CoV-2 infects blood monocytes to activate NLRP3 and AIM2 inflammasomes, pyroptosis and cytokine release. Preprint. Res Sq. 2021. https://doi.org/10.21203/rs.3.rs-153628/v1.

[49] Satıs H, Özger HS, Aysert Yıldız P, Hızel K, Gulbahar Ö, Erbas G, et al. Prognostic value of interleukin-18 and its association with other inflammatory markers and disease severity in COVID-19. Cytokine 2021;137:155302. https://doi.org/10.1016/j.cyto.2020.155302.

[50] Li S, Jiang L, Li X, Lin F, Wang Y, Li B, et al. Clinical and pathological investigation of patients with severe COVID-19. JCI Insight 2020;5:138070. https://doi.org/10.1172/jci.insight.138070.

[51] Paul O, Tao JQ, Litzky L, Feldman M, Montone K, Rajapakse C, et al. Vascular inflammation in lungs of patients with fatal coronavirus disease 2019 (COVID-19) infection: possible role for the NLRP3 inflammasome. Preprint. Res Sq 2021. https://doi.org/10.21203/rs.3.rs-842167/v1.

[52] Zhang J, Wu H, Yao X, Zhang D, Zhou Y, Fu B, et al. Pyroptotic macrophages stimulate the SARS-CoV-2-associated cytokine storm. Cell Mol Immunol 2021;18:1305–7. https://doi.org/10.1038/s41423-021-00665-0.

[53] Toldo S, Bussani R, Nuzzi V, Bonaventura A, Mauro AG, Cannatà A, et al. Inflammasome formation in the lungs of patients with fatal COVID-19. Inflamm Res 2021;70:7–10. https://doi.org/10.1007/s00011-020-01413-2.

[54] Gowda P, Patrick S, Joshi SD, Kumawat RK, Sen E. Glycyrrhizin prevents SARS-CoV-2 S1 and Orf3a induced high mobility group box 1 (HMGB1) release and inhibits viral replication. Cytokine 2021;142:155496. https://doi.org/10.1016/j.cyto.2021.155496.

[55] Chen L, Long X, Xu Q, Tan J, Wang G, Cao Y, et al. Elevated serum levels of S100A8/A9 and HMGB1 at hospital admission are correlated with inferior clinical outcomes in COVID-19 patients. Cell Mol Immunol 2020;17:992–4. https://doi.org/10.1038/s41423-020-0492-x.
[56] Ferreira AC, Soares VC, de Azevedo-Quintanilha IG, Dias S da SG, Fintelman-Rodrigues N, Sacramento CQ, et al. SARS-CoV-2 engages inflammasome and pyroptosis in human primary monocytes. Cell Death Dis 2021;7:43. https://doi.org/10.1038/s41420-021-00428-w.
[57] Zheng J, Wang Y, Li K, Meyerholz DK, Allamargot C, Perlman S. Severe acute respiratory syndrome coronavirus 2-induced immune activation and death of monocyte-derived human macrophages and dendritic cells. J Infect Dis 2021;223:785–95. https://doi.org/10.1093/infdis/jiaa753.
[58] Junqueira C, Crespo Â, Ranjbar S, Ingber J, Parry B, Ravid S, et al. SARS-CoV-2 infects blood monocytes to activate NLRP3 and AIM2 inflammasomes, pyroptosis and cytokine release. medRxiv 2021. https://doi.org/10.1101/2021.03.06.21252796.
[59] Pan P, Shen M, Yu Z, Ge W, Chen K, Tian M, et al. SARS-CoV-2 N protein promotes NLRP3 inflammasome activation to induce hyperinflammation. Nat Commun 2021;12:4664. https://doi.org/10.1038/s41467-021-25015-6.
[60] Theobald SJ, Simonis A, Georgomanolis T, Kreer C, Zehner M, Eisfeld HS, et al. Long-lived macrophage reprogramming drives spike protein-mediated inflammasome activation in COVID-19. EMBO Mol Med 2021;13:e14150. https://doi.org/10.15252/emmm.202114150.
[61] Sun X, Liu Y, Huang Z, Xu W, Hu W, Yi L, et al. SARS-CoV-2 non-structural protein 6 triggers NLRP3-dependent pyroptosis by targeting ATP6AP1. Cell Death Differ 2022;29(6):1240–54. https://doi.org/10.1038/s41418-021-00916-7.
[62] Amaral MP, Bortoluci KR. Caspase-8 and FADD: where cell death and inflammation collide. Immunity 2020;52:890–2. https://doi.org/10.1016/j.immuni.2020.05.008.
[63] Tummers B, Green DR. Caspase-8: regulating life and death. Immunol Rev 2017;277:76–89. https://doi.org/10.1111/imr.12541.
[64] Li S, Zhang Y, Guan Z, Li H, Ye M, Chen X, et al. SARS-CoV-2 triggers inflammatory responses and cell death through caspase-8 activation. Signal Transduct Target Ther 2020;5:235. https://doi.org/10.1038/s41392-020-00334-0.
[65] Karki R, Sharma BR, Tuladhar S, Williams EP, Zalduondo L, Samir P, et al. Synergism of TNF-α and IFN-γ triggers inflammatory cell death, tissue damage, and mortality in SARS-CoV-2 infection and cytokine shock syndromes. Cell 2021;184:149–168.e17. https://doi.org/10.1016/j.cell.2020.11.025.
[66] Shi J, Zhao Y, Wang Y, Gao W, Ding J, Li P, et al. Inflammatory caspases are innate immune receptors for intracellular LPS. Nature 2014;514:187–92. https://doi.org/10.1038/nature13683.
[67] Bibo-Verdugo B, Snipas SJ, Kolt S, Poreba M, Salvesen GS. Extended subsite profiling of the pyroptosis effector protein gasdermin D reveals a region recognized by inflammatory caspase-11. J Biol Chem 2020;295:11292–302. https://doi.org/10.1074/jbc.RA120.014259.
[68] Santos JC, Boucher D, Schneider LK, Demarco B, Dilucca M, Shkarina K, et al. Human GBP1 binds LPS to initiate assembly of a caspase-4 activating platform on cytosolic bacteria. Nat Commun 2020;11:3276. https://doi.org/10.1038/s41467-020-16889-z.
[69] Downs KP, Nguyen H, Dorfleutner A, Stehlik C. An overview of the non-canonical inflammasome. Mol Aspects Med 2020;76:100924. https://doi.org/10.1016/j.mam.2020.100924.
[70] Zanoni I, Tan Y, Di Gioia M, Broggi A, Ruan J, Shi J, et al. An endogenous caspase-11 ligand elicits interleukin-1 release from living dendritic cells. Science 2016;352:1232–6. https://doi.org/10.1126/science.aaf3036.
[71] Imai Y, Kuba K, Neely GG, Yaghubian-Malhami R, Perkmann T, van Loo G, et al. Identification of oxidative stress and Toll-like receptor 4 signaling as a key pathway of acute lung injury. Cell 2008;133:235–49. https://doi.org/10.1016/j.cell.2008.02.043.
[72] Fessler MB, Summer RS. Surfactant lipids at the host-environment interface. Metabolic sensors, suppressors, and effectors of inflammatory lung disease. Am J Respir Cell Mol Biol 2016;54:624–35. https://doi.org/10.1165/rcmb.2016-0011PS.
[73] Eltobgy M, Zani A, Kenney AD, Estfanous S, Kim E, Badr A, et al. Caspase-4/11 exacerbates disease severity in SARS-CoV-2 infection by promoting inflammation and thrombosis. Proc Natl Acad Sci U S A 2022;119(21). https://doi.org/10.1101/2021.09.24.461743. e2202012119.

[74] Pandey A, Shen C, Feng S, Man SM. Cell biology of inflammasome activation. Trends Cell Biol 2021;31:924–39. https://doi.org/10.1016/j.tcb.2021.06.010.

[75] Vora SM, Lieberman J, Wu H. Inflammasome activation at the crux of severe COVID-19. Nat Rev Immunol 2021;21:694–703. https://doi.org/10.1038/s41577-021-00588-x.

[76] Pereira B, Xu X-N, Akbar AN. Targeting inflammation and immunosenescence to improve vaccine responses in the elderly. Front Immunol 2020;11:583019. https://doi.org/10.3389/fimmu.2020.583019.

[77] Panda A, Qian F, Mohanty S, van Duin D, Newman FK, Zhang L, et al. Age-associated decrease in TLR function in primary human dendritic cells predicts influenza vaccine response. J Immunol 2010;184:2518–27. https://doi.org/10.4049/jimmunol.0901022.

[78] Connors J, Bell MR, Marcy J, Kutzler M, Haddad EK. The impact of immuno-aging on SARS-CoV-2 vaccine development. Geroscience 2021;43:31–51. https://doi.org/10.1007/s11357-021-00323-3.

[79] Sa Ribero M, Jouvenet N, Dreux M, Nisole S. Interplay between SARS-CoV-2 and the type I interferon response. PLoS Pathog 2020;16:e1008737. https://doi.org/10.1371/journal.ppat.1008737.

[80] Mazaleuskaya L, Veltrop R, Ikpeze N, Martin-Garcia J, Navas-Martin S. Protective role of Toll-like Receptor 3-induced type I interferon in murine coronavirus infection of macrophages. Viruses 2012;4:901–23. https://doi.org/10.3390/v4050901.

[81] Del Valle DM, Kim-Schulze S, Huang H-H, Beckmann ND, Nirenberg S, Wang B, et al. An inflammatory cytokine signature predicts COVID-19 severity and survival. Nat Med 2020;26:1636–43. https://doi.org/10.1038/s41591-020-1051-9.

[82] Arunachalam PS, Wimmers F, Mok CKP, Perera RAPM, Scott M, Hagan T, et al. Systems biological assessment of immunity to mild versus severe COVID-19 infection in humans. Science 2020;369:1210–20. https://doi.org/10.1126/science.abc6261.

[83] Konno Y, Kimura I, Uriu K, Fukushi M, Irie T, Koyanagi Y, et al. SARS-CoV-2 ORF3b is a potent interferon antagonist whose activity is increased by a naturally occurring elongation variant. Cell Rep 2020;32:108185. https://doi.org/10.1016/j.celrep.2020.108185.

[84] Gordon DE, Jang GM, Bouhaddou M, Xu J, Obernier K, White KM, et al. A SARS-CoV-2 protein interaction map reveals targets for drug repurposing. Nature 2020;583:459–68. https://doi.org/10.1038/s41586-020-2286-9.

[85] Banerjee AK, Blanco MR, Bruce EA, Honson DD, Chen LM, Chow A, et al. SARS-CoV-2 disrupts splicing, translation, and protein trafficking to suppress host defenses. Cell 2020;183:1325–1339.e21. https://doi.org/10.1016/j.cell.2020.10.004.

[86] Fajgenbaum DC, June CH. Cytokine storm. N Engl J Med 2020;383:2255–73. https://doi.org/10.1056/NEJMra2026131.

[87] Arango Duque G, Descoteaux A. Macrophage cytokines: involvement in immunity and infectious diseases. Front Immunol 2014;5. https://doi.org/10.3389/fimmu.2014.00491.

[88] Speyer CL, Ward PA. Role of endothelial chemokines and their receptors during inflammation. J Invest Surg 2011;24:18–27. https://doi.org/10.3109/08941939.2010.521232.

[89] Mangalmurti N, Hunter CA. Cytokine storms: understanding COVID-19. Immunity 2020;53:19–25. https://doi.org/10.1016/j.immuni.2020.06.017.

[90] Blanco-Melo D, Nilsson-Payant BE, Liu W-C, Uhl S, Hoagland D, Møller R, et al. Imbalanced host response to SARS-CoV-2 drives development of COVID-19. Cell 2020;181:1036–1045.e9. https://doi.org/10.1016/j.cell.2020.04.026.

[91] Yang L, Xie X, Tu Z, Fu J, Xu D, Zhou Y. Correction: the signal pathways and treatment of cytokine storm in COVID-19. Sig Transduct Target Ther 2021;6:326. https://doi.org/10.1038/s41392-021-00744-8.

[92] Schett G, Sticherling M, Neurath MF. COVID-19: risk for cytokine targeting in chronic inflammatory diseases? Nat Rev Immunol 2020;20:271–2. https://doi.org/10.1038/s41577-020-0312-7.

[93] Chowdhury MA, Hossain N, Kashem MA, Shahid MA, Alam A. Immune response in COVID-19: a review. Journal of Infection and Public Health 2020;13:1619–29. https://doi.org/10.1016/j.jiph.2020.07.001.

[94] Ruan Q, Yang K, Wang W, Jiang L, Song J. Clinical predictors of mortality due to COVID-19 based on an analysis of data of 150 patients from Wuhan, China. Intensive Care Med 2020;46:846–8. https://doi.org/10.1007/s00134-020-05991-x.

[95] Ramos-Casals M, Brito-Zerón P, López-Guillermo A, Khamashta MA, Bosch X. Adult haemophagocytic syndrome. The Lancet 2014;383:1503–16. https://doi.org/10.1016/S0140-6736(13)61048-X.

[96] Karakike E, Giamarellos-Bourboulis EJ. Macrophage activation-like syndrome: a distinct entity leading to early death in sepsis. Front Immunol 2019;10:55. https://doi.org/10.3389/fimmu.2019.00055.
[97] Huang C, Wang Y, Li X, Ren L, Zhao J, Hu Y, et al. Clinical features of patients infected with 2019 novel coronavirus in Wuhan, China. The Lancet 2020;395:497–506. https://doi.org/10.1016/S0140-6736(20)30183-5.
[98] Mehta P, McAuley DF, Brown M, Sanchez E, Tattersall RS, Manson JJ. COVID-19: consider cytokine storm syndromes and immunosuppression. The Lancet 2020;395:1033–4. https://doi.org/10.1016/S0140-6736(20)30628-0.
[99] Olbei M, Hautefort I, Modos D, Treveil A, Poletti M, Gul L, et al. SARS-CoV-2 causes a different cytokine response compared to other cytokine storm-causing respiratory viruses in severely ill patients. Front Immunol 2021;12:629193. https://doi.org/10.3389/fimmu.2021.629193.
[100] Perreau M, Suffiotti M, Marques-Vidal P, Wiedemann A, Levy Y, Laouénan C, et al. The cytokines HGF and CXCL13 predict the severity and the mortality in COVID-19 patients. Nat Commun 2021;12:4888. https://doi.org/10.1038/s41467-021-25191-5.
[101] Tay MZ, Poh CM, Rénia L, MacAry PA, Ng LFP. The trinity of COVID-19: immunity, inflammation and intervention. Nat Rev Immunol 2020;20:363–74. https://doi.org/10.1038/s41577-020-0311-8.
[102] Laing AG, Lorenc A, del Molino del Barrio I, Das A, Fish M, Monin L, et al. A dynamic COVID-19 immune signature includes associations with poor prognosis. Nat Med 2020;26:1623–35. https://doi.org/10.1038/s41591-020-1038-6.
[103] Chen G, Wu D, Guo W, Cao Y, Huang D, Wang H, et al. Clinical and immunological features of severe and moderate coronavirus disease 2019. Journal of Clinical Investigation 2020;130:2620–9. https://doi.org/10.1172/JCI137244.
[104] Herold T, Jurinovic V, Arnreich C, Lipworth BJ, Hellmuth JC, von Bergwelt-Baildon M, et al. Elevated levels of IL-6 and CRP predict the need for mechanical ventilation in COVID-19. J Allergy Clin Immunol 2020;146:128–136.e4. https://doi.org/10.1016/j.jaci.2020.05.008.
[105] Jones SA, Jenkins BJ. Recent insights into targeting the IL-6 cytokine family in inflammatory diseases and cancer. Nat Rev Immunol 2018;18:773–89. https://doi.org/10.1038/s41577-018-0066-7.
[106] Jordan SC. Innate and adaptive immune responses to SARS-CoV-2 in humans: relevance to acquired immunity and vaccine responses. Clin Exp Immunol 2021;204:310–20. https://doi.org/10.1111/cei.13582.
[107] Tanaka T, Narazaki M, Kishimoto T. IL-6 in inflammation, immunity, and disease. Cold Spring Harb Perspect Biol 2014;6:a016295. https://doi.org/10.1101/cshperspect.a016295.
[108] Arnold R, König B, Galatti H, Werchau H, König W. Cytokine (IL-8, IL-6, TNF-alpha) and soluble TNF receptor-I release from human peripheral blood mononuclear cells after respiratory syncytial virus infection. Immunology 1995;85:364–72.
[109] Rubin EJ, Longo DL, Baden LR. Interleukin-6 receptor inhibition in covid-19 — cooling the inflammatory soup. N Engl J Med 2021;384:1564–5. https://doi.org/10.1056/NEJMe2103108.
[110] Jones SA, Hunter CA. Is IL-6 a key cytokine target for therapy in COVID-19? Nat Rev Immunol 2021;21:337–9. https://doi.org/10.1038/s41577-021-00553-8.
[111] Xu X, Han M, Li T, Sun W, Wang D, Fu B, et al. Effective treatment of severe COVID-19 patients with tocilizumab. Proc Natl Acad Sci U S A 2020;117:10970–5. https://doi.org/10.1073/pnas.2005615117.
[112] Gupta S, Wang W, Hayek SS, Chan L, Mathews KS, Melamed ML, et al. Association between early treatment with tocilizumab and mortality among critically ill patients with COVID-19. JAMA Intern Med 2021;181:41–51. https://doi.org/10.1001/jamainternmed.2020.6252.
[113] The REMAP-CAP Investigators. Interleukin-6 receptor antagonists in critically ill patients with covid-19. N Engl J Med 2021;384:1491–502. https://doi.org/10.1056/NEJMoa2100433.
[114] Hermine O, Mariette X, Tharaux P-L, Resche-Rigon M, Porcher R, Ravaud P, et al. Effect of tocilizumab vs usual care in adults hospitalized with COVID-19 and moderate or severe pneumonia: a randomized clinical trial. JAMA Intern Med 2021;181:32. https://doi.org/10.1001/jamainternmed.2020.6820.
[115] Stone JH, Frigault MJ, Serling-Boyd NJ, Fernandes AD, Harvey L, Foulkes AS, et al. Efficacy of tocilizumab in patients hospitalized with covid-19. N Engl J Med 2020;383:2333–44. https://doi.org/10.1056/NEJMoa2028836.
[116] Veiga VC, Prats JAGG, Farias DLC, Rosa RG, Dourado LK, Zampieri FG, et al. Effect of tocilizumab on clinical outcomes at 15 days in patients with severe or critical coronavirus disease 2019: randomised controlled trial. BMJ 2021:n84. https://doi.org/10.1136/bmj.n84.

[117] Cron RQ, Caricchio R, Chatham WW. Calming the cytokine storm in COVID-19. Nat Med 2021;27:1674–5. https://doi.org/10.1038/s41591-021-01500-9.
[118] Gabay C, Lamacchia C, Palmer G. IL-1 pathways in inflammation and human diseases. Nat Rev Rheumatol 2010;6:232–41. https://doi.org/10.1038/nrrheum.2010.4.
[119] McElvaney OJ, McEvoy NL, McElvaney OF, Carroll TP, Murphy MP, Dunlea DM, et al. Characterization of the inflammatory response to severe COVID-19 illness. Am J Respir Crit Care Med 2020;202:812–21. https://doi.org/10.1164/rccm.202005-1583OC.
[120] Zhang W, Zhao Y, Zhang F, Wang Q, Li T, Liu Z, et al. The use of anti-inflammatory drugs in the treatment of people with severe coronavirus disease 2019 (COVID-19): the Perspectives of clinical immunologists from China. Clin Immunol 2020;214:108393. https://doi.org/10.1016/j.clim.2020.108393.
[121] Cauchois R, Koubi M, Delarbre D, Manet C, Carvelli J, Blasco VB, et al. Early IL-1 receptor blockade in severe inflammatory respiratory failure complicating COVID-19. Proc Natl Acad Sci USA 2020;117:18951–3. https://doi.org/10.1073/pnas.2009017117.
[122] the RCI-COVID-19 Study Group, Kooistra EJ, Waalders NJB, Grondman I, Janssen NAF, de Nooijer AH, et al. Anakinra treatment in critically ill COVID-19 patients: a prospective cohort study. Crit Care 2020;24:688. https://doi.org/10.1186/s13054-020-03364-w.
[123] Cavalli G, De Luca G, Campochiaro C, Della-Torre E, Ripa M, Canetti D, et al. Interleukin-1 blockade with high-dose anakinra in patients with COVID-19, acute respiratory distress syndrome, and hyperinflammation: a retrospective cohort study. Lancet Rheumatol 2020;2:e325–31. https://doi.org/10.1016/S2665-9913(20)30127-2.
[124] Katia F, Myriam DP, Ucciferri C, Auricchio A, Di Nicola M, Marchioni M, et al. Efficacy of canakinumab in mild or severe COVID-19 pneumonia. Immun Inflamm Dis 2021;9:399–405. https://doi.org/10.1002/iid3.400.
[125] Hiscott J, Nguyen T-LA, Arguello M, Nakhaei P, Paz S. Manipulation of the nuclear factor-κB pathway and the innate immune response by viruses. Oncogene 2006;25:6844–67. https://doi.org/10.1038/sj.onc.1209941.
[126] Robinson PC, Richards D, Tanner HL, Feldmann M. Accumulating evidence suggests anti-TNF therapy needs to be given trial priority in COVID-19 treatment. The Lancet Rheumatology 2020;2:e653–5. https://doi.org/10.1016/S2665-9913(20)30309-X.
[127] Li X, Maretzky T, Weskamp G, Monette S, Qing X, Issuree PDA, et al. iRhoms 1 and 2 are essential upstream regulators of ADAM17-dependent EGFR signaling. Proc Natl Acad Sci U S A 2015;112:6080–5. https://doi.org/10.1073/pnas.1505649112.
[128] Luo W-W, Li S, Li C, Zheng Z-Q, Cao P, Tong Z, et al. iRhom2 is essential for innate immunity to RNA virus by antagonizing ER- and mitochondria-associated degradation of VISA. PLoS Pathog 2017;13:e1006693. https://doi.org/10.1371/journal.ppat.1006693.
[129] Heurich A, Hofmann-Winkler H, Gierer S, Liepold T, Jahn O, Pohlmann S. TMPRSS2 and ADAM17 cleave ACE2 differentially and only proteolysis by TMPRSS2 augments entry driven by the severe acute respiratory syndrome coronavirus spike protein. J Virol 2014;88:1293–307. https://doi.org/10.1128/JVI.02202-13.
[130] Migliorini F, Torsiello E, Spiezia F, Oliva F, Tingart M, Maffulli N. Association between HLA genotypes and COVID-19 susceptibility, severity and progression: a comprehensive review of the literature. Eur J Med Res 2021;26:84. https://doi.org/10.1186/s40001-021-00563-1.
[131] Lin M, Tseng H-K, Trejaut JA, Lee H-L, Loo J-H, Chu C-C, et al. Association of HLA class I with severe acute respiratory syndrome coronavirus infection. BMC Med Genet 2003;4:9. https://doi.org/10.1186/1471-2350-4-9.
[132] Nguyen A, David JK, Maden SK, Wood MA, Weeder BR, Nellore A, et al. Human leukocyte antigen susceptibility map for severe acute respiratory syndrome coronavirus 2. J Virol 2020;94. https://doi.org/10.1128/JVI.00510-20.
[133] Ng MHL, Lau K, Li L, Cheng S, Chan WY, Hui PK, et al. Association of human-leukocyte-antigen class I (B*0703) and class II (DRB1*0301) genotypes with susceptibility and resistance to the development of severe acute respiratory syndrome. J Infect Dis 2004;190:515–8. https://doi.org/10.1086/421523.
[134] Zhou M, Xu D, Li X, Li H, Shan M, Tang J, et al. Screening and identification of severe acute respiratory syndrome-associated coronavirus-specific CTL epitopes. J Immunol 2006;177:2138–45. https://doi.org/10.4049/jimmunol.177.4.2138.

[135] Shkurnikov M, Nersisyan S, Jankevic T, Galatenko A, Gordeev I, Vechorko V, et al. Association of HLA class I genotypes with severity of coronavirus disease-19. Front Immunol 2021;12:641900. https://doi.org/10.3389/fimmu.2021.641900.

[136] Littera R, Campagna M, Deidda S, Angioni G, Cipri S, Melis M, et al. Human leukocyte antigen complex and other immunogenetic and clinical factors influence susceptibility or protection to SARS-CoV-2 infection and severity of the disease course. The Sardinian experience. Front Immunol 2020;11:605688. https://doi.org/10.3389/fimmu.2020.605688.

[137] Galluzzi L, Baehrecke EH, Ballabio A, Boya P, Bravo-San Pedro JM, Cecconi F, et al. Molecular definitions of autophagy and related processes. EMBO J 2017;36:1811–36. https://doi.org/10.15252/embj.201796697.

[138] Heckmann BL, Green DR. LC3-associated phagocytosis at a glance. J Cell Sci 2019;132:jcs222984. https://doi.org/10.1242/jcs.222984.

[139] Choi Y, Bowman JW, Jung JU. Autophagy during viral infection - a double-edged sword. Nat Rev Microbiol 2018;16:341–54. https://doi.org/10.1038/s41579-018-0003-6.

[140] Kumar A, Kumar P, Saumya KU, Giri R. Investigating the conformational dynamics of SARS-CoV-2 NSP6 protein with emphasis on non-transmembrane 91–112 & 231–290 regions. Microb Pathog 2021;161:105236. https://doi.org/10.1016/j.micpath.2021.105236.

[141] Klionsky DJ, Petroni G, Amaravadi RK, Baehrecke EH, Ballabio A, Boya P, et al. Autophagy in major human diseases. EMBO J 2021;40. https://doi.org/10.15252/embj.2021108863.

[142] Bonam SR, Muller S, Bayry J, Klionsky DJ. Autophagy as an emerging target for COVID-19: lessons from an old friend, chloroquine. Autophagy 2020;16:2260–6. https://doi.org/10.1080/15548627.2020.1779467.

[143] Gassen NC, Papies J, Bajaj T, Emanuel J, Dethloff F, Chua RL, et al. SARS-CoV-2-mediated dysregulation of metabolism and autophagy uncovers host-targeting antivirals. Nat Commun 2021;12:3818. https://doi.org/10.1038/s41467-021-24007-w.

[144] Bello-Perez M, Sola I, Novoa B, Klionsky DJ, Falco A. Canonical and noncanonical autophagy as potential targets for COVID-19. Cells 2020;9:E1619. https://doi.org/10.3390/cells9071619.

[145] Pehote G, Vij N. Autophagy augmentation to alleviate immune response dysfunction, and resolve respiratory and COVID-19 exacerbations. Cells 2020;9:E1952. https://doi.org/10.3390/cells9091952.

[146] Maity S, Saha A. Therapeutic potential of exploiting autophagy cascade against coronavirus infection. Front Microbiol 2021;12:675419. https://doi.org/10.3389/fmicb.2021.675419.

[147] Sargazi S, Sheervalilou R, Rokni M, Shirvaliloo M, Shahraki O, Rezaei N. The role of autophagy in controlling SARS-CoV-2 infection: an overview on virophagy-mediated molecular drug targets. Cell Biol Int 2021;45:1599–612. https://doi.org/10.1002/cbin.11609.

[148] Wang F, Tasset I, Cuervo AM, Muller S. In vivo remodeling of altered autophagy-lysosomal pathway by a phosphopeptide in lupus. Cells 2020;9:E2328. https://doi.org/10.3390/cells9102328.

[149] Tu X, Chong WP, Zhai Y, Zhang H, Zhang F, Wang S, et al. Functional polymorphisms of the CCL2 and MBL genes cumulatively increase susceptibility to severe acute respiratory syndrome coronavirus infection. J Infect 2015;71:101–9. https://doi.org/10.1016/j.jinf.2015.03.006.

[150] Ali YM, Ferrari M, Lynch NJ, Yaseen S, Dudler T, Gragerov S, et al. Lectin pathway mediates complement activation by SARS-CoV-2 proteins. Front Immunol 2021;12:714511. https://doi.org/10.3389/fimmu.2021.714511.

[151] Defendi F, Leroy C, Epaulard O, Clavarino G, Vilotitch A, Le Marechal M, et al. Complement alternative and mannose-binding lectin pathway activation is associated with COVID-19 mortality. Front Immunol 2021;12:742446. https://doi.org/10.3389/fimmu.2021.742446.

[152] Jarlhelt I, Nielsen SK, Jahn CXH, Hansen CB, Pérez-Alós L, Rosbjerg A, et al. SARS-CoV-2 antibodies mediate complement and cellular driven inflammation. Front Immunol 2021;12:767981. https://doi.org/10.3389/fimmu.2021.767981.

[153] Yu J, Yuan X, Chen H, Chaturvedi S, Braunstein EM, Brodsky RA. Direct activation of the alternative complement pathway by SARS-CoV-2 spike proteins is blocked by factor D inhibition. Blood 2020;136:2080–9. https://doi.org/10.1182/blood.2020008248.

[154] Singh J, Kar S, Hasnain SE, Ganguly S. SARS-CoV-2 ORF8 can fold into human factor 1 catalytic domain binding site on complement C3b: predict functional mimicry. bioRxiv 2020. https://doi.org/10.1101/2020.06.08.107011.

[155] Li L, Chen C. Contribution of acute-phase reaction proteins to the diagnosis and treatment of 2019 novel coronavirus disease (COVID-19). Epidemiol Infect 2020;148:e164. https://doi.org/10.1017/S095026882000165X.

[156] Hadjadj J, Yatim N, Barnabei L, Corneau A, Boussier J, Smith N, et al. Impaired type I interferon activity and inflammatory responses in severe COVID-19 patients. Science 2020;369:718–24. https://doi.org/10.1126/science.abc6027.
[157] Yan B, Freiwald T, Chauss D, Wang L, West E, Mirabelli C, et al. SARS-CoV-2 drives JAK1/2-dependent local complement hyperactivation. Sci Immunol 2021;6:eabg0833. https://doi.org/10.1126/sciimmunol.abg0833.
[158] Boussier J, Yatim N, Marchal A, Hadjadj J, Charbit B, El Sissy C, et al. Severe COVID-19 is associated with hyperactivation of the alternative complement pathway. J Allergy Clin Immunol 2021;S0091–6749(21):01761–9. https://doi.org/10.1016/j.jaci.2021.11.004.
[159] Ramlall V, Thangaraj PM, Meydan C, Foox J, Butler D, Kim J, et al. Immune complement and coagulation dysfunction in adverse outcomes of SARS-CoV-2 infection. Nat Med 2020;26:1609–15. https://doi.org/10.1038/s41591-020-1021-2.
[160] Yan B, Freiwald T, Chauss D, Wang L, West E, Bibby J, et al. SARS-CoV2 drives JAK1/2-dependent local and systemic complement hyper-activation. In: Review; 2020. https://doi.org/10.21203/rs.3.rs-33390/v1.
[161] Georg P, Astaburuaga-García R, Bonaguro L, Brumhard S, Michalick L, Lippert LJ, et al. Complement activation induces excessive T cell cytotoxicity in severe COVID-19. Cell 2022;185(3):493–512.e25. https://doi.org/10.1016/j.cell.2021.12.040. S0092867421015622.
[162] Holter JC, Pischke SE, de Boer E, Lind A, Jenum S, Holten AR, et al. Systemic complement activation is associated with respiratory failure in COVID-19 hospitalized patients. Proc Natl Acad Sci USA 2020;117:25018–25. https://doi.org/10.1073/pnas.2010540117.
[163] Cugno M, Meroni PL, Gualtierotti R, Griffini S, Grovetti E, Torri A, et al. Complement activation in patients with COVID-19: a novel therapeutic target. J Allergy Clin Immunol 2020;146:215–7. https://doi.org/10.1016/j.jaci.2020.05.006.
[164] Annane D, Heming N, Grimaldi-Bensouda L, Frémeaux-Bacchi V, Vigan M, Roux A-L, et al. Eculizumab as an emergency treatment for adult patients with severe COVID-19 in the intensive care unit: a proof-of-concept study. EClinicalMedicine 2020;28:100590. https://doi.org/10.1016/j.eclinm.2020.100590.
[165] Nanda A, Vura NVRK, Gravenstein S. COVID-19 in older adults. Aging Clin Exp Res 2020;32:1199–202. https://doi.org/10.1007/s40520-020-01581-5.
[166] Yan C, Gao H. New insights for C5a and C5a receptors in sepsis. Front Immun 2012;3. https://doi.org/10.3389/fimmu.2012.00368.
[167] Cyprian FS, Suleman M, Abdelhafez I, Doudin A, Masud Danjuma IM, Mir FA, et al. Complement C5a and clinical markers as predictors of COVID-19 disease severity and mortality in a multi-ethnic population. Front Immunol 2021;12:707159. https://doi.org/10.3389/fimmu.2021.707159.
[168] Huber S, Massri M, Grasse M, Fleischer V, Kellnerová S, Harpf V, et al. Systemic inflammation and complement activation parameters predict clinical outcome of severe SARS-CoV-2 infections. Viruses 2021;13:2376. https://doi.org/10.3390/v13122376.
[169] Gauchel N, Rieder M, Krauel K, Goller I, Jeserich M, Salzer U, et al. Complement system component dysregulation is a distinctive feature of COVID-19 disease: a prospective and comparative analysis of patients admitted to the emergency department for suspected COVID-19 disease. J Thromb Thrombolysis 2022;53(4):788–97. https://doi.org/10.1007/s11239-021-02617-x.
[170] Lafon E, Diem G, Witting C, Zaderer V, Bellmann-Weiler RM, Reindl M, et al. Potent SARS-CoV-2-specific T cell immunity and low anaphylatoxin levels correlate with mild disease progression in COVID-19 patients. Front Immunol 2021;12:684014. https://doi.org/10.3389/fimmu.2021.684014.
[171] Skendros P, Mitsios A, Chrysanthopoulou A, Mastellos DC, Metallidis S, Rafailidis P, et al. Complement and tissue factor–enriched neutrophil extracellular traps are key drivers in COVID-19 immunothrombosis. Journal of Clinical Investigation 2020;130:6151–7. https://doi.org/10.1172/JCI141374.
[172] Magro C, Mulvey JJ, Berlin D, Nuovo G, Salvatore S, Harp J, et al. Complement associated microvascular injury and thrombosis in the pathogenesis of severe COVID-19 infection: a report of five cases. Transl Res 2020;220:1–13. https://doi.org/10.1016/j.trsl.2020.04.007.
[173] Macor P, Durigutto P, Mangogna A, Bussani R, De Maso L, D'Errico S, et al. Multiple-organ complement deposition on vascular endothelium in COVID-19 patients. Biomedicines 2021;9:1003. https://doi.org/10.3390/biomedicines9081003.
[174] Magro CM, Mulvey J, Kubiak J, Mikhail S, Suster D, Crowson AN, et al. Severe COVID-19: a multifaceted viral vasculopathy syndrome. Ann Diagn Pathol 2021;50:151645. https://doi.org/10.1016/j.anndiagpath.2020.151645.

[175] Chen M, Jayne DRW, Zhao M-H. Complement in ANCA-associated vasculitis: mechanisms and implications for management. Nat Rev Nephrol 2017;13:359–67. https://doi.org/10.1038/nrneph.2017.37.

[176] Goodship THJ, Cook HT, Fakhouri F, Fervenza FC, Frémeaux-Bacchi V, Kavanagh D, et al. Atypical hemolytic uremic syndrome and C3 glomerulopathy: conclusions from a "kidney disease: improving global outcomes" (KDIGO) controversies conference. Kidney Int 2017;91:539–51. https://doi.org/10.1016/j.kint.2016.10.005.

[177] Chaturvedi S, Braunstein EM, Brodsky RA. Antiphospholipid syndrome: complement activation, complement gene mutations, and therapeutic implications. J Thromb Haemost 2021;19:607–16. https://doi.org/10.1111/jth.15082.

[178] Cugno M, Meroni PL, Gualtierotti R, Griffini S, Grovetti E, Torri A, et al. Complement activation and endothelial perturbation parallel COVID-19 severity and activity. J Autoimmun 2021;116:102560. https://doi.org/10.1016/j.jaut.2020.102560.

[179] Aiello S, Gastoldi S, Galbusera M, Ruggenenti PL, Portalupi V, Rota S, et al. C5a and C5aR1 are key drivers of microvascular platelet aggregation in clinical entities spanning from aHUS to COVID-19 [published correction appears in Blood Adv. 2022 May 10;6(9):2812]. Blood Adv 2022;6(3):866–81. https://doi.org/10.1182/bloodadvances.2021005246.

[180] Carvelli J, Demaria O, Vély F, Batista L, Chouaki Benmansour N, Fares J, et al. Association of COVID-19 inflammation with activation of the C5a-C5aR1 axis. Nature 2020;588:146–50. https://doi.org/10.1038/s41586-020-2600-6.

[181] Peffault de Latour R, Bergeron A, Lengline E, Dupont T, Marchal A, Galicier L, et al. Complement C5 inhibition in patients with COVID-19 - a promising target? Haematol 2020;105:2847–50. https://doi.org/10.3324/haematol.2020.260117.

[182] Gralinski LE, Sheahan TP, Morrison TE, Menachery VD, Jensen K, Leist SR, et al. Complement activation contributes to severe acute respiratory syndrome coronavirus pathogenesis. mBio 2018;9. https://doi.org/10.1128/mBio.01753-18.

[183] Jiang Y, Zhao G, Song N, Li P, Chen Y, Guo Y, et al. Blockade of the C5a–C5aR axis alleviates lung damage in hDPP4 -transgenic mice infected with MERS-CoV. Emerg Microb Infect 2018;7:1–12. https://doi.org/10.1038/s41426-018-0063-8.

[184] Diao B, Wang C, Tan Y, Chen X, Liu Y, Ning L, et al. Reduction and functional exhaustion of T cells in patients with coronavirus disease 2019 (COVID-19). Front Immunol 2020;11:827. https://doi.org/10.3389/fimmu.2020.00827.

[185] McEneny-King AC, Monteleone JPR, Kazani SD, Ortiz SR. Pharmacokinetic and pharmacodynamic evaluation of ravulizumab in adults with severe coronavirus disease 2019. Infect Dis Ther 2021;10:1045–54. https://doi.org/10.1007/s40121-021-00425-7.

[186] Merkel PA, Jayne DR, Wang C, Hillson J, Bekker P. Evaluation of the safety and efficacy of avacopan, a C5a receptor inhibitor, in patients with antineutrophil cytoplasmic antibody–associated vasculitis treated concomitantly with rituximab or cyclophosphamide/azathioprine: protocol for a randomized, double-blind, active-controlled, phase 3 trial. JMIR Res Protoc 2020;9:e16664. https://doi.org/10.2196/16664.

[187] Mastellos DC, Pires da Silva BGP, Fonseca BAL, Fonseca NP, Auxiliadora-Martins M, Mastaglio S, et al. Complement C3 vs C5 inhibition in severe COVID-19: early clinical findings reveal differential biological efficacy. Clin Immunol 2020;220:108598. https://doi.org/10.1016/j.clim.2020.108598.

[188] Risitano AM, Mastellos DC, Huber-Lang M, Yancopoulou D, Garlanda C, Ciceri F, et al. Complement as a target in COVID-19? Nat Rev Immunol 2020;20:343–4. https://doi.org/10.1038/s41577-020-0320-7.

[189] Urwyler P, Charitos P, Moser S, Heijnen IAFM, Trendelenburg M, Thoma R, et al. Recombinant human C1 esterase inhibitor (conestat alfa) in the prevention of severe SARS-CoV-2 infection in hospitalized patients with COVID-19: a structured summary of a study protocol for a randomized, parallel-group, open-label, multi-center pilot trial (PROTECT-COVID-19). Trials 2021;22:1. https://doi.org/10.1186/s13063-020-04976-x.

[190] Barkoff CM, Mousa SA. Pharmacotherapy in COVID 19: potential impact of targeting the complement system. Biomedicines 2020;9:11. https://doi.org/10.3390/biomedicines9010011.

[191] Noris M. The case of complement inhibitors. Advances in Biological Regulation 2021;81:100822. https://doi.org/10.1016/j.jbior.2021.100822.

[192] Afzali B, Noris M, Lambrecht BN, Kemper C. The state of complement in COVID-19. Nat Rev Immunol 2022;22(2):77–84. https://doi.org/10.1038/s41577-021-00665-1.

[193] Wu Z, McGoogan JM. Characteristics of and important lessons from the coronavirus disease 2019 (COVID-19) outbreak in China: summary of a report of 72 314 cases from the Chinese center for disease control and prevention. JAMA 2020;323:1239–42. https://doi.org/10.1001/jama.2020.2648.

[194] Guan W-J, Ni Z-Y, Hu Y, Liang W-H, Ou C-Q, He J-X, et al. Clinical characteristics of coronavirus disease 2019 in China. N Engl J Med 2020;382:1708–20. https://doi.org/10.1056/NEJMoa2002032.

[195] Wiersinga WJ, Rhodes A, Cheng AC, Peacock SJ, Prescott HC. Pathophysiology, transmission, diagnosis, and treatment of coronavirus disease 2019 (COVID-19): a review. JAMA 2020;324:782–93. https://doi.org/10.1001/jama.2020.12839.

[196] Donnelly CA, Ghani AC, Leung GM, Hedley AJ, Fraser C, Riley S, et al. Epidemiological determinants of spread of causal agent of severe acute respiratory syndrome in Hong Kong. Lancet 2003;361:1761–6. https://doi.org/10.1016/S0140-6736(03)13410-1.

[197] Assiri A, McGeer A, Perl TM, Price CS, Al Rabeeah AA, Cummings DAT, et al. Hospital outbreak of Middle East respiratory syndrome coronavirus. N Engl J Med 2013;369:407–16. https://doi.org/10.1056/NEJMoa1306742.

[198] Cotten M, Watson SJ, Kellam P, Al-Rabeeah AA, Makhdoom HQ, Assiri A, et al. Transmission and evolution of the Middle East respiratory syndrome coronavirus in Saudi Arabia: a descriptive genomic study. Lancet 2013;382:1993–2002. https://doi.org/10.1016/S0140-6736(13)61887-5.

[199] Hong K-H, Choi J-P, Hong S-H, Lee J, Kwon J-S, Kim S-M, et al. Predictors of mortality in Middle East respiratory syndrome (MERS). Thorax 2018;73:286–9. https://doi.org/10.1136/thoraxjnl-2016-209313.

[200] Chan JCK, Tsui ELH, Wong VCW, Hospital Authority SARS Collaborative Group. Prognostication in severe acute respiratory syndrome: a retrospective time-course analysis of 1312 laboratory-confirmed patients in Hong Kong. Respirology 2007;12:531–42. https://doi.org/10.1111/j.1440-1843.2007.01102.x.

[201] Lu L, Zhong W, Bian Z, Li Z, Zhang K, Liang B, et al. A comparison of mortality-related risk factors of COVID-19, SARS, and MERS: a systematic review and meta-analysis. J Infect 2020;81:e18–25. https://doi.org/10.1016/j.jinf.2020.07.002.

[202] Ren Y, He Q-Y, Fan J, Jones B, Zhou Y, Xie Y, et al. The use of proteomics in the discovery of serum biomarkers from patients with severe acute respiratory syndrome. Proteomics 2004;4:3477–84. https://doi.org/10.1002/pmic.200400897.

[203] Gu J, Korteweg C. Pathology and pathogenesis of severe acute respiratory syndrome. Am J Pathol 2007;170:1136–47. https://doi.org/10.2353/ajpath.2007.061088.

[204] Poon TCW, Pang RTK, Chan KCA, Lee NLS, Chiu RWK, Tong Y-K, et al. Proteomic analysis reveals platelet factor 4 and beta-thromboglobulin as prognostic markers in severe acute respiratory syndrome. Electrophoresis 2012;33:1894–900. https://doi.org/10.1002/elps.201200002.

[205] Biomarkers Definitions Working Group. Biomarkers and surrogate endpoints: preferred definitions and conceptual framework. Clin Pharmacol Ther 2001;69:89–95. https://doi.org/10.1067/mcp.2001.113989.

[206] Sproston NR, Ashworth JJ. Role of C-reactive protein at sites of inflammation and infection. Front Immunol 2018;9:754. https://doi.org/10.3389/fimmu.2018.00754.

[207] Ngwa DN, Agrawal A. Structure-function relationships of C-reactive protein in bacterial infection. Front Immunol 2019;10:166. https://doi.org/10.3389/fimmu.2019.00166.

[208] Bodman-Smith KB, Melendez AJ, Campbell I, Harrison PT, Allen JM, Raynes JG. C-reactive protein-mediated phagocytosis and phospholipase D signalling through the high-affinity receptor for immunoglobulin G (FcgammaRI). Immunology 2002;107:252–60. https://doi.org/10.1046/j.1365-2567.2002.01481.x.

[209] Ming DK, Myall AC, Hernandez B, Weiße AY, Peach RL, Barahona M, et al. Informing antimicrobial management in the context of COVID-19: understanding the longitudinal dynamics of C-reactive protein and procalcitonin. BMC Infect Dis 2021;21:932. https://doi.org/10.1186/s12879-021-06621-7.

[210] Keddie S, Ziff O, Chou MKL, Taylor RL, Heslegrave A, Garr E, et al. Laboratory biomarkers associated with COVID-19 severity and management. Clin Immunol 2020;221:108614. https://doi.org/10.1016/j.clim.2020.108614.

[211] Foulkes AS, Selvaggi C, Shinnick D, Lumish H, Kim E, Cao T, et al. Understanding the link between obesity and severe COVID-19 outcomes: causal mediation by systemic inflammatory response. J Clin Endocrinol Metab 2021:dgab629. https://doi.org/10.1210/clinem/dgab629.

[212] Bettini S, Bucca G, Sensi C, Dal Prà C, Fabris R, Vettor R, et al. Higher levels of C-reactive protein and ferritin in patients with overweight and obesity and SARS-CoV-2-related pneumonia. Obes Facts 2021;14:543–9. https://doi.org/10.1159/000517851.

[213] Dugué P-A, Hodge AM, Ulvik A, Ueland PM, Midttun Ø, Rinaldi S, et al. Association of markers of inflammation, the kynurenine pathway and B vitamins with age and mortality, and a signature of inflammaging. J Gerontol A Biol Sci Med Sci 2022;77(4):826–36. https://doi.org/10.1093/gerona/glab163. glab163.

[214] Villoteau A, Asfar M, Otekpo M, Loison J, Gautier J, Annweiler C, et al. Elevated C-reactive protein in early COVID-19 predicts worse survival among hospitalized geriatric patients. PLoS One 2021;16:e0256931. https://doi.org/10.1371/journal.pone.0256931.

[215] Luo X, Zhou W, Yan X, Guo T, Wang B, Xia H, et al. Prognostic value of C-reactive protein in patients with coronavirus 2019. Clin Infect Dis 2020;71:2174–9. https://doi.org/10.1093/cid/ciaa641.

[216] Danwang C, Endomba FT, Nkeck JR, Wouna DLA, Robert A, Noubiap JJ. A meta-analysis of potential biomarkers associated with severity of coronavirus disease 2019 (COVID-19). Biomark Res 2020;8:37. https://doi.org/10.1186/s40364-020-00217-0.

[217] Müller B, White JC, Nylén ES, Snider RH, Becker KL, Habener JF. Ubiquitous expression of the calcitonin-i gene in multiple tissues in response to sepsis. J Clin Endocrinol Metab 2001;86:396–404. https://doi.org/10.1210/jcem.86.1.7089.

[218] Assicot M, Gendrel D, Carsin H, Raymond J, Guilbaud J, Bohuon C. High serum procalcitonin concentrations in patients with sepsis and infection. Lancet 1993;341:515–8. https://doi.org/10.1016/0140-6736(93)90277-n.

[219] Müller B, Harbarth S, Stolz D, Bingisser R, Mueller C, Leuppi J, et al. Diagnostic and prognostic accuracy of clinical and laboratory parameters in community-acquired pneumonia. BMC Infect Dis 2007;7:10. https://doi.org/10.1186/1471-2334-7-10.

[220] Kamat IS, Ramachandran V, Eswaran H, Guffey D, Musher DM. Procalcitonin to distinguish viral from bacterial pneumonia: a systematic review and meta-analysis. Clin Infect Dis 2020;70:538–42. https://doi.org/10.1093/cid/ciz545.

[221] Gautam S, Cohen AJ, Stahl Y, Valda Toro P, Young GM, Datta R, et al. Severe respiratory viral infection induces procalcitonin in the absence of bacterial pneumonia. Thorax 2020;75:974–81. https://doi.org/10.1136/thoraxjnl-2020-214896.

[222] Richards O, Pallmann P, King C, Cheema Y, Killick C, Thomas-Jones E, et al. Procalcitonin increase is associated with the development of critical care-acquired infections in COVID-19 ARDS. Antibiotics (Basel) 2021;10:1425. https://doi.org/10.3390/antibiotics10111425.

[223] Hu R, Han C, Pei S, Yin M, Chen X. Procalcitonin levels in COVID-19 patients. Int J Antimicrob Agents 2020;56:106051. https://doi.org/10.1016/j.ijantimicag.2020.106051.

[224] Zhang L, Hou J, Ma F-Z, Li J, Xue S, Xu Z-G. The common risk factors for progression and mortality in COVID-19 patients: a meta-analysis. Arch Virol 2021;166:2071–87. https://doi.org/10.1007/s00705-021-05012-2.

[225] Mikami T, Miyashita H, Yamada T, Harrington M, Steinberg D, Dunn A, et al. Risk factors for mortality in patients with COVID-19 in New York city. J Gen Intern Med 2021;36:17–26. https://doi.org/10.1007/s11606-020-05983-z.

[226] Lippi G, Plebani M. Procalcitonin in patients with severe coronavirus disease 2019 (COVID-19): a meta-analysis. Clin Chim Acta 2020;505:190–1. https://doi.org/10.1016/j.cca.2020.03.004.

[227] Williams EJ, Mair L, de Silva TI, Green DJ, House P, Cawthron K, et al. Evaluation of procalcitonin as a contribution to antimicrobial stewardship in SARS-CoV-2 infection: a retrospective cohort study. J Hosp Infect 2021;110:103–7. https://doi.org/10.1016/j.jhin.2021.01.006.

[228] Hoffmann M, Kleine-Weber H, Schroeder S, Krüger N, Herrler T, Erichsen S, et al. SARS-CoV-2 cell entry depends on ACE2 and TMPRSS2 and is blocked by a clinically proven protease inhibitor. Cell 2020;181:271–280.e8. https://doi.org/10.1016/j.cell.2020.02.052.

[229] Qi F, Qian S, Zhang S, Zhang Z. Single cell RNA sequencing of 13 human tissues identify cell types and receptors of human coronaviruses. Biochem Biophys Res Commun 2020;526:135–40. https://doi.org/10.1016/j.bbrc.2020.03.044.

[230] De Smet V, Verhulst S, van Grunsven LA. Single cell RNA sequencing analysis did not predict hepatocyte infection by SARS-CoV-2. J Hepatol 2020;73:993–5. https://doi.org/10.1016/j.jhep.2020.05.030.

[231] Hikmet F, Méar L, Å E, Micke P, Uhlén M, Lindskog C. The protein expression profile of ACE2 in human tissues. Mol Syst Biol 2020;16:e9610. https://doi.org/10.15252/msb.20209610.

[232] Lagana SM, Kudose S, Iuga AC, Lee MJ, Fazlollahi L, Remotti HE, et al. Hepatic pathology in patients dying of COVID-19: a series of 40 cases including clinical, histologic, and virologic data. Mod Pathol 2020;33:2147–55. https://doi.org/10.1038/s41379-020-00649-x.

[233] Sonzogni A, Previtali G, Seghezzi M, Grazia Alessio M, Gianatti A, Licini L, et al. Liver histopathology in severe COVID 19 respiratory failure is suggestive of vascular alterations. Liver Int 2020;40:2110–6. https://doi.org/10.1111/liv.14601.

[234] Marjot T, Webb GJ, Barritt AS, Moon AM, Stamataki Z, Wong VW, et al. COVID-19 and liver disease: mechanistic and clinical perspectives. Nat Rev Gastroenterol Hepatol 2021;18:348–64. https://doi.org/10.1038/s41575-021-00426-4.

[235] Zhang Y, Zheng L, Liu L, Zhao M, Xiao J, Zhao Q. Liver impairment in COVID-19 patients: a retrospective analysis of 115 cases from a single centre in Wuhan city, China. Liver Int 2020;40:2095–103. https://doi.org/10.1111/liv.14455.

[236] Richardson S, Hirsch JS, Narasimhan M, Crawford JM, McGinn T, Davidson KW, et al. Presenting characteristics, comorbidities, and outcomes among 5700 patients hospitalized with COVID-19 in the New York city area. JAMA 2020;323:2052–9. https://doi.org/10.1001/jama.2020.6775.

[237] Fan Z, Chen L, Li J, Cheng X, Yang J, Tian C, et al. Clinical features of COVID-19-related liver functional abnormality. Clin Gastroenterol Hepatol 2020;18:1561–6. https://doi.org/10.1016/j.cgh.2020.04.002.

[238] Zhao D, Yao F, Wang L, Zheng L, Gao Y, Ye J, et al. A comparative study on the clinical features of coronavirus 2019 (COVID-19) pneumonia with other pneumonias. Clin Infect Dis 2020;71:756–61. https://doi.org/10.1093/cid/ciaa247.

[239] Malik P, Patel U, Mehta D, Patel N, Kelkar R, Akrmah M, et al. Biomarkers and outcomes of COVID-19 hospitalisations: systematic review and meta-analysis. BMJ Evid Based Med 2021;26:107–8. https://doi.org/10.1136/bmjebm-2020-111536.

[240] Phipps MM, Barraza LH, LaSota ED, Sobieszczyk ME, Pereira MR, Zheng EX, et al. Acute liver injury in COVID-19: prevalence and association with clinical outcomes in a large U.S. Cohort. Hepatology 2020;72:807–17. https://doi.org/10.1002/hep.31404.

[241] Zhou F, Yu T, Du R, Fan G, Liu Y, Liu Z, et al. Clinical course and risk factors for mortality of adult inpatients with COVID-19 in Wuhan, China: a retrospective cohort study. Lancet 2020;395:1054–62. https://doi.org/10.1016/S0140-6736(20)30566-3.

[242] Da BL, Kushner T, El Halabi M, Paka P, Khalid M, Uberoi A, et al. Liver injury in hospitalized patients with COVID-19 correlates with hyper inflammatory response and elevated IL-6. Hepatol Commun 2020;5(2):177–88. https://doi.org/10.1002/hep4.1631.

[243] Bloom PP, Meyerowitz EA, Reinus Z, Daidone M, Gustafson J, Kim AY, et al. Liver biochemistries in hospitalized patients with COVID-19. Hepatology 2021;73:890–900. https://doi.org/10.1002/hep.31326.

[244] Buckholz AP, Kaplan A, Rosenblatt RE, Wan D. Clinical characteristics, diagnosis, and outcomes of 6 patients with COVID-19 infection and rhabdomyolysis. Mayo Clin Proc 2020;95:2557–9. https://doi.org/10.1016/j.mayocp.2020.09.005.

[245] Cui H-J, Tong X-L, Li P, Hao Y-X, Chen X-G, Li A-G, et al. Serum hepatic enzyme manifestations in patients with severe acute respiratory syndrome: retrospective analysis. World J Gastroenterol 2004;10:1652–5. https://doi.org/10.3748/wjg.v10.i11.1652.

[246] Inoue M, Nakashima R, Enomoto M, Koike Y, Zhao X, Yip K, et al. Plasma redox imbalance caused by albumin oxidation promotes lung-predominant NETosis and pulmonary cancer metastasis. Nat Commun 2018;9:5116. https://doi.org/10.1038/s41467-018-07550-x.

[247] Huang J, Cheng A, Kumar R, Fang Y, Chen G, Zhu Y, et al. Hypoalbuminemia predicts the outcome of COVID-19 independent of age and co-morbidity. J Med Virol 2020;92:2152–8. https://doi.org/10.1002/jmv.26003.

[248] Aziz M, Fatima R, Lee-Smith W, Assaly R. The association of low serum albumin level with severe COVID-19: a systematic review and meta-analysis. Crit Care 2020;24:255. https://doi.org/10.1186/s13054-020-02995-3.

[249] Violi F, Cangemi R, Romiti GF, Ceccarelli G, Oliva A, Alessandri F, et al. Is albumin predictor of mortality in COVID-19? Antioxid Redox Signal 2021;35:139–42. https://doi.org/10.1089/ars.2020.8142.

[250] Xu Y, Yang H, Wang J, Li X, Xue C, Niu C, et al. Serum albumin levels are a predictor of COVID-19 patient prognosis: evidence from a single cohort in chongqing, China. Int J Gen Med 2021;14:2785–97. https://doi.org/10.2147/IJGM.S312521.

[251] Soeters PB, Wolfe RR, Shenkin A. Hypoalbuminemia: pathogenesis and clinical significance. JPEN J Parenter Enteral Nutr 2019;43:181–93. https://doi.org/10.1002/jpen.1451.
[252] Carter B, Collins JT, Barlow-Pay F, Rickard F, Bruce E, Verduri A, et al. Nosocomial COVID-19 infection: examining the risk of mortality. The COPE-Nosocomial Study (COVID in Older PEople). J Hosp Infect 2020;106:376–84. https://doi.org/10.1016/j.jhin.2020.07.013.
[253] Ciceri F, Castagna A, Rovere-Querini P, De Cobelli F, Ruggeri A, Galli L, et al. Early predictors of clinical outcomes of COVID-19 outbreak in Milan, Italy. Clin Immunol 2020;217:108509. https://doi.org/10.1016/j.clim.2020.108509.
[254] Long J, Luo Y, Wei Y, Xie C, Yuan J. The effect of cardiovascular disease and acute cardiac injury on fatal COVID-19: a meta-analysis. Am J Emerg Med 2021;48:128–39. https://doi.org/10.1016/j.ajem.2021.04.013.
[255] Deng G, Yin M, Chen X, Zeng F. Clinical determinants for fatality of 44,672 patients with COVID-19. Crit Care 2020;24:179. https://doi.org/10.1186/s13054-020-02902-w.
[256] Zhu Z, Wang M, Lin W, Cai Q, Zhang L, Chen D, et al. Cardiac biomarkers, cardiac injury, and comorbidities associated with severe illness and mortality in coronavirus disease 2019 (COVID-19): a systematic review and meta-analysis. Immun Inflamm Dis 2021;9:1071–100. https://doi.org/10.1002/iid3.471.
[257] Li C, Jiang J, Wang F, Zhou N, Veronese G, Moslehi JJ, et al. Longitudinal correlation of biomarkers of cardiac injury, inflammation, and coagulation to outcome in hospitalized COVID-19 patients. J Mol Cell Cardiol 2020;147:74–87. https://doi.org/10.1016/j.yjmcc.2020.08.008.
[258] Shi S, Qin M, Shen B, Cai Y, Liu T, Yang F, et al. Association of cardiac injury with mortality in hospitalized patients with COVID-19 in Wuhan, China. JAMA Cardiol 2020;5:802–10. https://doi.org/10.1001/jamacardio.2020.0950.
[259] Guo T, Fan Y, Chen M, Wu X, Zhang L, He T, et al. Cardiovascular implications of fatal outcomes of patients with coronavirus disease 2019 (COVID-19). JAMA Cardiol 2020;5:811–8. https://doi.org/10.1001/jamacardio.2020.1017.
[260] Stefanini GG, Chiarito M, Ferrante G, Cannata F, Azzolini E, Viggiani G, et al. Early detection of elevated cardiac biomarkers to optimise risk stratification in patients with COVID-19. Heart 2020;106:1512–8. https://doi.org/10.1136/heartjnl-2020-317322.
[261] Chung MK, Zidar DA, Bristow MR, Cameron SJ, Chan T, Harding CV, et al. COVID-19 and cardiovascular disease: from bench to bedside. Circ Res 2021;128:1214–36. https://doi.org/10.1161/CIRCRESAHA.121.317997.
[262] Guzik TJ, Mohiddin SA, Dimarco A, Patel V, Savvatis K, Marelli-Berg FM, et al. COVID-19 and the cardiovascular system: implications for risk assessment, diagnosis, and treatment options. Cardiovasc Res 2020;116:1666–87. https://doi.org/10.1093/cvr/cvaa106.
[263] Li L, Zhou Q, Xu J. Changes of laboratory cardiac markers and mechanisms of cardiac injury in coronavirus disease 2019. BioMed Res Int 2020;2020:7413673. https://doi.org/10.1155/2020/7413673.
[264] Thygesen K, Alpert JS, Jaffe AS, Chaitman BR, Bax JJ, Morrow DA, et al. Fourth universal definition of myocardial infarction (2018). Circulation 2018;138:e618–51. https://doi.org/10.1161/CIR.0000000000000617.
[265] Takeda S, Yamashita A, Maeda K, Maéda Y. Structure of the core domain of human cardiac troponin in the Ca(2+)-saturated form. Nature 2003;424:35–41. https://doi.org/10.1038/nature01780.
[266] Anderson PA, Malouf NN, Oakeley AE, Pagani ED, Allen PD. Troponin T isoform expression in humans. A comparison among normal and failing adult heart, fetal heart, and adult and fetal skeletal muscle. Circ Res 1991;69:1226–33. https://doi.org/10.1161/01.res.69.5.1226.
[267] Manocha KK, Kirzner J, Ying X, Yeo I, Peltzer B, Ang B, et al. Troponin and other biomarker levels and outcomes among patients hospitalized with COVID-19: derivation and validation of the HA2T2 COVID-19 mortality risk score. J Am Heart Assoc 2021;10:e018477. https://doi.org/10.1161/JAHA.120.018477.
[268] Kaufmann CC, Ahmed A, Kassem M, Freynhofer MK, Jäger B, Aicher G, et al. Improvement of outcome prediction of hospitalized patients with COVID-19 by a dual marker strategy using high-sensitive cardiac troponin I and copeptin. Clin Res Cardiol 2022;111(3):343–54. https://doi.org/10.1007/s00392-021-01970-4.
[269] Zwaenepoel B, Dhont S, Hoste E, Gevaert S, Schaubroeck H. The prognostic value of cardiac biomarkers and echocardiography in critical COVID-19. Front Cardiovasc Med 2021;8:752237. https://doi.org/10.3389/fcvm.2021.752237.

[270] Kinnunen P, Vuolteenaho O, Ruskoaho H. Mechanisms of atrial and brain natriuretic peptide release from rat ventricular myocardium: effect of stretching. Endocrinology 1993;132:1961–70. https://doi.org/10.1210/endo.132.5.8477647.

[271] Yasue H, Yoshimura M, Sumida H, Kikuta K, Kugiyama K, Jougasaki M, et al. Localization and mechanism of secretion of B-type natriuretic peptide in comparison with those of A-type natriuretic peptide in normal subjects and patients with heart failure. Circulation 1994;90:195–203. https://doi.org/10.1161/01.cir.90.1.195.

[272] Hunt PJ, Richards AM, Nicholls MG, Yandle TG, Doughty RN, Espiner EA. Immunoreactive amino-terminal pro-brain natriuretic peptide (NT-PROBNP): a new marker of cardiac impairment. Clin Endocrinol 1997;47:287–96. https://doi.org/10.1046/j.1365-2265.1997.2361058.x.

[273] Qin J-J, Cheng X, Zhou F, Lei F, Akolkar G, Cai J, et al. Redefining cardiac biomarkers in predicting mortality of inpatients with COVID-19. Hypertension 2020;76:1104–12. https://doi.org/10.1161/HYPERTENSIONAHA.120.15528.

[274] Ruscica M, Macchi C, Iodice S, Tersalvi G, Rota I, Ghidini S, et al. Prognostic parameters of in-hospital mortality in COVID-19 patients-An Italian experience. Eur J Clin Invest 2021;51:e13629. https://doi.org/10.1111/eci.13629.

[275] Zinellu A, Sotgia S, Fois AG, Mangoni AA. Serum CK-MB, COVID-19 severity and mortality: an updated systematic review and meta-analysis with meta-regression. Adv Med Sci 2021;66:304–14. https://doi.org/10.1016/j.advms.2021.07.001.

[276] Ma C, Tu D, Gu J, Xu Q, Hou P, Wu H, et al. The predictive value of myoglobin for COVID-19-related adverse outcomes: a systematic review and meta-analysis. Front Cardiovasc Med 2021;8:757799. https://doi.org/10.3389/fcvm.2021.757799.

[277] Antunes KH, Fachi JL, de Paula R, da Silva EF, Pral LP, dos Santos AÁ, et al. Microbiota-derived acetate protects against respiratory syncytial virus infection through a GPR43-type 1 interferon response. Nat Commun 2019;10:3273. https://doi.org/10.1038/s41467-019-11152-6.

[278] Hamming I, Timens W, Bulthuis MLC, Lely AT, Navis GJ, van Goor H. Tissue distribution of ACE2 protein, the functional receptor for SARS coronavirus. A first step in understanding SARS pathogenesis. J Pathol 2004;203:631–7. https://doi.org/10.1002/path.1570.

[279] null A, Al-Farabi MJ, Nugraha RA, Marsudi BA, Azmi Y. Biomarkers of endothelial dysfunction and outcomes in coronavirus disease 2019 (COVID-19) patients: a systematic review and meta-analysis. Microvasc Res 2021;138:104224. https://doi.org/10.1016/j.mvr.2021.104224.

[280] Liao D, Zhou F, Luo L, Xu M, Wang H, Xia J, et al. Haematological characteristics and risk factors in the classification and prognosis evaluation of COVID-19: a retrospective cohort study. Lancet Haematol 2020;7:e671–8. https://doi.org/10.1016/S2352-3026(20)30217-9.

[281] Favresse J, Lippi G, Roy P-M, Chatelain B, Jacqmin H, Ten Cate H, et al. D-dimer: preanalytical, analytical, postanalytical variables, and clinical applications. Crit Rev Clin Lab Sci 2018;55:548–77. https://doi.org/10.1080/10408363.2018.1529734.

[282] Polimeni A, Leo I, Spaccarotella C, Mongiardo A, Sorrentino S, Sabatino J, et al. Differences in coagulopathy indices in patients with severe versus non-severe COVID-19: a meta-analysis of 35 studies and 6427 patients. Sci Rep 2021;11:10464. https://doi.org/10.1038/s41598-021-89967-x.

[283] Chaudhary R, Garg J, Houghton DE, Murad MH, Kondur A, Chaudhary R, et al. Thromboinflammatory biomarkers in COVID-19: systematic review and meta-analysis of 17,052 patients. Mayo Clin Proc Innov Qual Outcomes 2021;5:388–402. https://doi.org/10.1016/j.mayocpiqo.2021.01.009.

[284] Zhao R, Su Z, Komissarov AA, Liu S-L, Yi G, Idell S, et al. Associations of D-dimer on admission and clinical features of COVID-19 patients: a systematic review, meta-analysis, and meta-regression. Front Immunol 2021;12:691249. https://doi.org/10.3389/fimmu.2021.691249.

[285] Löf A, Müller JP, Brehm MA. A biophysical view on von Willebrand factor activation. J Cell Physiol 2018;233:799–810. https://doi.org/10.1002/jcp.25887.

[286] Blasi A, von Meijenfeldt FA, Adelmeijer J, Calvo A, Ibañez C, Perdomo J, et al. In vitro hypercoagulability and ongoing in vivo activation of coagulation and fibrinolysis in COVID-19 patients on anticoagulation. J Thromb Haemost 2020;18:2646–53. https://doi.org/10.1111/jth.15043.

[287] Cotter AH, Yang S-JT, Shafi H, Cotter TM, Palmer-Toy DE. Elevated von Willebrand factor Antigen is an early predictor of mortality and prolonged length of stay for coronavirus disease 2019 (COVID-19) inpatients. Arch Pathol Lab Med 2022;146(1):34–7. https://doi.org/10.5858/arpa.2021-0255-SA.

[288] Sperk M, van Domselaar R, Rodriguez JE, Mikaeloff F, Sá Vinhas B, Saccon E, et al. Utility of proteomics in emerging and Re-emerging infectious diseases caused by RNA viruses. J Proteome Res 2020;19:4259–74. https://doi.org/10.1021/acs.jproteome.0c00380.

[289] Kimura Y, Nakai Y, Shin J, Hara M, Takeda Y, Kubo S, et al. Identification of serum prognostic biomarkers of severe COVID-19 using a quantitative proteomic approach. Sci Rep 2021;11:20638. https://doi.org/10.1038/s41598-021-98253-9.

[290] Klassen JL. Defining microbiome function. Nature Microbiology 2018;3:864–9. https://doi.org/10.1038/s41564-018-0189-4.

[291] Human Microbiome Project Consortium. Structure, function and diversity of the healthy human microbiome. Nature 2012;486:207–14. https://doi.org/10.1038/nature11234.

[292] Gill SR, Pop M, DeBoy RT, Eckburg PB, Turnbaugh PJ, Samuel BS, et al. Metagenomic analysis of the human distal gut microbiome. Science 2006;312:1355–9. https://doi.org/10.1126/science.1124234.

[293] Ostaff MJ, Stange EF, Wehkamp J. Antimicrobial peptides and gut microbiota in homeostasis and pathology. EMBO Mol Med 2013;5:1465–83. https://doi.org/10.1002/emmm.201201773.

[294] Proctor LM. The human microbiome project in 2011 and beyond. Cell Host Microbe 2011;10:287–91. https://doi.org/10.1016/j.chom.2011.10.001.

[295] Proctor L. Priorities for the next 10 years of human microbiome research. Nature 2019;569:623–5. https://doi.org/10.1038/d41586-019-01654-0.

[296] Reinold J, Farahpour F, Fehring C, Dolff S, Konik M, Korth J, et al. A pro-inflammatory gut microbiome characterizes SARS-CoV-2 infected patients and a reduction in the connectivity of an anti-inflammatory bacterial network associates with severe COVID-19. Front Cell Infect Microbiol 2021;11. https://doi.org/10.3389/fcimb.2021.747816.

[297] Sarkar A, Harty S, Moeller AH, Klein SL, Erdman SE, Friston KJ, et al. The gut microbiome as a biomarker of differential susceptibility to SARS-CoV-2. Trends Mol Med 2021;27:1115–34. https://doi.org/10.1016/j.molmed.2021.09.009.

[298] Dang AT, Marsland BJ. Microbes, metabolites, and the gut–lung axis. Mucosal Immunol 2019;12:843–50. https://doi.org/10.1038/s41385-019-0160-6.

[299] Budden KF, Gellatly SL, Wood DLA, Cooper MA, Morrison M, Hugenholtz P, et al. Emerging pathogenic links between microbiota and the gut–lung axis. Nat Rev Microbiol 2017;15:55–63. https://doi.org/10.1038/nrmicro.2016.142.

[300] Sencio V, Machado MG, Trottein F. The lung–gut axis during viral respiratory infections: the impact of gut dysbiosis on secondary disease outcomes. Mucosal Immunol 2021;14:296–304. https://doi.org/10.1038/s41385-020-00361-8.

[301] de Oliveira GLV, Oliveira CNS, Pinzan CF, de Salis LVV, Cardoso CR de B. Microbiota modulation of the gut-lung Axis in COVID-19. Front Immunol 2021;12. https://doi.org/10.3389/fimmu.2021.635471.

[302] Wu Y, Cheng X, Jiang G, Tang H, Ming S, Tang L, et al. Altered oral and gut microbiota and its association with SARS-CoV-2 viral load in COVID-19 patients during hospitalization. Npj Biofilms and Microbiomes 2021;7:61. https://doi.org/10.1038/s41522-021-00232-5.

[303] Yeoh YK, Zuo T, Lui GC-Y, Zhang F, Liu Q, Li AY, et al. Gut microbiota composition reflects disease severity and dysfunctional immune responses in patients with COVID-19. Gut 2021;70. https://doi.org/10.1136/gutjnl-2020-323020.

[304] Zuo T, Zhang F, Lui GCY, Yeoh YK, Li AYL, Zhan H, et al. Alterations in gut microbiota of patients with COVID-19 during time of hospitalization. Gastroenterology 2020;159(4):1302–1310.e5. https://doi.org/10.1053/j.gastro.2020.05.048.

[305] Iacob S, Iacob DG. Infectious threats, the intestinal barrier, and its trojan horse: dysbiosis. Front Microbiol 2019;10. https://doi.org/10.3389/fmicb.2019.01676.

[306] Giron LB, Dweep H, Yin X, Wang H, Damra M, Goldman AR, et al. Plasma markers of disrupted gut permeability in severe COVID-19 patients. Front Immunol 2021;12. https://doi.org/10.3389/fimmu.2021.686240.

[307] Saia RS, Giusti H, Luis-Silva F, Pedroso K de JB, Auxiliadora-Martins M, Morejón KML, et al. Clinical investigation of intestinal fatty acid-binding protein (I-FABP) as a biomarker of SARS-CoV-2 infection. Int J Infect Dis 2021;113:82–6. https://doi.org/10.1016/j.ijid.2021.09.051.

[308] Venzon M, Bernard-Raichon L, Klein J, Axelrad J, Hussey G, Sullivan A, et al. Gut microbiome dysbiosis during COVID-19 is associated with increased risk for bacteremia and microbial translocation. bioRxiv 2022. https://doi.org/10.1101/2021.07.15.452246.

[309] Sokol H, Contreras V, Maisonnasse P, Desmons A, Delache B, Sencio V, et al. SARS-CoV-2 infection in nonhuman primates alters the composition and functional activity of the gut microbiota. Gut Microb 2021;13:1893113. https://doi.org/10.1080/19490976.2021.1893113.

[310] Sencio V, Gallerand A, Gomes Machado M, Deruyter L, Heumel S, Soulard D, et al. Influenza virus infection impairs the gut's barrier properties and favors secondary enteric bacterial infection through reduced production of short-chain fatty acids. Infect Immun 2021;89. https://doi.org/10.1128/IAI.00734-20.

[311] Corrêa-Oliveira R, Fachi JL, Vieira A, Sato FT, Vinolo MAR. Regulation of immune cell function by short-chain fatty acids. Clinical & Translational Immunology 2016;5:e73. https://doi.org/10.1038/cti.2016.17.

[312] Vieira AT, Galvão I, Macia LM, Sernaglia ÉM, Vinolo MAR, Garcia CC, et al. Dietary fiber and the short-chain fatty acid acetate promote resolution of neutrophilic inflammation in a model of gout in mice. J Leukoc Biol 2017;101:275–84. https://doi.org/10.1189/jlb.3A1015-453RRR.

[313] Donovan C, Liu G, Shen S, Marshall JE, Kim RY, Alemao CA, et al. The role of the microbiome and the NLRP3 inflammasome in the gut and lung. J Leukoc Biol 2020;108:925–35. https://doi.org/10.1002/JLB.3MR0720-472RR.

[314] Macia L, Tan J, Vieira AT, Leach K, Stanley D, Luong S, et al. Metabolite-sensing receptors GPR43 and GPR109A facilitate dietary fibre-induced gut homeostasis through regulation of the inflammasome. Nat Commun 2015;6:6734. https://doi.org/10.1038/ncomms7734.

[315] Vieira AT, Galvão I, Amaral FA, Teixeira MM, Nicoli JR, Martins FS. Oral treatment with Bifidobacterium longum 5 1A reduced inflammation in a murine experimental model of gout. Benef Microbes 2015;6:799–806. https://doi.org/10.3920/BM2015.0015.

[316] Ziegler CGK, Allon SJ, Nyquist SK, Mbano IM, Miao VN, Tzouanas CN, et al. SARS-CoV-2 receptor ACE2 is an interferon-stimulated gene in human airway epithelial cells and is detected in specific cell subsets across tissues. Cell 2020;181:1016–1035.e19. https://doi.org/10.1016/j.cell.2020.04.035.

[317] Soni S, Jiang Y, Tesfaigzi Y, Hornick JL, Çataltepe S. Comparative analysis of ACE2 protein expression in rodent, non-human primate, and human respiratory tract at baseline and after injury: a conundrum for COVID-19 pathogenesis. PLoS One 2021;16:e0247510. https://doi.org/10.1371/journal.pone.0247510.

[318] Yang T, Chakraborty S, Saha P, Mell B, Cheng X, Yeo J-Y, et al. Gnotobiotic rats reveal that gut microbiota regulates colonic mRNA of Ace2 , the receptor for SARS-CoV-2 infectivity. Hypertension 2020;76. https://doi.org/10.1161/HYPERTENSIONAHA.120.15360.

[319] Chen R, Yu Y, Li W, Liu Y, Lu J, Chen F, et al. Gastrointestinal symptoms associated with unfavorable prognosis of COVID-19 patients: a retrospective study. Front Med 2020;7. https://doi.org/10.3389/fmed.2020.608259.

[320] Xu J, Chu M, Zhong F, Tan X, Tang G, Mai J, et al. Digestive symptoms of COVID-19 and expression of ACE2 in digestive tract organs. Cell Death Discovery 2020;6:76. https://doi.org/10.1038/s41420-020-00307-w.

[321] Koester ST, Li N, Lachance DM, Morella NM, Dey N. Variability in digestive and respiratory tract Ace2 expression is associated with the microbiome. PLoS One 2021;16:e0248730. https://doi.org/10.1371/journal.pone.0248730.

[322] Villapol S. Gastrointestinal symptoms associated with COVID-19: impact on the gut microbiome. Transl Res 2020;226:57–69. https://doi.org/10.1016/j.trsl.2020.08.004.

[323] Cruz CS, Ricci MF, Vieira AT. Gut microbiota modulation as a potential target for the treatment of lung infections. Front Pharmacol 2021;12. https://doi.org/10.3389/fphar.2021.724033.

[324] Zuo T, Liu Q, Zhang F, Lui GC-Y, Tso EY, Yeoh YK, et al. Depicting SARS-CoV-2 faecal viral activity in association with gut microbiota composition in patients with COVID-19. Gut 2021;70(2):276–84. https://doi.org/10.1136/gutjnl-2020-322294. gutjnl-2020.

[325] Lopez-Leon S, Wegman-Ostrosky T, Perelman C, Sepulveda R, Rebolledo PA, Cuapio A, et al. More than 50 long-term effects of COVID-19: a systematic review and meta-analysis. Sci Rep 2021;11:16144. https://doi.org/10.1038/s41598-021-95565-8.

[326] Bosco N, Noti M. The aging gut microbiome and its impact on host immunity. Gene Immun 2021;22:289–303. https://doi.org/10.1038/s41435-021-00126-8.

[327] Witkowski M, Weeks TL, Hazen SL. Gut microbiota and cardiovascular disease. Circ Res 2020;127:553–70. https://doi.org/10.1161/CIRCRESAHA.120.316242.

[328] Abenavoli L, Scarpellini E, Colica C, Boccuto L, Salehi B, Sharifi-Rad J, et al. Gut microbiota and obesity: a role for probiotics. Nutrients 2019;11:2690. https://doi.org/10.3390/nu11112690.

[329] Li W-Z, Stirling K, Yang J-J, Zhang L. Gut microbiota and diabetes: from correlation to causality and mechanism. World J Diabetes 2020;11:293–308. https://doi.org/10.4239/wjd.v11.i7.293.

[330] d'Ettorre G, Ceccarelli G, Marazzato M, Campagna G, Pinacchio C, Alessandri F, et al. Challenges in the management of SARS-CoV2 infection: the role of oral bacteriotherapy as complementary therapeutic strategy to avoid the progression of COVID-19. Front Med 2020;7. https://doi.org/10.3389/fmed.2020.00389.

[331] Ceccarelli G, Borrazzo C, Pinacchio C, Santinelli L, Pietro IG, Cavallari EN, et al. Oral bacteriotherapy in patients with COVID-19: a retrospective cohort study. Front Nutr 2021;7. https://doi.org/10.3389/fnut.2020.613928.

[332] He L-H, Ren L-F, Li J-F, Wu Y-N, Li X, Zhang L. Intestinal flora as a potential strategy to fight SARS-CoV-2 infection. Front Microbiol 2020;11. https://doi.org/10.3389/fmicb.2020.01388.

[333] Brüssow H. Host-modifying drugs against COVID -19: some successes, but not yet the breakthrough. Environ Microbiol 2021:1462–2920. https://doi.org/10.1111/1462-2920.15828. 15828.

[334] Russell CD, Millar JE, Baillie JK. Clinical evidence does not support corticosteroid treatment for 2019-nCoV lung injury. Lancet 2020;395:473–5. https://doi.org/10.1016/S0140-6736(20)30317-2.

[335] WHO Rapid Evidence Appraisal for COVID-19 Therapies (REACT) Working Group, Sterne JAC, Murthy S, Diaz JV, Slutsky AS, Villar J, et al. Association between administration of systemic corticosteroids and mortality among critically ill patients with COVID-19: a meta-analysis. JAMA 2020;324:1330–41. https://doi.org/10.1001/jama.2020.17023.

[336] Wagner C, Griesel M, Mikolajewska A, Mueller A, Nothacker M, Kley K, et al. Systemic corticosteroids for the treatment of COVID-19. Cochrane Database Syst Rev 2021;8:CD014963. https://doi.org/10.1002/14651858.CD014963.

[337] Salama C, Han J, Yau L, Reiss WG, Kramer B, Neidhart JD, et al. Tocilizumab in patients hospitalized with covid-19 pneumonia. N Engl J Med 2021;384:20–30. https://doi.org/10.1056/NEJMoa2030340.

[338] Soin AS, Kumar K, Choudhary NS, Sharma P, Mehta Y, Kataria S, et al. Tocilizumab plus standard care versus standard care in patients in India with moderate to severe COVID-19-associated cytokine release syndrome (COVINTOC): an open-label, multicentre, randomised, controlled, phase 3 trial. Lancet Respir Med 2021;9:511–21. https://doi.org/10.1016/S2213-2600(21)00081-3.

[339] Rosas IO, Bräu N, Waters M, Go RC, Hunter BD, Bhagani S, et al. Tocilizumab in hospitalized patients with severe covid-19 pneumonia. N Engl J Med 2021;384:1503–16. https://doi.org/10.1056/NEJMoa2028700.

[340] Della-Torre E, Campochiaro C, Cavalli G, De Luca G, Napolitano A, La Marca S, et al. Interleukin-6 blockade with sarilumab in severe COVID-19 pneumonia with systemic hyperinflammation: an open-label cohort study. Ann Rheum Dis 2020;79:1277–85. https://doi.org/10.1136/annrheumdis-2020-218122.

[341] Gritti G, Raimondi F, Bottazzi B, Ripamonti D, Riva I, Landi F, et al. Siltuximab downregulates interleukin-8 and pentraxin 3 to improve ventilatory status and survival in severe COVID-19. Leukemia 2021;35:2710–4. https://doi.org/10.1038/s41375-021-01299-x.

[342] Campochiaro C, Della-Torre E, Cavalli G, De Luca G, Ripa M, Boffini N, et al. Efficacy and safety of tocilizumab in severe COVID-19 patients: a single-centre retrospective cohort study. Eur J Intern Med 2020;76:43–9. https://doi.org/10.1016/j.ejim.2020.05.021.

[343] Salvarani C, Dolci G, Massari M, Merlo DF, Cavuto S, Savoldi L, et al. Effect of tocilizumab vs standard care on clinical worsening in patients hospitalized with COVID-19 pneumonia: a randomized clinical trial. JAMA Intern Med 2021;181:24–31. https://doi.org/10.1001/jamainternmed.2020.6615.

[344] Cremer PC, Abbate A, Hudock K, McWilliams C, Mehta J, Chang SY, et al. Mavrilimumab in patients with severe COVID-19 pneumonia and systemic hyperinflammation (MASH-COVID): an investigator initiated, multicentre, double-blind, randomised, placebo-controlled trial. Lancet Rheumatol 2021;3:e410–8. https://doi.org/10.1016/S2665-9913(21)00070-9.

[345] De Luca G, Cavalli G, Campochiaro C, Della-Torre E, Angelillo P, Tomelleri A, et al. GM-CSF blockade with mavrilimumab in severe COVID-19 pneumonia and systemic hyperinflammation: a single-centre, prospective cohort study. Lancet Rheumatol 2020;2:e465–73. https://doi.org/10.1016/S2665-9913(20)30170-3.

[346] Pupim L, Wang TS, Hudock K, Denson J, Fourie N, Hercilla Vasquez L, et al. LB0001 MAVRILIMUMAB improves outcomes in phase 2 trial IN NON-MECHANICALLY-VENTILATED patients with severe COVID-19 pneumonia and systemic hyperinflammation. Ann Rheum Dis 2021;80:198. https://doi.org/10.1136/annrheumdis-2021-eular.5012.

[347] Patel J, Beishuizen A, Ruiz XB, Boughanmi H, Cahn A, Criner GJ, et al. A randomized trial of otilimab in severe COVID-19 pneumonia (OSCAR). medRxiv 2021. https://doi.org/10.1101/2021.04.14.21255475.

[348] Fisher BA, Veenith T, Slade D, Gaskell C, Rowland M, Whitehouse T, et al. Namilumab or infliximab compared with standard of care in hospitalised patients with COVID-19 (CATALYST): a randomised, multicentre, multi-arm, multistage, open-label, adaptive, phase 2, proof-of-concept trial. Lancet Respir Med 2021. https://doi.org/10.1016/S2213-2600(21)00460-4. S2213260021004604.

[349] Temesgen Z, Assi M, Shweta FNU, Vergidis P, Rizza SA, Bauer PR, et al. GM-CSF neutralization with Lenzilumab in severe COVID-19 pneumonia: a case-cohort study. Mayo Clin Proc 2020;95:2382–94. https://doi.org/10.1016/j.mayocp.2020.08.038.

[350] Temesgen Z, Burger CD, Baker J, Polk C, Libertin CR, Kelley CF, et al. Lenzilumab in hospitalised patients with COVID-19 pneumonia (LIVE-AIR): a phase 3, randomised, placebo-controlled trial. Lancet Respir Med 2021;(21):S2213–600. https://doi.org/10.1016/S2213-2600(21)00494-X. 00494-X.

[351] Kyriazopoulou E, Panagopoulos P, Metallidis S, Dalekos GN, Poulakou G, Gatselis N, et al. An open label trial of anakinra to prevent respiratory failure in COVID-19. Elife 2021;10:e66125. https://doi.org/10.7554/eLife.66125.

[352] Kyriazopoulou E, Poulakou G, Milionis H, Metallidis S, Adamis G, Tsiakos K, et al. Early treatment of COVID-19 with anakinra guided by soluble urokinase plasminogen receptor plasma levels: a double-blind, randomized controlled phase 3 trial. Nat Med 2021;27:1752–60. https://doi.org/10.1038/s41591-021-01499-z.

[353] Tharaux P-L, Pialoux G, Pavot A, Mariette X, Hermine O, Resche-Rigon M, et al. Effect of anakinra versus usual care in adults in hospital with COVID-19 and mild-to-moderate pneumonia (CORIMUNO-ANA-1): a randomised controlled trial. Lancet Respir Med 2021;9:295–304. https://doi.org/10.1016/S2213-2600(20)30556-7.

[354] Caricchio R, Abbate A, Gordeev I, Meng J, Hsue PY, Neogi T, et al. Effect of canakinumab vs placebo on survival without invasive mechanical ventilation in patients hospitalized with severe COVID-19: a randomized clinical trial. JAMA 2021;326:230. https://doi.org/10.1001/jama.2021.9508.

[355] Galani I-E, Andreakos E. Impaired innate antiviral defenses in COVID-19: causes, consequences and therapeutic opportunities. Semin Immunol 2021;55:101522. https://doi.org/10.1016/j.smim.2021.101522.

[356] Galani IE, Triantafyllia V, Eleminiadou E-E, Koltsida O, Stavropoulos A, Manioudaki M, et al. Interferon-λ mediates non-redundant front-line antiviral protection against influenza virus infection without compromising host fitness. Immunity 2017;46:875–890.e6. https://doi.org/10.1016/j.immuni.2017.04.025.

[357] Schubert K, Karousis ED, Jomaa A, Scaiola A, Echeverria B, Gurzeler L-A, et al. SARS-CoV-2 Nsp1 binds the ribosomal mRNA channel to inhibit translation. Nat Struct Mol Biol 2020;27:959–66. https://doi.org/10.1038/s41594-020-0511-8.

[358] Lei X, Dong X, Ma R, Wang W, Xiao X, Tian Z, et al. Activation and evasion of type I interferon responses by SARS-CoV-2. Nat Commun 2020;11:3810. https://doi.org/10.1038/s41467-020-17665-9.

[359] Zheng Y, Zhuang M-W, Han L, Zhang J, Nan M-L, Zhan P, et al. Severe acute respiratory syndrome coronavirus 2 (SARS-CoV-2) membrane (M) protein inhibits type I and III interferon production by targeting RIG-I/MDA-5 signaling. Signal Transduct Target Ther 2020;5:299. https://doi.org/10.1038/s41392-020-00438-7.

[360] Miorin L, Kehrer T, Sanchez-Aparicio MT, Zhang K, Cohen P, Patel RS, et al. SARS-CoV-2 Orf6 hijacks Nup98 to block STAT nuclear import and antagonize interferon signaling. Proc Natl Acad Sci U S A 2020;117:28344–54. https://doi.org/10.1073/pnas.2016650117.

[361] Mu J, Fang Y, Yang Q, Shu T, Wang A, Huang M, et al. SARS-CoV-2 N protein antagonizes type I interferon signaling by suppressing phosphorylation and nuclear translocation of STAT1 and STAT2. Cell Discov 2020;6:65. https://doi.org/10.1038/s41421-020-00208-3.

[362] Wu J, Shi Y, Pan X, Wu S, Hou R, Zhang Y, et al. SARS-CoV-2 ORF9b inhibits RIG-I-MAVS antiviral signaling by interrupting K63-linked ubiquitination of NEMO. Cell Rep 2021;34:108761. https://doi.org/10.1016/j.celrep.2021.108761.

[363] Jiang H-W, Zhang H-N, Meng Q-F, Xie J, Li Y, Chen H, et al. SARS-CoV-2 Orf9b suppresses type I interferon responses by targeting TOM70. Cell Mol Immunol 2020;17:998–1000. https://doi.org/10.1038/s41423-020-0514-8.

[364] Han L, Zhuang M-W, Deng J, Zheng Y, Zhang J, Nan M-L, et al. SARS-CoV-2 ORF9b antagonizes type I and III interferons by targeting multiple components of the RIG-I/MDA-5-MAVS, TLR3-TRIF, and cGAS-STING signaling pathways. J Med Virol 2021;93:5376–89. https://doi.org/10.1002/jmv.27050.

[365] Xia H, Cao Z, Xie X, Zhang X, Chen JY-C, Wang H, et al. Evasion of type I interferon by SARS-CoV-2. Cell Rep 2020;33:108234. https://doi.org/10.1016/j.celrep.2020.108234.

[366] Galani I-E, Rovina N, Lampropoulou V, Triantafyllia V, Manioudaki M, Pavlos E, et al. Untuned antiviral immunity in COVID-19 revealed by temporal type I/III interferon patterns and flu comparison. Nat Immunol 2021;22:32–40. https://doi.org/10.1038/s41590-020-00840-x.

[367] Wang N, Zhan Y, Zhu L, Hou Z, Liu F, Song P, et al. Retrospective multicenter cohort study shows early interferon therapy is associated with favorable clinical responses in COVID-19 patients. Cell Host Microbe 2020;28:455–464.e2. https://doi.org/10.1016/j.chom.2020.07.005.

[368] Zhou Q, MacArthur MR, He X, Wei X, Zarin P, Hanna BS, et al. Interferon-α2b treatment for COVID-19 is associated with improvements in lung abnormalities. Viruses 2020;13:E44. https://doi.org/10.3390/v13010044.

[369] Hung IF-N, Lung K-C, Tso EY-K, Liu R, Chung TW-H, Chu M-Y, et al. Triple combination of interferon beta-1b, lopinavir-ritonavir, and ribavirin in the treatment of patients admitted to hospital with COVID-19: an open-label, randomised, phase 2 trial. Lancet 2020;395:1695–704. https://doi.org/10.1016/S0140-6736(20)31042-4.

[370] Monk PD, Marsden RJ, Tear VJ, Brookes J, Batten TN, Mankowski M, et al. Safety and efficacy of inhaled nebulised interferon beta-1a (SNG001) for treatment of SARS-CoV-2 infection: a randomised, double-blind, placebo-controlled, phase 2 trial. Lancet Respir Med 2021;9:196–206. https://doi.org/10.1016/S2213-2600(20)30511-7.

[371] Kalil AC, Mehta AK, Patterson TF, Erdmann N, Gomez CA, Jain MK, et al. Efficacy of interferon beta-1a plus remdesivir compared with remdesivir alone in hospitalised adults with COVID-19: a double-bind, randomised, placebo-controlled, phase 3 trial. Lancet Respir Med 2021;9:1365–76. https://doi.org/10.1016/S2213-2600(21)00384-2.

[372] Andreakos E, Tsiodras S. COVID-19: lambda interferon against viral load and hyperinflammation. EMBO Mol Med 2020;12:e12465. https://doi.org/10.15252/emmm.202012465.

[373] Feld JJ, Kandel C, Biondi MJ, Kozak RA, Zahoor MA, Lemieux C, et al. Peginterferon lambda for the treatment of outpatients with COVID-19: a phase 2, placebo-controlled randomised trial. Lancet Respir Med 2021;9:498–510. https://doi.org/10.1016/S2213-2600(20)30566-X.

[374] Jagannathan P, Andrews JR, Bonilla H, Hedlin H, Jacobson KB, Balasubramanian V, et al. Peginterferon Lambda-1a for treatment of outpatients with uncomplicated COVID-19: a randomized placebo-controlled trial. Nat Commun 2021;12:1967. https://doi.org/10.1038/s41467-021-22177-1.

[375] Guimarães PO, Quirk D, Furtado RH, Maia LN, Saraiva JF, Antunes MO, et al. Tofacitinib in patients hospitalized with covid-19 pneumonia. N Engl J Med 2021;385:406–15. https://doi.org/10.1056/NEJMoa2101643.

[376] Kalil AC, Patterson TF, Mehta AK, Tomashek KM, Wolfe CR, Ghazaryan V, et al. Baricitinib plus remdesivir for hospitalized adults with covid-19. N Engl J Med 2021;384:795–807. https://doi.org/10.1056/NEJMoa2031994.

[377] Marconi VC, Ramanan AV, de Bono S, Kartman CE, Krishnan V, Liao R, et al. Efficacy and safety of baricitinib for the treatment of hospitalised adults with COVID-19 (COV-BARRIER): a randomised, double-blind, parallel-group, placebo-controlled phase 3 trial. Lancet Respir Med 2021;9:1407–18. https://doi.org/10.1016/S2213-2600(21)00331-3.

[378] Liao J, Kapadia VS, Brown LS, Cheong N, Longoria C, Mija D, et al. The NLRP3 inflammasome is critically involved in the development of bronchopulmonary dysplasia. Nat Commun 2015;6:8977. https://doi.org/10.1038/ncomms9977.

[379] Coll RC, Robertson AAB, Chae JJ, Higgins SC, Muñoz-Planillo R, Inserra MC, et al. A small-molecule inhibitor of the NLRP3 inflammasome for the treatment of inflammatory diseases. Nat Med 2015;21:248–55. https://doi.org/10.1038/nm.3806.

[380] Marchetti C, Swartzwelter B, Gamboni F, Neff CP, Richter K, Azam T, et al. OLT1177, a β-sulfonyl nitrile compound, safe in humans, inhibits the NLRP3 inflammasome and reverses the metabolic cost of inflammation. Proc Natl Acad Sci USA 2018;115:E1530–9. https://doi.org/10.1073/pnas.1716095115.

[381] Bertinaria M, Gastaldi S, Marini E, Giorgis M. Development of covalent NLRP3 inflammasome inhibitors: chemistry and biological activity. Arch Biochem Biophys 2019;670:116–39. https://doi.org/10.1016/j.abb.2018.11.013.

[382] Li J, Wei Q, Li WX, McCowen KC, Xiong W, Liu J, et al. Metformin use in diabetes prior to hospitalization: effects on mortality in covid-19. Endocr Pract 2020;26:1166–72. https://doi.org/10.4158/EP-2020-0466.

[383] Xian H, Liu Y, Rundberg Nilsson A, Gatchalian R, Crother TR, Tourtellotte WG, et al. Metformin inhibition of mitochondrial ATP and DNA synthesis abrogates NLRP3 inflammasome activation and pulmonary inflammation. Immunity 2021;54:1463–1477.e11. https://doi.org/10.1016/j.immuni.2021.05.004.

[384] Ibrahim S, Lowe JR, Bramante CT, Shah S, Klatt NR, Sherwood N, et al. Metformin and covid-19: focused review of mechanisms and current literature suggesting benefit. Front Endocrinol 2021;12:587801. https://doi.org/10.3389/fendo.2021.587801.

[385] Magupalli VG, Negro R, Tian Y, Hauenstein AV, Di Caprio G, Skillern W, et al. HDAC6 mediates an aggresome-like mechanism for NLRP3 and pyrin inflammasome activation. Science 2020;369:eaas8995. https://doi.org/10.1126/science.aas8995.

[386] Reyes AZ, Hu KA, Teperman J, Wampler Muskardin TL, Tardif J-C, Shah B, et al. Anti-inflammatory therapy for COVID-19 infection: the case for colchicine. Ann Rheum Dis 2021;80:550–7. https://doi.org/10.1136/annrheumdis-2020-219174.

[387] Lopes MI, Bonjorno LP, Giannini MC, Amaral NB, Menezes PI, Dib SM, et al. Beneficial effects of colchicine for moderate to severe COVID-19: a randomised, double-blinded, placebo-controlled clinical trial. RMD Open 2021;7:e001455. https://doi.org/10.1136/rmdopen-2020-001455.

[388] Tardif J-C, Bouabdallaoui N, L'Allier PL, Gaudet D, Shah B, Pillinger MH, et al. Efficacy of colchicine in non-hospitalized patients with COVID-19. medRxiv 2021. https://doi.org/10.1101/2021.01.26.21250494.

[389] Liu X, Xia S, Zhang Z, Wu H, Lieberman J. Channelling inflammation: gasdermins in physiology and disease. Nat Rev Drug Discov 2021;20:384–405. https://doi.org/10.1038/s41573-021-00154-z.

[390] Hu JJ, Liu X, Xia S, Zhang Z, Zhang Y, Zhao J, et al. FDA-approved disulfiram inhibits pyroptosis by blocking gasdermin D pore formation. Nat Immunol 2020;21:736–45. https://doi.org/10.1038/s41590-020-0669-6.

[391] Humphries F, Shmuel-Galia L, Ketelut-Carneiro N, Li S, Wang B, Nemmara VV, et al. Succination inactivates gasdermin D and blocks pyroptosis. Science 2020;369:1633–7. https://doi.org/10.1126/science.abb9818.

[392] Mantero V, Abate L, Basilico P, Balgera R, Salmaggi A, Nourbakhsh B, et al. COVID-19 in dimethyl fumarate-treated patients with multiple sclerosis. J Neurol 2021;268:2023–5. https://doi.org/10.1007/s00415-020-10015-1.

[393] Jin Z, Du X, Xu Y, Deng Y, Liu M, Zhao Y, et al. Structure of Mpro from SARS-CoV-2 and discovery of its inhibitors. Nature 2020;582:289–93. https://doi.org/10.1038/s41586-020-2223-y.

[394] Olagnier D, Farahani E, Thyrsted J, Blay-Cadanet J, Herengt A, Idorn M, et al. SARS-CoV2-mediated suppression of NRF2-signaling reveals potent antiviral and anti-inflammatory activity of 4-octyl-itaconate and dimethyl fumarate. Nat Commun 2020;11:4938. https://doi.org/10.1038/s41467-020-18764-3.

[395] Kayagaki N, Warming S, Lamkanfi M, Vande Walle L, Louie S, Dong J, et al. Non-canonical inflammasome activation targets caspase-11. Nature 2011;479:117–21. https://doi.org/10.1038/nature10558.

[396] Rathinam VAK, Zhao Y, Shao F. Innate immunity to intracellular LPS. Nat Immunol 2019;20:527–33. https://doi.org/10.1038/s41590-019-0368-3.

[397] Wannamaker W, Davies R, Namchuk M, Pollard J, Ford P, Ku G, et al. (S)-1-((S)-2-{[1-(4-Amino-3-chloro-phenyl)-methanoyl]-amino}-3,3-dimethyl-butanoyl)-pyrrolidine-2-carboxylic acid ((2 R ,3 S)-2-ethoxy-5-oxo-tetrahydro-furan-3-yl)-amide (VX-765), an orally available selective interleukin (IL)-Converting enzyme/caspase-1 inhibitor, exhibits potent anti-inflammatory activities by inhibiting the release of IL-1β and IL-18. J Pharmacol Exp Ther 2007;321:509–16. https://doi.org/10.1124/jpet.106.111344.

[398] Xu X, Liu L, Wang Y, Wang C, Zheng Q, Liu Q, et al. Caspase-1 inhibitor exerts brain-protective effects against sepsis-associated encephalopathy and cognitive impairments in a mouse model of sepsis. Brain Behav Immun 2019;80:859–70. https://doi.org/10.1016/j.bbi.2019.05.038.

[399] Flores J, Noël A, Foveau B, Lynham J, Lecrux C, LeBlanc AC. Caspase-1 inhibition alleviates cognitive impairment and neuropathology in an Alzheimer's disease mouse model. Nat Commun 2018;9:3916. https://doi.org/10.1038/s41467-018-06449-x.

[400] McKenzie BA, Mamik MK, Saito LB, Boghozian R, Monaco MC, Major EO, et al. Caspase-1 inhibition prevents glial inflammasome activation and pyroptosis in models of multiple sclerosis. Proc Natl Acad Sci U S A 2018;115:E6065–74. https://doi.org/10.1073/pnas.1722041115.

[401] Jacotot É. [Caspase inhibition: from cellular biology and thanatology to potential clinical agents]. Med Sci 2020;36:1143–54. https://doi.org/10.1051/medsci/2020222.

[402] Plassmeyer M, Alpan O, Corley MJ, Premeaux TA, Lillard K, Coatney P, et al. Caspases and therapeutic potential of caspase inhibitors in moderate–severe SARS-CoV-2 infection and long COVID. Allergy 2022;77:118–29. https://doi.org/10.1111/all.14907.

[403] Linton SD, Aja T, Armstrong RA, Bai X, Chen L-S, Chen N, et al. First-in-Class Pan caspase inhibitor developed for the treatment of liver disease. J Med Chem 2005;48:6779–82. https://doi.org/10.1021/jm050307e.

[404] Garcia-Tsao G, Bosch J, Kayali Z, Harrison SA, Abdelmalek MF, Lawitz E, et al. Randomized placebo-controlled trial of emricasan for non-alcoholic steatohepatitis-related cirrhosis with severe portal hypertension. J Hepatol 2020;72:885–95. https://doi.org/10.1016/j.jhep.2019.12.010.

[405] Harrison SA, Goodman Z, Jabbar A, Vemulapalli R, Younes ZH, Freilich B, et al. A randomized, placebo-controlled trial of emricasan in patients with NASH and F1-F3 fibrosis. J Hepatol 2020;72:816–27. https://doi.org/10.1016/j.jhep.2019.11.024.

[406] Baker RE, Mahmud AS, Miller IF, Rajeev M, Rasambainarivo F, Rice BL, et al. Infectious disease in an era of global change. Nat Rev Microbiol 2022;20(4):193–205. https://doi.org/10.1038/s41579-021-00639-z.

[407] Saksena N, Bonam SR, Miranda-Saksena M. Immunopathogenesis of severe acute respiratory syndrome coronavirus-2: evolving knowledge and its current status. Explor Immunol 2021;1:61–79. https://doi.org/10.37349/ei.2021.00007.

[408] Merad M, Martin JC. Pathological inflammation in patients with COVID-19: a key role for monocytes and macrophages. Nat Rev Immunol 2020;20:355–62. https://doi.org/10.1038/s41577-020-0331-4.

[409] Zhou W, Wang W. Auto-antibodies against type I IFNs are associated with severe COVID-19 pneumonia. Signal Transduct Target Ther 2021;6:96. https://doi.org/10.1038/s41392-021-00514-6.

[410] Takahashi T, Ellingson MK, Wong P, Israelow B, Lucas C, Klein J, et al. Sex differences in immune responses that underlie COVID-19 disease outcomes. Nature 2020;588:315–20. https://doi.org/10.1038/s41586-020-2700-3.

[411] Adamczak D. The role of toll-like receptors and vitamin D in cardiovascular diseases—a review. IJMS 2017;18:2252. https://doi.org/10.3390/ijms18112252.

CHAPTER

4

The role of T cell immunity in COVID-19

Ulrik Stervbo[1] *and Nina Babel*[1,2]

[1]Center for Translational Medicine and Immune Diagnostics Laboratory, Medical Department I, Marien Hospital Herne, University Hospital of the Ruhr-University Bochum, Herne, Germany; [2]Charité—Universitätsmedizin Berlin, Humboldt-Universität zu Berlin, Berlin Center for Advanced Therapies, Berlin, Germany

Introduction

The adaptive immune system is divided into a humoral and a cellular arm and is important for the control and clearance of viral infections. Antibodies produced by B cells constitute the humoral arm, while the cellular arm is divided into two branches consisting of CD4+ helper T cells and CD8+ cytotoxic T cells. CD4+ T cells provide B cell help for affinity maturation to produce highly specific antibodies, which inhibit the binding of viruses to their entry molecules. The CD4+ helper T cells also help activate CD8+ T cells, which move on to eliminate infected cells and possess their own cytotoxic capabilities [1].

The role of T cells in the immune response against SARS-CoV-2 is evident from case studies on COVID-19 patients lacking B cells, either by agammaglobulinemia or pharmaceutical depletion. Two patients recovered from COVID-19 without the need for oxygen ventilation or intensive care and similar outcome were found in 31 patients with B-cell depletion therapy [2–5]. Though some fatal cases in B-cell deficient patients have also been reported, the data indicate that antibodies may not be essential to resolve COVID-19 [6]. In line with this notion are the observations that neutralizing antibody capacities do not correlate with disease severity [7–9].

Low CD4+ T cell count in uncontrolled HIV patients is associated with increased need for oxygen ventilation, admission to intensive care, and mortality during a SARS-CoV-2 infection [10]. Additionally, several reports on T cells in SARS-CoV-2 show detectable levels of SARS-CoV-2 reactive T cells after an infection [11–13]. Collectively, T cells have a central role in COVID-19, which is the subject of this chapter.

Autoimmunity, COVID-19, Post-COVID19 syndrome and COVID-19 vaccination
https://doi.org/10.1016/B978-0-443-18566-3.00021-9

Human corona virus

Viruses of the family *Coronaviridae* cause disease in humans and animals. Four of these (229E, NL63, OC43, and HKU1) are of the subfamily *Orthocoronavirinae* and are specific for humans. They typically infect only the upper respiratory tract and cause common cold-like symptoms [14]. In addition to these endemic coronaviruses, another three coronaviruses can replicate in the lower respiratory tract and can cause fatal pneumonia. These are the severe acute respiratory syndrome coronavirus (SARS-CoV-1), Middle East respiratory syndrome coronavirus (MERS), and the currently pandemic SARS-CoV-2.

Coronaviruses are enveloped, single-strand, positive-sense RNA viruses and with a genome size of 26–32 kb. The subfamily *Orthocoronavirinae* is subdivided into four genera Alpha-coronavirus, Beta-coronavirus, Gamma-coronavirus, and Delta-coronavirus. 229E and NL63 belong to the Alphacoronavirus and OC43 and HKU1 as well as MERS, SARS-CoV-1, and SARS-CoV-2 all belong to the Beta-coronavirus. Gamma- and Delta-coronaviruses infect mainly birds and pigs.

Human coronaviruses have a similar genome structure and protein organization (Fig. 4.1). About 2/3 of the entire genome is taken up by an open reading frame ORF1a/b, which encodes 16 nonstructural proteins (nsp1 through nsp16). The ORF1a and ORF1b are translated to the large polyproteins, commonly referred to as pp1a and pp1b, which are cleaved by papain-like cysteine protease (PLpro, which resides within nsp3) and 3C-like serine protease (3CLpro, also known as main protease Mpro, resides within nsp5) to produce nsps, including RNA-dependent RNA polymerases (RdRp, resides within nsp12) and helicase (Hel, resides within nsp13). The remaining 1/3 of the genome encodes four structural proteins: spike (S), envelope (E), membrane (M), and nucleocapsid (N). A hemagglutinin esterase (HE) protein also exists OC43 and HKU1.

The proteins commonly studied in the context of immune reaction are the S-, M-, and N-protein:

The S-protein has a molecular weight of 128–160 kDa before glycosylation and 150–200 kDa after N-linked glycosylation. The S-protein is inserted into the membrane as a homotrimer giving it its crown-like appearance and is the major determinant of host and tissue tropism. After binding to the entry receptor, the S-protein is cleaved to separate receptor-binding domain (RBD) and fusion domains of the S-protein. A second cleavage finally exposes the fusion peptide at the S2′, and fusion generally occurs within acidified endosomes [14].

In the case of SARS-CoV-2, the RBD is 214 amino acids long (spanning the residues 311–524 of the S-protein) and trophic for the angiotensin-converting enzyme 2 (ACE2). The polybasic sequence at the S1–S2 boundary is cleaved during maturation in the host cell, and only at the target cell is the S2′ site cleaved to expose the fusion peptide. The cleavage of S2′ is performed by the surface molecule transmembrane protease, serine 2 (TMPRSS2), or, after internalization into the endolysosomes, by cathepsins [17].

The S1 subunit (the N-terminal subunit) contains the receptor-binding domain (RBD) of SARS-CoV-2 and shares only 23%–25% identity with the endemic coronaviruses. Mutations in this region are particularly prone to generate new variants of concern and may

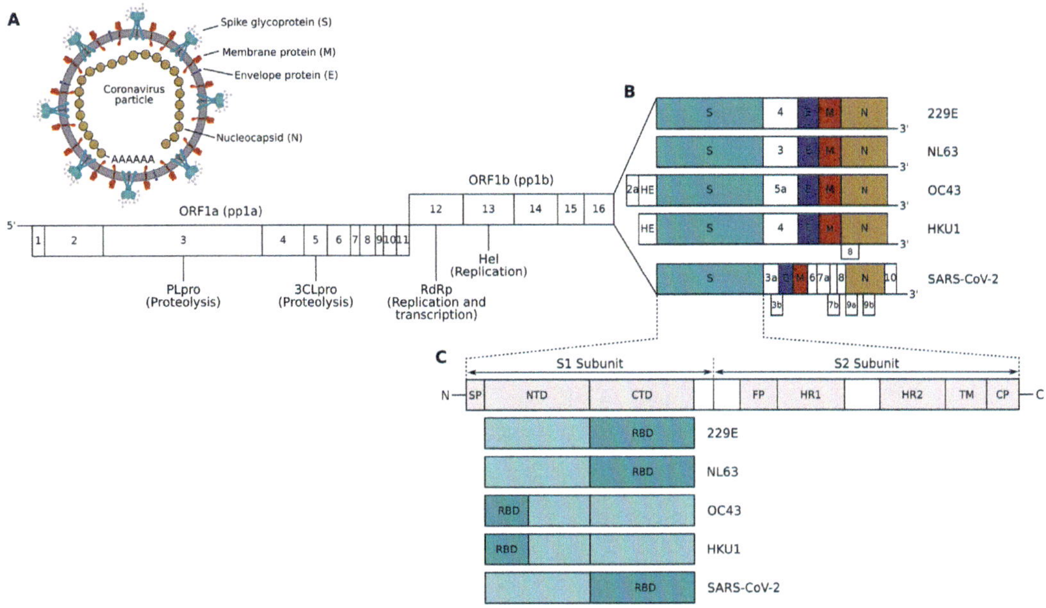

FIGURE 4.1 **Schematic representation of human corona virus's genome.** (A) The virus particle. (B) The genome of coronaviruses is a single-stranded RNA surrounded by Nucleocapsid (N) protein. The 5′-terminal ORF1a/b encodes the polyproteins 1a (pp1a) and pp1b. The polyproteins are cleaved by PLpro and 3CLpro to produce nonstructural proteins (nsps). Among the nsps are RdRp and Hel, which are involved in the transcription and replication. The remaining of the genome encodes the four structural proteins Spike (S), Membrane (M), Envelope (E), and Nucleocapsid (N). OC43 and HKU1 have in addition the hemagglutinin esterase (HE). (C) The S-protein consists of the S1 and S2 subunits. The S1 subunit contains a signal peptide (SP) and is further subdivided into the N-terminal and the C-terminal domain (NTD and CTD, respectively). The receptor-binding domain (RBD) is located within one of these domains. The S2 subunit includes the fusion peptide (FP), Heptated repeat 1 and 2 (HR1 and HR2), the transmembrane domain (TM), and a cytoplasmic peptide (CP). *The figure is adapted from Zhao X, Ding Y, Du J, Fan Y. 2020 update on human coronaviruses: one health, one world. Med Nov Technol Devices December 2020;8:100043. The schematic in A is adapted from SPQR10. Coronavirus virion structure.svg [Internet]. 2020. Available from: https://commons.wikimedia.org/wiki/File:Coronavirus_virion_structure.svg.*

result in immune escape [18]. The S2 subunit (the C-terminal subunit) of SARS-CoV-2 shares 33%–42% identity with the endemic coronaviruses [19].

The M-protein has a molecular weight of 25–30 kDa is the most abundant structural protein and possesses three transmembrane domains. The short N-terminal ectodomain of the M-protein is modified by O-linked glycosylation in OC43 and some animal coronaviruses. It forms a homodimer and interacts with other viral structural proteins to orchestrate the assembly of the coronavirus particle.

Peptides arising from an intracellular cleavage of proteins are presented on the surface of the cells in the context of the MHC and are thereby accessible to the T cell. This is opposed to antibodies that can bind directly to the S-protein on the surface of the virus. Since more COVID-19 patients may raise a T cell response against the M-protein compared to the S-protein, it is likely that infected cells produce large levels of this protein [20]. This in turn, makes the M-protein a relevant target for T cell-based vaccines.

The N-protein has a molecular weight of 43–50 kDa forms dimer and binds to the genomic RNA in a beads-on-a-string fashion, forming a helically symmetric nucleocapsid. The N-protein is phosphorylated by cellular kinase.

Preformed memory

One of the hallmarks of adaptive immunity is immunological memory. The activation of naïve a T cell when it first encounters its cognate antigen is slow and the barrier for activation is high. During the clearance of the pathogen, activated T cells gain memory of their activation, making later activation faster and easier, should the pathogen return. If a pathogen is sufficiently similar to the one originally creating the memory, the adaptive immune system may respond to this unseen pathogen as if it were already encountered. This transfer of recognition from one pathogen to the next is termed crossreactivity, and may, in the case of a truly novel pathogen like the SAR-CoV-2, represent a pool of preformed memory cells.

The frequency of SARS-CoV-2 cross-reactive T cells in unexposed individuals was a subject of great interest in the early phase of the pandemic since they could explain the frequent asymptomatic SARS-COV-2 infections and add to our understanding of the potential severity of the pandemic. Depending on origin, age, and methodological differences in the study design, 20%–80% of the unexposed prepandemic population were estimated to harbor T cells against at least one component of the SARS-CoV-2 [11,13,19–29]. This preformed T cell memory may be caused by repeated infections with endemic coronaviruses, but other pathogens are also possible [19,22–24,30]. For instance, Loyal and coworkers nicely demonstrated the existence of an immunodominant peptide located within the fusion peptide domain of the S-protein (spanning the residues 816–830), which was recognized by CD4+ T cells in 20% of unexposed individuals, 50%–60% of SARS-CoV-2 convalescents, and 97% of BNT162b2-vaccinated individuals [24].

Given its potential for vaccine development, the S-protein was the focus of immunological evaluation. However, we and others also noted extensive immunogenic properties of N- and M-protein of the SARS-CoV-2 [11,20,29]. CD4+ T cells specific for SARS-CoV-2 M-protein were found in 30% of unexposed donors (i.e. samples frozen before the pandemic) while N-protein reactive CD4+ T cells were found in 10% of unexposed donors [20]. In this particular study, 40% of the unexposed donors had CD4+ T cells against the S-protein. Antigen-specific CD8+ T cells were found in 20% of the unexposed donors for either of the M-, N-, or S-protein [20].

The effect of the preformed memory in the response to a SARS-CoV-2 infection is subject to some debate [31]. Some protection against infection has been observed for T cells against N-and M-, but not S-protein [32]. It is, however, more likely that the preformed memory against SARS-CoV-2 can have a beneficial effect on COVID-19 and in vaccine response [24,33,34]. This view is challenged by some observations, where the preformed memory is of low avidity and associated with severe COVID-19 [22]. Preformed memory is, in general, a double-edged sword that may direct cells to a suboptimal or aberrant response as shown for H1N1 influenza [35].

T cells in the early infection

The cytokine environment

There is mounting evidence that events early in the SARS-CoV-2 infection can affect the severity of the disease. An impaired type I interferon (IFN) response can result in an uncontrolled viral infection [36]. In line with this, neutralizing autoantibodies against type I IFN (IFN-α and IFN-ω) was associated with severe COVID-19 [37]. Neutralizing IFN-I autoantibodies were found in 10.2% (101/987) of patients with life-threatening COVID-19, compared to a total absence in patients (663) with asymptomatic or mild COVID-19, and only in 0.33% (4/1227) of unexposed donors [37]. Similarly, 3.5% (23/659) of patients with severe COVID-19 had deleterious variants in loci involved in TLR3-and IRF7-dependent IFN-I signaing [38]. The observation, of increased blood concentrations of IFN-α in some patients with severe COVID-19, makes the timing of the cytokines release a possible important factor [39]. This is supported by findings, that TGFβ levels had a faster dynamic in patients with severe COVID-19, which strongly limits early NK cell function [40]. In contrast, early and transient increases in monocytes and NK cells were found in patients with moderate disease courses [41].

Type 1 IFN are important molecules in initiating an immune response as they induce the expression of costimulatory molecules and the major histocompatibility complex II (MHC-II) on antigen-presenting cells. These in turn activate both CD4+ and CD8+ T cells. In addition, type I IFN also acts directly on CD4+ and CD8+ T cells and promote their expansion and differentiation [42].

Cytokines like interleukin-6 (IL-6), IL-8, and tumor necrosis factor (TNF) are associated with severe COVID-19 [43]. In general, an increased IL-6 and decreased Type I IFN is an inappropriate inflammatory response associated with severe disease [44]. Pyroptosis is usually seen with cytopathic viruses, including SARS-CoV-2 [45]. Although programmed and controlled, it is a highly inflammatory form of cell death and may contribute to the high levels of IL-6 and TNF observed in patients with severe COVID [45]. In fact, aberrant cytokine levels might render T cells irresponsive to SARS-CoV-2 [42].

Several studies report a higher viral load in the upper respiratory tract on the admission of patients later developing severe COVID-19 [46–48]. Although a compelling explanation, a meta-analysis of 34 studies found that a similar number of reports either approved or opposed the association between viral load and COVID-19 severity [49].

Lymphopenia

Lymphopenia is a common feature of many viral respiratory infections. However, in contrast to other infections, where the lymphopenia is rapidly recovered, COVID-19-associated lymphopenia is more severe and longer-lasting and is associated with severe disease [50–53]. In addition, T cell populations seem more affected by COVID-19-associated lymphopenia [54]. The lymphopenia may be explained by recruitment to the respiratory tract [21,55,56]. However, single-cell RNA-sequencing of lung tissue and bronchoalveolar lavage fluid found that the infiltration is not excessive [55,56].

High levels of proinflammatory cytokines such as IL-6 or TNF as well as proapoptotic molecules like FAS and TNF also contribute to lymphopenia [57–59]. Finally, cell death triggered by infection of immune cells by SARS-CoV-2 cannot be ruled out [60].

Collectively, the initial cytokine environment might influence the number of T cells, as well as the type of T cell response generated in COVID-19.

Disease severity and T cells

Dynamics of T cells in COVID-19

Compared to the innate immune system, the adaptive immune system reacts slow to infections, and it takes 6–10 days to generate a sufficient T cell response after infection, which can facilitate viral clearance Given the existence of preformed memory and the fact that the exact time of SARS-CoV-2 infection is unknown, it is difficult at best to determine the timespan from infection to the appearance of appropriate T cell response. Both CD4+ and CD8+ T cells specific for components of SARS-CoV-2 have been detected 2–4 days after the onset of symptoms [12,29,61]. Although measurable CD8+ T cells have been reported detectable on day 1 after symptoms onset [62]. In fact, smaller studies showed a strong association between early induction of CD4+ T cells and mild COVID-19 [12,61]. These observations were confirmed in a larger study with 229 patients [39].

In contrast to the association between early T cell induction and mild COVID-19, late and weak induction of SARS-CoV-2 specific T cells is associated with severe or fatal COVID-19 [11,12,19,63]. Interestingly, titers of neutralizing antibodies do not correlate with disease severity [7–9]. T cells slowly decline after clearing of the SARS-CoV-2 but remain detectable for at least 6–8 months [64].

The number of distinct epitopes (the epitope breadth) recognized by the T cells might be limited [31]. In line with this, early T cell response is directed against different epitopes in different viral proteins [12,29,65]. Whether the magnitude of this response does not associate with disease severity is unclear [20,66].

Though the negative association between T cells and disease is compelling, some reports demonstrate a proportionality to the disease severity [20,29,67]. Most of these studies have small cohorts, but in one with 203 patients, no association between T cells and disease severity was found [68]. Collectively, this demonstrates the heterogeneity of the immunological COVID-19 manifestations.

T cell functionality

Activated CD4+ T cells in COVID-19 patients have a Th1 signature as evident by production of IFN-γ, TNF, and IL-2 [12,13,19,20]. SARS-CoV-2 reactive CD8+ were found to express cytotoxic molecules like IFN-γ, granzyme B, perforin, and CD107a [12,13,20,62].

We and others have evaluated the T cell response in COVID-19 toward the ubiquitous S-protein, but also against the M and N-proteins of the SARS-CoV-2 virus [20,69]. In general, a larger proportion of T cells specific for the M-protein produced IFN-γ compared to cells specific for S- or N-protein. In elderly patients with a higher risk for severe COVID-19, a lower frequency of T cells produced IFN-γ while an increased frequency produced IL-2 [69]. In another report, a shift from bifunctional CD4+ T cells producing IFN-γ/IL-2 or IFN-γ/TNF to IL-2/TNF was observed with increased COVID-19 severity [20]. The shift was most prominent for T cells reactive to the S-protein, but also for T cells against M- and N-protein. This lack of a clear and robust Th1 induction in patients with severe COVID-19 has been termed "immunological misfiring" [39].

CD4+ T cells reactive to the S-protein of SARS-CoV-2 were found in 65% of unexposed renal transplant patients (RTx) patients, and 80% harbored S-protein specific CD8+ T cells [70]. This is within the range of previous observations for the healthy population [20,21]. In line with this, the CD4+ response against S-, M-, and N-protein had a similar magnitude throughout the disease course in a pancreas-kidney transplant patient with COVID-19 [71]. For CD8+T cells, a clear immune dominance of N-protein was observed. This observation is in line with others, where the magnitude and functional characteristics of SARS-CoV-2-reactive T cells were comparable between COVID-19 patients with and without transplants [72–74].

Collectively, an early and robust Th1 response seems to favor a mild COVID-19, whereas a severe disease course is marked by delayed T cell activation, with a potentially inappropriate cytokine signature.

TCR signature in COVID-19

The T cell receptor (TCR) is a heterodimeric surface molecule that endows the T cell with its antigen specificity. The receptor is created through somatic recombination of the variable (V) and joining (J) segment genes (and diversity [D] for beta chains; Fig. 4.2). Three hypervariable regions complementarity determining regions (CDR) exist in the TCR. While CDR1 and two are coded within the V-gene, the CDR3 - which sits between the V-region and the J-region - is created by random insertion and deletion of nucleotides. It is this randomness of the CDR3, which gives rise to the large variation of the TCR. In fact, up to 10^{15} different TCRs can be created though only up to 10^{10} (or 10 clones or each TCR) may exist at the same time [75,76].

Given the importance of TCRs in the immune reaction, much effort has gone into collecting and making available COVID-relevant TCR data [77,78]. Utilizing these resources, characteristic motifs of the CDR3 sequence in convalescent COVID-19 patients have been identified,

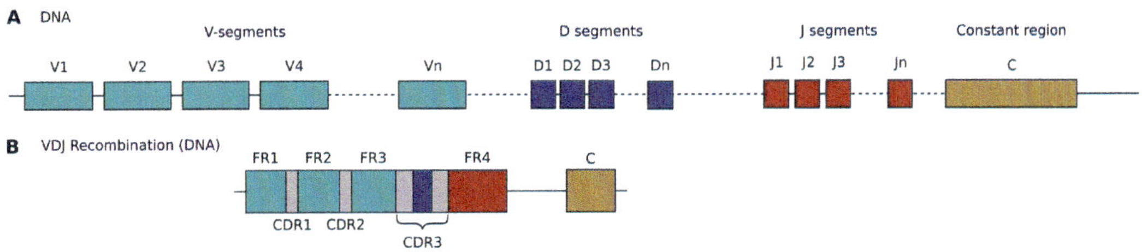

FIGURE 4.2 **T cell receptor recombination.** Schematic representation of TCR recombination. The process is similar for both the α and β chains, with the exception that only the TCR β chain contains D-genes.

paving the way for an approved TCR-based diagnostic test [79–81]. TCRs with SARS-CoV-2 signatures can be identified in repertoires of unexposed individuals, indicating that these are preexpanded [26,82]. Using a reverse epitope discovery approach on public single-cell TCR data, SARS-CoV-2 S-protein specific clusters were identified and validated in a cohort before and after vaccine with ChAdOx1-S [83]. These findings make a prejab evaluation of the vaccine efficacy possible.

Few reports exist on the dynamics of the TCR repertoire in COVID19. However, these reports agree, that diversity in patients with severe disease course is decreased compared to patients with a mild COVID19 [84–86]. This results in fewer clusters of similar TCRs and a lower number of TCRs shared between clusters [84]. The avidity of the antigen-specific TCRs in these clusters was not evaluated and it is therefore not possible to determine if the decrease in diversity is the result of the cause of the disease course.

Conclusion

The image arising after the collective and intense research into the role of T cells in COVID-19 is summarized in Fig. 4.3. Differences in the ability of the innate immunity to assert control very early on in the infection in the upper respiratory tract may lead to a higher load in the lower respiratory tract. This leads to an immunopathogenesis signified by lymphopenia and the accumulation of immune cells in the lung tissue [21,87]. The immunopathogenesis is more extensive and widespread in patients who develop severe COVID-19. In addition, the initial dysfunctional environment may lead to a skew in the imprinting expanding T cells, changing their cytokine profile and further aggravating the immunopathogenesis.

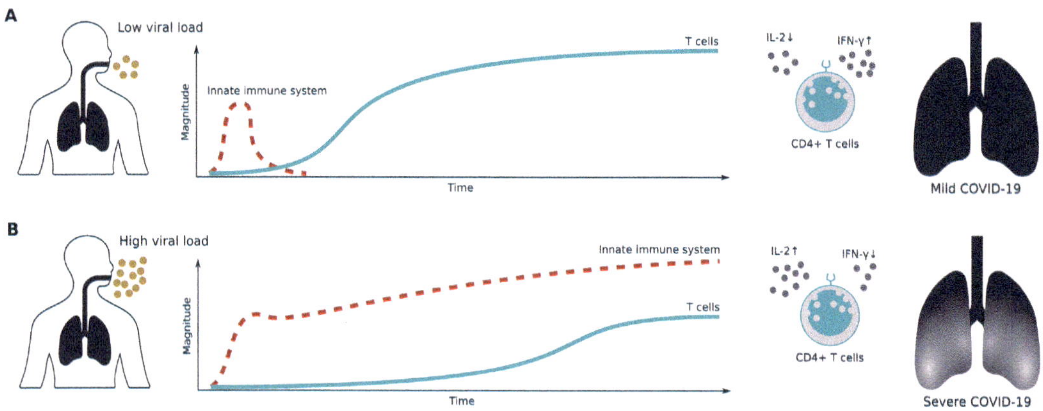

FIGURE 4.3 **Overview of T cells in COVID-19.** (A) An early control of the virus replication limits the T cell lymphopenia, why a large pool of T cells—including cross-reactive memory cells—further controls the infection, leading to mild and maybe even asymptomatic COVID-19. (B) An early rise in SARS-CoV-2 viral load severely reduces the T cell pool, causing an imbalance in the cytokine environment. This leads to a delayed adaptive immune response with a skewed cytokine profile. Consequently, severe COVID-19 ensures.

References

[1] Oh DY, Fong L. Cytotoxic CD4+ T cells in cancer: expanding the immune effector toolbox. Immunity December 2021;54(12):2701–11.

[2] Montero-Escribano P, Matías-Guiu J, Gómez-Iglesias P, Porta-Etessam J, Pytel V, Matias-Guiu JA. Anti-CD20 and COVID-19 in multiple sclerosis and related disorders: a case series of 60 patients from Madrid, Spain. Mult Scler Relat Disord July 2020;42:102185.

[3] Novi G, Mikulska M, Briano F, Toscanini F, Tazza F, Uccelli A, et al. COVID-19 in a MS patient treated with ocrelizumab: does immunosuppression have a protective role? Mult Scler Relat Disord July 2020;42:102120.

[4] Safavi F, Nourbakhsh B, Azimi AR. B-cell depleting therapies may affect susceptibility to acute respiratory illness among patients with multiple sclerosis during the early COVID-19 epidemic in Iran. Mult Scler Relat Disord August 2020;43:102195.

[5] Soresina A, Moratto D, Chiarini M, Paolillo C, Baresi G, Focà E, et al. Two X-linked agammaglobulinemia patients develop pneumonia as COVID-19 manifestation but recover. In: Eigenmann P, editor. Pediatr Allergy Immunol. 31(5); July 2020. p. 565–9.

[6] Ponsford MJ, Shillitoe BMJ, Humphreys IR, Gennery AR, Jolles S. COVID-19 and X-linked agammaglobulinemia (XLA) – insights from a monogenic antibody deficiency. Curr Opin Allergy Clin Immunol December 2021;21(6):525–34.

[7] Dan JM, Mateus J, Kato Y, Hastie KM, Yu ED, Faliti CE, et al. Immunological memory to SARS-CoV-2 assessed for up to 8 months after infection. Science February 5, 2021;371(6529):eabf4063.

[8] Piccoli L, Park Y-J, Tortorici MA, Czudnochowski N, Walls AC, Beltramello M, et al. Mapping neutralizing and immunodominant sites on the SARS-CoV-2 spike receptor-binding domain by structure-guided high-resolution serology. Cell November 12, 2020;183(4):1024–1042.e21.

[9] Robbiani DF, Gaebler C, Muecksch F, Lorenzi JCC, Wang Z, Cho A, et al. Convergent antibody responses to SARS-CoV-2 in convalescent individuals. Nature August 2020;584(7821):437–42.

[10] Braunstein SL, Lazar R, Wahnich A, Daskalakis DC, Blackstock OJ. Coronavirus disease 2019 (COVID-19) infection among people with human immunodeficiency virus in New York city: a population-level analysis of linked surveillance data. Clin Infect Dis June 15, 2021;72(12):e1021–9.

[11] Grifoni A, Weiskopf D, Ramirez SI, Mateus J, Dan JM, Moderbacher CR, et al. Targets of T cell responses to SARS-CoV-2 coronavirus in humans with COVID-19 disease and unexposed individuals. Cell June 25, 2020;181(7):1489–1501.e15.

[12] Rydyznski Moderbacher C, Ramirez SI, Dan JM, Grifoni A, Hastie KM, Weiskopf D, et al. Antigen-specific adaptive immunity to SARS-CoV-2 in acute COVID-19 and associations with age and disease severity. Cell November 12, 2020;183(4):996–1012.e19.

[13] Sekine T, Perez-Potti A, Rivera-Ballesteros O, Strålin K, Gorin J-B, Olsson A, et al. Robust T cell immunity in convalescent individuals with asymptomatic or mild COVID-19. Cell October 1, 2020;183(1):158–168.e14.

[14] Fehr AR, Perlman S. Coronaviruses: an overview of their replication and pathogenesis. Methods Mol Biol Clifton NJ 2015;1282:1–23.

[15] Zhao X, Ding Y, Du J, Fan Y. 2020 update on human coronaviruses: one health, one world. Med Nov Technol Devices December 2020;8:100043.

[16] SPQR10. Coronavirus virion structure.svg [Internet]. 2020. Available from: https://commons.wikimedia.org/wiki/File:Coronavirus_virion_structure.svg.

[17] Jackson CB, Farzan M, Chen B, Choe H. Mechanisms of SARS-CoV-2 entry into cells. Nat Rev Mol Cell Biol January 2022;23(1):3–20.

[18] Harvey WT, Carabelli AM, Jackson B, Gupta RK, Thomson EC, Harrison EM, et al. SARS-CoV-2 variants, spike mutations and immune escape. Nat Rev Microbiol July 2021;19(7):409–24.

[19] Braun J, Loyal L, Frentsch M, Wendisch D, Georg P, Kurth F, et al. SARS-CoV-2-reactive T cells in healthy donors and patients with COVID-19. Nature November 12, 2020;587(7833):270–4.

[20] Thieme CJ, Anft M, Paniskaki K, Blazquez-Navarro A, Doevelaar A, Seibert FS, et al. Robust T cell response toward spike, membrane, and nucleocapsid SARS-CoV-2 proteins is not associated with recovery in critical COVID-19 patients. Cell Rep Med September 22, 2020;1(6):100092.

[21] Anft M, Paniskaki K, Blazquez-Navarro A, Doevelaar A, Seibert FS, Hölzer B, et al. COVID-19-Induced ARDS is associated with decreased frequency of activated memory/effector T cells expressing CD11a(+). Mol Ther J Am Soc Gene Ther December 2, 2020;28(12):2691–702.

[22] Bacher P, Rosati E, Esser D, Martini GR, Saggau C, Schiminsky E, et al. Low-avidity CD4+ T cell responses to SARS-CoV-2 in unexposed individuals and humans with severe COVID-19. Immunity December 2020;53(6):1258–1271.e5.

[23] Le Bert N, Tan AT, Kunasegaran K, Tham CYL, Hafezi M, Chia A, et al. SARS-CoV-2-specific T cell immunity in cases of COVID-19 and SARS, and uninfected controls. Nature August 1, 2020;584(7821):457–62.

[24] Loyal L, Braun J, Henze L, Kruse B, Dingeldey M, Reimer U, et al. Cross-reactive CD4+ T cells enhance SARS-CoV-2 immune responses upon infection and vaccination. Science October 8, 2021;374(6564):eabh1823.

[25] Mateus J, Grifoni A, Tarke A, Sidney J, Ramirez SI, Dan JM, et al. Selective and cross-reactive SARS-CoV-2 T cell epitopes in unexposed humans. Science October 2, 2020;370(6512):89–94.

[26] Minervina AA, Komech EA, Titov A, Bensouda Koraichi M, Rosati E, Mamedov IZ, et al. Longitudinal high-throughput TCR repertoire profiling reveals the dynamics of T-cell memory formation after mild COVID-19 infection. Elife January 5, 2021;10:e63502.

[27] Nelde A, Bilich T, Heitmann JS, Maringer Y, Salih HR, Roerden M, et al. SARS-CoV-2-derived peptides define heterologous and COVID-19-induced T cell recognition. Nat Immunol January 2021;22(1):74–85.

[28] Shomuradova AS, Vagida MS, Sheetikov SA, Zornikova KV, Kiryukhin D, Titov A, et al. SARS-CoV-2 epitopes are recognized by a public and diverse repertoire of human T cell receptors. Immunity December 2020;53(6):1245–1257.e5.

[29] Weiskopf D, Schmitz KS, Raadsen MP, Grifoni A, Okba NMA, Endeman H, et al. Phenotype and kinetics of SARS-CoV-2–specific T cells in COVID-19 patients with acute respiratory distress syndrome. Sci Immunol June 26, 2020;5(48):eabd2071.

[30] Stervbo U, Rahmann S, Roch T, Westhoff TH, Babel N. Epitope similarity cannot explain the pre-formed T cell immunity towards structural SARS-CoV-2 proteins. Sci Rep December 2020;10(1):18995.

[31] Grifoni A, Sidney J, Vita R, Peters B, Crotty S, Weiskopf D, et al. SARS-CoV-2 human T cell epitopes: adaptive immune response against COVID-19. Cell Host Microbe July 2021;29(7):1076–92.

[32] Kundu R, Narean JS, Wang L, Fenn J, Pillay T, Fernandez ND, et al. Cross-reactive memory T cells associate with protection against SARS-CoV-2 infection in COVID-19 contacts. Nat Commun December 2022;13(1):80.

[33] Lipsitch M, Grad YH, Sette A, Crotty S. Cross-reactive memory T cells and herd immunity to SARS-CoV-2. Nat Rev Immunol November 2020;20(11):709–13.

[34] Mallajosyula V, Ganjavi C, Chakraborty S, McSween AM, Pavlovitch-Bedzyk AJ, Wilhelmy J, et al. CD8+ T cells specific for conserved coronavirus epitopes correlate with milder disease in patients with COVID-19. Sci Immunol July 29, 2021;6(61):eabg5669.

[35] Nienen M, Stervbo U, Mölder F, Kaliszczyk S, Kuchenbecker L, Gayova L, et al. The role of pre-existing cross-reactive central memory CD4 T-cells in vaccination with previously unseen influenza strains. Front Immunol 2019;10:593.

[36] Wang X, Xu G, Liu X, Liu Y, Zhang S, Zhang Z. Multiomics: unraveling the panoramic landscapes of SARS-CoV-2 infection. Cell Mol Immunol October 2021;18(10):2313–24.

[37] Bastard P, Rosen LB, Zhang Q, Michailidis E, Hoffmann H-H, Zhang Y, et al. Autoantibodies against type I IFNs in patients with life-threatening COVID-19. Science October 23, 2020;370(6515):eabd4585.

[38] Zhang Q, Bastard P, Liu Z, Le Pen J, Moncada-Velez M, Chen J, et al. Inborn errors of type I IFN immunity in patients with life-threatening COVID-19. Science October 23, 2020;370(6515):eabd4570.

[39] Lucas C, Wong P, Klein J, Castro TBR, Silva J, Sundaram M, et al. Longitudinal analyses reveal immunological misfiring in severe COVID-19. Nature August 2020;584(7821):463–9.

[40] Witkowski M, Tizian C, Ferreira-Gomes M, Niemeyer D, Jones TC, Heinrich F, et al. Untimely TGFβ responses in COVID-19 limit antiviral functions of NK cells. Nature December 9, 2021;600(7888):295–301.

[41] Bolouri H, Speake C, Skibinski D, Long SA, Hocking AM, Campbell DJ, et al. The COVID-19 immune landscape is dynamically and reversibly correlated with disease severity. J Clin Invest February 1, 2021;131(3):e143648.

[42] King C, Sprent J. Dual nature of type I interferons in SARS-CoV-2-induced inflammation. Trends Immunol April 2021;42(4):312–22.

[43] Del Valle DM, Kim-Schulze S, Huang H-H, Beckmann ND, Nirenberg S, Wang B, et al. An inflammatory cytokine signature predicts COVID-19 severity and survival. Nat Med October 2020;26(10):1636–43.

[44] Blanco-Melo D, Nilsson-Payant BE, Liu W-C, Uhl S, Hoagland D, Møller R, et al. Imbalanced host response to SARS-CoV-2 drives development of COVID-19. Cell May 2020;181(5):1036–1045.e9.

[45] Ferreira AC, Soares VC, de Azevedo-Quintanilha IG, Dias S da SG, Fintelman-Rodrigues N, Sacramento CQ, et al. SARS-CoV-2 engages inflammasome and pyroptosis in human primary monocytes. Cell Death Dis March 1, 2021;7(1):1–12.

[46] Boyapati A, Wipperman MF, Ehmann PJ, Hamon S, Lederer DJ, Waldron A, et al. Baseline severe acute respiratory syndrome viral load is associated with coronavirus disease 2019 severity and clinical outcomes: post hoc analyses of a phase 2/3 trial. J Infect Dis December 1, 2021;224(11):1830–8.

[47] Magleby R, Westblade LF, Trzebucki A, Simon MS, Rajan M, Park J, et al. Impact of severe acute respiratory syndrome coronavirus 2 viral load on risk of intubation and mortality among hospitalized patients with coronavirus disease 2019. Clin Infect Dis December 6, 2021;73(11):e4197–205.

[48] Pujadas E, Chaudhry F, McBride R, Richter F, Zhao S, Wajnberg A, et al. SARS-CoV-2 viral load predicts COVID-19 mortality. Lancet Respir Med September 2020;8(9):e70.

[49] Dadras O, Afsahi AM, Pashaei Z, Mojdeganlou H, Karimi A, Habibi P, et al. The relationship between COVID-19 viral load and disease severity: a systematic review. Immun Inflamm Dis December 2021;13:iid3.580.

[50] Chen G, Wu D, Guo W, Cao Y, Huang D, Wang H, et al. Clinical and immunological features of severe and moderate coronavirus disease 2019. J Clin Invest May 1, 2020;130(5):2620–9.

[51] Diao B, Wang C, Tan Y, Chen X, Liu Y, Ning L, et al. Reduction and functional exhaustion of T cells in patients with coronavirus disease 2019 (COVID-19). Front Immunol 2020;11:827.

[52] Guan W, Ni Z, Hu Y, Liang W, Ou C, He J, et al. Clinical characteristics of coronavirus disease 2019 in China. N Engl J Med April 30, 2020;382(18):1708–20.

[53] Tan L, Wang Q, Zhang D, Ding J, Huang Q, Tang Y-Q, et al. Lymphopenia predicts disease severity of COVID-19: a descriptive and predictive study. Signal Transduct Target Ther March 27, 2020;5(1):33.

[54] Chen Z, John Wherry E. T cell responses in patients with COVID-19. Nat Rev Immunol September 2020;20(9):529–36.

[55] Liao M, Liu Y, Yuan J, Wen Y, Xu G, Zhao J, et al. Single-cell landscape of bronchoalveolar immune cells in patients with COVID-19. Nat Med June 2020;26(6):842–4.

[56] Wichmann D, Sperhake J-P, Lütgehetmann M, Steurer S, Edler C, Heinemann A, et al. Autopsy findings and venous thromboembolism in patients with COVID-19: a prospective cohort study. Ann Intern Med August 18, 2020;173(4):268–77.

[57] Giamarellos-Bourboulis EJ, Netea MG, Rovina N, Akinosoglou K, Antoniadou A, Antonakos N, et al. Complex immune dysregulation in COVID-19 patients with severe respiratory failure. Cell Host Microbe June 10, 2020;27(6):992–1000.e3.

[58] Mathew D, Giles JR, Baxter AE, Oldridge DA, Greenplate AR, Wu JE, et al. Deep immune profiling of COVID-19 patients reveals distinct immunotypes with therapeutic implications. Science September 4, 2020;369(6508):eabc8511.

[59] Mazzoni A, Salvati L, Maggi L, Capone M, Vanni A, Spinicci M, et al. Impaired immune cell cytotoxicity in severe COVID-19 is IL-6 dependent. J Clin Invest September 1, 2020;130(9):4694–703.

[60] Ren X, Wen W, Fan X, Hou W, Su B, Cai P, et al. COVID-19 immune features revealed by a large-scale single-cell transcriptome atlas. Cell November 11, 2021;184(23):5838.

[61] Tan AT, Linster M, Tan CW, Le Bert N, Chia WN, Kunasegaran K, et al. Early induction of functional SARS-CoV-2-specific T cells associates with rapid viral clearance and mild disease in COVID-19 patients. Cell Rep February 2021;34(6):108728.

[62] Schulien I, Kemming J, Oberhardt V, Wild K, Seidel LM, Killmer S, et al. Characterization of pre-existing and induced SARS-CoV-2-specific CD8+ T cells. Nat Med January 2021;27(1):78–85.

[63] Zhou R, To KK-W, Wong Y-C, Liu L, Zhou B, Li X, et al. Acute SARS-CoV-2 infection impairs dendritic cell and T cell responses. Immunity October 13, 2020;53(4):864–877.e5.

[64] Bertoletti A, Tan AT, Le Bert N. The T-cell response to SARS-CoV-2: kinetic and quantitative aspects and the case for their protective role. Oxf Open Immunol January 6, 2021;2(1):iqab006.

[65] Tarke A, Sidney J, Kidd CK, Dan JM, Ramirez SI, Yu ED, et al. Comprehensive analysis of T cell immunodominance and immunoprevalence of SARS-CoV-2 epitopes in COVID-19 cases. Cell Rep Med February 16, 2021;2(2):100204.

[66] Peng Y, Mentzer AJ, Liu G, Yao X, Yin Z, Dong D, et al. Broad and strong memory CD4+ and CD8+ T cells induced by SARS-CoV-2 in UK convalescent individuals following COVID-19. Nat Immunol November 2020;21(11):1336–45.

[67] Schub D, Klemis V, Schneitler S, Mihm J, Lepper PM, Wilkens H, et al. High levels of SARS-CoV-2–specific T cells with restricted functionality in severe courses of COVID-19. JCI Insight October 15, 2020;5(20):e142167.
[68] Nielsen SS, Vibholm LK, Monrad I, Olesen R, Frattari GS, Pahus MH, et al. SARS-CoV-2 elicits robust adaptive immune responses regardless of disease severity. EBioMedicine June 2021;68:103410.
[69] Sattler A, Angermair S, Stockmann H, Heim KM, Khadzhynov D, Treskatsch S, et al. SARS-CoV-2-specific T cell responses and correlations with COVID-19 patient predisposition. J Clin Invest December 1, 2020;130 (12):6477–89.
[70] Anft M, Blazquez-Navarro A, Stervbo U, Skrzypczyk S, Witzke O, Wirth R, et al. Detection of pre-existing SARS-CoV-2-reactive T cells in unexposed renal transplant patients. J Nephrol August 2021;34(4):1025–37.
[71] Babel N, Anft M, Blazquez-Navarro A, Doevelaar AAN, Seibert FS, Bauer F, et al. Immune monitoring facilitates the clinical decision in multifocal COVID-19 of a pancreas-kidney transplant patient. Am J Transplant November 2020;20(11):3210–5.
[72] Candon S, Guerrot D, Drouot L, Lemoine M, Lebourg L, Hanoy M, et al. T cell and antibody responses to SARS-CoV-2: experience from a French transplantation and hemodialysis center during the COVID-19 pandemic. Am J Transplant Off J Am Soc Transplant Am Soc Transpl Surg February 2021;21(2):854–63.
[73] Favà A, Donadeu L, Sabé N, Pernin V, González-Costello J, Lladó L, et al. SARS-CoV-2-specific serological and functional T cell immune responses during acute and early COVID-19 convalescence in solid organ transplant patients. Am J Transplant Off J Am Soc Transplant Am Soc Transpl Surg August 2021;21(8):2749–61.
[74] Thieme CJ, Blazquez-Navarro A, Safi L, Kaliszczyk S, Paniskaki K, Neumann IE, et al. Impaired humoral but substantial cellular immune response to variants of concern B1.1.7 and B.1.351 in hemodialysis patients after vaccination with BNT162b2. J Am Soc Nephrol JASN November 2021;32(11):2725–7.
[75] Nikolich-Žugich J, Slifka MK, Messaoudi I. The many important facets of T-cell repertoire diversity. Nat Rev Immunol February 2004;4(2):123–32.
[76] Lythe G, Callard RE, Hoare RL, Molina-París C. How many TCR clonotypes does a body maintain? J Theor Biol January 2016;389:214–24.
[77] Corrie BD, Marthandan N, Zimonja B, Jaglale J, Zhou Y, Barr E, et al. iReceptor: a platform for querying and analyzing antibody/B-cell and T-cell receptor repertoire data across federated repositories. Immunol Rev July 2018;284(1):24–41.
[78] Nolan S, Vignali M, Klinger M, Dines JN, Kaplan IM, Svejnoha E, et al. A large-scale database of T-cell receptor beta (TCRβ) sequences and binding associations from natural and synthetic exposure to SARS-CoV-2 [Cited 2022 Jan 14]. Research Square 2020. https://doi.org/10.21203/rs.3.rs-51964.
[79] Sheridan C. COVID-19 testing turns to T cells. Nat Biotechnol May 2021;39(5):533–4.
[80] Snyder TM, Gittelman RM, Klinger M, May DH, Osborne EJ, Taniguchi R, et al. Magnitude and dynamics of the T-cell response to SARS-CoV-2 infection at both individual and population levels [Cited 2022 Jan 14]. medRxiv 2020. https://doi.org/10.1101/2020.07.31.20165647. 07.31.20165647.
[81] Wang Y, Duan F, Zhu Z, Yu M, Jia X, Dai H, et al. Analysis of TCR repertoire by high-throughput sequencing indicates the feature of T cell immune response after SARS-CoV-2 infection. Cells December 27, 2021;11(1):68.
[82] Simnica D, Schultheiß C, Mohme M, Paschold L, Willscher E, Fitzek A, et al. Landscape of T-cell repertoires with public COVID-19-associated T-cell receptors in pre-pandemic risk cohorts. Clin Transl Immunol January 2021;10(9):e1340.
[83] Pogorelyy MV, Rosati E, Minervina AA, Scheffold A, Franke A, Bacher P, et al. Resolving SARS-CoV-2 CD4+ T cell specificity via reverse epitope discovery. Cell Reports Medicine 2022;3(8):100697.
[84] Chang C-M, Feng P, Wu T-H, Alachkar H, Lee K-Y, Chang W-C. Profiling of T Cell repertoire in SARS-CoV-2-infected COVID-19 patients between mild disease and pneumonia. J Clin Immunol August 2021;41(6):1131–45.
[85] Park JJ, Lee KAV, Lam SZ, Chen S. T cell receptor repertoire signatures associated with COVID-19 severity [Cited 2022 Jan 14]. bioRxiv 2021. https://doi.org/10.1101/2021.11.30.470640. 11.30.470640.
[86] Zhang F, Gan R, Zhen Z, Hu X, Li X, Zhou F, et al. Adaptive immune responses to SARS-CoV-2 infection in severe versus mild individuals. Signal Transduct Target Ther December 2020;5(1):156.
[87] Sette A, Crotty S. Adaptive immunity to SARS-CoV-2 and COVID-19. Cell February 2021;184(4):861–80.

CHAPTER

5

Laboratory characteristics of cytokine storm syndrome in COVID-19 infection

Olga Y. Tkachenko, Margarita Y. Pervakova and Sergey V. Lapin

Laboratory for Diagnostics of Autoimmune Diseases, Center for Molecular Medicine, Saint Petersburg Pavlov State Medical University, Saint Petersburg, Russia

Cytokine storm or cytokine release syndrome: definition and features

Inflammation is a universal protective mechanism that activates in response to a pathogen invasion. In some pathologies, the immune system inability to eliminate pathogen can lead to its overstimulation and cytokine storm syndrome (CSS) development [1]. This severe condition is characterized by overwhelming systemic inflammation and hemodynamic instability, leading to a multiple organ dysfunction syndrome (MODS) and fatal outcomes in many cases. Common manifestations include sustained fever, splenomegaly, hepatomegaly with liver dysfunction, lymphadenopathy, coagulopathy, cytopenia, skin rash, and variable neurologic symptoms [2]. The documented conditions causing CSS are hemophagocytic lymphohistiocytosis (HLH), septic shock (SS), toxin-mediated shock syndrome (e.g., staph toxic shock), some acute viral infections, and graft versus host disease [3].

The main cytokine classes include interleukins, interferons, chemokines, mesenchymal growth factors, the tumor necrosis factor (TNF) family, and adipokines. Cytokines are secreted biologically active molecules that regulate cell growth and metabolism, as well as cellular interactions through their specific binding to certain receptors and subsequent induction of intracellular signaling. There exists cytokines that are involved in adaptive immunity (IL-2 and IL-4), proinflammatory cytokines and interleukins (interferon-I, -II and -III; IL-1, IL-6, and IL-17; and TNF-α) and antiinflammatory cytokines (e.g., IL-10). In response to

Autoimmunity, COVID-19, Post-COVID19 syndrome and COVID-19 vaccination
https://doi.org/10.1016/B978-0-443-18566-3.00005-0

stressful internal processes (such as cancer or microbial infection), host cells secrete cytokines that play a very important role in reprogramming cellular metabolism as a defense response [4]. Interferons, interleukins, chemokines, and TNF α are the main components involved in the development of the CSS.

Cytokines affect nearly every biological process, including embryonic development, disease pathogenesis, nonspecific and specific response to antigen, changes in cognitive functions and aging [5]. Under a pathogen invasion, cytokines serve as intercellular messengers in the immune system, integrating function of several cell types into a coherent immune response, targeted to eliminate infectious agent [6]. In the process of an innate immune response, the production and secretion of cytokines occurs due to the nonspecific stimulation of pattern-recognition receptors (PRRs), which detect distinct evolutionarily conserved structures on pathogens, termed pathogen-associated molecular patterns (PAMPs). These receptors are based in antigen-presenting cells (APCs), such as granulocytes, macrophages, and dendritic cells (DCs), where they are located on the cell surface, in endosomes or in cytoplasm according to the receptor subclass [7]. It is considered that key proinflammatory cytokines in different hyperinflammatory states are IFN-γ, TNF, IL-1β, IL-6, IL-10, and IL-18, and their metabolic effects explain most of manifestations, appearing during CSS development.

In March 2020, the World Health Organization announced a pandemic of new coronavirus disease 2019 (COVID-19), which in most severe cases was characterized by pulmonary infiltration, accompanied by CSS [8]. According to recent data, impaired clearance of SARS-CoV-2 due to its genetic characteristics and virulence factors, delayed, and weakened interferon response to SARS-CoV-2 in the early stages of the disease, increased nettosis and pyroptosis induced by the virus created background for a severe course of viral infection complicated by CSS syndrome [9–11]. A distinctive feature of CSS was an uncontrolled and dysfunctional immune response associated with constant activation of lymphocytes and macrophages, which produced large number of cytokines, causing CSS. Many clinical features of CS can be explained by the effects of proinflammatory cytokines such as interferon (INF)-gamma, TNF, interleukin (IL) -1, IL-6, and IL-18 [12–17].

The severity of COVID-19 is associated with robust systemic inflammatory response that can initiate a CSS including circulating cytokines and chemokines, such as IL-1α, IL-1β, IL-2, IL-7, IL-6, IL-8, IL-10, TNF, interferon (IFN)-γ, granulocyte colony-stimulating factor (G-CSF), IFN-inducible protein-10 (IP-10), CCL2 (monocyte chemotactic protein [MCP]-1), CCL3 (macrophage inflammatory protein one alpha [MIP1α]), CXC-chemokine ligand 10 (CXCL10), etc. [18–21]. Features of CSS and pathogenesis of COVID-19 have been proposed to be a consequence of immune hyperactivity and/or a failure to resolve the inflammatory response because of ongoing viral replication or immune dysregulation [22]. On the one hand, a correlation was found between viral load in the nasopharynx and levels of cytokines (e.g., IFN-α, IFN-γ and TNF). On the other hand, CSS associated with reduced cytotoxic CD4 + and CD8 + T cells, NK cells, memory T cells and regulatory T cells, B cells [23,24]. Probably CSS during COVID-19 is the result of a defective (or delayed) first line of defense, followed by persistent hypercytokinemia and dysfunctional T-cell response. This consequences in impaired clearance of apoptotic cells or infected/activated macrophages, increased viral replication, followed by IL-18/IFN-γ synthesis, activating macrophages, resulting in the release of multiple cytokines, hemophagocytosis, coagulopathy, and ARDS. An unbalanced immune response in COVID-19 illustrates by a weak production of type I interferons (IFN-Is) [25]. Antagonism occurs at various phases in IFN signaling pathway, including by preventing pattern recognition by the viral RNA recognizing receptor (RRR), by preventing RRR signaling via TBK1/nuclear factor κB kinase-subunit-ε inhibitor (IKKε), TRAF3 and IRF3, preventing downstream interferon signaling through STAT1; and promoting host mRNA degradation and inhibiting host protein translation. Antagonism of the interferon response promotes viral replication, which leads to an increase in the release of pyroptosis products, which can further cause aberrant inflammatory reactions [26].

Clinical examples of cytokine storm syndrome

The term CSS was frequently used to describe the severe course of a number of diseases that led to an uncontrolled inflammatory response. Initially CSS was described as a part of excessive inflammatory response in graft versus host disease (GvHD) in 1993, and further the term was adopted for severe cases of viral and bacterial infections [27]. Pathological immune activation may occur under infectious, iatrogenic triggers or malignancies, and usually requires some latent or diagnosed preexisting conditions, such as genetic immune defects, prolonged immunosuppression, or chronic aberrant immune activity like in rheumatic diseases and persistent infections. Since the avian influenza epidemic in 2003–08 with high mortality rate, this term has become widespread [28]. Since the pandemic was recognized COVID-19-associated CSS development has become the major health problem [8].

The documented conditions, leading to CSS, also include genetically mediated immunological disorders, such as hemophagocytic lymphohistiocytosis (HLH) and its particular variant—macrophage activation syndrome (MAS), but also bacterial sepsis, toxin-mediated shock syndrome, some viral infections, Kawasaki disease, thrombocytopenic purpura [29]. Occasionally the term CSS is used to refer «cytokine release syndrome» (CRS), which occurs in result of targeted antitumor therapy (e.g., anti-CD19 CAR T-cell therapy), though this condition is considered to affect distinct immunological pathway and may be delayed until days or weeks after treatment [30]. Clinical examples of CSS presents in Table 5.1.

Although CSS and sepsis can cause deep endothelial activation and disseminated intravascular coagulation, some patients with primary immune-mediated vasculopathies develop syndromes similar to CSS (fever, disseminated intravascular coagulation, and organ dysfunction). This is perhaps best described in *Kawasaki disease* [31]. A significant proportion of patients with *thrombotic thrombocytopenic purpura* often develop characteristic signs of CSS such as prolonged fever, hemodynamic instability, central nervous system involvement, and coagulopathy.

Clinical signs of CSS include persistent fever, splenomegaly, hepatomegaly with liver dysfunction, lymphadenopathy, coagulopathy, cytopenia, skin rash, and various neurological symptoms. Symptoms of CSS are difficult to distinguish from those caused by underlying diseases [4,32–36]. Observation of patients with pathology associated with CSS is critical for the diagnosis of this condition. All signs are nonspecific in themselves, however, a combination of clinical symptoms and laboratory manifestations, their severity and changes over time

TABLE 5.1 Clinical examples of cytokine storm syndrome.

Disease/Condition	Damaging factor
Primary hemophagocytic lymphohistiocytosis	Mutations in genes PRF1, UNC13D or MUNC13-4, STX11 and STXBP2, UNC18B
Secondary HLH in the presence of malignant neoplasms, infections, autoimmune or autoinflammatory pathologies	Difficulty eliminating an infectious agent with a weakened T-cell response; cytokines produced by tumor cells, etc.
Macrophage activation syndrome	Disruption of perforin-mediated target cell lysis
Sepsis and septic shock	Lipopolysaccharide and other microbial components
Cytokine release syndrome (post-CAR-T cell therapy)	Hyperactivation of antigen-presenting cells upon infusion of antitumor T cells
Kawasaki disease and other primary vascular causes of CSS	Superantigen (viruses and bacteria)

underlie the diagnosis of CSS. Comparison of clinical and laboratory characteristics of different types of CSS is shown in Table 5.2.

Prognostic value of cytokine measurement in COVID-19

In a number of studies of cytokines in COVID-19, it was shown that in patients with severe COVID-19 and those who died from this infection, the levels of cytokines such as IL-1β, IL-2 and its soluble receptor, IL-6, IL-8, IL-17, IL-18, TNF-α, monocyte chemoattractant protein 1 (MCP1 or CCL2), macrophage inflammatory protein 1-alpha (MIP-1α or CCL3)), as well as the antiinflammatory cytokine IL-10, were significantly higher than in the group of patients with milder forms of SARS-CoV-2 [16,37].

During the first wave of coronavirus epidemic that developed in St. Petersburg, Russia, late spring of 2020 we collected serum samples, clinical data, and disease outcomes of 226 patients hospitalized in clinics of Pavlov State Medical University with viral pneumonia (CT severity score ≥2). In all COVID-19 patients, a SARS-CoV-2 nucleic acid sample was confirmed by PCR using samples from oropharyngeal swabs before hospitalization (Table 5.3). All serum samples were obtained at the time of hospitalization. This study was approved by the local ethics committee of Pavlov First Saint Petersburg State Medical University. The studied cohort of COVID-19 pneumonia included 138 (61%) men and 88 (39%) women, whose mean age was 56.82 ± 13.9 (from 23 to 87 years old). Any of the patients were vaccinated at that time. All examined patients had fever above 38°C, cough (158 [69.9%]), pain and chest pressure (31 [13,7%]). Diarrhea (11 [25%]) and anosmia (18.5 [42%]) were more common among patients with a favorable course of COVID-19.

In our cohort IL-1b, IL-2, IL-6, IL-8, IL-10, IL-18, TNF-a, IFNα, IFNy were measured with ELISA. The concentrations of IL-2, IL-1b, TNF-α, and IL-8 in patients with COVID-19-associated pneumonia were significantly higher than in healthy donors, but no differences

TABLE 5.2 Comparison of clinical and laboratory characteristics of CSS.

Characteristics	Primary HLH	Post CAR-T cell therapy	Sepsis	Macrophage activation syndrome	COVID-19
Clinical	Fever; Hepatosplenomegaly; Hepatobiliary dysfunction; Generalized lymphadenopathy; Coagulopathy; Neurologic symptoms; Headache; Cognitive changes; Focal neurologic deficits; Seizure	Fever; hypotension; Hypoxia; Malaise; Anorexia; Myalgias; Tachycardia; Widened pulse pressure; Capillary leak syndrome; Renal impairment; Hepatic failure; DIC; Multiorgan dysfunction;	Fever (more than 38.5°C) or hypothermia (less than 36°C); Hypotension; tachycardia; Tachypnea; Rigors; altered mental status; Mottled skin on inspection; petechiae; diaphoresis; Respiratory (cough, hemoptysis at el.); Gastrointestinal (abdominal distention on inspection, abdominal pain et al.); Genitourinary (costovertebral tenderness and suprapubic pain on palpatio, caginal discharge, or bleeding); Skin and soft tissue (erythema and/or edema, lymphadenopathy, wounds, ulcerations et al.); Meningismus; septic arthritis; endocarditis;	Fever hepatosplenome-galy, lymphadenopathy Hemorrhages (purpura, easy bruising, mucosal bleeding) Rash Central nervous system manifestations (lethargy, irritability, disorientation, headache, seizures, and coma)	Fever; Hypotension; Hypoxia; ARDS; Cardiomyopathy; Multi-organ dysfunction; Thrombosis;
Laboratory	Cytopenia (2 lineages in the peripheral blood); hypofibrinogenemia; ↑Ferritin; Hypertriglyceridemia; Hyperbilirubinemia; ↑ ALT, AST; ↑Cell count and/or protein content in CSF; ↑sCD25; ↑sCD163; Low or absent natural killer cell activity;	↑CRP; ↑↑Ferritin; ↑D dimer; ↑Fibrinogen; ↑Triglycerides;	↑↑↑WBC; ↓ Platelet; ↑Glucose; ↑Creatinine; ↑ ALT, AST; ↑Serum lactate; ↑Procalcitonin; blood, urine, stool, sputum, skin, cerebrospinal fluid cultures;	Pancytopenia; Hypofibrinogenemia; ↑ ALT, AST; Hypertriglyceridemia,; ↑↑↑ ferritin; Coagulopathy; Hyponatremia; Hyperfibrinogenemia (and low ESR)	Leukopenia/ lymphopenia/anemia; Thrombocytopenis (or Tr-cytosis); ↑CRP; Hyperferritinemia; Hypoalbminemia; Cytolysis (transaminases, direct bilirubin, and ammonia) ↑Alkaline phosphatase; ↑Triglycerides; CSF pleocytosis; ↑D-dimer; Hyperfibrinogenemia (and low ESR)

TABLE 5.3 Demographic and clinical characteristics of COVID-19 patients (n = 226).

Characteristics	All patients (n = 226)	Recovery (n = 190)	Death (n = 36)	*P* value
Demographic				
Age 0–45 years, % (n)	17.8 (41)	18.9 (36)	8.3 (3)	ns
Age 45–65 years,% (n)	50.4 (114)	52.6 (100)	30.5 (11)	0,01
Age 65–85 years,% (n)	31.4 (71)	26.8 (51)	58.3 (21)	< 0,0005
Men, %,n)	61.0 (138)	60.5 (115)	63.8 (23)	ns
BMI (kg/m^2), median (25–75th)	29.41 (8–33)	29.7 (2–34)	27.9 (24.9–31.96)	ns
Clinical symptoms				
Fever (°C), median (25–75th)	38.9	39.0	38.8	ns
Cough, % (n)	69.9 (158)	70.5 (134)	66.6 (24)	< 0,0001
Pain/tightness in the chest, % (n)	13,731)	13,1 (25)	16,6(6)	NS
Diarrhea, % (n)	11 (25)	12.1 (23)	5.55 (2)	Nns
Anosmia, % (n)	18.58 (42)	21.57 (41)	2.7 (1)	0,01
CT severity score (Estimation of lung parenchymal involvement)				
CT-2, moderate (25-50%)	42.47 (96)	44.2 (84)	33.3 (12)	0,02
CT-3, severe (50-75%)	39.8 (90)	41.5 (79)	30.5 (11)	0,02
CT-4, critical (>75%)	6.19 (14)	14.2 (27)	33.3 (12)	0,01
SpO2,%,median (25–75th)	89.5 (84–94)	91 (86–94)	81(70–87.5)	< 0,0001
NEWS2 >4, median (25–75th)	6 (3–7)	5 (3–7)	7 (6–8)	< 0,0001

were found between the deceased and surviving patients. In our study, the patients who died were more likely to have initially elevated concentrations of IL-6, IL-10, IL-18, and PCT than recovered patients (Fig. 5.1).

Clinical significance of cytokine concentration was confirmed by a number of studies. It was known that IL-6 is synthesized by T-lymphocytes, fibroblasts, endothelial cells, monocytes and was an important mediator during the acute phase response in sepsis and other infections [38]. It was found that this cytokine is elevated in both severe and mild COVID-19, while it has a direct correlation with the volume of the affected lung tissue in patients with ARDS. E. Giofoni et al. (2020) showed that PZ IL-6 25 pg/mL in blood is an independent risk factor for the progression of severe COVID-19 [39]. In another study, IL-6 levels> 80 pg/mL were associated with the need for mechanical ventilation [40].

Several studies have shown that the concentration of IL-18 in the blood has a significant correlation with the severity of COVID-19 and damage to vital organs [41]. Noteworthy is the fact that the increase in blood levels of IL-18, due to the activation of NLRP3/

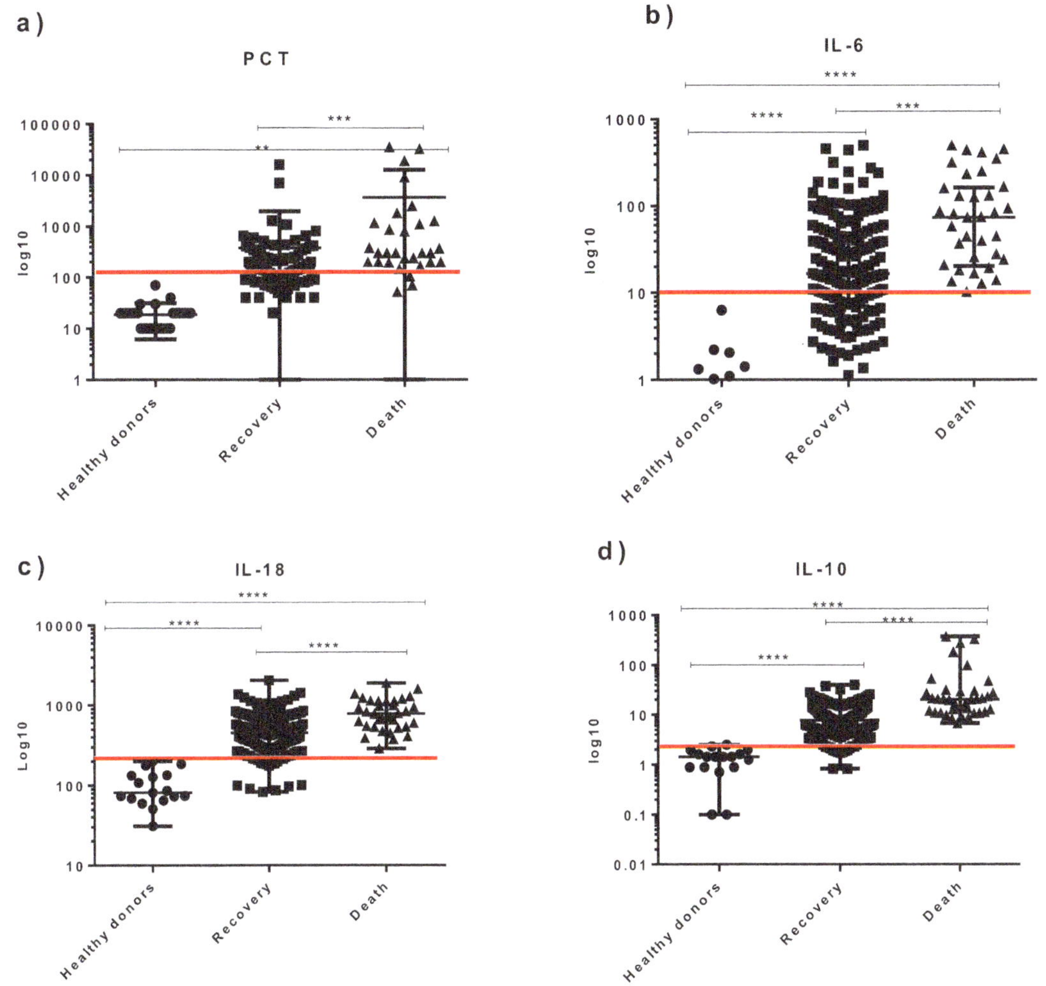

FIGURE 5.1 Concentration of procalcitonin (a, PCT), interleukin 6 (b,IL-6), interleukin 18 (c,IL18), interleukin 10 (d,IL10) in healthy individuals, recovered and deceased patients with COVID-19-associated pneumonia. Cytokine concentrations are presented in ng/mL on vertical axis as log10. Notes: IL-6—interleukin 6, IL-18—interleukin 18, IL-10—interleukin 10, PCT—procalcitonin.

inflammasome, is characteristic of both COVID-19 and autoinflammatory diseases. In the cohort we studied, in those who died the concentration of IL-18 was significantly higher than in those patients who survived. It was noted that the levels of IL-18 in our study had correlations with the severity of respiratory failure, the degree of lung damage according to CT data, as well as the NEWS and SOFA scores.

A unique feature of COVID-19 is an increase in the level of IL-10 in patients with severe disease [14,42,43]. It should be noted that IL-10 is also one of the key cytokines in sepsis and systemic inflammatory processes. On the one hand, the induction of IL-10 synthesis at the initial stage of COVID-19 inhibits cellular immunity. However, as the production of endogenous IL-10 increases, as in endotoxemia and sepsis, IL-10 can enhance the hyperinflammatory response [44]. The results of our study indicate that IL-10, according to the ROC analysis, is a more informative indicator of a poor prognosis in patients with COVID-19-associated pneumonia compared to other biomarkers.

Many studies have shown that an increased PCT level is significantly associated with the severity of COVID-19 [13,45,46]. It is assumed that the cascade of inflammatory reactions triggered by the coronavirus through the release of proinflammatory cytokines such as IL-1b and IL-6 can induce the release of PCT in patients even without bacterial coinfection. A meta-analysis showed that the severe form of COVID-19 can be distinguished from the moderate one by a slightly higher PCT (by 0.2 ng/mL). In our cohort, the procalcitonin level of 0.32 ng/mL or higher was recorded in almost half of the patients who died, which confirms its high predictive value. An increase in both CRP and PCT may be associated not only with a huge inflammatory process, but also with a higher incidence of bacterial superinfections among critically ill patients with COVID-19 (up to 50% among deceased patients).

Immunological patterns of secondary hemophagocytic lymphohistiocytosis, bacterial sepsis, and COVID-19

Secondary HLH (sHLS) and sepsis are both typical hyperinflammatory diseases associated with CSS. Some common features were found in CSS caused by COVID-19 and sHLH due to the severity of their clinical course, frequent lungs involvement [6], and similar immunological profile including elevated IL-1β, IL-2, IL-8, IL-10, IL-17, TNF-α, IFN-γ et al. [7]. Furthermore, both COVID-19 and HLH also has common immunological and clinical characteristics with septic shock (SS), caused by bacterial infection [8,9]. Although an elevation of many inflammatory parameters is essential for all mentioned conditions, some of them could be combined and serve as patterns, reflecting immunopathological characteristics of underlying diseases.

There were also available retrospective collections of 49 samples from patients with secondary hemophagocytic syndrome and 52 samples from patient with septic shock collected a year before. Serum samples and clinical data of 39 sHLH and 47 SS consecutive fatal cases that had been collected within 2018–2019 years were analyzed retrospectively and compared to fatal COVID-19 group. The median number of days from admission and taking blood until the end point was 6.0 days in sHLH and 1.0 day in SS. 7-day and 28-day CFRs consisted 50.0% and 75.0% in sHLH, and 95.4% and 100.0% in SS, respectively. The sHLH diagnosis was established with the use of HLH-2004 criteria [12] and H-Score [13]. The median number of points was 5.0 (4.0–6.0) by HLH-2004 criteria and 227 (178.5–256.0) by H-Score. The diagnosis of sepsis was established according to ACCP/SCCM sepsis criteria and confirmed based on the positive blood culture result in 57.45% (27/47) cases [14]. The median value on the Sequential Organ Failure Assessment (SOFA) Score in SS patients consisted 12.0 points. Assessing the risk of developing a severe course of COVID-19 has evaluated using previously developed National Early Warning Score 2 (NEWS2). The median value on National Early Warning Score 2 (NEWS2) Score in fatal COVID-19 patients consisted seven points.

Serum samples, demographic, and clinical data were collected from 37 lethal cases of COVID-19, 39 retrospective fatal cases sHLH and 47 retrospective fatal SS (Table 5.4). Secondary HPS with hyperferrininemia was related to hemato-oncology diseases, and in over half of septic patients the microbial agent was known. The samples came from patients during last two weeks of the disease before death.

Serum cytokine levels in patients with fatal COVID-19, SS, and sHLH are presented in a Table 5.5:

Hypercytokinemia is essential component of systemic inflammation and by itself is not specific for any definite pathology; however, the proportions of certain parameters may vary depending on the pathogen type, underlying disease, and patient's individual features. It was noticed, that WBC rate [47], CRP [48], and PCT values [49] are typically higher, while NPT and ferritin are lower in bacterial infections compared to viral [50]. The novel concept divides infectious pathogens into intracellular and extracellular due to their ability to affect different PPRs and induce different inflammatory pathways [7]. In particular, Slaats J et al. have proposed IL-1/IL-6/CRP pattern for extracellular pathogen-induced response and IL-18/ferritin pattern for intracellular pathogen-induced response [51]. In this view, CSS may be considered as a condition prevalently induced by extracellular parasites, though the cases of intracellular sepsis were also reported [52]. Meanwhile, hyperinflammation in sHLH is

TABLE 5.4 Demographic parameters of patients with fatal COVID-19, SS, and sHLH outcomes.

	Secondary hemophagocytic syndrome (N = 39)	**Bacterial sepsis and septic shock (N = 47)**	**Pneumonia COVID-19 (N = 36)**
Study	**Retrospective, 2018–19**	**Retrospective, 2018–19**	**Prospective, 2020**
Age, median	58.0	65.0	69.0
Gender (m/f)	19/20	30/17	24/13
Etiology	• Hemato-oncology: 71.8% • Infections(Leishmania spp., HIV, Epstein–Barr virus): 15.4% • Idiopathic: 12.8%	• Klebsiella pheumoniae: 21.3% • Staphylococcus spp: 19.2% • Acinetobacter baumannii: 10.6% • Pseudomonas aeruginosa: 6.4% • Streptococci spp.: 6.4% • Others—6.3%	SARS-CoV-2: 100.0%
Cause of death	• Poly-organic failure: 61.6% • Oncology progression: 33.3% • Stroke: 5.13%	• Polyorganic failure: 100.0%	• ARDS: 73.0% • Poly-organ failure 21.6% • Heart attack 5.4%
Therapy	Chemotherapy (etoposide), IVIG, cyclosporin A, steroids	Antibiotics	Anticytokine treatment, Jak inhibitors, steroids,

Note: AMI, Acute Myocardial Infarction; *ARDS*, Acute Respiratory Distress Syndrome; *COVID-19*, coronavirus disease 2019; *MODS*, Multiple Organ Dysfunction Syndrome; *SARS-CoV-2*, Severe Acute Respiratory Syndrome Coronavirus 2; *sHLH*, secondary Hemophagocytic Lymphohistiocytosis; *SS*, Septic Shock (caused by bacteria).

TABLE 5.5 Cytokine levels in patients with fatal COVID-19, SS, and sHLH outcomes.

Parameter	Donor values	sHLH	SS	COVID-19	sHLH/ SS	sHLH/ COVID-19	SS/ COVID-19
IL-1β, pg/mL,median (25–75th)	0.20 (0.10–0.87)	0.13 (0.1–1.47)	0.36 (0.11–19.95)	0.88 (0.15–1.67)	ns	ns	ns
IL-2, pg/mL,median (25–75th)	0.15 (0.10–0.20)	1.46 (0.32–43.07)	0.01 (0.01–0.14)	0.07 (0.01–0.18)	*	ns	ns
IL-6, pg/mL,median (25–75th)	0.63 (0.25–1.37)	24.23 (7.91–122.90)	99.80 (16.94–512.3)	75.27 (24.30–166.1)	**	**	ns
IL-8, pg/mL,median (25–75th)	2.90 (2.21–3.98)	141.3 (74.31–343.5)	498.1 (80.47–643.2)	23.78 (14.86–32.28)	ns	****	****
IL-10, pg/mL,median (25–75th)	1.43 (0.89–1.79)	64.70 (17.90–236.8)	42.33 (15.87–500.0)	20.00 (11.16–29.80)	ns	*	*
IL-17A, pg/mL,median (25–75th)	4.85 (0.19–21.57)	51.32 (6.89–101.5)	8.11 (0.21–30.53)	31.95 (30.29–33.66)	*	ns	ns
IL-18, pg/mL,median (25–75th)	81.40 (67.06–133.80)	2690.0 (2042.0–2741.0)	1575.0 (942.4–2368.0)	783.9 (537.4–1117.0)	*	****	****
IFN-γ, pg/mL,median (25–75th)	0.20 (0.10–0.52)	35.24 (21.00–55.62)	19.35 (11.02–36.61)	4.55 (0.21–10.19)	*	****	*
TNF-α, pg/mL,median (25–75th)	0.71 (0.30–1.04)	36.90 (22.13–60.73)	19.33 (9.58–37.62)	3.77 (2.17–6.11)	ns	**	*

Note: P values for each pair are presented as ns ($P > 0.04$, not significant), *($P < 0.05$), ** ($P < 0.01$), *** ($P < 0.001$), and **** ($P < 0.0001$). *COVID-19*, coronavirus disease 2019; *sHLH*, secondary Hemophagocytic Lymphohistiocytosis; *SS*, Septic Shock (caused by bacteria). The groups were compared by Kruskal–Wallis one-way analysis of variance and Dunn's pairwise posttest.

triggered by either intracellular infectious agents (viral, bacterial, or protozoan) or malignancies [53] and inflated in result of genetic defect of CD8+T-cells or natural killers [54]. Both viruses and malignancies are known to activate IFN-γ mediated cell immunity [55]. The distributions of inflammatory biomarkers in deceased patients with COVID-19, sHLH, and SS and in different COVID-19 outcomes (fatal v/s nonfatal) are presented in Figs. 5.2–5.3 .

Considering the chart in a Fig. 5.2, it was noted that each hyperinflammatory condition had distinct increased and decreased parameters, suggesting that this imbalance may be a better differentiating marker compared to a set of the most increased parameters. Figs. 5.2 and 5.3 illustrated that despite deceased COVID-19 patients had significantly higher IL-6, IL-8, IL-10, IL-18, PCT, CRP, and NPT levels compared to survived, some of these parameters were lower compared to SS and sHLH. In particular, patients with COVID-19 had the lowest IFN-γ median concentration compared to other fatal conditions, what can be explained by the fact that SARS-CoV-2 is able to suppress both interferon types I and II expression in monocytes and epithelial cells [27,28].

Although both COVID-19 and sHLH were provoked by intracellular pathogens, the pattern of COVID-19 was more similar to SS. In particular, deceased patients with COVID-19 and SS had comparable IL-6, ferritin, %GF, and NLR values. Recently NLR was identified as an

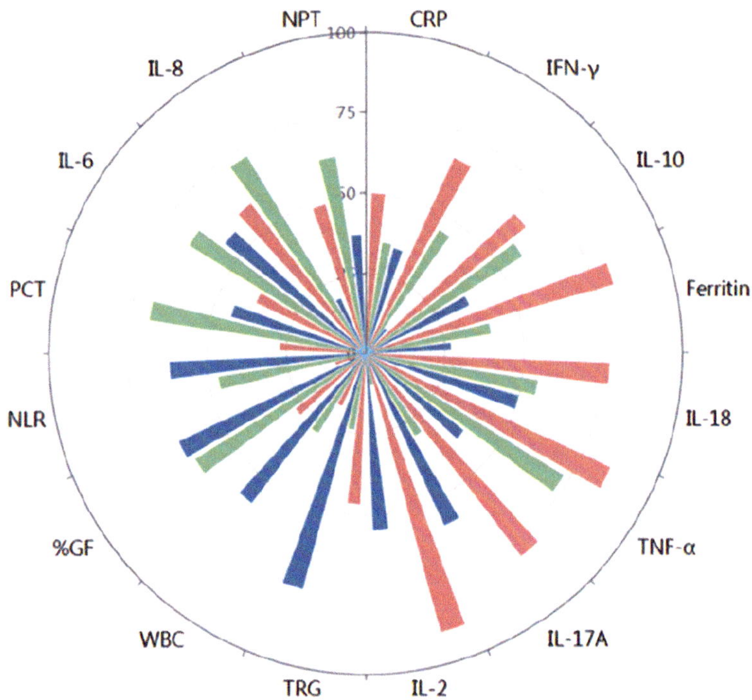

FIGURE 5.2 Rose Plote describing inflammatory parameters in patients with fatal COVID-19, sHLH, and SS outcomes. Median values of laboratory parameters are transformed into percentile values of these parameters in total group of patients with fatal conditions.

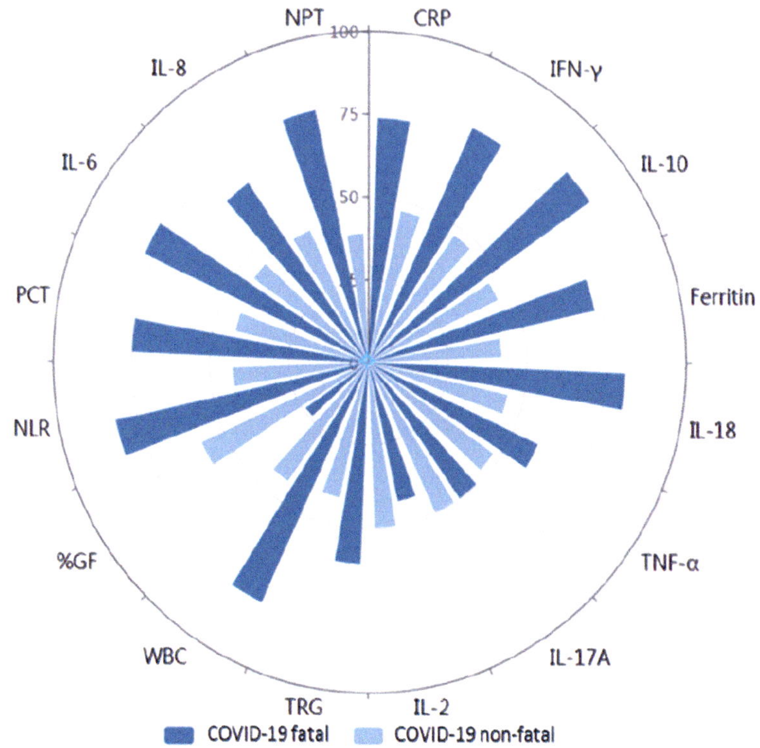

FIGURE 5.3 Rose Plot describing inflammatory parameters in patients with fatal and nonfatal COVID-19 outcomes. Median values of laboratory parameters are transformed into percentile values of these parameters in total COVID-19 group. *Note: %GF*, the percent of Glycosylated Ferritin fraction; *COVID-19*, coronavirus disease 2019; *CRP*, C-reactive protein; *NLR*, Neutrophil to Lymphocyte ratio; *NPT*, neopterin; *PCT*, procalcitonin; *sHLH*, secondary Hemophagocytic Lymphohistiocytosis; *SS*, Septic Shock (caused by bacteria); *TRG*, triglycerides; *WBC*, White Blood Cells.

independent risk factor for critical illness in patients with COVID-19 infection (with a threshold value of 3.13 in early stage) [29], and in the current study deceased COVID-19 patients demonstrated its highest level. Revealed disproportions in COVID-19 included high IL-6, IL-17A, WBC, NLR, and low IFN-γ, TNF-α, IL-8, IL-2 concentrations that seemed to be the sign of its unfavorable course. Previously Bert NL and al. reported an imbalanced response in symptomatic COVID-19 patients with elevated IL-6, TNF-α, IL-1β, and IL-10, but decreased IL-2 and IFN-γ production, whereas asymptomatic patients had proportionally high IL-2 and IFN-γ levels [30]. Nevertheless, both decreased [31] and increased [32] IFN-γ levels in severe COVID-19 compared to its mild form were reported. Low IL-2 and IFN-γ levels most likely reflected cytotoxic immunity suppression, while an activation of IL-6/IL-17 pathway with subsequent neutrophil recruitment may play the role of an alternative mechanism of antiviral defense. Recent studies revealed a range of effects of these cells, aimed at eliminating intracellular pathogens via binding their extracellular forms by neutrophil extracellular traps [33], shuttling to the lymph nodes and presenting to lymphocytes [34], expression chemokines for macrophages and T-lymphocytes [4], etc.

As it was said above, hyperinflammation is a result of immune system inability to eliminate pathogen that also manifests as imbalanced response. Each fatal condition has demonstrated some immunological pattern: high IL-6/NLR and low IFN-γ/TNF-α in COVID-19; high IL-8/IL-6 and low IL-17A/IL-2/sTfR in SS; high IL-18/ferritin/IL-17A and low IL-6/PCT/NLR%GF in sHLH.

Cytokine storm syndrome score for disease prognosis

Predicting the course of COVID-19 infection is of fundamental importance for the timely and adequate distribution of treatment efforts in the face of limited time and material resources caused by the massive admission of patients. A significant number of new clinical algorithms and models have been proposed to solve this problem. A number of studies have evaluated the use of previously developed clinical scales for assessing the risk of developing a severe course, including the pneumonia severity index (PSI), the CURB-65 and CRB-65 pneumonia severity scores, A-DROP and SMART-COP, the severity rating score patient NEWS2, sequential assessment of organ failure qSOFA, and criteria for systemic inflammatory response syndrome [56]. Thus, the NEWS2 scale was superior to qSOFA and other scales in terms of predicting the critical course in hospitalized patients [57]. New scales for assessing the severity of COVID-19 were also developed, based on demographic data, the presence of concomitant diseases, instrumental studies, saturation, and laboratory parameters [56]. A large-scale study of the informativeness of this approach was carried out in China, where the area under the ROC curve of the clinical risk scale was 0.88 (95% CI, 0.85–0.91), and when validated it was also 0.88 (95% CI, 0.84–0.93). The American 10-point scale for assessing the severity of COVID-19, including age, oxygen saturation, blood pressure, blood urea, CRP, and international normalized ratio, showed similar prognostic indicators [58]. Despite the decisive role of cytokines and the development of CSS, they are not included in risk stratification algorithms due to the inaccessibility of their routine measurement in most clinical laboratories.

Since IL-6, IL-10, IL-18, and PCT were associated with disease severity and death, these indicators were integrated into a 12-point scale called the CSS score. The f ranges of IL-6, IL-18, IL-10, PCT, and the corresponding score are presented in Table 5.4. Cut-off of these ranges was established on the basis of ROC analysis. The cut-off between low and medium levels were determined on the basis of the concentrations of the studied laboratory parameters and were characterized by a sensitivity of 60% and a specificity of 75%, and values between the medium and high levels—a sensitivity of 40% and a specificity of 90%. The CSS score represents the sum of IL-6, IL-10, IL-18, and PCT scores (Table 5.6), from 0 to 12. Patients who score 6 points or more have a high risk of an unfavorable outcome of the disease. According to the ROC analysis, the area under the curve for the CSS score was superior to for each of the four markers separately (AUC 0.90 (95% CI 0.84–0.95), $P < 0.001$).

To assess the prognosis of the outcome of the disease, we carried out an analysis of laboratory data, which revealed significant differences between patients who died from COVID-19 and those who survived (Table 5.3). Thus, among patients with a poor outcome, the following were significantly more frequent: leukocytosis (26 patients [72%] versus 55 [28.9%]; $P < 0.001$), as well as lymphopenia (25 [69.4%] patients versus 69 [36%]; $P < 0.001$). The average number of leukocytes and neutrophils in deceased patients was

TABLE 5.6 Cytokine storm syndrome score.

	Score = 0	Score = 1	Score = 2	Score = 3
Biomarkers	Normal range	Borderline increase	Moderately increase	Ultimately high
IL-6, pg/mL	0–10	10–40	40–100	>100
IL-18, pg/mL	0–300	300–650	650–1000	>1000
IL-10,pg/mL	0–5	5–10	10–30	>30
PCT, pg/mL	0–0.25	0.25–0.99	1.0–2.0	>2.0

Notes: IL-10, interleukin 10; *IL-18*, interleukin 18; *IL-6*, interleukin 6; *PCT*, procalcitonin; The score of cytokine storm is a 12-point score that includes different levels of concentrations of IL-6, IL-18, IL-10, PCT. Scores from one to three correspond to normal, borderline, medium and high level of these biomarkers. A value of **six and more points** is associated with a high risk of unfavorable outcome.

significantly higher, and the average number of lymphocytes and platelets was significantly lower than in recovered patients (Table 5.2). There was also a significant difference in the levels of a number of biochemical and coagulation parameters. It should be noted that 16 (44%) of 36 deceased patients and 53 (27%) of 190 recovered patients had a D-dimer concentration above 1000 ng/mL. The levels of C-reactive protein and ferritin in the blood in deceased patients was significantly higher than in the group of recovered individuals (60 vs 144 mg/L and 605 vs 1243 μg/L, $P < 0.0005$, respectively).

To compare the predictive value of the CSS score and other pro-inflammatory and other biomarkers, ROC curves of the levels of D-dimer, neutrophils, C-reactive protein, ferritin, and LDH were constructed (Fig. 5.4). The area under the curve was the largest for CSS score and amounted to 0.90 (0,85- 0,96) with sensitivity of 83.33% (62.62-95.26) and specificity 84.48% (78.23–89.52). For the diagnosis of critical COVID-19, the area under the curve for

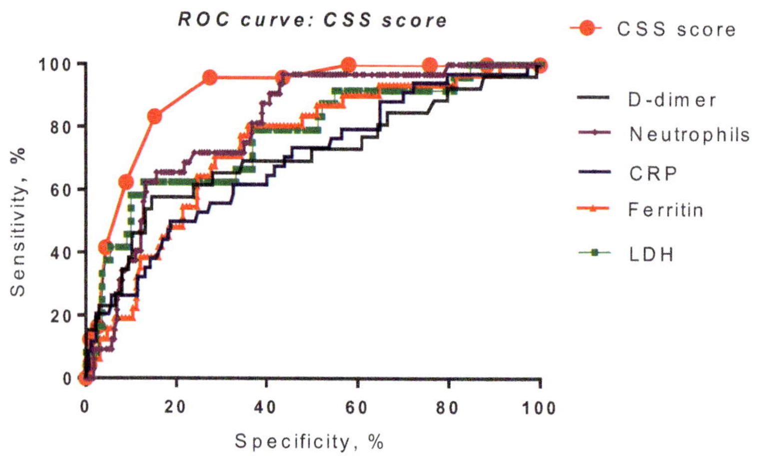

FIGURE 5.4 ROC curves of tCSS score, C-reactive protein, lactate hydrogenase, ferritin, D-dimer, neutrophils for predicting the critical course of COVID-19. Notes: *CRP*, C-reactive protein; *CSS*, cytokine storm syndrome; *LDH*, lactatdehydrogenase.

neutrophils was 0.80 (0.73-0.88), for LDH - 0.77 (0.66–0.88), for D-dimer—0.70 (0.57–0.82). Proinflammatory markers such as CRP and ferritin showed an area under the ROC curve of 0.69 (0.59–0.78) and 0.74 (0.64–0.83), respectively.

Validation of cytokine storm syndrome score and its clinical relationship

To validate the CSS score and to prove its prognostic significance, we have also tested samples of 121 patient collected during second wave of the epidemic that happened in St. Petersburg, Russia, during the winter of 2020. There were 48 hospitalized patients with COVID-19 pneumonia not required ICU and 80 hospitalized patients with COVID-19 severe and critical pneumonia.

To identify patients at risk of death in the validation cohort, the integration of markers into the CSS score showed a relatively high sensitivity (78.79%, 95% CI% 0.61–0.91) and significantly increased the specificity (81.12%, 95% CI 71.24–88.80). Clinical sensitivity of CSS score (≥6 points) for fatal outcomes was 78.79% and specificity of 81.12% (Table 5.7). The CSS score positively and statistically significantly correlates with the NEWS2 (0.56, $P < 0.05$), the duration of oxygen therapy ($R = 4.49$, $P < 0.05$) and the degree of lung damage based on CT results (3.48, $P < 0.05$).

Thus, we have confirmed the predictive value of the CSS score in relation to the risk of an unfavorable prognosis of the course of COVID-19. The combined prognostic capabilities of IL-6, IL-18, IL-10, and PCT, integrated into CSS score, can help identify patients at high risk of death in COVID-19-associated pneumonia. Important clinical issue of COVID-19 pneumonia is the relationship between severe disease and older age and the number of comorbidities.

TABLE 5.7 Diagnostic test evaluation of IL-6, IL-10, IL-18, PCT, cytokine storm syndrome score.

Marker	Cut-off	P	Sensitivity, % (95% CI)	Specificity, % (95% CI)	Odds ratio (95% CI)	Relative risk (95% CI)	PPV (95% CI)	NPV (95% CI)
IL-6 (pg/mL)	16.53	< 0.0001	94.23 (79.77–99.26)	52.0 (42.96–64.00)	18.28 (4.11–81.33)	10.63 (2.66–42.34)	0.44 (0.32 –0.56)	0.95 (0.85 –0.99)
IL-18 (pg/mL)	535.9	0.0235	75.76 (0.57–0.88)	47.06 (36.13–58.13)	2.77 (1.12–6.85)	2.14 (1.05–4.34)	0.35 (0.24 –0.48)	0.83 (0.69 –0.92)
IL-10 (pg/mL)	17.45	< 0.0001	78.79 (0.61–0.91)	74.12 (0.63–0.83)	10.64 (4.04–27.94)	5.41 (2.56–11.46)	0.54 (0.39 –0.68)	0.90 (0.80 –0.95)
PCT (pg/mL)	0.56	< 0.0001	45.71 (28.83–63.35)	87.06 (78.02 93.36)	5.66 (2.26–14.20)	2.90 (1.74–4.82)	0.59 (0.38 –0.77)	0.79 (0.69 –0.87)
CSS score	>6	< 0.0001	78.79 (61.09–0.91)	81.1 (71.2–88.84)	16.02 (5.90–43.38) 5.914 to 43.38	6.71 (3.19–14.16)	0.62 (0.45 –0.76)	0.88 (0.82 –0.96)

Note: NPV, negative predictive value; *PPV*, positive predictive value; *CSS*, cytokine storm syndrome.

We have studied the prevalence of comorbidity, that was found in 70% among hospitalized patients, while hypertension (HD) was observed in 57.8% (n = 130), coronary heart disease (IHD)—in 27% (n = 61), diabetes mellitus (DM)—in 16.2% (n = 36), chronic heart failure (CHF)—in 8.6% (n = 19). About 9.6% (n = 21) of patients had oncological diseases in the active stage, and 3.7% (n = 8) had chronic kidney disease. It should be noted that a high incidence of comorbidities was observed in critically ill patients, as well as in the group of patients with fatal outcome (Fig. 5.5). Chronic kidney disease, coronary heart disease, and cancer were directly correlated with number of deaths.

The number of deaths of patients under 45 years old was 3 (7.31%), from 45 to 65 years old—12 (10.5%), while the largest number of deaths was observed in the group of patients aged 65–85 years (21 [58, 3%]). Body mass index (BMI) in 42% of cases exceeded 30 kg/m^2. BMI in women was 33.0 ± 1.4 kg/m^2 and was significantly ($P < 0.01$) higher than the average BMI in men (29.3 ± 0.7 kg/m^2). We have found the association between CSS score and age group and the presence of life threating comorbidities (Fig. 5.6).

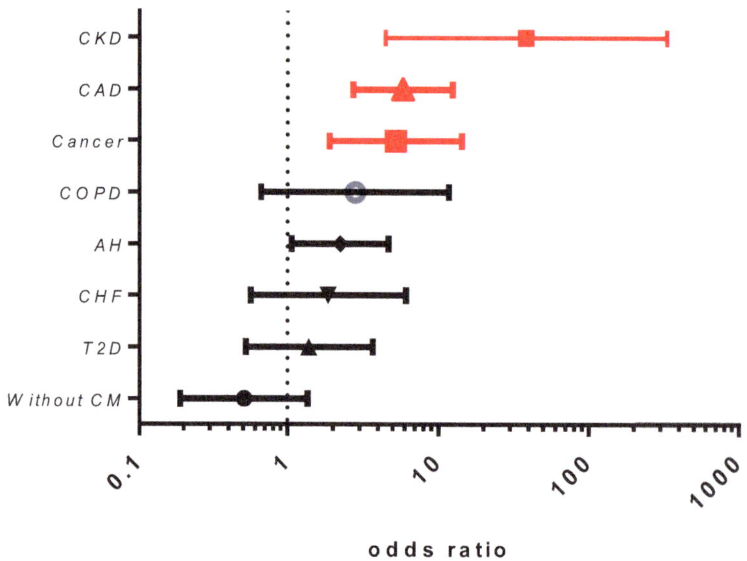

FIGURE 5.5 Forest graph showing the relationship of various comorbidities and the risk of death. On the ordinate axis comorbidities represent, on logarithmic axis—odds ratio of the risks of death. Groups of comorbidity with the highest odds ratios are highlighted in red. Note: *AH*, arterial hypertension; *CAD*, coronary artery disease; *CHF*, congestive heart failure; *CKD*, chronic kidney disease; *CM*, comorbidity; *COPD*, chronic obstructive pulmonary disease; *T2D*, type 2 diabetes.

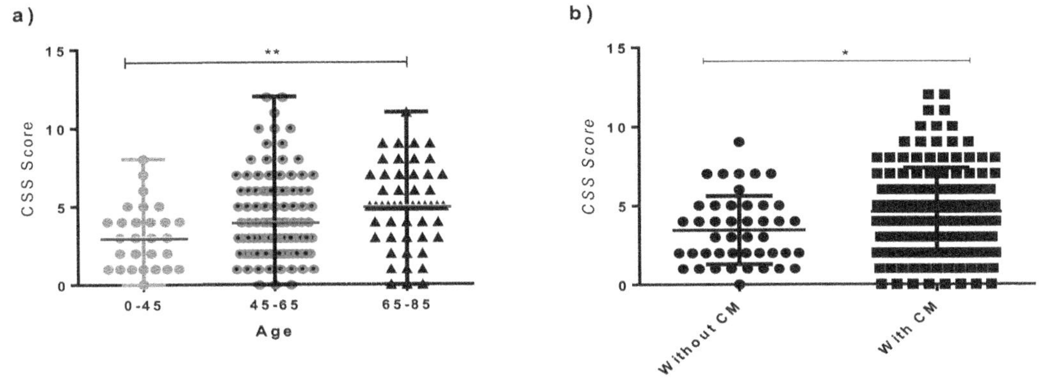

FIGURE 5.6 Relationship between SCC score points and age (A) and presence of life threating comorbidities (B) *Notes: CM*, comorbidities; *CSS*, cytokine storm syndrome.

Conclusion remarks

- COVID19 in characterized by unique pattern of proinflammatory cytokine synthesis including IL-18/ferritin and IL-17A; IL-6/CRP and IL-8/TNFa/procalcitonin; IL-10/ lymphopenia;
- Profiles of cytokines and laboratory biomarkers resemble both sepsis and hemophagocytic (MAS) syndrome;
- Levels of proinflammatory monocytic cytokines are higher in patients further transferred to ICU for pulmonary support and are associated with high mortality;
- Cytokine storm parameters are higher in patients belonging to risk groups (higher age and with higher number of comorbidities);
- Integrated Cytokine Storm Score can help to predict most severe cases of COVID-19 disease.

References

[1] Tisoncik JR, Korth MJ, Simmons CP, Farrar J, Martin TR, Katze MG. Into the eye of the cytokine storm. Microbiol Mol Biol Rev 2012;76(1):16–32. https://journals.asm.org/doi/10.1128/MMBR.05015-11.

[2] Cron RQ, Behrens EM. Cytokine Storm Syndrome. Cham: Springer International Publishing; 2019. http://link.springer.com/10.1007/978-3-030-22094-5.

[3] Nazinitsky A, Rosenthal KS. Cytokine storms. Infect Dis Clin Pract 2010;18(3):188–92. https://journals.lww.com/00019048-201005000-00011.

[4] Minoia F, Davì S, Horne A, Demirkaya E, Bovis F, Li C, et al. Clinical features, treatment, and outcome of macrophage activation syndrome complicating systemic juvenile idiopathic arthritis: a multinational, multicenter study of 362 patients. Arthritis Rheumatol 2014 г;66(11):3160–9. https://doi.org/10.1002/art.38802.

[5] Dinarello CA. Historical insights into cytokines. Eur J Immunol 2007;37(S1):S34–45. https://onlinelibrary.wiley.com/doi/10.1002/eji.200737772.

[6] Ray A. Cytokines and their role in health and disease: a brief overview. MOJ Immunol [Интернет] 2016;4(2). https://medcraveonline.com/MOJI/cytokines-and-their-role-in-health-and-disease-a-brief-overview.html.

[7] Mogensen TH. Pathogen recognition and inflammatory signaling in innate immune defenses. Clin Microbiol Rev. 2009;22(2):240–73.

[8] Canedo-Marroquín G, Saavedra F, Andrade CA, Berrios RV, Rodríguez-Guilarte L, Opazo MC, et al. SARS-CoV-2: immune response elicited by infection and development of vaccines and treatments. Front Immunol 2020;11. https://www.frontiersin.org/articles/10.3389/fimmu.2020.569760/full.

[9] Snijder EJ, van der Meer Y, Zevenhoven-Dobbe J, Onderwater JJM, van der Meulen J, Koerten HK, et al. Ultrastructure and origin of membrane vesicles associated with the severe acute respiratory syndrome coronavirus replication complex. J Virol 2006;80(12):5927–40. https://jvi.asm.org/content/80/12/5927.

[10] Dias Junior AG, Sampaio NG, Rehwinkel J. A balancing act: MDA5 in antiviral immunity and autoinflammation. Trends Microbiol 2019;27(1):75–85. http://www.ncbi.nlm.nih.gov/pubmed/30201512.

[11] Barnes BJ, Adrover JM, Baxter-Stoltzfus A, Borczuk A, Cools-Lartigue J, Crawford JM, et al. Targeting potential drivers of COVID-19: neutrophil extracellular traps. J Exp Med 2020;217(6). https://rupress.org/jem/article/doi/10.1084/jem.20200652/151683/Targeting-potential-drivers-of-COVID19-Neutrophil.

[12] Grasselli G, Zangrillo A, Zanella A, Antonelli M, Cabrini L, Castelli A, et al. Baseline characteristics and outcomes of 1591 patients infected with SARS-CoV-2 admitted to ICUs of the lombardy region, Italy. JAMA 2020;323(16):1574. https://jamanetwork.com/journals/jama/fullarticle/2764365.

[13] Zhang J, Dong X, Cao Y, Yuan Y, Yang Y, Yan Y, et al. Clinical characteristics of 140 patients infected with SARS-CoV-2 in Wuhan, China. Allergy 2020;75(7):1730–41. https://onlinelibrary.wiley.com/doi/10.1111/all.14238.

[14] Huang C, Wang Y, Li X, Ren L, Zhao J, Hu Y, et al. Clinical features of patients infected with 2019 novel coronavirus in Wuhan, China. Lancet (London, England) 2020;395(10223):497–506. https://www.ncbi.nlm.nih.gov/pmc/articles/PMC7278637/.

[15] Mehta P, McAuley DF, Brown M, Sanchez E, Tattersall RS, Manson JJ. COVID-19: consider cytokine storm syndromes and immunosuppression. Lancet 2020;395(10229):1033–4. https://linkinghub.elsevier.com/retrieve/pii/S0140673620306280.

[16] McGonagle D, Sharif K, O'Regan A, Bridgewood C. The role of cytokines including interleukin-6 in COVID-19 induced pneumonia and macrophage activation syndrome-like disease. Autoimmun Rev 2020;19(6):102537. http://www.ncbi.nlm.nih.gov/pubmed/32251717.

[17] Jamilloux Y, Henry T, Belot A, Viel S, Fauter M, El Jammal T, et al. Should we stimulate or suppress immune responses in COVID-19? Cytokine and anti-cytokine interventions. Autoimmun Rev 2020;19(7):102567. https://linkinghub.elsevier.com/retrieve/pii/S1568997220301294.

[18] Del Valle DM, Kim-Schulze S, Huang H-H, Beckmann ND, Nirenberg S, Wang B, et al. An inflammatory cytokine signature predicts COVID-19 severity and survival. Nat Med 2020;26(10):1636–43. https://www.nature.com/articles/s41591-020-1051-9.

[19] Chen Y, Wang J, Liu C, Su L, Zhang D, Fan J, et al. IP-10 and MCP-1 as biomarkers associated with disease severity of COVID-19. Mol Med 2020;26(1):97. https://molmed.biomedcentral.com/articles/10.1186/s10020-020-00230-x.

[20] Azzout M, Dietrich C, Machavoine F, Gastineau P, Bottier A, Lezmi G, et al. IL-33 enhances IFNγ and TNFα production by human MAIT cells: a new pro-Th1 effect of IL-33. Int J Mol Sci 2021;22(19):10602. https://www.mdpi.com/1422-0067/22/19/10602.

[21] Ye Q, Wang B, Mao J. The pathogenesis and treatment of the 'Cytokine Storm' in COVID-19. J Infect 2020;80(6):607–13. https://linkinghub.elsevier.com/retrieve/pii/S0163445320301651.

[22] Fajgenbaum DC, June CH. Cytokine storm. Longo DL, редактор. N Engl J Med 2020;383(23):2255–73. http://www.nejm.org/doi/10.1056/NEJMra2026131.

[23] Qi C, Zhou L, Hu Z, Zhang S, Yang S, Tao Y, et al. Dysregulation of immune response in patients with coronavirus 2019 (COVID-19) in Wuhan, China. Clin Infect Dis 2020;71(15):762–8. https://academic.oup.com/cid/article/71/15/762/5803306.

[24] Wang F, Nie J, Wang H, Zhao Q, Xiong Y, Deng L, et al. Characteristics of peripheral lymphocyte subset alteration in COVID-19 pneumonia. J Infect Dis 2020;221(11):1762–79. https://academic.oup.com/jid/article/221/11/1762/5813618.

[25] Sa Ribero M, Jouvenet N, Dreux M, Nisole S. Interplay between SARS-CoV-2 and the type I interferon response. Stapleford K, редактор. PLOS Pathog 2020;16(7):e1008737. https://dx.plos.org/10.1371/journal.ppat.1008737.

[26] Bourdon M, Manet C, Montagutelli X. Host genetic susceptibility to viral infections: the role of type I interferon induction. Genes Immun 2020;21(6–8):365–79. http://www.nature.com/articles/s41435-020-00116-2.

[27] Ferrara JL, Abhyankar S, Gilliland DG. Cytokine storm of graft-versus-host disease: a critical effector role for interleukin-1. Transplant Proc 1993;25(1 Pt 2):1216–7. http://www.ncbi.nlm.nih.gov/pubmed/8442093.

[28] Us D. Cytokine storm in avian influenza. Mikrobiyol Bul. 2008;42(2):365–80.

[29] Rodríguez-Pintó I, Espinosa G, Cervera R. The catastrophic antiphospholipid Syndrome. B: antiphospholipid antibody Syndrome. 2015. p. 249–62. c.

[30] Porter D, Frey N, Wood PA, Weng Y, Grupp SA. Grading of cytokine release syndrome associated with the CAR T cell therapy tisagenlecleucel. J Hematol Oncol 2018;11(1):35.

[31] Sharma C, Ganigara M, Galeotti C, Burns J, Berganza FM, Hayes DA, et al. Multisystem inflammatory syndrome in children and Kawasaki disease: a critical comparison. Nat Rev Rheumatol 2021;17(12):731–48. https://www.nature.com/articles/s41584-021-00709-9.

[32] Janka GE. Familial and acquired hemophagocytic lymphohistiocytosis. Annu Rev Med 2012;63(1):233–46. http://www.annualreviews.org/doi/10.1146/annurev-med-041610-134208.

[33] Haddad E, Sulis ML, Jabado N, Blanche S, Fischer A, Tardieu M. Frequency and severity of central nervous system lesions in hemophagocytic lymphohistiocytosis. Blood 1997;89(3):794–800. https://doi.org/10.1182/blood.V89.3.794.

[34] Jovanovic A, Kuzmanovic M, Kravljanac R, Micic D, Jovic M, Gazikalovic S, et al. Central nervous system involvement in hemophagocytic lymphohistiocytosis: a single-center experience. Pediatric Neurology 2014;50(3):233–7. https://doi.org/10.1016/j.pediatrneurol.2013.10.014.

[35] Parodi A, Davì S, Pringe AB, Pistorio A, Ruperto N, Magni-Manzoni S, et al. Macrophage activation syndrome in juvenile systemic lupus erythematosus: a multinational multicenter study of thirty-eight patients. Arthritis & Rheumatism 2009;60(11):3388–99. https://doi.org/10.1002/art.24883.

[36] Gavand PE, Serio I, Arnaud L, Costedoat-Chalumeau N, Carvelli J, Dossier A, et al. Clinical spectrum and therapeutic management of systemic lupus erythematosus-associated macrophage activation syndrome: a study of 103 episodes in 89 adult patients. Autoimmun Rev 2017;16(7):743–9. https://doi.org/10.1016/j.autrev.2017.05.010.

[37] Xie Y, Wang Z, Liao H, Marley G, Wu D, Tang W. Epidemiologic, clinical, and laboratory findings of the COVID-19 in the current pandemic: systematic review and meta-analysis. BMC Infect Dis 2020;20(1):640. https://doi.org/10.1186/s12879-020-05371-2. https://bmcinfectdis.biomedcentral.com/articles/10.1186/s12879-020-05371-2.

[38] Song J, Park DW, Moon S, Cho H-J, Park JH, Seok H, et al. Diagnostic and prognostic value of interleukin-6, pentraxin 3, and procalcitonin levels among sepsis and septic shock patients: a prospective controlled study according to the Sepsis-3 definitions. BMC Infect Dis 2019;19(1):968.

[39] Grifoni E, Valoriani A, Cei F, Lamanna R, Gelli AMG, Ciambotti B, et al. Interleukin-6 as prognosticator in patients with COVID-19. J Infect 2020;81(3):452–82. https://linkinghub.elsevier.com/retrieve/pii/S0163445320303881.

[40] Herold T, Jurinovic V, Arnreich C, Lipworth BJ, Hellmuth JC, von Bergwelt-Baildon M, et al. Elevated levels of IL-6 and CRP predict the need for mechanical ventilation in COVID-19. J Allergy Clin Immunol 2020;146(1):128–136.e4.

[41] Satıs H, Özger HS, Aysert Yıldız P, Hızel K, Gulbahar Ö, Erbas G, et al. Prognostic value of interleukin-18 and its association with other inflammatory markers and disease severity in COVID-19. Cytokine 2021;137:155302. https://linkinghub.elsevier.com/retrieve/pii/S1043466620303185.

[42] Lu L, Zhang H, Dauphars DJ, He Y-W. A potential role of interleukin 10 in COVID-19 pathogenesis. Trends Immunol 2021;42(1):3–5. https://linkinghub.elsevier.com/retrieve/pii/S1471490620302568.

[43] Diao B, Wang C, Tan Y, Chen X, Liu Y, Ning L, et al. Reduction and functional exhaustion of T cells in patients with coronavirus disease 2019 (COVID-19). Front Immunol 2020;11:827. https://www.frontiersin.org/article/10.3389/fimmu.2020.00827/full.

[44] Han H, Ma Q, Li C, Liu R, Zhao L, Wang W, et al. Profiling serum cytokines in COVID-19 patients reveals IL-6 and IL-10 are disease severity predictors. Emerg Microbes Infect 2020;9(1):1123–30. https://www.tandfonline.com/doi/full/10.1080/22221751.2020.1770129.

[45] Wang D, Hu B, Hu C, Zhu F, Liu X, Zhang J, et al. Clinical characteristics of 138 hospitalized patients with 2019 novel coronavirus-infected pneumonia in Wuhan, China. JAMA 2020;323(11):1061–9. http://www.ncbi.nlm.nih.gov/pubmed/32031570.

[46] Zhou F, Yu T, Du R, Fan G, Liu Y, Liu Z, et al. Clinical course and risk factors for mortality of adult inpatients with COVID-19 in Wuhan, China: a retrospective cohort study. Lancet 2020;395(10229):1054–62. http://www.ncbi.nlm.nih.gov/pubmed/32171076.

[47] Korppi M, Kröger L, Laitinen M. White blood cell and differential counts in acute respiratory viral and bacterial infections in children. Scand J Infect Dis. 1993;25(4):435–40.
[48] Korppi M, Kröger L. C-reactive protein in viral and bacterial respiratory infection in children. Scand J Infect Dis. 1993;25(2):207–13.
[49] Delevaux I. Can procalcitonin measurement help in differentiating between bacterial infection and other kinds of inflammatory processes? Ann Rheum Dis. 2003;62(4):337–40.
[50] Ip M, Rainer TH, Lee N, Chan C, Chau SSL, Leung W, et al. Value of serum procalcitonin, neopterin, and C-reactive protein in differentiating bacterial from viral etiologies in patients presenting with lower respiratory tract infections. Diagn Microbiol Infect Dis. 2007;59(2):131–6.
[51] Slaats J, ten Oever J, van de Veerdonk FL, Netea MG. IL-1β/IL-6/CRP and IL-18/ferritin: distinct inflammatory programs in infections. Bliska JB, редактор. PLOS Pathog. 2016;12(12):e1005973.
[52] Mckinlay AW, White N, Buxton D, Inglis JM, Johnson FWA, Kurtz JB, et al. Severe Chlamydia psittaci sepsis in pregnancy. QJM An Int J Med. 1985;57(1):689–96.
[53] Karlsson T. Secondary haemophagocytic lymphohistiocytosis: experience from the uppsala university hospital. Ups J Med Sci 2015;120(4):257–62.
[54] de Saint Basile G, Moshous D, Fischer A. Genetics and Pathogenesis of Hemophagocytic Lymphohistiocytosis. B: histiocytic disorders. Cham: Springer International Publishing; 2018. p. 197–214.
[55] Gujar S, Pol JG, Kim Y, Lee PW, Kroemer G. Antitumor benefits of antiviral immunity: an underappreciated aspect of oncolytic virotherapies. Trends Immunol. март 2018 г;39(3):209–21.
[56] Liang W, Liang H, Ou L, Chen B, Chen A, Li C, et al. Development and validation of a clinical risk score to predict the occurrence of critical illness in hospitalized patients with COVID-19. JAMA Intern Med 2020;180(8):1081. http://118.126.104.170/.
[57] Myrstad M, Ihle-Hansen H, Tveita AA, Andersen EL, Nygård S, Tveit A, et al. National Early Warning Score 2 (NEWS2) on admission predicts severe disease and in-hospital mortality from Covid-19 - a prospective cohort study. Scand J Trauma Resusc Emerg Med 2020;28(1):66. https://pubmed.ncbi.nlm.nih.gov/32660623/.
[58] Altschul DJ, Unda SR, Benton J, de la Garza Ramos R, Cezayirli P, Mehler M, et al. A novel severity score to predict inpatient mortality in COVID-19 patients. Sci Rep 2020;10(1):16726. http://www.nature.com/articles/s41598-020-73962-9.

CHAPTER

6

COVID-19: the impact of the cytokine storm on the immune-neuroendocrine system

Luis J. Jara[1], *Caroline I. Gutierrez-Melgarejo*[2], *Irvin Ordoñez-González*[3], *Berenice López-Zamora*[4], *Maria F. Galaviz-Sánchez*[2], *Gabriela Medina*[5,6], *María Pilar Cruz-Domínguez*[6,7] *and Olga Vera-Lastra*[6,8]

[1]Rheumatology Division, Instituto Nacional de Rehabilitación "Luis Guillermo Ibarra Ibarra", México City, México; [2]Centro de Investigación Clínica GRAMEL, México City, México; [3]Universidad Veracruzana, Facultad de Medicina, Veracruz, México; [4]Instituto Politécnico Nacional, Escuela Superior de Medicina, Campus Casco de Santo Tomás, Sección de Estudios de Posgrado e Investigación, México City, México; [5]Translational Research Unit, Hospital de Especialidades "Dr. Antonio Fraga Mouret" Centro Médico Nacional La Raza, Instituto Mexicano del Seguro Social, México City, México; [6]Division of Postgraduate Studies, Faculty of Medicine, Universidad Nacional Autónoma de México, México City, México; [7]Direction of Education and Research, Hospital de Especialidades "Dr. Antonio Fraga Mouret" Centro Médico Nacional La Raza, Instituto Mexicano del Seguro Social, México City, México; [8]Internal Medicine Department, Hospital de Especialidades "Dr. Antonio Fraga Mouret" Centro Médico Nacional La Raza, Instituto Mexicano del Seguro Social, México City, México

Introduction

Since December 2019, when the new pandemic caused by the SARS-CoV-2 virus, called COVID-19 infection, appeared, vulnerable groups of patients (20%) with the following independent risk factors have been identified: individuals over 65 years of age, patients with comorbidities such as obesity, arterial hypertension, diabetes, cancer, autoimmune diseases, smoking,

Autoimmunity, COVID-19, Post-COVID19 syndrome and COVID-19 vaccination
https://doi.org/10.1016/B978-0-443-18566-3.00033-5

asthma, and others comorbidities. The main characteristic of these vulnerable groups infected by SARS-CoV-2 is the rapid evolution to acute respiratory distress syndrome (ARDS) caused by viral infection and cytokine storm syndrome. This fact is responsible for the high morbidity and mortality of these patients and must be treated effectively and in a timely manner [1,2].

The term "cytokine storm" was first proposed in 1993 by Ferrara et al. in order to explain the Graft versus Host Diseases (GVHD), the major complication of allogeneic bone marrow transplantation. Evidence from 28 years ago indicated that this severe complication was caused by the dysregulated production of cytokines by T cells and other inflammatory cells. In this way, inflammatory cytokines act as mediators of acute GVHD, and these alterations of the complex cytokine network and the interactions with transplanted tissue can trigger a true "cytokine storm syndrome" with subsequent cellular damage [3,4]. Previously, in 1991, Chatenaud et al. [5], observed that after infusion of anti-CD3 monoclonal antibodies for the treatment and prevention of GVHD, patients and experimental models developed a transient systemic clinical picture that they called "Cytokine release syndrome" very similar to "Cytokine Storm Syndrome"; therefore, these terms can be used synonymously. These inflammatory syndromes are characterized by an overactivation of the cells of the immune system with hyper release of cytokines and are life-threatening. Cytokine storm syndrome and cytokine release syndrome have been described in infections caused by any agent, during experimental treatments, cancer, autoimmune diseases, and monogenic diseases [6]. During the pandemic, we have learned that COVID-19 infection is a systemic viral infection that affects multiple organs, apparatus, and systems and that leads to functional alterations and structural damage both in the acute phase and in the postCOVID-19 phase [7,8].

The term immune-neuroendocrine system was first proposed by Besedovsky H and Sorkin [9] in 1977 in order to incorporate the functioning of the self-regulated immune system into a comprehensive response in coordination with the endocrine system and the central nervous system (CNS), configuring an immune-neuroendocrine network. This hypothesis is based on the existence of afferent and efferent pathways present in the immuno-neuroendocrine structures. These immune-neuroendocrine responses are produced as a consequence of antigenic stimulation and under situations of molecular, physical, chemical, and emotional stress. Bidirectional communication between the immune, endocrine and the CNS has been demonstrated in these situations. This communication is based on the synthesis and release of hormones, neuropeptides, neurotransmitters, and cytokines by all three systems. These messengers will fulfill their defense function, interacting with receptors for these molecules present in the cells that make up the immune-neuroendocrine system. This comprehensive and bidirectional response, observed under stress situations, has a solid molecular basis and has been demonstrated in experimental models and in humans. The quality and intensity of this response is directly related to the type and magnitude of the environmental factor, as well as age, sex, reproductive status, and genetic factors. Therefore, an alteration in the immune-neuroendocrine response participates in the development of autoimmune diseases, as has been demonstrated in experimental models and in humans. The immuno-neuroendocrine response to stress, including the activation of the sympathetic and parasympathetic nervous system, aims to slow down the innate/inflammatory immune response at the local and systemic level and restore molecular homeostasis. In this regard, multiple evidence indicate that the CNS regulates this innate immune response [10–12]. The activated immune cells process peripheral information before sending it to the brain and releases various products, especially cytokines, which transmit information to the brain, which processes it through the tripartite synapse made up of neurons, microglia, and astrocytes. The processed information, depending on the intent of the information, may or not generate a neuroendocrine response. These findings have led to the hypothesis that the immune system is a sensory organ that responds to the regulatory mechanisms of the CNS inhibiting or stimulating the immune system [13].

COVID-19 infection, the cytokine storm and the immuno-neuroendocrine system

The immuno-neuroendocrine interaction is activated by stress factors such as infections, autoimmune diseases, or trauma. The main stress response systems are: 1. The hypothalamic–pituitary–adrenal axis (HPA). 2. The hypothalamic–pituitary–thyroid axis (HPT). 3.The hypothalamic–pituitary–gonadal axis (HPG). 4. Prolactin/growth hormone system, and 5. The autonomic nervous system. The immuno-neuroendocrine interaction is activated by stress factors such as infections, autoimmune diseases, or trauma [14,15].

Recent evidence shows that COVID-19 infection can affect the immune-neuroendocrine system, both in its invasion stage to different organs and tissues, and probably in the recovery stage. This damage is caused by viral infection and/or cytokine storm [2,16]. Next, we will discuss the devastating effect of SARS-CoV-2 infection and cytokine storm on the immune-neuroendocrine system.

The hypothalamic–pituitary–adrenal axis (HPA), COVID-19 infection, and cytokine storm

The main axis of the immune-neuroendocrine response to stress is the HPA. Therefore, the interaction between viral infections, cytokines, and HPA axis activation is of great importance. For example, HIV infection is associated with activation of HPA, with glucocorticoid release. Multiple alterations of the HPA axis have been described in HIV patients, ranging from subclinical adrenal insufficiency to complete adrenal insufficiency. Another important finding in patients with HIV is high blood levels of cortisol, with elevated or decreased levels of ACTH, suggesting a direct action of the virus or cytokines on HPA, changes in steroidogenesis that lead to increased production of cortisol, or antiretroviral treatment [17,18].

During a viral infection, proinflammatory cytokines, synthesized and released as a consequence of the activation of the immune system, act on the three levels of action of HPA: hypothalamus, with CRH release, pituitary, with ACTH release, and adrenal glands, with synthesis and cortisol release. The presence of receptors for cytokines in HPA cells favors the integration of bidirectional immuno-neuroendocrine communication. If the stimulus persists, there may be independent mechanisms in the three levels of HPA, due to the direct action of proinflammatory cytokines. An important aspect to consider is that the magnitude of the immune-neuroendocrine response can be specific for each virus [19,20].

The impact of COVID-19 infection on HPA has been little studied. Severely ill patients for a long time develop adrenocortical dysfunction. This clinical picture is called "critical illness-related corticosteroid insufficiency" (CIRCI). This CIRCI syndrome has been described in septicemia, severe pneumonia, and ARDS and is associated with biological markers of inflammation and activation of the coagulation cascade, similar to that observed in COVID-19 infection [21–23]. In this regard, a retrospective study analyzed the effect of SARS-CoV-2 infection on the adrenal cortex. Their findings showed that ACE2 and TMPRSS2 are localized in adrenocortical cells. In addition, the cortisol levels are lower in critically ill patients with COVID-19 as compared to those of non-COVID-19 critically ill patients. Most of the patients met the criteria for the diagnosis of CIRCI [24]. The first study to analyze the HPA axis was carried out in 28 patients with COVID-19 and different degrees of severity of the infection. Peripheral blood levels of plasma cortisol, ACTH, and dehydroepiandrosterone sulfate were determined in all patients. Hormone levels are correlated with the severity of the COVID-19 infection. The results of this study showed that a significant number of seriously ill patients with COVID-19 had low levels of cortisol and ACTH consistent with central adrenal insufficiency [25]. A recent study analyzed the hormonal profile of patients with COVID-19. Of 235 patients studied, 14% had severe disease and 5.5% died. The results of this study demonstrate adrenal insufficiency, low T3, and low TSH syndrome and hyperprolactinemia in COVID-19 hospitalized patients [26].

Finally, there is pathologic evidence of the changes that COVID-19 (in patients that had a severe disease) can cause on HPA axis. An autopsy study of COVID 19 revealed that different patients presented: necrosis, ischemic, cortical lipid degeneration, hemorrhage, focal adrenalitis, vascular thrombosis, and focal inflammation. In other autopsy study, it was founded the SARS genome in hypothalamic neurons [27,28].

Taking all this evidence together, there is no doubt about the devastating effect of COVID-19 infection on the HPA axis, especially in seriously ill patients. Therefore, a decrease in plasma cortisol can be considered a biomarker of severe COVID-19 infection.

In relation to long COVID-19, defined as the persistence of fatigue and cognitive dysfunction after 3 months of negativization of the molecular swab test, a recent study suggests that, long COVID symptoms could be explained by an adrenal insufficiency, demonstrated by salivary cortisol determination, due to a COVID-19 action on adrenal glands and by an iatrogenic side effect of high glucocorticoid therapy during the COVID-19 infection [29]. New prospective studies will be necessary to know the effect of long or post-COVID-19, on the HPA axis.

The hypothalamic—pituitary—thyroid axis (HPT), COVID-19 infection, and cytokine storm

The anatomic location of the thyroid is contiguous to the upper airways, which is a main entrance site of corona viruses. In an in vitro study, it was shown that ACE-2 is expressed in follicular cells of the thyroid, which makes them a strong target for the entry of SARS-CoV-2. Accordingly, throughout the pandemic, cases of patients with SARS-CoV-2 infection diagnosed with typical painful subacute thyroiditis have been reported [30].

During SARS-CoV-2 with cytokine storm phase, increased concentrations of interleukins, and in particular interleukin 6 (IL-6) were observed, that lead to thyrotoxicosis, with alteration of thyroid hormone transporting proteins, and altered secretion of TSH in pituitary cells, resulting in abnormal functional parameters of the thyroid. There is a decrease in the concentration of free T3, which is correlated with an increase in pro-inflammatory cytokines, normal or moderately decreased free T4, and normal or decreased TSH. These abnormalities are described as "low T3 syndrome" or "euthyroid disease syndrome" (abnormalities of thyroid function parameters reported in non—thyroid-related conditions). These abnormalities in thyroid function tests are generally transient and do not require specific treatment. During follow-up, the cytokine storm syndrome can cause a prolonged dysregulation of the immune system, leading to autoimmune disorders such as antiphospholipid syndrome, thrombocytopenia, hemolytic anemia, Guillain-Barré syndrome, Graves' disease, and, chronic autoimmune thyroiditis [31].

In a cohort study where 456 hospitalized patients from three London hospitals with clinical suspicion of COVID-19 were included. TSH and FT4 (free T4) levels were routinely evaluated, 334 of them had a confirmed diagnosis of COVID-19, and 122 did not. The authors found of confirmed COVID-19 patients, 86% were euthyroid, while only a minority were subclinical hypothyroid (5.1%) or open hypothyroid (0.6%) and 2.4% had suspected secondary hypothyroidism. No patient received a diagnosis of subclinical or overt thyrotoxicosis. The authors observed slightly lower TSH and FT4 levels among COVID-19 patients compared to those without COVID-19, even within the normal range. In addition, lower levels of TSH and FT4 were observed in patients with fatal disease and in those admitted to the ICU. A significant inverse relationship between C-reactive protein and cortisol levels and TSH levels was observed in COVID-19 patients. In a subset of patients in whom previous assessments of TSH and FT4 levels were available, a slight reduction in TSH and FT4 levels was observed in patients with COVID-19, but not in those without COVID-19. Finally, among 55 patients in whom an assessment of thyroid function parameters was performed before admission, at the time of admission and after a median follow-up of 79 days, the results showed that the thyroid function parameters returned to baseline levels after recovery from COVID-19. The authors concluded that there was no evidence of a COVID-19-related thyroiditis/thyrotoxicosis in their cohort, but that their findings are more indicative of a non-thyroidal illness (NTI) syndrome [32].

Wei L et al. [33] conducted a study to evaluate any possible injury to the thyroid gland caused by SARS in tissue samples obtained from five SARS autopsies and found that the follicular architecture was altered and showed distortion, dilation, and collapse. No cells other than calcitonin positive were detected in the SARS thyroid and both parafollicular and follicular cells were injured. This may provide an explanation for both the low serum triiodothyronine and thyroxine levels associated with SARS patients. Apoptosis may play a role in the pathogenesis of SARS-associated coronavirus infection in the thyroid gland.

Feghali K et al. [34] presented three cases of patients who developed autoimmune thyroid disease, such as profound hypothyroidism and Graves' disease, at 6 and 8 weeks after COVID-19 infection, respectively. They suggest that the temporal relationship between COVID-19 infection and the manifestations of autoimmune thyroid disease in the patients described here raises the question of the combined effects of COVID-19 on the immune system and the thyroid gland. Most reported case series of hyperthyroidism during active COVID-19 infection suggested that a destructive viral thyroiditis contributed to clinical presentation of subacute thyroiditis, with prompt symptomatic improvement with steroids (prednisone) and resolution of biochemical abnormalities (TSH normalization). A recent study analyzed the prevalence of thyroid disease in 191 patients hospitalized for COVID-19 infection, without known thyroid disease. Around 15% of patients with mild to moderate COVID-19 had thyroid dysfunction due to a direct effect of SARS-CoV-2 or the inflammatory state caused by the cytokine storm [35].

New prospective studies will be necessary to know the effect of long or post-COVID-19 COVID_19, on the HPT axis.

The hypothalamic–pituitary–gonadal axis (HPG), COVID-19 infection, and cytokine storm

The HPG axis plays an important role within the immune-neuroendocrine system; therefore, it is of interest to know the influence that COVID-19 infection has on HPG axis.

Extensive cohorts of patients recovered from severe COVID-19 infection have demonstrated low androgens levels such testosterone, Sertoli cell dysfunction, and spermatogenesis disruption around 8–12 weeks after disease onset, directly affecting the fertility of survivors [36,37].

An important point is the disruption of the HPG axis caused by the coronavirus, what propitiates a testicular atrophy breaking steroidogenesis and spermatogenesis, altering the reproductive health and the appearance of sexual disorders as erectile dysfunction of patient survivors of COVID-19 disease, causing infertility in many cases [38].

On the other hand, in women SARS-CoV-2 damages ovaries and interrupts oogenesis by binding to angiotensin, leading to infertility [39].

The late impact on posthospital COVID-19 patients goes beyond the respiratory condition, SARS-CoV-2 reduces angiotensin levels by altering the regulation of spermatogenesis in severe conditions, in addition to high levels of luteinizing hormone manifesting hypothyroidism hypogonadotropic, demonstrating that SARS-CoV-2 is able to suppress the HPG axis [40].

Studies with postmortem testicular biopsies demonstrate the presence of SARS-CoV-2 infection and its involvement in spermatogenesis, exposing degenerated germ cells in the seminiferous tubules, triggering an autoimmune response that contributes to viral orchitis and therefore testicular damage [41].

Hypercortisolism (>744 nmol/L) caused by the pathological stress of the COVID-19 disease during the acute phase is found to be a prognostic biomarker of the severity of the disease because it is associated with an increase in mortality and a survival reduction. COVID-19 patients receiving glucocorticoids may have with hypogonadism [42].

The acute respiratory syndrome caused by COVID-19 infection and cytokine storm is more frequent in men than in women. These clinical findings have made it possible to propose that testosterone may be a risk factor for the development of the cytokine storm. In this regard, a recent systematic review of the literature indicates that low testosterone levels in elderly men with COVID-19 are a risk factor for a worse prognosis and mortality [43].

For all these reasons, we recommend a comprehensive gonadal function and reproductive evaluation in all patients recovered from COVID-19 infection, including gonadotropins and sex steroid hormones.

The autonomic nervous system: sympathetic and parasympathetic, COVID-19 infection, and cytokine storm

The autonomic nervous system is composed of three main branches: The sympathetic, parasympathetic, and enteric nervous system systems. These systems are fundamental components of the immune-neuroendocrine response, which has a connection with the immune system that is activated after any kind of stress situation, including infections. In this way, the neuroendocrine system expands the concept of the autonomic nervous system. Under stress situations, the interaction between the immune system and the autonomic nervous system is mediated by the activated vagus nerve, which inhibits cytokine production and the inflammatory process [44,45].

One of the hormones that is involved in the sympathetic system (SS) is epinephrine (EPI), this hormone is able to make several changes when the body is under stress situations, for example, it can increase sweating, cardiac rate, serum glucose levels, hepatic breakdown of lipids to free fatty acids and it also can activate platelets and stimulate renin–angiotensin–aldosterone system. On the other side, the effects of parasympathetic system (PS) are decreased when an individual is under stress conditions. The manifestations of the PS inhibition are similar to the manifestations of the activation of the SS. Pro-inflammatory cytokines such as IL6 and TNFα not only stimulate the HPA axis, but also stimulate the release of EPI [45].

Several diseases like diabetes mellitus, hypertension, and chronic kidney disease have an association with the sympathetic activity; these patients have a worse outcome when they get infected by SARS COV2 because of the increased sympathetic activity [46].

Within the examples that try to prove the involvement of SS and NS in COVID-19 are hyperglycemia, the glucose presents high levels in some of the patients that have a severe outcome; hypokalemia that it is associated with a high mortality [45]. A recent study shows that patients with severe COVID-19 present greater alterations of the autonomic nervous system, manifested by greater alterations in autonomic dysfunction, demonstrated by heart rate variability (HRV), than mild patients. Therefore, HRV measurements can be used as a noninvasive predictor for clinical outcome [47].

Central nervous system, cytokine storm, and COVID-19

Since the beginning of the pandemic, evidence has been sought of how COVID-19 invades different systems in the human body. At the moment, it is known that SARS-CoV-2 is transmitted from person to person through infectious droplets resulting from the respiratory fluxes of the infected population.

The infection of this virus toward the different cell groups occurs when SARS-CoV-2 enters the human body through the upper respiratory tract through the olfactory route, which at its entrance meets the cavity nasal and anatomical structures such as the nasal mucosa, the olfactory bulb, and the lamina cribosa. At the moment, it is known that the way the virus enters is important since the way it enters will determine the reach to the CNS. Cytokine storm makes the blood–brain barrier more permeable, thus facilitating the entry of the SARS-CoV-2 virus to the brain and can infect neurons, astrocytes, and microglia [2,48].

SARS-CoV-2 reaches the CNS through the olfactory mucosa where the dendrites of the olfactory sensory neurons project toward the nasal cavity and the axons exit through the cribriform plate toward the olfactory bulb [49], subsequently. It is through the union of Protein S1 with ACE two which are expressed in ACE2 is expressed in oligodendrocytes, astrocytes, neurons, and monocytes/macrophages [50], which causes the release of proinflammatory cytokines typical of the "Cytokine Storm" which inevitably leads to overwhelming systemic inflammation [51] and causing the release of IL-1, IL-2, IL-4, IL-6, IL-8, IL-9, IL-10, IL-18, IFN−γ, and TNF-α [51]. This neurotropism causes the following manifestations at the CNS level: headaches, dizziness, disorientation, delirium, epilepsy, intraventricular hemorrhage and even cerebral vascular events [2]. In this way, SARS-CoV-2 reaches the brain stem and causes cytopathy

[50] which requires greater energy expenditure and neuronal death as a result, this explains why the sense of smell is altered in patients with COVID-19 and the way in which the CNS is accessed [49] presenting itself as a wide range of diseases [53] that involve the CNS which range from anosmia, which is mostly the initial symptom, to cerebrovascular accidents.

Another way in which the virus enters the cerebrospinal fluid (CSF) is by reaching the olfactory nerve and the bulb, leading to demyelinating lesions [39]. In addition, changes have been found resulting from hypoxia in the CNS causing cerebral infarcts, probably caused by microthrombi [54].

In a brain autopsy analysis, the highest viral RNA load for SARS-CoV-2 was found in the olfactory mucosa below the cribriform plate [49] and in a case series of 110 patients performed by tissue analysis. In patients who died from COVID-19, it was found that SARS-CoV-2 reaches the CNS in only 53% and evidence of the presence of cytotoxic T lymphocytes in the brain and cerebellum was found in 79% of them, as well as evidence of SARS-CoV-2 to the histopathological study of the Frontal Lobe in 39% [52], also finding Astrogliosis and Microgliosis. At the moment, the presence of SARS-CoV-2 has been demonstrated in CSF or brain due to encephalopathy associated with the septic state in which these outcomes result from the cytokine storm produced by the inflammatory state. A wide range of neurological manifestations, as well as histopathological findings, have been described so far, which suggest that damage to the CNS by COVID-19 probably has multiple pathogenic mechanisms: endothelitis, coagulopathy, sepsis encephalopathy, among others [54]. Oxytocin is a neurohormone produced in

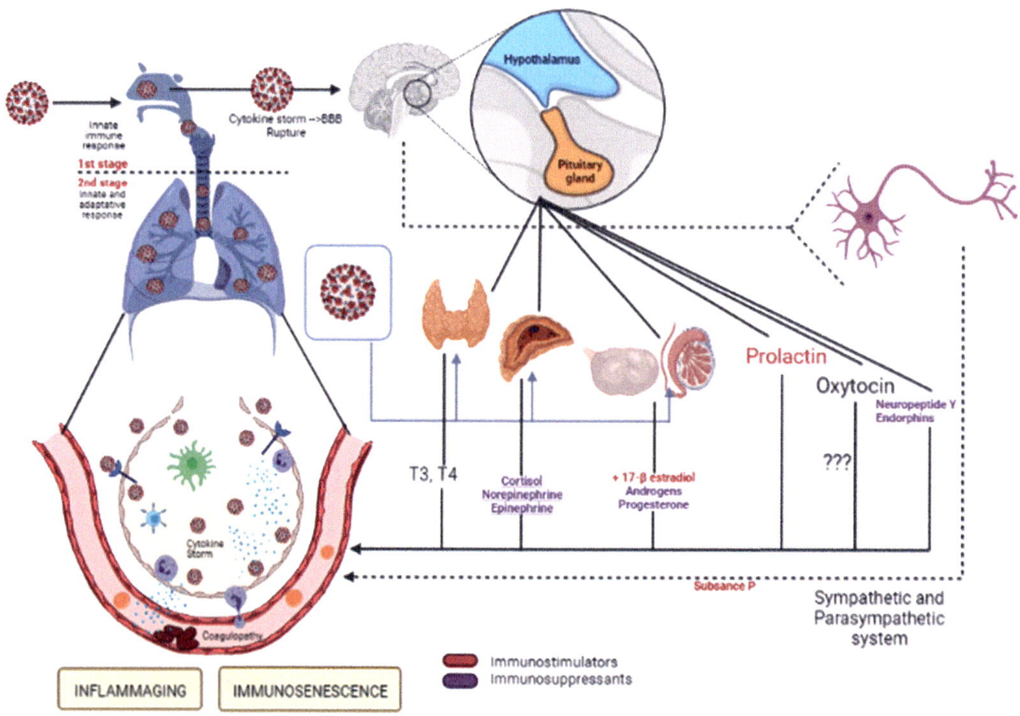

FIGURE 6.1 Interaction between COVID-19 infection and immune-neuroendocrine system. The cytokine storm has a devastating effect on HPA, HPT, HPG, prolactin/growth hormone system, and the autonomic nervous system. Oxytocin, a hormone release by the posterior pituitary, could be a direct antiviral effect against SARS-CoV-2.

the hypothalamus and secreted from the posterior pituitary gland. Several studies have shown that it has the ability to inhibit the inflammatory/immune-neuroendocrine response. Therefore, oxytocin could have a direct anti SARS-CoV-2 effect [55].

With all the aforementioned, we can deduce that there is no clear and direct evidence that SARS-CoV-2 causes alterations in brain tissue, but rather because of the cytokine storm caused by the viral infection, so it is imperative to give it the importance necessary for brain autopsies in patients who died from COVID-19.

In summary:

1. From the beginning of the SARS-CoV-2 virus infection, the neuroendocrine immune system responds according to the characteristics of the individual age, gender, comorbidities.
2. If the infection progresses to the cytokine storm, the immune-neuroendocrine system and its stress response axes will be attacked by the cytokine storm and/or by the virus itself (Fig. 6.1).
3. The long-term consequences of the cytokine storm's effect on the neuroendocrine immune system are currently unknown.

Conclusions

1. The immune-neuroendocrine system is activated under stress situations and other alarm situations, in order to protect ourselves.
2. During COVID-19 infection, a large number of infected patients are subjected to intense stress, which leads to activation of the neuroendocrine immune system.
3. If the SARS-CoV2 infection progresses to the invasion phase, the immune-neuroendocrine system is directly affected by the SARS-CoV2 virus or cytokine storm.
4. The long-term effect of COVID-19 infection on the neuroendocrine immune system is unknown and should be investigated.

References

[1] Moore JB, June CH. Cytokine release syndrome in severe COVID-19. Science 2020;368(6490):473–4. https://doi.org/10.1126/science.abb8925.

[2] Jara LJ, López-Zamora B, Ordoñez-González I, et al. The immune-neuroendocrine system in COVID-19, advanced age and rheumatic diseases. Autoimmun Rev 2021;20(11):102946. https://doi.org/10.1016/j.autrev.2021.102946.

[3] Ferrara JL, Abhyankar S, Gilliland DG. Cytokine storm of graft-versus-host disease: a critical effector role for interleukin-1. Transplant Proc February 1993;25(1 Pt 2):1216–7.

[4] Ferrara JL. Cytokine dysregulation as a mechanism of graft versus host disease. CurrOpinImmunol October 1993;5(5):794–9. https://doi.org/10.1016/0952-7915(93)90139-j.

[5] Chatenoud L, Ferran C, Bach JF. The anti-CD3-induced syndrome: a consequence of massive in vivo cell activation. Curr Top Microbiol Immunol 1991;174:121–34. https://doi.org/10.1007/978-3-642-50998-8_9.

[6] Fajgenbaum DC, June CH. Cytokine storm. N Engl J Med 2020;383(23):2255–73. https://doi.org/10.1056/NEJMra2026131.

[7] Temgoua MN, Endomba FT, Nkeck JR, Kenfack GU, Tochie JN, &Essouma M. Coronavirus disease 2019 (COVID-19) as a multi-systemic disease and its impact in low- and middle-income countries (LMICs). SN

comprehensive clinical medicine. Advance online publication; 2020. p. 1–11. https://doi.org/10.1007/s42399-020-00417-7.
[8] Nalbandian A, Sehgal K, Gupta A, et al. Post-acute COVID-19 syndrome. Nat Med 2021;27(4):601–15. https://doi.org/10.1038/s41591-021-01283-z.
[9] Besedovsky H, Sorkin E. Network of immune-neuroendocrine interactions. Clin Exp Immunol 1977;27(1):1–12.
[10] Wilder RL. Neuroendocrine-immune system interactions and autoimmunity. Annu Rev Immunol 1995;13:307–38. https://doi.org/10.1146/annurev.iy.13.040195.001515.
[11] Besedovsky HO, del Rey A. Immune-neuro-endocrine interactions: facts and hypotheses. Endocr Rev 1996;17(1):64–102. https://doi.org/10.1210/edrv-17-1-64.
[12] Sternberg EM. Neural regulation of innate immunity: a coordinated nonspecific host response to pathogens. Nat Rev Immunol 2006;6(4):318–28. https://doi.org/10.1038/nri1810.
[13] Besedovsky HO. The immune system as a sensorial system that can modulate brain functions and reset homeostasis. Ann N Y Acad Sci February 2019;1437(1):5–14. https://doi.org/10.1111/nyas.13935.
[14] Sharif K, Watad A, Coplan L, Lichtbroun B, Krosser A, Lichtbroun M, Bragazzi NL, Amital H, Afek A, Shoenfeld Y. The role of stress in the mosaic of autoimmunity: an overlooked association. Autoimmun Rev October 2018;17(10):967–83. https://doi.org/10.1016/j.autrev.2018.04.005.
[15] Jara LJ, Navarro C, Medina G, Vera-Lastra O, Blanco F. Immune-neuroendocrine interactions and autoimmune diseases. Clin Dev Immunol 2006 ;13(2–4):109–23. https://doi.org/10.1080/17402520600877059.
[16] Diep PT, de Kok V. Could oxytocin reduce autoimmune disease in COVID-19? Autoimmun Rev November 2021;16:102994. https://doi.org/10.1016/j.autrev.2021.102994.
[17] Chrousos GP, Zapanti ED. Hypothalamic-pituitary-adrenal axis in HIV infection and disease. EndocrinolMetab-Clin North Am 2014;43(3):791–806.
[18] Zapanti E, Terzidis K, Chrousos G. Dysfunction of the hypothalamic-pituitary-adrenal axis in HIV infection and disease. Hormones (Basel) 2008;7(3):205–16.
[19] Silverman M, Pearce B, Biron C, Miller A. Immune Modulation of the hypothalamic-pituitary-adrenal (HPA) axis during viral infection. Viral Immunol 2005;18(1):41–78.
[20] Pérez AR, Bottasso O, Savino W. The impact of infectious diseases upon neuroendocrine circuits. Neuroimmunomodulation 2009;16:96–105.
[21] Peeters B, Meersseman P, Vander Perre S, Wouters PJ, Vanmarcke D, Debaveye Y, Billen J, Vermeersch P, Langouche L, Van den Berghe G. Adrenocortical function during prolonged critical illness and beyond: a prospective observational study. Intensive Care Med October 2018;44(10):1720–9. https://doi.org/10.1007/s00134-018-5366-7. Epub 2018 Sep. 13.
[22] Annane D, Pastores SM, Arlt W, Balk RA, Beishuizen A, Briegel J, Carcillo J, Christ-Crain M, Cooper MS, Marik PE, GU M, Olsen KM, Rochwerg B, Rodgers SC, Russell JA, Van den Berghe G. Critical illness-related corticosteroid insufficiency (CIRCI): a narrative review from a multispecialty task force of the society of critical care medicine (SCCM) and the European society of intensive care medicine (ESICM). Intensive Care Med December 2017;43(12):1781–92. https://doi.org/10.1007/s00134-017-4914-x. Epub 2017 Sep. 21.
[23] Yuan Y, Sun C, Tang X, Cheng C, Mombaerts L, Wang M, Hu T, Sun C, Guo Y, Li X, Xu H, Ren T, Xiao Y, Xiao Y, Zhu H, Wu H, Li K, Chen C, Liu Y, Liang Z, Cao Z, Zhang HT, ChPaschaldis I, Liu Q, Goncalves J, Zhong Q, Yan L. Development and validation of a prognostic risk score system for COVID-19 inpatients: a multi-center retrospective study in China. Engineering (Beijing) November 2020;28. https://doi.org/10.1016/j.eng.2020.10.013 [Epub ahead of print].
[24] Mao Y, Xu B, Guan W, Xu D, Li F, Ren R, Zhu X, Gao Y, Jiang L. The adrenal cortex, an underestimated site of SARS-CoV-2 infection. Front Endocrinol January 8, 2021;11:593179. https://doi.org/10.3389/fendo.2020.593179.
[25] Alzahrani AS, Mukhtar N, Aljomaiah A, Aljamei H, Bakhsh A, Alsudani N, Elsayed T, Alrashidi N, Fadel R, Alqahtani E, Raef H, Butt MI, Sulaiman O. TheImpact of COVID-19 viral infection on the hypothalamic-pituitary-adrenal Axis. Endocr Pract February 2021;27(2):83–9. https://doi.org/10.1016/j.eprac.2020.10.014. Epub 2020 Dec 15. PMID: 33554871.
[26] Kumar B, Gopalakrishnan M, Garg MK, Purohit P, Banerjee M, Sharma P, Khichar S, Kothari N, Bhatia P, Nag VL, Misra S. Endocrine dysfunction among patients with COVID-19: a single-center experience from a tertiary hospital in India. Indian J EndocrinolMetab 2021 ;25(1):14–9. https://doi.org/10.4103/ijem.IJEM_577_20. Epub 2021 Jul 21.
[27] Freire Santana M, Borba MGS, Baía-da-Silva DC, Val F, Alexandre MAA, Brito-Sousa JD, Melo GC, Queiroga MVO, Leão Farias ME, Camilo CC, Naveca FG, Xavier MS, Monteiro WM, Augusto PivotoJoão G,

Hajjar LA, Ordi J, Lacerda MVG, Ferreira LCL. Case report: adrenal pathology findings in severe COVID-19: an autopsy study. Am J Trop Med Hyg October 2020;103(4):1604–7.

[28] Gu J, Gong E, Zhang B, Zheng J, Gao Z, Zhong Y, Zou W, Zhan J, Wang S, Xie Z, Zhuang H, Wu B, Zhong H, Shao H, Fang W, Gao D, Pei F, Li X, He Z, Xu D, Shi X, Anderson VM, Leong AS. Multiple organ infection and the pathogenesis of SARS. J Exp Med August 1, 2005;202(3):415–24.

[29] Salzano C, Saracino G, Cardillo G. Possible adrenal involvement in long COVID syndrome. Medicina (Kaunas) October 11, 2021;57(10):1087. https://doi.org/10.3390/medicina57101087.

[30] Li MY, Li L, Zhang Y, Wang XS. Expression of the SARS-CoV-2 cell receptor gene Ace2 in a wide variety of human tissues. Infect Dis Poverty 2020;9(1):45. https://doi.org/10.1186/S40249-020-00662-X.

[31] Caron P. Thyroid disorders and SARS-CoV-2 infection: from pathophysiological mechanism to patient management. Ann Endocrinol 2020;81(5):507–10. https://doi.org/10.1016/j.ando.2020.09.001.

[32] Khoo B, Tan T, Clarke SA, et al. ThyroidFunctionBefore, during, and after COVID-19. J ClinEndocrinolMetab 2021;106(2):e803–11. https://doi.org/10.1210/clinem/dgaa830.

[33] Wei L, Sun S, Xu CH, et al. Pathologyofthethyroid in severe acute respiratorysyndrome. Hum Pathol 2007;38(1):95–102. https://doi.org/10.1016/j.humpath.2006.06.011.

[34] Feghali K, Atallah J, Norman C. Manifestations of thyroid disease post COVID-19 illness: report of Hashimoto thyroiditis, Graves' disease, and subacute thyroiditis. J Clin Transl Endocrinol Case Rep 2021;22:100094. https://doi.org/10.1016/j.jecr.2021.100094.

[35] Lui DTW, Lee CH, Chow WS, Lee ACH, Tam AR, Fong CHY, Law CY, Leung EKH, To KKW, Tan KCB, Woo YC, Lam CW, Hung IFN, Lam KSL. Thyroid dysfunction in relation to immune profile, disease status, and outcome in 191 patients with COVID-19. J Clin Endocrinol Metab January 23, 2021;106(2):e926–35. https://doi.org/10.1210/clinem/dgaa813. PMID: 33141191.

[36] Moreno-Perez O, Merino E, Alfayate R, Torregrosa ME, Andres M, León-Ramirez JE. Male pituitary–gonadal axis dysfunction in post-acute COVID-19 syndrome—prevalence and associated factors: a Mediterranean case series. Clin Endocrinol 2021:1–10.

[37] Aboelnaga MM, Abdelrazek A, Abdullah N, El Shaer M. Late impact of COVID-19 pneumonia on testosterone levels in recovered, post-hospitalized male patients. J Endocrinol Metab 2021;11(3–4):76–82.

[38] Selvaraj K, Ravichandran S, Krishnan S, Radhakrishnan RK, Manickam N, Kandasamy M. Testicular atrophy and hypothalamic pathology in COVID-19: possibility of the incidence of male infertility and HPG Axis Abnormalities. Reprod Sci October 2021;28(10):2735–42. https://doi.org/10.1007/s43032-020-00441-x. Epub 2021 Jan 7.

[39] Markiewicz-Gospodarek A, Wdowiak P, Czeczelewski M, Forma A, Flieger J, Januszewski J, Radzikowska-Büchner E, et al. The impact of SARS-CoV-2 infection on fertility and female and male reproductive systems. J Clin Med 2021;10:4520.

[40] Sengupta P, Dutta S. COVID-19 and hypogonadism: secondary immune responses rule-over endocrine mechanisms. Hum Fertil January 2021;13:1–6. https://doi.org/10.1080/14647273.2020.1867902 [Epub ahead of print].

[41] Ma X, Guan C, Chen R, Wang Y, Feng S, Wang R, et al. Pathological and molecular examinations of postmortem testis biopsies reveal SARS-CoV-2 infection in the testis and spermatogenesis damage in COVID-19 patients. Cell Mol Immunol 2021;18:487–9.

[42] Tan T, Khoo B, Mills EG, Phylactou M, Patel B, Eng PC, et al. Association between high serum total cortisol concentrations andmortality from COVID-19. Lancet Diabetes Endocrinol 2020;8:659–60.

[43] Giagulli VA, Guastamacchia E, Magrone T, Jirillo E, Lisco G, De Pergola G, Triggiani V. Worse progression of COVID-19 in men: is testosterone a key factor? Andrology January 2021;9(1):53–64. https://doi.org/10.1111/andr.12836. Epub 2020 Jun 28.

[44] Kenney MJ, Ganta CK. Autonomic nervous system and immune system interactions. Compr Physiol July 2014;4(3):1177–200.

[45] Goldstein DS. The extended autonomic system, dyshomeostasis, and COVID-19. Clin Auton Res August 2020;30(4):299–315.

[46] Del Rio R, Marcus NJ, Inestrosa NC. Potential role of autonomic dysfunction in covid-19 morbidity and mortality. Front Physiol October 2020;16.

[47] Pan Y, Yu Z, Yuan Y, Han J, Wang Z, Chen H, Wang S, Wang Z, Hu H, Zhou L, Lai Y, Zhou Z, Wang Y, Meng G, Yu L, Jiang H. Alteration of autonomic nervous system is associated with severity and outcomes in patients with COVID-19. Front Physiol May 19, 2021;12:630038. https://doi.org/10.3389/fphys.2021.630038.

[48] Mehta S, Bhandari S, Mehta S. Brain autopsies in fatal COVID-19 and postulated pathophysiology: more puzzling than a Rubik's cube. J Clin Pathol September 2021;74(9):612–3. https://doi.org/10.1136/jclinpath-2020-206967. Epub 2020 Sep. 9.

[49] Meinhardt J, Radke J, Dittmayer C, Franz J, Thomas C, Mothes R, Laue M, Schneider J, Brünink S, Greuel S, Lehmann M, Hassan O, Aschman T, Schumann E, Chua RL, Conrad C, Eils R, Stenzel W, Windgassen M, Rößler L, Goebel HH, Gelderblom HR, Martin H, Nitsche A, Schulz-Schaeffer WJ, Hakroush S, Winkler MS, Tampe B, Scheibe F, Körtvélyessy P, Reinhold D, Siegmund B, Kühl AA, Elezkurtaj S, Horst D, Oesterhelweg L, Tsokos M, Ingold-Heppner B, Stadelmann C, Drosten C, Corman VM, Radbruch H, Heppner FL. Olfactory transmucosal SARS-CoV-2 invasion as a port of central nervous system entry in individuals with COVID-19. Nat Neurosci February 2021;24(2):168–75. https://doi.org/10.1038/s41593-020-00758-5. Epub 2020 Nov 30.

[50] Singh H, Singh A, Khan AA, Gupta V. Immune mediating molecules and pathogenesis of COVID-19-associated neurological disease. Microb Pathog September 2021;158:105023. https://doi.org/10.1016/j.micpath.2021.105023. Epub 2021 Jun 4.

[51] Thepmankorn P, Bach J, Lasfar A, Zhao X, Souayah S, Chong ZZ, Souayah N. Cytokine storm induced by SARS-CoV-2 infection: the spectrum of its neurological manifestations. Cytokine February 2021;138:155404. https://doi.org/10.1016/j.cyto.2020.155404. Epub 2020 Dec 11.

[52] Matschke J, Lütgehetmann M, Hagel C, Sperhake JP, Schröder AS, Edler C, et al. Neuropathology of patients with COVID-19 in Germany: a post-mortem case series. Lancet Neurol November 2020;19(11):919–29. https://doi.org/10.1016/S1474-4422(20)30308-2.

[53] Glatzel M. Neuropathology of COVID-19: where are the neuropathologists? Brain Pathol July 2020;30(4):729. https://doi.org/10.1111/bpa.12871.

[54] Maury A, Lyoubi A, Peiffer-Smadja N, de Broucker T, Meppiel E. Neurological manifestations associated with SARS-CoV-2 and other coronaviruses: a narrative review for clinicians. Rev Neurol (Paris) 2021 Jan-Feb;177(1–2):51–64. https://doi.org/10.1016/j.neurol.2020.10.001.

[55] Diep PT, de Kok V. Could oxytocin reduce autoimmune disease in COVID-19? Autoimmun Rev 2022;21(2):102994. https://doi.org/10.1016/j.autrev.2021.102994.

CHAPTER

7

Genetic predisposition to COVID-19 and post-COVID syndrome

Anna Malkova[1,2]

[1]Ariel University, Ariel, Israel; [2]Saint Petersburg State University, Saint Petersburg, Russia

Introduction

Coronavirus infection is a highly contagious disease affected already 250 million people over the whole world. Unfortunately, around 20% of coronavirus-infected patients progress to the development of viral pneumonia, while some of them are likely to develop a very severe form of the disease. The life-threatening complications of the disease include cardiovascular disorders and systemic inflammatory response, which leads to the development of acute respiratory distress syndrome (ARDS) [1]. Moreover, up to 60% of patients have post-COVID complications, such as autoimmune, endocrinal, neurological disorders [2]. Recently the predisposing factors of susceptibility, severe course of the disease, are the actual problem in COVID prevention programs. The aim of this work is to analyze genetic predisposition to Sars-Cov2 infection, a severe form of the COVID-19 and post-COVID syndrome (PCS).

Genetic predisposing factors in COVID-19

The X chromosome—gender

COVID-19 may be associated with worse outcomes in males than in females [3]. Such differences can be explained by different immunoregulatory functions of estrogen and testosterone [4]. By activating the estrogen receptor, estrogens regulate the development of immune cells and the pathways of the immune system response against infections (and autoantigens), which leads to B-cell-mediated adaptive immunity and the production of specific antibodies [5,6]. It can explain the higher level of SARS-CoV-2 IgG antibodies at an early stage of infection among women [7,8].

Autoimmunity, COVID-19, Post-COVID19 syndrome and COVID-19 vaccination
https://doi.org/10.1016/B978-0-443-18566-3.00014-1

During the innate immune response, estrogen also activates its receptor on monocytes, macrophages, and neutrophils, inducing the production of pro-inflammatory cytokines (IL-12, TNF-α) and chemokines (CCL2) [5,6]. These pro-inflammatory mediators activate lymphocytes and alveolar macrophages with increased production of type I and III interferons (IFN), which is important for reducing the production of viral titers [9]. Conversely, testosterone has an immunosuppressive effect and does not significantly affect inflammatory and reparative immune functions [10].

Expression of ACE2 and related proteins

ACE is believed to have a protective function against lung damage; therefore, damage of cells expressing ACE2 can lead to a loss of ACE2 protective function [11]. Overexpression of human ACE2 has been shown to increase the severity of the disease in a mouse model of SARS-CoV infection [12] and injection of SARS-CoV spike protein in mice exacerbated lung damage [13]. Thus it can be assumed that the severity of lung damage is due to cell lysis after virus and reduction of ACE2-dependent reparative capacity of the lung tissue [14].

The results of various studies indicate the association between the degree of expression and the types of configuration of ACE2 and related proteins in susceptibility to SARS-CoV-2 and predisposition to severe disease [14]. Several works showed a correlation between high ACE2 expression and the severe course of the disease, which was also more frequently observed in men [15–17].

The polymorphisms of the ACE2 gene also proved to be important for severe course of COVID-19 [18]. Two specific ACE2 alleles (i.e., rs73635825 and rs143936283) showed a low binding affinity of the entire SARS-CoV-2 S-protein, so viral attachment decreased and potential resistance to infection was reported [19].

Among ACE2-related proteins, significant genetic characteristics were revealed. Polymorphisms in TMPRSS2 gene, encoding transporter protein for ACE2, have been shown to be strongly associated with the susceptibility and severity of COVID-19 [20,21] with higher expression in males [19]. Patients with wild-type or naïve ACE2 and TMPRSS2 expression have a severe form [22]. The researcher also revealed polymorphisms p.Arg514-Gly detected in patients with cardiovascular and pulmonary complications in the African/African-American population.

Association between the overexpression of the SLC6A20 gene located at the 3p21.31 locus and encoding the sodium/imino-acid (proline) transporter 1 (SIT1) for ACE2 with the more severe course of COVID-19 was found [23], Rs2271616:G>T allele was found to be associated with susceptibility (Table 7.1) [24].

TABLE 7.1 Specifics of ACE2 and related proteins expression and susceptibility to COVID-19.

ACE2	TMPRSS2	SLC6A20
High expression rs2285666 allele rs73635825 allele rs143936283 allele	p.Val160Met allele	Rs2271616:G > T allele

Expression of pro-inflammatory proteins and its receptors

A relationship between the severe course of the disease and the features of the 3p21.31 locus [23], other genes coding inflammatory cytokines were described in several studies and evaluated in meta-analyses [24,25] (Table 7.2).

TABLE 7.2 The expression of pro-inflammatory proteins and its receptors and susceptibility to different forms of COVID-19.

		Specifics in COVID		
The gene	**The function of the encoded protein**	**Susceptibility**	**Severe course**	**Protection**
CXCR6	Regulates the specific location of lung tissue-resident-memory CD8+ T cell		Decreased expression rs10490770:T > C allele	
TLR7	The innate immune response against coronaviruses with the IFN-γ production		Decreased expression	
IFNAR2	Induces antiviral response		Decreased expression	
OAS1, 3	Degradation of viral RNA and activate antiviral responses in nonclassical monocytes and T-cell subsets		Decreased expression	
IL10RB	Induces IL-10 pathway with antiinflammatory functions in T-cell subsets		Increased expression	
CCR9	Expression is induced in the early stages of airway inflammation		SNP	
DTX1	Regulates NOTCH activity in naive B cells		rs2010604 allele	
ERAP2	The final modification of antigens for presentation by MHC-I molecules		rs150892504 allele	
IFITM3	Enhances the accumulation of CD8+ T cells in airways to promote mucosal immune cell persistence		Homozygous inheritance of the rs12252 allele	
TYK2	Regulates the endocytic trafficking of cytokine receptors	rs74956615:T > A allele	rs34536443:G > C allele	
PPP1R15A	Regulates cytokine production in stimulated dendritic cells	rs4801778 and rs11541192:G > A alleles		
DPP9	Plays a role in antigen maturation, cell migration, and cell adhesion		rs2109069:G > A allele	
FOXP4	Necessary for normal T cell cytokine recall responses to an antigen		rs1886814:A > C allele	
KANSL1	The acetylation of nucleosomal histone H4 on several lysine residues			rs1819040:T > A allele

- CXCR6 gene

The gene encodes chemokine receptor 6 with the CXC motif (CXCR6), which regulates the specific location of lung tissue-resident-memory CD8+ T cells, specific against respiratory system pathogens, including influenza viruses [26] and plays a role in chemokine signaling [27]. In the patients with severe COVID-19, decreased expression of the CXCR6 gene and the SNP polymorphism rs10490770:T > C were found [24,26].

- CCR9 gene

The gene encodes a homeostatic and inflammatory chemokine receptor (CCR9), involved in the pathogenesis of pneumonia of various origins and its expression is induced in the early stages of airway inflammation. CCR9 and its ligand CCL25 have been shown to play an important role in modulating the recruitment of eosinophils and lymphocytes in the early stages of inflammation [28]. The polymorphism of the gene was found in patients with severe infection [26].

- ERAP2 gene

The gene encodes metalloaminopeptidase involved in the final modification of antigens for presentation by MHC-I molecules [29]. The SNP rs150892504 allele was associated with an increased risk of death in COVID-19.

- TLR7 gene

The gene encodes toll-like receptor 7. A small study of four clinical cases of severe coronavirus infection found loss-of-function variants in X-chromosomal encoding the TLR7 gene in patients and their relatives. It was correlated with a decrease in the type I interferon (IFN) signaling in peripheral blood mononuclear cells from patients, decreased production of IFN-γ, IFN type II [30]. According to fundamental researches, the X chromosomal TLR7 gene is associated with the maintenance of the innate immune response against coronaviruses [31]

- IFITM3 gene

The gene encodes interferon-induced transmembrane protein 3 (IFITM3), which enhances the accumulation of CD8+ T cells in airways to promote mucosal immune cell persistence [32,33]. This protein is considered to participate in the viral invasion and be associated with COVID-19 severity and cytokine release syndrome [34]. The homozygous inheritance of the rs12252 allele of the gene may contribute to severe disease [35].

- TYK2 gene

The gene encodes the tyrosine kinase 2 (TYK2), which regulates the endocytic trafficking of cytokine receptors [36]. Allele rs74956615:T > A is associated with COVID-19 susceptibility, while rs34536443:G > C (p.Pro1104Ala) with for critical illness and hospitalization [24]

- PPP1R15A gene

The gene encodes protein phosphatase one subunit Ppp1r15a/GADD34 (PPP1R15A), which regulates cytokine production in stimulated dendritic cells. SNP rs4801778 and rs11541192:G > A were associated with COVID-19 susceptibility [24].

- DPP9 gene

The gene encodes DPP9 dipeptidyl peptidase 9 (DPP9), which plays a role in antigen maturation, cell migration, and cell adhesion [37]. An intronic variant rs2109069:G > A was positively correlated with critical illness, was previously reported to be risk-increasing for interstitial lung disease [24].

- FOXP4 gene

The gene encodes Forkhead box transcription factors 4, which is expressed in both thymocytes and peripheral CD4(+) and CD8(+) T cells and is dispensable for T cell development, but necessary for normal T cell cytokine recall responses to an antigen following pathogenic infection [38]. The allele rs1886814:A > C was found as a factor of an increased risk of severe COVID [24].

- KANSL1 gene

The gene encodes KAT8 regulatory NSL complex subunit 1, which is involved in the acetylation of nucleosomal histone H4 and can regulate transcription [39]. The intronic variants (1q22) and rs1819040:T > A were assumed as protective factors against hospitalization due to COVID-19 [24].

However, all these studies evaluated gene expression in general, though the impact of COVID-19-risk variants on gene expression in specific cell types plays a key role in COVID-19 pathogenesis. Therefore, the research group of Schmiedel et al. [40] performed a large study based on meta-analyses of GWAS, eQTLs (DICE database), chromatin accessibility profiles of 13 different immune cell types and 2 cell types in activated conditions, and 3D cis-interactome maps. They found the association between the risk of severe COVID-19 and the changes in the following genes:

- Reduced expression of the gene encoding interferon receptor 2 (IFNAR2) in multiple immune cells;
- Reduced expression of two interferon-inducible genes: OAS1 in nonclassical monocytes and OAS3 in T-cell subsets. OAS1 and OAS3 encode for the oligoadenylate synthase family of proteins that degrade viral RNA and activate antiviral responses;
- Increased expression of the gene IL10RB, encoding IL-10 receptor beta, in NK cells and T-cell subsets.

Also as the risk factors of the severe form of the diseases were revealed the following genes:

- The genes ACBD4, ARL17A, and LRRC37A2 in follicular helper T cells, helper T cells 2, and helper T cells 1/17;
- The gene DTX1 encoding an ubiquitin ligase Deltex1 that regulates NOTCH activity in naive B cells;
- The gene of CXCR6 in follicular helper T cells;
- The gene of CCR9 in naive regulatory T cells.

HLA-genotypes

HLA-genotypes play one of the most important roles in immune response; therefore, studies on its association with susceptibility to COVID-19 are conducted mostly in every country (Table 7.2). The results of different analyses of HLA-genes based on PCR, next-generation sequencing (NGS), programming are presented on Table 7.3.

As is seen in the table, the results obtained are contradictory. However, according to the data published we can assume, that HLA-A*02 Genotype can be associated with a protective function, while genotypes HLA-DRB1*08, HLA-A*25, HLA-B*15 with a genetic predisposition to Sars-Cov-2 infection and Genotypes HLA-A*01, HLA-C*1, 4, HLA-DQA1*01 with the severe form of the COVID-19. Data on the diagnostic significance of HLA-DRB1*03, 04 have shown contradictory results. The meta-analysis showed the genotype HLA-B*15:03 as a predisposition factor to infection [25].

Recently there are several works on the binding capacity of MHC-molecules and virus peptides. The study conducted in Spain revealed that patients with mild/asymptomatic form possessed HLA Class I genotypes, which have a significant statistical affinity for a greater number of viral peptides, especially HLA-A*02, C*01 [51]. According to Nguyen et al. [41] MHC-A*02:02, -B*15:03, -C*12:03 have the greatest ability to present highly conserved SARS-CoV-2 peptides. Meanwhile, the researchers found that HLA-A*24:02 or HLA-A*11:01 have a larger capacity to present SARS-CoV-2 antigens, which can make these genotypes protective against severe infection. On the other side, the big research based on Allele Frequency Net Database, World Health Organization (WHO) coronavirus disease (COVID-2019) situation reports, HLA-peptide binding prediction algorithms, the Immune Epitope Database and Analysis Resource for different 19 countries didn't reveal any significant differences between countries in total confirmed cases and deaths caused by COVID-19 and HLA-C, -DPB1, or -DQB1 alleles, while HLA-A*02:01 was highest in countries with highest mortality and morbidity [52].

ABO

ABO blood groups were also studied as the predisposition factor to COVID-19, and the results published are contradictory, which can be explained by population particularities [53]. The blood group A was considered to increase the risk of COVID-19 infection and mortality, while the blood group O with a decreased risk in several reports [54–58]. These findings were confirmed by the study of Gérard et al., according to whom the blood groups B and O were less associated with COVID-19 [59].

However, some recent articles reported on a higher risk of infection in individuals with blood group B [59], lower risk with blood group AB and no association between blood group and the risk of severe infection [60].

Predisposition to PCS

According to different classifications, there are several types of PCS: symptoms that persist after recovery from acute SARS-CoV-2 infection, symptoms resulting from damage to

TABLE 7.3 The studies published on association of HLA-genotypes and susceptibility to COVID-19.

Author, year	Material	Method	HLA genotypes with a possible protective function	Predisposing HLA genotypes
Nguyen et al. [41]	FASTA-formatted protein sequence data	Programming	MHC-A*02:02, -B*15:03, −C*12:03	HLA-B*46:01 MHC-A*25:01, C*01:02
Copley et al. [42]	Database UniProt	Programming	HLA- DQA1*03:01, DQB1*03:01, DRB1*04:01, DRB4*01:01, DPA1*01:03, DPB1*04:01	HLA-DQA1*01:01, DQA1*05:01, DQB1*05:03, DQB1*02:01, DRB1*03:01, DRB3*01:01, DPA1*02:01, DPB1*01:01
Wang et al. [43]	China, n = 82	NGS		HLA-C*07:29, B*15:27
Severe Covid-19 GWAS group [23]	Spain, Italy, n = 1980	Global Screening Array (GSA)	No association	
Littera et al. [44]	Italy, healthy controls n = 619, COVID-19 patients n = 182	PCR-SSP	HLA-A*02:05, B*58:01, C*07:01, DRB1*03:01	HLA- A*30:02, B*14:02, C*04:01 C*08:02, DRB1*08:01
Shkurnikov et al. [45]	Russia, n = 79	NGS + programming for peptide binding	HLA-A*02:01, 03:01	HLA-A*01:01
Correale et al. [46]	Italy, n = 120,926	Analysis of database	HLA-B*14, B*18, and B*49	HLA-A*25, B*08, B*44, B*15:01, B*51, C*01, and C*03
Fischer et al. [46]	Germany, n = 157	PCR, NGS	HLA- B*35:01, DRB1*01:01, DRB1*03:01	HLA- B*15:01, DQB1*03:2
Langton et al. [47]	UK, hospitalized n = 49, asymptomatic n = 69	NGS		HLA-DRB1*04:01 asymptomatic form
Naemi et al. [48]	Saudi Arabia, mild/moderate n = 106, severe/critical n = 29, asymptomatic or negative n = 135	SSO-PCR	HLA-C*16	HLA-A*01, B*56, DRB1*08
Novelli et al. [49]	Italy, severe or extremely severe n = 99, reference group = 1017	NGS		HLA-DRB1*15:01, -DQB1*06:02 and -B*27:07
Warren et al. [50]	Canada, COVID-19 positive n = 100, negative patients n = 26	HLA prediction software		HLA-DPA1*02:02 HLA-A*11:01, C*04:01, DQA1*01:02-severe

multiple organs, such as the heart, lung, kidneys, skin, and nervous system, consequences of COVID-19 treatment or prolonged hospitalization, and novel symptoms or syndromes that arise after mild or asymptomatic infection [61–63].

Because the virus infection is accompanied with autoimmune reaction, some PCS complications might be connected with autoimmune inflammation damaging the endocrinal, nerve system [64]. The recent analysis of PCS after mild/asymptomatic forms of the disease showed that such complications are more characteristic for women, which are in general more predisposed to autoimmune reactions and less to severe course of the disease [65]. It can be assumed that the genetic predisposing factors can be genotypes HLA-A*02:01 and HLA-A*03:01, associated with a low probability of developing a severe form of COVID-19 [45], and HLA-DRB1*04: 01 associated with asymptomatic infection [47].

Conclusions

According to data published in original studies, meta-analysis, reviews [24,25,66], we can assume that predisposition to the infection, severe course, or PCS can be based on several factors (Fig. 7.1):

- ACE2 and related proteins expression: high expression or polymorphisms of ACE2, TMPRSS2, SLC6A20
- Individual characteristic of the immune system: changed expression of different genes in multiple immune cells (IFNAR2, CXCR6, OAS1 and OAS3, IL10RB, DTX1, CCR9, TLR7, ERAP2, IFITM3, TYK2, PPP1R15A, DPP9, FOXP4, KANSL1) HLA-genotypes (HLA-

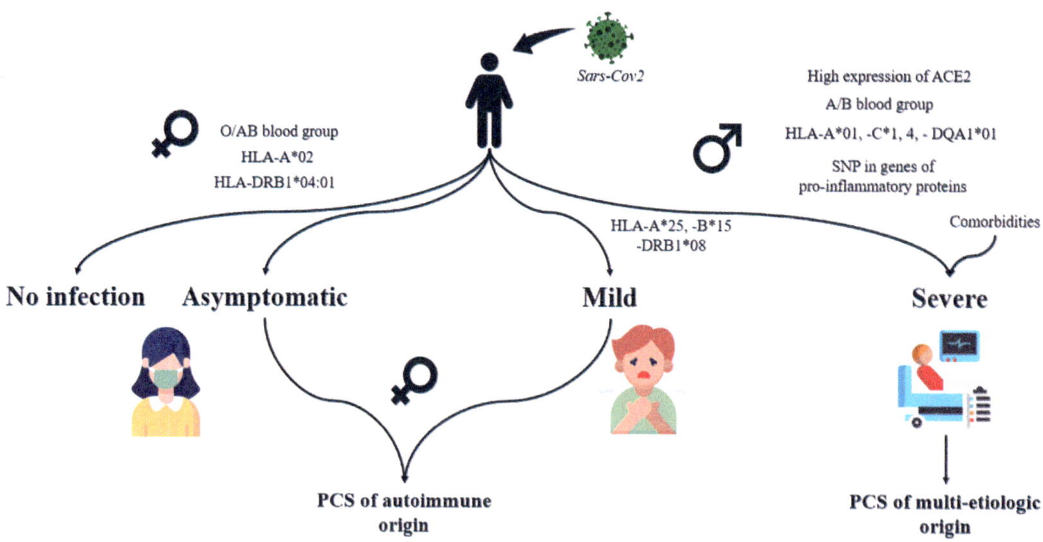

FIGURE 7.1 The potential genetic factors predisposing to different forms of COVID-19 and post-COVID syndrome.

DRB1*08, HLA-A*25, HLA-B*15—genetic predisposition, HLA-A*01, HLA-C*1, 4, HLA-DQA1*01—severe course)

- Gender (male are predisposed to infection and severe course, while women to PCS)
- ABO genotype: A/B—predisposition, O/AB—protective

The analysis performed showed contradictory data, which can be explained by variability of population studied, different research protocols (number of patients, inclusion and exclusion criteria, etc.). It is obvious that predisposition can be predicted not only with genetic factors, but also with knowledge about comorbidities, and the virus strain, which makes this scientific area actual for the whole period of Sars-Cov2 circulation among humans.

References

[1] Wu Z, McGoogan JM. Characteristics of and important lessons from the coronavirus disease 2019 (COVID-19) outbreak in China: summary of a report of 72314 cases from the Chinese center for disease control and prevention. J Am Med Assoc 2020;323(13):1239–42. https://doi.org/10.1001/jama.2020.2648.

[2] Carod-Artal FJ. Post-COVID-19 syndrome: epidemiology, diagnostic criteria and pathogenic mechanisms involved. Rev Neurol 2021;72:384–96. https://doi.org/10.33588/RN.7211.2021230.

[3] Lakbar I, Luque-Paz D, Mege JL, Einav S, Leone M. COVID-19 gender susceptibility and outcomes: a systematic review. PLoS One 2020;15. https://doi.org/10.1371/JOURNAL.PONE.0241827.

[4] Furman D, Hejblum BP, Simon N, Jojic V, Dekker CL, Thiebaut R, Tibshirani RJ, Davis MM. Systems analysis of sex differences reveals an immunosuppressive role for testosterone in the response to influenza vaccination. Proc Natl Acad Sci USA 2014;111(2):869–74.

[5] Hughes GC, Choubey D. Modulation of autoimmune rheumatic diseases by oestrogen and progesterone. Nat Rev Rheumatol 2014;10(12):740–51. https://doi.org/10.1038/nrrheum.2014.144.

[6] Taneja V. Sex hormones determine immune response. Front Immunol 2018;9:1931. https://doi.org/10.3389/fimmu.2018.01931.

[7] The Novel Coronavirus Pneumonia Emergency Response Epidemiology Team China CDC. The epidemiological characteristics of an outbreak of 2019 novel coronaviurs diseases. Vital Surveill 2020;41(2):145–51.

[8] Zeng F, Dai C, Cai P, Wang J, Xu L, Li J, Hu G, Wang L. A comparison study of SARS-CoV-2 IgG antibody between male and female COVID-19 patients: a possible reason underlying different outcome between gender. J Med Virol 2020;92(10):2050–4. https://doi.org/10.1101/2020.03.26.20040709.

[9] Channappanavar R, Fett C, Mack M, Ten Eyck PP, Meyerholz DK, Perlman S. Sex-based differences in susceptibility to severe acute respiratory syndrome coronavirus infection. J Immunol 2017;198(10):4046–53. https://doi.org/10.4049/jimmunol.1601896.

[10] Straub RH CM, Bijlsma JW, Masi A. Role of neuroendocrine and neuroimmune mechanisms in chronic inflammatory rheumatic diseases-The 10-year update. Semin Arthritis Rheum 2013;43(3):392–404.

[11] Imai Y, Kuba K, Penninger JM. Angiotensin-converting enzyme 2 in acute respiratory distress syndrome. Cell Mol Life Sci 2007;64(15):2006–12. https://doi.org/10.1007/s00018-007-6228-6.

[12] Yang XH QC, Deng W, Tong Z, Liu YX, Zhang LF, Zhu H, Gao H, Huang L, Liu YL, Ma CM, Xu YF, Ding MX, Deng HK, Qin CYang XH, Deng W, Tong Z, Liu YX, Zhang LF, Zhu H, Gao H, Huang L, Liu YL, Ma CM, Xu YF, Ding MX, Deng HK. Mice transgenic for human angiotensin-converting enzyme 2 provide a model for SARS coronavirus infection. Comp Med 2007;57(5):450–9.

[13] Imai Y, Kuba K, Rao S, Huan Y, Guo F, Guan B, Yang P, Sarao R, Wada T, Leong-Poi H, Crackower MA, Fukamizu A, Hui CC, Hein L, Uhlig S, Slutsky AS, Jiang C, Penninger JM. Angiotensin-converting enzyme 2 protects from severe acute lung failure. Nature 2005;436(7047):112–6. https://doi.org/10.1038/nature03712.

[14] Kuba K, Imai Y, Rao S, Gao H, Guo F, Guan B, Huan Y, Yang P, Zhang Y, Deng W, Bao L, Zhang B, Liu G, Wang Z, Chappell M, Liu Y, Zheng D, Leibbrandt A, Wada T, Slutsky AS, Liu D, Qin C, Jiang C, Penninger JM. A crucial role of angiotensin converting enzyme 2 (ACE2) in SARS coronavirus-induced lung injury. Nat Med 2005;11(8):875–9. https://doi.org/10.1038/nm1267.

[15] Zhao Y, Zhao Z, Wang Y, Zhou Y, Ma Y, Zuo W. Single-cell RNA expression profiling of ACE2, the receptor of SARS-CoV-2. Am J Respir Crit Care Med 2020;202(5):756–9. https://doi.org/10.1164/rccm.202001-0179LE.

[16] Baker SA, Kwok S, Berry GJ, Montine TJ. Angiotensin-converting enzyme 2 (ACE2) expression increases with age in patients requiring mechanical ventilation. PLoS One 2021;16:e0247060. https://doi.org/10.1371/JOURNAL.PONE.0247060.

[17] Devaux CA, Rolain JM, Raoult D. ACE2 receptor polymorphism: susceptibility to SARS-CoV-2, hypertension, multi-organ failure, and COVID-19 disease outcome. J Microbiol Immunol Infect 2020;53:425–35. https://doi.org/10.1016/J.JMII.2020.04.015.

[18] Fakhouri EW, Peterson SJ, Kothari J, Alex R, Shapiro JI, Abraham NG. Genetic polymorphisms complicate covid-19 therapy: pivotal role of ho-1 in cytokine storm. Antioxidants 2020;9:1–23. https://doi.org/10.3390/antiox9070636.

[19] Gemmati D, Bramanti B, Serino ML, Secchiero P, Zauli G, Tisato V. COVID-19 and individual genetic susceptibility/receptivity: role of ACE1/ACE2 genes, immunity, inflammation and coagulation. might the double x-chromosome in females be protective against SARS-COV-2 compared to the single x-chromosome in males? Int J Mol Sci 2020;21. https://doi.org/10.3390/ijms21103474.

[20] Hoffmann M, Kleine-Weber H, Schroeder S, Krüger N, Herrler T, Erichsen S, Schiergens TS, Herrler G, Wu NH, Nitsche A, Müller MA, Drosten C, Pöhlmann S. SARS-CoV-2 cell entry depends on ACE2 and TMPRSS2 and is blocked by a clinically proven protease inhibitor. Cell 2020;181(2):271–80. https://doi.org/10.1016/j.cell.2020.02.052. e8.

[21] Fujikura K, Uesaka K. Genetic variations in the human severe acute respiratory syndrome coronavirus receptor ACE2 and serine protease TMPRSS2. J Clin Pathol 2021;74:307–13. https://doi.org/10.1136/jclinpath-2020-206867.

[22] Hou Y, Zhao J, Martin W, Kallianpur A, Chung MK, Jehi L, Sharifi N, Erzurum S, Eng C, Cheng F. New insights into genetic susceptibility of COVID-19: an ACE2 and TMPRSS2 polymorphism analysis. BMC Med 2020;18:1–8. https://doi.org/10.1186/s12916-020-01673-z.

[23] Severe Covid-19 GWAS Group KT, Ellinghaus D, Degenhardt F, Bujanda L, Buti M, Albillos A, Invernizzi P, Fernández J, Prati D, Baselli G, Asselta R, Grimsrud MM, Milani C, Aziz F, Kässens J, May S, Wendorff M, Wienbrandt L, Uellendahl-Werth F, Zheng T, Yi X. Genomewide association study of severe covid-19 with respiratory failure. N Engl J Med 2020;383(16):1522–34. https://doi.org/10.1056/nejmoa2020283.

[24] Initiative COVID-19 Host Genetics, Mapping the human genetic architecture of COVID-19. Nature. (n.d.). https://doi.org/10.1038/s41586-021-03767-x.

[25] SeyedAlinaghi SA, Mehrtak M, MohsseniPour M, Mirzapour P, Barzegary A, Habibi P, Moradmand-Badie B, Afsahi AM, Karimi A, Heydari M, Mehraeen E, Dadras O, Sabatier JM, Voltarelli F. Genetic susceptibility of COVID-19: a systematic review of current evidence. Eur J Med Res 2021;26:46. https://doi.org/10.1186/s40001-021-00516-8.

[26] Wein AN, McMaster SR, Takamura S, Dunbar PR, Cartwright EK, Hayward SL, McManus DT, Shimaoka T, Ueha S, Tsukui T, Masumoto T, Kurachi M, Matsushima K, Kohlmeier JE. CXCR6 regulates localization of tissue-resident memory CD8 T cells to the airways. J Exp Med 2019;216(12):2748–62. https://doi.org/10.1084/jem.20181308.

[27] Xiao G, Wang X, Wang J, Zu L, Cheng G, Hao M, Sun X, Xue Y, Lu J, Wang J. CXCL16/CXCR6 chemokine signaling mediates breast cancer progression by pERK1/2-dependent mechanisms. Oncotarget 2015;6:14165–78. https://doi.org/10.18632/oncotarget.3690.

[28] Cervantes-Barragan L, Züst R, Weber F, Spiegel M, Lang KS, Akira S, Thiel V, Ludewig B. Control of coronavirus infection through plasmacytoid dendritic-cell- derived type I interferon. Blood 2007;109(3):1131–7. https://doi.org/10.1182/blood-2006-05-023770.

[29] Lu C, Gam R, Pandurangan AP, Gough J. Genetic risk factors for death with SARS-CoV-2 from the UK Biobank. medRxiv 2020. https://doi.org/10.1101/2020.07.01.20144592. 2020.07.01.20144592.

[30] Van Der Made CI, Simons A, Schuurs-Hoeijmakers J, Van Den Heuvel G, Mantere T, Kersten S, Van Deuren RC, Steehouwer M, Van Reijmersdal SV, Jaeger M, Hofste T, Astuti G, Corominas Galbany J, Van Der Schoot V, Van Der Hoeven H, Hagmolen Of Ten Have W, Klijn E, Van Den Meer C, Fiddelaers J, De Mast Q, Bleeker-Rovers CP, Joosten LAB, Yntema HG, Gilissen C, Nelen M, Van Der Meer JWM, Brunner HG, Netea MG, Van De Veerdonk FL, Hoischen A. Presence of genetic variants among young men with severe COVID-19. J Am Med Assoc 2020;324(7):663–73. https://doi.org/10.1001/jama.2020.13719.

[31] Moreno-Eutimio MA, López-Macías C, Pastelin-Palacios R. Bioinformatic analysis and identification of single-stranded RNA sequences recognized by TLR7/8 in the SARS-CoV-2, SARS-CoV, and MERS-CoV genomes. Microb Infect 2020;22:226–9. https://doi.org/10.1016/j.micinf.2020.04.009.

[32] Brass AL, Huang IC, Benita Y, John SP, Krishnan MN, Feeley EM, Ryan BJ, Weyer JL, van der Weyden L, Fikrig E, Adams DJ, Xavier RJ, Farzan M, Elledge SJ. The IFITM proteins mediate cellular resistance to influenza A H1N1 virus, west nile virus, and dengue virus. Cell 2009. https://doi.org/10.1016/j.cell.2009.12.017.

[33] Wakim LM, Gupta N, Mintern JD, Villadangos JA. Enhanced survival of lung tissue-resident memory CD8 + T cells during infection with influenza virus due to selective expression of IFITM3. Nat Immunol 2013. https://doi.org/10.1038/ni.2525.

[34] Dai Y-J, Zhang W-N, Wang W-D, He S-Y, Liang C-C, Wang D-W. Two potential novel SARS-CoV-2 entries, TMPRSS2 and IFITM3, in healthy individuals and cancer patients. SSRN Electron J 2020. https://doi.org/10.2139/ssrn.3564377.

[35] Zhang Y, Qin L, Zhao Y, Zhang P, Xu B, Li K, Liang L, Zhang C, Dai Y, Feng Y, Sun J, Hu Z, Xiang H, Knight JC, Dong T, Jin R. Interferon-induced transmembrane protein-3 genetic variant rs12252-C is associated with disease severity in COVID-19. J Infect Dis 2020;222(1):34–7.

[36] Cendrowski J, Mamińska A, Miaczynska M. Endocytic regulation of cytokine receptor signaling. Cytokine Growth Factor Rev 2016;32:63–73. https://doi.org/10.1016/j.cytogfr.2016.07.002.

[37] Ross B, Krapp S, Augustin M, Kierfersauer R, Arciniega M, Geiss-Friedlander R, Huber R. Structures and mechanism of dipeptidyl peptidases 8 and 9, important players in cellular homeostasis and cancer. Proc Natl Acad Sci USA 2018;115:E1437–45. https://doi.org/10.1073/pnas.1717565115.

[38] Wiehagen KR, Corbo-Rodgers E, Li S, Staub ES, Hunter CA, Morrisey EE, Maltzman JS. Foxp4 is dispensable for T cell development, but required for robust recall responses. PLoS One 2012;7. https://doi.org/10.1371/journal.pone.0042273.

[39] Zollino M, Orteschi D, Murdolo M, Lattante S, Battaglia D, Stefanini C, Mercuri E, Chiurazzi P, Neri G, Marangi G. Mutations in KANSL1 cause the 17q21.31 microdeletion syndrome phenotype. Nat Genet 2012;44:636–8. https://doi.org/10.1038/ng.2257.

[40] Schmiedel BJ, Chandra V, Rocha J, Gonzalez-Colin C, Bhattacharyya S, Madrigal A, Ottensmeier CH, Ay F, Vijayanand P. COVID-19 genetic risk variants are associated with expression of multiple genes in diverse immune cell types. bioRxiv 2020;12. https://doi.org/10.1038/s41467-021-26888-3. 2020.12.01.407429.

[41] Nguyen A, David JK, Maden SK, Wood MA, Weeder BR, Nellore A, Thompson RF. Human leukocyte antigen susceptibility map for SARS-CoV-2. J Virol 2020;94(13):e00510–20. https://doi.org/10.1128/JVI.00510-20.

[42] Copley HC, Gragert L, Leach AR, Kosmoliaptsis V. Influence of HLA class II polymorphism on predicted cellular immunity against SARS-CoV-2 at the population and individual level. Front Immunol 2021;12:2791. https://doi.org/10.3389/FIMMU.2021.669357/BIBTEX.

[43] Wang W, Zhang W, Zhang J, He J, Zhu F. Distribution of HLA allele frequencies in 82 Chinese individuals with coronavirus disease-2019 (COVID-19). HLA 2020;96(2):194–6. https://doi.org/10.1111/tan.13941.

[44] Littera DS, Campagna M, Angioni FD, Cipri S, Melis M, Santus LSS, Lai A, Porcella R, Rassu MF, Scioscia KM, Schirru D, Cordeddu W, Serra CM, Ragatzu P, Del Giacco DS, Restivo A, Orrù OG, Palimodde A, Perra R, Conti OS, Balestrieri C, Serra PA, Marongiu CL. Human leukocyte antigen Complex and other immunogenetic and clinical factors influence susceptibility or protection to SARS-CoV-2 infection and severity of the disease course. The Sardinian experience. Front Immunol 2020;11:605688. https://doi.org/10.3389/fimmu.2020.605688.

[45] Shkurnikov M, Nersisyan S, Jankevic T, Galatenko A, Gordeev I, Vechorko V, Tonevitsky A. Association of HLA class I genotypes with severity of coronavirus disease-19. Front Immunol 2021;12. https://doi.org/10.3389/FIMMU.2021.641900.

[46] Correale P, Mutti L, Pentimalli F, Baglio G, Saladino RE, Sileri P, Giordano A. HLA-B*44 and C*01 prevalence correlates with Covid19 spreading across Italy. Int J Mol Sci 2020;21:1–12. https://doi.org/10.3390/IJMS21155205.

[47] Langton DJ, Bourke SC, Lie BA, Reiff G, Natu S, Darlay R, Burn J, Echevarria C. The influence of HLA genotype on the severity of COVID-19 infection. HLA 2021;98:14–22. https://doi.org/10.1111/TAN.14284.

[48] Naemi FMA, Al-adwani S, Al-khatabi H, Al-nazawi A. Frequency of HLA alleles among COVID-19 infected patients: preliminary data from Saudi Arabia. Virology 2021;560:1–7. https://doi.org/10.1016/J.VIROL.2021.04.011.

[49] Novelli A, Andreani M, Biancolella M, Liberatoscioli L, Passarelli C, Colona VL, Rogliani P, Leonardis F, Campana A, Carsetti R, Andreoni M, Bernardini S, Novelli G, Locatelli F. HLA allele frequencies and susceptibility to COVID-19 in a group of 99 Italian patients. HLA 2020;96:610–4. https://doi.org/10.1111/TAN.14047.

[50] Warren RL, Birol I. Retrospective in silico HLA predictions from COVID-19 patients reveal alleles associated with disease prognosis. medRxiv 2020. https://doi.org/10.1101/2020.10.27.20220863.

[51] Iturrieta-Zuazo I, Rita CG, García-Soidán A, de Malet Pintos-Fonseca A, Alonso-Alarcón N, Pariente-Rodríguez R, Tejeda-Velarde A, Serrano-Villar S, Castañer-Alabau JL, Nieto-Gañán I. Possible role of HLA class-I genotype in SARS-CoV-2 infection and progression: a pilot study in a cohort of Covid-19 Spanish patients. Clin Immunol 2020;219. https://doi.org/10.1016/J.CLIM.2020.108572.

[52] Tomita Y, Ikeda T, Sato R, Sakagami T. Association between HLA gene polymorphisms and mortality of COVID-19: an in silico analysis, Immunity. Inflamm Dis 2020;8:684–94. https://doi.org/10.1002/iid3.358.

[53] Liu N, Zhang T, Ma L, Zhang H, Wang H, Wei W, Pei H, Li H. The impact of ABO blood group on COVID-19 infection risk and mortality: a systematic review and meta-analysis. Blood Rev 2021;48. https://doi.org/10.1016/j.blre.2020.100785.

[54] Wu Y, Feng Z, Li P, Yu Q. Relationship between ABO blood group distribution and clinical characteristics in patients with COVID-19. Clin Chim Acta 2020;509:220–3. https://doi.org/10.1016/J.CCA.2020.06.026.

[55] Göker H, Aladağ-Karakulak E, Demiroğlu H, Ayaz CM, Büyükasik Y, İnkaya AC, Aksu S, Sayinalp N, Haznedaroğlu İC, Uzun Ö, Akova M, Özcebe O, Ünal S. The effects of blood group types on the risk of COVID-19 infection and its clinical outcome. Turk J Med Sci 2020;50:679–83. https://doi.org/10.3906/SAG-2005-395.

[56] Li J, Wang X, Chen J, Cai Y, Deng A, Yang M. Association between ABO blood groups and risk of SARS-CoV-2 pneumonia. Br J Haematol 2020;190:24–7. https://doi.org/10.1111/BJH.16797.

[57] Zietz M, Zucker J, Tatonetti NP. Testing the association between blood type and COVID-19 infection, intubation, and death. medRxiv 2020. https://doi.org/10.1101/2020.04.08.20058073.

[58] Zhao J, Yang Y, Huang H, Li D, Gu D, Lu X, Zhang Z, Liu L, Liu T, Liu Y, He Y, Sun B, Wei M, Yang G, Wang X, Zhang L, Zhou X, Xing M, Wang PG. Relationship between the ABO blood group and the coronavirus disease 2019 (COVID-19) susceptibility. Clin Infect Dis 2021;73:328–31. https://doi.org/10.1093/CID/CIAA1150.

[59] Gérard C, Maggipinto G, Minon JM. COVID-19 and ABO blood group: another viewpoint. Br J Haematol 2020;190:e93–4. https://doi.org/10.1111/bjh.16884.

[60] Almadhi MA, Abdulrahman A, Alawadhi A, Rabaan AA, Atkin S, AlQahtani M. The effect of ABO blood group and antibody class on the risk of COVID-19 infection and severity of clinical outcomes. Sci Rep 2021;11:1–5. https://doi.org/10.1038/s41598-021-84810-9.

[61] Amenta EM, Spallone A, Rodriguez-Barradas MC, Sahly HME, Atmar RL, Kulkarni PA. Postacute covid-19: an overview and approach to classification. Open Forum Infect Dis 2020;7. https://doi.org/10.1093/ofid/ofaa509.

[62] Ceravolo MG, Arienti C, de Sire A, Andrenelli E, Negrini F, Lazzarini SG, Patrini M, Negrini S. Rehabilitation and COVID-19: the Cochrane Rehabilitation 2020 rapid living systematic review. Eur J Phys Rehabil Med 2020;56:642–51. https://doi.org/10.23736/S1973-9087.20.06501-6.

[63] Post-COVID Conditions. CDC (n.d.). https://www.cdc.gov/coronavirus/2019-ncov/long-term-effects/index.html (accessed September 30, 2021).

[64] Ehrenfeld M, Tincani A, Andreoli L, Cattalini M, Greenbaum A, Kanduc D, Alijotas-Reig J, Zinserling V, Semenova N, Amital H, Shoenfeld Y. Covid-19 and autoimmunity. Autoimmun Rev 2020;19:102597. https://doi.org/10.1016/j.autrev.2020.102597.

[65] Malkova A, Kudryavtsev I, Starshinova A, Kudlay D, Zinchenko Y, Glushkova A, Yablonskiy P, Shoenfeld Y. Post COVID-19 syndrome in patients with asymptomatic/mild form. Pathogens 2021;10:1408. https://doi.org/10.3390/PATHOGENS10111408. 10 (2021) 1408.

[66] Malkova A, Kudlay D, Kudryavtsev I, Starshinova A, Yablonskiy P, Shoenfeld Y. Immunogenetic predictors of severe covid-19. Vaccines 2021;9:1–13. https://doi.org/10.3390/vaccines9030211.

CHAPTER

8

Molecular mimicry and SARS-CoV-2

Eirini I. Rigopoulou[1], Arad Dotan[2,3], Georgios Efthymiou[1], Efthymios Dardiotis[4], Yehuda Shoenfeld[2,5] and Dimitrios P. Bogdanos[1]

[1]Faculty of Medicine, School of Health Sciences, University of Thessaly, Larissa, Greece; [2]Zabludowicz Center for Autoimmune Diseases, Sheba Medical Center, Ramat Gan, Israel; [3]Sackler Faculty of Medicine, Tel Aviv University, Tel Aviv, Israel; [4]Department of Neurology, Faculty of Medicine, School of Health Sciences, University of Thessaly, Larissa, Greece; [5]Tel Aviv University, Tel Aviv, Israel

The plethora of immune-mediated phenomena and autoimmune disorders induced by or following COVID-19 (and/or SARS-VoV-2 vaccination) has led several authors around the globe to suggest (some of those in a very bold manner) that the virus and the immune response it initiates is instrumental for the induction of autoimmunity and overt autoimmune diseases [1–4]. Moreover, several long-lasting post-COVID-19 disorders have been considered autoimmune in nature [5]. Lastly, several manifestations developed by COVID-19 imitate full-blown autoimmune diseases [6,7].

Upon infection, several viruses can induce the de novo development of autoantibodies, and this is also the case for SARS-CoV-2, mostly in severe cases [2,8]. These autoantibodies are directed against a plethora of known autoantigens, newly identified human proteins but also against cytokines, such as interferons and may influence disease's outcome [2,9]. How these autoantibodies arise has been the focus of intense research [10]. As for other autoantibodies, the most well-described mechanism for the induction of viral-triggered autoimmunity related to SARS-CoV-2 has been considered that of molecular mimicry [2,11,12] (Figs. 8.1 and 8.2).

The concept of molecular mimicry and its relevance to autoimmunity

The mechanism of molecular mimicry has been proposed widely for the induction of organ-specific and non–organ-specific autoantibodies [11,13–16]. Others include bystander polyclonal activation and viral persistence, mainly with epitope spreading. It is quite

Autoimmunity, COVID-19, Post-COVID19 syndrome and COVID-19 vaccination
https://doi.org/10.1016/B978-0-443-18566-3.00026-8

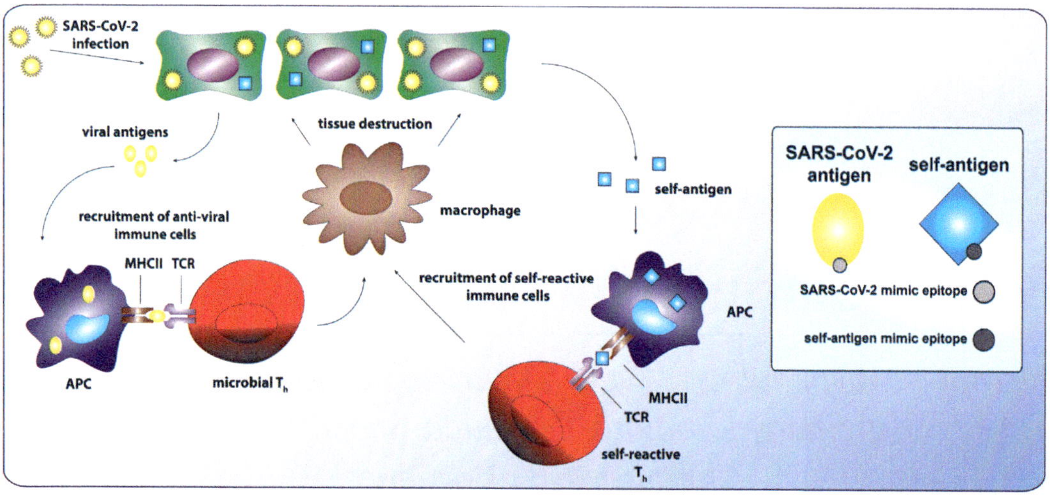

FIGURE 8.1 **Molecular mimicry as a mechanism of SARS-CoV-2 induced autoimmunity.** Following SARS-CoV-2 infection, activated T helper (microbial T_h) mediates the viral clearance. In the case of molecular mimicry, cross-reactive T cells recognize both the viral epitope and a self-epitope. The release of self-antigens and their uptake by antigen presenting cells (APC) induces autoimmune tissue destruction. Abbreviations: MHCII, major histocompatibility complex type II; TCR, T cell receptor.

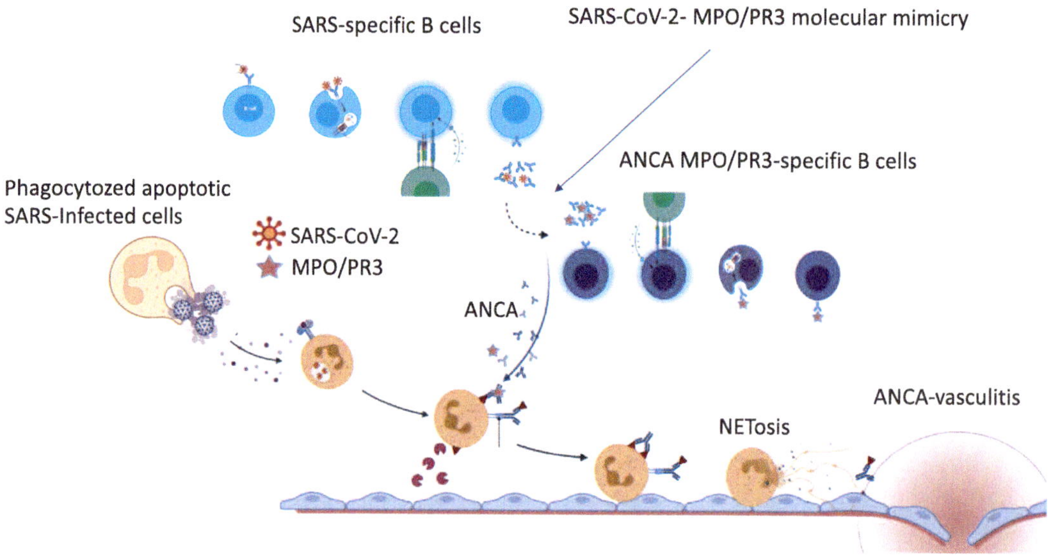

FIGURE 8.2 **Molecular mimicry as a mechanism of SARS-CoV-2 induced ANCA-vasculitis: a hypothesis.** Following SARS-CoV-2 infection, B-cells are activated and by antigen-specific antibodies against immunodominant SARS-CoV-2 epitopes are initiated. In case of molecular mimicry with ANCA autoantigens such as MPO or PR3, autoantibodies targeting MPO or PR3 mimics are induced leading to a perpetuation of an autoimmune cascade, including NETosis, provoking full-blown ANCA vasculitis. In another interrelated mechanism, SARS-CoV-2 infected apoptotic host cells are phagocytized by neutrophils, and internalized viral antigens are de novo inducing SARS-CoV-2-specific immune responses, including those against SARS-CoV-2 epitopes which mimic MPO or PR3 antigens. These phenomena may also induce ANCA-vasculitis.

straightforward to envisage how molecular mimicry can elicit autoreactive responses [15,17]. The major concept of the mechanism is simple and clear. Molecular mimicry is nothing more and nothing less than a shared immunologic epitope between a pathogen and the host [11] (Fig. 8.1). This implies per se the existence of "similar antigenic structures shared by molecules from dissimilar genes or by other protein products" [18]. Immune responses to the one can elicit immune responses to the other, a phenomenon known as immunological cross-reactivity [14].

When an organism (the host), in our case a human, is infected, the immune system is activated in an attempt to control the virus. Activation of the immune system leads to the induction of antigen-specific humoral and cellular immune responses against specific viral proteins [15]. Regarding T cells, the epitopes recognized by CD4 and CD8 are short-length amino acid sequences. In the case of antiviral antibodies, the epitopic regions are predominantly conformational polypeptidyl sequences rather than short peptides of few amino acids.

Irrespectively, of whether we are considering molecular mimicry at the antibody or at the cellular level, it appears that several, specific viral sequences (or sequences from other pathogens) share a high degree of amino acid similarities with self-proteins and fulfill the criteria for antigenic mimicry at the B-cell or T-cell level as they have extensively been described over the years [17–19]. If this amino acid similarity concerns epitopes of the virus and the self, it can be the impetus of antigenic mimicry. It immediately implies that antibodies or T cells, which recognize this viral sequence it may also cross-recognize the self-epitopes, just because of the amino acid homology shared by the two antigenic proteins.

The consequence of this phenomenon has is tremendous for the understanding of the pathogenesis of autoimmune diseases. If responses against the virus are predominantly relate to the viral protein which is homologous to self, its time an infection takes place, the generation of antiviral antibodies against this viral epitope could also initiate, most precisely, cross-react with the homologous self-autoepitope. Initiation of autoantibodies (irrespectively of the trigger) may lead to the induction of autoimmune phenomena and clinically evident autoimmune disease (Fig. 8.2).

Several examples of molecular mimicry as the leading mechanism triggering autoimmunity have been described in the past. For example, patients with rheumatic fever due to group A beta-hemolytic streptococci develop antibodies, which can cross-recognize antigens on heart and joint tissues [20]. Cardiac myosin has been the target of antibodies specifically reacting with the M protein of streptococci and immunization with specific viral M peptides can induce rheumatic heart disease in murine models of the disease. Another classical example of molecular mimicry is that of Guillain-Barré Syndrome (GBS) [21].

Such examples of cross-reactive epitopes have been described in a plethora of experimental diseases, as well as in autoimmune diseases of relevance to human beings [22].

Early studies investigating the role of molecular mimicry have noted that monoclonal antibodies raised against specific viral proteins could also react with cellular proteins [23]. A large study has shown that approximately one in 20 monoclonal antibodies developed against viral proteins could also react with self-proteins, suggesting that viral epitopes and self-epitopes were targets of cross-reactive antibodies.

The concept of T-cell mimicry is similar to that of B-cell mimicry, but it is less easy to understand, as we will discuss later [19,24]. A seminal study by Oldstone and Fujinami showed that the hepatitis B virus DNA polymerase and myelin basic protein share a 6-mer in common and that the viral peptide if is injected to rabbits can induce experimental autoimmune encephalomyelitis, which is the animal model of multiple sclerosis [25]. We have described several hepatitis B surface antigen mimics of myelin antigens that could act as potential targets of antiviral antibodies during infection or even during vaccination, to prevent from the infection [26]. Molecular mimicry and immunological cross-reactivity has been the mechanism most frequently cited, as the likely cause of vaccine-induced autoimmunity, but solid evidence in support of this has not been obtained [27,28].

Molecular mimicry has been studied not only as a tool to explain how autoimmunity may arise following infection of susceptible individuals, but also as an instrument for modern immunology to discover more perplexed pathogen–host interactions, as well as to discover new autoantigens linked with autoimmune diseases [27,29–34].

Over the years, it has been elegantly shown by our group and several others that B cells and T cell cross-reactive immune responses involving pathogens and autoantigens are very frequent [11,13–15,17,18,25,26,29,33–41]. As it very common, it has been extremely likely that there is an increased risk that the response to an infecting agent will also attack the host causing autoimmunity. A permutation of the current theme "one viral agent-one human autoantigen" is that describing the "multiple hit" scenario of molecular mimicry, which describes a series of subsequent or concurrent infections with two or more pathogens all of which share antigenic mimicry with a specific autoepitope [42–44]. In that case, the totality of infections and the immune responses they are initiating increase the number of the hits, that is, accelerate the number of viral-specific and their host mimics effector T cells or cross-reactive antibodies leading to the perpetuation of autoimmunity and the precipitation of the immune attack against the host. The mimics could be from the same pathogen or different pathogens and may originate from viruses and microbes, as long as they fulfill the criterion, which justifies their ability to be targeted by cross-reactive B cells (antibodies) and/or T-cells [11]. As it has been noted before, the induction of cross-reactivity does not require evidence that the pathogen (i.e., the virus) replicate within the cell, as the instructor for the induction of autoimmunity is the immune response against self-mimicking viral agents rather than the virus itself (a phenomenon also known as "hit-and-run") [11]. Also, molecular mimicry could indeed be only one piece of the puzzle, that is, only one of the mechanisms which are needed for an autoimmune disease to appear in a susceptible individual, others participating long before or after the initiation of autoimmune disease over the long incubation period needed for the overt disease to appear (at times it may takes few decades) [45].

Tools to study molecular mimicry

Antigenic mimicry is instrumental for the initiation of cross-reactive T cells and antibodies [46]. Antibodies against a pathogen may cross-react against self-epitope, if the epitopes are stereotactically indistinguishable, that is, if the antigenic surfaces are to be similar. To understand that, we need to get as an example the case of a B-cell epitope, which consisted of a short linearized sequence. Several computerized programs such as that of BLAST can compare the amino acid composition of two proteins and provide results regarding amino acid sequence similarities. However, most B-cell epitopes are conformational and lengthy.

No need of identical or homologous amino acid sequence similarity is needed as long as their antigenic surfaces in a three-dimensional manner are similar. In that case, irrespectively of the degree of amino acid similarity, molecular mimicry is operated and immunological cross-reactivity is induced [46]. This is of paramount importance for the understanding of the studies so far conducted in SARS-CoV-2 and COVID-19, as hundreds of pairs of homologous viral/self-proteins have been reported. Most of those have been based on amino acid alignment comparisons between SARS-CoV-2 and human proteins using the Basic Local Alignment Search Tool (BLAST) platform of the National Center for Biotechnology Information (NCBI). BLAST is useful but not always successful in providing a meticulous assessment of the extent of homologous sequences as it may miss identical amino acid sequences shared in common by nonhomologous regions of the compared proteins, as well as mimics of non-peptidic and discontinuous protein epitopes [47].

This chapter highlights the studies so far conducted, which assess the likely role of molecular mimicry between SARS-CoV-2 and self-antigens in the induction of autoantibodies and autoimmunity in general.

Bioinformatic approaches investigating the role of SARS-CoV-2-related autoimmunity by molecular mimicry

A search in PubMed library using as keywords the terms "molecular mimicry," "SARS," and "autoimmune" produces 54 hits (end of January 2021). Out of those, 22 represent review articles. Most papers assess the potential role of molecular mimicry based on bioinformatic analysis.

Darja Kanduc and her group were probably the very first to pay meticulous attention to the existence of mimics between SARS-CoV-2 and human proteins. In one of their very first studies, Kanduc and Shoenfeld used 7-meric sequences as probes to test for potential overlaps with SARS-CoV-2 spike glycoproteins and mammalian proteomes. Initially, the authors calculated that the probability of the occurrence in two proteins of just one 7-mer equals to $\sim 20^{-7}$. (1 out of 1,280,000,000) and that the same probability of just one hexapeptide is equal to $\sim 20^{-6}$ (or 1 out of 64,000,000). They were able to identify more than 300 human proteins which share a 6-mer with SARS-CoV-2 spike glycoproteins and more than 25 of those shared a 7-mer [48]. In another study, the same investigators reported that 230 out of the 733 6-mers composing 233 published SARS-COv-2 epitopes appeared in 460 human proteins, some more than once [49]. Several of those originated from human proteins relevant to neurologic, pulmonary, cardiac, cancerous, and autoimmune disorders. Another study found 41 5-mers from SARS-CoV-2 spike glycoprotein to be shared with 27 human proteins related to oogenesis, uterine receptivity, decidualization, and placentation of potential relevance to which may contribute to female infertility [50]. Out of those 27, 23 were known SARS-CoV-2 spike glycoprotein immunodominant epitopes [50]. A bioinformatics analysis has claimed that peptide mimicries are common between SARS-CoV-2 and human proteome, as well as between human proteome and other pathogens but appear infrequent between eat the heptapeptide level are common between pathogens and primates [51]. The study of molecular mimicry must be based on immunodominant epitopes of SARS-CoV-2, especially if those are meticulously

TABLE 8.1 Representative bioinformatically predicted epitopes of SARS-CoV-2 structural proteins.

Epitope	SARS-CoV-2 protein	Position	Aa length	Reference
LDSKTQ	Protein S–	110–115	6	[69]
EYVSQPFLM	Protein S–	169–177	9	[70]
SETKCTLKSF	Protein S–	297–306	10	[70]
YNSASFSTFKCYGVSPTKLNDLCFT	Protein S–	369–393	25	[71]
ELLHAPATVCGPKKSTNLVKN	Protein S–	516–536	21	[71]
IPIGAGICASY	Protein S–	664–674	11	[70]
LADAGFIKQYGDCLG	Protein S–	828–842	15	[71]
TLVKQLSSNFGAISSVLNDI	Protein S–	961–980	20	[72]
QQLIRAAEIRASANLAATKM	Protein S–	1010–1029	20	[72]
KEELDKYFKNHTSPDVDLGD	Protein S–	1149–1168	20	[72]
EVAKNLNESL	Protein S–	1188–1197	10	[70]
VMVTIMLCCMTSCCSCLKGC	Protein S–	1228–1247	20	[72]
SRGGSQASSRSSSRSR	Protein N–	176–191	16	[12]
QQQQGQTVTKKSAAEASKKP	Protein N–	239–258	20	[72]
RRGPEQTQGNFGDQELIRQG	Protein N–	276–295	20	[72]
LPQRQKKQ	Protein N–	382–389	8	[12]
KQLQQSMSSADS	Protein N–	405–416	12	[70]
RTRSMWSFNPETN	Protein M–	105–117	13	[70]
PLLESELVIGAVILRGHLRI	Protein M–	132–151	20	[70]
NYKLNTDHSSSSDNIA	Protein M–	203–218	18	[70]
SVLLFLAFVVFLLVT	Protein E–	16–30	15	[70]

assessed (e.g., see Table 8.1). Ourselves have identified several of those viral/self-mimicking sequences potentially implicated in viral-triggered autoimmune phenomena (Tables 8.2–8.5).

Molecular mimicry has even been considered instrumental for the induction of cytokine storm related to SARS-CoV-2 infection [52]. The most profound consideration for the induction of autoimmunity by molecular mimicry is that concerning the *de novo* appearance of autoantibodies [2,8,53,54]. Among the numerous clinical autoimmune phenomena and disorders linked to SARS-CoV-2, either due to vaccination or most frequently due to infection, is GBS [55]. GBS and anti-phospholipid syndrome (APS) will be used as two typical examples from the very many disorders that have been linked with SARS-CoV-2, via molecular mimicry.

TABLE 8.2 Representative alignments between human protein sequences and SARS-CoV-2 protein S epitope sequences.

Human protein			SARS-CoV-2 protein S	
Protein	Position	Sequence	Position	Sequence
Ankyrin–	3444–3448	LDSKT–	110–114	LDSKT
Homeobox protein DLX-3–	72–78	NGLAGTG–	544–550	NGLTGTG
Selenoprotein I–	366–371	VKQLSS–	963–968	VKQLSS
Protein kintoun–	769–775	NLNESVI–	1192–1198	NLNESLI
Exportin 7–	541–547	TGCCSCL–	1238–1244	TSCCSCLS

TABLE 8.3 Representative alignments between human protein sequences and SARS-CoV-2 protein N epitope sequences.

Human protein			SARS-CoV-2 protein N	
Protein	Position	Sequence	Position	Sequence
Arg protein tyrosine kinase-binding protein–	247–253	SSRSSSR–	183–189	SSRSSSR
Retinoblastoma-like protein 2–	819–824	QGQSVT–	242–247	QGQTVT
Dynein heavy chain 14, axonemal–	416–421	QELIRQ–	289–293	QELIRQ
Gamma-aminobutyric acid (GABA) A receptor, beta 3–	336–341	PQRQKK–	383–388	PQRQKK
Codanin-1–	260–265	KQLQQS–	405–410	KQLQQS

TABLE 8.4 Representative alignments between human protein sequences and SARS-CoV-2 protein M epitope sequences.

Human protein			SARS-CoV-2 protein M	
Protein	Position	Sequence	Position	Sequence
Olfactory receptor 4C46–	204–210	ICLLNFA–	32–38	ICLLQFA
Aconitase–	507–512	FNPETN–	112–117	FNPETN
Melanocortin 5 receptor–	56–62	LVIGAIV–	138–144	LVIGAVI
Spermatogenesis-associated protein 1–	27–32	NYKLNT–	203–208	NYKLNT
NOX5 protein–	133–140	ADGNGAIT–	2–9	ADSNGTIT

TABLE 8.5 Representative alignments between human protein sequences and SARS-CoV-2 protein E epitope sequences.

Human protein			SARS-CoV-2 protein E	
Protein	Position	Sequence	Position	Sequence
NRCAM protein–	95–101	TGTLIIN–	9–15	TGTLIVN
Cytochrome P450-IIB–	4–10	SVLLFLA–	16–22	SVLLFLA
ADAMTS-like 1–	13–18	LLFLAF–	18–23	LLFLAF
SLC7A13 protein–	333–338	LLVTLG–	27–32	LLVTLA
AGBL3 protein–	146–151	FVYSRV–	57–62	YVYSRV

SARS-CoV-2, molecular mimicry, and Guillain–Barré syndrome

More than 100 case reports and cases series of various types of GBS, the most prominent being acute inflammatory demyelinating polyneuropathy, have been reported in the literature related to previous SARS-CoV-2 infection. Most cases of SARS-CoV-2 infection and COVID-19 preceded GBS onset by up to 4 weeks [56–58]. Up to 10% of the reported case series had IgG SARS-CoV-2 antibodies and only a minority of those (3.81%) of those had anti-ganglioside antibodies against various gangliosides, such as GM1, GD1a, GT1a, GM2, and GQ1b [57].

Keddie et al. not only reported lack of epidemiological evidence linking SARS-CoV-2 and GBS, but also found not significant amino acid similarity between SARS-CoV-2 proteins and human proteins of relevance to GBS, that could justify a mechanism of molecular mimicry in motion. There BLAST searches included spike/surface, envelope, membrane, and nucleocapsid phosphoprotein of SARS-CoV-2. The only exception for a similarity that could make sense was that of a pentapeptide (VVVNA) that was found in the viral ORF1ab/ORF1a polyprotein and the human mono-ADP-ribosyltransferase (PARP14).Others have used a different approach being able to identify likely mimics that could explain post-COVID-19 induced GBS, like the similarities shared between human heat shock and chaperones with SARS-CoV-2 proteins [59,60]. Though some of the shared sequences appear to correspond to immunoreactive epitopes, their immunoreactivity has not been tested in sera of cells from SARS-CoV-2-linked GBS [59].

SARS-CoV-2, molecular mimicry, and anti-phospholipid syndrome (APS)

The exceptionally high prevalence of thromboembolic events in COVID-19 patients, implicating both arterial and venous circulation, has led authors to methodically assess their clinical and pathological features concluding that COVID-19 thrombosis shares a lot in common with APS. It has become apparent, though, that antiphospholipid antibodies in COVID-19 are distinctive from those detectable in APS, in terms of their epitope specificity [61]. Nevertheless, the *de novo* induction of APS-related autoantibodies in COVID-19 has led several investigators to suggest that SARS-mediated APS like disorder, via molecular mimicry and subsequent immune-mediated endothelial dysfunction, could credibly explain how thrombogenesis appears in COVID-19 [62–64]. BLAST and LALIGN searches were employed to identify and analyze SARS-CoV-2 and human blood proteins related to coagulopathies [63]. SARS-CoV-2 appears to exhibit amino acid similarity with various mimicry human blood proteins at a rate, which is significantly higher than the control virus average [63]. Similarities between SARS-CoV-2 replicase 1a or spike protein and platelet phosphodiesterases or Rh blood group proteins were those mostly seen. Several matching sets were also found between these two SARS-CoV-2 proteins and prothrombin, complement C3, C4, and C5 [63].

When the overall SARS-CoV-2 proteome is analyzed, an extensive number of exhibits similarities to serum albumin, clotting factors, platelet phosphodiesterases, Rh blood group proteins, prothrombin, VWF, Factor IX, Factor Xa, ADAMTS13, and CD55/DAF was noted [63]. None of those mimics was tested for immunological cross-reactivity in biomaterial from infected patients.

SARS-CoV-2 vaccination and autoimmunity

It is logical to assume that molecular mimicry could be a major contributor of vaccine-induced immune-mediated phenomena. That assumption has long been regarded as a potential threat for vaccines based on whole antigens, or large polypeptides capable of inducing immune-responses against dozens or even hundreds of mimicking self-epitopes of relevance to autoimmunity [21,22,26,27,33,65]. Indeed, *emerging evidence has suggested that newly developed autoimmune manifestations including GBS and VITT, as well as other organ and nonorgan-specific autoimmune diseases, such as IgA nephropathy, autoimmune liver diseases, and several other organ-specific and nonorgan-specific autoimmune diseases is likely associated with or de novo induced by COVID-19 vaccines [2]. Mimicry is to blame at some extent also in that case.* For example, homologies between SARS-CoV-2 spike protein and platelet factor 4/heparin have been found, raising concerns as to whether vaccination may induce autoantibodies, but these SARS-CoV-2 epitopic regions appear not to be cross-recognized by anti-PF4 antibodies or *vice versa* [2,66]. The extent by which molecular mimicry induced by vaccination may contribute to vaccine-induced autoimmune phenomena raises concerns, especially in view of the fact that all the current vaccines are based on immunization with the full protein rather than immunodominant polypeptides. The fact that immunity raised against the virus appears to last for a limited period (up to 6 months) may prevent from long-lasting unwanted consequences of antiviral immune responses raised against mimicking selfproteins.

SARS-CoV-2 and evidence of immunological cross-reactivity

Vojdani A and his coauthors have provided intriguing findings suggesting that various monoclonal or polyclonal antibodies specific for SARS-CoV-2 specifically react with various selfantigens [67,68]. Among various antigenic preparations, mitochondria, microsomes, myosin, actin, insulin-R, GAD-65, thyroid peroxidase, and many others were targeted by monoclonal antibodies specific for SARS-CoV-2 [67,68]. Another study has failed to provide confirmatory data [8].

Conclusions

Meticulous data regarding the assessment of mimicking peptide sets and the level of cross-reactivity at the B-cell and T-cell levels are limited, and this is one of the major pitfalls of the current status of emerging research.

Most data are based on the investigation and report of amino acid homologies between the virus and selfproteins rather evidence of immunological cross-reactivity by studies using sera or peripheral blood mononuclear cells and this is a severe limitation. However, data are continuously provided and very soon, we will have specific answers to most of the assumed links between the virus and specific autoimmune diseases.

References

[1] Chen Y, Xu Z, Wang P, et al. New-onset autoimmune phenomena post-COVID-19 vaccination. Immunology 2021;165.
[2] Dotan A, Muller S, Kanduc D, David P, Halpert G, Shoenfeld Y. The SARS-CoV-2 as an instrumental trigger of autoimmunity. Autoimmun Rev 2021;20(4):102792.
[3] Elrashdy F, Tambuwala MM, Hassan SS, et al. Autoimmunity roots of the thrombotic events after COVID-19 vaccination. Autoimmun Rev 2021;20(11):102941.
[4] Zacharias H, Dubey S, Koduri G, D'Cruz D. Rheumatological complications of Covid 19. Autoimmun Rev 2021;20(9):102883.
[5] Anaya JM, Rojas M, Salinas ML, et al. Post-COVID syndrome. A case series and comprehensive review. Autoimmun Rev 2021;20(11):102947.
[6] Matucci-Cerinic M, Hughes M, Taliani G, Kahaleh B. Similarities between COVID-19 and systemic sclerosis early vasculopathy: a "viral" challenge for future research in scleroderma. Autoimmun Rev 2021;20(10):102899.
[7] Gkoutzourelas A, Bogdanos DP, Sakkas LI. Kawasaki disease and COVID-19. Mediterr J Rheumatol 2020;31(Suppl. 2):268–74.
[8] Damoiseaux J, Dotan A, Fritzler MJ, et al. Autoantibodies and SARS-CoV2 infection: the spectrum from association to clinical implication: report of the 15th Dresden symposium on autoantibodies. Autoimmun Rev 2021;21(3):103012.
[9] Bastard P, Rosen LB, Zhang Q, et al. Autoantibodies against type I IFNs in patients with life-threatening COVID-19. Science 2020;370(6515).
[10] Redwan EM, Alghamdi MF, El-Aziz TMA, et al. The mechanism behind flaring/triggering of autoimmunity disorders associated with COVID-19. Autoimmun Rev 2021;20(10):102909.
[11] Oldstone MB. Molecular mimicry and immune-mediated diseases. Faseb J 1998;12(13):1255–65.
[12] Ahmed SF, Quadeer AA, McKay MR. Preliminary identification of potential vaccine targets for the COVID-19 coronavirus (SARS-CoV-2) based on SARS-CoV immunological studies. Viruses 2020;12(3).
[13] Albert LJ, Inman RD. Molecular mimicry and autoimmunity. N Engl J Med 1999;341(27):2068–74.
[14] Bogdanos DP, Choudhuri K, Vergani D. Molecular mimicry and autoimmune liver disease: virtuous intentions, malign consequences. Liver 2001;21(4):225–32.
[15] Bogdanos DP, Mieli-Vergani G, Vergani D. Virus, liver and autoimmunity. Dig Liver Dis 2000;32(5):440–6.
[16] Gkoutzourelas A, Barmakoudi M, Bogdanos DP. A bioinformatics analysis reveals novel pathogens as molecular mimicry triggers of systemic sclerosis. Mediterr J Rheumatol 2020;31(1):50–70.
[17] Oldstone MB. Molecular mimicry, microbial infection, and autoimmune disease: evolution of the concept. Curr Top Microbiol Immunol 2005;296:1–17.

[18] Cusick MF, Libbey JE, Fujinami RS. Molecular mimicry as a mechanism of autoimmune disease. Clin Rev Allergy Immunol 2012;42(1):102–11.
[19] Wucherpfennig KW. Structural basis of molecular mimicry. J Autoimmun 2001;16(3):293–302.
[20] Guilherme L, Kalil J, Cunningham M. Molecular mimicry in the autoimmune pathogenesis of rheumatic heart disease. Autoimmunity 2006;39(1):31–9.
[21] Israeli E, Agmon-Levin N, Blank M, Chapman J, Shoenfeld Y. Guillain-Barre syndrome–a classical autoimmune disease triggered by infection or vaccination. Clin Rev Allergy Immunol 2012;42(2):121–30.
[22] Blank M, Krause I, Fridkin M, et al. Bacterial induction of autoantibodies to beta2-glycoprotein-I accounts for the infectious etiology of antiphospholipid syndrome. J Clin Invest 2002;109(6):797–804.
[23] Srinivasappa J, Saegusa J, Prabhakar BS, et al. Molecular mimicry: frequency of reactivity of monoclonal antiviral antibodies with normal tissues. J Virol 1986;57(1):397–401.
[24] Wucherpfennig KW. Mechanisms for the induction of autoimmunity by infectious agents. J Clin Invest 2001;108(8):1097–104.
[25] Oldstone MB. Molecular mimicry and autoimmune disease. Cell 1987;50(6):819–20.
[26] Bogdanos DP, Smith H, Ma Y, Baum H, Mieli-Vergani G, Vergani D. A study of molecular mimicry and immunological cross-reactivity between hepatitis B surface antigen and myelin mimics. Clin Dev Immunol 2005;12(3):217–24.
[27] Polymeros D, Tsiamoulos ZP, Koutsoumpas AL, et al. Bioinformatic and immunological analysis reveals lack of support for measles virus related mimicry in Crohn's disease. BMC Med 2014;12:139.
[28] Koutsoumpas A, Polymeros D, Tsiamoulos Z, et al. Peculiar antibody reactivity to human connexin 37 and its microbial mimics in patients with Crohn's disease. J Crohns Colitis 2011;5(2):101–9.
[29] Oldstone MB. Molecular mimicry as a mechanism for the cause and a probe uncovering etiologic agent(s) of autoimmune disease. Curr Top Microbiol Immunol 1989;145:127–35.
[30] Polymeros D, Bogdanos DP, Day R, Arioli D, Vergani D, Forbes A. Does cross-reactivity between mycobacterium avium paratuberculosis and human intestinal antigens characterize Crohn's disease? Gastroenterology 2006;131(1):85–96.
[31] Baum H, Brusic V, Choudhuri K, Cunningham P, Vergani D, Peakman M. MHC molecular mimicry in diabetes. Nat Med 1995;1(5):388.
[32] Gregorio GV, Choudhuri K, Ma Y, et al. Mimicry between the hepatitis C virus polyprotein and antigenic targets of nuclear and smooth muscle antibodies in chronic hepatitis C virus infection. Clin Exp Immunol 2003;133(3):404–13.
[33] Bogdanos DP, Rigopoulou EI. Self-mimicking autoimmune domains of hepatitis C virus core antigen. Vaccine 2006;24(37–39):6173–4.
[34] Bogdanos DP, Rigopoulou EI. Viral/self-mimicry and immunological cross-reactivity as a trigger of hepatic C virus associated autoimmune diabetes. Diabetes Res Clin Pract 2007;77(1):155–6.
[35] Bogdanos DP, Baum H, Grasso A, et al. Microbial mimics are major targets of crossreactivity with human pyruvate dehydrogenase in primary biliary cirrhosis. J Hepatol 2004;40(1):31–9.
[36] Bogdanos DP, Baum H, Gunsar F, et al. Extensive homology between the major immunodominant mitochondrial antigen in primary biliary cirrhosis and *Helicobacter pylori* does not lead to immunological cross-reactivity. Scand J Gastroenterol 2004;39(10):981–7.
[37] Bogdanos DP, Baum H, Sharma UC, et al. Antibodies against homologous microbial caseinolytic proteases P characterise primary biliary cirrhosis. J Hepatol 2002;36(1):14–21.
[38] Bogdanos DP, Lenzi M, Okamoto M, et al. Multiple viral/self immunological cross-reactivity in liver kidney microsomal antibody positive hepatitis C virus infected patients is associated with the possession of HLA B51. Int J Immunopathol Pharmacol 2004;17(1):83–92.
[39] Bogdanos DP, Pares A, Baum H, et al. Disease-specific cross-reactivity between mimicking peptides of heat shock protein of Mycobacterium gordonae and dominant epitope of E2 subunit of pyruvate dehydrogenase is common in Spanish but not British patients with primary biliary cirrhosis. J Autoimmun 2004;22(4):353–62.
[40] Fujinami RS, Oldstone MB. Molecular mimicry as a mechanism for virus-induced autoimmunity. Immunol Res 1989;8(1):3–15.
[41] Oldstone MB. Virus-induced autoimmunity: molecular mimicry as a route to autoimmune disease. J Autoimmun 1989;2(Suppl. 1):187–94.
[42] Vergani D, Bogdanos DP, Baum H. Unusual suspects in primary biliary cirrhosis. Hepatology 2004;39(1):38–41.

[43] Koutsoumpas AL, Smyk DS, Bogdanos DPE. Coli induced experimental model of primary biliary cirrhosis: at last. Int J Hepatol 2014;2014:848373.
[44] Smyk DS, Koutsoumpas AL, Mytilinaiou MG, Rigopoulou EI, Sakkas LI, Bogdanos DP. *Helicobacter pylori* and autoimmune disease: cause or bystander. World J Gastroenterol 2014;20(3):613–29.
[45] Getts DR, Chastain EM, Terry RL, Miller SD. Virus infection, antiviral immunity, and autoimmunity. Immunol Rev 2013;255(1):197–209.
[46] Quaratino S, Thorpe CJ, Travers PJ, Londei M. Similar antigenic surfaces, rather than sequence homology, dictate T-cell epitope molecular mimicry. Proc Natl Acad Sci U S A 1995;92(22):10398–402.
[47] Pertsemlidis A, Fondon 3rd JW. Having a BLAST with bioinformatics (and avoiding BLASTphemy). Genome Biol 2001;2(10). REVIEWS2002.
[48] Kanduc D, Shoenfeld Y. Molecular mimicry between SARS-CoV-2 spike glycoprotein and mammalian proteomes: implications for the vaccine. Immunol Res 2020;68(5):310–3.
[49] Kanduc D. From anti-SARS-CoV-2 immune responses to COVID-19 via molecular mimicry. Antibodies 2020;9(3).
[50] Dotan A, Kanduc D, Muller S, Makatsariya A, Shoenfeld Y. Molecular mimicry between SARS-CoV-2 and the female reproductive system. Am J Reprod Immunol 2021;86(6):e13494.
[51] Kanduc D. Lack of molecular mimicry between nonhuman primates and infectious pathogens: the possible genetic bases. Glob Med Genet 2021;8(1):32–7.
[52] Kanduc D. From anti-SARS-CoV-2 immune response to the cytokine storm via molecular mimicry. Antibodies 2021;10(4).
[53] Halpert G, Shoenfeld Y. SARS-CoV-2, the autoimmune virus. Autoimmun Rev 2020;19(12):102695.
[54] Chen C, Amelia A, Ashdown GW, Mueller I, Coussens AK, Eriksson EM. Risk surveillance and mitigation: autoantibodies as triggers and inhibitors of severe reactions to SARS-CoV-2 infection. Mol Med 2021;27(1):160.
[55] Lima M, Siokas V, Aloizou AM, et al. Unraveling the possible routes of SARS-COV-2 invasion into the central nervous system. Curr Treat Options Neurol 2020;22(11):37.
[56] Freire M, Andrade A, Sopena B, et al. Guillain Barre syndrome associated with COVID-19- lessons learned about its pathogenesis during the first year of the pandemic, a systematic review. Autoimmun Rev 2021;20(8):102875.
[57] Tawakul AA, Al-Doboke AW, Altayyar SA, Alsulami SA, Alfahmi AM, Nooh RT. Guillain-Barre syndrome in the COVID-19 pandemic. Neurol Int 2021;14(1):34–48.
[58] Zito A, Alfonsi E, Franciotta D, et al. COVID-19 and guillain-barre syndrome: a case report and review of literature. Front Neurol 2020;11:909.
[59] Lucchese G, Floel A. SARS-CoV-2 and Guillain-Barre syndrome: molecular mimicry with human heat shock proteins as potential pathogenic mechanism. Cell Stress Chaperones 2020;25(5):731–5.
[60] Lucchese G, Floel A. Guillain-Barre syndrome, SARS-CoV-2 and molecular mimicry. Brain 2021;144(5):e43.
[61] Borghi MO, Beltagy A, Garrafa E, et al. Anti-phospholipid antibodies in COVID-19 are different from those detectable in the anti-phospholipid syndrome. Front Immunol 2020;11:584241.
[62] Tung ML, Tan B, Cherian R, Chandra B. Anti-phospholipid syndrome and COVID-19 thrombosis: connecting the dots. Rheumatol Adv Pract 2021;5(1):rkaa081.
[63] Root-Bernstein R. COVID-19 coagulopathies: human blood proteins mimic SARS-CoV-2 virus, vaccine proteins and bacterial co-infections inducing autoimmunity: combinations of bacteria and SARS-CoV-2 synergize to induce autoantibodies targeting cardiolipin, cardiolipin-binding proteins, platelet factor 4, prothrombin, and coagulation factors. Bioessays 2021;43(12):e2100158.
[64] Carnevale S, Giovanetti M, Benvenuto D, Ciccozzi M, Broccolo F. Is molecular mimicry between hPF4 and SARS-CoV-2 spike protein a potential basis for autoimmune responses in vaccinated and naturally infected patients? Semin Thromb Hemost 2022. https://doi.org/10.1055/s-0041-1742092Letter.
[65] Dotan A, Shoenfeld Y. Perspectives on vaccine induced thrombotic thrombocytopenia. J Autoimmun 2021;121:102663.
[66] Greinacher A, Selleng K, Mayerle J, et al. Anti-platelet factor 4 antibodies causing VITT do not cross-react with SARS-CoV-2 spike protein. Blood 2021;138(14):1269–77.
[67] Vojdani A, Kharrazian D. Potential antigenic cross-reactivity between SARS-CoV-2 and human tissue with a possible link to an increase in autoimmune diseases. Clin Immunol 2020;217:108480.
[68] Vojdani A, Vojdani E, Kharrazian D. Reaction of human monoclonal antibodies to SARS-CoV-2 proteins with tissue antigens: implications for autoimmune diseases. Front Immunol 2020;11:617089.

[69] Zheng M, Song L. Novel antibody epitopes dominate the antigenicity of spike glycoprotein in SARS-CoV-2 compared to SARS-CoV. Cell Mol Immunol 2020;17(5):536–8.

[70] Grifoni A, Sidney J, Zhang Y, Scheuermann RH, Peters B, Sette A. A sequence homology and bioinformatic approach can predict candidate targets for immune responses to SARS-CoV-2. Cell Host Microbe 2020;27(4):671–680 e672.

[71] Bhattacharya M, Sharma AR, Patra P, et al. Development of epitope-based peptide vaccine against novel coronavirus 2019 (SARS-COV-2): immunoinformatics approach. J Med Virol 2020;92(6):618–31.

[72] Lyons-Weiler J. Pathogenic priming likely contributes to serious and critical illness and mortality in COVID-19 via autoimmunity. J Transl Autoimmun 2020;3:100051.

CHAPTER

9

In silico study of molecular mimicry between SARS-CoV-2 and neutrophil extracellular traps composition in granulocyte-rich supernatants of patients with systemic lupus erythematosus and lupus nephritis

Yekbun Adiguzel[1] *and Yehuda Shoenfeld*[2,3]

[1]Department of Medical Biology, School of Medicine, Atilim University, Kizilcasar Mah, Incek, Golbasi, Ankara, Turkey; [2]Zabludowicz Center for Autoimmune Diseases, Sheba Medical Center, Ramat Gan, Israel; [3]Tel Aviv University, Tel Aviv, Israel

Introduction

COVID-19 pandemic is a global crisis with devastating effects. The genetic make-up of the people providing resistance or susceptibility to a severe form of the disease is critical for the disease outcome. Immune responses of infected individuals to the SARS-CoV-2 protein sequences with similar regions in human proteins can result in an autoimmune reaction [1–7]. There are studies alluding to an association of different HLA alleles [8–11] and coronavirus-sourced epitopes [12], including SARS-CoV-2 [13]. Warren and Birol [14] reported the identification of HLA class I allele A*24:02 by transcriptome sequencing of bronchoalveolar lavage fluid samples in four of a total number of five individuals from China, who had COVID-19. A study conducted

Autoimmunity, COVID-19, Post-COVID19 syndrome and COVID-19 vaccination
https://doi.org/10.1016/B978-0-443-18566-3.00017-7

in Italy [15,16] revealed the association of HLA-DRB1*06:02, -DQB1*15:01, and -B*27:07 in 99 individuals affected by severe or extremely severe COVID-19. Nguyen et al. [17] searched an association of the worldwide distribution of HLA-A, -B, and -C alleles with the severity of COVID-19. HLA-B*46:01 possibly correlates with an elevated severity of the SARS-CoV diseases [18]. HLA-B*07:03 [19,20], and HLA-DRB1*12:02 are leading to susceptibility to SARS [20,21]. Further, binding affinities of 9mer and 15mer peptides of SARS-CoV-2 to 17,805 HLA alleles (9360 class I and 8445 class II) were predicted [22]. Total 368,145 peptides with a strong binding affinity to an allele under study, and epitope-sets representatives of most of the population (i.e., 90%) in 57 countries, were identified. Another study [23] combined prediction results of two different prediction tools [24,25] and estimated binding affinities of 8–11mer peptides of SARS-CoV-2 to 79 HLA class I alleles. SARS-CoV-2 peptides' binding prediction results were compared with that of the SARS-CoV and HCoV-OC43 structural proteins. Putative T cell epitopes of SARS-CoV and SARS-CoV-2 were predicted [26] together with binding affinities to 13 HLA class I alleles, and the study also included a population-level analysis [23]. It was a genome-wide association study. As Chakravarty [27] pointed out, such association studies do not identify (or emphasize) rare alleles, which can underestimate the risk posed by such alleles.

Immune-related disease severity of COVID-19 is established, yet multifaceted [28–33]. Regarding autoimmunity, critically ill patients with COVID-19 [34] displayed "hallmarks of extrafollicular B cell activation as previously described in autoimmune settings." Kawasaki disease, autoimmune cytopenia, Guillain-Barré syndrome, and the antiphospholipid syndrome were noticeable in patients with COVID-19 [35]. COVID-19-associated thrombosis is related to secondary antiphospholipid antibody syndrome [36]. Cerebrospinal fluid findings of patients with COVID-19 indicated autoimmunity [37]. Autoantibodies against type I IFNs in cases of serious COVID-19 were reported [38]. Autoimmune diseases following SARS-CoV-2 infections include antineutrophil cytoplasmic antibodies-associated vasculitis [39]. Further, the possible involvement of autoimmunity in COVID-19 [40–45] leads to suggestions on the related therapeutic approaches [46–48].

In terms of autoimmunity with the involvement of molecular mimicry, even an early hypothesis mentioned molecular mimicry as a mechanism that could act through e.g., overexpression of the antistress proteins and the development of an immune response to those self-proteins due to similarities between them and the SARS-CoV-2 proteins [49]. Other than that, Kanduc and Shoenfeld [50–52] studied molecular mimicry in COVID-19 pathogenesis. They pointed at the autoimmune reaction risk due to shared peptides, highlighted the importance of developing vaccines with peptides specific to the virus, and possible distinct outcomes of testing vaccines under development on animals, compared to testing them on humans. Indeed, several authors have published studies involving the severity of COVID-19 and molecular mimicry as a possible mechanism of autoimmunity upon SARS-CoV-2 infection [53–60]. Molecular mimicry map of SARS-CoV-2 is present [61], and earlier studies [62] served as the basis for listing autoimmune-associated MHC class I and class II alleles [61,63–67].

Neutrophil extracellular traps (NETs) increase thrombosis in the case of autoimmune diseases [68]. Several studies (e.g. Refs. [69–76]) focused on anti-neutrophil cytoplasmic antibodies. NETs exist also in the pathogenesis of COVID-19 [67,77–79]. NET granules can be early markers of post-COVID syndrome [80]. Blood myeloperoxidase-DNA, a serum marker of circulating NETs, is a potential biomarker of early response to SARS-CoV-2 infection [81], and elastase and augmented innate immunity are involved in multi-visceral manifestations of

SARS-CoV-2 [82]. Inhibition of NETs' formation can be a possible means of treatment, considering the devastating effects of NETs in COVID-19 [67,77–79,82–84]. In relation, we looked for a possible molecular mimicry between peptides of SARS-CoV-2 and the NETs-associated 148 proteins, which were reported to be significantly expressed in NETs induced in neutrophils derived from the blood supernatant samples of patients with systemic lupus erythematosus (SLE) and lupus nephritis (LN) [85]. Peptides of SARS-CoV-2 both similar to one of those human proteins and have affinities to the same HLA supertype representatives as those binding strongly to their similar human peptides, can be a potential risk factor for NETs-related autoimmune disease pathogenicity, based on molecular mimicry, in susceptible individuals infected with SARS-CoV-2.

Materials and methods

Blastp searches

Selected NETs related proteins included 148 proteins, which were reported [85] to be significantly expressed in 'ex-vivo' induced NETs composition in cell suspensions obtained from granulocyte-rich blood supernatants of patients with SLE and LN. Protein (s1) sequences with single-letter amino acid codes were obtained from UniProt [86] and NCBI [87] in fasta format (s2). Blastp [88] searches were performed at NCBI. For blastp searches, parameters (algorithm-options) were as follows: Max target sequences 250; no automatic adjustment for short sequences; expect threshold 29,000; word size two; max matches in a query range 0; matrix either pam 30 or pam 70; gap costs 9.1, 7.2, and 14.2, separately, for pam30 matrix, and 10.1, 8.2, and 11.2, separately, for pam70 matrix; and no filter or masking. Searches were limited to SARS-CoV-2 (taxid:2697049). The resulting alignment text files (s3–s14) of input sequences were analyzed using MS Office Excel. Alignment results with less than 50% identity and redundant results were eliminated, and one sequence ID of each aligned subject sequence was retained (s15, s16). A pivot table was generated (s17) to make an input list of query and subject sequences for predicting binding strengths to HLA supertype representatives. Associated queries and subjects with less than eight amino acids were excluded from the input list.

HLA binding predictions

The input list for HLA-binding prediction was in fasta format (s18), with alphanumeric codes as input sequence names. The purpose of the predictions was to determine query-subject pairs with strong binding affinities to the same HLA alleles within the HLA supertype representatives (HLA-A*01:01, HLA-A*02:01, HLA-A*03:01, HLA-A*24:02, HLA-A*26:01, HLA-B*07:02, HLA-B*08:01, HLA-B*15:01, HLA-B*27:05, HLA-B*39:01, HLA-B*40:01, HLA-B*58:01). NetMHCcons and NetCTLpan were the prediction tools. NetMHCcons v1.1 [89] predicts HLA affinities. It integrates NetMHC v4.0 [90,91], PickPocket v1.1 [92], and NetMHCpan v4.1 [93]. NetCTLpan (v1.1 [94] and v1.2 [95]) predicts epitopes of cytotoxic T lymphocytes. Predictions were performed using all peptide lengths and the default parameters for the remaining options (s19–s23). Strong binding (SB) predictions by NetMHCcons and epitope predictions by NetCTLpan were deemed significant. Epitope pairs with less than five matching amino acids or less than 50% identity were eliminated.

Proteins' features and network images

Features of the identified proteins with predicted epitope pairs were summarized using NCBI Entrez [96], UniProtKB/Swiss Prot [86], MalaCards [97,98], and SuperPathways [99], obtained through GeneCards [100]. Network images were prepared with the MalaCards diseases and the SuperPathways information, using Cytoscape [101] version 3.8.2 running with Java 11.0.6.

Results and discussion

Table 9.1 presents the results of the HLA-binding predictions following the blastp searches of 148 proteins. The first human protein in Table 9.1, antigen KI-67 [85] appears in the files as UPI0002065088 (due to the obsolete entry of the protein.)

Table 9.1 is an extensive list displaying potential epitope pairs sourced from selected human proteins and SARS-CoV-2. That list is inspected for the number of unique query epitopes, subject epitopes, human proteins, and their length percentages associated with each HLA (Fig. 9.1). Fig. 9.2 presents similar analysis results for the number of unique HLAs, query epitopes, and subject epitopes, associated with each human protein. The term unique refers to the presence of any difference. Therefore, overlapping query or subject sequences are included. Interactions of the overlapping sequences with the HLA alleles can differ. Query and subject (epitopes) mentioned in the remaining discussion are unique sequences and can include overlaps.

Fig. 9.1 reveals that HLA-A*24:02 is predicted to bind strongly to a relatively high number of subject sequences, while the number of associated human proteins and queries is low. This discrepancy is because the SARS-CoV-2 envelope protein's several slightly varying sequences of the same part remain SB. Accordingly, Fig. 9.2 shows that part (MYSYVTEELPQLI) of S-formylglutathione hydrolase reveals an association with the highest number of (i.e., 8) unique subject sequences (MYSFVSEEIGTLI, MYSFVSEETGALI, MYSFVSEETGMLI, MYSFVSEETGTLI, MYSFVSEETGTLL, MYSFVSEETSTLI, MYSFVSEETVTLI, MYSFVTEETGTLI). It may be indicative of a pertaining pathology despite viral evolution.

Fig. 9.1 also demonstrates that HLA-A*02:01 is predicted to bind strongly to a relatively higher number of queries and subjects, while the associated human protein is rather less. This observation is related to the presence of more queries in a comparatively lower number of inspected human proteins, which is due to including overlapping sequences. This is the case especially for the cysteine-rich secretory protein 3 (Fig. 9.2), as the main source of this observation (Fig. 9.1) with six overlapped epitope pairs having affinity to HLA-A*02:01 (Table 9.1). It can make HLA-A*02:01 serotypes more vulnerable due to epitopes sourced by cysteine-rich secretory protein 3, upon infection with SARS-CoV-2. This interpretation is based on a higher likelihood of ending up in peptides with affinities to a certain allele after proteasomal degradation when overlapping sequences retain affinity to the allele. In relation, cysteine-rich secretory protein 3 revealed the highest fold-change with decreased protein levels in COVID-19 patients [65].

Total human protein length percentages are also presented in Fig. 9.1. That value is expected to be correlated with the number of human protein query sequences. Consequently, observations are more than expected in the case of HLA-A*01:01, HLA-A*02:01, and HLA-

TABLE 9.1 SARS-CoV-2 proteins that align with 36 proteins significantly expressed in NETs induced in samples of SLE and LN, and with peptides SB to the same HLA allele and/or as epitope (E) of the same HLA allele. These epitope pairs have at least five matching amino acids and 50% identity.

Length of human protein	Human protein	Query (sourced by human protein)	Subject (sourced by SARS-CoV-2 protein)	SARS-CoV-2 protein	Allele	Tool
3255	UPI0002065088	SEETNTEIVECIL	SEETGTLIVNSVL	Envelope protein, partial	HLA-B*40:01	NetMHCcons
360	Ficolin-1	MFLNMFTL	FLAMITLA	ORF7a protein, partial	HLA-A*02:01	NetCTLpan
		FLHIKNLPA	FLHVNYVPA	Surface glycoprotein	HLA-A*02:01	NetCTLpan
		RRMDGSVDFY	GRVDGRVDLF	ORF1ab polyprotein	HLA-B*27:05	NetCTLpan
		IMFLNMFTL	ILFLAMITL	ORF7a protein, partial	HLA-A*02:01	NetMHCcons
		RRMDGSVDF	RVDGQVDLF	ORF1ab polyprotein	HLA-A*01:01	NetCTLpan
		RRMDGSVDF	SRVDGQVDL	ORF1ab polyprotein	HLA-B*39:01	NetCTLpan
416	Protocadherin-15	ALAFIIILCCIPAI	FLAFVVFLLVILAI	Envelope protein	HLA-A*02:01	NetMHCcons
		IPAILVVL	ILAILTAL	Envelope protein	HLA-A*02:01	NetCTLpan
		ALLALAFIIIL	LLFLAFVVFLL	Envelope protein	HLA-A*02:01	NetCTLpan
		ALLALAFIIIL	LLSLAFVVFLL	Envelope protein	HLA-A*02:01	NetCTLpan
158	High mobility group protein B1	KMSSYAFF	KMSSYSLF	ORF1ab polyprotein	HLA-A*24:02	NetCTLpan

(Continued)

TABLE 9.1 SARS-CoV-2 proteins that align with 36 proteins significantly expressed in NETs induced in samples of SLE and LN, and with peptides SB to the same HLA allele and/or as epitope (E) of the same HLA allele. These epitope pairs have at least five matching amino acids and 50% identity.—cont'd

Length of human protein	Human protein	Query (sourced by human protein)	Subject (sourced by SARS-CoV-2 protein)	SARS-CoV-2 protein	Allele	Tool
		KMSSYAFF	KMSSYSLF	ORF1ab polyprotein	HLA-B*15:01	NetCTLpan/ NetMHCcons
		KMSSYAFF	KMSSYSLF	ORF1ab polyprotein	HLA-B*58:01	NetCTLpan
54	AF4/FMR2 family member 3 (fragment)	ILNQRNDSL	ILKQANNSL	ORF1ab polyprotein, partial	HLA-B*08:01	NetCTLpan
134	High mobility group protein B2 (fragment)	KMSSYAFF	KMSSYSLF	ORF1ab polyprotein	HLA-A*24:02	NetCTLpan
		KMSSYAFF	KMSSYSLF	ORF1ab polyprotein	HLA-B*15:01	NetCTLpan/ NetMHCcons
307	Helix-destabilizing protein	ATVEEVDAAM	DTVEEVLSEA	ORF1ab polyprotein	HLA-A*26:01	NetCTLpan
1551	Protein-tyrosine-phosphatase (fragment)	ERLKPYVAAQL	ERLKPFAAETL	ORF1ab polyprotein, partial	HLA-B*39:01	NetCTLpan
		IVIAILLF	IVNSVLLF	Envelope protein, partial	HLA-B*58:01	NetCTLpan
		ERLKPYVAAQL	RLKPFAAETLK	ORF1ab polyprotein, partial	HLA-A*03:01	NetCTLpan
1059	E3 ubiquitin-protein ligase MYCBP2 (fragment)	RWLGPRITF	HRNAPRITF	Nucleocapsid phosphoprotein, partial	HLA-B*27:05	NetCTLpan
		NRWLGPRITF	NQRNAPRITF	Nucleocapsid phosphoprotein, partial	HLA-B*15:01	NetCTLpan

		NRWLGPRITF	NQRNGPRITF	Nucleocapsid phosphoprotein, partial	HLA-B*15:01	NetCTLpan
		RWLGPRITF	QRNAPRITF	Nucleocapsid phosphoprotein, partial	HLA-B*27:05	NetCTLpan
		RWLGPRITF	QRNGPRITF	Nucleocapsid phosphoprotein, partial	HLA-B*27:05	NetCTLpan
285	Tropomyosin alpha-3 chain	EEIKILTDKL	EEIKFLTENL	ORF1a polyprotein	HLA-B*40:01	NetCTLpan
276	Cysteine-rich secretory protein 3	FPAMTLFPVLL	FLAFLLFPVLI	ORF7b	HLA-A*02:01	NetCTLpan
		AMTLFPVLLFLV	FLAFLLFPVLIM	ORF7b	HLA-A*02:01	NetMHCcons
		FPAMTLFPVL	FLLFPVLIML	ORF7b	HLA-A*02:01	NetCTLpan
		TLFPVLLFLV	FLLFPVLIML	ORF7b	HLA-A*02:01	NetMHCcons
		MTLFPVLLF	LFPVLIMLI	ORF7b	HLA-A*24:02	NetCTLpan
		MTLFPVLLF	LLFPVLIML	ORF7b	HLA-A*02:01	NetCTLpan
		FPAMTLFPVL	LLFPVLIMLI	ORF7b	HLA-A*02:01	NetCTLpan
		TLFPVLLFLV	LLFPVLIMLI	ORF7b	HLA-A*02:01	NetMHCcons
89	Barrier-to-autointegration factor	HRDFVAEPM	HTDFSSEIM	ORF1a polyprotein	HLA-A*01:01	NetCTLpan
98	Cystatin-B	LTLSNYQTNK	KRHTFSNYQH	ORF1ab polyprotein	HLA-B*27:05	NetCTLpan

(Continued)

TABLE 9.1 SARS-CoV-2 proteins that align with 36 proteins significantly expressed in NETs induced in samples of SLE and LN, and with peptides SB to the same HLA allele and/or as epitope (E) of the same HLA allele. These epitope pairs have at least five matching amino acids and 50% identity.—cont'd

Length of human protein	Human protein	Query (sourced by human protein)	Subject (sourced by SARS-CoV-2 protein)	SARS-CoV-2 protein	Allele	Tool
650	Isoform H14 of myeloperoxidase	LTSFVDASMVY	HTQFVDMSMTY	ORF1ab polyprotein	HLA-A*01:01	NetCTLpan/ NetMHCcons
		LTSFVDASMVY	HTQFVDMSMTY	ORF1ab polyprotein	HLA-A*26:01	NetCTLpan
		LTSFVDASMVY	HTQFVDMSMTY	ORF1ab polyprotein	HLA-B*58:01	NetCTLpan
		LTSFVDASMVY	NLHTQFVDMSM	ORF1ab polyprotein	HLA-B*08:01	NetCTLpan
		TSFVDASMVY	TQFVDMSMTY	ORF1ab polyprotein	HLA-B*15:01	NetCTLpan
87	Acyl-CoA-binding protein	GTSKEDAMKAY	GTSSGDATTAY	ORF1ab polyprotein(, partial)	HLA-A*01:01	NetCTLpan/ NetMHCcons
		GTSKEDAMKAY	GTSSGDATTAY	ORF1ab polyprotein(, partial)	HLA-A*26:01	NetCTLpan
		GTSKEDAMKAY	GTSSGDATTAY	ORF1ab polyprotein(, partial)	HLA-B*15:01	NetCTLpan
1085	Isoform 2 of Thrombospondin-1	LELRGLRTI	RELRTIKVF	ORF1a polyprotein	HLA-B*40:01	NetCTLpan
		LELRGLRTI	SLRELRTIK	ORF1a polyprotein	HLA-A*03:01	NetCTLpan
		LELRGLRTIV	SLRELRTIKV	ORF1a polyprotein	HLA-B*08:01	NetCTLpan
		LELRGLRTI	SLRGVRTIK	ORF1a polyprotein	HLA-A*03:01	NetCTLpan

267	Neutrophil elastase	LGRNRGIASVL	AMRNAGIAGVL	ORF1ab polyprotein	HLA-B*07:02	NetCTLpan
		GRNRGIASVL	MRNAGIAGVL	ORF1ab polyprotein	HLA-B*27:05	NetCTLpan
		GRNRGIASVL	MRNAGIAGVL	ORF1ab polyprotein	HLA-B*39:01	NetCTLpan
255	Cathepsin G	NRNVNPVAL	IRSVYPVAL	ORF1ab polyprotein	HLA-B*27:05	NetCTLpan
		NRNVNPVAL	IRSVYPVAL	ORF1ab polyprotein	HLA-B*39:01	NetCTLpan/NetMHCcons
		RNRNVNPVAL	RIRSVYPVAL	ORF1ab polyprotein	HLA-B*07:02	NetCTLpan
		RNRNVNPVAL	RIRSVYPVAL	ORF1ab polyprotein	HLA-B*08:01	NetCTLpan
282	S-formylglutathione hydrolase	MYSYVTEELPQLI	MYSFVSEEIGTLI	Envelope protein	HLA-A*24:02	NetMHCcons
		MYSYVTEELPQLI	MYSFVSEETGALI	Envelope protein	HLA-A*24:02	NetMHCcons
		MYSYVTEELPQLI	MYSFVSEETGMLI	Envelope protein	HLA-A*24:02	NetMHCcons
		MYSYVTEELPQLI	MYSFVSEETGTLI	Envelope protein	HLA-A*24:02	NetMHCcons
		MYSYVTEELPQLI	MYSFVSEETGTLL	Envelope protein	HLA-A*24:02	NetMHCcons
		MYSYVTEELPQLI	MYSFVSEETSTLI	Envelope protein	HLA-A*24:02	NetMHCcons
		MYSYVTEELPQLI	MYSFVSEETVTLI	Envelope protein	HLA-A*24:02	NetMHCcons
		MYSYVTEELPQLI	MYSFVTEETGTLI	Envelope protein	HLA-A*24:02	NetMHCcons

(Continued)

TABLE 9.1 SARS-CoV-2 proteins that align with 36 proteins significantly expressed in NETs induced in samples of SLE and LN, and with peptides SB to the same HLA allele and/or as epitope (E) of the same HLA allele. These epitope pairs have at least five matching amino acids and 50% identity.—cont'd

Length of human protein	Human protein	Query (sourced by human protein)	Subject (sourced by SARS-CoV-2 protein)	SARS-CoV-2 protein	Allele	Tool
715	Eosinophil peroxidase	LTSFVDASMVY	HTQFVDMSMTY	ORF1a polyprotein	HLA-A*01:01	NetCTLpan/ NetMHCcons
		LTSFVDASMVY	HTQFVDMSMTY	ORF1a polyprotein	HLA-A*26:01	NetCTLpan
		LTSFVDASMVY	HTQFVDMSMTY	ORF1a polyprotein	HLA-B*58:01	NetCTLpan
		LTSFVDASMVY	NLHTQFVDMSM	ORF1a polyprotein	HLA-B*08:01	NetCTLpan
		FVDASMVY	TQFVDMSM	ORF1a polyprotein	HLA-B*39:01	NetCTLpan
		TSFVDASMVY	TQFVDMSMTY	ORF1a polyprotein	HLA-B*15:01	NetCTLpan
967	Aminopeptidase N	FAYQNTIY	FAFPFTIY	ORF10 protein, partial	HLA-B*15:01	NetCTLpan
		FAYQNTIY	FAFPFTIY	ORF10 protein, partial	HLA-B*58:01	NetCTLpan
		HTFAYQNTIY	NVFAFPFTIY	ORF10 protein, partial	HLA-A*01:01	NetCTLpan
		HTFAYQNTIY	NVFAFPFTIY	ORF10 protein, partial	HLA-A*26:01	NetCTLpan
586	Lamin-B1	KIGDTSVSY	KIGDKSVYY	ORF1a polyprotein	HLA-A*03:01	NetCTLpan
187	Phosphatidylethanolamine-binding protein 1	DISSGTVLSDY	DIAANTVLWDY	ORF1ab polyprotein, partial	HLA-A*01:01	NetCTLpan

		DISSGTVLSDY	DIAANTVLWDY	ORF1ab polyprotein, partial	HLA-A*26:01	NetCTLpan/NetMHCcons
		DISSGTVLSDY	DIASNTVIWDY	ORF1ab polyprotein	HLA-A*01:01	NetCTLpan
		DISSGTVLSDY	DIASNTVIWDY	ORF1ab polyprotein	HLA-A*26:01	NetCTLpan/NetMHCcons
		DISSGTVLSDY	DISANTVIWDY	ORF1ab polyprotein	HLA-A*26:01	NetCTLpan/NetMHCcons
		ISSGTVLSDY	IAANTVLWDY	ORF1ab polyprotein	HLA-B*58:01	NetCTLpan
		ISSGTVLSDY	IASNTVIWDY	ORF1ab polyprotein	HLA-B*58:01	NetCTLpan
		ISSGTVLSDY	ISANTVIWDY	ORF1ab polyprotein	HLA-A*01:01	NetCTLpan/NetMHCcons
		ISSGTVLSDY	ISANTVIWDY	ORF1ab polyprotein	HLA-B*58:01	NetCTLpan
1960	Myosin-9	VELDNVTGL	LQAENVTGL	ORF1ab polyprotein	HLA-A*02:01	NetCTLpan
		VELDNVTGL	LQAENVTGL	ORF1ab polyprotein	HLA-B*39:01	NetCTLpan
		VELDNVTGL	LQVENVTGL	ORF1ab polyprotein	HLA-B*39:01	NetCTLpan
199	Transgelin-2	GTNRGASQAGMTGY	GSSRGTSPARMAGY	Nucleocapsid phosphoprotein, partial	HLA-A*01:01	NetMHCcons
		ASQAGMTGY	TSPARMAGY	Nucleocapsid phosphoprotein, partial	HLA-A*26:01	NetCTLpan

(Continued)

TABLE 9.1 SARS-CoV-2 proteins that align with 36 proteins significantly expressed in NETs induced in samples of SLE and LN, and with peptides SB to the same HLA allele and/or as epitope (E) of the same HLA allele. These epitope pairs have at least five matching amino acids and 50% identity.—cont'd

Length of human protein	Human protein	Query (sourced by human protein)	Subject (sourced by SARS-CoV-2 protein)	SARS-CoV-2 protein	Allele	Tool
380	Vasodilator-stimulated phosphoprotein	FRVVGRKM	FRVIGHSM	ORF1a polyprotein	HLA-B*27:05	NetCTLpan
		FRVVGRKM	FRVIGHSM	ORF1a polyprotein	HLA-B*39:01	NetCTLpan
127	Nuclear transport factor 2	IYIDASCL	AYIDNSSL	ORF1a polyprotein	HLA-A*24:02	NetCTLpan
		RTQLGAIY	RTDLMAAY	ORF1ab polyprotein	HLA-A*01:01	NetCTLpan/ NetMHCcons
		RTQLGAIY	RTDLMAAY	ORF1ab polyprotein	HLA-B*58:01	NetCTLpan
103	Histone H4	TVTAMDVVY	TVTSTDVVY	ORF1ab polyprotein	HLA-A*01:01	NetCTLpan
		TVTAMDVVY	TVTSTDVVY	ORF1ab polyprotein	HLA-A*26:01	NetCTLpan
		VTAMDVVY	VTSTDVVY	ORF1ab polyprotein	HLA-B*58:01	NetCTLpan
241	Glutathione S-transferase omega-1	IWPWFERL	KWPWFIWL	Surface glycoprotein	HLA-A*24:02	NetCTLpan
		IWPWFERL	KWPWYIRL	Surface glycoprotein	HLA-A*24:02	NetCTLpan
		YLIWPWFERL	YIKWPWFIWL	Surface glycoprotein	HLA-B*08:01	NetCTLpan
		YLIWPWFERL	YIKWPWYIRL	Surface glycoprotein	HLA-B*08:01	NetCTLpan

		YLIWPWFERL	YIKWPWYNWL	Surface glycoprotein	HLA-B*08:01	NetCTLpan
		YLIWPWFERL	YIKWPWYSWL	Surface glycoprotein	HLA-B*08:01	NetCTLpan
		YLIWPWFERL	YMKWPWYIWL	Surface glycoprotein	HLA-A*02:01	NetCTLpan
		YLIWPWFERL	YMKWPWYIWL	Surface glycoprotein	HLA-B*08:01	NetCTLpan
911	NF-X1-type zinc finger protein NFXL1	DEVAVELSL	DEVAIDLSL	ORF1ab polyprotein	HLA-B*40:01	NetCTLpan
		EVAVELSL	EVAIDLSL	ORF1ab polyprotein	HLA-A*26:01	NetCTLpan
341	DnaJ homolog subfamily C member 22	ISLSSMVNFY	ASISAMVRMY	ORF1a polyprotein	HLA-A*01:01	NetCTLpan
		ISLSSMVNFY	ASISAMVRMY	ORF1a polyprotein	HLA-B*15:01	NetCTLpan
		LSSMVNFYI	ISAMVRMYI	ORF1a polyprotein	HLA-B*58:01	NetCTLpan/ NetMHCcons
		LSSMVNFY	LSAMVRMY	ORF1ab polyprotein	HLA-A*01:01	NetMHCcons
4596	Dynein axonemal heavy chain 5	EVSPLATSL	EVTPLGTWL	Nucleocapsid phosphoprotein	HLA-A*26:01	NetCTLpan
		LEVSPLATSL	MEVTPLGTWL	Nucleocapsid phosphoprotein	HLA-B*40:01	NetMHCcons
		MAQMGLEVSPL	MSRIGMEVTPL	Nucleocapsid phosphoprotein	HLA-B*07:02	NetCTLpan
		MAQMGLEVSPL	MSRIGMEVTPL	Nucleocapsid phosphoprotein	HLA-B*08:01	NetCTLpan
		AQMGLEVSPL	SRIGMEVTPL	Nucleocapsid phosphoprotein	HLA-B*27:05	NetCTLpan
		AQMGLEVSPL	SRIGMEVTPL	Nucleocapsid phosphoprotein	HLA-B*39:01	NetCTLpan/ NetMHCcons

(Continued)

TABLE 9.1 SARS-CoV-2 proteins that align with 36 proteins significantly expressed in NETs induced in samples of SLE and LN, and with peptides SB to the same HLA allele and/or as epitope (E) of the same HLA allele. These epitope pairs have at least five matching amino acids and 50% identity.—cont'd

Length of human protein	Human protein	Query (sourced by human protein)	Subject (sourced by SARS-CoV-2 protein)	SARS-CoV-2 protein	Allele	Tool
1722	Isoform 4 of kinesin-like protein KIF20B	SIKFSVWVSF	ISAGFSLWVY	ORF1ab polyprotein	HLA-A*01:01	NetCTLpan
		SIKFSVWVSF	ISAGFSLWVY	ORF1ab polyprotein	HLA-A*26:01	NetCTLpan
		SIKFSVWVSF	ISAGFSLWVY	ORF1ab polyprotein	HLA-B*15:01	NetCTLpan/ NetMHCcons
		SIKFSVWVSF	ISAGFSLWVY	ORF1ab polyprotein	HLA-B*58:01	NetCTLpan
		SIKFSVWVSF	MISAGFSLWV	ORF1ab polyprotein	HLA-A*02:01	NetCTLpan
		MANSIKFSVW	MMISAGFSLW	ORF1ab polyprotein	HLA-B*58:01	NetMHCcons
		NMANSIKFSVWV	NMMISAGFSLWV	ORF1ab polyprotein	HLA-A*02:01	NetMHCcons
1451	Isoform 6 of membrane-associated guanylate kinase, WW, and PDZ domain-containing protein 1	FLKRGDGSV	FLKRGDKSV	ORF1a polyprotein	HLA-B*08:01	NetCTLpan
		GVVSTVVQPY	VVSPVMEPIY	ORF3a protein	HLA-A*01:01	NetCTLpan
2541	Talin-1	FTLDFGDY	FTLEKGIY	Surface glycoprotein(, partial)	HLA-A*26:01	NetMHCcons
		KSFTLDFGDYQDGYY	KSFTLEKGIYQTSNF	Surface glycoprotein(, partial)	HLA-B*58:01	NetMHCcons

		KSFTLDFGDY	KSFTVEKGIY	Surface glycoprotein(, partial)	HLA-B*58:01	NetCTLpan
5142	Protein piccolo	APVSTDNTF	LIITTDNTF	Surface glycoprotein	HLA-B*15:01	NetCTLpan
		APVSTDNTF	QMITTDNTF	Surface glycoprotein	HLA-B*15:01	NetCTLpan
		SSVATPTPSTF	TSIATPTNFTI	Surface glycoprotein	HLA-B*58:01	NetCTLpan

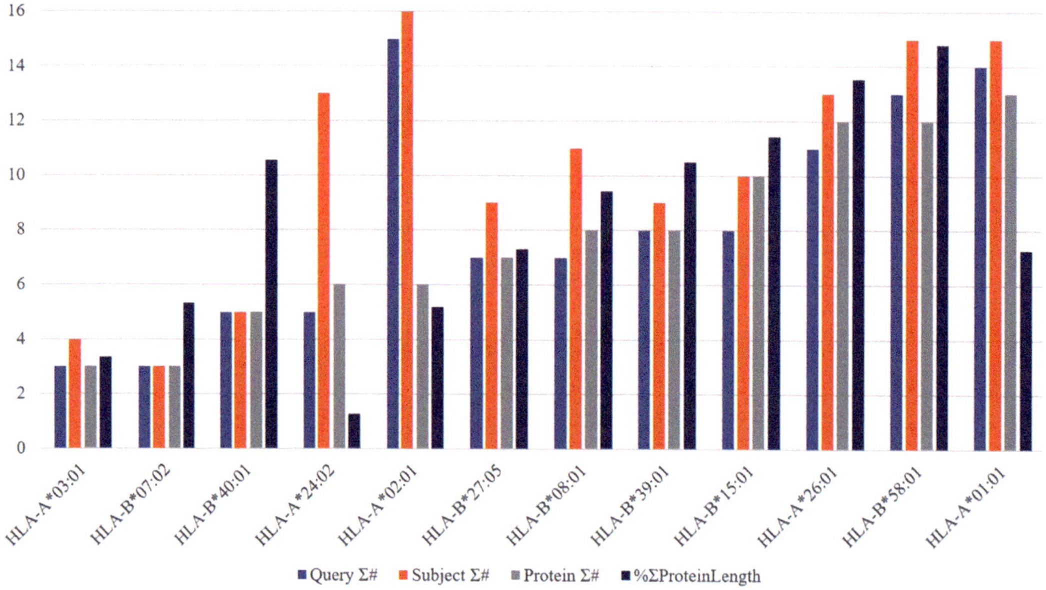

FIGURE 9.1 Numbers of unique query epitopes, subject epitopes, human proteins, and their length percentages, associated with each HLA. (Displayed according to the increasing number of human proteins.)

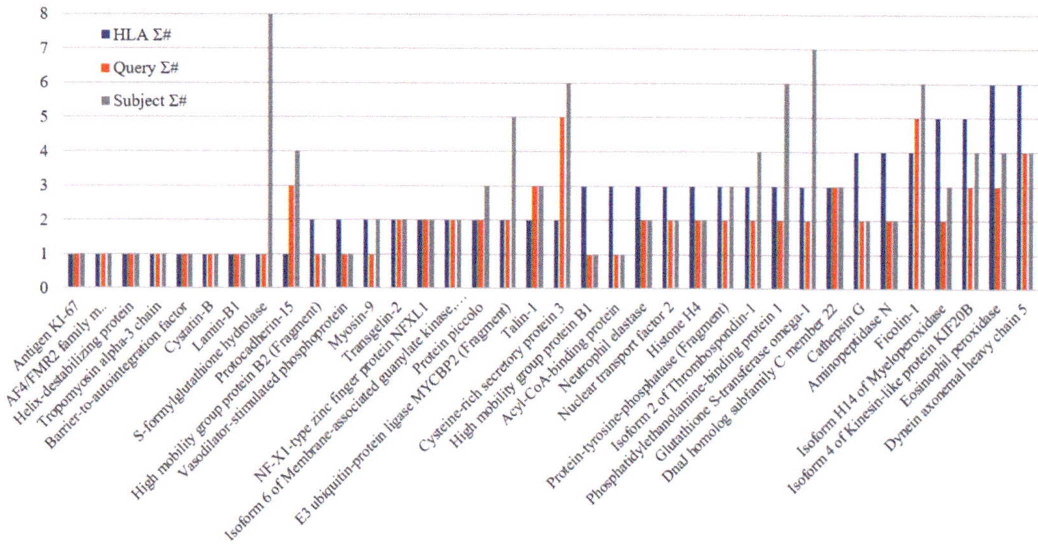

FIGURE 9.2 Numbers of unique HLA alleles, query epitopes, and subject epitopes, associated with each human protein. (Displayed according to the increasing number of HLA alleles. Antigen KI-67: UPI0002065088.)

A*24:02, while they are less than expected in the case of HLA-B*40:01 and HLA-B*07:02. According to Fig. 9.2, as mentioned, part of S-formylglutathione hydrolase reveals an association with the highest number of subjects. It was among the downregulated xenobiotic metabolism-PXR signaling pathway-related enzymes in the liver of patients with COVID-19 [102,103]. Further, parts of cysteine-rich secretory protein 3 and ficolin-1 reveal associations with the highest numbers of queries. Cysteine-rich secretory protein 3 is already mentioned. Ficolin-1 associates with the highest number of (i.e., 3) different SARS-CoV-2 proteins (Fig. 9.3), and its associated pathway, i.e., the lectin pathway, is activated intensely in COVID-19 [104]. Fig. 9.2 further reveals that eosinophil peroxidase and dynein axonemal heavy chain 5 are associated with the highest number of HLA alleles.

We also looked at the association of individual human proteins under investigation with each HLA allele (SI-Table 9.1), and of the individual HLA alleles with each human protein (SI-Table 9.2). Fig. 9.4 schematizes these associations. Fig. 9.4 and SI-Table 9.1 display that predictions reveal affinity of:

- HLA-A*01:01 to parts of thirteen proteins
- Both HLA-A*26:01 and HLA-B*58:01 to parts of twelve proteins
- HLA-B*15:01 to parts of ten proteins
- Both HLA-B*08:01 and HLA-B*39:01 to parts of eight proteins
- HLA-B*27:05 to parts of seven proteins
- Both HLA-A*02:01 and HLA-A*24:02 to parts of six proteins
- HLA-B*40:01 to parts of five proteins
- Both HLA-A*03:01 and HLA-B*07:02 to parts of three proteins

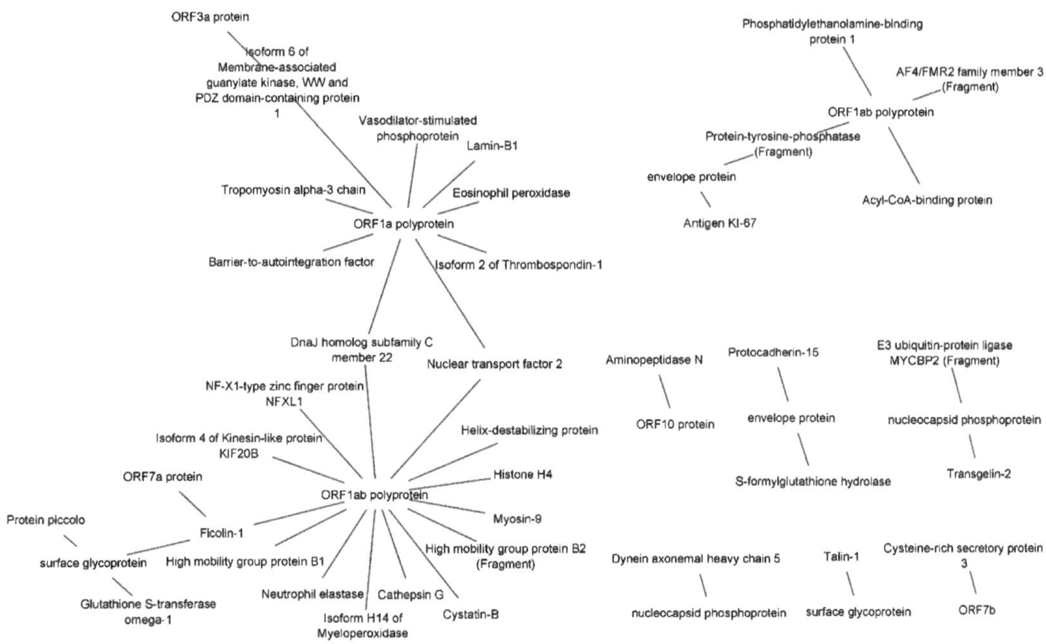

FIGURE 9.3 Associations between 36 human proteins identified here and the SARS-CoV-2 proteins. (Prepared using Cytoscape 3.8.2 running with Java 11.0.6. SARS-CoV-2 proteins are blue-colored.)

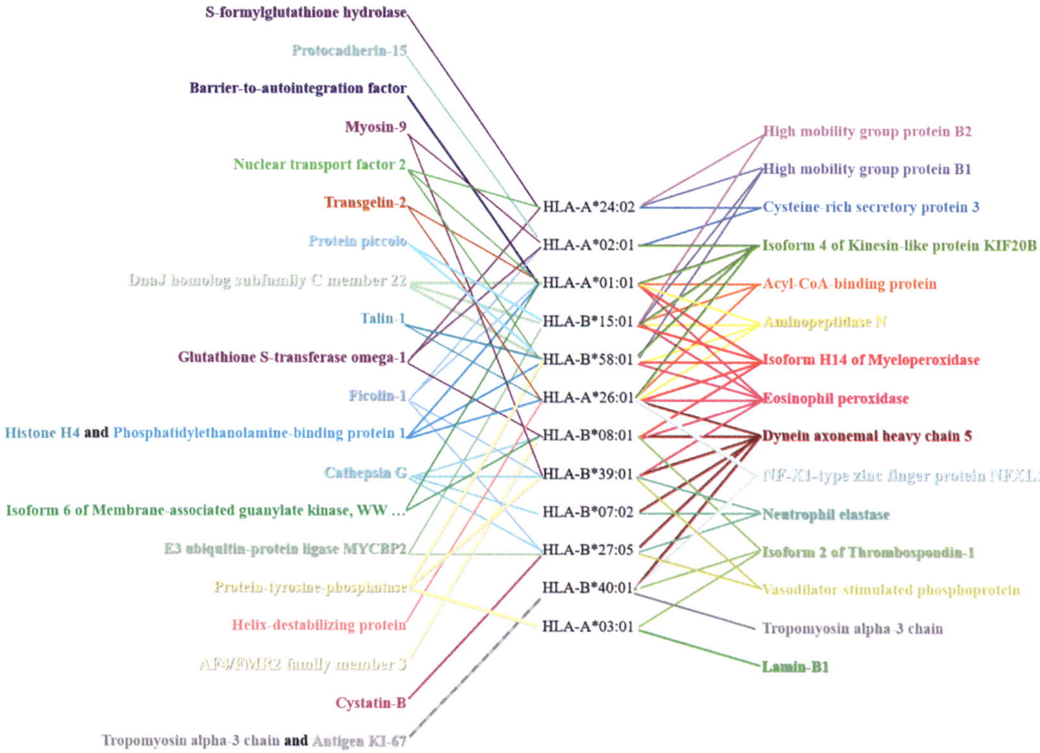

FIGURE 9.4 Associations between 36 human proteins and HLA alleles of interest. Human proteins and lines associating them with the HLA alleles are color-coded. Tropomyosin alpha-3 chain and antigen KI-67 are associated with the same proteins, such as the histone H4 and the phosphatidylethanoamine-binding protein.

Proteins associated with the highest number of different alleles

As mentioned, two proteins contain peptides SB to the highest number of different HLA supertype representatives. One of those two proteins is *eosinophil peroxidase*. Its peptides are SB to HLA-A*01:01, HLA-A*26:01, HLA-B*08:01, HLA-B*15:01, HLA-B*58:01, and HLA-B*39:01. Highest number of different proteins are SB to these alleles. Association per allele ranges from 8 to 13 different proteins, with an average of 10.5 ± 2.2. The remaining alleles revealed affinity to parts of 5.0 ± 1.7 different proteins on average, ranging from three to seven. Other proteins with predicted SB peptides to those six alleles are as follows:

- *Isoform H14 myeloperoxidase* peptides SB to all except HLA-B*39:01.
- *Aminopeptidase N* has peptides SB to all except HLA-B*08:01 and HLA-B*39:01.
- *Isoform 4 of Kinesin-like protein KIF20B* peptides SB to all except HLA-B*08:01 and HLA-B*39:01, and further has peptides SB to HLA-A*02:01, which is not among those six alleles.
- *Acyl-CoA-binding protein* peptides SB to HLA-A*01:01, HLA-A*26:01, and HLA-B*15:01.
- *DnaJ homolog subfamily C member 22* peptides SB to HLA-A*01:01, HLA-B*15:01, and HLA-B*58:01.

- *Histone H4* peptides SB to HLA-A*01:01, HLA-A*26:01, and HLA-B*58:01.
- *Phosphatidylethanolamine-binding protein 1* peptides SB to HLA-A*01:01, HLA-A*26:01, and HLA-B*58:01.
- *Dynein axonemal heavy chain 5* is the other protein with peptides SB to the highest number of different HLA supertype representatives. Among those, HLA-A*26:01, HLA-B*08:01, and HLA-B*39:01 are the alleles common to that of *eosinophil peroxidase,* and the remaining three alleles are HLA-B*07:02, HLA-B*27:05, and HLA-B*40:01.

A total number of seven proteins among 36 proteins have no peptides SB to those six alleles. These proteins are not SB to more than two different HLA supertype representatives. Their names and the associated alleles are *cystatin-B* (HLA-B*27:05), *cystein-rich secretory protein 3* (HLA-A*02:01 and HLA-A*24:02), *lamin-B1* (HLA-A*03:01), *protocadherin-15* (-HLA-A*02:01), *S-formylglutathione hydrolase* (HLA-A*24:02), *tropomyosin alpha-3 chain* (HLA-B*40:01), and *antigen KI-67* (HLA-B*40:01).

This study versus HLA association studies of disease severity

Note that the results of this study cannot be correlated directly with the HLA association studies of COVID-19 disease severity [8–11]. Those studies tend to explain the observed relations with differing binding propensities of the HLA alleles to the SARS-CoV-2 peptides, proportional to the protection. Here, this work aimed to identify potential alleles with affinities to the similar peptides of SARS-CoV-2 and NETs-proteins. These peptides are only a subset of HLA-binding SARS-CoV-2 peptides. An allele associated with severe disease would expectedly have a lower binding propensity to the SARS-CoV-2 peptides. Such an allele would be associated with a lower number of queries and subjects here as well. Therefore, HLA-A*03:01 and HLA-B*07:02 are associated with the smallest number of query and subject sequences (Fig. 9.1). In support, HLA-A*03:01 is a related risk factor [11] while HLA-B*07:02 is among the top HLA alleles associated with admission to the intensive care unit [9]. A similar interpretation is not necessarily valid for the HLA alleles binding to a higher number of SARS-CoV-2 peptides, considering the favorable effects of a higher immune response and the adverse effects of a possible autoimmune reaction. Among those, alleles with lower affinities to the SARS-CoV-2 peptide similar of the human peptides, or alleles with affinities to such human proteins with lower expression levels, or fewer criticalities, can be advantageous. In relation, host-pathogen evolution and pathogen coevolution could be working toward diminished autoimmune responses involving molecular mimicry [105].

General features of the identified proteins

- *Antigen KI-67* is a nuclear protein, associated with cellular proliferation.
- *Ficolin-1* recognizes sugar moieties of pathogen-associated molecular patterns on microbes, activating the complement system, the lectin pathway. It can also activate monocytes.
- *Protocadherin-15* is crucial to the maintenance of normal functioning of the retina and cochlea.

- *High mobility group protein B1* is a nonhistone, nuclear DNA-binding protein. Its immune-related roles involve promoting the host inflammatory response to sterile and infectious signals, involving in the coordination and integration of innate and adaptive immune responses, activating TLR9-mediated immune responses, mediating autophagy, acting as danger-associated molecular pattern molecules leading to elevated immune responses at tissue injury, and activating autoreactive B cells. Its disulfide form is released from apoptotic cells and promotes immunological tolerance. Inflammatory events including SLE involve higher serum levels of it. It is critical for the entry of human coronavirus NL63/HCoV-NL63, SARS-CoV, and SARS-CoV-2, and increase by SARS-CoV-2 infection.
- *AF4/FMR2 family member 3 (fragment)* is a tissue-restricted nuclear transcriptional activator and is preferentially expressed in lymphoid tissue.
- *High mobility group protein B2* is chromatin-associated and has immune-related functions like the high mobility group protein B1. It associates with rheumatoid arthritis.
- *Helix destabilizing protein* is among heterogeneous nuclear ribonucleoproteins. It can affect Hepatitis C virus RNA replication and possibly interacts with SARS-CoV nucleoprotein.
- *Protein-tyrosine-phosphatase* is a receptor-type signaling protein.
- *E3 ubiquitin-protein ligase MYCBP2* takes a role in nervous system development and regulates autophagy, and (cAMP and mTOR) signaling pathways.
- *Tropomyosin alpha-3 chain* is an actin-binding protein that stabilizes actin filaments. Other than several forms of myopathies, familial hemiplegic migraine, and different types of allergies are among 39 diseases associated with its gene, TPM3.
- *Cysteine-rich secretory protein 3* is present in the reproductive tracts, with different functions in males and females.
- *Barrier-to-autointegration factor* proteins protect retroviruses from intramolecular integration and endorse intermolecular integration into the host genome.
- *Cystatin* has *endopeptidase inhibitor activity.*
- *Isoform H14 of myeloperoxidase* is a heme protein. It is synthesized during myeloid differentiation; is a major component of neutrophil azurophilic granules; overexpressed in monocytes, neutrophils, and nasal epithelium. Several autoimmune diseases are among 192 diseases associated with its gene, MPO.
- *Acyl-CoA-binding protein* is a conserved protein that can bind to acyl-Coenzyme A esters; can also displace diazepam bound to the type A gamma-aminobutyric acid receptors at the brain synapses.
- *Isoform 2 of thrombospondin-1* is a glycoprotein mediating intercellular interactions and cellular interactions with the matrix; can bind heparin and calcium.
- *Neutrophil elastase* is a serine protease and can hydrolyze many proteins, other than elastin. Vasculitis, autoimmune vasculitis, SLE, rheumatoid arthritis, and several forms of neutropenia are among 99 diseases associated with its gene, ELANE.
- *Cathepsin* is a peptidase S1 protein family member and is an antimicrobial protein present in azurophil granules of neutrophilic polymorphonuclear leukocytes. It is overexpressed in neutrophils and nasal epithelium. Vasculitis, inflammatory bowel disease, SLE, rheumatoid arthritis, and immune deficiency disease are among 30 diseases for its gene, CTSG.

- *S-formylglutathione hydrolase* is a serine hydrolase.
- *Eosinophil peroxidase* is released at sites of parasitic infection or allergen stimulation. Besides asthma, several allergies are among 36 diseases associated with its gene, EPX.
- *Aminopeptidase N* is a membrane-bound zinc metalloprotease and takes part in the final digestion of peptides in the small intestine. It is a receptor for the HCoV-229E alphacoronavirus and other nonhuman coronaviruses, and probably involves cleavage of peptides bound to major histocompatibility complex class II molecules. Autoimmune disease is listed among 33 diseases associated with its gene, ANPEP.
- *Lamin-B1* is among two B-type lamin proteins and is a component of the nuclear lamina.
- *Phosphatidylethanolamine-binding protein 1* modulates multiple signaling pathways, and can be cleaved further into active peptides.
- *Myosin-9* is a nonmuscle myosin.
- *Transgelin-2* is like the transgelin protein. It is an early marker of differentiated smooth muscle and can bind to actin filaments.
- *Vasodilator-stimulated phosphoprotein* associates with the actin filament formation and regulates actin dynamics, including actin dynamics in platelets. Thrombosis is among 11 diseases associated with its gene, VASP.
- *Nuclear transport factor 2* is a cytosolic factor that facilitates *protein transport into the nucleus.*
- *Histone H14* is a basic nuclear protein and is required for nucleosome formation.
- *Glutathione S-transferase omega-1* is functioning in the xenobiotics' and carcinogens' metabolism.
- *NF-X1-type zinc finger protein NFXL1* has *DNA binding transcription factor activity* and *proximal promoter DNA-binding transcription repressor activity.*
- *DnaJ homolog subfamily C member 22* can bind to *unfolded proteins* and *chaperones.*
- *Dynein axonemal heavy chain 5* is part of the microtubule-associated motor protein complex, which generates force in the cilia.
- *Isoform 4 of kinesin-like protein KIF20B* is a plus-end-directed motor enzyme, needed for the completion of cytokinesis.
- *Isoform 6 of membrane-associated guanylate kinase, WW, and PDZ domain-containing protein 1* can take part in intercellular junctions as a scaffold protein.
- *Talin-1* is a cytoskeletal protein that can bind to actin. Combined (T and B cell) immunodeficiency is present among five diseases associated with its gene, TLN1.
- *Protein piccolo* is a presynaptic cytoskeletal matrix part, most of these proteins are DNA interacting proteins, structural proteins, actin-binding proteins, and proteinases, peptidases.

SARS-CoV-2 and COVID-19-related features of the identified proteins

In addition to the above summary, *cysteine-rich secretory protein 3* revealed the highest fold-change with decreased levels in COVID-19 patients [65]. In our study, it revealed associations with the highest numbers of query-epitopes, like *ficolin-1*, which is additionally related to the highest number of (i.e., 3) different SARS-CoV-2 proteins. *Ficolin-1* can be a therapeutic target for autoimmune diseases [106]. The lectin pathway, to which it belongs, is activated intensely in COVID-19 [104]. The lectin complement system can be linking SARS-CoV-2 with Kawasaki Disease [107]. Another protein, *high mobility group protein B2* is binding to the (rapidly spreading) G614 spike protein of SARS-CoV-2, compared to D614 spike protein of SARS-CoV-2 [108]. *Helix-destabilizing protein* (*heterogeneous nuclear ribonucleoprotein A1*) has an affinity to the nucleocapsid protein of SARS coronavirus [63]. Also, the gene encoding heterogeneous nuclear ribonucleoprotein A1 is mentioned under the intermediate genes linked to endothelial dysfunction and vascular remodeling, in integrated network analysis for identifying new genes associated with SARS-CoV-2 [64]. *Myeloperoxidase* is among the autoantigens increased in the bloods of patients with SARS-CoV-2 infection [66] and associated with NETs in COVID-19 [67]. The concentration of *neutrophil elastase* in blood was correlated with increased neutrophil stimulation in the case of COVID-19 [82]. *Cathepsin G* was significantly elevated in the lungs of SARS-CoV-2 infected macaques [83] and it was among the upregulated proteins in nasopharyngeal swabs of patients with COVID-19 [84]. As mentioned earlier, *S-formylglutathione hydrolase* is among the downregulated xenobiotic metabolism-PXR signaling pathway-related enzymes in the liver of patients with COVID-19 [102,103]. It revealed an association with the highest number of subject epitope sequences here. CD13, also known as *aminopeptidase N* or membrane alanyl aminopeptidase [109], is the receptor of α-coronavirus HCoV-229E [110]. It is significantly elevated in the serum samples of patients with COVID-19 compared to healthy controls [111]. Also, CD13 is overexpressed in patients with Parkinson's disease, and this association was suggested to be an explanation for their higher COVID-19 susceptibility [112]. Expression of CD13 increased in CD13low and CD10low immature neutrophils in the intensive care unit patients with COVID-19 [113]. *Eosinophil peroxidase* was higher in mice exposed to viral RNA, as an experimental model of COVID-19 [114]. This protein and *dynein axonemal heavy chain 5* are two proteins with peptides SB to the highest number of different HLA supertype representatives. The latter was listed among proteins with considerable similarity to immunogenic SARS-CoV-2 peptides [115]. Authors stated that the respective T cells should have been under negative selection, and aberrant immune responses in the form of immunopathology or autoimmunity in the future, may otherwise be the case.

Wang et al. [116–119] conducted a study revealing the autoantigenome from six cell lines (HFL1 human fetal lung fibroblasts, HS-Sultan B lymphoblasts, Wil2-NS B-lymphoblasts, A549 lung epithelial cells, Jurkat T-lymphoblasts, and HEp-2 fibroblasts) as the proteins with the propensity to become autoantigens upon SARS-CoV-2 infection. Eight of the identified proteins in our study are present there as well. Those proteins are

- *High mobility group protein B1* (in HFL1 cells [116,119])
- *Heterogeneous nuclear ribonucleoprotein A1* (in all except A549 cells [119])
- *Tropomyosin alpha-3 chain* (in all cell lines [119])
- *Thrombospondin-1* (in HFL1 cells [116,119])
- *Lamin-B1* (in HFL1 cells [116,119], Wil2-NS B-lymphoblasts, Jurkat T-lymphoblasts [119])
- *Myosin-9* (in all except HS-Sultan B lymphoblasts and Jurkat T-lymphoblasts [119])
- *Histone H4* (in all cell lines [119])
- *Talin-1* (in all except Jurkat T-lymphoblasts and HEp-2 fibroblasts [119])

A systematic analysis of the diseases associated with the 36 identified proteins and the SuperPathways involved by these 36 proteins is performed using the data, wherever available. There are many closely related diseases, which are considered distinct (Fig. 9.5, SI-Table 9.3). Antigen KI-67 associates with the highest number of diseases ([220], MalaCards/GeneCards), while it associates with three pathways (DNA damage, neuroscience, and primary focal segmental glomerulosclerosis). It also associates with one HLA allele (HLA-B*40:01) and these can infer that either the pathways or the HLA allele in question, or both, lead to a higher disease susceptibility when there are aberrations in these proteins and/or their expression levels.

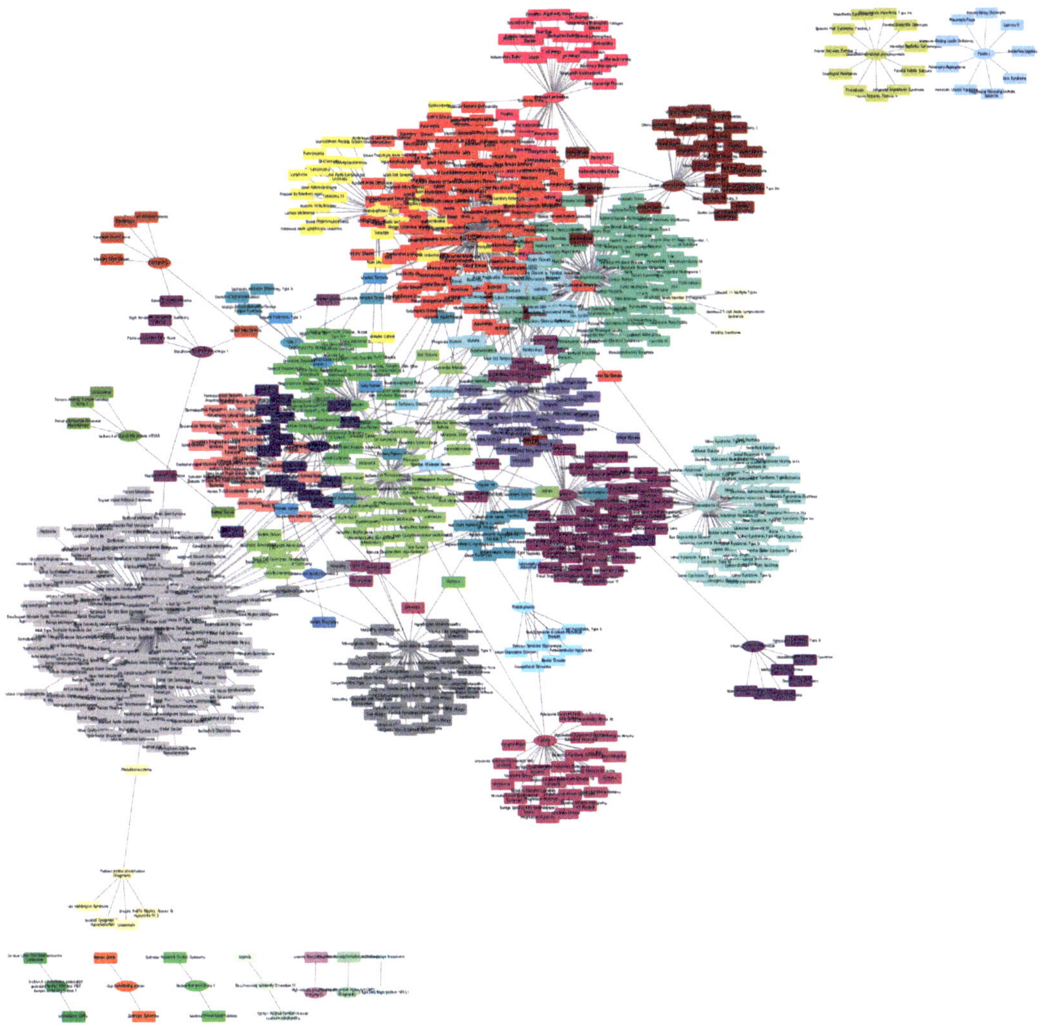

FIGURE 9.5 Associations between 36 human proteins identified here and diseases. Disease information is from MalaCards under GeneCards. (Prepared using Cytoscape 3.8.2 running with Java 11.0.6. Source nodes in oval shapes are human proteins. The image is color-coded.)

The disease associated with the highest number of proteins among 36 identified proteins is disease of the mental health (SI-Table 9.3). SuperPathway with the highest number of associated human proteins among the identified proteins is the innate immune system (SI-Table 9.4, Fig. 9.6). Yet, frequent representation of the well-studied proteins, diseases, and pathways can generate bias. Keeping this fact in mind, SuperPathways associated with the highest

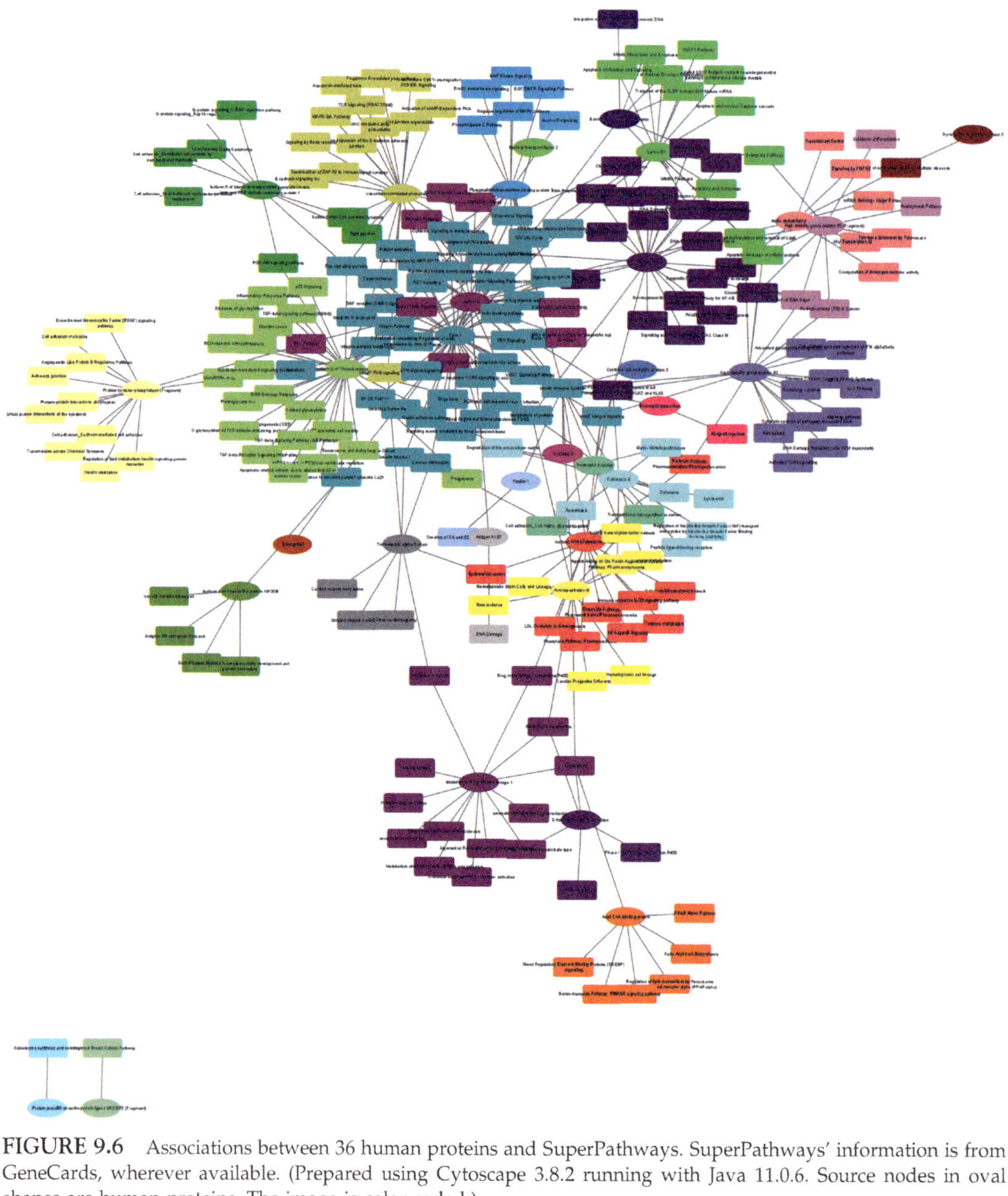

FIGURE 9.6 Associations between 36 human proteins and SuperPathways. SuperPathways' information is from GeneCards, wherever available. (Prepared using Cytoscape 3.8.2 running with Java 11.0.6. Source nodes in oval shapes are human proteins. The image is color-coded.)

number of proteins among the 32 proteins with SuperPathway information are innate immune system, activated PKN1 stimulates the transcription of androgen receptor-regulated genes KLK2 and KLK3 (*shortened as "activated PKN1 stimulated KLK2 and KLK3"*), and signaling by GPCR. Innate immune system associates with thirteen proteins and each of the other two SuperPathways associates with six proteins. The SuperPathways innate immune system and activated PKN1 stimulated KLK2 and KLK3 including neutrophil degranulation and NET formation. *Ficolin-1, cysteine-rich secretory protein 3, cystatin-B, eosinophil peroxidase, aminopeptidase N, high mobility group protein B1, isoform H14 of myeloperoxidase, neutrophil elastase,* and *cathepsin G* proteins associate with the innate immune system and include neutrophil degranulation among the contained pathways. The latter four proteins associate with the activated PKN1 stimulated KLK2 and KLK3 as well. Since they associate with two SuperPathways including neutrophil degranulation among the contained pathways, those four proteins can be suggested to have a stronger involvement in a possible NET pathology through molecular mimicry in susceptible individuals with COVID-19. Those proteins were mentioned while discussing SARS-CoV-2 and COVID-19-related features of the identified proteins. Possible susceptibility would be higher if a higher number of those proteins are predicted to have an affinity to the same HLA allele. Accordingly, *high mobility group protein B1* and *isoform H14 of myeloperoxidase* both associate with HLA-B*15:01, *isoform H14 of myeloperoxidase* and *cathepsin G* both associate with HLA-B*08:01, and *cathepsin G* and *neutrophil elastase* both associate with HLA-B*07:02, HLA-B*27:05, and HLA-B*39:01.

Things-to-improve

Amendments of this work can involve the following to derive additional information: Sequences with less than eight aa peptide-length could not be predicted. Their predictions can be performed by including a certain number of upstream and/or downstream amino acids of the respective sequences. This is done (Table 9.2) but the results are yet to be implemented in the present analysis. Those predictions revealed six new human and SARS-CoV-2 epitope pairs of the same HLA allele, wherein only one of those includes the same protein and allele combination as that in Table 9.1.

Searches, predictions, and following analysis can be improved by varying respective parameters, in addition to expanding the inputs. Most importantly, predictions for the other class I alleles, and class II alleles can be done. Accordingly, NetMHCII-2.3 [120] was applied to estimate the binding of peptides to autoimmunity-associated class II alleles [61,62] available at NetMHCII-2.3. Predictions were performed for similar peptides with 13−17 aa lengths and the results were obtained as epitopes with exclusively 13−17 aa lengths (Table 9.3). Those predictions revealed 14 new human and SARS-CoV-2 epitope pairs of the same class II allele, associated with autoimmune diseases, including systemic lupus erythematosus. Predictions for the other class I and class II alleles would lead to new results. Experimental, and clinical work must support these findings, and this work can be evaluated and studied further in relation to the antimitochondrial antibodies [121].

TABLE 9.2 SARS-CoV-2 proteins that align with six proteins significantly expressed in NETs induced in samples of SLE and LN, and with peptides either WB or SB to the same HLA allele and/or as epitope (E) of the same HLA allele. These epitope pairs have at least five matching amino acids and 62.5% identity. Results were obtained by working on the respective similar sequences with less than eight aa, manually, by including a few upstream and/or downstream amino acids.

Human protein	Query epitope[a]	Subject epitope[a]	SARS-CoV-2 protein	Allele
Histone H4	YEETRGVL (SB, E)	GETLGVLV (SB, E)	ORF1ab, ORF1a polyproteins	HLA-B*40:01
		GETRGVLV (WB)	ORF1a polyprotein	
MIX23	WMQSELNV (WB)	WMQSEFRV (WB)	Surface glycoprotein	HLA-A*02:01
Cysteine-rich secretory protein 3	LLFLVAGL (WB)	FLLFLVLI (SB)	ORF7b	HLA-A*02:01
Mast cell-expressed membrane protein 1	KILEVLQK (SB)	NLLEILQK (WB)	ORF1ab, ORF1a polyproteins	HLA-A*03:01
Cathepsin G	LLLLAFLL (WB)	FLAFLLFL (SB)	ORF7b	HLA-A*02:01
	LLAFLLPT (WB)			
Vimentin	HEEEIQEL (SB, E)	RQEEVQEL (WB)	ORF7a	HLA-B*40:01
		RQEEIQEL (WB, E)		

[a]*Query epitope sourced by human protein and subject epitope sourced by SARS-CoV-2 protein. Affinities wrote in parenthesis followed by the epitope sequences, wherein SB: strong binding and WB: weak binding (predicted by NetMHCcons), E: epitope (predicted by NetCTLpan).*

TABLE 9.3 SARS-CoV-2 proteins that align with 14 proteins significantly expressed in NETs induced in samples of SLE and LN, and with peptides SB to the same class II allele. The allele associated with the autoimmune disease is written bold in carriers and systemic lupus erythematosus is also written in bold to highlight. To include in the table, the number of matching aa in the possible epitope pairs (*not indicated*) is checked only for the epitopes of subject-peptides that can be paired with a different query-peptide than the query-peptide in the inputs. Also, such a subject-epitope is not included in the table when the original subject-epitope is included.

Human protein	Query epitope[a]	Subject epitope[a]	SARS-CoV-2 protein	Allele	Disease
Ficolin-1	DRGYFLSGWHTIY	ANYFLCWHTICYD	ORF3a protein	HLA-DPA1*01:03-**DPB1*04:02**	Type 1 diabetes
	RGYFLSGWHTIYL	NYFLCWHTICYDY			
	GYFLSGWHTIYLP	YFLCWHTICYDYC			
	LDRGYFLSGWHTIY	DANYFLCWHTICYD			
	DRGYFLSGWHTIYL	ANYFLCWHTICYDY			
	RGYFLSGWHTIYLP	NYFLCWHTICYDYC			
Protocadherin-15	FIIILCCIPAILV	VFLLVTLAILTAL	Envelope protein	HLA-**DQA1*01:02**-DQB1*05:01	**Systemic lupus erythematosus**
	IIILCCIPAILVV	VVFLLVTLAILTAL			
	FIIILCCIPAILVV				
	IIILCCIPAILVVL				
Serpin I2	VLKSFFSAISEKK	CKSAFYILPSIIS	ORF1ab polyprotein	HLA-**DRB1*04:01**	Multiple sclerosis
	LKSFFSAISEKKQ	KSAFYILPSIISN			
	KSFFSAISEKKQE	SAFYILPSIISNK			
	VLKSFFSAISEKKQE	AFYILPSIISNKK			
		KCKSAFYILPSIISN			
		CKSAFYILPSIISNK			
		KSAFYILPSIISNKK			
		SAFYILPSIISNKKQ			
		AFYILPSIISNKKQE			
60S ribosomal protein L3	CVVMAAVSLSPAS	DAVIKTLQPVSEL	ORF1ab polyprotein	HLA-**DQA1*01:02**-DQB1*05:01	**Systemic lupus erythematosus**
	VVMAAVSLSPASA				
	VMAAVSLSPASAR				
	NQVFGQDEMIDVI	PTKVTFGDDTMIE	ORF1ab polyprotein	HLA-DPA1*01:03-**DPB1*04:02**	Type 1 diabetes
	VNQVFGQDEMIDVI	TKVTFGDDTMIEV			
	NQVFGQDEMIDVIG	KVTFGDDTMIEVQ			
		PTKVTFGDDTMIEV			
		TKVTFGDDTMIEVQ			

(Continued)

TABLE 9.3 SARS-CoV-2 proteins that align with 14 proteins significantly expressed in NETs induced in samples of SLE and LN, and with peptides SB to the same class II allele. The allele associated with the autoimmune disease is written bold in carriers and systemic lupus erythematosus is also written in bold to highlight. To include in the table, the number of matching aa in the possible epitope pairs (*not indicated*) is checked only for the epitopes of subject-peptides that can be paired with a different query-peptide than the query-peptide in the inputs. Also, such a subject-epitope is not included in the table when the original subject-epitope is included.—cont'd

Human protein	Query epitope[a]	Subject epitope[a]	SARS-CoV-2 protein	Allele	Disease
Helix-destabilizing protein	RGFGFVTYATVEE	RGFGASVEEVLSE	ORF1ab polyprotein	HLA-**DQA1*05:01-DQB1*02:01**	Graves' disease
	GFGFVTYATVEEV	GFGASVEEVLSEA			
	RGFGFVTYATVEEV	RGFGDTVEEVLSE			
	RGFGFVTYATVEEVD	RGFGYSVEEVLSE			
	GFGFVTYATVEEVDA	GFGYSVEEVLSEA			
	FGFVTYATVEEVDAA	RGFGASVEEVLSEA			
	GFVTYATVEEVDAAM	RGFGYSVEEVLSEA			
	RGFGFVTYATVEEVDA	RGFGASVEEVLSEAR			
		GFGASVEEVLSEARQ			
		RGFGYSVEEVLSEAR			
		GFGYSVEEVLSEARQ			
		RGFGASVEEVLSEARQ			
		RGFGYSVEEVLSEARQ			
Protein-tyrosine-phosphatase	ILIVIAILLFKRK	IFLIVAAIVFKRK	ORF7a protein	HLA-DPA1*02:01-**DPB1*05:01**	Graves' disease
Glyceraldehyde-3-phosphate dehydrogenase	ALQNIIPASTGAA	PLNIIPLTTAAXX	ORF1a polyprotein, ORF1ab polyprotein	HLA-**DQA1*05:01-DQB1*03:02**	Graves' disease, multiple sclerosis
		LNIIPLTTAAXXM			
		NIIPLTTAAXXMV			
	GALQNIIPASTGA	CVPLNIIPLTTAA	ORF1a polyprotein, ORF1ab polyprotein	HLA-**DQA1*05:01-**DQB1*03:03	Graves' disease
	ALQNIIPASTGAA	VPLNIIPLTTAAK			
	LQNIIPASTGAAK	PLNIIPLTTAAKL			
	QNIIPASTGAAKA	LNIIPLTTAAKLM			
	NIIPASTGAAKAV	PLNIIPLTTAAKX			
	IIPASTGAAKAVG	LNIIPLTTAAKXM			
	RGALQNIIPASTGA	VPLNIIPLTTAAX			
	GALQNIIPASTGAA	PLNIIPLTTAAXX			

TABLE 9.3 SARS-CoV-2 proteins that align with 14 proteins significantly expressed in NETs induced in samples of SLE and LN, and with peptides SB to the same class II allele. The allele associated with the autoimmune disease is written bold in carriers and systemic lupus erythematosus is also written in bold to highlight. To include in the table, the number of matching aa in the possible epitope pairs (*not indicated*) is checked only for the epitopes of subject-peptides that can be paired with a different query-peptide than the query-peptide in the inputs. Also, such a subject-epitope is not included in the table when the original subject-epitope is included.—cont'd

Human protein	Query epitope[a]	Subject epitope[a]	SARS-CoV-2 protein	Allele	Disease
	ALQNIIPASTGAAK	LNIIPLTTAAXXM			
	LQNIIPASTGAAKA	NIIPLTTAAXXMV			
	QNIIPASTGAAKAV	IIPLTTAAXXMVV			
	NIIPASTGAAKAVG	CXPLNIIPLTTAA			
	IIPASTGAAKAVGK	XPLNIIPLTTAAK			
	GALQNIIPASTGAAK	GCVPLNIIPLTTAA			
	ALQNIIPASTGAAKA	CVPLNIIPLTTAAK			
	LQNIIPASTGAAKAV	VPLNIIPLTTAAKL			
	QNIIPASTGAAKAVG	PLNIIPLTTAAKLM			
	NIIPASTGAAKAVGK	LNIIPLTTAAKLMV			
		CVPLNIIPLTTAAX			
		VPLNIIPLTTAAXX			
		PLNIIPLTTAAXXM			
		LNIIPLTTAAXXMV			
		NIIPLTTAAXXMVV			
		IIPLTTAAXXMVVI			
		IPLTTAAXXMVVIP			
		PLNIIPXTTAAKLM			
		GCXPLNIIPLTTAA			
		CXPLNIIPLTTAAK			
		XPLNIIPLTTAAKL			
		VPLNIIPLTTAAKLM			
		VPLNIIPLTTAAKXM			
		PLNIIPLTTAAKXMV			
		XPLNIIPLTTAAKLM			

(*Continued*)

TABLE 9.3 SARS-CoV-2 proteins that align with 14 proteins significantly expressed in NETs induced in samples of SLE and LN, and with peptides SB to the same class II allele. The allele associated with the autoimmune disease is written bold in carriers and systemic lupus erythematosus is also written in bold to highlight. To include in the table, the number of matching aa in the possible epitope pairs (*not indicated*) is checked only for the epitopes of subject-peptides that can be paired with a different query-peptide than the query-peptide in the inputs. Also, such a subject-epitope is not included in the table when the original subject-epitope is included.—cont'd

Human protein	Query epitope[a]	Subject epitope[a]	SARS-CoV-2 protein	Allele	Disease
Isoform 2 of Thrombospondin-1	VLELRGLRTIVTT	LKTLLSLRGVRTI	ORF1a polyprotein	HLA-**DQA1*01:02**-DQB1*05:01	**Systemic lupus erythematosus**
	LELRGLRTIVTTL	KTLLSLRGVRTIK			
	ELRGLRTIVTTLQ	TLLSLRGVRTIKV			
	LRGLRTIVTTLQD	DNLKTLLSLRGVRT			
	SMVLELRGLRTIVT	NLKTLLSLRGVRTI			
	MVLELRGLRTIVTT	LKTLLSLRGVRTIK			
	VLELRGLRTIVTTL	KTLLSLRGVRTIKV			
	LELRGLRTIVTTLQ	TLLSLRGVRTIKVF			
	ELRGLRTIVTTLQD	DNLKTLLSLRGVRTI			
	LRGLRTIVTTLQDS	NLKTLLSLRGVRTIK			
	SMVLELRGLRTIVTT	LKTLLSLRGVRTIKV			
	MVLELRGLRTIVTTL	KTLLSLRGVRTIKVF			
	VLELRGLRTIVTTLQ	DNLKTLLSLRGVRTIKV			
	LELRGLRTIVTTLQD				
	SSMVLELRGLRTIVTTL				
	SMVLELRGLRTIVTTLQ				
	MVLELRGLRTIVTTLQD				
	VLELRGLRTIVTTLQDS				
	LELRGLRTIVTTLQDSI				
	SSMVLELRGLRTI	LKTLLSLRGVRTI	ORF1a polyprotein	HLA-**DQA1*05:01**-DQB1*04:02	Graves' disease
	SMVLELRGLRTIV	KTLLSLRGVRTIK			
	MVLELRGLRTIVT	TLLSLRGVRTIKV			
	VLELRGLRTIVTT	LLSLRGVRTIKVF			
	LSSMVLELRGLRTI	LSLRGVRTIKVFT			
	SSMVLELRGLRTIV	NLKTLLSLRGVRTI			
	SMVLELRGLRTIVT	LKTLLSLRGVRTIK			

TABLE 9.3 SARS-CoV-2 proteins that align with 14 proteins significantly expressed in NETs induced in samples of SLE and LN, and with peptides SB to the same class II allele. The allele associated with the autoimmune disease is written bold in carriers and systemic lupus erythematosus is also written in bold to highlight. To include in the table, the number of matching aa in the possible epitope pairs (*not indicated*) is checked only for the epitopes of subject-peptides that can be paired with a different query-peptide than the query-peptide in the inputs. Also, such a subject-epitope is not included in the table when the original subject-epitope is included.—cont'd

Human protein	Query epitope[a]	Subject epitope[a]	SARS-CoV-2 protein	Allele	Disease
	MVLELRGLRTIVTT	KTLLSLRGVRTIKV			
	SMVLELRGLRTIVTT	TLLSLRGVRTIKVF			
	MVLELRGLRTIVTTL	LLSLRGVRTIKVFT			
	SSMVLELRGLRTIVTT	LSLRGVRTIKVFTT			
	SMVLELRGLRTIVTTL	SLRGVRTIKVFTTV			
	MVLELRGLRTIVTTLQ	LLSLRGVRTIKVFTT			
	ELSSMVLELRGLRTIVT	LSLRGVRTIKVFTTV			
	LSSMVLELRGLRTIVTT	TLLSLRGVRTIKVFTT			
	SSMVLELRGLRTIVTTL	LLSLRGVRTIKVFTTV			
	SMVLELRGLRTIVTTLQ	LSLRGVRTIKVFTTVD			
	MVLELRGLRTIVTTLQD	DNLKTLLSLRGVRTIKV			
		NLKTLLSLRGVRTIKVF			
		LKTLLSLRGVRTIKVFT			
		KTLLSLRGVRTIKVFTT			
		TLLSLRGVRTIKVFTTV			
		LLSLRGVRTIKVFTTVD			
		LSLRGVRTIKVFTTVDN			
	LELRGLRTIVTTLQ	KTLLSLRELRTIKV TLLSLRELRTIKVF	ORF1a polyprotein	HLA-**DRB1*04:04**	Multiple sclerosis
S-formylglutathione hydrolase	MYSYVTEELPQLI	MYSFVSEEIGTLI MYSFVSEETVTLI	Envelope protein	HLA-**DQA1*0501-DQB1*02:01**	Graves' disease
Vasodilator-stimulated phosphoprotein	RATVMLYDDGNKR ATVMLYDDGNKRW SRATVMLYDDGNKR RATVMLYDDGNKRW	TSRTVYDDGARRV SRTVYDDGARRVW TSRTVYDDGARRVW	ORF1ab polyprotein	**HLA-DRB1*03:01**	**Systemic lupus erythematosus,** multiple sclerosis, graves' disease

(Continued)

TABLE 9.3 SARS-CoV-2 proteins that align with 14 proteins significantly expressed in NETs induced in samples of SLE and LN, and with peptides SB to the same class II allele. The allele associated with the autoimmune disease is written bold in carriers and systemic lupus erythematosus is also written in bold to highlight. To include in the table, the number of matching aa in the possible epitope pairs (*not indicated*) is checked only for the epitopes of subject-peptides that can be paired with a different query-peptide than the query-peptide in the inputs. Also, such a subject-epitope is not included in the table when the original subject-epitope is included.—cont'd

Human protein	Query epitope[a]	Subject epitope[a]	SARS-CoV-2 protein	Allele	Disease
Histone HIST2H3PS2	ELLIRKLPFQRLV	ESNKKFLPFQQFG	Surface glycoprotein	HLA-DPA1*02:01-**DPB1*05:01**	Graves' disease
	LLIRKLPFQRLVR	SNKKFLPFQQFGR			
DnaJ homolog subfamily C member 22	LVALISLSSMVNF	LVQLAPISAMVRM	ORF1a polyprotein, ORF1ab polyprotein	HLA-**DQA1*01:02**-DQB1*05:01	**Systemic lupus erythematosus**
	LVALISLSSMVNFY	LVQMASISAMVRM			
	LVALISLSSMVNFYI	LVQLAPISAMVRMY			
		LVQMASISAMVRMY			
		LVQLAPISAMVRMYI			
		LVQMAPLSAMVRMYI			
Isoform 6 of membrane-associated guanylate kinase, WW and PDZ domain-containing protein 1	GGSGVVSTVVQPY	GGSSGVVNPVMEP	ORF3a protein	HLA-**DQA1*05:01-DQB1*03:02**	Graves' disease, multiple sclerosis
	GSGVVSTVVQPYD	GSSGVVNPVMEPI			
	SGVVSTVVQPYDV	SSGVVNPVMEPIY			
	GGGSGVVSTVVQPY	GSSGVVNPVVEPI			
	GGSGVVSTVVQPYD	SSGVVNPVVEPIY			
	GSGVVSTVVQPYDV	GGSSGVVNPVMEPI			
	GGGSGVVSTVVQPYD	GSSGVVNPVMEPIY			
	GGSGVVSTVVQPYDV	SSGVVNPVMEPIYD			
		GSSGVVNPVVEPIY			
		GSSGVVNSVMEPIY			
		SSGVVNSVMEPIYD			
		GSSGVVSPVMEPIY			
		SSGVVSPVMEPIYD			
		GGSSGVVNPVMEPIY			
	GGSGVVSTVVQPY	GSSGVVSPVMEPI	ORF3a protein	HLA-**DQA1*05:01**-DQB1*03:04	Graves' disease
	GGSGVVSTVVQPYD	GSSGVVSPVMEPIY			
Protein piccolo	NGVVYSSVATPTP	NSVAYSNTSIATP			

TABLE 9.3 SARS-CoV-2 proteins that align with 14 proteins significantly expressed in NETs induced in samples of SLE and LN, and with peptides SB to the same class II allele. The allele associated with the autoimmune disease is written bold in carriers and systemic lupus erythematosus is also written in bold to highlight. To include in the table, the number of matching aa in the possible epitope pairs (*not indicated*) is checked only for the epitopes of subject-peptides that can be paired with a different query-peptide than the query-peptide in the inputs. Also, such a subject-epitope is not included in the table when the original subject-epitope is included.—cont'd

Human protein	Query epitope[a]	Subject epitope[a]	SARS-CoV-2 protein	Allele	Disease
	NGVVYSSVATPTPS	NSVAYSNTSIATPT	Surface glycoprotein	HLA-**DQA1*05:01-DQB1*03:02**	Graves' disease, multiple sclerosis
	GVVYSSVATPTPST	SVAYSNTSIATPTN			
	VVYSSVATPTPSTF	VAYSNTSIATPTNF			
	NGVVYSSVATPTP	NSVAYSNTSIATP	Surface glycoprotein	HLA-**DQA1*05:01-**DQB1*03:03	Graves' disease
	NGVVYSSVATPTPS	NSVAYSNTSIATPT			
	GVVYSSVATPTPST	SVAYSNTSIATPTN			
	VVYSSVATPTPSTF	VAYSNTSIATPTNF			
	NGVVYSSVATPTPSTF	NSVAYSNTSIATPTNF			
	GVVYSSVATPTPSTFA	SVAYSNTSIATPTNFT			
	VVYSSVATPTPSTFAI	VAYSNTSIATPTNFTI			
	VYSSVATPTPSTFAIT	NSVAYSNTSIATPTNFT			
	YSSVATPTPSTFAITT	SVAYSNTSIATPTNFTI			
	SSVATPTPSTFAITTQ	VAYSNTSIATPTNFTIS			
	NGVVYSSVATPTPSTFA	AYSNTSIATPTNFTISV			
	GVVYSSVATPTPSTFAI				
	VVYSSVATPTPSTFAIT				
	VYSSVATPTPSTFAITT				
	YSSVATPTPSTFAITTQ				
	QPLMIAPVSTDNT	YEPLIITTDNTFV	Surface glycoprotein	HLA-**DQA1*01:02-**DQB1*05:01	**Systemic lupus erythematosus**
		EPLIITTDNTFVS			
	LMIAPVSTDNTFAVS	FYEPLIITTDNTFVS	Surface glycoprotein	HLA-**DRB1*03:01**	**Systemic lupus erythematosus,** multiple sclerosis, graves' disease
	PLMIAPVSTDNTFAVS	FYEPQMITTDNTFVS			
		NFYEPLIITTDNTFVS			

[a] *Query epitope sourced by human protein and subject epitope sourced by SARS-CoV-2 protein.*

Conclusion

HLA supertype representative alleles can bear autoimmunity risk with NETs-pathology, through molecular mimicry, but individuals with HLA-A*01:01 serotypes may be at higher risk and HLA-A*02:01 serotypes can be at greater risk than expected if infected with SARS-CoV-2.

Data availability

Data cited in *Materials and Methods* are available [122] at shorturl.at/lAE89 (shortened at shorturl.at).

Appendix

SI-TABLE 9.1 Individual associations of identified human proteins with different HLA alleles. HLA alleles are in bold, followed by the associated human proteins. The ordering of the list is primarily downwards and then rightwards, according to the allele names.

HLA-A*01:01	**HLA-B*08:01 (continues)**
Acyl-CoA-binding protein	Eosinophil peroxidase
Aminopeptidase N	Glutathione S-transferase omega-1
Barrier-to-autointegration factor	Isoform 2 of Thrombospondin-1
DnaJ homolog subfamily C member 22	Isoform 6 of membrane-associated guanylate kinase, WW and PDZ domain-containing protein 1
Eosinophil peroxidase	Isoform H14 of myeloperoxidase
Ficolin-1	**HLA-B*15:01**
Histone H4	Acyl-CoA-binding protein
Isoform 4 of kinesin-like protein KIF20B	Aminopeptidase N
Isoform 6 of membrane-associated guanylate kinase, WW and PDZ domain-containing protein 1	DnaJ homolog subfamily C member 22
Isoform H14 of myeloperoxidase	E3 ubiquitin-protein ligase MYCBP2 (fragment)
Nuclear transport factor 2	Eosinophil peroxidase
Phosphatidylethanolamine-binding protein 1	High mobility group protein B1
Transgelin-2	High mobility group protein B2 (fragment)
HLA-A*02:01	Isoform 4 of kinesin-like protein KIF20B

SI-TABLE 9.1 Individual associations of identified human proteins with different HLA alleles. HLA alleles are in bold, followed by the associated human proteins. The ordering of the list is primarily downwards and then rightwards, according to the allele names.—cont'd

HLA-A*01:01	**HLA-B*08:01 (continues)**
Cysteine-rich secretory protein 3	Isoform H14 of myeloperoxidase
Ficolin-1	Protein piccolo
Glutathione S-transferase omega-1	**HLA-B*27:05**
Isoform 4 of kinesin-like protein KIF20B	Cathepsin G
Myosin-9	Cystatin-B
Protocadherin-15	Dynein axonemal heavy chain 5
HLA-A*03:01	E3 ubiquitin-protein ligase MYCBP2 (fragment)
Isoform 2 of Thrombospondin-1	Ficolin-1
Lamin-B1	Neutrophil elastase
Protein-tyrosine-phosphatase (fragment)	Vasodilator-stimulated phosphoprotein
HLA-A*24:02	**HLA-B*39:01**
Cysteine-rich secretory protein 3	Cathepsin G
Glutathione S-transferase omega-1	Dynein axonemal heavy chain 5
High mobility group protein B1	Eosinophil peroxidase
High mobility group protein B2 (fragment)	Ficolin-1
Nuclear transport factor 2	Myosin-9
S-formylglutathione hydrolase	Neutrophil elastase
HLA-A*26:01	Protein-tyrosine-phosphatase (fragment)
Acyl-CoA-binding protein	Vasodilator-stimulated phosphoprotein
Aminopeptidase N	**HLA-B*40:01**
Dynein axonemal heavy chain 5	Dynein axonemal heavy chain 5
Eosinophil peroxidase	Isoform 2 of Thrombospondin-1
Helix-destabilizing protein	NF-X1-type zinc finger protein NFXL1
Histone H4	Tropomyosin alpha-3 chain
Isoform 4 of kinesin-like protein KIF20B	Antigen KI-67 (UPI0002065088)
Isoform H14 of myeloperoxidase	**HLA-B*58:01**
NF-X1-type zinc finger protein NFXL1	Aminopeptidase N
Phosphatidylethanolamine-binding protein 1	DnaJ homolog subfamily C member 22
Talin-1	Eosinophil peroxidase

(Continued)

SI-TABLE 9.1 Individual associations of identified human proteins with different HLA alleles. HLA alleles are in bold, followed by the associated human proteins. The ordering of the list is primarily downwards and then rightwards, according to the allele names.—cont'd

HLA-A*01:01	**HLA-B*08:01 (continues)**
Transgelin-2	High mobility group protein B1
HLA-B*07:02	Histone H4
Cathepsin G	Isoform 4 of kinesin-like protein KIF20B
Dynein axonemal heavy chain 5	Isoform H14 of myeloperoxidase
Neutrophil elastase	Nuclear transport factor 2
HLA-B*08:01	Phosphatidylethanolamine-binding protein 1
AF4/FMR2 family member 3 (fragment)	Protein piccolo
Cathepsin G	Protein-tyrosine-phosphatase (fragment)
Dynein axonemal heavy chain 5	Talin-1

SI-TABLE 9.2 Individual associations of HLA alleles with the identified human protein. Human proteins are in bold, followed by the associated HLA alleles. Descending order of the list is primarily downwards and then rightwards, according to the number of associated alleles.

Eosinophil peroxidase	**Nuclear transport factor 2**	**Transgelin-2**
HLA-A*01:01	HLA-A*01:01	HLA-A*01:01
HLA-A*26:01	HLA-A*24:02	HLA-A*26:01
HLA-B*08:01	HLA-B*58:01	**E3 ubiquitin-protein ligase MYCBP2 (fragment)**
HLA-B*15:01	**DnaJ homolog subfamily C member 22**	HLA-B*15:01
HLA-B*39:01	HLA-A*01:01	HLA-B*27:05
HLA-B*58:01	HLA-B*15:01	**Protein piccolo**
Dynein axonemal heavy chain 5	HLA-B*58:01	HLA-B*15:01
HLA-A*26:01	**High mobility group protein B1**	HLA-B*58:01
HLA-B*07:02	HLA-A*24:02	**Isoform 6 of membrane-associated guanylate kinase, WW, and PDZ domain-containing protein 1**
HLA-B*08:01	HLA-B*15:01	HLA-A*01:01
HLA-B*27:05	HLA-B*58:01	HLA-B*08:01

SI-TABLE 9.2 Individual associations of HLA alleles with the identified human protein. Human proteins are in bold, followed by the associated HLA alleles. Descending order of the list is primarily downwards and then rightwards, according to the number of associated alleles.—cont'd

Eosinophil peroxidase	**Nuclear transport factor 2**	**Transgelin-2**
HLA-B*39:01	**Neutrophil elastase**	**Talin-1**
HLA-B*40:01	HLA-B*07:02	HLA-A*26:01
Isoform 4 of kinesin-like protein KIF20B	HLA-B*27:05	HLA-B*58:01
HLA-A*01:01	HLA-B*39:01	**Myosin-9**
HLA-A*02:01	**Acyl-CoA-binding protein**	HLA-A*02:01
HLA-A*26:01	HLA-A*01:01	HLA-B*39:01
HLA-B*15:01	HLA-A*26:01	**Cysteine-rich secretory protein 3**
HLA-B*58:01	HLA-B*15:01	HLA-A*02:01
Isoform H14 of myeloperoxidase	**Isoform 2 of Thrombospondin-1**	HLA-A*24:02
HLA-A*01:01	HLA-A*03:01	**NF-X1-type zinc finger protein NFXL1**
HLA-A*26:01	HLA-B*08:01	HLA-A*26:01
HLA-B*08:01	HLA-B*40:01	HLA-B*40:01
HLA-B*15:01	**Protein-tyrosine-phosphatase (fragment)**	**Tropomyosin alpha-3 chain**
HLA-B*58:01	HLA-A*03:01	HLA-B*40:01
Aminopeptidase N	HLA-B*39:01	**Lamin-B1**
HLA-A*01:01	HLA-B*58:01	HLA-A*03:01
HLA-A*26:01	**Glutathione S-transferase omega-1**	**S-formylglutathione hydrolase**
HLA-B*15:01	HLA-A*02:01	HLA-A*24:02
HLA-B*58:01	HLA-A*24:02	**AF4/FMR2 family member 3 (fragment)**
Cathepsin G	HLA-B*08:01	HLA-B*08:01
HLA-B*07:02	**Histone H4**	**Barrier-to-autointegration factor**
HLA-B*08:01	HLA-A*01:01	HLA-A*01:01
HLA-B*27:05	HLA-A*26:01	**Cystatin-B**
HLA-B*39:01	HLA-B*58:01	HLA-B*27:05
Ficolin-1	**High mobility group protein B2 (fragment)**	**Antigen KI-67 (UPI0002065088)**

(*Continued*)

SI-TABLE 9.2 Individual associations of HLA alleles with the identified human protein. Human proteins are in bold, followed by the associated HLA alleles. Descending order of the list is primarily downwards and then rightwards, according to the number of associated alleles.—cont'd

Eosinophil peroxidase	**Nuclear transport factor 2**	**Transgelin-2**
HLA-A*01:01	HLA-A*24:02	HLA-B*40:01
HLA-A*02:01	HLA-B*15:01	**Protocadherin-15**
HLA-B*27:05	**Vasodilator-stimulated phosphoprotein**	HLA-A*02:01
HLA-B*39:01	HLA-B*27:05	**Helix-destabilizing protein**
Phosphatidylethanolamine-binding protein 1	HLA-B*39:01	HLA-A*26:01
HLA-A*01:01	**Transgelin-2**	
HLA-A*26:01	HLA-A*01:01	
HLA-B*58:01	HLA-A*26:01	

SI-TABLE 9.3 Individual associations of diseases with the identified human protein. Diseases are in bold, followed by the associated human proteins. Descending order of the list is primarily downwards and then rightwards, according to the number of associated human proteins.

Diseases associated proteins	**Amelanotic melanoma**	**Reticulate acropigmentation of kitamura**
Disease of mental health	Cathepsin	E3 ubiquitin-protein ligase MYCBP2 (Fragment)
Barrier-to-autointegration factor	Isoform 2 of Thrombospondin-1	**Visceral heterotaxy**
Helix-destabilizing protein	**B-lymphoblastic leukemia/Lymphoma**	Dynein axonemal heavy chain 5
High mobility group protein B1	Aminopeptidase N	**Reticulosarcoma**
Histone H4	Isoform H14 of Myeloperoxidase	Aminopeptidase N
Isoform H14 of Myeloperoxidase	**Collagenous colitis**	**Vitreoretinopathy, neovascular inflammatory**
Protein piccolo	Eosinophil peroxidase	Isoform 2 of Thrombospondin-1
Tropomyosin alpha-3 chain	Isoform H14 of Myeloperoxidase	**Retinal detachment**
Lung cancer	**Body Mass index quantitative trait locus 11**	High mobility group protein B1
Aminopeptidase N	Isoform 2 of Thrombospondin-1	**Whim syndrome 1**

SI-TABLE 9.3 Individual associations of diseases with the identified human protein. Diseases are in bold, followed by the associated human proteins. Descending order of the list is primarily downwards and then rightwards, according to the number of associated human proteins.—cont'd

Diseases associated proteins	**Amelanotic melanoma**	**Reticulate acropigmentation of kitamura**
Antigen KI-67	Myosin-9	Neutrophil elastase
High mobility group protein B1	**Appendicitis**	**Nephroma**
Isoform 2 of Thrombospondin-1	High mobility group protein B1	Antigen KI-67
Isoform H14 of Myeloperoxidase	Isoform H14 of Myeloperoxidase	**Wilson disease**
Phosphatidylethanolamine-binding protein 1	**Breast adenocarcinoma**	S-formylglutathione hydrolase
Retinitis pigmentosa	Antigen KI-67	**Myxopapillary ependymoma**
Dynein axonemal heavy chain 5	Isoform 2 of Thrombospondin-1	Antigen KI-67
Histone H4	**Bacterial pneumonia**	**Y-linked deafness**
Lamin-B1	High mobility group protein B1	Protocadherin-15
Protocadherin-15	Neutrophil elastase	**Retinitis pigmentosa-deafness syndrome**
Tropomyosin alpha-3 chain	**Dementia**	Protocadherin-15
Type 2 diabetes mellitus	Cystatin	**Zellweger syndrome**
High mobility group protein B1	Helix-destabilizing protein	Acyl-CoA-binding protein
Isoform 2 of Thrombospondin-1	**Barrett'S adenocarcinoma**	**Nose disease**
Isoform H14 of Myeloperoxidase	Glutathione S-transferase omega-1	Eosinophil peroxidase
Myosin-9	Transgelin-2	**Reynolds syndrome**
Neutrophil elastase	**Bronchopneumonia**	Lamin-B1
Inflammatory bowel disease	Isoform H14 of Myeloperoxidase	**Kawasaki disease**
Cathepsin	Neutrophil elastase	Neutrophil elastase
Eosinophil peroxidase	**Rhabdoid meningioma**	**Epithelial recurrent erosion dystrophy**
High mobility group protein B1	Antigen KI-67	Nuclear transport factor 2
Isoform H14 of Myeloperoxidase	**Synovitis**	**Loeffler endocarditis**
Neutrophil elastase	High mobility group protein B1	Eosinophil peroxidase
Colorectal cancer	**Small cell carcinoma**	**Esophagus adenocarcinoma**

(*Continued*)

SI-TABLE 9.3 Individual associations of diseases with the identified human protein. Diseases are in bold, followed by the associated human proteins. Descending order of the list is primarily downwards and then rightwards, according to the number of associated human proteins.—cont'd

Diseases associated proteins	Amelanotic melanoma	Reticulate acropigmentation of kitamura
Antigen KI-67	Antigen KI-67	Transgelin-2
Helix-destabilizing protein	**Oral leukoplakia**	**Mucocutaneous leishmaniasis**
High mobility group protein B1	Antigen KI-67	Nuclear transport factor 2
Isoform 2 of Thrombospondin-1	**Usher syndrome, type ih**	**Essential thrombocythemia**
Isoform H14 of Myeloperoxidase	Protocadherin-15	Isoform H14 of Myeloperoxidase
Rheumatoid arthritis	**Orbital cancer**	**Lens disease**
Cathepsin	Antigen KI-67	Myosin-9
High mobility group protein B1	**Nasal cavity lymphoma**	**Exanthem**
Isoform H14 of Myeloperoxidase	Antigen KI-67	Isoform H14 of Myeloperoxidase
Neutrophil elastase	**Orbital granuloma**	**Malignant fibrous histiocytoma**
Systemic lupus erythematosus	Isoform H14 of Myeloperoxidase	Antigen KI-67
Cathepsin	**Spinocerebellar ataxia 36**	**Exocrine pancreatic insufficiency**
High mobility group protein B1	Cystatin	Neutrophil elastase
Isoform H14 of Myeloperoxidase	**Neurilemmomatosis**	**Microscopic Colitis**
Neutrophil elastase	Barrier-to-autointegration factor	Isoform 6 of membrane-associated guanylate kinase, WW and PDZ domain-containing protein 1
Respiratory failure	**Tuberculum sellae meningioma**	**Extrahepatic cholestasis**
Aminopeptidase N	Antigen KI-67	Isoform H14 of Myeloperoxidase
Eosinophil peroxidase	**Osteogenesis imperfecta, type Xiv**	**Myeloperoxidase deficiency**
Isoform H14 of Myeloperoxidase	Dynein axonemal heavy chain 5	Isoform H14 of Myeloperoxidase
Neutrophil elastase	**Vestibular gland benign neoplasm**	**Extrapulmonary tuberculosis**
Prostate cancer	Antigen KI-67	Protocadherin-15
Antigen KI-67	**Osteogenesis imperfecta, type Xvi**	**Large cell neuroendocrine carcinoma**
Cysteine-rich secretory protein 3	Vasodilator-stimulated phosphoprotein	Antigen KI-67
Isoform 2 of Thrombospondin-1	**Scleral disease**	**End stage renal disease**

SI-TABLE 9.3 Individual associations of diseases with the identified human protein. Diseases are in bold, followed by the associated human proteins. Descending order of the list is primarily downwards and then rightwards, according to the number of associated human proteins.—cont'd

Diseases associated proteins	**Amelanotic melanoma**	**Reticulate acropigmentation of kitamura**
Phosphatidylethanolamine-binding protein 1	Isoform H14 of Myeloperoxidase	Myosin-9
Microcephaly	**Osteopoikilosis**	**Leukodystrophy**
Cystatin	Barrier-to-autointegration factor	Lamin-B1
Lamin-B1	**Sinonasal undifferentiated carcinoma**	**Eye degenerative disease**
Protein piccolo	Antigen KI-67	Protocadherin-15
Protocadherin-15	**Otitis externa**	**Lymphoma**
Lung disease	Neutrophil elastase	Aminopeptidase N
Cathepsin	**Spinal canal and spinal cord meningioma**	**Eyelid carcinoma**
High mobility group protein B1	Antigen KI-67	Protocadherin-15
Isoform H14 of Myeloperoxidase	**Otitis media**	**Mastoiditis**
Neutrophil elastase	Isoform H14 of Myeloperoxidase	Isoform H14 of Myeloperoxidase
Glomerulonephritis	**Status asthmaticus**	**Fabry disease**
Cathepsin	Neutrophil elastase	Isoform H14 of Myeloperoxidase
Isoform H14 of Myeloperoxidase	**Otopalatodigital syndrome spectrum disorder**	**Meninges sarcoma**
Myosin-9	S-formylglutathione hydrolase	Antigen KI-67
Neutrophil elastase	**Thrombosis**	**Familial expansile osteolysis**
Malaria	Vasodilator-stimulated phosphoprotein	Vasodilator-stimulated phosphoprotein
Cathepsin	**Ovarian cancer**	**Mixed oligodendroglioma-astrocytoma**
Isoform 2 of Thrombospondin-1	Isoform 2 of Thrombospondin-1	Antigen KI-67
Isoform H14 of Myeloperoxidase	**Urinary tract papillary transitional cell benign neoplasm**	**Familial febrile seizures**
Neutrophil elastase	Antigen KI-67	Vasodilator-stimulated phosphoprotein

(Continued)

SI-TABLE 9.3 Individual associations of diseases with the identified human protein. Diseases are in bold, followed by the associated human proteins. Descending order of the list is primarily downwards and then rightwards, according to the number of associated human proteins.—cont'd

Diseases associated proteins	Amelanotic melanoma	Reticulate acropigmentation of kitamura
Granulomatosis with polyangiitis	**Ovarian endometrioid stromal sarcoma**	**Erysipelas**
Cathepsin	Antigen KI-67	Neutrophil elastase
High mobility group protein B1	**Vaccinia**	**Familial hemiplegic migraine**
Isoform H14 of Myeloperoxidase	Barrier-to-autointegration factor	Tropomyosin alpha-3 chain
Neutrophil elastase	**Ovary sarcoma**	**Joubert syndrome 1**
Heart disease	Antigen KI-67	Dynein axonemal heavy chain 5
Dynein axonemal heavy chain 5	**X-linked alport syndrome**	**Familial hypercholesterolemia**
Isoform 2 of Thrombospondin-1	Myosin-9	Isoform H14 of Myeloperoxidase
Isoform H14 of Myeloperoxidase	**Pacinian tumor**	**Epilepsy**
Neutrophil elastase	Antigen KI-67	Cystatin
Immune deficiency disease	**Rhinitis**	**Familial partial lipodystrophy**
Barrier-to-autointegration factor	Eosinophil peroxidase	Barrier-to-autointegration factor
Cathepsin	**Neuroendocrine tumor**	**Lattice corneal dystrophy**
Helix-destabilizing protein	Antigen KI-67	Helix-destabilizing protein
High mobility group protein B1	**Secondary progressive multiple sclerosis**	**Familial retinoblastoma**
Diabetes mellitus	Helix-destabilizing protein	S-formylglutathione hydrolase
High mobility group protein B1	**Pancreatitis**	**Ectopic pregnancy**
Isoform 2 of Thrombospondin-1	Neutrophil elastase	Cysteine-rich secretory protein 3
Isoform H14 of Myeloperoxidase	**Sialolithiasis**	**Fanconi anemia, complementation group I**
Neutrophil elastase	Transgelin-2	Isoform 4 of kinesin-like protein KIF20B
Bronchiectasis	**Pancytopenia**	**Lingual-facial-buccal dyskinesia**
Cathepsin	Aminopeptidase N	Cystatin
Dynein axonemal heavy chain 5	**Skin melanoma**	**Farmer'S lung**
Isoform H14 of Myeloperoxidase	Antigen KI-67	Neutrophil elastase
Neutrophil elastase	**Papillary carcinoma**	**Lung leiomyosarcoma**
Acute promyelocytic leukemia	Antigen KI-67	Antigen KI-67
Aminopeptidase N	**Soft tissue sarcoma**	**Fasciitis**

SI-TABLE 9.3 Individual associations of diseases with the identified human protein. Diseases are in bold, followed by the associated human proteins. Descending order of the list is primarily downwards and then rightwards, according to the number of associated human proteins.—cont'd

Diseases associated proteins	**Amelanotic melanoma**	**Reticulate acropigmentation of kitamura**
Cathepsin	Antigen KI-67	Myosin-9
Isoform H14 of Myeloperoxidase	**Papillary thyroid microcarcinoma**	**Major depressive disorder**
Neutrophil elastase	Antigen KI-67	Protein piccolo
Adult respiratory distress syndrome	**Spinal meningioma**	**Febrile seizures, familial, 2**
Cathepsin	Antigen KI-67	Vasodilator-stimulated phosphoprotein
High mobility group protein B1	**Papilloma**	**Marginal corneal ulcer**
Isoform H14 of Myeloperoxidase	Antigen KI-67	Isoform H14 of Myeloperoxidase
Neutrophil elastase	**Splenic artery aneurysm**	**Febrile seizures, familial, 4**
Breast cancer	Isoform H14 of Myeloperoxidase	Vasodilator-stimulated phosphoprotein
Antigen KI-67	**Papilloma of choroid plexus**	**Mediastinitis**
Isoform 2 of Thrombospondin-1	Antigen KI-67	Isoform H14 of Myeloperoxidase
Myosin-9	**Subacute bacterial endocarditis**	**Fibrosarcoma**
Tropomyosin alpha-3 chain	Isoform H14 of Myeloperoxidase	Isoform 2 of Thrombospondin-1
Primary hyperoxaluria	**Neuromuscular disease**	**Melon allergy**
Barrier-to-autointegration factor	Lamin-B1	Tropomyosin alpha-3 chain
Histone H4	**T-cell lymphoblastic leukemia/Lymphoma**	**Fibrous histiocytoma**
Lamin-B1	Helix-destabilizing protein	Antigen KI-67
Thrombocytopenia	**Parametritis**	**Dysentery**
High mobility group protein B1	Isoform H14 of Myeloperoxidase	Isoform H14 of Myeloperoxidase
Isoform 2 of Thrombospondin-1	**Toxic shock syndrome**	**Fibrous meningioma**
Myosin-9	High mobility group protein B1	Antigen KI-67
Severe congenital neutropenia	**Paranasal sinus cancer**	**Epithelial-stromal tgfbi dystrophy**
Cathepsin	Transgelin-2	Helix-destabilizing protein

(*Continued*)

SI-TABLE 9.3 Individual associations of diseases with the identified human protein. Diseases are in bold, followed by the associated human proteins. Descending order of the list is primarily downwards and then rightwards, according to the number of associated human proteins.—cont'd

Diseases associated proteins	**Amelanotic melanoma**	**Reticulate acropigmentation of kitamura**
Isoform H14 of Myeloperoxidase	**Ureter small cell carcinoma**	**Fish allergy**
Neutrophil elastase	Antigen KI-67	Tropomyosin alpha-3 chain
Peritonitis	**Nephrotic syndrome**	**Mononeuritis of upper limb and mononeuritis multiplex**
Cathepsin	Myosin-9	Isoform H14 of Myeloperoxidase
Isoform H14 of Myeloperoxidase	**Usher syndrome, type ic**	**Focal cortical dysplasia, type Ii**
Neutrophil elastase	Protocadherin-15	High mobility group protein B1
Periodic fever, familial, autosomal dominant	**Paraquat Poisoning**	**Multisystem proteinopathy**
Cathepsin	High mobility group protein B1	Helix-destabilizing protein
Isoform H14 of Myeloperoxidase	**Usher syndrome, Type Iiia**	**Focal segmental glomerulosclerosis**
Neutrophil elastase	Protocadherin-15	Myosin-9
Pneumonia	**Parasagittal meningioma**	**Esophageal adenoid cystic carcinoma**
High mobility group protein B1	Antigen KI-67	Antigen KI-67
Isoform H14 of Myeloperoxidase	**Vascular disease**	**Follicular adenoma**
Neutrophil elastase	Isoform H14 of Myeloperoxidase	Antigen KI-67
Vasculitis	**Parasitic helminthiasis infectious disease**	**Ischemic fasciitis**
Cathepsin	Eosinophil peroxidase	Myosin-9
Isoform H14 of Myeloperoxidase	**Vulvar disease**	**Folliculotropic mycosis fungoides**
Neutrophil elastase	Antigen KI-67	Antigen KI-67
Pulmonary disease, chronic obstructive	**Parathyroid adenoma**	**Juvenile rheumatoid Arthritis**
Cathepsin	Antigen KI-67	High mobility group protein B2 (fragment)
Isoform H14 of Myeloperoxidase	**Oral cavity cancer**	**Food allergy**
Neutrophil elastase	Isoform H14 of Myeloperoxidase	Eosinophil peroxidase
Pulmonary fibrosis, idiopathic	**Parathyroid carcinoma**	**Keratoconus**

SI-TABLE 9.3 Individual associations of diseases with the identified human protein. Diseases are in bold, followed by the associated human proteins. Descending order of the list is primarily downwards and then rightwards, according to the number of associated human proteins.—cont'd

Diseases associated proteins	**Amelanotic melanoma**	**Reticulate acropigmentation of kitamura**
High mobility group protein B1	Antigen KI-67	Cathepsin
Isoform H14 of Myeloperoxidase	**Rheumatic fever**	**Fragile X-associated tremor/ataxia syndrome**
Neutrophil elastase	Ficolin-1	Helix-destabilizing protein
Muscular dystrophy	**Parkinson disease, late-onset**	**Lactose intolerance**
Barrier-to-autointegration factor	Glutathione S-transferase omega-1	Aminopeptidase N
Helix-destabilizing protein	**Nut midline carcinoma**	**Frontal convexity meningioma**
Lamin-B1	Histone H4	Antigen KI-67
Leukemia, acute lymphoblastic	**Pasteurellosis**	**Larynx cancer**
AF4/FMR2 family member 3 (Fragment)	Neutrophil elastase	Antigen KI-67
Aminopeptidase N	**Sclerosing cholangitis**	**Frontal lobe neoplasm**
Isoform H14 of Myeloperoxidase	Isoform H14 of Myeloperoxidase	Antigen KI-67
Inflammatory myofibroblastic tumor	**Patulous eustachian tube**	**Leiomyoma**
Antigen KI-67	Isoform H14 of Myeloperoxidase	Antigen KI-67
Helix-destabilizing protein	**Sella turcica neoplasm**	**Frontotemporal dementia**
Tropomyosin alpha-3 chain	Antigen KI-67	Helix-destabilizing protein
Gastroesophageal reflux	**Pediatric systemic lupus Erythematosus**	**Ectodermal dysplasia 10b, hypohidrotic/Hair/ Tooth type, autosomal recessive**
Antigen KI-67	High mobility group protein B1	Isoform H14 of Myeloperoxidase
Isoform H14 of Myeloperoxidase	**Shrimp allergy**	**Frontotemporal dementia and/or amyotrophic lateral sclerosis 1**
Neutrophil elastase	Tropomyosin alpha-3 chain	Helix-destabilizing protein
Leukemia, acute myeloid	**Pelger-Huet anomaly**	**Epilepsy, Myoclonic Juvenile**
Aminopeptidase N	Lamin-B1	Cystatin
Histone H4	**Sickle cell disease**	**Fundus dystrophy**

(*Continued*)

SI-TABLE 9.3 Individual associations of diseases with the identified human protein. Diseases are in bold, followed by the associated human proteins. Descending order of the list is primarily downwards and then rightwards, according to the number of associated human proteins.—cont'd

Diseases associated proteins	**Amelanotic melanoma**	**Reticulate acropigmentation of kitamura**
Isoform H14 of Myeloperoxidase	Isoform 2 of Thrombospondin-1	Protocadherin-15
Gingivitis	**Pelvic inflammatory disease**	**Leukoplakia**
Cathepsin	Isoform H14 of Myeloperoxidase	Antigen KI-67
Isoform H14 of Myeloperoxidase	**Skin carcinoma**	**Endocarditis**
Neutrophil elastase	Isoform 2 of Thrombospondin-1	Eosinophil peroxidase
Myeloid sarcoma	**Pericardium disease**	**Lipoprotein quantitative trait locus**
Aminopeptidase N	Isoform H14 of Myeloperoxidase	Isoform H14 of Myeloperoxidase
Isoform H14 of Myeloperoxidase	**Skull base meningioma**	**Endocrine organ benign neoplasm**
Phosphatidylethanolamine-binding protein 1	Antigen KI-67	Antigen KI-67
Hemorrhagic disease	**Myoclonus**	**Distal arthrogryposis**
Isoform H14 of Myeloperoxidase	Cystatin	Tropomyosin alpha-3 chain
Myosin-9	**Smooth muscle tumor**	**Dyslexia**
Neutrophil elastase	Antigen KI-67	Dynein axonemal heavy chain 5
Myocardial infarction	**Periodontitis**	**Lupus erythematosus**
High mobility group protein B1	Neutrophil elastase	High mobility group protein B1
Isoform 2 of Thrombospondin-1	**Specific language impairment**	**Gastrointestinal stromal tumor**
Isoform H14 of Myeloperoxidase	NF-X1-type zinc finger protein NFXL1	Antigen KI-67
Chronic rhinitis	**Peripheral artery disease**	**Macrothrombocytopenia and granulocyte inclusions with or without nephritis or sensorineural hearing loss**
Dynein axonemal heavy chain 5	Isoform H14 of Myeloperoxidase	Myosin-9
Eosinophil peroxidase	**Spinal cord melanoma**	**Gemistocytic astrocytoma**
Isoform H14 of Myeloperoxidase	Antigen KI-67	Antigen KI-67
Chronic granulomatous disease	**Peritoneal mesothelioma**	**Male infertility**

SI-TABLE 9.3 Individual associations of diseases with the identified human protein. Diseases are in bold, followed by the associated human proteins. Descending order of the list is primarily downwards and then rightwards, according to the number of associated human proteins.—cont'd

Diseases associated proteins	**Amelanotic melanoma**	**Reticulate acropigmentation of kitamura**
Cathepsin	High mobility group protein B1	Dynein axonemal heavy chain 5
Isoform H14 of Myeloperoxidase	**Spindle cell thymoma**	**Gingival disease**
Neutrophil elastase	Antigen KI-67	Neutrophil elastase
Cholangitis, primary sclerosing	**Myoepithelioma**	**Mannose-binding lectin Deficiency**
Cathepsin	Antigen KI-67	Ficolin-1
Isoform H14 of Myeloperoxidase	**Spitz nevus**	**Endometrial adenocarcinoma**
Neutrophil elastase	Antigen KI-67	Antigen KI-67
Asthma	**Peters-plus syndrome**	**Mast-cell leukemia**
Eosinophil peroxidase	Isoform 2 of Thrombospondin-1	Isoform H14 of Myeloperoxidase
Isoform H14 of Myeloperoxidase	**Squamous cell carcinoma**	**Glanzmann thrombasthenia 1**
Neutrophil elastase	Antigen KI-67	Isoform 2 of Thrombospondin-1
Chronic kidney disease	**Petroclival meningioma**	**Maxillary sinusitis**
High mobility group protein B1	Antigen KI-67	Isoform H14 of Myeloperoxidase
Isoform H14 of Myeloperoxidase	**Stiff skin syndrome**	**Gliofibroma**
Myosin-9	Isoform 2 of Thrombospondin-1	Antigen KI-67
Bladder cancer	**Phagocyte bactericidal dysfunction**	**Melanoma**
Antigen KI-67	Cathepsin	Isoform 2 of Thrombospondin-1
Isoform 2 of Thrombospondin-1	**Submandibular gland cancer**	**Gliosarcoma**
Isoform 4 of kinesin-like protein KIF20B	High mobility group protein B1	Antigen KI-67
Alzheimer disease	**Neutropenia, severe congenital, 1, autosomal dominant**	**Melioidosis**
Glutathione S-transferase omega-1	Neutrophil elastase	High mobility group protein B1
Isoform H14 of Myeloperoxidase	**Necrotizing sialometaplasia**	**Glomangiomatosis**

(*Continued*)

SI-TABLE 9.3 Individual associations of diseases with the identified human protein. Diseases are in bold, followed by the associated human proteins. Descending order of the list is primarily downwards and then rightwards, according to the number of associated human proteins.—cont'd

Diseases associated proteins	Amelanotic melanoma	Reticulate acropigmentation of kitamura
Phosphatidylethanolamine-binding protein 1	Antigen KI-67	Antigen KI-67
Burkitt lymphoma	**Physical disorder**	**Meningeal melanocytoma**
Helix-destabilizing protein	Dynein axonemal heavy chain 5	Antigen KI-67
Isoform 2 of Thrombospondin-1	**Tetrasomy 21**	**Disease by infectious agent**
Lamin-B1	Aminopeptidase N	Aminopeptidase N
Cystic fibrosis	**Pilomyxoid astrocytoma**	**Meningothelial meningioma**
Cathepsin	Antigen KI-67	Antigen KI-67
Isoform H14 of Myeloperoxidase	**Thyroid gland follicular carcinoma**	**Glossopharyngeal nerve disease**
Neutrophil elastase	Antigen KI-67	Isoform H14 of Myeloperoxidase
Proctitis	**Pineal gland cancer**	**Microcephaly, autosomal dominant**
Eosinophil peroxidase	Antigen KI-67	Lamin-B1
Isoform H14 of Myeloperoxidase	**Transitional cell carcinoma**	**Glycoproteinosis**
Sarcoma, synovial	Antigen KI-67	Cystatin
Antigen KI-67	**Pineal region meningioma**	**Microvascular complications of diabetes 5**
Barrier-to-autointegration factor	Antigen KI-67	Isoform 2 of Thrombospondin-1
Renal cell carcinoma, nonpapillary	**Oligodendroglioma**	**Goodpasture syndrome**
Antigen KI-67	Antigen KI-67	Isoform H14 of Myeloperoxidase
Isoform 2 of Thrombospondin-1	**Pituitary apoplexy**	**Migraine, familial hemiplegic, 1**
Netherton syndrome	High mobility group protein B1	Tropomyosin alpha-3 chain
Cathepsin	**Urethral benign neoplasm**	**Granular cell tumor**
Neutrophil elastase	Antigen KI-67	Antigen KI-67
Ulcerative colitis	**Pituitary carcinoma**	**Monocytic leukemia**
Cathepsin	Antigen KI-67	Isoform H14 of Myeloperoxidase
Isoform H14 of Myeloperoxidase	**Usher syndrome type 2**	**Endometrial cancer**
Neural tube defects	Protocadherin-15	Antigen KI-67

SI-TABLE 9.3 Individual associations of diseases with the identified human protein. Diseases are in bold, followed by the associated human proteins. Descending order of the list is primarily downwards and then rightwards, according to the number of associated human proteins.—cont'd

Diseases associated proteins	**Amelanotic melanoma**	**Reticulate acropigmentation of kitamura**
Lamin-B1	**Pituitary gland disease**	**Motor neuron disease**
Transgelin-2	Antigen KI-67	Helix-destabilizing protein
Rare genetic deafness	**Usher syndrome, type if**	**Graves' disease**
Myosin-9	Protocadherin-15	Isoform H14 of Myeloperoxidase
Protocadherin-15	**Plasma protein metabolism disease**	**Multiple cranial nerve palsy**
Neutropenia	Neutrophil elastase	Isoform H14 of Myeloperoxidase
Isoform H14 of Myeloperoxidase	**Usher syndrome, Type IIC**	**Gray platelet syndrome**
Neutrophil elastase	Protocadherin-15	Myosin-9
Retinal disease	**Plasmacytoma**	**Muscular atrophy**
High mobility group protein B1	Antigen KI-67	Helix-destabilizing protein
Protocadherin-15	**Usher syndrome, Type IJ**	**Greenberg dysplasia**
Nonsyndromic deafness	Protocadherin-15	Lamin-B1
Myosin-9	**Plasmodium falciparum malaria**	**Myasthenic syndrome, congenital, 22**
Protocadherin-15	Isoform 2 of Thrombospondin-1	Barrier-to-autointegration factor
Skin disease	**Variola minor**	**Griscelli syndrome, type 3**
Isoform 2 of Thrombospondin-1	Isoform 4 of kinesin-like protein KIF20B	Phosphatidylethanolamine-binding protein 1
Isoform H14 of Myeloperoxidase	**Platelet glycoprotein iv deficiency**	**Myeloid leukemia**
Noonan syndrome 1	Isoform 2 of Thrombospondin-1	Isoform H14 of Myeloperoxidase
Histone H4	**Optic nerve sheath meningioma**	**Haemophilus meningitis**
Protocadherin-15	Antigen KI-67	Antigen KI-67
Vascular cancer	**Pleurisy**	**Ischemia**
Aminopeptidase N	Isoform H14 of Myeloperoxidase	Isoform H14 of Myeloperoxidase
Isoform 2 of Thrombospondin-1	**Vitelliform macular dystrophy**	**Disseminated eosinophilic collagen disease**

(*Continued*)

SI-TABLE 9.3 Individual associations of diseases with the identified human protein. Diseases are in bold, followed by the associated human proteins. Descending order of the list is primarily downwards and then rightwards, according to the number of associated human proteins.—cont'd

Diseases associated proteins	**Amelanotic melanoma**	**Reticulate acropigmentation of kitamura**
Onchocerciasis	Myosin-9	Eosinophil peroxidase
Eosinophil peroxidase	**Pneumoconiosis**	**Isolated congenital breast hypoplasia/aplasia**
Neutrophil elastase	High mobility group protein B1	Protein-tyrosine-phosphatase (Fragment)
Pulmonary fibrosis	**Wilms tumor 1**	**Endometrial disease**
Isoform H14 of Myeloperoxidase	Isoform 2 of Thrombospondin-1	Isoform H14 of Myeloperoxidase
Neutrophil elastase	**Neutropenia, severe congenital, X-linked**	**Juvenile pilocytic astrocytoma**
Orofacial cleft	Neutrophil elastase	Antigen KI-67
Antigen KI-67	**Y-linked monogenic disease**	**Hemangioma, capillary infantile**
Myosin-9	Protocadherin-15	Myosin-9
Recessive dystrophic epidermolysis bullosa	**Neutrophilic dermatosis, acute febrile**	**Kartagener syndrome**
High mobility group protein B1	Isoform H14 of Myeloperoxidase	Dynein axonemal heavy chain 5
Isoform 2 of Thrombospondin-1	**Rhabdoid cancer**	**Hemangiopericytoma, malignant**
Pancreatic cancer	Barrier-to-autointegration factor	Antigen KI-67
High mobility group protein B1	**Polyarteritis nodosa**	**Keratoacanthoma**
Isoform 2 of Thrombospondin-1	Isoform H14 of Myeloperoxidase	Antigen KI-67
Myxofibrosarcoma	**Rhabdomyosarcoma**	**Hemochromatosis type 2**
Antigen KI-67	Antigen KI-67	Neutrophil elastase
Isoform 2 of Thrombospondin-1	**Polycythemia vera**	**Keratocystic odontogenic tumor**
Papillon-lefevre syndrome	Isoform H14 of Myeloperoxidase	Antigen KI-67
Cathepsin	**Nasal cavity disease**	**Hemochromatosis, type 1**
Neutrophil elastase	Eosinophil peroxidase	Isoform H14 of Myeloperoxidase
Retinoblastoma	**Polymorphous low-grade adenocarcinoma**	**Kinsship syndrome**
High mobility group protein B1	Antigen KI-67	AF4/FMR2 family member 3 (Fragment)

SI-TABLE 9.3 Individual associations of diseases with the identified human protein. Diseases are in bold, followed by the associated human proteins. Descending order of the list is primarily downwards and then rightwards, according to the number of associated human proteins.—cont'd

Diseases associated proteins	**Amelanotic melanoma**	**Reticulate acropigmentation of kitamura**
S-formylglutathione hydrolase	**Right atrial isomerism**	**Hemolytic uremic syndrome, atypical 1**
Paranasal sinus disease	Dynein axonemal heavy chain 5	Ficolin-1
Dynein axonemal heavy chain 5	**Pontocerebellar hypoplasia**	**Large cell carcinoma with rhabdoid phenotype**
Isoform H14 of Myeloperoxidase	Protein piccolo	Antigen KI-67
Sensorineural hearing loss	**Schizophrenia**	**Early myoclonic encephalopathy**
Myosin-9	Protocadherin-15	Cystatin
Protocadherin-15	**Pontocerebellar hypoplasia, type 3**	**Laryngeal squamous cell carcinoma**
Pheochromocytoma	Protein piccolo	Antigen KI-67
Antigen KI-67	**Scleritis**	**Henoch-schoenlein purpura**
Protein-tyrosine-phosphatase (Fragment)	Isoform H14 of Myeloperoxidase	Isoform H14 of Myeloperoxidase
Tonsillitis	**Postaxial acrofacial dysostosis**	**Lateral sclerosis**
Aminopeptidase N	Dynein axonemal heavy chain 5	Helix-destabilizing protein
Isoform H14 of Myeloperoxidase	**Sebaceous breast carcinoma**	**Hepatic Coma**
Myopathy	Antigen KI-67	Acyl-CoA-binding protein
Helix-destabilizing protein	**Post-cardiac arrest syndrome**	**Leber plus disease**
Tropomyosin alpha-3 chain	High mobility group protein B1	Isoform H14 of Myeloperoxidase
Usher syndrome	**Secretory meningioma**	**Endometrial hyperplasia**
Myosin-9	Antigen KI-67	Antigen KI-67
Protocadherin-15	**Posterior uveal melanoma**	**Leiomyosarcoma**
Pollen allergy	Isoform 2 of Thrombospondin-1	Antigen KI-67
Eosinophil peroxidase	**Obstructive hydrocephalus**	**Endometrial stromal sarcoma**
Isoform H14 of Myeloperoxidase	Antigen KI-67	Helix-destabilizing protein

(*Continued*)

SI-TABLE 9.3 Individual associations of diseases with the identified human protein. Diseases are in bold, followed by the associated human proteins. Descending order of the list is primarily downwards and then rightwards, according to the number of associated human proteins.—cont'd

Diseases associated proteins	Amelanotic melanoma	Reticulate acropigmentation of kitamura
Vernal conjunctivitis	**Predominantly cortical thymoma**	**Leprosy 3**
Eosinophil peroxidase	Antigen KI-67	Ficolin-1
Isoform H14 of Myeloperoxidase	**Severe congenital neutropenia 1**	**Endometrial stromal tumor**
Primary ciliary dyskinesia	Neutrophil elastase	Helix-destabilizing protein
Dynein axonemal heavy chain 5	**Pre-malignant neoplasm**	**Leukemia, acute monocytic**
Neutrophil elastase	Antigen KI-67	Isoform H14 of Myeloperoxidase
Rapidly progressive glomerulonephritis	**Shwachman-diamond syndrome 1**	**Hereditary elliptocytosis**
Isoform H14 of Myeloperoxidase	Neutrophil elastase	Isoform 2 of Thrombospondin-1
Neutrophil elastase	**Premature menopause**	**Epilepsy with generalized tonic-clonic seizures**
Hypereosinophilic syndrome	Isoform 2 of Thrombospondin-1	Cystatin
Eosinophil peroxidase	**Sickle cell anemia**	**Hereditary spherocytosis**
Isoform H14 of Myeloperoxidase	Isoform H14 of Myeloperoxidase	Isoform 2 of Thrombospondin-1
Malignant astrocytoma	**Primary autosomal recessive microcephaly**	**Leukocyte adhesion deficiency, type iii**
Antigen KI-67	Isoform 4 of kinesin-like protein KIF20B	Talin-1
Isoform 2 of Thrombospondin-1	**Silicosis**	**Herpes simplex Encephalitis**
Inner ear disease	High mobility group protein B1	Neutrophil elastase
Isoform H14 of Myeloperoxidase	**Primary biliary Cholangitis**	**Leukodystrophy, demyelinating, adult-onset, autosomal dominant**
Protocadherin-15	Ficolin-1	Lamin-B1
Emery-dreifuss muscular dystrophy	**Situs inversus**	**High grade ependymoma**
Barrier-to-autointegration factor	Dynein axonemal heavy chain 5	Antigen KI-67
Lamin-B1	**Night blindness, congenital stationary, type 1a**	**Leukostasis**

SI-TABLE 9.3 Individual associations of diseases with the identified human protein. Diseases are in bold, followed by the associated human proteins. Descending order of the list is primarily downwards and then rightwards, according to the number of associated human proteins.—cont'd

Diseases associated proteins	**Amelanotic melanoma**	**Reticulate acropigmentation of kitamura**
Mixed phenotype acute leukemia	Glutathione S-transferase omega-1	Isoform H14 of Myeloperoxidase
Aminopeptidase N	**Occupational dermatitis**	**High grade glioma**
Isoform H14 of Myeloperoxidase	Protein piccolo	Antigen KI-67
Emery-dreifuss muscular dystrophy 1, X-linked	**Myopathy, centronuclear, 1**	**Lipodystrophy, familial partial, type 5**
Barrier-to-autointegration factor	Tropomyosin alpha-3 chain	Lamin-B1
Lamin-B1	**Skull base cancer**	**Holt-Oram Syndrome**
Idiopathic interstitial pneumonia	Antigen KI-67	Histone H4
Isoform 2 of Thrombospondin-1	**Nonencapsulated sclerosing carcinoma**	**Liver leiomyosarcoma**
Neutrophil elastase	Lamin-B1	Antigen KI-67
Emery-dreifuss muscular dystrophy 2, autosomal dominant	**Sleeping sickness**	**Human T-cell leukemia virus type 2**
Barrier-to-autointegration factor	Myosin-9	Helix-destabilizing protein
Lamin-B1	**Progeroid syndrome**	**Loiasis**
Leukemia, chronic myeloid	Barrier-to-autointegration factor	Eosinophil peroxidase
Isoform H14 of Myeloperoxidase	**Smarca4-deficient sarcoma of thorax**	**Endomyocardial fibrosis**
Neutrophil elastase	Barrier-to-autointegration factor	Eosinophil peroxidase
Eosinophil peroxidase deficiency	**Progressive myoclonus epilepsy**	**Double outlet right ventricle**
Eosinophil peroxidase	Cystatin	Dynein axonemal heavy chain 5
Isoform H14 of Myeloperoxidase	**Snail allergy**	**Hydrops of gallbladder**
Melanoma, uveal	Tropomyosin alpha-3 chain	Aminopeptidase N
High mobility group protein B1	**Progressive myoclonus epilepsy 1a**	**Lung meningioma**
Isoform 2 of Thrombospondin-1	Cystatin	Antigen KI-67

(*Continued*)

SI-TABLE 9.3 Individual associations of diseases with the identified human protein. Diseases are in bold, followed by the associated human proteins. Descending order of the list is primarily downwards and then rightwards, according to the number of associated human proteins.—cont'd

Diseases associated proteins	Amelanotic melanoma	Reticulate acropigmentation of kitamura
Extrinsic allergic alveolitis	**Solitary fibrous tumor/ Hemangiopericytoma**	**Endophthalmitis**
Isoform H14 of Myeloperoxidase	Antigen KI-67	High mobility group protein B1
Neutrophil elastase	**Progressive myoclonus epilepsy 4**	**Lymphoblastic lymphoma**
Muscular dystrophy, congenital, lmna-related	Cystatin	Isoform H14 of Myeloperoxidase
Barrier-to-autointegration factor	**Sphenoorbital meningioma**	**Hyperinsulinemic hypoglycemia**
Lamin-B1	Antigen KI-67	Histone H4
Gastric cancer	**Progressive myoclonus epilepsy 7**	**Lymphoplasmacyte-rich meningioma**
Antigen KI-67	Cystatin	Antigen KI-67
Isoform 2 of Thrombospondin-1	**Spinal cancer**	**Hyperinsulinemic hypoglycemia, familial, 1**
Hypertension, essential	Antigen KI-67	Histone H4
Isoform H14 of Myeloperoxidase	**Progressive relapsing multiple Sclerosis**	**Macular degeneration, age-related, 1**
Myosin-9	Ficolin-1	Isoform 2 of Thrombospondin-1
Gastroenteritis	**Spinal disease**	**Hyperinsulinemic hypoglycemia, familial, 2**
Aminopeptidase N	Antigen KI-67	Histone H4
Eosinophil peroxidase	**Proliferative fasciitis**	**Ductal carcinoma in situ**
Disseminated intravascular coagulation	Myosin-9	Antigen KI-67
High mobility group protein B1	**Spinal muscular atrophy**	**Hyperoxaluria, primary, type I**
Neutrophil elastase	Helix-destabilizing protein	Histone H4
Dystonia	**Proliferative glomerulonephritis**	**Episodic pain syndrome, familial, 3**
Cystatin	Isoform H14 of Myeloperoxidase	Vasodilator-stimulated phosphoprotein
Lamin-B1	**Spinocerebellar ataxia 2**	**Hyperoxaluria, primary, type ii**
Kidney disease	Helix-destabilizing protein	Tropomyosin alpha-3 chain
High mobility group protein B1	**Myopathy, centronuclear, 2**	**Malignant pheochromocytoma**

SI-TABLE 9.3 Individual associations of diseases with the identified human protein. Diseases are in bold, followed by the associated human proteins. Descending order of the list is primarily downwards and then rightwards, according to the number of associated human proteins.—cont'd

Diseases associated proteins	**Amelanotic melanoma**	**Reticulate acropigmentation of kitamura**
Myosin-9	Tropomyosin alpha-3 chain	Antigen KI-67
Dilated cardiomyopathy	**Spinocerebellar ataxia, autosomal recessive 8**	**Hyperoxaluria, primary, type iii**
Talin-1	Lamin-B1	S-formylglutathione hydrolase
Tropomyosin alpha-3 chain	**Prostate stromal sarcoma**	**Mantle cell lymphoma**
Leukocyte adhesion deficiency, type I	Antigen KI-67	Antigen KI-67
Isoform H14 of Myeloperoxidase	**Spitzoid melanoma**	**Hypersensitivity reaction type iii disease**
Talin-1	Tropomyosin alpha-3 chain	Isoform H14 of Myeloperoxidase
Hemangioma	**Protein-energy malnutrition**	**Mast cell neoplasm**
Antigen KI-67	Isoform H14 of Myeloperoxidase	Cathepsin
Myosin-9	**Squamous cell bile duct carcinoma**	**Hypersensitivity vasculitis**
Mast-cell sarcoma	Antigen KI-67	Isoform H14 of Myeloperoxidase
Aminopeptidase N	**Psammomatous meningioma**	**Epithelial malignant thymoma**
Isoform H14 of Myeloperoxidase	Antigen KI-67	Antigen KI-67
Hepatocellular carcinoma	**Staphylococcal toxic shock Syndrome**	**Encephalopathy**
Antigen KI-67	High mobility group protein B1	Cystatin
Glutathione S-transferase omega-1	**Pseudoachondroplasia**	**Maxillary sinus cancer**
Middle ear disease	Isoform 2 of Thrombospondin-1	Transgelin-2
Dynein axonemal heavy chain 5	**Stickler syndrome**	**Hypertrophic cardiomyopathy**
Isoform H14 of Myeloperoxidase	Protocadherin-15	Tropomyosin alpha-3 chain
Hereditary angioedema	**Pseudosarcomatous fibromatosis**	**Meckel syndrome, type 1**
Isoform H14 of Myeloperoxidase	Myosin-9	Dynein axonemal heavy chain 5

(*Continued*)

SI-TABLE 9.3 Individual associations of diseases with the identified human protein. Diseases are in bold, followed by the associated human proteins. Descending order of the list is primarily downwards and then rightwards, according to the number of associated human proteins.—cont'd

Diseases associated proteins	**Amelanotic melanoma**	**Reticulate acropigmentation of kitamura**
Neutrophil elastase	**Stroke, ischemic**	**Hypohidrotic ectodermal dysplasia autosomal recessive**
Multiple sclerosis	High mobility group protein B1	Cystatin
Helix-destabilizing protein	**Psoriasis**	**Meier-Gorlin syndrome 1**
Lamin-B1	Neutrophil elastase	Histone H4
Hereditary angioedema with normal C1inh	**Subleukemic leukemia**	**Ichthyosis, congenital, autosomal recessive 9**
Isoform H14 of Myeloperoxidase	Isoform H14 of Myeloperoxidase	Antigen KI-67
Neutrophil elastase	**Psoriasis 15**	**Melanoma in congenital melanocytic nevus**
Myelodysplastic syndrome	Neutrophil elastase	Antigen KI-67
Aminopeptidase N	**Supratentorial cancer**	**Idiopathic Edema**
Isoform H14 of Myeloperoxidase	Antigen KI-67	Isoform H14 of Myeloperoxidase
Hutchinson–gilford progeria syndrome	**Pulmonary artery leiomyosarcoma**	**Melanotic neurilemmoma**
Barrier-to-autointegration factor	Antigen KI-67	Antigen KI-67
Lamin-B1	**Synovium cancer**	**Eosinophilic gastritis**
Myeloproliferative neoplasm	Barrier-to-autointegration factor	Eosinophil peroxidase
Aminopeptidase N	**Pulmonary Aspergilloma**	**Melnick-needles syndrome**
Isoform H14 of Myeloperoxidase	Ficolin-1	S-formylglutathione hydrolase
Acute pancreatitis	**Tanycytic ependymoma**	**Idiopathic Neutropenia**
Isoform H14 of Myeloperoxidase	Antigen KI-67	High mobility group protein B1
Neutrophil elastase	**Pulmonary blastoma**	**Membranous nephropathy**
Bronchitis	Antigen KI-67	Isoform H14 of Myeloperoxidase
Isoform H14 of Myeloperoxidase	**Temporal arteritis**	**Ileitis**
Neutrophil elastase	Isoform H14 of Myeloperoxidase	Isoform H14 of Myeloperoxidase
Breast disease	**Myopathy, congenital, with fiber-type disproportion**	**Meninges hemangiopericytoma**

SI-TABLE 9.3 Individual associations of diseases with the identified human protein. Diseases are in bold, followed by the associated human proteins. Descending order of the list is primarily downwards and then rightwards, according to the number of associated human proteins.—cont'd

Diseases associated proteins	**Amelanotic melanoma**	**Reticulate acropigmentation of kitamura**
Antigen KI-67	Tropomyosin alpha-3 chain	Antigen KI-67
Isoform 2 of Thrombospondin-1	**Nemaline myopathy**	**Digenic disease**
Aspergillosis	Tropomyosin alpha-3 chain	Protocadherin-15
Eosinophil peroxidase	**Pulmonary embolism**	**Meningioma, familial**
Neutrophil elastase	Isoform H14 of Myeloperoxidase	Antigen KI-67
Cardiomyopathy, dilated, 1h	**Thrombotic thrombocytopenic purpura**	**Immune-complex glomerulonephritis**
Barrier-to-autointegration factor	Isoform 2 of Thrombospondin-1	Isoform H14 of Myeloperoxidase
Lamin-B1	**Pulmonary emphysema**	**Mesenchymal cell neoplasm**
Acute proliferative glomerulonephritis	Neutrophil elastase	Tropomyosin alpha-3 chain
Cathepsin	**Oculopharyngeal muscular dystrophy**	**Immunodeficiency 39**
Isoform H14 of Myeloperoxidase	Helix-destabilizing protein	Neutrophil elastase
Anca-associated Vasculitis	**Pulmonary eosinophilia**	**Microcephaly 26, primary, autosomal dominant**
High mobility group protein B1	Eosinophil peroxidase	Lamin-B1
Isoform H14 of Myeloperoxidase	**Tracheal lymphoma**	**Myiasis**
Autism	Antigen KI-67	DnaJ homolog subfamily C member 22
Isoform 2 of Thrombospondin-1	**Non-invasive bladder papillary urothelial neoplasm**	**Microcystic meningioma**
Protocadherin-15	Antigen KI-67	Antigen KI-67
Bronchial disease	**Transitional meningioma**	**Myoclonic epilepsy of lafora**
Eosinophil peroxidase	Antigen KI-67	Cystatin
Neutrophil elastase	**Myoclonus Epilepsy**	**Microscopic Polyangiitis**
Autoimmune disease	Cystatin	Isoform H14 of Myeloperoxidase
Aminopeptidase N	**Nemaline myopathy 1**	**Dysferlinopathy**

(Continued)

SI-TABLE 9.3 Individual associations of diseases with the identified human protein. Diseases are in bold, followed by the associated human proteins. Descending order of the list is primarily downwards and then rightwards, according to the number of associated human proteins.—cont'd

Diseases associated proteins	**Amelanotic melanoma**	**Reticulate acropigmentation of kitamura**
Isoform H14 of Myeloperoxidase	Tropomyosin alpha-3 chain	Isoform 2 of Thrombospondin-1
Allergic rhinitis	**Pulmonary hemosiderosis**	**Mid-dermal Elastolysis**
Eosinophil peroxidase	Isoform H14 of Myeloperoxidase	Neutrophil elastase
Isoform H14 of Myeloperoxidase	**Unverricht-lundborg syndrome**	**Myelophthisic anemia**
Autoimmune vasculitis	Cystatin	Aminopeptidase N
Isoform H14 of Myeloperoxidase	**Pulmonary hypertension**	**Migraine with or without aura 1**
Neutrophil elastase	Neutrophil elastase	Tropomyosin alpha-3 chain
Chorioamnionitis	**Ureterocele**	**Myh-9 related disease**
High mobility group protein B1	Protein-tyrosine-phosphatase (Fragment)	Myosin-9
Neutrophil elastase	**Pulmonary vein stenosis**	**Mixed endometrial stromal and smooth muscle tumor**
Autosomal dominant nonsyndromic deafness	Antigen KI-67	Antigen KI-67
Myosin-9	**Urinary schistosomiasis**	**Inclusion body myopathy with paget disease of bone and frontotemporal dementia**
Protocadherin-15	Eosinophil peroxidase	Helix-destabilizing protein
Anaplastic astrocytoma	**Purulent acute otitis media**	**Epithelioid inflammatory myofibroblastic sarcoma**
Antigen KI-67	Isoform H14 of Myeloperoxidase	Tropomyosin alpha-3 chain
Isoform 2 of Thrombospondin-1	**Nephrosclerosis**	**Infertility**
Autosomal dominant non-syndromic sensorineural deafness type dfna	Isoform H14 of Myeloperoxidase	Dynein axonemal heavy chain 5
Myosin-9	**Pustular Psoriasis**	**Mononeuritis multiplex**
Protocadherin-15	Neutrophil elastase	Isoform H14 of Myeloperoxidase
Acute megakaryocytic leukemia	**Usher syndrome, type I**	**Eosinophilic gastroenteritis**
Aminopeptidase N	Protocadherin-15	Eosinophil peroxidase

SI-TABLE 9.3 Individual associations of diseases with the identified human protein. Diseases are in bold, followed by the associated human proteins. Descending order of the list is primarily downwards and then rightwards, according to the number of associated human proteins.—cont'd

Diseases associated proteins	**Amelanotic melanoma**	**Reticulate acropigmentation of kitamura**
Isoform H14 of Myeloperoxidase	**Pustulosis palmaris et Plantaris**	**Mononeuropathy**
Autosomal recessive nonsyndromic deafness	Neutrophil elastase	Isoform H14 of Myeloperoxidase
Myosin-9	**Usher syndrome, type id**	**Inflammatory bowel disease 4**
Protocadherin-15	Protocadherin-15	Eosinophil peroxidase
Breast ductal carcinoma	**Nephrogenic adenoma of the urethra**	**Mouth disease**
Antigen KI-67	Antigen KI-67	High mobility group protein B1
Isoform 2 of Thrombospondin-1	**Usher syndrome, type ig**	**Inflammatory diarrhea**
Autosomal recessive non-syndromic sensorineural deafness type dfnb	Protocadherin-15	Isoform H14 of Myeloperoxidase
Myosin-9	**Rare Deafness**	**Mucoepidermoid carcinoma**
Protocadherin-15	Protocadherin-15	Antigen KI-67
Aleukemic leukemia cutis	**Usher syndrome, type iia**	**Ectodermal dysplasia 1, hypohidrotic, X-linked**
Aminopeptidase N	Protocadherin-15	Isoform H14 of Myeloperoxidase
Isoform H14 of Myeloperoxidase	**Nestor-guillermo progeria syndrome**	**Epithelioid trophoblastic tumor**
Crescentic glomerulonephritis	Barrier-to-autointegration factor	Antigen KI-67
Cathepsin	**Usher syndrome, type iid**	**Inguinal Hernia**
Isoform H14 of Myeloperoxidase	Protocadherin-15	Neutrophil elastase
Allergic disease	**Reactive arthritis**	**Muscle tissue disease**
Eosinophil peroxidase	Isoform H14 of Myeloperoxidase	Lamin-B1
Isoform H14 of Myeloperoxidase	**Usher syndrome, type iiib**	**Epidural spinal canal neoplasm**
Deafness, autosomal recessive	Protocadherin-15	Antigen KI-67
Myosin-9	**Nonsyndromic hearing loss**	**Elane-related Neutropenia**

(Continued)

SI-TABLE 9.3 Individual associations of diseases with the identified human protein. Diseases are in bold, followed by the associated human proteins. Descending order of the list is primarily downwards and then rightwards, according to the number of associated human proteins.—cont'd

Diseases associated proteins	**Amelanotic melanoma**	**Reticulate acropigmentation of kitamura**
Protocadherin-15	Protocadherin-15	Neutrophil elastase
Buschke-ollendorff syndrome	**Usher syndrome, type Ik**	**Intermediate congenital nemaline myopathy**
Barrier-to-autointegration factor	Protocadherin-15	Tropomyosin alpha-3 chain
Lamin-B1	**Relapsing-remitting multiple sclerosis**	**Myalgic encephalomyelitis/Chronic fatigue Syndrome**
Acute leukemia	Helix-destabilizing protein	Talin-1
Aminopeptidase N	**Van maldergem syndrome**	**Interstitial nephritis, karyomegalic**
Isoform H14 of Myeloperoxidase	Protein-tyrosine-phosphatase (Fragment)	Vasodilator-stimulated phosphoprotein
Alpha-1-antitrypsin deficiency	**Non-syndromic intellectual disability**	**Myasthenic syndrome, congenital, 5**
Isoform H14 of Myeloperoxidase	Barrier-to-autointegration factor	Vasodilator-stimulated phosphoprotein
Neutrophil elastase	**Optic nerve neoplasm**	**Intracranial berry aneurysm**
Blood coagulation disease	Antigen KI-67	High mobility group protein B1
Isoform H14 of Myeloperoxidase	**Renal hypertension**	**Myelofibrosis**
Myosin-9	Myosin-9	Isoform H14 of Myeloperoxidase
Chronic endophthalmitis	**Neonatal period electroclinical syndrome**	**Intravascular fasciitis**
Cathepsin	Cystatin	Myosin-9
Neutrophil elastase	**Non-syndromic X-linked intellectual disabilit**	**Elephantiasis**
Blood platelet disease	Protein piccolo	Neutrophil elastase
Isoform H14 of Myeloperoxidase	**Vestibular disease**	**Intraventricular meningioma**
Myosin-9	Protocadherin-15	Antigen KI-67

SI-TABLE 9.4 Individual associations of SuperPathways with the identified human proteins containing SuperPathway information. SuperPathways are in bold, followed by the associated proteins. Descending order of the list is primarily downwards and then rightwards, according to the number of associated proteins.

Innate immune system	**Benzene metabolism**
Aminopeptidase N	Isoform H14 of myeloperoxidase
Cathepsin G	**Allograft rejection**
Cystatin-B	Eosinophil peroxidase
Cysteine-rich secretory protein 3	**DNA double strand break response**
Eosinophil peroxidase	Histone H4
Ficolin-1	**NF-kappaB signaling**
High mobility group protein B1	Isoform H14 of myeloperoxidase
Isoform H14 of myeloperoxidase	**DNA double-strand break repair**
Myosin-9	Histone H4
Neutrophil elastase	**Creation of C4 and C2 activators**
Phosphatidylethanolamine-binding protein 1	Ficolin-1
Talin-1	**Cell adhesion molecules**
Vasodilator-stimulated phosphoprotein	Protein-tyrosine-phosphatase (fragment)
Activated PKN1 stimulates transcription of AR (androgen receptor) regulated genes KLK2 and KLK3	**Phospholipase-C pathway**
Cathepsin G	Phosphatidylethanolamine-binding protein 1
High mobility group protein B1	**Cell adhesion_Cadherin-mediated cell adhesion**
Histone H4	Protein-tyrosine-phosphatase (fragment)
Isoform H14 of myeloperoxidase	**Activation of cAMP-Dependent PKA**
Myosin-9	Vasodilator-stimulated phosphoprotein
Neutrophil elastase	**E-cadherin signaling in keratinocytes**
Signaling by GPCR	Vasodilator-stimulated phosphoprotein
Helix-destabilizing protein	**Regulation of lipid metabolism insulin signaling-generic cascades**
Histone H4	Protein-tyrosine-phosphatase (fragment)
Isoform 2 of Thrombospondin-1	**ECM-receptor interaction**
Myosin-9	Isoform 2 of Thrombospondin-1
Phosphatidylethanolamine-binding protein 1	**SALM protein interactions at the synapses**
Talin-1	Protein-tyrosine-phosphatase (fragment)

(Continued)

SI-TABLE 9.4 Individual associations of SuperPathways with the identified human proteins containing SuperPathway information. SuperPathways are in bold, followed by the associated proteins. Descending order of the list is primarily downwards and then rightwards, according to the number of associated proteins.—cont'd

Innate immune system	**Benzene metabolism**
HIV life cycle	**Ectoderm differentiation**
Barrier-to-autointegration factor	High mobility group protein B2 (fragment)
Isoform 2 of Thrombospondin-1	**Aurora B signaling**
Lamin-B1	Phosphatidylethanolamine-binding protein 1
Phosphatidylethanolamine-binding protein 1	**EGF receptor (ErbB1) signaling pathway**
Talin-1	Talin-1
Metabolism of proteins	**Stabilization and expansion of the E-cadherin adherens junction**
Aminopeptidase N	Vasodilator-stimulated phosphoprotein
Cathepsin G	**EGF/EGFR signaling pathway**
Histone H4	Phosphatidylethanolamine-binding protein 1
Isoform 2 of Thrombospondin-1	**mRNA splicing - major pathway**
Talin-1	Helix-destabilizing protein
Cytoskeletal signaling	**Cell adhesion_Cell-matrix glycoconjugates**
Lamin-B1	Neutrophil elastase
Myosin-9	**Negative regulation of MAPK pathway**
Nuclear transport factor 2	Phosphatidylethanolamine-binding protein 1
Talin-1	**EPHA forward signaling**
Vasodilator-stimulated phosphoprotein	Myosin-9
Developmental biology	**O-linked glycosylation**
Histone H4	Isoform 2 of Thrombospondin-1
Myosin-9	**Cell adhesion_Endothelial cell contacts by junctional mechanisms**
Phosphatidylethanolamine-binding protein 1	Isoform 6 of membrane-associated guanylate kinase, WW and PDZ domain-containing protein 1
Talin-1	**Coregulation of androgen receptor activity**
Vasodilator-stimulated phosphoprotein	Helix-destabilizing protein
amb2 integrin signaling	**ErbB1 downstream signaling**
High mobility group protein B1	Phosphatidylethanolamine-binding protein 1
Isoform H14 of myeloperoxidase	**Paxillin-dependent events mediated by a4b1**

SI-TABLE 9.4 Individual associations of SuperPathways with the identified human proteins containing SuperPathway information. SuperPathways are in bold, followed by the associated proteins. Descending order of the list is primarily downwards and then rightwards, according to the number of associated proteins.—cont'd

Innate immune system	**Benzene metabolism**
Neutrophil elastase	Talin-1
Talin-1	**Cell adhesion_Endothelial cell contacts by non-junctional mechanisms**
Metabolism	Isoform 6 of membrane-associated guanylate kinase, WW and PDZ domain-containing protein 1
Acyl-CoA-binding protein	**Phase I biotransformations, non P450**
Aminopeptidase N	S-formylglutathione hydrolase
Glutathione S-transferase omega-1	**Etoposide pathway, pharmacokinetics/ Pharmacodynamics**
S-formylglutathione hydrolase	Isoform H14 of myeloperoxidase
Ras signaling pathway	**PKMTs methylate histone lysines**
Isoform 2 of Thrombospondin-1	Histone H4
Isoform 6 of membrane-associated guanylate kinase, WW and PDZ domain-containing protein 1	**Factors involved in megakaryocyte development and platelet production**
Talin-1	Isoform 4 of kinesin-like protein KIF20B
Vasodilator-stimulated phosphoprotein	**PPAR alpha pathway**
Response to elevated platelet cytosolic Ca2+	Acyl-CoA-binding protein
Isoform 2 of Thrombospondin-1	**Fatty Acyl-CoA biosynthesis**
Isoform 4 of kinesin-like protein KIF20B	Acyl-CoA-binding protein
Talin-1	**Proteoglycans in cancer**
Transgelin-2	Isoform 2 of Thrombospondin-1
Mitotic prophase	**Fc gamma R-mediated phagocytosis**
Barrier-to-autointegration factor	Vasodilator-stimulated phosphoprotein
Histone H4	**Regulation of insulin-like growth factor (IGF) transport and uptake by insulin-like growth factor binding proteins (IGFBPs)**
Lamin-B1	Cathepsin G
Degradation of the extracellular matrix	**Fluid shear stress and atherosclerosis**
Cathepsin G	Glutathione S-transferase omega-1
Isoform 2 of Thrombospondin-1	**Arsenate detoxification I (glutaredoxin)**
Neutrophil elastase	Glutathione S-transferase omega-1

(*Continued*)

SI-TABLE 9.4 Individual associations of SuperPathways with the identified human proteins containing SuperPathway information. SuperPathways are in bold, followed by the associated proteins. Descending order of the list is primarily downwards and then rightwards, according to the number of associated proteins.—cont'd

Innate immune system	Benzene metabolism
Chromatin regulation/Acetylation	**Activated TLR4 signaling**
High mobility group protein B1	High mobility group protein B1
High mobility group protein B2 (fragment)	**RIG-I/MDA5 mediated induction of IFN-alpha/beta pathways**
Histone H4	High mobility group protein B1
RET signaling	**Gastric cancer**
Isoform 2 of Thrombospondin-1	Glutathione S-transferase omega-1
Phosphatidylethanolamine-binding protein 1	**Selenium micronutrient network**
Talin-1	Isoform H14 of myeloperoxidase
Cell cycle, mitotic	**Gastric cancer network 1**
Barrier-to-autointegration factor	Isoform 4 of kinesin-like protein KIF20B
Histone H4	**Shigellosis**
Lamin-B1	Talin-1
C-MYB transcription factor network	**Cell cycle checkpoints**
Aminopeptidase N	Histone H4
Isoform H14 of myeloperoxidase	**Development endothelin-1/EDNRA signaling**
Neutrophil elastase	Talin-1
Primary focal segmental glomerulosclerosis FSGS	**Amebiasis**
Antigen KI-67	Cathepsin G
Myosin-9	**Signaling events mediated by HDAC class III**
Talin-1	Histone H4
CDK-mediated phosphorylation and removal of Cdc6	**Golgi-to-ER retrograde transport**
High mobility group protein B1	Isoform 4 of kinesin-like protein KIF20B
High mobility group protein B2 (fragment)	**Striated muscle contraction**
Lamin-B1	Tropomyosin alpha-3 chain
Integrin pathway	**GPCR pathway**
Isoform 2 of Thrombospondin-1	Talin-1
Myosin-9	**Apoptosis-related network due to altered Notch3 in ovarian cancer**

SI-TABLE 9.4 Individual associations of SuperPathways with the identified human proteins containing SuperPathway information. SuperPathways are in bold, followed by the associated proteins. Descending order of the list is primarily downwards and then rightwards, according to the number of associated proteins.—cont'd

Innate immune system	**Benzene metabolism**
Talin-1	Isoform 2 of Thrombospondin-1
Sertoli-sertoli cell junction dynamics	**G-protein signaling_H-RAS regulation pathway**
Isoform 6 of membrane-associated guanylate kinase, WW and PDZ domain-containing protein 1	Isoform 6 of membrane-associated guanylate kinase, WW and PDZ domain-containing protein 1
Myosin-9	**Myometrial relaxation and contraction pathways**
Vasodilator-stimulated phosphoprotein	Glutathione S-transferase omega-1
Apoptotic cleavage of cellular proteins	**G-protein signaling_Rap1A regulation pathway**
High mobility group protein B1	Isoform 6 of membrane-associated guanylate kinase, WW and PDZ domain-containing protein 1
High mobility group protein B2 (fragment)	**Nectin adhesion pathway**
Lamin-B1	Talin-1
Tight junction	**Adherens junction**
Isoform 6 of membrane-associated guanylate kinase, WW and PDZ domain-containing protein 1	Protein-tyrosine-phosphatase (fragment)
Myosin-9	**Class I MHC mediated antigen processing and presentation**
Vasodilator-stimulated phosphoprotein	Vasodilator-stimulated phosphoprotein
Focal adhesion	**Granzyme-A pathway**
Isoform 2 of Thrombospondin-1	High mobility group protein B2 (fragment)
Talin-1	**O-glycosylation of TSR domain-containing proteins**
Vasodilator-stimulated phosphoprotein	Isoform 2 of Thrombospondin-1
Glutathione metabolism	**Hematopoietic cell lineage**
Aminopeptidase N	Aminopeptidase N
Glutathione S-transferase omega-1	**Advanced glycosylation endproduct receptor signaling**
S-formylglutathione hydrolase	High mobility group protein B1
Actin nucleation by ARP-WASP complex	**Cell junction organization**
Myosin-9	Vasodilator-stimulated phosphoprotein
Talin-1	**p53 signaling**
Vasodilator-stimulated phosphoprotein	Isoform 2 of Thrombospondin-1
Peptide hormone metabolism	**Angiogenesis (CST)**

(Continued)

SI-TABLE 9.4 Individual associations of SuperPathways with the identified human proteins containing SuperPathway information. SuperPathways are in bold, followed by the associated proteins. Descending order of the list is primarily downwards and then rightwards, according to the number of associated proteins.—cont'd

Innate immune system	**Benzene metabolism**
Aminopeptidase N	Isoform 2 of Thrombospondin-1
Cathepsin G	**Pathways affected in adenoid cystic carcinoma**
Matrix metalloproteinases	Isoform 6 of membrane-associated guanylate kinase, WW and PDZ domain-containing protein 1
Cathepsin G	**HIV transcription elongation**
Neutrophil elastase	Helix-destabilizing protein
Signaling by rho GTPases	**Brain-derived neurotrophic factor (BDNF) signaling pathway**
Histone H4	Protein-tyrosine-phosphatase (fragment)
Myosin-9	**Human T-cell leukemia virus 1 infection**
Cardiac conduction	Talin-1
Talin-1	**Carbon metabolism**
Tropomyosin alpha-3 chain	S-formylglutathione hydrolase
Oncogenic MAPK signaling	**Viral carcinogenesis**
Phosphatidylethanolamine-binding protein 1	Histone H4
Talin-1	**B cell receptor signaling pathway (sino)**
Activation of DNA fragmentation factor	Talin-1
High mobility group protein B1	**Benzodiazepine pathway, pharmacodynamics**
High mobility group protein B2 (fragment)	Acyl-CoA-binding protein
Platinum pathway, pharmacokinetics/ pharmacodynamics	**Phenytoin pathway, pharmacokinetics**
High mobility group protein B1	Isoform H14 of myeloperoxidase
Isoform H14 of myeloperoxidase	**Immune response IL-23 signaling pathway**
Cellular senescence (REACTOME)	Isoform H14 of myeloperoxidase
Histone H4	**Cardiac muscle contraction**
Lamin-B1	Tropomyosin alpha-3 chain
Transcriptional misregulation in cancer	**Inflammatory response pathway**
Isoform H14 of myeloperoxidase	Isoform 2 of Thrombospondin-1
Neutrophil elastase	**Cytosolic sensors of pathogen-associated DNA**
cGMP-PKG signaling pathway	High mobility group protein B1

SI-TABLE 9.4 Individual associations of SuperPathways with the identified human proteins containing SuperPathway information. SuperPathways are in bold, followed by the associated proteins. Descending order of the list is primarily downwards and then rightwards, according to the number of associated proteins.—cont'd

Innate immune system	**Benzene metabolism**
Tropomyosin alpha-3 chain	**Syndecan-4-mediated signaling events**
Vasodilator-stimulated phosphoprotein	Isoform 2 of Thrombospondin-1
Mitotic metaphase and anaphase	**Cardiac progenitor differentiation**
Barrier-to-autointegration factor	Aminopeptidase N
Lamin-B1	**TCR signaling (REACTOME)**
Adhesion	Vasodilator-stimulated phosphoprotein
Protein-tyrosine-phosphatase (fragment)	**PPAR signaling pathway**
Talin-1	Acyl-CoA-binding protein
Pathways in cancer	**Telomere extension by telomerase**
Glutathione S-transferase omega-1	Helix-destabilizing protein
Tropomyosin alpha-3 chain	**Protein-protein interactions at synapses**
Cytochrome P450 - arranged by substrate type	Protein-tyrosine-phosphatase (fragment)
Glutathione S-transferase omega-1	**TGF-beta signaling pathway (KEGG)**
S-formylglutathione hydrolase	Isoform 2 of Thrombospondin-1
PI3K-akt signaling pathway	**Apoptotic pathways in synovial fibroblasts**
Isoform 2 of Thrombospondin-1	Histone H4
Isoform 6 of membrane-associated guanylate kinase, WW and PDZ domain-containing protein 1	**Autophagy - animal**
Cytokine signaling in immune system	High mobility group protein B1
Phosphatidylethanolamine-binding protein 1	**Regulation of actin dynamics for phagocytic cup formation**
Talin-1	Myosin-9
Semaphorin interactions	**Bladder cancer**
Myosin-9	Isoform 2 of Thrombospondin-1
Talin-1	**Regulation of lipid metabolism by peroxisome proliferator-activated receptor alpha (PPARalpha)**
Agents acting on the renin-angiotensin system pathway, pharmacodynamics	Acyl-CoA-binding protein
Aminopeptidase N	**Translocation of ZAP-70 to immunological synapse**
Cathepsin G	Vasodilator-stimulated phosphoprotein

(Continued)

SI-TABLE 9.4 Individual associations of SuperPathways with the identified human proteins containing SuperPathway information. SuperPathways are in bold, followed by the associated proteins. Descending order of the list is primarily downwards and then rightwards, according to the number of associated proteins.—cont'd

Innate immune system	Benzene metabolism
Immune response CCR3 signaling in eosinophils	**Aquaporin-mediated transport**
Myosin-9	Vasodilator-stimulated phosphoprotein
Talin-1	**Chemical carcinogenesis - receptor activation**
Cytoskeleton remodeling regulation of actin cytoskeleton by rho GTPases	Glutathione S-transferase omega-1
Myosin-9	**Aldosterone synthesis and secretion**
Talin-1	Protein piccolo
Transport of the SLBP independent mature mRNA	**VEGF signaling pathway**
Barrier-to-autointegration factor	Talin-1
Lamin-B1	**RhoGDI pathway**
Defensins	Myosin-9
Cathepsin G	**Autophagy pathway**
Neutrophil elastase	High mobility group protein B1
Meiosis	**RNA polymerase II transcription initiation and promoter clearance**
Histone H4	Histone H4
Lamin-B1	**Malaria**
DNA damage/Telomere stress induced senescence	Isoform 2 of Thrombospondin-1
Histone H4	**Salmonella infection (KEGG)**
Lamin-B1	Myosin-9
Neuroscience	**MAP kinase signaling**
Aminopeptidase N	Phosphatidylethanolamine-binding protein 1
Antigen KI-67	**Deregulated CDK5 triggers multiple neurodegenerative pathways in alzheimers disease models**
DREAM repression and dynorphin expression	Lamin-B1
Lamin-B1	**MAPK-erk pathway**
Talin-1	Vasodilator-stimulated phosphoprotein
PAK pathway	**Ascorbate recycling (cytosolic)**
Myosin-9	Glutathione S-transferase omega-1
Protein-tyrosine-phosphatase (fragment)	**Chromatin organization**

SI-TABLE 9.4 Individual associations of SuperPathways with the identified human proteins containing SuperPathway information. SuperPathways are in bold, followed by the associated proteins. Descending order of the list is primarily downwards and then rightwards, according to the number of associated proteins.—cont'd

Innate immune system	**Benzene metabolism**
Drug metabolism - cytochrome P450	Histone H4
Glutathione S-transferase omega-1	**Signaling by FGFR2**
Isoform H14 of myeloperoxidase	Helix-destabilizing protein
Pathways of neurodegeneration - multiple diseases	**Blood-brain barrier and immune cell transmigration: VCAM-1/CD106 signaling**
Dynein axonemal heavy chain 5	Vasodilator-stimulated phosphoprotein
Helix-destabilizing protein	**Development angiotensin activation of ERK**
Endometrial cancer	Talin-1
Isoform H14 of myeloperoxidase	**MET promotes cell motility**
Tropomyosin alpha-3 chain	Isoform 2 of Thrombospondin-1
Phagosome	**Signaling by robo receptor**
Isoform 2 of Thrombospondin-1	Vasodilator-stimulated phosphoprotein
Isoform H14 of myeloperoxidase	**Apoptosis and survival caspase cascade**
EPH-ephrin signaling	Lamin-B1
Myosin-9	**Signaling events mediated by focal adhesion kinase**
Talin-1	Talin-1
Platelet activation	**Apoptosis modulation and signaling**
Talin-1	Lamin-B1
Vasodilator-stimulated phosphoprotein	**Development NOTCH1-mediated pathway for NF-KB activity modulation**
ERK signaling	Histone H4
Myosin-9	**Metabolism of water-soluble vitamins and cofactors**
Talin-1	Glutathione S-transferase omega-1
Retinoblastoma (RB) in cancer	**Sterol regulatory element-binding proteins (SREBP) signaling**
High mobility group protein B1	Acyl-CoA-binding protein
High mobility group protein B2 (fragment)	**MicroRNAs in cancer**
Gene expression	Isoform 2 of Thrombospondin-1
Helix-destabilizing protein	**Sweet taste signaling**
Histone H4	Myosin-9

(Continued)

SI-TABLE 9.4 Individual associations of SuperPathways with the identified human proteins containing SuperPathway information. SuperPathways are in bold, followed by the associated proteins. Descending order of the list is primarily downwards and then rightwards, according to the number of associated proteins.—cont'd

Innate immune system	Benzene metabolism
Signaling by moderate kinase activity BRAF mutants	**miRNA targets in ECM and membrane receptors**
Phosphatidylethanolamine-binding protein 1	Isoform 2 of Thrombospondin-1
Talin-1	**Chromosome maintenance**
Granzyme pathway	Histone H4
High mobility group protein B2 (fragment)	**Telomere C-strand (lagging strand) synthesis**
Lamin-B1	High mobility group protein B1
Smooth muscle contraction	**Angiopoietin like protein 8 regulatory pathway**
Talin-1	Protein-tyrosine-phosphatase (fragment)
Tropomyosin alpha-3 chain	**TGF-beta receptor signaling (WikiPathways)**
Hematopoietic stem cells and lineage-specific markers	Isoform 2 of Thrombospondin-1
Aminopeptidase N	**Insulin resistance**
Isoform H14 of myeloperoxidase	Protein-tyrosine-phosphatase (fragment)
Initiation of nuclear envelope reformation	**TGF-beta signaling pathway (WikiPathways)**
Barrier-to-autointegration factor	Isoform 2 of Thrombospondin-1
Lamin-B1	**Integrated breast cancer pathway**
Signaling by Wnt	E3 ubiquitin-protein ligase MYCBP2 (fragment)
Histone H4	**TNFR1 pathway**
Platinum drug resistance	Lamin-B1
Glutathione S-transferase omega-1	**Integration of viral DNA into host genomic DNA**
Oxytocin signaling pathway	Barrier-to-autointegration factor
Myosin-9	**Translational control**
Dilated cardiomyopathy	Helix-destabilizing protein
Tropomyosin alpha-3 chain	**Integrin alphaIIb beta3 signaling**
RhoA signaling pathway	Talin-1
Talin-1	**Transmission across chemical synapses**
Diseases of glycosylation	Protein-tyrosine-phosphatase (fragment)
Isoform 2 of Thrombospondin-1	**Apoptosis and autophagy**
Necroptosis	Lamin-B1

SI-TABLE 9.4 Individual associations of SuperPathways with the identified human proteins containing SuperPathway information. SuperPathways are in bold, followed by the associated proteins. Descending order of the list is primarily downwards and then rightwards, according to the number of associated proteins.—cont'd

Innate immune system	Benzene metabolism
High mobility group protein B1	**Unfolded protein response (UPR)**
DNA damage	Talin-1
Antigen KI-67	**Integrins in angiogenesis**
Peptide ligand-binding receptors	Talin-1
Cathepsin G	**Vesicle-mediated transport**
DNA damage response	Isoform 4 of kinesin-like protein KIF20B
Isoform 2 of Thrombospondin-1	**LDL oxidation in atherogenesis**
Regulation of actin cytoskeleton	Isoform H14 of myeloperoxidase
Myosin-9	**Lysosome**
DNA damage response (only ATM dependent)	Cathepsin G
High mobility group protein B1	**IL-2 pathway**
Senescence and autophagy in cancer	High mobility group protein B1
Isoform 2 of Thrombospondin-1	

References

[1] Kohm AK, Fuller KG, Miller SD. Mimicking the way to autoimmunity: an evolving theory of sequence and structural homology. Trends Microbiol 2003;11:101–5.

[2] Lule S, Colpak AI, Balci-Peynircioglu B, Gursoy-Ozdemir Y, Peker S, Kalyoncu U, et al. Behcet Disease serum is immunoreactive to neurofilament medium which share common epitopes to bacterial HSP-65, a putative trigger. J Autoimmun 2017;84:87–96.

[3] Negi S, Singh H, Mukhopadhyay A. Gut bacterial peptides with autoimmunity potential as environmental trigger for late onset complex diseases: in-silico study. PLoS One 2017;12:e0180518.

[4] Trost B, Lucchese G, Stufano A, Bickis M, Kusalik A, Kanduc D. No human protein is exempt from bacterial motifs, not even one. Self Nonself 2010;1:328–34.

[5] Vellozzi C, Iqbal S, Broder K. Guillain-Barre syndrome, influenza, and influenza vaccination: the epidemiologic evidence. Clin Infect Dis 2014;58:1149–55.

[6] Yuki N. Ganglioside mimicry and peripheral nerve disease. Muscle Nerve 2007;35:691–711.

[7] Zabriskie JB, Freimer EH. An immunological relationship between the group. A streptococcus and mammalian muscle. J Exp Med 1966;124:661–78.

[8] Fischer JC, Schmidt AG, Bölke E, Uhrberg M, Keitel V, Feldt T, et al. Association of HLA genotypes, AB0 blood type and chemokine receptor 5 mutant CD195 with the clinical course of COVID-19. Eur J Med Res 2021;1(26):107.

[9] Weiner J, Suwalski P, Holtgrewe M, Rakitko A, Thibeault C, Müller M, et al. Increased risk of severe clinical course of COVID-19 in carriers of HLA-C*04:01. EClinicalMedicine 2021;40:101099.

[10] Gutiérrez-Bautista JF, Rodriguez-Nicolas A, Rosales-Castillo A, López-Ruz MÁ, Martín-Casares AM, Fernández-Rubiales A, et al. Study of HLA-A;-B;-C;-DRB1 and -DQB1 polymorphisms in COVID-19 patients. J Microbiol Immunol Infect 2021;S1684–1182(21). 00183-3.

[11] Alnaqbi H, Tay GK, Jelinek HF, Francis A, Alefishat E, E l Haj Chehadeh S, et al. HLA repertoire of 115 UAE nationals infected with SARS-CoV-2. Hum Immunol 2021;S0198−8859(21). 00211-1.

[12] Sylvester-Hvid C, Morten N, Lamberth K, Røder G, Justesen S, Lundegaard C, et al. SARS CTL vaccine candidates;HLA supertype-, genome-wide scanning and biochemical validation. Tissue Antigens 2004;63(5):395−400.

[13] Liu J, Wu P, Gao F, Qi J, Kawana-Tachikawa A, Xie J, et al. Novel immunodominant peptide presentation strategy: a featured HLA-A*2402-restricted cytotoxic T-lymphocyte epitope stabilized by intrachain hydrogen bonds from Severe Acute Respiratory Coronavirus nucleocapsid protein. J Virol 2010;84(22):11849−57.

[14] Warren RL, Birol I. HLA predictions from the bronchoalveolar lavage fluid and blood samples of eight COVID-19 patients at the pandemic onset. Bioinform 2021;36(21):5271−3.

[15] Novelli A, Andreani M, Biancolella M, Liberatoscioli L, Passarelli C, Colona VL, et al. HLA allele frequencies and susceptibility to COVID-19 in a group of 99 Italian patients. HLA 2020;96(5):610−4.

[16] Tavasolian F, Rashidi M, Hatam GR, Jeddi M, Hosseini AZ, Mosawi SH, et al. HLA, immune response, and susceptibility to COVID-19. Front Immunol 2021;11:601886.

[17] Nguyen A, David JK, Maden SK, Wood MA, Weeder BR, Nellore A, et al. Human leukocyte antigen susceptibility map for severe acute respiratory syndrome coronavirus 2. J Virol 2020;94(13):e00510−20.

[18] Lin M, Tseng HK, Trejaut JA, Lee HL, Loo JH, Chu CC, et al. Association of HLA class I with severe acute respiratory syndrome coronavirus infection. BMC Med Genet 2003;4:9.

[19] Ng MH, Lau KM, Li L, Cheng SH, Chan WY, Hui PK, et al. Association of human-leukocyte-antigen class I (B*0703) and class II (DRB1*0301) genotypes with susceptibility and resistance to the development of severe acute respiratory syndrome. J Infect Dis 2004;190(3):515−8.

[20] Alicia SM. HLA studies in the context of coronavirus outbreaks. Swiss Med Wkly 2020;150:w20248.

[21] Keicho N, Itoyama S, Kashiwase K, Phi NC, Long HT, Ha LD, et al. Association of human leukocyte antigen class II alleles with severe acute respiratory syndrome in the Vietnamese population. Hum Immunol 2009;70(7):527−31.

[22] Campbell KM, Steiner G, Wells DK, Ribas A, Kalbasi A. Prioritization of SARS-CoV-2 epitopes using a pan-HLA and global population inference approach. BioRxiv [Preprint] June 29, 2020. https://doi.org/10.1101/2020.03.30.016931.

[23] La Porta CA, Zapperi S. Estimating the binding of Sars-CoV-2 peptides to HLA class I in human subpopulations using artificial neural networks. Cell Syst 2020;11:412−7.

[24] Jurtz V, Paul S, Andreatta M, Marcatili P, Peters B, Nielsen M. NetMHCpan-4.0: improved peptide−MHC class I interaction predictions integrating eluted ligand and peptide binding affinity data. J Immunol 2017;199(9):3360−8.

[25] O'Donnell TJ, Rubinsteyn A, Bonsack M, Riemer AB, Laserson U, Hammerbacher J. MHCflurry: open-source class I MHC binding affinity prediction. Cell Syst 2018;7(1):129−32.

[26] Trolle T, Nielsen M. NetTepi: an integrated method for the prediction of T cell epitopes. Immunogenetics 2014;66(7−8):449−56.

[27] Chakravarty S. COVID-19: the effect of host genetic variations on host − virus interactions. J Proteome Res 2021;20(1):139−53.

[28] Atyeo C, Fischinger S, Zohar T, Slein MD, Burke J, Loos C, et al. Distinct early serological signatures track with SARS-CoV-2 survival. Immunity 2020;53:524−32.

[29] Kaneko N, Kuo HH, Boucau J, Farmer JR, Allard-Chamard H, Mahajan VS, et al. Loss of Bcl-6-expressing T follicular helper cells and germinal centers in COVID-19. Cell 2020;183:1−15.

[30] Kuri-Cervantes L, Pampena MB, Meng W, Rosenfeld AM, Ittner CA, Weisman AR, et al. Comprehensive mapping of immune perturbations associated with severe COVID-19. Sci Immunol 2020;5:eabd7114.

[31] Laing AG, Lorenc A, del Molino del Barrio I, Das A, Fish M, Monin L, et al. A dynamic COVID-19 immune signature includes associations with poor prognosis. Nat Med 2020;26:1623−35.

[32] Lucas C, Wong P, Klein J, Castro TB, Silva J, Sundaram M, et al. Longitudinal analyses reveal immunological misfiring in severe COVID-19. Nature 2020;584:463−9.

[33] Mathew D, Giles JR, Baxter AE, Oldridge DA, Greenplate AR, Wu JE, et al. Deep immune profiling of COVID-19 patients reveals distinct immunotypes with therapeutic implications. Science 2020;369:eabc8511.

[34] Woodruff MC, Ramonell RP, Cashman KS, Nguyen DC, Saini AS, Haddad NS, et al. Extrafollicular B cell responses correlate with neutralizing antibodies and morbidity in COVID-19. Nat Immunol 2020;21:1506−16.

[35] Rodríguez Y, Novelli L, Rojas M, De Santis M, Acosta-Ampudia Y, Monsalve DM, et al. Autoinflammatory and autoimmune conditions at the crossroad of COVID-19. J Autoimmun 2020;114:102506.
[36] Cavalli E, Bramanti A, Ciurleo R, Tchorbanov AI, Giordano A, Fagone P, et al. Entangling COVID-19 associated thrombosis into a secondary antiphospholipid antibody syndrome: diagnostic and therapeutic perspectives (Review). Int J Mol Med 2020;46(3):903–12.
[37] Lucchese G. Cerebrospinal fluid findings in COVID-19 indicate autoimmunity. Lancet Microbe 2020;1:e242.
[38] Bastard P, Rosen LB, Zhang Q, Michailidis E, Hoffmann HH, Zhang Y, et al. Autoantibodies against type I IFNs in patients with life-threatening COVID-19. Science 2020;370. eabd4585.
[39] Uppal NN, Kello N, Shah HH, Khanin Y, De Oleo IR, Epstein E, et al. De novo ANCA-associated vasculitis with glomerulonephritis in COVID-19. Kidney Int Rep 2020;5(11):2079–83.
[40] Ryabkova VA, Churilov LP, Shoenfeld Y. Influenza infection;SARS;MERS and COVID-19: cytokine storm—the common denominator and the lessons to be learned. Clin Immunol 2021;223. 108652.
[41] David P, Shoenfeld Y. The smell in COVID-19 infection: diagnostic opportunities. Isr Med Assoc J 2020;22(7):401–3.
[42] Cavalli E, Petralia MC, Basile MS, Bramanti A, Bramanti P, Nicoletti F, et al. Transcriptomic analysis of COVID19 lungs and bronchoalveolar lavage fluid samples reveals predominant B cell activation responses to infection. Int J Mol Med 2020;46(4):1266–73.
[43] Dotan A, Muller S, Kanduc D, David P, Halpert G, Shoenfeld Y. The SARS-CoV-2 as an instrumental trigger of autoimmunity. Autoimmun Rev 2021;20(4):102792.
[44] Ehrenfeld M, Tincani A, Andreoli L, Cattalini M, Greenbaum A, Kanduc D, et al. Covid-19 and autoimmunity. Autoimmun Rev 2020;8(19):102597.
[45] Halpert G, Shoenfeld Y. SARS-CoV-2, the autoimmune virus. Autoimmun Rev 2020;19(2):102695.
[46] Rojas M, Rodríguez Y, Monsalve DM, Acosta-Ampudia Y, Camacho B, Gallo JE, et al. Convalescent plasma in Covid-19: possible mechanisms of action. Autoimmun Rev 2020;19(7). 102554.
[47] Perricone C, Bartoloni E, Bursi R, Cafaro G, Guidelli GM, Shoenfeld Y, et al. COVID-19 as part of the hyperferritinemic syndromes: the role of iron depletion therapy. Immunol Res 2020;68(4):213–24.
[48] Shoenfeld Y. Corona (COVID-19) time musings: our involvement in COVID-19 pathogenesis;diagnosis;treatment and vaccine planning. Autoimmun Rev 2020;19(6):102538.
[49] Cappello F, Gammazza AM, Dieli F, de Macario EC, Macario AJ. Does SARS-CoV-2 trigger stress-induced autoimmunity by molecular mimicry? A hypothesis. J Clin Med 2020;9:2038.
[50] Kanduc D, Shoenfeld Y. On the molecular determinants of the SARS-CoV-2 attack. Clin Immunol 2020;215:108426.
[51] Kanduc D, Shoenfeld Y. Medical, genomic, and evolutionary aspects of the peptide sharing between pathogens, primates, and humans. Global Med Genet 2020;7:64–7.
[52] Kanduc D, Shoenfeld Y. Molecular mimicry between SARS-CoV-2 spike glycoprotein and mammalian proteomes: implications for the vaccine. Immunol Res 2020;68:310–3.
[53] Kanduc D. From anti-SARS-CoV-2 immune responses to COVID-19 via molecular mimicry. Antibodies 2020;9:33.
[54] Lucchese G, Flöel A. Molecular mimicry between SARS-CoV-2 and respiratory pacemaker neurons. Autoimmun Rev 2020;19:102556.
[55] Lucchese G, Flöel A. SARS-CoV-2 and Guillain-Barré syndrome: molecular mimicry with human heat shock proteins as potential pathogenic mechanism. Cell Stress Chaperones 2020;25:731–5.
[56] Angileri F, Legare S, Gammazza AM, de Macario EC, Macario AJ, Cappello F. Molecular mimicry may explain multi-organ damage in COVID-19. Autoimmun Rev 2020;19:102591.
[57] Vojdani A, Kharrazian D. Potential antigenic cross-reactivity between SARS-CoV-2 and human tissue with a possible link to an increase in autoimmune diseases. Clin Immunol 2020;217:108480.
[58] Lyons-Weiler J. Pathogenic priming likely contributes to serious and critical illness and mortality in COVID-19 via autoimmunity. J Transl Autoimmun 2020;3:100051.
[59] Adiguzel Y. Molecular mimicry between SARS-CoV-2 and human proteins. Autoimmun Rev 2021;20:102791.
[60] Adıgüzel Y. Molecular mimicry with Nsp11 protein of SARS-CoV-2 in individuals with HLA-B*15:01 allele. Turk J Immunol 2021;9(2):95–104.
[61] An H, Eun M, Yi J, Park J. CRESSP: a comprehensive pipeline for prediction of immunopathogenic SARS-CoV-2 epitopes using structural properties of proteins. Brief Bioinform 2022;23(2):bbac056.

[62] Matzaraki V, Kumar V, Wijmenga C, Zhernakova A. The MHC locus and genetic susceptibility to autoimmune and infectious diseases. Genome Biol 2017;18:76.

[63] Luo H, Chen Q, Chen J, Chen K, Shen X, Jian H. The nucleocapsid protein of SARS coronavirus has a high binding affinity to the human cellular heterogeneous nuclear ribonucleoprotein A1. FEBS (Fed Eur Biochem Soc) Lett 2005;579:2623–8.

[64] Pavel A, del Giudice G, Federico A, Di Lieto A, Kinaret PAS, Serra A, et al. Integrated network analysis reveals new genes suggesting COVID-19 chronic effects and treatment. Briefings Bioinf 2021;22(2):1430–41.

[65] Geyer PE, Arend FM, Doll S, Louiset ML, Winter SV, Müller-Reif JB, et al. High-resolution serum proteome trajectories in COVID-19 reveal patient-specific seroconversion. EMBO Mol Med 2021;13:e14167.

[66] Sharif-Askari NS, Sharif-Askari FS, Ahmed SBM, Hannawi S, Hamoudi R, Hamid Q, et al. Enhanced expression of autoantigens during SARS-CoV-2 viral infection. Front Immunol 2021;12:2271.

[67] Zuo Y, Yalavarthi S, Shi H, Gockman K, Zuo M, Madison JA, et al. Neutrophil extracellular traps in COVID-19. JCI Insight 2020;5(11):e138999.

[68] Roldan EQ, Biasiotto G, Magro P, Zanella I. The possible mechanisms of action of 4-aminoquinolines (chloroquine/hydroxychloroquine) against Sars-Cov-2 infection (COVID-19): a role for iron homeostasis? Pharmacol Res 2020;158:104904.

[69] Kaplan MJ, Radic M. Neutrophil extracellular traps (NETs): double-edged swords of innate immunity. J Immunol 2012;189(6):2689–95.

[70] Brinkmann V, Zychlinsky A. Neutrophil extracellular traps: is immunity the second function of chromatin? J Cell Biol 2012;198(5):773–83.

[71] Papayannopoulos V. Neutrophil extracellular traps in immunity and disease. Nature Reviews 2018;18:134–47.

[72] Vorobjeva NV, Chernyak BV. NETosis: molecular mechanisms, role in physiology and pathology. Biochemistry (Moscow) 2020;85(10):1178–90.

[73] Panda R, Krieger T, Hopf L, Renné T, Haag F, Röber N, et al. Neutrophil extracellular traps contain selected antigens of anti-neutrophil cytoplasmic antibodies. Front Immunol 2017;8:439.

[74] Brinkmann V. Neutrophil extracellular traps in the second decade. J Innate Immun 2018;10:414–21.

[75] Petretto A, Bruschi M, Pratesi F, Croia C, Candiano G, Ghiggeri G, et al. Neutrophil extracellular traps (NET) induced by different stimuli: a comparative proteomic analysis. PLoS One 2019;14(7):e0218946.

[76] Yipp BG, Kubes P. NETosis: how vital is it? Blood 2013;122(16):2784–94.

[77] Yaqinuddin A, Kvietys P, Kashir J. Role of neutrophil extracellular traps in acute lung injury. Respir Investig 2020;58:419–20.

[78] Leppkes M, Knopf J, Naschberger E, Lindemann A, Singh J, Hermann I, et al. Vascular occlusion by neutrophil extracellular traps in COVID-19. EBioMedicine 2020;58:102925.

[79] Tomar B, Anders HJ, Desai J, Mulay SR. Neutrophils and neutrophil extracellular traps drive necroinflammation in COVID-19. Cells 2020;9:1383.

[80] Sawadogo SA, Dighero-Kemp B, Ouédraogo DD, Hensley L, Sakandé J. How NETosis could drive "post COVID-19 syndrome" among survivors. Immunol Lett 2020;228:35–7.

[81] Guéant JL, Fromonot J, Guéant-Rodriguez RM, Lacolley P, Guieu R, Regnault V. Blood myeloperoxidase-DNA, a biomarker of early response to SARS-CoV-2 infection. Allergy 2020;76(3):893–6.

[82] Guéant JL, Rodriguez-Gueant RM, Fromonot J, Oussalah A, Louis H, Chery C, et al. Elastase and exacerbation of neutrophil innate immunity are involved in multi- visceral manifestations of COVID- 19. Allergy 2021;76(6):1846–58.

[83] Rosa BA, Ahmed M, Singh DK, Choreño-Parra JA, Cole J, Jiménez-Álvarez LA, et al. IFN signaling and neutrophil degranulation transcriptional signatures are induced during SARS-CoV-2 infection. Commun Biol 2021;4:290.

[84] Akgun E, Tuzuner MB, Sahin B, Kilercik M, Kulah C, Cakiroglu HN, et al. Proteins associated with neutrophil degranulation are upregulated in nasopharyngeal swabs from SARS-CoV-2 patients. PLoS One 2020;15(10):e0240012.

[85] Bruschi M, Petretto A, Santucci L, Vaglio A, Pratesi F, Migliorini P, et al. Neutrophil extracellular traps protein composition is specific for patients with Lupus nephritis and includes methyl-oxidized αenolase (methionine sulfoxide 93). Sci Rep 2019;9:7934.

[86] The UniProt Consortium. UniProt: a worldwide hub of protein knowledge. Nucleic Acids Res 2019;47:D506–15.

[87] NCBI Resource Coordinators. Database resources of the national center for biotechnology information. Nucleic Acids Res 2017;46:D8–13.
[88] Altschul SF, Madden TL, Schäffer AA, Zhang J, Zhang Z, Miller W, et al. Gapped BLAST and PSI-BLAST: a new generation of protein database search programs. Nucleic Acids Res 1997;25:3389–402.
[89] Karosiene E, Lundegaard C, Lund O, Nielsen M. NetMHCcons: a consensus method for the major histocompatibility complex class I predictions. Immunogenetics 2012;64(3):177–86.
[90] Andreatta M, Nielsen M. Gapped sequence alignment using artificial neural networks: application to the MHC class I system. Bioinformatics 2016;32(4):511–7.
[91] Nielsen M, Lundegaard C, Worning P, Lauemoller SL, Lamberth K, Buus S, et al. Reliable prediction of T-cell epitopes using neural networks with novel sequence representations. Protein Sci 2003;12:1007–17.
[92] Zhang H, Lund O, Nielsen M. The PickPocket method for predicting binding specificities for receptors based on receptor pocket similarities: application to MHC-peptide binding. Bioinformatics 2009;25(10):1293–9.
[93] Reynisson B, Alvarez B, Paul S, Peters B, Nielsen M. NetMHCpan-4.1 and NetMHCIIpan-4.0: improved predictions of MHC antigen presentation by concurrent motif deconvolution and integration of MS MHC eluted ligand data. Nucleic Acids Res 2020;48(W1):W449–54.
[94] Stranzl T, Larsen MV, Lundegaard C, Nielsen M. NetCTLpan. Pan-specific MHC class I pathway epitope predictions. Immunogenetics 2020;62(6):357–68.
[95] Larsen MV, Lundegaard C, Lamberth K, Buus S, Lund O, Nielsen M. Large-scale validation of methods for cytotoxic T-lymphocyte epitope prediction. BMC Bioinf 2007;8:424.
[96] Brown GR, Hem V, Katz KS, Ovetsky M, Wallin C, Ermolaeva O, et al. Gene: a gene-centered information resource at NCBI. Nucleic Acids Res 2015;43:D36–42.
[97] Rappaport S, Fishilevich S, Nudel R, Twik M, Belinky F, Plaschkes I, et al. Rational confederation of genes and diseases: NGS interpretation via GeneCards, MalaCards and VarElect. Biomed Eng Online 2017;16:72.
[98] Rappaport N, Twik M, Plaschkes I, Nudel R, Iny Stein T, Levitt J, et al. MalaCards: an amalgamated human disease compendium with diverse clinical and genetic annotation and structured search. Nucleic Acids Res 2017;45:D877–87.
[99] Belinky F, Nativ N, Stelzer G, Zimmerman S, Iny Stein T, Safran M, et al. PathCards: multi-source consolidation of human biological pathways. Database 2015;2015:bav006.
[100] Stelzer G, Rosen R, Plaschkes I, Zimmerman S, Twik M, Fishilevich S, et al. The GeneCards suite: from gene data mining to disease genome sequence analysis. Curr Protoc Bioinform 2016;54. 1.30.1–1.30.33.
[101] Shannon P, Markiel A, Ozier O, Baliga NS, Wang JT, Ramage D, et al. Cytoscape: a software environment for integrated models of biomolecular interaction networks. Genome Res 2003;13(11):2498–504.
[102] Nie X, Qian L, Sun R, Huang B, Dong X, Xiao Q, et al. Multi-organ proteomic landscape of COVID-19 autopsies. Cell 2021;184(3):775–91.
[103] Nie X, Qian L, Sun R, Huang B, Dong X, Xiao Q, et al. Multi-organ proteomic landscape of COVID-19 autopsies. Cell 2021;184:775–91.
[104] Malaquias MAS, Gadotti AC, Motta-Junior JDS, Martins APC, Azevedo MLV, Benevides APK, et al. The role of the lectin pathway of the complement system in SARS-CoV-2 lung injury. Transl Res 2021;231:55–63.
[105] Adiguzel Y. Peptides of *H. sapiens* and P. falciparum that are predicted to bind strongly to HLA-A*24:02 and homologous to a SARS-CoV-2 peptide. Acta Trop 2021;221:106013.
[106] Katayama M, Ota K, Nagi-Miura N, Ohno N, Yabuta N, Nojima H, et al. Ficolin-1 is a promising therapeutic target for autoimmune diseases. Int Immunol 2018;31(1):23–32.
[107] Anastasia P, Sofia G, Linda K, Steven S. Does the lectin complement pathway link Kawasaki Disease and SARS-CoV-2. Front Immunol 2021;11:3674.
[108] Bamberger C, Pankow S, Martínez-Bartolomé S, Diedrich J, Park R, Yates III J. The host interactome of spike expands the tropism of SARS-CoV-2. BioRxiv [Preprint] February 16, 2021. https://doi.org/10.1101/2021.02.16.431318.
[109] Lu C, Amin MA, Fox DA. CD13/Aminopeptidase N is a potential therapeutic target for inflammatory disorders. J Immunol 2020;204(1):3–11.
[110] Nomura R, Kiyota A, Suzaki E, Kataoka K, Ohe Y, Miyamoto K, et al. Human coronavirus 229E binds to CD13 in rafts and enters the cell through caveolae. J Virol 2004;78(16):8701–8.

[111] Tsou E, Sule G, Gurrea Rubio M, Amin M, Zuo Y, Knight J, et al. Identification of CD13 as a potential cause for SARS-CoV-2-triggered hyperinflammation and thrombosis [abstract]. Arthritis Rheumatol 2020;72(Suppl. 10).

[112] Lowes H, Robertson F, Pyle A, Hussain R, Coxhead J, Yarnall AJ, et al. The human coronavirus receptor ANPEP (CD13) is overexpressed in Parkinson's Disease. Mov Disord 2020;35(12):2134–6.

[113] Peyneau M, Granger V, Wicky PH, Khelifi-Touhami D, Timsit JF, Lescure FX, et al. Innate immune deficiencies in patients with COVID-19. MedRxiv [Preprint] March 31, 2021. https://doi.org/10.1101/2021.03.29.21254560.

[114] Gebremeskel S, Schanin J, Coyle KM, Butuci M, Luu T, Brock EC, et al. Mast cell and eosinophil activation are associated with COVID-19 and TLR-mediated viral inflammation: implications for an anti-Siglec-8 antibody. Front Immunol 2021;12:641.

[115] Buckley PR, Lee CH, Pereira Pinho M, Ottakandathil Babu R, Woo J, Antanaviciute A, et al. HLA-dependent variation in SARS-CoV-2 CD8+ T cell cross-reactivity with human coronaviruses. Immunology 2022;166(1):78–103.

[116] Wang JY, Zhang W, Roehrl VB, Roehrl MW, Roehrl MH. An autoantigen atlas from human lung HFL1 cells offers clues to neurological and diverse autoimmune manifestations of COVID-19. Front Immunol 2022;13:831849.

[117] Wang JY, Zhang W, Roehrl MW, Roehrl VB, Roehrl MH. An Autoantigen-ome from HS-Sultan B-Lymphoblasts offers a molecular map for investigating autoimmune sequelae of COVID-19. BioRxiv [Preprint] April 6, 2021. https://doi.org/10.1101/2021.04.05.438500.

[118] Wang JY, Zhang W, Roehrl MW, Roehrl VB, Roehrl MH. An autoantigen profile of human A549 lung cells reveals viral and host etiologic molecular attributes of autoimmunity in COVID-19. J Autoimmun 2021;120:102644.

[119] Wang JY, Roehrl MW, Roehrl VB, Roehrl MH. A master autoantigen-ome links alternative splicing, female predilection, and COVID-19 to autoimmune diseases. J Transl Autoimmun 2022;5:100147.

[120] Jensen KK, Andreatta M, Marcatili P, Buus S, Greenbaum JA, Yan Z, et al. Improved methods for predicting peptide binding affinity to MHC class II molecules. Immunology 2018;154:394–406.

[121] Baum H. Mitochondrial antigens, molecular mimicry and autoimmune disease. Biochim Biophys Acta 1995;1271:111–21.

[122] Adiguzel Y. Adiguzel-Shoenfeld_Dataset1. Mendeley Data; 2021. V1.x.

CHAPTER

10

COVID-19 and the hyperferritinemic syndromes

G. Zandman-Goddard and M. Tocut

Department of Internal Medicine C, Wolfson Medical Center; Sackler Faculty of Medicine, Tel Aviv University, Tel Aviv, Israel

Elevated serum ferritin levels in inflammatory processes are due to release from damaged tissues, increased synthesis, or decreased clearance. H-ferritin has an immunomodulatory function and pro-inflammatory activity leading to the induction and expression of IL-1β.

Ferritin synthesis by hepatocytes is induced by IL-1, IL-6, and TNF-a. Ferritin may be secreted by hepatocytes and also macrophages. Macrophage activation could actively contribute to ferritin production. Ferritin may be an early marker of inflammatory reactions.

Underlying conditions in hyperferritinemia without an associated iron overload include metabolic syndrome and obesity, insulin resistance/diabetes mellitus, excessive alcohol consumption, inflammatory and infectious conditions (septic shock, COVID-19), malignancy (solid and hematological), and benign hyperferritinemia. Importantly, patients with immune-mediated syndromes (primary and secondary hemophagocytic histiocytosis-HLH, Adult-Onset Still's Disease-AOSD) and autoimmune diseases may have high levels of ferritin [1,2].

In a previous study of ours, we evaluated 403 patients for hyperferritinemia in various autoimmune diseases. Elevated titers of ferritin were found in 23% of SLE patients, 15% of patients with dermatomyositis, 8% of multiple sclerosis patients, and 4% of rheumatoid arthritis patients [3]. Elevated levels were also associated with SLE disease severity [4].

Some diseases are characterized by very elevated ferritin levels and have been termed as the hyperferritinemic syndromes. The hyperferritinemic syndromes include macrophage activation syndrome (MAS), AOSD, catastrophic antiphospholipid syndrome (CAPS), and septic shock. All these entities are associated with elevated levels of ferritin and life-threatening disease due to a cytokine storm leading to multiorgan failure. These diseases respond to similar therapies: corticosteroids, intravenous immunoglobulin-IVIG, plasma exchange, and biologics [5].

Autoimmunity, COVID-19, Post-COVID19 syndrome and COVID-19 vaccination
https://doi.org/10.1016/B978-0-443-18566-3.00035-9

MAS is a life-threatening complication of inflammatory/autoimmune diseases. A secondary form is also known as familial hemophagocytic histiocytosis (FHLH). The syndrome is characterized by activation of macrophages in the spleen, bone marrow, and lymph nodes. MAS may occur in patients with autoimmune diseases or can mimic the onset of an autoimmune disease. For example, one study investigated the prediction of MAS in 75 childhood SLE (cSLE) patients. Elevated ferritin levels (>699 mg/dL) were the best sole discriminator between MAS and non-MAS patients. This diagnostic marker improved sensitivity and specificity [6]. The benefit of evaluating ferritin levels as a marker for secondary MAS was confirmed in other studies. Elevated ferritin levels (>627 mg/L) provided 89% specificity and 95% sensitivity. Fever and elevated ferritin levels (>500 mg/L) decreased time to diagnosis from 8.4 to 2.8 days. A significant reduction in mortality rates (25%–6.7%) was demonstrated with the early initiation of treatment [7]. Secondary MAS requires additional treatment including: IVIG, anakinra (anti IL-1 antibody), and calcineurin inhibitors.

Severe COVID-19 is characterized by an immune dysregulation leading to the development of a cytokine storm and not as a direct result of viral infection. A cytokine storm is present in the setting of an elevation in circulating cytokines, systemic inflammatory symptoms, and secondary organ failure (renal/hepatic). Many different etiologies may lead to the development of a cytokine storm: autoimmune diseases, auto-inflammatory disorders, secondary MAS, iatrogenic, and pathogen-induced-COVID-19 [8].

The cytokine storm appears during the third phase of COVID-19 infection. Activation of the storm may also originate within the lungs. The cytokine release is similar to what is described in the hyperferritinemic syndromes and is the result of overstimulation of the immune system, release of the pro-inflammatory cytokines, IL-1 and interferon (IFN), which further lead to a cascade of inflammation. The successive occurrences of acute lung injury, abnormal alterations in vascular hemostasis, and cytokine-mediated tissue damage can eventually result in mortality. Viral infection can induce antiviral responses in neighboring cells as well as recruit innate and adaptive immune cells: Macrophages, dendritic cells, T cells, B cells, and NK cells lead to self-amplifying inflammatory cascade in a positive feedback loop manner [9].

Hyperferritinemia, molecular, and epigenetic factors contribute to the evolution of COVID-19 infection and an exaggerated inflammatory response [10–12].

Furthermore, patients with COVID-19 may develop multisystem inflammatory syndrome (MIS). MIS is more common in children (MIS-C) while it has also been reported but less often in adults (MIS-A). MIS does not follow severe disease as in MAS. Lymphopenia and thromboembolic events are more common. MIS is characterized by a distinct genetic signature that is overexpressed leading to the upregulation of IL-1B, CASP1, IL-10, slow down-regulation of TLR8, NOD9, and down-regulation of IL-6, FOXP3, perforin, and IFN-I inducible genes. It may be difficult to differentiate MAS from MIS because they may share in common clinical and laboratory findings. The clinical manifestations are persistent fever and multiorgan involvement. The shared laboratory findings are hyperferritinemia, pancytopenia, lymphopenia, and hypercoagulopathy. However, MAS follows severe disease, is an entity that develops in autoimmune diseases, infections, and malignancy, and is defined by a different cytokine profile.

Therapy for severe COVID-19 is yet to be established. Corticosteroids are beneficial while anticytokine treatment remains controversial. Treatment with IVIG can lead to normalization of gene signaling expression.

Hyperferritinemia may predict the outcome of COVID-19 patients in the ICU. One study investigated ferritin levels in 100 intensive care unit (ICU) patients with COVID-19 pneumonia. The patients were divided into three groups according to disease severity: moderate (n-17), severe (n-40), and critical (n-43). Ferritin levels were evaluated with other markers and cytokines: IL-6, IL-8, IL-10, TNF-α, CRP. Ferritin levels were highest in the critical patients. The median ferritin level was 3.4 times higher in patients who died compared to those that survived. Hyperferritinemia was an independent predictor of in-hospital mortality ($P = .013$). High ferritin levels were a better predictor of mortality than CRP and procalcitonin. Other studies confirm that hyperferritinemia is associated with mortality. The average concentration of ferritin in severe cases was 800 mg/L. The ferritin level in nonsurvivors was 1400 mg/L. The combination of ferritin levels and CRP may provide better results in the prediction of in-hospital mortality [13].

COVID-19 severity is associated with a rapid onset of respiratory failure and the need for assisted ventilation. Consecutive ferritin levels may predict the need for ventilation support. The aim of one longitudinal study was to determine the need for ventilation support in 269 COVID-19 patients, utilizing consecutive measurement of ferritin and CRP levels over 28 days. The investigators evaluated the daily degree of hyperinflammation (HI) to the escalation of the patient status and requirement for mechanical ventilation. HI included ferritin >1500 mg/L and an elevated CRP that doubled during hospitalization. HI started to develop 5 days before ventilatory support, and the majority of patients (74%) requiring respiratory support met the criteria of HI [14].

One of the many questions that remain is whether therapies for hyperferritinemic syndromes are also beneficial for severe COVID-19 patients. As in the hyperferritinemic syndrome, IVIG may be beneficial and lead to a reduction in ferritin levels. Specific IVIG (sIVIG)-immunoglobulins derived from patients that have recovered from COVID-19 and specific and concentrated IVIG (scIVIG)-specific anti-COVID-19 antibodies derived from immunoglobulins from recovered corona infection patients may be beneficial in COVID-19 cytokine storm [15]. IL-6 inhibition with IV tocilizumab (Actemra) used in CAPS and HLH remains controversial as therapy for severe COVID-19. Other potential therapeutic targets to control cytokines storms in COVID-19 are as follows: JAK inhibitor (baricitinib), IFN-γ inhibitor, TNF-α inhibitor, colchicine, blood purification therapy, and stem cell therapy. Perhaps, a combination of antiviral and antiinflammatory therapy for severe COVID-19 will be the most effective [16].

In conclusion, severe COVID-19 disease should be included in the hyperferritinemic syndromes because it is a distinct entity to those that have been previously described. Elevated ferritin levels are associated with the hyperinflammatory mechanisms of COVID-19 disease. Escalating concentrations of ferritin may be a marker for rapidly worsening of COVID-19 disease and the need for assisted ventilation. Meanwhile, the impact of various therapies (steroids, IVIG, IL-6 and IL-I inhibitors, and IFNγ inhibitors) is yet to be established.

References

[1] Sandnes M, Ulvik RJ, Vorland M, Reikvam H. Hyperferritinemia- A clinical overview. J Clin Med 2021;10:2008.
[2] Zandman-Goddard G, Shoenfeld Y. Ferritin in autoimmune diseases. Autoimmun Rev 2007;6:457–63.
[3] Orbach H, Zandman-Goddard G, Amital H, Barak V, Szekanecz Z, Szucs G, et al. Novel biomarkers in autoimmune diseases. Ann NY Acad Sci 2007;1109:385–400.
[4] Zandman-Goddard G, Shoenfeld Y. Hyperferritinemia in autoimmunity. Isr Med Assoc J 2008;10:83–4.
[5] Rosaria C, Zandman-Goddard G, Meyron-Holtz EG, D'Cruz DP, Shoenfeld Y. The hyperferritinemic syndrome. BMC Med 2013;11:185.
[6] Gerstein M, Borgia RE, Dominguez D, Feldman BM, Liao F, Levy DM, et al. Predicting MAS in childhood SLE patients at diagnosis. J Rheumatol 2021;48:1450–7.
[7] Smitherman EA, Cron RQ. Hyperferritinemia wins again. J Rheumatol 2021;48:1355–7.
[8] Faigenbaum DC, June CH. Cytokine storm. N Engl J Med 2020;383:2252–73.
[9] Tang L, Yin Z, Hu Y, Mei H. Controlling the cytokine storm is vital in COVID-19. Front Immunol 2020;11:570993.
[10] Colafrancesco S, Allessandri C, Conti F, Priori R. COVID-19 gone bad: a new character in the spectrum of the hyperferritinemic syndrome? Autoimmun Rev 2020;19:1–5.
[11] Mahroum N, Alghory KZ, Alwani A, Seida R, Alrais M, Shoenfeld Y. Ferritin-from iron, through inflammation and autoimmunity, to COVID-19. J Autoimmun 2022;126:102778.
[12] Qin C, Zhou L, Hu Z, Zhang S, Yang S, Tao Y, et al. Dysregulation of immune response in patients with coronavirus 2019 (COVID-19) in Wuhan, China. Clin Infect Dis 2020;71:762–8.
[13] Deng F, Zhang L, Lyu L, Lu Z, Gao D, Ma X, et al. Increased levels of ferritin on admission predicts ICU mortality in patients with COVID-19. Med Clin 2021;156:324–31.
[14] Manson JJ, Crooks C, Naja M, Ledlie A, Goulden B, Liddle T, et al. COVID-19-associated hyperinflammation and escalation of patient care. Lancet Rheumatol 2020;2:e594–602.
[15] Danieli MG, Piga MA, Paladini A, Longhi E, Mezzanotte C, Moroncini G, Shoenfeld Y. Intravenous immunoglobulin as an important adjunct in the prevention and therapy of coronavirus 2019 disease. Scand J Immunol 2021;94:e13101.
[16] Ruscitti P, Berardicurti O, Di Benedetto P, Ciprani P, Iagnocco A, Shoenfeld Y, et al. Severe COVID-19, another piece in the puzzle of the hyperferritinemic syndrome. Front Immunol 2020;11:1130.

CHAPTER

11

SARS-CoV-2 and microbiome: pathology, implications and therapeutic options

Maria V. Sankova[1], *Vladimir N. Nikolenko*[1,2], *Sergey V. Sankov*[1] and *Mikhail Y. Sinelnikov*[1,3,4]

[1]First Moscow State Medical University named after I.M. Sechenov (Sechenov University), Moscow, Russia; [2]Lomonosov Moscow State University, Moscow, Russia; [3]Research Institute of Human Morphology, Moscow, Russia; [4]Russian Scientific Centre of Surgery named after academician B.V. Petrovsky, Moscow, Russia

The ongoing SARS-CoV-2 pandemic has strained healthcare systems worldwide. The multidisciplinary approach to the treatment of COVID-19 is currently the most supported. Within this approach, special attention is directed toward the microbiome and it's role in the formation of local barrier immunity. Most of the body's immune responses are carried out at the level of mucous membranes and mucosa-associated lymphoid tissue (MALT). These structures constantly interact with pathogenic microorganisms and serve as the first line of defense against invading pathogens [1]. The most significant place in this structured system of organic barriers is occupied by the intestines, which represent the largest area of contact with the external environment and contain nearly 80% of all immunocompetent cells [2,3]. One of the main components of its natural defense is the normal intestinal microbiota, the total number of different microorganisms which reach over 10^{15}, which is almost twice the number of the body's own cells [4,5]. The qualitative and quantitative composition of the natural intestinal microbiome is relatively stable: for example, 90% of all intestinal inhabitants are considered the "main microflora", represented by anaerobic bacteria of the genera Bifidobacterium and Bacteroides; 10% is made up of associated microflora, which consists mainly of aerobic bacteria: lactobacilli, *Escherichia coli*, enterococci, etc.; about 0.01% is represented by transient microflora, including random types of microorganisms, among which are clostridia, staphylococci, proteus, viruses, fungi, and others [6,7].

Autoimmunity, COVID-19, Post-COVID19 syndrome and COVID-19 vaccination
https://doi.org/10.1016/B978-0-443-18566-3.00023-2

The microbiome, intestinal ecosystem, and immunoresistance: uniquely balanced

The spatial interaction between the intestinal microbiota and intestinal immune cells has a special organization that supports the action of both innate and acquired defense reactions (Fig. 11.1). The first layer facing the intestinal lumen consists mainly of mucus and can be divided into an outer, less dense, sublayer abundantly populated with commensals, and an inner sublayer containing high concentrations of antimicrobial peptides and secretory immunoglobulin-A (IgA), which makes it virtually impermeable to pathogenic microorganisms [8]. An important role of the intestinal microbiota located directly within the intestinal lumen is to increase colonization resistance due to the production of lactic acid, bacteriocins, hydrogen peroxide, lysozymes, antibiotics, and other antimicrobial factors that prevent adhesion, growth, and invasion of opportunistic flora [9,10].

The second level of defense is represented by a monolayer of intestinal epithelial cells originating from temporarily amplified cells, which in turn give rise to undifferentiated stem cells [11,12]. The goblet cells located here produce mucin, which prevents the invasion of pathogens, and local neuroendocrine cells regulate intestinal motility, acidity, digestion, the blood supply to the mucous membrane, and cell proliferation [13–15]. According to the latest data, normal microbiota can influence the secretory function of these cells and control intestinal metabolism [14,16–18]. Paneth cells play a special protective role in this layer, by creating within the intestinal lumen high concentrations of antimicrobial peptides lysozymes, α-defensins, RegIIIβ and RegIIIγ lectins, secretory phospholipase A2, angiogenin four, and α1-antitrypsin [19].

Intestinal immune cells

A very important cell type, which is present at the level of the epithelial layer is the specific microfold Multifold cells or M-cells. Their main function is the controlled transfer of antigen material of the intestinal microbiota from the intestinal lumen via transcytosis to macrophages, dendritic cells, and T- and B-lymphocytes. By realizing this function, they regulate cellular and humoral immune response mechanisms. Due to a thin glycocalyx, they actively absorb the apical surface of macromolecules, transport them as endosomes through their cytoplasm and, through exocytosis, hand them over to immunocompetent cells located both in the pockets of M-cells and in isolated lymphoid nodules and Peyer's patches located in the lamina propria and related to the third layer of the intestinal wall [20]. The presence of commensals promotes the synthesis and accumulation of prointerline-1 and prointerlein-18 in macrophages, which significantly accelerate immune response to pathogens [21,22]. It was found that constant presentation of microflora particles to cells of innate immunity promotes the development of barrier immunity and the maintenance of the immune system in a state of initial activation, which allows, if necessary, to effectively and quickly respond to aggression [8,23,24].

Activated B-lymphocytes differentiate into plasma cells, which produce IgA. When passing through epithelial cells, IgA attaches a secretory component that protects it from proteolysis, allowing it to emerge on the surface of mucous membranes in the form of secretory

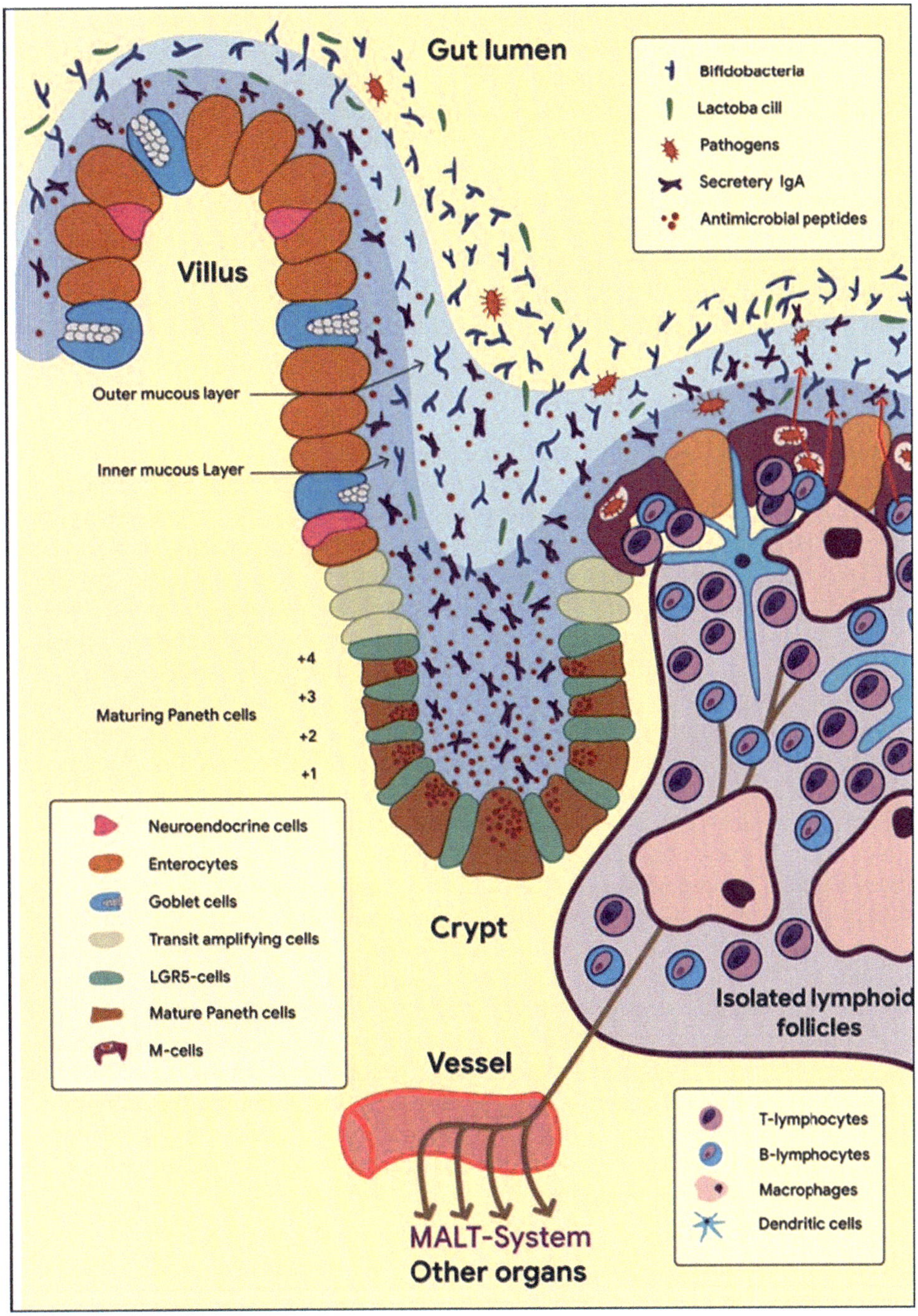

FIGURE 11.1 Spatial interaction between the intestinal microbiota and intestinal immune cells. The normal microflora, located within the intestinal lumen exerts direct antipathogenic activity, increasing the colonization defense mechanisms. It can also be seen constantly stimulating immunocompetent cells at different levels and, thus, maintaining the MALT-system in a readiness state for a quick response to the invasion of all pathogens, including RNA-containing viruses, including SARS-CoV-2.

immunoglobulin-A (sIgA), providing local antibacterial and antiviral protection. The antiinflammatory effect of sIgA is realized due to the inactivation of phagocyte chemotaxis and inhibition of proinflammatory cytokine synthesis [7]. Both B- and T-lymphocytes of MALT initiate acquired immunity and are closely associated with regional lymphatic formations, in which the immune response becomes generalized. MALT lymphocytes continuously migrate from one compartment of the mucosal immune system to another (homing effect), creating simultaneous activations of immune response in all mucous surfaces, regardless of the localization of the antigenic stimulus, and thereby providing global protection of all barrier tissues [21,25–28]. Evidence of the effects of intestinal microbiota on general immunological reactivity is seen by the ability of variable bacteria of the normal flora to enhance the immunogenicity of vaccines by specific stimulation of antibody formation [29,30].

Signal pattern recognizing receptors

The biological material of symbionts is well recognized by specific signal Pattern Recognizing Receptors - sPRR (Toll-like and Nod-like receptors), expressed by intestinal epithelial cells, Paneth cells and innate immune cells [19]. This close interaction is necessary for stimulation of mucus production, antimicrobial peptides, and secretory IgA, and for tightening intercellular contacts and reducing the permeability of the intestinal epithelial layer [22,24,31]. The presence of normal intestinal microbiota is necessary to mediate the shift in T-helpers-2/T-helpers-1 ratio toward the latter, preventing the development of proallergenic reactions [32–34]. The antiinflammatory effect of intestinal microbiota is thereby realized through constant stimulation of commensal-specific regulatory T-lymphocytes (TRegs), producing the antiinflammatory cytokine - interleukin-10 [22,35–37]. More so, there is evidence that polysaccharides of anaerobic bacteria, by binding to Toll-like receptors of innate immune cells, block their proinflammatory activity [38].

Constant stimulation of sPRR receptors by intestinal microbiota plays an important role in the formation of a local pool of T-helpers-17, which are responsible for the regulation of neutrophil activity via the MALT system and the process of switching antibody classes in B-lymphocytes [21,31,39]. It was found that obligate intestinal bacteria are involved in the promotion of immune response against viral infections, influencing the maturation of virus-specific CD4+ and CD8+ T-cell subpopulations [5,27,40,41]. Due to the phenomenon of molecular mimicry and the presence of receptors acquired from the host's epithelium, the microflora is capable of intercepting and excreting viruses with the appropriate ligands [6]. Thus, symbiotic microorganisms increase the colonization resistance of intestinal mucosa and carry out direct antipathogenic activity [5,40,42,43]. Strengthening the antiviral response and increasing resistance to viral infections is especially important in the pathogenesis of the SARS-CoV-2 infection during the ongoing pandemic in order to mediate an adequate immune response during the development of COVID-19 [44,45].

Microbiome functions

The **synthetic, metabolic, and homeostatic functions** of the microbiome, which affect the activity of all organs and systems, are of great importance in increasing the body's immunoresistance. Symbiotic commensals provide valuable vitamins (B1, B2, B3, B5, B6, B8, B9, B12, C, K), essential amino acids, and coenzymes (tocopherrols, b-alanine), which are necessary for metabolic reactions and maintaining homeostasis [6,46]. The microbiome's **secretion function** is realized by secreting hormones (estrogens), biologically active substances, and signaling molecules, the microbiome participates in the regulation of internal organ function and the central nervous system. Thus, γ-aminobutyric acid, produced by intestinal flora, is a vital neurotransmitter involved in central inhibition [47]. Organic acids obtained in the process of noral microbiota metabolism create an acidic environment in the intestine, which prevents the reproduction of pathogens and promotes better absorption of vitamin D, calcium, and iron [48].

The metabolic role of intestinal microbiota includes the fermentation of undigested food components, which is referred to as **symbiotic digestion** [Belizário JE, Faintuch J, Garay-Malpartida M., 2018]. Proteolytic microorganisms (Bacteroides, normal *Escherichia coli*) process proteins, and saccharolytic anaerobes (Bifidobacterium) aim for monosaccharide fragments, which, during subsequent fermentation, turn into low molecular weight fatty acids, the utilization of which in the Krebs cycle leads to the formation of a universal energy substrate for the heart, brain, kidneys, muscles and other tissues [49–51]. It has been proven that these short-chain fatty acids reduce inflammation, and stabilize glucose and blood lipids [51]. The obligate microflora of the large intestine provides the final hydrolysis of proteins, saponification of fats, and fermentation of high molecular weight carbohydrates that were not absorbed in the small intestine [49].

The intestinal microbiota promotes the **production of enzymes** involved in the metabolism of proteins, fats, carbohydrates, cholesterol, bile acids, and urea, which is of great importance in the maintenance of carbohydrate, lipid, and nitrogen metabolism [51–54]. More so, the microbiota is involved in the **inactivation of biologically active components**, in particular alkaline phosphatase, trypsin, and enterokinase [55]. Several representatives of normal microflora perform the **biotransformation function**, by transforming foreign substances - xenobiotics - into nontoxic products that are safely removed from the body. Symbionts are also capable of accumulating significant amounts of various exogenous toxins and metabolites, including nitrates, amines, phenols, histamine, mercaptan, mutagenic steroids, heavy metals, formaldehydes, and several poisons (**reservoir function**), thus protecting enterocytes and other organs from the effects of damaging factors and carcinogens [48,56].

Obligate microorganisms maintain optimal physicochemical homeostatic parameters in the intestinal epithelium, including differentiated pH values, redox potential, and rheological characteristics [2]. Importantly, they are involved in maintaining the ionic balance through active absorption of monocarboxylic acids, which are closely associated with the transport of sodium ions [57]. Methane-forming bacteria, using carbon dioxide and hydrogen for their metabolism, are involved in the regulation of gas formation, a vital aspect of normal intestinal homeostasis [6,58]. As can be seen, the normal intestinal microbiota functions as a unique ecosystem and a complex metabolic organ, which provides the required amount and profile of final metabolites for the macroorganism, neutralizes toxic exogenous and endogenous substrates, regulates the functioning of local organs and systems, maintaining its homeostasis and immunoresistance, which is of particular importance during the SARS-CoV-2 pandemic.

Gut microbiome dysbiosis and SARS-CoV-2

Intestinal dysbiosis is a syndrome characterized by persistent changes in the qualitative and/or quantitative composition of the intestinal microflora with the subsequent development of immunological and metabolic disorders [59,60]. The most significant reasons for the development of this condition include infectious diseases, surgical interventions, antibacterial and radiation therapy, and the use of hormones and cytostatics. Serious risk factors for intestinal dysbiosis are unbalanced and irregular nutrition, stresses of various origins, disturbed biorhythms, decreased immune status, and chronic diseases of internal organs [6,58,59,61]. Over 90% of the world's inhabitants, to 1° or another, suffer from dysbiosis [62,63], which is considered a pathogenetic link in the development of a variety of pathological processes in the human body [64]. During the SARS-CoV-2 pandemic, changes in physical activity and diet, together with the stress regarding the new coronavirus infection, lead to a sharp increase in local disturbances in the balance of intestinal microbiota [65,66].

Any dysbiotic changes in the intestinal microbiota lead to a decrease in the production of mucus, antimicrobial peptides, and secretory IgA. Following a steady decrease in the number of normal bacteria in the intestine, the colonization of mucous membranes by opportunistic flora increases [67]. Thinning of the protective barrier is accompanied by damage to enterocytes and increased intestinal permeability [68]. These changes are accompanied by a weakening of the MALT barrier function and the creation of conditions for the invasion of pathogens. Considering also that all MALT compartments are closely interconnected due to selective homing, an immune imbalance in one part of this system leads to the disruption of all the others [31].

Dysbiosis and immune modulation of microbiota

It has been shown that the health of intestinal microbiota affects the susceptibility to the new coronavirus infection [69]. Changes in the normal composition of the intestinal microbiota can also be the cause of an insufficient immune response during vaccination against SARS-CoV-2 [30]. In elderly patients, the violation of eubiotic ratios of microbial species occurs naturally due to a decrease in the number of beneficial bacteria such as Bifidobacterium, Bacteroides, and Lactobacillus, and an increase in the number of facultative anaerobes [70–72], which significantly reduces immunoresistance to viral infections. In this regard, it is important to provide microbiota correction in elderly patients, who are more at risk of severe COVID-19 [73].

Disturbances in the composition of the intestinal microbiota are accompanied by the dysregulation of T-cell adaptive immunity, manifested both by a decrease in the production of biologically active substances and sPRR-induced release of proinflammatory cytokines that cause the development or decompensation of immune-mediated diseases such as inflammatory bowel disease, bronchial asthma, rheumatoid arthritis, allergies, type II diabetes mellitus and obesity [31], which complicate the course of SARS-CoV-2 infection [74]. Microbiota imbalance leads to the development of chronic concomitant diseases, which can be considered as an underlying cause of more severe COVID-19 [75]. Disruption of the normal composition of intestinal microbiota is associated with increased reactivity of the hypothalamic-pituitary-adrenal system, and a decrease in stress resistance and the manifestation. depressive disorders [76]. Violation of the activating tolerogenic effect of normal microflora on MALT leads to a significant decrease in antiviral protection and resistance to viral infections, which is a serious risk factor for SARS-CoV-2 infection during a pandemic [77].

SARS-CoV-2 and microbiota

SARS-CoV-2 is a single-stranded RNA virus of positive polarity, which belongs to the Coronaviridae family, genus Betacoronavirus [78]. Infection occurs when the pathogen enters the epithelial cells of the upper respiratory tract and gastrointestinal tract, on the surface of which a large number of receptors for angiotensin-converting enzyme type 2 (ACE2) are localized [79]. The separation of the S-spike spike protein into S1 and S2 by serine (TMPRSS2) and furin (FURIN) proteases is required for the attachment of the virion to the ACE-2 receptor on the cell membrane [80]. After the attachment of the S1 domain to the ACE-2 receptor, the S2 domain attaches to the outer side of the apical membrane of the epithelial cell, and the viral RNA enters the cell via endocytosis [81]. It has been established that the further course COVID-19 is largely determined by the actual state of both nonspecific defense mechanisms and a specific adaptive immune response [82]. Intestinal dysbiosis and associated disorders in the immune status are important risk factors. Multiple replications of SARS-CoV-2 and the release of virions from cells are accompanied by host cell death. Blocking ACE-2 receptors by a high viral load further impairs the body's ability to create a stable and balanced immune response. The high expression of ACE2 in the intestinal tract makes the small and large intestines very susceptible to SARS-CoV-2 infection. It has been shown that the number of these receptors increases significantly with age, which may cause a more severe course of SARS-CoV-2 infection in the elderly [83].

By blocking the ACE2 receptor, SARS-CoV-2 significantly reduces its expression in organs and tissues (Fig. 11.2). As a result, on the one hand, there is an accumulation of angiotensin-II (AT-II) and bradykinin (BK), which contribute to an increase in the overproduction of proinflammatory cytokines and the development of a "cytokine storm"; on the other hand, a decrease in the concentration of angiotensin 1-7 (AT 1-7) is accompanied by a weakening of its antiinflammatory, antifibrotic, and antithrombotic effects [84]. The combination of hyperinflammation and coagulopathy causes apoptosis of infected enterocytes, a violation of the intestinal barrier and an increase of systemic bacterial lipopolysaccharides, a decrease in surfactant synthesis, and alveolar edema with the development of acute respiratory distress syndrome, generalized endothelial dysfunction, and mass formation of microthrombi [85].

According to clinical and experimental studies, ACE2 controls the expression of B^0AT1, a sodium-dependent neutral amino acid transporter that is located on the apical membrane of enterocytes and is involved in the Na+-associated absorption of neutral amino acids. Impaired absorption of tryptophan leads to decreased release of antimicrobial peptides and, consequently, to significant changes in the microbiota, potentiating intestinal inflammation [65]. Rapid reproduction of opportunistic and pathogenic microbes promotes their translocation through the intestinal wall with the development of endogenous infection [55]. Increased intestinal permeability and microbial dysbiosis further may contribute to a cytokine storm in patients with SARS-CoV-2 [65]. These findings are consistent with clinical observations indicating the relationship between the severity of intestinal dysbiosis, the occurrence of complications in SARS-CoV-2, and the severity of the post-COVID period [77].

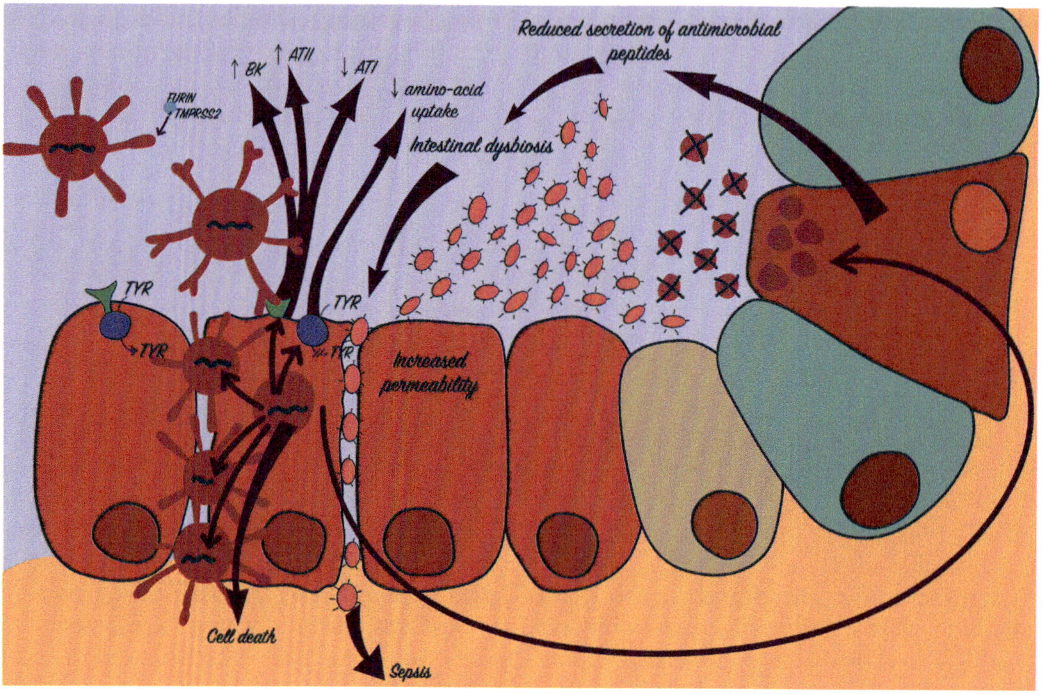

FIGURE 11.2 Cascade of reactions resulting from SARS-CoV-2 blocking of ACE2 receptor and penetrating intestinal epithelial cells. ACE2 receptor blockade during SARS-CoV-2 introduction into the cells is accompanied by accumulation of angiotensin-II (AT-II) and bradykinin (BK), contributing to the proinflammatory cytokine hyperproduction, and a decrease in the concentration of angiotensin 1-7 (AT 1-7) with antiinflammatory and antithrombotic effects. In addition, tryptophan absorption is impaired, leading to the blocked release of antimicrobial peptides. Increased intestinal permeability and rapid multiplication of pathogenic microbes create conditions for their translocation through the intestinal wall with the development of endogenous infection and 'cytokine storm' in patients with SARS-CoV-2.

In conclusion, the maintenance of the number, composition, and functional activity of the intestinal microbiota is a vital aspect of normal physiological homesotasis. The proven influence of the intestinal microbiota on immune adaptation and resistance to infection, including viral infections, indicates the importance of intestinal microbiota evaluation and correction during the SARS-CoV-2 pandemic.

Microbiome and therapeutic options in SARS-CoV-2 pandemic

The proven effect of dysbiotic disorders on the level of postvaccination immunity, the likelihood of infection with SARS-CoV-2, and the risk of severe disease indicate the importance of intestinal microbiota in the prevention of complications and overall infection risk. The fundamental factor in the stability of the intestinal microflora is a diet that includes regular consumption of probiotic foods.

Probiotic foods: microbiome restoration and supplementation

Bioproducts with selected strains of normal human microflora are referred to as probiotic foods [86]. Such foods include sour milk products containing probiotic microorganisms and their metabolites. Probiotics contribute to the preservation and restoration of the microbiome. The advantages of fermented milk drinks include the presence of an optimal ratio of trace elements and amino acids, their better assimilation, and the presence of lactic acid bacteria, which have a positive effect on the physiological functions of the body [87].

A popular probiotic drink is **kefir**, which combines two types of fermentations (lactic acid and alcoholic) during preparation, leading to a significant increase in the microbial content, their important metabolites, and vitamins. Kefir is based on kefir fungi, which are a symbiotic formation, including lactic acid bacteria, yeast, and acetic acid bacteria [88]. Lactobacilli occupy a special place in increasing the body's immunoresistance. The variety of lactobacilli included in kefir very much depends on the manufacturer, but in all samples, the constant components are Lactobacillus kefiranofaciens, Lactobacillus kefiri, Lactobacillus rhamnosus, Lactobacillus paracasei, and Lactobacilli plantarum. It has been established that each of these microorganisms has its own characteristics and range of action, which determines the spectrum of therapeutic value of the entire food product. Lactobacillus kefiri is characterized by a high level of antimicrobial activity against gram-positive and gram-negative pathogens [89], cholesterol-metabolic activity [90], and immunomodulatory activity [91]. Lactobacillus kefiranofaciens play an important role in antiallergic mechanisms [92].

The most studied type of probiotic lactobacillus in kefir culture – Lactobacillus rhamnosus – is especially relevant during the SARS-CoV-2 pandemic, as its strains have been shown to promote epithelial cell regeneration and protect the intestinal epithelial barrier from pathogen penetration [93]. Lipoteichoic acids found on the cell wall of these symbionts are important effector molecules in stimulating not only local intestinal immunocytes but also effector cells of the respiratory tract, which plays an important role in the prevention of respiratory infections [94]. It should be noted that these lactobacilli actively synthesize essential amino acids, vitamins K, D, and group B vitamins promote the absorption of iron and calcium, maintain overall immunoresistance, and by producing linoleic acid reduces the accumulation of adipose tissue in the body and contribute to weight loss [6].

Lactobacilli plantarum found in probiotics are able to maintain the concentration of omega-3 fatty acids, vitamins, and antioxidants [95]. Regular consumption of Lactobacillus paracasei, characterized by the ability to correct the formation of a protective mucous barrier, is considered an effective strategy for increasing resistance to viral infection [96]. The lactic acid flora of kefir is also represented by lactococci and leuconostococci, which exhibit pronounced antibacterial activity [97]. An obligatory component of the kefir fungus is acetic acid bacteria – Acetobacter, which in the presence of yeast increases the antibiotic properties of kefir [98]. The balanced effect of yeast, lactic acid, and acetic acid bacteria supports the intestinal microflora and immunity, prevents infection, and suppresses the spread of the virus in the body, which is especially important during the SARS-CoV-2 pandemic [45,99].

The composition of **bifikefir** is distinguished by the additional presence of Bifidobacteria bifidum, which plays a role in restoring the balance of intestinal microflora and normalization of the digestive function of the intestines, activates metabolic processes, modulates the innate immune response of the macroorganism and increases its immunoresistance [100]. Strains of

Bifidobacterium adolescentis are also added to biokefir. They produce gamma-aminobutyric acid in the human gastrointestinal tract and play a key role in the prevention of anxiety and depressive disorders [101], the frequency of which increased significantly during the SARS-CoV-2 pandemic [102]. In addition, these probiotic microorganisms show high potential for enhancing local immune defenses by stimulating macrophages [103].

The beneficial properties of **fermented yogurt** are a result of fermentation of pasteurized chilled milk containing lactic acid streptococci (Streptococcus lactis and Streptococcus cremoris), the main fermentation product of which is lactic acid, which determines the pronounced antagonistic activity against opportunistic and pathogenic microflora [104]. Lactobacillus delbrueckii spp. Bulgaricus is also present in yogurt, the daily intake of which has been shown to prevent viral infection even in elderly patients with a weakened immune system by stimulating increased production of IgA in saliva [105]. Furthermore, yogurt is rich in B-group vitamins, trace elements such as calcium, magnesium, phosphorus, sodium and potassium, contains omega-3 and omega-6 fatty polyunsaturated acids, and easily digestible valuable amino acids – valine, lysine, cysteine, arginine, and tryptophan, which increases the body's immunoresistance [106].

The technology for the production of **fermented baked milk** differs from the production of yogurt only in that baked milk is used initially. Nevertheless, preliminary heat treatment of milk makes it possible to increase the concentration of proteins, fatty components, macro- and microelements in the final product. As a result of this process, melanoidins are formed, which, in addition to the formation of a specific taste, aroma, and color, play the role of protective colloids that remove toxins and have antioxidant and antimicrobial properties [107]. Varenets is a fermented milk product made from baked milk and cream, in which starter cultures of Streptococcus thermophilic are used, which has a pronounced immunomodulatory effect on human peripheral blood mononuclear cells, and Lactobacillus helveticus, which increases the humoral immune response and the immune response of barrier tissues, both in young and in elderly people [108,109].

A unique representative of fermented milk products is **acidophilus**, which is obtained by adding lactic acid streptococci and acidophilus bacillus to whole milk [110]. Lactobacillus acidophilus, unlike many probiotic microorganisms, is resistant to the acidic environment of the stomach and to the action of many antibiotics, and therefore provides longer suppression of pathogenic and opportunistic flora and contributes to the restoration of intestinal microbiota even during antibiotic therapy. According to research, Lactobacillus acidophilus has an immunomodulatory effect, increasing the production of antibodies and activating phagocytosis. In addition, they take part in the synthesis of vitamin K, and correction of lipid and carbohydrate metabolism, which plays an important role in the immune homeostasis of the macroorganism [111]. The high content of beneficial nutrients makes acidophilus extremely valuable for children during the SARS-CoV-2 pandemic. The use of both Lactobacillus acidophilus and Streptococcus thermophilic strains is often used in probiotic milk preparations for children up to 3 years of age [112]. The combination of Lactobacillus acidophilus with Bifidobacterium animalis subsp. lactis BB-12 is used to create fermented milk, which has been shown to increase the viscosity of the intestinal mucin layer, sIgA production, and resistance to viral infections [113]. Subjects with type II diabetes mellitus, are recommended to systematically consume yoghurts containing probiotic strains of Lactobacillus acidophilus and Bifidobacterium animalis subsp. lactis BB-12, as their regular intake decreases total cholesterol and low-density serum lipoprotein, which may help reduce risk factors for cardiovascular disease [114]. Consequently, these benefits are also seen in COVID-19 treatment [115].

Traditional fermented milk products are giving way to new probiotics developed specifically to improve the immune system and digestion. Lactobacillus rhamnosus became the basis of such new products [116]. The products of the French concern "Actimel" contain beneficial lactobacilli – Lactobacillus casei, the regular use of which reduces the manifestations of stress and improves the mood of patients who have previously shown symptoms of depression [117]. Daily intake of these probiotic microorganisms reduces insulin resistance, correcting symptoms of type II diabetes [118], and reducing the frequency and duration of upper respiratory tract infections by immune system modulation [119]. A functional fermented milk drink "Imunele" is known for the combination of Lactobacillus casei and Lactobacillus rhamnosus with a mutually reinforcing effect [6].

The undisputed leader in terms of production volume and importance in maintaining the microbiome are **yoghurts**, based on Streptococcus thermophilus and Lactobacillus delbrueckii spp. bulgaricus, which are characterized by prebiotic, immunostimulating, and cholesterol-lowering activity [120]. The series of fermented milk yoghurts "Activia" of the French corporation Danone deserves special attention, as Bifidobacterium animalis subsp, lactis BB-12 strains are additionally used in their starter culture, the regular intake of which increases the body's resistance to viral infections [121]. Numerous studies have established their positive effect on lipid metabolism [122], glucose tolerance [114], and immunoresistance [113]. Inclusion of these yoghurts in daily diet helps reduce the risk of obesity and metabolic syndrome [123].

In the manufacture of **sour cream**, the cream is subjected to lactic acid fermentation with the participation of a combination of starter cultures including Streptococcus thermophilus and Lactococcus lactis [124]. The entry of Lactococcus lactis strains into the intestinal microflora has a strong immunomodulatory effect on plasmacytoid dendritic cells, potentially important for antiviral immunity [125]. Due to the presence of highly digestible proteins, trace elements, and vitamins, sour cream is especially useful in patients with compromised immune systems [126].

Cottage cheese products also contain valuable bacteria which can be suggested for prebiotic treatment. Bacteria from cottage cheese products produce antibacterial substrates, short-chain fatty acids, polysaccharides, antioxidants, nucleic acids, lipo- and glycoproteins, vitamins, various enzymes and lectins, amino acids, growth and coagulation factors, defensin-like and signaling molecules [127]. The inclusion of these active substances in a healthy diet helps complement the function of normal intestinal microbiota and is currently considered an alternative to the use of live microorganisms for correction of dysbiosis in persons with immunosuppressive status during the SARS-CoV-2 pandemic [117].

For the fermentation of **curd** products, the following lactobacilli are used - Lactococcus lactis, Streptococcus thermophilus, Bifidobacterium bifidum, and Propionibakterium freudenreichii, each of which contributes in its own wat to the restoration of healthy intestinal microbiota and correction of immune status [128]. The most useful transient bacteria are Propionibacterium freudenreichii, the exometabolites of which are B-group vitamins, antimicrobial factors, linoleic acid conjugates, exoenzymes, and antimutagenic factors, as well as bifidogenic factors—growth stimulators of bifidobacteria, which have a healing and immunomodulatory effect [129]. Recently, probiotic developers have been focusing their attention on the production of **probiotic cheeses**, as they are characterized by such valuable properties as high protein content, absence of lactose, and relatively long shelf life [130].

Non-dairy probiotic products are becoming increasingly popular [29]. Lactic acid fermentation, used in salting and pickling, is an important way to preserve fruits and vegetables, which at the same time become sources of natural probiotics [131]. One of the most popular and oldest traditional products in this category is **sauerkraut**, which in the process of fermentation is enriched with active substrates of microorganism metabolism, organic acids, and vitamins [132]. Of the probiotic microorganisms at the initial stages of fermentation, Leuconostoc mesenteroides predominate in the medium, which contributes to a decrease in the mass of abdominal fat [133], correction of blood glucose levels [134] and lipid spectrum indicators [135], which is especially important in the ongoing SARS-CoV-2 pandemic.

The traditional Korean **kimchi** is fermented vegetables seasoned with pepper, garlic, and ginger, made primarily from cabbage [136]. Regular consumption of this fermented product is associated with numerous health benefits, including reducing obesity, insulin resistance, and cholesterol levels, correcting blood pressure, and strengthening the immune system [137]. The inclusion in the diet of a Japanese traditional **miso-soup** made by fermenting soybeans, wheat, and rice with a special type of Aspergillus oryzae mold, increases the bioavailability of coenzyme Q10, which is a fat-soluble antioxidant and is involved in energy production [138].

The therapeutic effect of a Japanese fermented soy product, **natto**, containing the bacterial strain Bacillus subtilis, is primarily associated with its immunomodulatory effect, the availability of antimicrobial peptides, digestive enzymes, and vitamins [139]. A similar fermented soy product from Indonesia is called **tempeh**, and contains the fungal culture Rhizopus oligosporus and is popular as a substitute for high protein meat. It has been shown that tempeh consumption reduces the risk of metabolic syndrome [140].

Kvass is a popular fermented drink, based on bread leaven, which includes three types of lactobacilli: Lactobacillus casei, Lactobacillus asidophilus, Lactobacillus plantarum and baker's pressed yeast *Saccharomyces cerevisiae*, which are not a component of natural intestinal microbiota but are valuable for their antipathogenic action [141,142]. **Kombucha** is another important nondairy probiotic which is based on lactic acid fermentation and acetic bacteria, fungi, and yeast. Studies have proven the pronounced immunostimulant, antioxidant and antimicrobial properties of kombuch [143].

All fermented foods have been found to correct the composition of intestinal microbiota, while most provide decreased duration and frequency of infectious processes, enhance antioxidant, antiinflammatory, and immune responses, and may help reduce the risks associated with SARS-CoV-2 infection [144].

The role of probiotics in pathology correction

In order to preserve the intestinal microbiota under the influence of stress factors and to restore it in case of dysbiosis, specific dosages have been suggested for different symbionts, which are optimal in providing a positive effect on the physiological, metabolic, and immune reactions of the body. Currently, depending on the composition and pharmacological activity, several generations of probiotic drugs are distinguished, which have proven clinical efficacy and safety [6]. The range of therapeutic effects of these drugs is determined by the types of microorganisms included in them. In clinical practice, the most appropriate approach is a differentiated one, taking into account the severity of the dysbiotic condition, comorbidities, and the age of the patients [145].

Numerous studies have shown that in children, the predominant species of bifidobacteria in the intestine are Bifidobacteria infantis, Bifidobacteria bifidum, Bifidobacterium breve, and Bifidobacteria longum [70,146–149]. These anaerobes are one of the first to colonize the gastrointestinal tract in healthy infants, therefore, to increase the immunoresistance of children during the SARS-CoV-2 pandemic, especially infants, probiotic drugs containing these bifidobacteria are of choice (Table 11.1).

Bifidobacteria infantis are found in large quantities in breast milk and adapt well to the infant GI tract due to their ability to consume complex milk carbohydrates, improve intestinal barrier function and accelerate the maturation of the immune response [150]. They were shown to be effective at protecting a child in the early years of his life from pathogens and reducing diarrhea incidence [151], which recently is often the first symptom of SARS-CoV-2 infection [152]. It has been proven that in bottle-fed infants, these symbionts at the end of the fourth week of treatment increased the production of sIgA, which increases mucosal immune competence and is essential in protecting against viral infections [153].

There is evidence that indole-3-lactic acid, a metabolic product of Bifidobacteria infantis, has pleiotropic protective effects on immature enterocytes including antiinflammatory and antiviral in preterm infants [154] that are at risk for SARS-CoV-2 infection [155]. The decrease in the abundance of these probiotic microorganisms correlates with increased intestinal inflammation [156]. It was also established that a high rate of Bifidobacteria infantis colonization is associated with a low risk of atopic diseases in children [149]. In children with allergies, the level of Bifidobacteria adolescentis, is increased, which Bifidobacteria infantis is scarce [146].

A common component of probiotics for children is Bifidobacteria bifidum, which significantly increases colonization resistance of infant's gut due to their sortase-dependent pili and transaldolase that not only contribute to its establishment but also display immunomodulatory activity [157–159]. An interesting fact is that the drinking of these symbionts programs the immune system in infancy and creates a protective barrier that specifically acts against possible bacterial infections [100].

It has been shown that strains of these microorganisms can cause increased production of cytokine IL-17 [160]. Bifidobacteria bifidum administration in low birth weight infants enhances humoral immunity, significantly increasing serum IgG and intestinal sIgA levels [161]. It is noteworthy that the cleavage of mucin by strains of Bifidobacteria bifidum causes an increase in mucus secretion and restoration of the mucous membrane, which strengthens the epithelial barrier [162]. By maintaining the balance of the intestinal microflora, these symbionts modulate the infants' innate immune response and increase their immunoresistance to viral infections [100]. By regulating gut microbiota, Bifidobacteria bifidum reduce milk allergy in infants [163].

Bifidobacteria bifidum have the ability to metabolize human milk oligosaccharides and can be prescribed to children in the form of a mono-component probiotic [164,165]. Interestingly, a probiotic intervention in children may be crucial in terms of preventing the establishment of a dysbiotic microbiota with its associated negative health implications [166]. Sorbed Bifidobacterium bifidum are very effective in correcting pathogenic microbiota as they

TABLE 11.1 Probiotics of choice for children in SARS-CoV-2 pandemic.

Ingredients	Drug name
B. bifidum	Bifidumbacterin (Russia) tablets, capsules, lyophilizate for oral and topical use, powder for oral and topical use, vaginal suppositories Bifidumbacterin dry (Russia) lyophilizate for preparation of solution for oral and topical use Bifidumbacterin 1000 (Russia) tablets Bifidumbacterium bifidum-SM (Russia) powder for oral use Bifidobacterium bifidum (Russia) powder for oral use BifoVir (Russia) oral powder/lyophilizate for oral and topical use Lifepack Probiotics (France) capsules
B. bifidum sorbed on activated carbon	Probifor (Russia) capsules, powder for oral use Bifidumbacterin forte (Russia) capsules, powder for oral use Biosorb-Bifidum (Russia) powder for oral use
B. lactis (BB-12)	Linex for children (Slovenia) powder for oral use in sachet
L. acidophilus	Atsilakt (Russia) tablets, powder, lyophilizate for oral and topical use, vaginal suppositories Lactobacterin (Russia) lyophilizate for oral and topical use, vaginal suppositories Narine (Armenia) powder for oral use, capsules, tablets Nature's Bounty Acidophilus Probiotic (USA) capsules Vitaflor (Russia) lozenges, powder for oral use, lyophilizate for oral and topical use
B. bifidum, B. longum	Bifidum BAG (Russia) solution for oral use Bifilong (Russia) lyophilizate for oral use
B. bifidum, B. breve, B. infantis	Bifidum-multi-1 (Russia) capsules
B. bifidum, B. breve, B. infantis, B. longum	Bifidum-multi-2 (Russia) capsules
B. bifidum, L. acidophilus	Infloran Bern (Switzerland) capsules
B. longum, L. acidophilus	Omniflora (Germany) capsules
B. bifidum, B. longum, L. acidophilus	Наринэ Форте (Армения) powder for oral use, capsules, tablets
B. bifidum, L. acidophilus, L. bulgaricus	Sinerlac (France) capsules
B. bifidum, B. longum, B. lactis, B. breve, B. infantis, L. gasseri, L. rhamnosus	Kyolic, Kyo-Dophilus, Multi 9 Probiotic (USA) capsules
B. bifidum, L. acidophilus	Infloran Bern (Switzerland) capsules

TABLE 11.1 Probiotics of choice for children in SARS-CoV-2 pandemic.—cont'd

Ingredients	Drug name
B. longum, L. acidophilus	Omniflora (Germany) capsules
B. bifidum, B. longum, L. acidophilus	Наринэ Форте (Armenia) powder for oral use, capsules, tablets
B. bifidum, B. longum, L. gasseri	Kyolic, Kyo-Dophilus, Daily Probiotic (USA) capsules Kyolic, Kyo-Dophilus, Kids Probiotic (USA) tablets
B. bifidum, B. longum, B. lactis, B. breve, B. infantis, L. gasseri, L. rhamnosus	Kyolic, Kyo-Dophilus, Multi 9 Probiotic (USA) capsules
B. bifidum + lysozyme	Bifiliz (Russia) lyophilizate for oral and topical use, suppositories
B. bifidum + fructo-oligosaccharides + sunflower oil triglyceride mixture	Liveo baby (Latvia) powder and oil solution for suspension preparation
B. lactis, L. acidophilus + palm oil + fructooligosaccharides + skim milk powder	Normobact Junior (Israel) tablets
B. longum + hydrolyzate-soybean medium	Soy-bifidum (Russia) solution for oral use
B. longum + fructooligosaccharides, xylitol + C	Fine bifido jelly (Japan) gel
B. longum + Q10 + B3	Lactoflorene Cholesterol (Italy) powder for oral use
B. lactis + sunflower oil, antioxidants DL-alpha tocopherol, and citric acid, sucrose	Linex for children (Denmark) drops for oral use
L. acidophilus + C	Biobacton (Russia) solution for oral use, vaginal suppositories
L. acidophilus + kefir fungus polysaccharide	Acipol (Russia) capsules
L. acidophilus + lysozyme	Kipatsid (Russia) tablets
L. acidophilus + apple fruit	Vitadophilus (USA) powder for oral use
L. acidophilus + fructooligosaccharides	VPLAB Duobact (UK) capsules
L. acidophilus + barley wort	Lactofor (Russia) solution for oral use
L. acidophilus + Plantaginis seeds, Sterculia platanifolia leaves, Sennae leaves (Cassia Tora), Rosae fruits, Frangula, Chlorella, Aloe vera leaves, beta-carotene, papain, Júglans régia leaves, garlic bulbs, rice bran oil extract	Nutri-Cleanse Vitamax (USA) capsules
L. acidophilus + natural cow's milk, skim milk powder, whole milk powder + Zn + Fe	Narine F-balance (Russia) liquid for oral use
B. longum, B. breve + lactulose	RatioNutriLife Bifidobacteria (Japan) capsules
B. bifidum, L. acidophilus + fructooligosaccharides	Liveo children (Latvia) powder for oral use

(Continued)

TABLE 11.1 Probiotics of choice for children in SARS-CoV-2 pandemic.—cont'd

Ingredients	Drug name
B. bifidum, L. acidophilus + lactose + hyaluronic acid	Gialakt (Russia) capsules
B. lactis, L. rhamnosus GG + B1 + B6 + isomaltose; xylitol; fructooligosaccharides	Bifiform Baby (Italy) powder for oral use, tablets
B. longum, L. rhamnosus + DL- alpha tocopherol acetate	Acipol Baby (Spain) oil suspension
B. breve, L. rhamnosus + corn oil	Kids Preema Duo (Italy) children drop for oral use
B. bifidum, B. longum, L. gasseri, + A + B1 + B2 + B5 + B6 + B7 + B9 + B12 + E + C + D3 + Ca + Fe + Zn	Bion 3 Kid (Austria) tablets
B. lactis, L. acidophilus, L. reuteri + lactoferrin + fructooligosaccharides	NATUMA bactoflor baby (Italy) drops for oral use
B. longum, B. breve, L. acidophilus + colostrum (from cattle), rice bran, fructooligosaccharides	ChildLife, Probiotics with Colostrum (USA) tablets
B. longum, L. acidophilus, L. plantarum, + Zn + lactoferrin + inulin	NATUMA bactoflor kids (Italy) powder for oral use in sachet
B. longum, B. infantis, L. rhamnosus, L.acidophilus + C	Primadophilus Children's (USA) powder for oral use
B. bifidum, B. longum, B. infantis, B. breve, L. rhamnosus, L. plantarum + maltose, fructooligosaccharides, glucose	Neobiotic Lactobalance Baby (Korea) powder for oral use in sachet
B. bifidum, B. longum, B. breve, B. infantis, L. acidophilus, L. plantarum, L. casei + oligofructose + inulin + B1 + B2 + B4 + B5 + B6 + B7 + B9 + B12 + E + C + Zn + Se	Normospectrum Junior (Russia) capsules Normospectrum Baby (Russia) capsules
B. bifidum, B. longum, B. lactis, L. acidophilus, L. casei, L. paracasei, L. plantarum, L. rhamnosus, L. salivarius + fructooligosaccharides, oligofructose	Maxilak Baby (Poland) powder for oral use in sachet
Bifidobacterium BB-12, L. paracasei, Streptococcus thermophilic + fructooligosaccharides	Florok Baby (Denmark) powder for oral use in sachet
B. longum, B. breve, B. infantis, L. acidophilus, L. casei, L. rhamnosus, Streptococcus thermophilus + fructooligosaccharides	Buck-Set Baby (UK) powder for oral use in sachet
Probiotic B. infantis, B. bifidum, B. longum, B. breve, L. casei, L. acidophilus, L. rhamnosus + **prebiotic** inulin, fibregam, lactulose, vitamins B + beta-glucan + **metabiotic** lysates of Propionibacterium freudenreichii and Propionibacterium arabinosum	Panbiolact Kids (Russia) capsules
Probiotics L. acidophilus + **prebiotic** sorbitol, lactose, papain + **enzyme** amylase	Acidophilus-Jura N (Germany) powder for oral use

colonize the intestinal mucosa well, adsorb and remove endo- and exotoxins, replacing pathogenic bacteria and their metabolic products from the body. It has been shown that the use of Bifidobacterium bifidum reduces the duration of the diarrheal syndrome and improves the well-being of patients with SARS-CoV-2 [167].

Bifidobacteria breve is predominantly found in infant microbiota, and have high antimicrobial activity against different pathogens [168]. They are known to be selective consumers of human milk oligosaccharides [169]. Research results indicate that these symbionts have a strictly controlled system of gene transcription regulation in the management of this metabolic process, which promotes the digestion of plant-derived carbohydrates [170].

Bifidobacteria breve supplementation promotes microbiome correction in preterm infants [171]. These probiotic microorganisms exhibit immunostimulating properties, are characterized by antimicrobial activity and do not exhibit signs of transmissible antibiotic resistance. They are prescribed for diarrhea intestinal colic, celiac disease, variety of allergic and neurological disorders. Bifidobacteria breve is also used to prevent infections in premature infants that occur during antibiotic treatment or chemotherapy [172,173]. Researcher shows Amoxicillin-Clavulanic Acid Resistance in these strains of bifidobacteria [174]. Other authors identified a gene homologous to the rRNA methylase genes, which confers resistance to erythromycin and clindamycin [175].

Bifidobacteria longum, also present in the intestine, is distinguished by a wide variety of glycosyl hydrolases capable of metabolizing carbohydrates, ranging from milk oligosaccharides to vegetable carbs, which may explain their competitive advantage over other bacteria and long-term stability in the gut microbiome [147,176–179]. This culture of bacteria has been identified to possess high acid resistance, adhesive and immunomodulatory properties [180]. Lactose and bovine milk oligosaccharides synergistically stimulate the growth of these microorganisms [181,182]. There is evidence that food allergy in children, and in particular IgE-mediated allergy to milk, is caused by changes in the composition and functionality of intestinal microbiota and a decrease in titers of Bifidobacteria infantis, Bifidobacterium breve, and Bifidobacteria longum [183].

Probiotic microorganisms are known to increase resistance to common viral infections as well as reduce the incidence of acute respiratory tract infections include [121]. It has been proven that several symbionts are able to inhibit the activity of several pathogenic microorganisms: *Escherichia coli*, Bacillus cereus, *Enterococcus faecalis*, Shigella sonnei, *Salmonella enterica*, *Clostridium perfringens*, *Clostridium difficile*, Listeria monocytogenes, *Pseudomonas aeruginosa*, and Candida albicans [184]. A randomized, double-blind, placebo-controlled trial showed that Bifidobacterium lactis BB-12 has therapeutic efficacy in the correction of infant colic. At the same time, an increase in the number of bifidobacteria correlates with an increase in butyrate and sIgA, as well as with a decrease in fecal calprotectin levels, which is a marker of intestinal inflammation [185]. Other authors have established a pronounced Bifidobacteria lactis BB-12 ability to colonize infant microbiota. The addition of dairy oligosaccharides further enhances their engraftment, suggesting a strong symbiotic effect [186]. It has been proven that Bifidobacteria lactis BB-12 supplementation benefits low birth weight infants [187]. It was also shown that Bifidobacterium lactis Bb12 enhances intestinal antibody response in infants, which is especially relevant in preventing SARS-CoV-2 infection [188].

The dominant species of lactobacillus in the intestines of children is Lactobacillus acidophilus, which modulates immune responses and improves intestinal resistance to pathogens.

These beneficial microorganisms ferment glucose with the formation of hydrogen peroxide, lactic and acetic acids, which help maintain a low acidity environment and inhibit the growth and reproduction of pathogenic microorganisms [184]. Lactobacillus acidophilus has been shown to alleviate β-lactoglobulin-induced allergic inflammation [189]. By producing bacteriocins—acidophyllin and lactocidin, they affect the balance of bacteria in the human intestine, reduce the likelihood of gastrointestinal infections, support digestion and improve the absorption of minerals, which plays an important role in the immune homeostasis of children [6]. According to recent data, children treated with Lactobacillus acidophilus, zink, and vitamins A, D, and C showed a reduced risk of upper airway infection [190].

The combination of bifidobacteria and lactobacilli species prevailing in the children's intestine is of great importance for increasing the spectrum and synergism of their activity. Thus, the combination of Bifidobacteria lactis BB-12 with Lactobacillus rhamnosus opens a broader window of opportunity in the prevention of inflammatory conditions, including eczema [191]. The same microorganisms are effective in the prevention of diarrheal syndrome in children with severe malnutrition [192]. The oral administration of probiotic formulas containing both Bifidobacterium longum and Lactobacillus acidophilus significantly improves the course of rotavirus infection, reducing fever duration, frequency of diarrhea, and vomiting [193]. The mixture of Bifidobacterium lactis, Lactobacillus rhamnosus, and Lactobacillus acidophilus results in even shorter diarrhea durations and quicker rehabilitation [194]. Probiotics containing Lactobacillus helveticus, Bifidobacterium infantis, and Bifidobacterium bifidum significantly increase the efficacy of standard diarrhea treatment regardless of etiology and improve iron metabolism in anemic patients [195]. More so, the combination of Bifidobacterium longum, Bifidobacterium infantis, and Lactobacillus acidophilus has been shown to be effective in the prevention of intestinal dysbiosis in preterm infants [196].

Several studies demonstrated a decrease in upper respiratory infection frequency and severity in children taking Lactobacillus acidophilus and Bidfidobacterium lactis [197]. The introduction of Lactobacillus acidophilus and Bifidobacterium bifidum for preterm infants is associated with a decreased incidence of necrotizing enterocolitis and late-onset sepsis [198–200]. Observational reports indicate that a mixture of Bifidobacteria lactis BB-12 and Enterococcus faecium statistically decreases atopy symptoms [201].

Numerous studies have shown that each symbiont possesses a unique set of characteristics that affect the human body (Table 11.2). Currently, complex biological products that combine live bacteria, **prebiotics** (compounds that stimulate their growth and vital activity), and **metabiotics** (the products of their metabolism) are vital components of therapy. The identification of pathogenic and opportunistic enterobacteria in the microbiome dictates the need to choose drugs that also contain **bioenteroseptics**, represented by living microorganisms that are not found in the normal human microbiota, but are capable of eliminating opportunistic microbiota. Concomitant diseases of the gastrointestinal tract with enzyme deficiency require treatment with **cobiotics**—preparations that additionally include various types of digestive enzymes, which act to improve the absorption of carbohydrates, lipids, and proteins in the small intestine [202]. A consortium of bacteria of the human microbiome, which has been proven to influence the correction of a certain syndrome, is the basis for a **bioprobiotics** complex with targeted action.

TABLE 11.2 Distinctive therapeutic effects of probiotic microorganisms.

	↑ resistance to viral infections, incl. SARS-CoV-2	↑postvaccination immunity	↓production of cytokines, incl. in SARS-CoV-2	↓ duration and severity of respiratory infections, incl. SARS-CoV-2	↓ the likelihood and duration of diarrheal syndrome, incl. in SARS-CoV-2	Correction of lipid profile	correction of glucose tolerance & metabolic syndromre	correction of anxiety-depressive disorders	prevention and correction of allergic reactions
B. bifidum	■				■				
B. longum	■				■	■	■	■	
B. lactis BB-12	■					■	■		
L. acidophilus	■			■	■	■	■		
L. rhamnosus	■	■		■	■		■		
L. plantarum	■		■	■		■			
L. paracasei	■								
Escherichia coli	■								
B. adolescentis					■			■	
B. breve							■	■	■
L. casei	■						■		
L. fermentum	■	■							
L. helveticus	■								■
L. reuteri			■		■				
Ent. faecium	■								
Str. thermophilus	■								
L. bulgaricus	■								
Lactococcus lactis	■			■	■				

Modulation of the immune response through microbiota correction

During the SARS-CoV-2 pandemic, bioprobiotics are especially important, as they can have a modulating effect on the immune system. The most effective bioprobiotics are combinations of lacto- and bifidobacteria, which are used not only to correct cellular immunity but also to reduce the risk and severity of viral infections [6]. Probiotic microorganisms that increase immunoresistance include Bifidobacterium bifidum, Bifidobacterium longum, Bifidobacterium lactis BB-12, Lactobacillus acidophilus, Lactobacillus rhamnosus, Lactobacilli plantarum, Lactobacillus paracasei, Lactobacillus casei, Lactobacillus fermentum, Lactobacillus helveticus, Lactobacillus bulgaricus, *Escherichia coli*, Enterococcus faecium, Streptococcus thermophilus, and Lactococcus lactis.

The immunomodulatory and prophylactic effects of Bifidobacterium bifidum probiotic strain have been proven in influenza infections [203]. The complex mixture of polysaccharides produced by this bacterium may differentially regulate the host immunity, either enhancing immunity or inducing immune tolerance [204–207]. It has been established that probiotics containing Bifidobacterium longum modulate not only T-cell and dendritic cell phenotypes [208], but also the systemic immune response toward both IgE production and regulation of Th1/Th2 balance [209]. Intranasal Bifidobacterium longum protects against viral-induced lung inflammation [210]. Daily Bifidobacterium lactis BB-12 consumption enhances polymorphonuclear cell phagocytic capacity and natural killer cell activity [211].

Lactobacillus acidophilus ranks first among lactobacilli in its immunomodulatory effect, which is realized through an increase in antibody production and activation of phagocytosis [212]. Lipoteichoic acids and unmethylated CpG oligonucleotides of the cell walls of Lactobacillus rhamnosus and Lactobacillus plantarum are the most important effector molecules in immunomodulation. These symbionts have a stimulating effect not only locally on intestinal immunocytes, but also systemically—on the effector cells of the respiratory tract, therefore they are intended for the prevention of respiratory infections [94,213]. Lactobacillus paracasei are able to effectively restore the intestinal microflora and mucous barrier that protects the body from all pathogens [96].

Lactobacillus helveticus administration improves humoral and mucosal immune response in both young and elderly adults [108,214]. Daily intake of Lactobacillus casei reduces the incidence and duration of upper respiratory tract infections [119]. Lactobacillus fermentum is an excellent candidate for the development of probiotics aimed at regulation of immune response to pathogen invasion [215]. Studies have shown that daily intake of Lactobacillus bulgaricus helps prevent viral infections in elderly pateitns with weakened immunity by increasing salivary IgA production [105].

The nonpathogenic strain of *Escherichia coli* is used to strengthen the barrier function of the intestinal epithelium, which is carried out through the release of antimicrobial substances and the synthesis of a fixing protein that promotes the formation of strong intercellular contacts between intestinal mucosa cells [216]. In combination with obligate probionts, opportunistic bacteria Enterococcus faecium significantly enhances the intestinal barrier function and helps protect against penetration of pathogenic microorganisms and their toxins [217]. Scientific studies show the strong action of Streptococcus thermophilus on human mononuclear cells, promoting an array of antiinflammatory properties [109]. Oral administration of Lactococcus lactis has potent immunomodulatory effects on plasmacytoid dendritic cells, potentially relevant to antiviral immunity [125]. Table 11.3 presents probiotics containing representatives of human intestinal microflora with a proven ability to enhance the activity of various parts of the immune system involved in antiviral response.

Postvaccination immunity modulation through microbiota correction

Lactobacillus rhamnosus and Lactobacillus fermentum have been shown to increase the immunogenicity of vaccines. The intake of these lactobacilli in association with vaccination significantly increased the titer of specific antibodies and the rate of seroconversion, which may be used to increase the effectiveness of COVID-19 vaccines [30,218,219]. Table 11.4 presents the probiotic drugs of choice for enhancing the production of post-vaccination immunity.

TABLE 11.3 Probiotics with proven immunomodulatory activity to enhance antiviral immunity.

Ingredients	Drug name
B. lactis, L. acidophilus, L. paracasei, L. rhamnosus, L. reuteri, L. casei + fructooligosaccharides	Synbiotics Vision Bio-In Probiotics & Prebiotics (France) powder for oral use in sachet
B. bifidum, B. lactis, L. acidophilus, L. paracasei, L. plantarum, L. rhamnosus, L. salivarius + fructooligosaccharides, inulin	Rioflora (Netherlands, Germany) capsules
B. bifidum, B. lactis, L. acidophilus, L. salivarius, L. plantarum, L. rhamnosus, L. reuteri + fructooligosaccharides + Chamomile extract + C + Zn	Synbiotics Vision Bio-In for Respiratory System (France) powder for oral use in sachet
B. bifidum, B. longum, L. acidophilus, L. plantarum, L. casei, L. rhamnosus, L. salivarius + C	Flora, Super 8 Hi-Potency Probiotic (Canada) capsules
B. lactis, L. acidophilus, L. casei, L. plantarum, L. salivarius, L. rhamnosus, L. reuteri + fructooligosaccharides + Urtíca extract + B5	Synbiotics Vision Bio-In for Hyper Sensivity (France) powder for oral use in sachet
B. bifidum, B. longum, B. 1actis, L. acidophilus, L. rhamnosus, Streptococcus thermophiles + C	Neobiotic Lactobalance (Korea) capsules
B. bifidum, B. infantis, B. lactis, L. acidophilus, L. casei; L. plantarum, Streptococcus thermophilus + C + inulin	Synbiotic Premium (Russia) capsules
B. bifidum, B. lactis, B. infantis, L. acidophilus, L. casei, L. plantarum, Streptococcus thermophiles + C + inulin	Probiotic + prebiotic Sinobactin Premium (Canada) capsules
B. longum, B. breve, L. acidophilus, L. rhamnosus, L. casei, L. bulgaricus, Streptococcus thermophilus + inulin	Multiflora Anti-Age Evalar (Russia) capsules
B. bifidum, B. longum. B. breve, B. adolescentis, L. acidophilus, L.casei, L.plantarum, Streptococcus thermophilus + kim milk, gelatose, lactulose + C	Synbiotic renewal (Russia) capsules
L. casei, L. paracasei, L. rhamnosus, L. reuteri, L. acidophilus, Streptococcus thermophiles + fructooligosaccharides + Ca + Mg + D3	Synbiotics Vision Bio-In Bonecare (France) powder for oral use in sachet
B. bifidum, B. animalis, L. acidophilus, L. helveticus, Lactococcus lactis, Streptococcus thermophilus, Propionibacterium freudenreichii ssp. shermanii +A + B1 + B2 + B3 + B5 + B6 + B7 + B9 + C + E + K + D + inulin, dry powder from natural juices	Evitalia-bifid (Russia) tablets
B. bifidum, B. animalis, L. acidophilus, L.helveticus, Lactococcus lactis, Streptococcus thermophilus, Propionibacterium freudenreichii ssp. shermanii + inulin, lactulose	Bifidum Evitalia (Russia) capsules
Probiotic B. infantis, B. bifidum, B. longum, B. breve, L. casei, L. acidophilus, L. rhamnosus + **prebiotic** inulin, fibregam, lactulose, vitamins B + beta-glucan + **metabiotic** lysates of Propionibacterium freudenreichii and Propionibacterium arabinosum	Panbiolact Kids (Russia) capsules
Bioenteroseptic Bacillus subtilis + **probiotic** L acidophilus, L. paracasei, L. casei, L. bulgaricus, L. rhamnosus, L. plantarum, L. salivarius + **prebiotic** microcrystalline cellulose	Enzymedica, Pro-Bio (USA) capsules

(*Continued*)

TABLE 11.3 Probiotics with proven immunomodulatory activity to enhance antiviral immunity.—cont'd

Ingredients	Drug name
Probiotic B. bifidum, B. lactis, L. casei, L. plantarum, L. bulgaricus, L. acidophilus, Propionibacterium freudenreichii + **prebiotic** from Jerusalem artichoke tuber powder (inulin) + B2 + B3 + B10 + cysteine + **enzymes** lactase, papain	Panbiolact (Russia) capsules
Bioenteroseptic Bacillus subtilis + **probiotic** L acidophilus, L. paracasei, L. bulgaricus, L. rhamnosus, L. plantarum, L. casei, L. salivarius + **enzymes** amylase, glucoamylase, lipase, protease, cellulase, alpha-galactosidase, lactase, maltase, xylanase, invertase, pectinase, hemicellulase	Enzymedica, Digest + Probiotics (USA) capsules
Bioenteroseptic Bacillus subtilis + **probiotic** L acidophilus, L. paracasei, L. bulgaricus, L. rhamnosus, L. plantarum, L. casei, L. salivarius + **enzymes** amylase, glucoamylase, lipase, protease, cellulase, alpha-galactosidase, lactase, maltase xylanase, invertase, pectinase	Enzymedica, Digest Basic + Probiotics (USA) capsules
Probiotic L. acidophilus, L. rhamnosus, L. casei, L. gasseri, L. plantarum, L. bulgaricus, L. salivarius, L. paracasei + **enzymes** amylase, protease, glucoamylase, alpha-galactosidase, cellulase, lipase, lactase, beta-glucanase, maltase, xylanase, invertase, pectinase, hemicellulase	Enzymedica, Digest + Gold Probiotics (USA) capsules
B. bifidum, B. longum, B. lactis, L. acidophilus, L. plantarum, L. salivarius, L. rhamnosus, L. casei + inulin + microcrystalline cellulose	Nutrition Now, PB 8 (USA) capsules
B. lactis, B. longum, L.acidophilus, L. paracasei, L. plantarum, L. salivarius, Lactococcus lactis, Streptococcus thermophiles + fructooligosaccharides, inulin	Rioflora Immuno (Netherlands, Germany) capsules
B. bifidum, B. longum, L. acidophilus, L. casei, L, plantarum, Lactococcus lactis, L. rhamnosus, L.reuteri, + Fructooligosaccharides, Acai Berry Extract Powder + C	Synbiotics Vision Bio-In with antioxydants (France) powder for oral use in sachet
B. bifidum, B. longum, B. lactis, L. acidophilus, L. casei, L. paracasei, L. plantarum, L. rhamnosus, L. salivarius + fructooligosaccharides, oligofructose	Maxilak Baby (Poland) powder for oral use in sachet
B. bifidum, B. longum, B. breve, L. acidophilus, L. plantarum, Lactococcus lactis, L. rhamnosus, L. casei, L. paracasei + L-leucine	Sports Research, Daily Probiotics (USA) capsules
B. bifidum, B. longum, B. lactis, B. breve, L. acidophilus, L. plantarum, L. paracasei, L. casei, L. brevis, L. rhamnosus, L. salivarius + microcrystalline cellulose, fructooligosaccharides	Healthy BIOM, High Potency Probiotics (USA) capsules
B. bifidum, B. longum, B. breve, L. helveticus, L. rhamnosus, Lactococcus lactis, L. casei, L. plantarum, Streptococcus thermophiles + oligofructose + olive oil + C	Maxilak (Poland) capsules
B. longum, B. lactis, B. breve, L. acidophilus, L. plantarum, L. salivarius, L. casei, L. rhamnosus, L. paracasei, Streptococcus thermophilus + microcrystalline cellulose, fructooligosaccharides	Now, Probiotic-10 (USA) Capsules
B. longum, B. lactis, B. breve, L. acidophilus, L. plantarum, L. casei, L. rhamnosus, L. salivarius, L.paracasei, Streptococcus thermophilus + microcrystalline cellulose, fructooligosaccharides	Lake Avenue Nutrition Probiotic (USA) Capsules

TABLE 11.3 Probiotics with proven immunomodulatory activity to enhance antiviral immunity.—cont'd

Ingredients	Drug name
B. longum, B. lactis, B. breve, L. acidophilus, L. plantarum, L. casei, L. rhamnosus, L.salivarius, L. paracasei, Streptococcus thermophilus + microcrystalline cellulose, fructooligosaccharides, Aloe barbadensis leaf	Now Foods, Aloe 10,000 Probiotics (USA) Capsules
B. bifidum, B. longum, B. breve, L. helveticus, L. casei, L. rhamnosus, L. plantarum, Lactococcus lactis, Streptococcus thermophilus + fructooligosaccharides + B1 + B2 + B6	Lacidoforte (Bulgaria) capsules
Probiotic L. acidophilus, L. plantarum, L. casei, L. salivarius, L. rhamnosus, L. helveticus, B. bifidum, B. lactis, B. breve, B. longum + **prebiotic** green papaya, apple pectin, ginger, fennel seeds, kelp, nori, wakame, Méntha piperíta leaf, inulin + **enzymes** amylase, glucoamylase, lipase, protease, invertase, maltase, cellulase, bromelain, lactase, papain	Zenwise Health, Daily Digestive Enzymes (USA) capsules
Probiotic L. acidophilus, L. plantarum, L. casei, L. salivarius, L. rhamnosus, L. helveticus, B. bifidum, B. lactis, B. breve, B. longum + **prebiotik** microcrystalline cellulose, inulin, fruit green papaya, apple pectin, ginger, turmeric, fennel seeds, kelp, nori, wakame Méntha piperíta leaf + **enzymes** amylase, glucoamylase, lipase, protease, invertase, maltase, cellulase, bromelain, lactase, papain	Zenwise Health, Daily Digestive Enzymes with Prebiotics and Probiotics (USA) capsules
B. longum, B. lactis, B. breve, B. infantis, L.acidophilus, L. brevis, L. bulgaricus, L. casei, L. fermentum, L. helveticus, L. plantarum, Streptococcus thermophiles + Saccharide, Prunus domestica L., Spinacia oleracea L., Lycium chinense Mill., Lentinula Eldodes, Brassica rapa var. Perviridis, Ficus carica L., V.ashei Reade, V.australe Small, Myrica rubra, Citrus junos, Agaricus blazei, Grifola frondosa, Hizikia fusiforme, Undaria pinnatifida, Laminaria japonica	Dr. Ohhra Probiotics (Japan) capsules
B. bifidum, B. longum, B. breve, L. acidophilus, L.helveticus, L. rhamnosus, L. plantarum, L. casei, Lactococcus lactis, Streptococcus thermophilus + galactooligosaccharides	Bificin (USA) capsules
B. bifidum, B. longum, B. breve, L. acidophilus, L. helveticus, L. rhamnosus, L. casei, L. plantarum, Lactococcus lactis, Streptococcus thermophilus + galactooligosaccharides	Synbiotic Vitateka (probiotic + prebiotic) (USA) capsules
B. bifidum, B. longum, B. breve, L. helveticus, L. rhamnosus, L. casei, L. plantarum, L. acidophilus, Lactococcus lactis, Streptococcus thermophilus + oligofructose	Linebact Maxi synbiotic (USA) capsules
B. bifidum, B. longum, B. adolescentis, L. acidophilus, L. casei, L. helveticus, L. bulgaricus, L. plantarum, Lactococcus lactis, Streptococcus thermophiles, Propionibacterium freudenreichii + red beet juice, enzyme-protein complex of fermented skim milk	Unibacter (Russia) capsules
B. bifidum, B. longum, B. adolescentis, L. acidophilus, L.casei, L. bulgaricus, L. helveticus, L. plantarum, Lactococcus lactis, Lactococcus cremoris, Lactococcus diacetilactis, Streptococcus thermophilus, Propionibacterium shermanii, Propionibacterium arabinosum + skim pasteurized milk mixture	Santa Rus-B (Russia) capsules

(*Continued*)

TABLE 11.3 Probiotics with proven immunomodulatory activity to enhance antiviral immunity.—cont'd

Ingredients	Drug name
Bioenteroseptic Bacillus coagulans + **probiotic** L. acidophilus, B. lactis, L. plantarum, L. casei, Lactococcus lactis, L. bulgaricus, L. rhamnosus, L. brevis, B. bifidum, Streptococcus thermophiles + **prebiotic** microcrystalline cellulose, fructooligosaccharides, whole Acai berry concentrate	Nature's Plus, Ultra Probiotics, (USA) capsules
Bioenteroseptic Saccharomyces boulardii + **probiotic** L acidophilus, L. rhamnosus, L. reuteri, L. brevis, L. bulgaricus, L. helveticus, B. bifidum, B. lactis, B. longum, Pediococcus acidilactici, Pediococcus pentosaceus, Propionibacterium freudenreichii, Streptococcus thermophiles + **prebiotic** microcrystalline cellulose, polysaccharides complex from Lessonia nigrescens, inulin, rice extract + **enzymes** of lactic acid bacteria – L. fermentum	Probulin, Total Care Probiotic (USA) capsules
B. bifidum, B. breve, B. longum, B. lactis, L. acidophilus, L. casei, L. paracasei, L. plantarum, L. rhamnosus, L. helveticus, Streptococcus thermophilus + fructooligosaccharides	Mirrolla Synbiotic MAX (Russia) capsules
B. bifidum, B. longum, B. infantis, B. breve, L. acidophilus, L. casei, L. plantarum, L. rhamnosus, L. helveticus, L. salivarius, L. fermentum, L. bulgaricus, Lactococcus lactis, Streptococcus thermophiles	Buck-Set Forte (UK/Russia) capsules
Bioenteroseptic Bacillus coagulans + **probiotic** L. acidophilus, L. plantarum, L. reuteri, B. longum, B. lactis, L. casei, L. salivarius, L. brevis, B. bifidum, B. animalis, L. mesenteroides, S thermophiles, P. acidilactici, L. fermentum, L. rhamnosus, L. gasseri, L. paracasei, B. breve, Lactococcus lactis, L. bulgaricus, L. helveticus, L. crispatus, B. adolescentis. B. infantis, Pediococcus pentosaceus + **prebiotic** Green Banana, Organic Acacia, Chicory	Nature's Plus, GI Natural Probiotic Mega, (USA) capsules

Metabolic syndrome correction with probiotics

The creation of a recombinant strain of Lactobacillus plantarum expressing the SARS-CoV-2 spike protein is a promising research area, which may provide a promising oral vaccine candidate [220]. The intranasal administration of these lactobacilli significantly enchanced specific mucosal IgA antibodies in the respiratory and intestinal tract that indicates that they are capable of inducing humoral immune response and could be used as a mucosal vaccine candidate against the SARS-CoV-2 infection [221]. Additionally, novel oral vaccines based on self-amplifying RNA lipid nanparticles, transfected in Lactobacillus plantarum have been proposed, which increased the production of IgG and IgA SARS-COV-2 neutralizing antibodies [222].

It is well established that such comorbid pathologies as obesity, impaired lipid and carbohydrate metabolism are risk factors for severe COVID-19 and lethal outcome [223–233]. As such, special attention should be paid to correction of metabolic disorders during the SARS-CoV-2 pandemic. It has been shown that the use of certain probiotic microorganisms contributes to the normalization of lipid and glucose metabolism. Specifically, Bifidobacterium

TABLE 11.4 Probiotics of choice for enhancing post-vaccination immunity to SARS-CoV-2.

Ingredients	Drug name
L. rhamnosus	Gefilus Basic (Finland) capsules Lactobacillus rhamnosus-SM (Russia) powder for oral use in sachet
L. rhamnosus + fructooligosaccharides	Normobact L (Poland) powder for oral use
L. rhamnosus + B1 + B2 + B6 + Zn	Complinex Immuno Probiotic (Slovenia) capsules
L. rhamnosus + fructooligosaccharides + Na and K salt complex	Normobact Aquabalans (Italy) powder for oral use
L. rhamnosus + глюкоза + Na and K salt complex	REGIDRON BIO (Italy) powder for oral use
L. rhamnosus + A + B1 + B2 + B4 + B5 + B6 + B7 + B9 + B12 + E + C + D3 + Ca + Fe + Mg + I + Mn + Cr + Se + Zn	Multi-tabs Immuno Plus (Italy) tablets
L. rhamnosus + D3, refined and unrefined olive oil, medium chain triglycerides	PRO Bifid Malysh (Croatia) drops for oral use
L. rhamnosus + Na and K salt complex + fructose	NATUMA floractive (Italy) powder for oral use in sachet
L. rhamnosus + inulin from Cichorium root	Culturelle, Digestive Daily Probiotic (USA) capsules
L. rhamnosus + larch arabinogalactan, blue agave inulin, fructooligosaccharides (from Cichorium root)	Lake Avenue Nutrition, Digestive Support Probiotic (США) capsules
L. rhamnosus, **L. helveticus**	Lacidofil (Poland) capsules
L. plantarum, **L. fermentum**, L.casei	Bio Long Life Lactobacterin liquid concentrate of Lactobacilli (Russia) solution for oral use
B. bifidum, B. adolescentis, L. bulgaricus, **L. rhamnosus**, L. sakei, immobilized on activated biopolymers (pectin, cellulose) + лактулоза + B1 + B2 + B6 + C	Duopik (Ukraine) powder for oral use
B. longum, B. lactis, **B. breve**, B. infantis, L.acidophilus, L. brevis, L. bulgaricus, L. casei, **L. fermentum, L. helveticus**, L. plantarum, Streptococcus thermophiles + Saccharide, Prunus domestica L., Spinacia oleracea L., Lycium chinense Mill., Lentinula Eldodes, Brassica rapa var. Perviridis, Ficus carica L., V.ashei Reade, V.australe Small, Myrica rubra, Citrus junos, Agaricus blazei, Grifola frondosa, Hizikia fusiforme, Undaria pinnatifida, Laminaria japonica	Dr. Ohhra Probiotics (Japan) capsules
B. bifidum, B. longum, B. infantis, **B. breve**, L. acidophilus, L. casei, L. plantarum, **L. rhamnosus**, **L. helveticus**, L. salivarius, **L. fermentum**, L. bulgaricus, Lactococcus lactis, Streptococcus thermophiles	Buck-Set Forte (UK/Russia) capsules
bioenteroseptic Bacillus coagulans + **probiotic** L. acidophilus, L. plantarum, L. reuteri, B. longum, B. lactis, L. casei, L. salivarius, L. brevis, B. bifidum, B. animalis, L. mesenteroides, S thermophiles, P. acidilactici, L. fermentum, **L. rhamnosus**, L. gasseri, L. paracasei, B. breve, Lactococcus lactis, L. bulgaricus, **L. helveticus**, L. crispatus, B. adolescentis. B. infantis, Pediococcus pentosaceus + **prebiotic** Green Banana, Organic Acacia, Chicory	Nature's Plus, GI Natural Probiotic Mega, (USA) capsules

longum has been shown to reduce blood cholesterol levels, and normalize impaired flucose tolerance through linoleic acid activity [6]. Regular intake of Bifidobacterium lactis BB-12 is also accompanied by a positive effect on both lipid metabolism [122], and glucose tolerance [114]. Lactobacillus acidophilus is also actively involved in the correction of lipid and carbohydrate metabolism [111,114].

Lactobacillus plantarum strains improve vascular endothelial function and decrease systemic inflammation [234]. Their unique ability to separate glycine and taurine from bile acids leads to their elimination and correction of lipid metabolism [235]. Lactobacillus rhamnosus has been shown to reduce obesity risks by producing a conjugated form of linoleic acid [236]. Bifidobacterium breve has also been shown to be effective in obesity treatment [237]. Lactobacillus casei is shown to attenuate several symptoms of type 2 diabetes, including fasting blood glucose, postprandial blood glucose, glucose intolerance, and insulin resistance [118]. Probiotics containing the maximum complex of beneficial bacteria and to a greater extent aimed at correcting metabolic syndrome are presented in Table 11.5.

Impact of COVID-19 on mental health and the role of microbiota

Numerous studies show a significant deterioration in mental health of the population during the SARS-CoV-2 pandemic [238–240]. Fear of coronavirus infection, a continuous flow of negative information, prolonged isolation and the need for constant compliance with sanitary and hygienic requirements leads to an increase in fear and anxiety in society, which is confirmed by data from a number of studies in Russia [241], Japan [242], China [243,244], Spain [245], USA [239,246] and Italy [246]. The complex of identified psychological disorders associated with the impact of the pandemic of the new coronavirus infection was isolated as the **COVID-19 stress syndrome** [247]. Chronic stress condition can negatively affect the course of other chronic conditions [248]. The impact of SARS-CoV-2 infection on mental health is alarming, as it is not uncommon to result in depressive disorders [249,250].

Bifidobacteria and lactobacilli are able to metabolize glutamate (an excitatory neurotransmitter) into gamma-aminobutyric acid, which is involved in the processes of inhibition of the central nervous system. Under the influence of this mediator, the energy processes of the brain are activated, the metabolic activity of nerual tissues increases, the utilization of glucose by the brain improves and blood supply increases. As such, gamma-aminobutyric acid has been shown to correct anxiety-depressive disorders and improve sleep quality [251]. In clinical studies, antidepressant action has been confirmed in Bifidobacterium longum, Bifidobacterium breve and Bifidobacterium adolescentis. Indeed, it was found that B. longum consumption is associated with reduced stress and improved memory [252]. Bifidobacterium breve strains show considerable anxiolytic and antidepressant effects, suggesting novel avenues for therapeutic strategies towards treating anxiety-depressive disorders [172]. Bifidobacterium adolescentis are distinguished by high metabolic activity and might represent a model gamma-aminobutyric acid producer in the human gastrointestinal tract, which highlights their potential in gut-brain axis interaction and antidepressant action [101]. Such probiotic microorganisms with antidepressant action, called psychobiotics, are discussed in Table 11.6.

TABLE 11.5 Probiotics of choice in correction of metabolic syndrome.

Ingredients	Drug name
Polyprobiotics (5) + Prebiotics	
B. bifidum, B. longum, B. lactis, B.breve, L. acidophilus, L. rhamnosus + palm oil, fish gelatin (tilapia), glycerin, soy lecithin, pectin	Nature's Way, Probiotic Pearls Complete (USA) capsules
B. bifidum, B. longum, L. acidophilus, L. plantarum, L. casei, L. rhamnosus, L. salivarius + C	Flora, Super 8 Hi-Potency Probiotic (Canada) capsules
B. lactis, L. acidophilus, L. casei, L. plantarum, L. salivarius, L. rhamnosus, L. reuteri + fructooligosaccharides + Urtíca extract + B5	Synbiotics Vision Bio-In for Hyper Sensivity (France) powder for oral use in sachet
B. bifidum, B. longum, B. breve, B. infantis, L. acidophilus, L. plantarum, L. casei + oligofructose + inulin + B1 + B2 + B4 + B5 + B6 + B7 + B9 + B12 + E + C + Zn + Se	Normospectrum (Russia) capsules Normospectrum Forte (Russia) capsules Normospectrum Junior (Russia) capsules Normospectrum Baby (Russia) capsules
B. bifidum, B. longum, L. acidophilus, L. casei, L, plantarum, L. lactis, L. rhamnosus, L. reuteri, + Fructooligosaccharides, Acai Berry Extract Powder + C	Synbiotics Vision Bio-In with antioxydants (France) powder for oral use in sachet
B. longum, B. breve, L. acidophilus, L. rhamnosus, L. casei, L. bulgaricus, Streptococcus thermophilus + inulin	Multiflora Anti-Age Evalar (Russia) capsules
B. longum, B. breve, B. infantis, L. acidophilus, L. casei, L. rhamnosus, Streptococcus thermophilus + fructooligosaccharides	Buck-Set Baby (UK) powder for oral use in sachet
B. bifidum, B. longum. B. breve, B.adolescentis, L. acidophilus, L.casei, L.plantarum, Streptococcus thermophilus + kim milk,gelatose, lactulose + C	Synbiotic renewal (Russia) capsules
B. bifidum, B. longum, B. breve,L. helveticus, L. rhamnosus, L. lactis, L. casei, L. plantarum,Streptococcus thermophiles + oligofructose + olive oil +C	Maxilak (Poland) capsules
B. bifidum, B. longum, B. breve, L. helveticus, L. casei, L. rhamnosus, L. plantarum, Lactococcus lactis, Streptococcus thermophilus + fructooligosaccharides + B1 + B2 + B6	Lacidoforte (Bulgaria) capsules
bioenteroseptic Bacillus coagulans + **probiotic** L. acidophilus, B. lactis, L. plantarum, L. casei, Lactococcus lactis, L. bulgaricus, L. rhamnosus, L. brevis, B. bifidum, Streptococcus thermophiles + **prebiotic** microcrystalline cellulose, fructooligosaccharides, whole Acai berry concentrate	Nature's Plus, Ultra Probiotics, (USA) capsules
Probiotic B. infantis, B. bifidum, B. longum, B. breve, L. casei, L. acidophilus, L. rhamnosus + **prebiotic** inulin, fibregam, lactulose, vitamins B + beta-glucan + **metabiotic** lysates of Propionibacterium freudenreichii and Propionibacterium arabinosum	Panbiolact Kids (Russia) capsules

(Continued)

TABLE 11.5 Probiotics of choice in correction of metabolic syndrome.—cont'd

Ingredients	Drug name
Polyprobiotics (6) + Prebiotics	
B. bifidum, B. longum, B. lactis, L. acidophilus, L. plantarum, L. salivarius, L. rhamnosus, L. casei + inulin + microcrystalline cellulose	Nutrition Now, PB 8 (USA) capsules
B. bifidum, B. longum, B. lactis, L. acidophilus, L. casei, L. paracasei, L. plantarum, L. rhamnosus, L. salivarius + fructooligosaccharides, oligofructose	Maxilak Baby (Poland) powder for oral use in sachet
B. bifidum, B. longum, B. breve, L. acidophilus, L. plantarum, L. lactis, L. rhamnosus, L. casei, L. paracasei + L-leucine	Sports Research, Daily Probiotics (USA) capsules
B. longum, B. lactis, B. breve, B. infantis, L.acidophilus, L. brevis, L. bulgaricus, L. casei, L. fermentum, L. helveticus, L. plantarum, Streptococcus thermophiles + Saccharide, Prunus domestica L., Spinacia oleracea L., Lycium chinense Mill., Lentinula Eldodes, Brassica rapa var. Perviridis, Ficus carica L., V.ashei Reade, V.australe Small, Myrica rubra, Citrus junos, Agaricus blazei, Grifola frondosa, Hizikia fusiforme, Undaria pinnatifida, Laminaria japonica	Dr. Ohhra Probiotics (Japan) capsules
B. bifidum, B. longum, B. breve, L. acidophilus, L.helveticus, L. rhamnosus, L. plantarum, L. casei, Lactococcus lactis, Streptococcus thermophilus + galactooligosaccharides	Bificin (USA) capsules
B. bifidum, B. longum, B. breve, L. acidophilus, L. helveticus, L. rhamnosus, L. casei, L. plantarum, Lactococcus lactis, Streptococcus thermophilus + galactooligosaccharides	Synbiotic Vitateka (probiotic + prebiotic) (USA) capsules
B. bifidum, B. longum, B. breve, L. helveticus, L. rhamnosus, L. casei, L. plantarum, L. acidophilus, Lactococcus lactis, Streptococcus thermophilus + oligofructose	Linebact Maxi synbiotic (USA) capsules
Probiotic L. acidophilus, L. plantarum, L. casei, L. salivarius, L. rhamnosus, L. helveticus, B. bifidum, B. lactis, B. breve, B. longum + **prebiotic** green papaya, apple pectin, ginger, fennel seeds, kelp, nori, wakame, Méntha piperíta leaf, inulin + **enzymes** amylase, glucoamylase, lipase, protease, invertase, maltase, cellulase, bromelain, lactase, papain	Zenwise Health, Daily Digestive Enzymes (USA) capsules
Polyprobiotics (7) + Prebiotics	
B. bifidum, B. longum, B. lactis, B. breve, L. acidophilus, L. plantarum, L. paracasei, L. casei, L. brevis, L. rhamnosus, L. salivarius + microcrystalline cellulose, fructooligosaccharides	Healthy BIOM, High Potency Probiotics (USA) capsules
B. longum, B. lactis, B. breve, L. acidophilus, L. plantarum, L. salivarius, L. casei, L. rhamnosus, L. paracasei, Streptococcus thermophilus + microcrystalline cellulose, fructooligosaccharides	Now, Probiotic-10 (USA) Capsules
B. longum, B. lactis, B. breve, L. acidophilus, L. plantarum, L. casei, L. rhamnosus, L. salivarius, L.paracasei, Streptococcus thermophilus + microcrystalline cellulose, fructooligosaccharides	Lake Avenue Nutrition Probiotic (USA) Capsules

TABLE 11.5 Probiotics of choice in correction of metabolic syndrome.—cont'd

Ingredients	Drug name
B. longum, B. lactis, B. breve, L. acidophilus, L. plantarum, L. casei, L. rhamnosus, L.salivarius, L. paracasei, Streptococcus thermophilus + microcrystalline cellulose, fructooligosaccharides, Aloe barbadensis leaf	Now Foods, Aloe 10,000 Probiotics (USA) Capsules
B. bifidum, B. breve, B. longum, B. lactis, L. acidophilus, L. casei, L. paracasei, L. plantarum, L. rhamnosus, L. helveticus, Streptococcus thermophilus + fructooligosaccharides	Mirrolla Synbiotic MAX (Russia) capsules
bioenteroseptic Bacillus coagulans + **probiotic** L. acidophilus, L. plantarum, L. reuteri, B. longum, B. lactis, L. casei, L. salivarius, L. brevis, B. bifidum, B. animalis, L. mesenteroides, S thermophiles, P. acidilactici, L. fermentum, L. rhamnosus, L. gasseri, L. paracasei, B. breve, Lactococcus lactis, L. bulgaricus, L. helveticus, L. crispatus, B. adolescentis. B. infantis, Pediococcus pentosaceus + **prebiotic** Green Banana, Organic Acacia, Chicory	Nature's Plus, GI Natural Probiotic Mega, (USA) capsules
Probiotic L. acidophilus, L. plantarum, L. casei, L. salivarius, L. rhamnosus, L. helveticus, B. bifidum, B. lactis, B. breve, B. longum + **prebiotik** microcrystalline cellulose, inulin, fruit green papaya, apple pectin, ginger, turmeric, fennel seeds , kelp, nori, wakame Méntha piperíta leaf + **enzymes** amylase, glucoamylase, lipase, protease, invertase, maltase, cellulase, bromelain, lactase, papain	Zenwise Health, Daily Digestive Enzymes with Prebiotics and Probiotics (USA) capsules

TABLE 11.6 Probiotics of choice for correcting anxiety-depressive disorders during SARS-CoV-2 pandemic.

Ingredients	Drug name
B. bifidum, **B.longum, B.adolescentis, B.breve** + lactitol, glucose	Probioflor BAG-Bifido (Russia) capsules
B. bifidum, **B.longum. B. breve, B.adolescentis**, L. acidophilus, L.casei, L.plantarum, Streptococcus thermophilus + kim milk, gelatose, lactulose + C	Synbiotic renewal (Russia) capsules
Probiotic B. breve, L. acidophilus, L. casei, L. salivarius, L. rhamnosus, Propionibacterium freudenreichii + **metabiotic** lysate mix **B. adolescentis, B. longum**, L. bulgaricus, Streptococcus thermophilus + **prebiotic** inulin	Panbiolact De-Fem (Russia) capsules
bioenteroseptic Bacillus coagulans + **probiotic** L. acidophilus, L. plantarum, L. reuteri, **B. longum**, B. lactis, L. casei, L. salivarius, L. brevis, B. bifidum, B. animalis, L. mesenteroides, S thermophiles, P. acidilactici, L. fermentum, L. rhamnosus, L. gasseri, L. paracasei, **B. breve**, Lactococcus lactis, L. bulgaricus, L. helveticus, L. crispatus, **B. adolescentis**. B. infantis, Pediococcus pentosaceus + **prebiotic** Green Banana, Organic Acacia, Chicory	Nature's Plus, GI Natural Probiotic Mega, (USA) capsules

Hyperreactive reactions and microbiota

Patients with hyperreactive allergic conditions require special attnetion during the SARS-CoV-2 pandemic due to their predisposition to acute respiratory infections [253–255]. It has been established that persistent hyperreactive inflammation weakens the immune system and causes interferon type I depletion, which leads to a weakened antiviral response [256,257]. Moreover, allergic comorbidity is associated with more severe SARS-CoV-2 clinical outcomes [253,258,259]. Most hyperreactive conditions are linked to compositional and functional changes in gut microbiota that affect oral tolerance through interaction of microbial molecules with pattern recognition receptors on immune cells [260–262].

In recent years probiotics have gained widespread attention as a preventive and therapeutic treatment for hyperreactive conditions, including allergic reactions [262–264]. Bifidobacterium breve and Lactobacillus helveticus are considered especially promising in correction of chronic allergic conditions. Bifidobacterium breve is involved in modulation of anti-allergic processes by IL-33/ST2 signaling [265,266]. More so, B. breve plays a role in sppresion of T-helper type 2 immune responses and modulating the systemic Th1/Th2 balance [267]. The enzymatic activity of Lactobacillus helveticus is beneficial for the host, as it increases the breakdown of allergens, suppresses eosinophil production [108,214,268]. Probiotics containing combinations of microorganisms involved in antihyperreactive and antiallergenic action are presented in Table 11.7.

SARS-CoV-2 associated respiratory syndrome and microbiome

The SARS-CoV-2 virus primarily enters via epithelial cells of the alveoli, making pulmonary cells the primary target and promoting the well-known respiratory syndrome [82,269]. The degree of damage to pulmonary tissues largely determines the clinical progression of COVID-19 [270–272]. Currently, probiotics are discussed as a factor in slowing the progression of COVID-19 progression through pulmonary protection [273–275].

It has been proven that the use of a special strain of Lactobacillus plantarum in the treatment of respiratory tract infections helps reduce the duration of inflammation [276]. In addition, this probiotic has demonstrated efficacy similar to the action of antibiotics against pneumococcus and Staphylococcus aureus, which often complicate viral infections [276]. The results of other authors showed that Lactobacillus plantarum significantly inhibits SARS-CoV-2 replication and production of reactive oxygen species (ROS). Lactobacillus plantarum has therefore been suggested as a prevention agent, complicating the binding of ss-RNA during replication of SARS-CoV-2 [277].

Lactococcus lactis, a bacteria capable of synthetizing bacteriocin nisin, has a pronounced antagonistic activity against most pathogenic gram-positive bacteria (staphylococci, micrococci, bacilli, clostridia) [278]. Moreover, its lipopeptide lactococcin Gb demonstrates immunomodulatory activity and ability to bind to the spike protein and receptor molecule to competitively inhibit SARS-CoV-2 interaction with host epithelial cells expressing ACE2 [279]. Antimicrobial peptides glycocin F (from Lactococcus lactis) and lactococcine G (from Lactobacillus plantarum) have high affinities to bind to SARS-CoV-2 viral proteins, promoting its elimination [280].

TABLE 11.7 Probiotics of choice for correcting allergy manifestations.

Ingredients	Drug name
B. bifidum, B. longum, B. infantis, B. breve, L. acidophilus, L. casei, L. plantarum, L. rhamnosus, L. helveticus, L. salivarius, L. fermentum, L. bulgaricus, Lactococcus lactis, Streptococcus thermophiles	Buck-Set Forte (UK/ Russia) capsules
B. bifidum, B. longum, B. breve,L. helveticus, L. rhamnosus, Lactococcus lactis, L. casei, L. plantarum, Streptococcus thermophiles + oligofructose + olive oil + C	Maxilak (Poland) capsules
B. bifidum, B. breve, B. longum, B. lactis, L. acidophilus, L. casei, L. paracasei, L. plantarum, L. rhamnosus, L. helveticus, Streptococcus thermophilus + fructooligosaccharides	Mirrolla Synbiotic MAX (Russia) capsules
B. longum, B. lactis, B. breve, B. infantis, L.acidophilus, L. brevis, L. bulgaricus, L. casei, L. fermentum, L. helveticus, L. plantarum, Streptococcus thermophiles + Saccharide, Prunus domestica L., Spinacia oleracea L., Lycium chinense Mill., Lentinula Eldodes, Brassica rapa var. Perviridis, Ficus carica L., V.ashei Reade, V.australe Small, Myrica rubra, Citrus junos, Agaricus blazei, Grifola frondosa, Hizikia fusiforme, Undaria pinnatifida, Laminaria japonica	Dr. Ohhra Probiotics (Japan) capsules
B. bifidum, B. longum, B. breve, L. acidophilus, L.helveticus, L. rhamnosus, L. plantarum, L. casei, Lactococcus lactis, Streptococcus thermophilus + galactooligosaccharides	Bificin (USA) capsules
B. bifidum, B. longum, B. breve, L. acidophilus, L. helveticus, L. rhamnosus, L. casei, L. plantaru Lactococcus lactis, Streptococcus thermophilus + galactooligosaccharides	Synbiotic Vitateka (probiotic + prebiotic) (USA) capsules
B. bifidum, B. longum, B. breve, L. helveticus, L. rhamnosus, L. casei, L. plantarum, L. acidophilus, Lactococcus lactis, Streptococcus thermophilus + oligofructose	Linebact Maxi synbiotic (USA) capsules
B. bifidum, B. longum, B. breve, L. helveticus, L. casei, L. rhamnosus, L. plantarum, Lactococcus lactis, Streptococcus thermophilus + fructooligosaccharides + B1 + B2 + B6	Lacidoforte (Bulgaria) capsules
metabiotic peptides of B. breve, L. helveticus, L. plantarum, Propionibacterium freudenreichii + **enzymes** glutathione, superoxide dismutase + **prebiotic** L-rarnitine, hesperidin, C, Zn, succinic acid, cysteine, coenzyme Q10, lipoic acid, Mn, Cu	Mega Pro Age (Russia) powder for oral use in sachet
Probiotic L. acidophilus, L. plantarum, L. casei, L. salivarius, L. rhamnosus, L. helveticus, B. bifidum, B. lactis, B. breve, B. longum + **prebiotic** green papaya, apple pectin, ginger, fennel seeds, kelp, nori, wakame, Méntha piperíta leaf, inulin + **enzymes** amylase, glucoamylase, lipase, protease, invertase, maltase, cellulase, bromelain, lactase, papain	Zenwise Health, Daily Digestive Enzymes (USA) capsules
Probiotic L. acidophilus, L. plantarum, L. casei, L. salivarius, L. rhamnosus, L. helveticus, B. bifidum, B. lactis, B. breve, B. longum + **prebiotik** microcrystalline cellulose, inulin, fruit green papaya, apple pectin, ginger, turmeric, fennel seeds, kelp, nori, wakame Méntha piperíta leaf + **enzymes** amylase, glucoamylase, lipase, protease, invertase, maltase, cellulase, bromelain, lactase, papain	Zenwise Health, Daily Digestive Enzymes with Prebiotics and Probiotics (USA) capsules

Oral administration of Lactobacillus acidophilus significantly decreases pulmonary bacterial load and severity of viral infections [212]. It was also shown that administration of this probiotic stimulates and modulates the respiratory immune system [281]. Lactobacillus rhamnosus is distinguished by a special ability to produce antimicrobial factors reuterin, lactocidin, plantaricin, and lactolin [2]. The ability of these microorganisms to enhance type I interferons and antiviral factors in the respiratory tract, stimulate Th1 response, antibody production, regulate inflammation and coagulation actiity during the course of viral infections helps reduce tissue damage and preserve pulmonary function, indicating their potential to favorably influence the immune response against the SARS-CoV-2 virus [282]. Complexes containing these probiotic microorganisms are shown in Table 11.8.

Gastrointestinal pathology and COVID-19

When infected with SARS-CoV-2, in addition to respiratory symptoms, almost half of patients have intestinal distress [152,275,283–285]. Gastrointestinal symptoms are the second most common in COVID-19 [286,287]. These findings suggest that the intestinal tract serves as a locus of high viral activity and replication, mainly due to ACE-2 expression in the intestinal epithelium [288–292]. Patients suffering from chronic gastrointestinal diseases are considered to be at moderate-to-high risk of SARS-CoV-2 infection, implying the importance of microbiota dysbiosis in disease pathogenesis [293]. Importantly, antibioitcs prescribed to treat COVID-19 complications cause a wide variety of intestinal pathology [84]. Hospitalized COVID-19 patients with diarrhea showed an increase in the titer of opportunistic flora and a decrease in the population of beneficial bacteria. Moreover, the severity of dysbiosis correlated with the severity of COVID-19 and viral load [294].

Currently, probiotics play a decisive role in the treatment of diarrheal syndrome in SARS-CoV-2. Combined preparations containing highly adhesive symbiotic strains should be used. Among bifidobacteria, sorbed Bifidobacterium bifidum proved clinical efficacy, the use of which significantly improved the well-being of patients with SARS-CoV-2 and reduced the duration of diarrheal syndrome [167] Research shows that these symbionts relieve the diarrhea symptoms by significantly reducing stool water content, restoring villi structure in the jejunum and ameliorating fecal short-chain fatty acid content [295]. Oral Bifidobacterium bifidum administration palliated diarrhea partly through protection against virus-induced lesions and mucosal protective factors [296].

Bifidobacteria longum proved to be effective at reducing virus-induced diarrhea by preventing the interaction of viruses and host cells due to produced low-molecular weight and non-protein components [151,297]. Bifidobacteria longum can prevent antibiotic associated diarrhoea since they have antibiotic resistance due to the presence of ABC-type multidrug efflux systems [298]. The 11-mer peptide, derived from Bifidobacteria longum, has been identified as an antiviral agent both in vivo and in vitro [299]. Bifidobacterium adolescentis shows potential to strengthen host defense against gastrointestinal infection via stimulation of macrophage activity [103]. These probiotics significantly decrease diarrhea and exhibit protective effects through enhancing tight junction protein and mucin expression, decreasing pro-inflammatory cytokines and increasing anti-inflammatory molecule content [300].

TABLE 11.8 Probiotics of choice for reducing viral (including SARS-CoV-2) respiratory syndrome severity.

Ingredients	Drug name
L.acidophilus, L.casei, L. plantarum, Lactococcus lactis + lactitol, glucose	Probioflor Bag-lacto (Russia) capsules
B. bifidum, B. longum, B. breve,L. helveticus, L. rhamnosus, Lactococcus lactis, L. casei, L. plantarum,Streptococcus thermophiles + oligofructose + olive oil + C	Maxilak (Poland) capsules
B. bifidum, B. longum, B. breve, L. helveticus, L. casei, L. rhamnosus, L. plantarum, Lactococcus lactis, Streptococcus thermophilus + fructooligosaccharides + B1 + B2 + B6	Lacidoforte (Bulgaria) capsules
B. lactis, B. longum, L.acidophilus, L. paracasei, L. plantarum, L. salivarius, Lactococcus lactis, Streptococcus thermophiles + fructooligosaccharides, inulin	Rioflora Immuno (Netherlands, Germany) capsules
B. lactis, B. longum, L.acidophilus, L. paracasei, L. plantarum, L. salivarius, Lactococcus lactis, Streptococcus thermophiles + fructooligosaccharides, inulin	Rioflora Immuno (Netherlands, Germany) capsules
B. bifidum, B. longum, B. adolescentis, L. acidophilus, L. casei, L. helveticus, L. bulgaricus, L. plantarum, Lactococcus lactis, Streptococcus thermophiles, Propionibacterium freudenreichii + red beet juice, enzyme-protein complex of fermented skim milk	Unibacter (Russia) capsules
B. bifidum, B. longum, L. acidophilus, L. casei, L, plantarum, Lactococcus lactis, L. rhamnosus, L.reuteri, + Fructooligosaccharides, Acai Berry Extract Powder + C	Synbiotics Vision Bio-In with antioxydants (France) powder for oral use in sachet
B. bifidum, B. longum, B. adolescentis, L. acidophilus, L.casei, L. bulgaricus, L. helveticus, L. plantarum, Lactococcus lactis, Lactococcus cremoris, Lactococcus diacetilactis, Streptococcus thermophilus, Propionibacterium shermanii, Propionibacterium arabinosum + skim pasteurized milk mixture	Santa Rus-B (Russia) capsules
B. bifidum, B. longum, B. infantis, B. breve, L. acidophilus, L. casei, L. plantarum, L. rhamnosus, L. helveticus, L. salivarius, L. fermentum, L. bulgaricus, Lactococcus lactis, Streptococcus thermophiles	Buck-Set Forte (UK/Russia) capsules
B. bifidum, B. longum, B. breve, L. acidophilus, L.helveticus, L. rhamnosus, L. plantarum, L. casei, Lactococcus lactis, Streptococcus thermophilus + galactooligosaccharides	Bificin (USA) capsules
B. bifidum, B. longum, B. breve, L. acidophilus, L. helveticus, L. rhamnosus, L. casei, L. plantaru Lactococcus lactis, Streptococcus thermophilus + galactooligosaccharides	Synbiotic Vitateka (probiotic + prebiotic) (USA) capsules
B. bifidum, B. longum, B. breve, L. helveticus, L. rhamnosus, L. casei, L. plantarum, L. acidophilus, Lactococcus lactis, Streptococcus thermophilus + oligofructose	Linebact Maxi synbiotic (USA) capsules

(Continued)

TABLE 11.8 Probiotics of choice for reducing viral (including SARS-CoV-2) respiratory syndrome severity.—cont'd

Ingredients	Drug name
bioenteroseptic Bacillus coagulans + **probiotic** L. acidophilus, L. plantarum, L. reuteri, B. longum, B. lactis, L. casei, L. salivarius, L. brevis, B. bifidum, B. animalis, L. mesenteroides, S thermophiles, P. acidilactici, L. fermentum, L. rhamnosus, L. gasseri, L. paracasei, B. breve, Lactococcus lactis, L. bulgaricus, L. helveticus, L. crispatus, B. adolescentis. B. infantis, Pediococcus pentosaceus + **prebiotic** Green Banana, Organic Acacia, Chicory	Nature's Plus, GI Natural Probiotic Mega, (USA) capsules
bioenteroseptic Bacillus coagulans + **probiotic** L. acidophilus, B. lactis, L. plantarum, L. casei, Lactococcus lactis, L. bulgaricus, L. rhamnosus, L. brevis, B. bifidum, Streptococcus thermophiles + **prebiotic** microcrystalline cellulose, fructooligosaccharides, whole Acai berry concentrate	Nature's Plus, Ultra Probiotics, (USA) capsules

Lactobacillus acidophilus supplementation is shown to be effective and safe in the treatment of acute and chronic diarrhea, including antibiotic-associated diarrhea, even in immunocompromised patients [301]. Lactobacillia rhamnosus has shown the ability to prevent the course of acute diarrhea associated with viral and bacterial infections [302]. The pronounced antidiarrheal activity of these commensals is due to the upregulation of TLR3 gene expression [303]. Probiotics containing Lactobacillus rhamnosus, Bifidobacterium bifidum and Bifidobacterium longum have been shown to be effective in treating diarrhea associated with SARS-CoV-2 and in preventing hospital-acquired diarrhea in patients who received a single antibiotic [304].

The antidiarrheal activity of Lactobacillus reuteri containing probiotics is due to its ability to produce a broad-spectrum antibiotic - reuterin, which has a strong inhibitory effect on a wide range of pathogenic microorganisms, including gram-negative and gram-positive bacteria [305]. The effectiveness of this probiotic microorganism in the treatment of diarrhea has been shown in numerous studies [306–310]. Lactococcus lactis synthesize the bacteriocin nisin, which exhibits antagonistic activity against most pathogenic gram-positive bacteria—staphylococci, micrococci, bacilli, clostridia [278]. Probiotic complexes with an antidiarrheal effect, are presented in Table 11.9.

The role of the microbiome in SARS-CoV-2 associated cytokine storm

The cytokine storm is an immunopathological reaction of the human body to the SARS-CoV-2 virus, characterized by hypercytokinemia and the development of life-threatening conditions including acute respiratory syndrome, multiple organ failure, and coagulopathy [311–314]. An association between intestinal microbiota composition and the susceptibility of some patients to develop severe COVID-19 has been shown by several studies [315–318].

TABLE 11.9 Probiotics of choice for reducing diarrhea syndrome in SARS-CoV-2 patients.

Ingredients	Drug name
B. bifidum, B. lactis, L. acidophilus, L. salivarius, L. plantarum, L. rhamnosus, L. reuteri + fructooligosaccharides + Chamomile extract + C + Zn	Synbiotics Vision Bio-In for Respiratory System (France) powder for oral use in sachet
B. bifidum, B. longum, L. acidophilus, L. plantarum, L. casei, L. rhamnosus, L. salivarius + C	Flora, Super 8 Hi-Potency Probiotic (Canada) capsules
B. bifidum, B. longum, B. lactis, L. acidophilus, L. plantarum, L. salivarius, L. rhamnosus, L. casei + inulin + microcrystalline cellulose	Nutrition Now, PB 8 (USA) capsules
B. bifidum, B. longum, B. lactis, L. acidophilus, L. casei, L. paracasei, L. plantarum, L. rhamnosus, L. salivarius + fructooligosaccharides, oligofructose	Maxilak Baby (Poland) powder for oral use in sachet
B. bifidum, B. longum, B. lactis, B. breve, L. acidophilus, L. plantarum, L. paracasei, L. casei, L. brevis, L. rhamnosus, L. salivarius + microcrystalline cellulose, fructooligosaccharides	Healthy BIOM, High Potency Probiotics (USA) capsules
B. bifidum, B.longum. B. breve, B.adolescentis, L. acidophilus, L.casei, L.plantarum, Streptococcus thermophilus + kim milk, gelatose, lactulose + C	Synbiotic renewal (Russia) capsules
B. bifidum, B. longum, B. breve,L. helveticus, L. rhamnosus, Lactococcus lactis, L. casei, L. plantarum, Streptococcus thermophiles + oligofructose + olive oil +C	Maxilak (Poland) capsules
B. bifidum, B. breve, B. longum, B. lactis, L. acidophilus, L. casei, L. paracasei, L. plantarum, L. rhamnosus, L. helveticus, Streptococcus thermophilus + fructooligosaccharides	Mirrolla Synbiotic MAX (Russia) capsules
B. bifidum, B. longum, B. breve, L. helveticus, L. casei, L. rhamnosus, L. plantarum, Lactococcus lactis, Streptococcus thermophilus + fructooligosaccharides + B1 + B2 + B6	Lacidoforte (Bulgaria) capsules
B. bifidum, B. longum, B. infantis, B. breve, L. acidophilus, L. casei, L. plantarum, L. rhamnosus, L. helveticus, L. salivarius, L. fermentum, L. bulgaricus, Lactococcus lactis, Streptococcus thermophiles	Buck-Set Forte (UK/Russia) capsules
B. bifidum, B. longum, B. breve, L. acidophilus, L.helveticus, L. rhamnosus, L. plantarum, L. casei, Lactococcus lactis, Streptococcus thermophilus + galactooligosaccharides	Bificin (USA) capsules
B. bifidum, B. longum, B. breve, L. acidophilus, L. helveticus, L. rhamnosus, L. casei, L. plantaru Lactococcus lactis, Streptococcus thermophilus + galactooligosaccharides	Synbiotic Vitateka (probiotic + prebiotic) (USA) capsules
B. bifidum, B. longum, B. breve, L. helveticus, L. rhamnosus, L. casei, L. plantarum, L. acidophilus, Lactococcus lactis, Streptococcus thermophilus + oligofructose	Linebact Maxi synbiotic (USA) capsules

(*Continued*)

TABLE 11.9 Probiotics of choice for reducing diarrhea syndrome in SARS-CoV-2 patients.—cont'd

Ingredients	Drug name
B. bifidum, B. longum, B. adolescentis, L. acidophilus, L. casei, L. helveticus, L. bulgaricus, L. plantarum, Lactococcus lactis, Streptococcus thermophiles, Propionibacterium freudenreichii + red beet juice, enzyme-protein complex of fermented skim milk	Unibacter (Russia) capsules
B. bifidum, B. longum, B. adolescentis, L. acidophilus, L.casei, L. bulgaricus, L. helveticus, L. plantarum, Lactococcus lactis, Lactococcus cremoris, Lactococcus diacetilactis, Streptococcus thermophilus, Propionibacterium shermanii, Propionibacterium arabinosum + skim pasteurized milk mixture	Santa Rus-B (Russia) capsules
B. bifidum, B. longum, L. acidophilus, L. casei, L, plantarum, Lactococcus lactis, L. rhamnosus, L.reuteri + Fructooligosaccharides, Acai Berry Extract Powder + C	Synbiotics Vision Bio-In with antioxydants (France) powder for oral use in sachet
B. bifidum, B. longum, B. breve, L. acidophilus, L. plantarum, Lactococcus lactis, L. rhamnosus, L. casei, L. paracasei + L-leucine	Sports Research, Daily Probiotics (USA) capsules
Bioenteroseptic Bacillus coagulans + **probiotic** L. acidophilus, L. plantarum, L. reuteri, B. longum, B. lactis, L. casei, L. salivarius, L. brevis, B. bifidum, B. animalis, L. mesenteroides, S thermophiles, P. acidilactici, L. fermentum, L. rhamnosus, L. gasseri, L. paracasei, B. breve, Lactococcus lactis, L. bulgaricus, L. helveticus, L. crispatus, B. adolescentis. B. infantis, Pediococcus pentosaceus + **prebiotic** Green Banana, Organic Acacia, Chicory	Nature's Plus, GI Natural Probiotic Mega, (USA) capsules
Probiotic L. acidophilus, L. plantarum, L. casei, L. salivarius, L. rhamnosus, L. helveticus, B. bifidum, B. lactis, B. breve, B. longum + **prebiotic** green papaya, apple pectin, ginger, fennel seeds, kelp, nori, wakame, Méntha piperíta leaf, inulin + **enzymes** amylase, glucoamylase, lipase, protease, invertase, maltase, cellulase, bromelain, lactase, papain	Zenwise Health, Daily Digestive Enzymes (USA) capsules
Probiotic L. acidophilus, L. plantarum, L. casei, L. salivarius, L. rhamnosus, L. helveticus, B. bifidum, B. lactis, B. breve, B. longum + **prebiotik** microcrystalline cellulose, inulin, fruit green papaya, apple pectin, ginger, turmeric, fennel seeds, kelp, nori, wakame Méntha piperíta leaf + **enzymes** amylase, glucoamylase, lipase, protease, invertase, maltase, cellulase, bromelain, lactase, papain	Zenwise Health, Daily Digestive Enzymes with Prebiotics and Probiotics (USA) capsules
Bioenteroseptic Saccharomyces boulardii + **probiotic** L acidophilus, L. rhamnosus, L. reuteri, L. brevis, L. bulgaricus, L. helveticus, B. bifidum, B. lactis, B. longum, Pediococcus acidilactici, Pediococcus pentosaceus, Propionibacterium freudenreichii, Streptococcus thermophiles + **prebiotic** microcrystalline cellulose, polysaccharides complex from Lessonia nigrescens, inulin, rice extract + **enzymes** of lactic acid bacteria − L. fermentum	Probulin, Total Care Probiotic (USA) capsules

TABLE 11.10 Probiotics of choice for cytokine storm prevention.

Ingredients	Drug name
L. rhamnosus, L. reuteri	Lactogin (Croatia) capsules
L. reuteri + sucrose, sunflower oil, triglyceride oil	BioGaia (Sweden) probiotic drops for baby
L. reuteri + sucrose, sunflower oil, medium-chain caprylic triglycerides + D3	BioGaia (Sweden) probiotic drops for babies with vitamin D3
L. reuteri + sucrose, xylitol	BioGaia (Sweden) tablets
L. reuteri + medium-chain triglycerides	Maxilak Baby (Poland) drops for oral use
L. reuteri + sunflower oil	BioAmicus Probiotics Lactobacillus (Canada) drops for oral use
L. reuteri + sunflower oil + D3	BioAmicus Probiotics Lactobacillus with vitamin D3 (Canada) drops for oral use
L. reuteri Protectis + plant oils derivatives	Rela Life (Sweden) drops for oral use
L. acidophilus, L. rhamnosus, L. reuteri + fructooligosaccharides	Nature's Way, Primadophilus Reuteri Superior Probiotic (USA) capsules
L. acidophilus, L. plantarum, L. rhamnosus, L. reuteri, L. gasseri + fructooligosaccharides + Vaccinium macrocarpon extract + D-mannose	Synbiotics Vision Bio-In for Women's Health (France) powder for oral use in sachet
L. salivarius, L. paracasei, L. rhamnosus, L. reuteri, L. brevis + fructooligosaccharides + L-lysine + D3	Synbiotics Vision Bio-In for Oral Care (France) powder for oral use in sachet
B. lactis, L. acidophilus, L. reuteri + lactoferrin + fructooligosaccharides	NATUMA bactoflor baby (Italy) drops for oral use
B. bifidum, B. lactis, L. acidophilus, L. plantarum, L. reuteri + fructooligosaccharides + Cucurbita seed extract + E + Zn + lycopene	Synbiotics Vision Bio-In for Men's Health (France) powder for oral use in sachet
B. lactis, L. acidophilus, L. paracasei, L. rhamnosus, L. reuteri, L. casei + fructooligosaccharides	Synbiotics Vision Bio-In Probiotics & Prebiotics (France) powder for oral use in sachet
B. bifidum, B. lactis, L. acidophilus, L. salivarius, L. plantarum, L. rhamnosus, L. reuteri + fructooligosaccharides + Chamomile extract + C + Zn	Synbiotics Vision Bio-In for Respiratory System (France) powder for oral use in sachet
B. lactis, L. acidophilus, L. casei, L. plantarum, L. salivarius, L. rhamnosus, L. reuteri + fructooligosaccharides + Urtíca extract + B5	Synbiotics Vision Bio-In for Hyper Sensivity (France) powder for oral use in sachet
B. bifidum, B. longum, L. acidophilus, L. casei, L, plantarum, L. lactis, L. rhamnosus, L.reuteri, + Fructooligosaccharides, Acai Berry Extract Powder + C	Synbiotics Vision Bio-In with antioxydants (France) powder for oral use in sachet
B. bifidum, B. longum, B. lactis, B. breve, B. infantis, L. gasseri, L. plantarum, **L. reuteri**, L. salivarius + sunflower oil	BioAmicus Probiotics Complete (Canada) drops for oral use

(Continued)

TABLE 11.10 Probiotics of choice for cytokine storm prevention.—cont'd

Ingredients	Drug name
L. casei, L. paracasei, L. rhamnosus, L. reuteri, L. acidophilus, Streptococcus thermophiles + fructooligosaccharides + Ca + Mg + D3	Synbiotics Vision Bio-In Bonecare (France) powder for oral use in sachet
Bioenteroseptic Bacillus coagulans + **probiotic** L. acidophilus, L. plantarum, L. reuteri, B. longum, B. lactis, L. casei, L. salivarius, L. brevis, B. bifidum, B. animalis, L. mesenteroides, S thermophiles, P. acidilactici, L. fermentum, L. rhamnosus, L. gasseri, L. paracasei, B. breve, Lactococcus lactis, L. bulgaricus, L. helveticus, L. crispatus, B. adolescentis. B. infantis, Pediococcus pentosaceus + **prebiotic** Green Banana, Organic Acacia, Chicory	Nature's Plus, GI Natural Probiotic Mega, (USA) capsules
Bioenteroseptic Saccharomyces boulardii + **probiotic** L acidophilus, L. rhamnosus, L. reuteri, L. brevis, L. bulgaricus, L. helveticus, B. bifidum, B. lactis, B. longum, Pediococcus acidilactici, Pediococcus pentosaceus, Propionibacterium freudenreichii, Streptococcus thermophiles + **prebiotic** microcrystalline cellulose, polysaccharides complex from Lessonia nigrescens, inulin, rice extract + **enzymes** of lactic acid bacteria – L. fermentum	Probulin, Total Care Probiotic (USA) capsules

Probiotics, as potential immunomodulatory agents, are proposed to improve the host's response to viral infection [205]. Normal microbiota bacteria have the potential to ameliorate the onset of the cytokine storm through a differential effect on pro- and antiinflammatory cytokines [319]. Lactobacilli plantarum and Lactobacillus reuteri are known to suppress plasma concentrations of inflammatory cytokines [276]. Lactobacillus reuteri reduces the production of proinflammatory cytokines while promoting the development of regulatory T cells. With the ability to strengthen the intestinal barrier, colonization of these commensals can reduce microbial translocation from the intestinal lumen into tissues [320,321]. Probiotics containing these symbionts are shown in Table 11.10.

Metabiotics: novel treatment strategies

Patients with a damaged intestinal barrier and concomitant immunodeficiency require the restoration of the intestinal microbiome visa metabiotics—a new generation of biological products containing not the microorganisms themselves, but the products of their metabolism. The most important components of metabiotics are the structural components of probiotic bacteria themselves, antibacterial substrates, short-chain fatty organic acids, polysaccharides, antioxidants, nucleic acids, lipo- and glycoproteins, vitamins, enzymes and lectins, amino acids, growth and coagulation factors, signaling molecules. The use of these active substances, which perform the functions of normal intestinal microbiota, is currently considered an alternative to the use of living microorganisms and a promising direction for the safe correction of dysbiotic disorders in immunocompromised patients [127,322]. Modern metabiotics are presented in Table 11.11.

Conclusion

The complex nature of intestinal homeostasis is defined by the intricate relationships formed between resident microflora, transient microorganisms and pathogens, and human tissues and cells. The SARS-CoV-2 virus leads to a cascade of pathological changes, which are stalled by both human immune system resources and symbiotic microorganisms, which enhance immune response and act as a figurative shield, receiving a portion of the viral load onto itself. The positive capabilities of the intestinal microbiome are numerous, yet modern lifestyle most often leads to dysbiosis, in which the positive aspects of the microbiome are outweighed by the negative effects of pathogenic flora. In dysbiosis, patients often lack valuable intestinal protection and immune support, which leads to more severe responses to viral infections. A wide variety of probiotics exists, which can significantly improve the outcome of SARS-CoV-2 infection in different clinical and age-related groups. The benefits of symbiotic and opportunistic microflora underline the importance of probiotic supplementation, yet further research is required to evaluate the clinical efficacy of supportive probiotic administration in the treatment or prevention of COVID-19. Nonetheless, the translational benefits of microbiome corrective therapy are thoroughly described in the literature and are in detail presented in this chapter. Understanding the importance of the intestinal microbiome is key to the formation of a proper individualized approach to patient management.

TABLE 11.11 Metabiotics.

Ingredients	Drug name
Germfree aqueous substrates of metabolites Escherichia coli, Streptococcus faecalis, L. acidophilus, L.helveticus	Hilak forte (Germany) drops for oral use
Metabolites of the cell-free culture fluid of Bacillus subtilis bacteria	Bactistatin (Russia) capsules
Probiotic bacteria metabolites analogs: lactic acid, succinic acid, formic acid, L-lysine hydrochloride, L-glutamic acid, L-valine, L-methionine, L-alanine, L-leucine, glycine, L-aspartic acid	Aktoflor-S (Russia) solution for oral use
Fermentation extract of L.curvatus, L.casei, L.acidophilus, L. plantarum, L. fermentum, L.salivarius, L.brevis, L.rhamnosus, fermented on soy milk, citric acid, lactic acid, mineral water	Daigo (Япония) liquid for oral use in sachet
Metabolites Lactobacillus reuteri	Helinorm (Russia) capsules
Metabolic product metafiltrates of B. adolescentis, L. acidophilus, L. salivarius, L. helveticus, Propionibacterium freudenreichii + lactulose	T8 MOVIO (Cyprus) liquid for oral use
Inulin + butyric acid + microcrystalline cellulose	Zakofalk NMX (Germany) tablets

References

[1] Shi N, Li N, Duan X, Niu H. Interaction between the gut microbiome and mucosal immune system. Mil Med Res April 27, 2017;4:14. https://doi.org/10.1186/s40779-017-0122-9. PMID: 28465831; PMCID: PMC5408367.

[2] Оганезова ИА. Кишечная микробиота и иммунитет: иммуномодулирующие эффекты. Lactobacillus rhamnosus GG//РМЖ 2018;26(9):39–44. – С.

[3] Fenton TM, Jørgensen PB, Niss K, Rubin SJS, Mörbe UM, Riis LB, Da Silva C, Plumb A, Vandamme J, Jakobsen HL, Brunak S, Habtezion A, Nielsen OH, Johansson-Lindbom B, Agace WW. Immune profiling of human gut-associated lymphoid tissue identifies a role for isolated lymphoid follicles in priming of region-specific immunity. Immunity March 17, 2020;52(3). https://doi.org/10.1016/j.immuni.2020.02.001. 557-570.e6. Epub 2020 Mar 10. PMID: 32160523; PMCID: PMC7155934.

[4] Belkaid Y, Harrison OJ. Homeostatic immunity and the microbiota. Immunity April 18, 2017;46(4):562–76. https://doi.org/10.1016/j.immuni.2017.04.008. PMID: 28423337; PMCID: PMC5604871.

[5] Maschirow L, Suttorp N, Opitz B. Microbiota-dependent regulation of antimicrobial immunity in the lung. Am J Respir Cell Mol Biol September 2019;61(3):284–9. https://doi.org/10.1165/rcmb.2019-0101TR. PMID: 31059654.

[6] Ардатская МД, Бельмер СВ, Добрица ВП, Захаренко СМ, Лазебник ЛБ, Минушкин ОН, Орешко ЛС, Ситкин СИ, Ткаченко ЕИ, Суворов АН, Чавкин АИ, Шендеров БА. Дисбиоз (дисбактериоз) кишечника: современное состояние проблемы, комплексная диагностика и лечебная коррекция. Лкспериментальная и клиническая гастроэнтерология 2015;5(117):13–50. – С.

[7] Sánchez-Salguero ES, Santos-Argumedo L. La asociación de la microbiota humana con la inmunoglobulina A y su participación en la respuesta inmunológica [Human microbiota association with immunoglobulin A and its participation in immune response]. Rev Alerg Mex 2018 ;65(3):264–78. https://doi.org/10.29262/ram.v65i3.519. Spanish. PMID: 30176205.

[8] Chang CS, Kao CY. Current understanding of the gut microbiota shaping mechanisms. J Biomed Sci August 21, 2019;26(1):59. https://doi.org/10.1186/s12929-019-0554-5. PMID: 31434568; PMCID: PMC6702754.

[9] Ducarmon QR, Zwittink RD, Hornung BVH, van Schaik W, Young VB, Kuijper EJ. Gut microbiota and colonization resistance against bacterial enteric infection. Microbiol Mol Biol Rev June 5, 2019;83(3):e00007–19. https://doi.org/10.1128/MMBR.00007-19. PMID: 31167904; PMCID: PMC6710460.

[10] Leshem A, Liwinski T, Elinav E. Immune-microbiota interplay and colonization resistance in infection. Mol Cell May 21, 2020;78(4):597–613. https://doi.org/10.1016/j.molcel.2020.03.001. Epub 2020 Mar 23. PMID: 32208169.

[11] Blanpain C, Fuchs E. Stem cell plasticity. Plasticity of epithelial stem cells in tissue regeneration. Science June 13, 2014;344(6189):1242281. https://doi.org/10.1126/science.1242281. Epub 2014 Jun 12. Review.

[12] Okumura R, Takeda K. Roles of intestinal epithelial cells in the maintenance of gut homeostasis. Exp Mol Med May 26, 2017;49(5):e338. https://doi.org/10.1038/emm.2017.20. PMID: 28546564; PMCID: PMC5454438.

[13] Cox HM. Neuroendocrine peptide mechanisms controlling intestinal epithelial function. Curr Opin Pharmacol December 2016;31:50–6. https://doi.org/10.1016/j.coph.2016.08.010. Epub 2016 Sep 3. PMID: 27597736.

[14] Knoop KA, Newberry RD. Goblet cells: multifaceted players in immunity at mucosal surfaces. Mucosal Immunol November 2018;11(6):1551–7. https://doi.org/10.1038/s41385-018-0039-y. Epub 2018 Jun 4. PMID: 29867079.

[15] Zhang M, Wu C. The relationship between intestinal goblet cells and the immune response. Biosci Rep October 30, 2020;40(10). https://doi.org/10.1042/BSR20201471. BSR20201471. PMID: 33017020; PMCID: PMC7569202.

[16] Dockray GJ. Enteroendocrine cell signalling via the vagus nerve. Curr Opin Pharmacol 2013;13:954–8. https://doi.org/10.1016/j.coph.2013.09.007.

[17] Bauer PV, Hamr SC, Duca FA. Regulation of energy balance by a gut-brain axis and involvement of the gut microbiota. Cell Mol Life Sci CMLS 2016;73:737–55. https://doi.org/10.1007/s00018-015-2083-z.

[18] Obrenovich M, Sankar Chittoor Mana T, Rai H, Shola D, Sass C, McCloskey B, Levison BS. Recent findings within the microbiota–gut–brain–endocrine metabolic interactome. Pathol Lab Med Int 2017;9:21–30. https://doi.org/10.2147/PLMI.S121487.

[19] Nikolenko VN, Oganesyan MV, Sankova MV, Bulygin KV, Vovkogon AD, Rizaeva NA, Sinelnikov MY. Paneth cells: maintaining dynamic microbiome-host homeostasis, protecting against inflammation and cancer. Bioessays March 2021;43(3):e2000180. https://doi.org/10.1002/bies.202000180. Epub 2020 Nov 27. PMID: 33244814.

[20] Ohno H. Intestinal M cells. J Biochem February 2016;159(2):151–60. https://doi.org/10.1093/jb/mvv121. Epub 2015 Dec 3. PMID: 26634447; PMCID: PMC4892784.

[21] Brown RL, Clarke TB. The regulation of host defences to infection by the microbiota. Immunology January 2017;150(1):1–6. https://doi.org/10.1111/imm.12634. Epub 2016 Aug 9. PMID: 27311879; PMCID: PMC5221693.

[22] Maldonado Galdeano C, Cazorla SI, Lemme Dumit JM, Vélez E, Perdigón G. Beneficial effects of probiotic consumption on the immune system. Ann Nutr Metab 2019;74(2):115–24. https://doi.org/10.1159/000496426. Epub 2019 Jan 23. PMID: 30673668.

[23] Thaiss CA, Zmora N, Levy M, Elinav E. The microbiome and innate immunity. Nature July 7, 2016;535(7610):65–74. https://doi.org/10.1038/nature18847. PMID: 27383981.

[24] Zheng D, Liwinski T, Elinav E. Interaction between microbiota and immunity in health and disease. Cell Res June 2020;30(6):492–506. https://doi.org/10.1038/s41422-020-0332-7. Epub 2020 May 20. PMID: 32433595; PMCID: PMC7264227.

[25] Pearson C, Uhlig HH, Powrie F. Lymphoid microenvironments and innate lymphoid cells in the gut. Trends Immunol June 2012;33(6):289–96. https://doi.org/10.1016/j.it.2012.04.004. Epub 2012 May 10. PMID: 22578693.

[26] Druzd D, Matveeva O, Ince L, Harrison U, He W, Schmal C, Herzel H, Tsang AH, Kawakami N, Leliavski A, Uhl O, Yao L, Sander LE, Chen CS, Kraus K, de Juan A, Hergenhan SM, Ehlers M, Koletzko B, Haas R, Solbach W, Oster H, Scheiermann C. Lymphocyte circadian clocks control lymph node trafficking and adaptive immune responses. Immunity January 17, 2017;46(1):120–32. https://doi.org/10.1016/j.immuni.2016.12.011. Epub 2017 Jan 10. PMID: 28087238; PMCID: PMC5263259.

[27] Sumida H. Dynamics and clinical significance of intestinal intraepithelial lymphocytes. Immunol Med September 2019;42(3):117–23. https://doi.org/10.1080/25785826.2019.1658516. Epub 2019 Aug 27. PMID: 31453756.

[28] Allie SR, Randall TD. Resident memory B cells. Viral Immunol May 2020;33(4):282–93. https://doi.org/10.1089/vim.2019.0141. Epub 2020 Feb 5. PMID: 32023188; PMCID: PMC7247033.

[29] Starovoitova S. Non-dairy functional food products enriched probiotic microorganisms as an alternative way delivery of probiotics to microorganisms (Doctoral dissertation). 2020.

[30] Długońska H, Grzybowski M. Personalized vaccination? II. The role of natural microbiota in a vaccine-induced immunity. Wiad Parazytol 2011;57(2):71–6. PMID: 21682089.

[31] Козлов ИГ. Микробиота, мукозальный иммунитет и антибиотики: тонкости взаимодействия. РМЖ 2018;8(1):19–27. – С.

[32] McCoy KD, Ronchi F, Geuking MB. Host-microbiota interactions and adaptive immunity. Immunol Rev September 2017;279(1):63–9. https://doi.org/10.1111/imr.12575. PMID: 28856735.

[33] Zhao Q, Elson CO. Adaptive immune education by gut microbiota antigens. Immunology May 2018;154(1):28–37. https://doi.org/10.1111/imm.12896. Epub 2018 Feb 8. PMID: 29338074; PMCID: PMC5904715.

[34] Wang L, Zhu L, Qin S. Gut microbiota modulation on intestinal mucosal adaptive immunity. J Immunol Res October 2019;3(2019):4735040. https://doi.org/10.1155/2019/4735040. PMID: 31687412; PMCID: PMC6794961.

[35] Ferreira LMR, Muller YD, Bluestone JA, Tang Q. Next-generation regulatory T cell therapy. Nat Rev Drug Discov October 2019;18(10):749–69. https://doi.org/10.1038/s41573-019-0041-4. Epub 2019 Sep 20. PMID: 31541224; PMCID: PMC7773144.

[36] Savage PA, Klawon DEJ, Miller CH. Regulatory T cell development. Annu Rev Immunol April 26, 2020;38:421–53. https://doi.org/10.1146/annurev-immunol-100219-020937. Epub 2020 Jan 28. PMID: 31990619.

[37] Rana J, Biswas M. Regulatory T cell therapy: current and future design perspectives. Cell Immunol October 2020;356:104193. https://doi.org/10.1016/j.cellimm.2020.104193. Epub 2020 Aug 12. PMID: 32823038.

[38] Jiang F, Meng D, Weng M, Zhu W, Wu W, Kasper D, Walker WA. The symbiotic bacterial surface factor polysaccharide A on Bacteroides fragilis inhibits IL-1β-induced inflammation in human fetal enterocytes via toll receptors 2 and 4. PLoS One March 9, 2017;12(3):e0172738. https://doi.org/10.1371/journal.pone.0172738. PMID: 28278201; PMCID: PMC5344356.

[39] Wan Z, Zhou Z, Liu Y, Lai Y, Luo Y, Peng X, Zou W. Regulatory T cells and T helper 17 cells in viral infection. Scand J Immunol May 2020;91(5):e12873. https://doi.org/10.1111/sji.12873. Epub 2020 Mar 10. PMID: 32090360.

[40] Калюжин ОВ. Пробиотики как современные средства укрепления противоинфекционной иммунной защиты: миф или реальность? РМЖ 2012;20(28):1395–401. – C.

[41] Ruane D, Brane L, Reis BS, Cheong C, Poles J, Do Y, Zhu H, Velinzon K, Choi JH, Studt N, Mayer L, Lavelle EC, Steinman RM, Mucida D, Mehandru S. Lung dendritic cells induce migration of protective T cells to the gastrointestinal tract. J Exp Med August 26, 2013;210(9):1871–88. https://doi.org/10.1084/jem.20122762. Epub 2013 Aug 19. PMID: 23960190; PMCID: PMC3754860.

[42] Shelly A, Gupta P, Ahuja R, Srichandan S, Meena J, Majumdar T. Impact of microbiota: a paradigm for evolving herd immunity against viral diseases. Viruses October 10, 2020;12(10):1150. https://doi.org/10.3390/v12101150. PMID: 33050511; PMCID: PMC7599628.

[43] Baghbani T, Nikzad H, Azadbakht J, Izadpanah F, Haddad Kashani H. Dual and mutual interaction between microbiota and viral infections: a possible treat for COVID-19. Microb Cell Factories November 26, 2020;19(1):217. https://doi.org/10.1186/s12934-020-01483-1. PMID: 33243230; PMCID: PMC7689646.

[44] Belojevic G, Prasher D. Music of microbiota against SARS CoV-2. Noise Health 2019 ;21(100):97. https://doi.org/10.4103/nah.NAH_45_20. PMID: 32655062; PMCID: PMC7532784.

[45] Dhar D, Mohanty A. Gut microbiota and Covid-19- possible link and implications. Virus Res August 2020;285:198018. https://doi.org/10.1016/j.virusres.2020.198018. Epub 2020 May 13. PMID: 32430279; PMCID: PMC7217790.

[46] Rowland I, Gibson G, Heinken A, Scott K, Swann J, Thiele I, Tuohy K. Gut microbiota functions: metabolism of nutrients and other food components. Eur J Nutr February 2018;57(1):1–24. https://doi.org/10.1007/s00394-017-1445-8. Epub 2017 Apr 9. PMID: 28393285; PMCID: PMC5847071.

[47] Strandwitz P. Neurotransmitter modulation by the gut microbiota. Brain Res August 15, 2018;1693(Pt B):128–33. https://doi.org/10.1016/j.brainres.2018.03.015. PMID: 29903615; PMCID: PMC6005194.

[48] Чурса РВ, Месникова ИЛ, Микша ЯС. Кишечная микрофлора: роль в поддержании здоровья и развитии патологии, возможности коррекции : учеб.-метод. пособие. Минск : БГМУ 2017;36.

[49] Костюкевич ОИ, Былова НА, Симбирцева АС. Роль кишечной микробиоты в развитии заболеваний печени и желчевыводящих путей. РМЖ 2016;24(11):713–20. – C.

[50] Hu J, Lin S, Zheng B, Cheung PCK. Short-chain fatty acids in control of energy metabolism. Crit Rev Food Sci Nutr May 24, 2018;58(8):1243–9. https://doi.org/10.1080/10408398.2016.1245650. Epub 2017 Jun 12. PMID: 27786539.

[51] He J, Zhang P, Shen L, Niu L, Tan Y, Chen L, Zhao Y, Bai L, Hao X, Li X, Zhang S, Zhu L. Short-chain fatty acids and their association with signalling pathways in inflammation, glucose and lipid metabolism. Int J Mol Sci September 2, 2020;21(17):6356. https://doi.org/10.3390/ijms21176356. PMID: 32887215; PMCID: PMC7503625.

[52] Ramírez-Pérez O, Cruz-Ramón V, Chinchilla-López P, Méndez-Sánchez N. The role of the gut microbiota in bile acid metabolism. Ann Hepatol November 2017;16(Suppl. 1: s3–105.):s15–20. https://doi.org/10.5604/01.3001.0010.5494. PMID: 29080339.

[53] Lopes RCSO, Balbino KP, Jorge MP, Ribeiro AQ, Martino HSD, Alfenas RCG. Modulation of intestinal microbiota, control of nitrogen products and inflammation by pre/probiotics in chronic kidney disease: a systematic review. Nutr Hosp April 27, 2018;35(3):722–30. https://doi.org/10.20960/nh.1642. English. PMID: 29974784.

[54] Le Roy T, Lécuyer E, Chassaing B, Rhimi M, Lhomme M, Boudebbouze S, Ichou F, Haro Barceló J, Huby T, Guerin M, Giral P, Maguin E, Kapel N, Gérard P, Clément K, Lesnik P. The intestinal microbiota regulates host cholesterol homeostasis. BMC Biol November 27, 2019;17(1):94. https://doi.org/10.1186/s12915-019-0715-8. PMID: 31775890; PMCID: PMC6882370.

[55] Крамарь ЛВ, Крамарь ОГ. Современная стратегия коррекции нарушений кишечной микробиоты при дисбактериозе кишечника. Лекарственный вестник 2015;9(3):50–6. – C.

[56] Nichols RG, Peters JM, Patterson AD. Interplay between the host, the human microbiome, and drug metabolism. Hum Genom June 11, 2019;13(1):27. https://doi.org/10.1186/s40246-019-0211-9. PMID: 31186074; PMCID: PMC6558703.

[57] Rao MC. Physiology of electrolyte transport in the gut: implications for disease. Compr Physiol June 12, 2019;9(3):947–1023. https://doi.org/10.1002/cphy.c180011. PMID: 31187895.

[58] Wang J, Li F, Tian Z. Role of microbiota on lung homeostasis and diseases. Sci China Life Sci December 2017;60(12):1407–15. https://doi.org/10.1007/s11427-017-9151-1. Epub 2017 Oct 9. PMID: 29019144; PMCID: PMC7089139.
[59] Weiss GA, Hennet T. Mechanisms and consequences of intestinal dysbiosis. Cell Mol Life Sci August 2017;74(16):2959–77. https://doi.org/10.1007/s00018-017-2509-x. Epub 2017 Mar 28. PMID: 28352996.
[60] Sommer F, Anderson JM, Bharti R, Raes J, Rosenstiel P. The resilience of the intestinal microbiota influences health and disease. Nat Rev Microbiol October 2017;15(10):630–8. https://doi.org/10.1038/nrmicro.2017.58. Epub 2017 Jun 19. PMID: 28626231.
[61] Biedermann L, Rogler G. The intestinal microbiota: its role in health and disease. Eur J Pediatr February 2015;174(2):151–67. https://doi.org/10.1007/s00431-014-2476-2. Epub 2015 Jan 7. PMID: 25563215.
[62] Чорошилова ИА, Гранитов ВМ. Пробиотики в терапии вирусных гепатитов. Бюллетень медицинской науки 2016;1(5):16–9.
[63] Grace E, Shaw C, Whelan K, Andreyev HJ. Review article: small intestinal bacterial overgrowth–prevalence, clinical features, current and developing diagnostic tests, and treatment. Aliment Pharmacol Ther October 2013;38(7):674–88. https://doi.org/10.1111/apt.12456. Epub 2013 Aug 20. PMID: 23957651.
[64] Гурова ММ, Чавкин АИ. Место метабиотиков в коррекции дисбиоза кишечника. Вопросы практической педиатрии 2018;13(2):70–6. – С.
[65] Naumenko NV, Potoroko IY, Kalinina IV, Nenasheva AV, Botvinnikova VV. Possibilities of regulating stress-protective activity of food products to improve immunity under the conditions of the COVID-19 pandemic. Human. Sport. Medicine 2020;20(S1):116–27. https://doi.org/10.14529/hsm20s115 (in Russ.).
[66] Scartoni FR, Sant'Ana LO, Murillo-Rodriguez E, Yamamoto T, Imperatori C, Budde H, Vianna JM, Machado S. Physical exercise and immune system in the elderly: implications and importance in COVID-19 pandemic period. Front Psychol November 19, 2020;11:593903. https://doi.org/10.3389/fpsyg.2020.593903. PMID: 33329256; PMCID: PMC7711129.
[67] Hill DA, Siracusa MC, Abt MC, Kim BS, Kobuley D, Kubo M, Kambayashi T, Larosa DF, Renner ED, Orange JS, Bushman FD, Artis D. Commensal bacteria-derived signals regulate basophil hematopoiesis and allergic inflammation. Nat Med March 25, 2012;18(4):538–46. https://doi.org/10.1038/nm.2657. PMID: 22447074; PMCID: PMC3321082.
[68] Macfarlane S. Antibiotic treatments and microbes in the gut. Environ Microbiol April 2014;16(4):919–24. https://doi.org/10.1111/1462-2920.12399. Epub 2014 Jan 29. PMID: 24471523.
[69] Gou W, Fu Y, Yue L, Chen G, Cai X, Shuai M, Zheng J-S. Gut microbiota may underlie the predisposition of healthy individuals to COVID-19. medRxiv 2020:1–44. https://doi.org/10.1101/2020.04.22.20076091.
[70] Kato K, Odamaki T, Mitsuyama E, Sugahara H, Xiao JZ, Osawa R. Age-related changes in the composition of gut Bifidobacterium species. Curr Microbiol August 2017;74(8):987–95. https://doi.org/10.1007/s00284-017-1272-4. Epub 2017 Jun 8. PMID: 28593350; PMCID: PMC5486783.
[71] Maynard C, Weinkove D. The gut microbiota and ageing. Subcell Biochem 2018;90:351–71. https://doi.org/10.1007/978-981-13-2835-0_12. PMID: 30779015.
[72] Kim S, Jazwinski SM. The gut microbiota and healthy aging: a mini-review. Gerontology 2018;64(6):513–20. https://doi.org/10.1159/000490615. Epub 2018 Jul 19. PMID: 30025401; PMCID: PMC6191326.
[73] Liu K, Chen Y, Lin R, Han K. Clinical features of COVID-19 in elderly patients: a comparison with young and middle-aged patients. J Infect June 2020;80(6):e14–8. https://doi.org/10.1016/j.jinf.2020.03.005. Epub 2020 Mar 27. PMID: 32171866; PMCID: PMC7102640.
[74] Yang J, Zheng Y, Gou X, Pu K, Chen Z, Guo Q, Ji R, Wang H, Wang Y, Zhou Y. Prevalence of comorbidities and its effects in patients infected with SARS-CoV-2: a systematic review and meta-analysis. Int J Infect Dis May 2020;94:91–5. https://doi.org/10.1016/j.ijid.2020.03.017. Epub 2020 Mar 12. PMID: 32173574; PMCID: PMC7194638.
[75] Ejaz H, Alsrhani A, Zafar A, Javed H, Junaid K, Abdalla AE, Abosalif KOA, Ahmed Z, Younas S. COVID-19 and comorbidities: deleterious impact on infected patients. J Infect Public Health December 2020;13(12):1833–9. https://doi.org/10.1016/j.jiph.2020.07.014. Epub 2020 Aug 4. PMID: 32788073; PMCID: PMC7402107.
[76] Комарова ОН, Чавкин АИ. Взаимосвязь стресса, иммунитета и кишечной микробиоты. Педиатрическая фармакология 2020;17(1):18–24. – С.
[77] Yeoh YK, Zuo T, Lui GC, Zhang F, Liu Q, Li AY, Chung AC, Cheung CP, Tso EY, Fung KS, Chan V, Ling L, Joynt G, Hui DS, Chow KM, Ng SSS, Li TC, Ng RW, Yip TC, Wong GL, Chan FK, Wong CK, Chan PK, Ng SC.

Gut microbiota composition reflects disease severity and dysfunctional immune responses in patients with COVID-19. Gut April 2021;70(4):698–706. https://doi.org/10.1136/gutjnl-2020-323020. Epub 2021 Jan 11. PMID: 33431578; PMCID: PMC7804842.

[78] Hu B, Guo H, Zhou P, Shi ZL. Characteristics of SARS-CoV-2 and COVID-19. Nat Rev Microbiol March 2021;19(3):141–54. https://doi.org/10.1038/s41579-020-00459-7. Epub 2020 Oct 6. PMID: 33024307; PMCID: PMC7537588.

[79] Mönkemüller K, Fry L, Rickes S. COVID-19, coronavirus, SARS-CoV-2 and the small bowel. Rev Esp Enferm Dig May 2020;112(5):383–8. https://doi.org/10.17235/reed.2020.7137/2020. PMID: 32343593.

[80] Yan R, Zhang Y, Li Y, Xia L, Guo Y, Zhou Q. Structural basis for the recognition of SARS-CoV-2 by full-length human ACE2. Science March 27, 2020;367(6485):1444–8. https://doi.org/10.1126/science.abb2762. Epub 2020 Mar 4. PMID: 32132184; PMCID: PMC7164635.

[81] Ou X, Liu Y, Lei X, Li P, Mi D, Ren L, Guo L, Guo R, Chen T, Hu J, Xiang Z, Mu Z, Chen X, Chen J, Hu K, Jin Q, Wang J, Qian Z. Characterization of spike glycoprotein of SARS-CoV-2 on virus entry and its immune cross-reactivity with SARS-CoV. Nat Commun March 27, 2020;11(1):1620. https://doi.org/10.1038/s41467-020-15562-9. Erratum in: Nat Commun. 2021 Apr 1;12(1):2144. PMID: 32221306; PMCID: PMC7100515.

[82] Harrison AG, Lin T, Wang P. Mechanisms of SARS-CoV-2 transmission and pathogenesis. Trends Immunol December 2020;41(12):1100–15. https://doi.org/10.1016/j.it.2020.10.004. Epub 2020 Oct 14. PMID: 33132005; PMCID: PMC7556779.

[83] Vuille-Dit-Bille RN, Liechty KW, Verrey F, Guglielmetti LC. SARS-CoV-2 receptor ACE2 gene expression in small intestine correlates with age. Amino Acids July 2020;52(6–7):1063–5. https://doi.org/10.1007/s00726-020-02870-z. Epub 2020 Jul 5. PMID: 32627059; PMCID: PMC7335412.

[84] Мосина ЛМ, Суркова ЕЮ, Гераськин АЕ, Полозова ЛИ. Патогенетические механизмы прямого и опосредованного поражения кишечника у больных коронавирусной инфекцией, вызванной вирусом SARS-COV-2. Современные проблемы науки и образования 2021. – № 2. – URL: датаобращенияhttps://science-education.ru/ru/article/view?id=30754(дата обращения: 27.11.2021 .

[85] Russell MW, Moldoveanu Z, Ogra PL, Mestecky J. Mucosal immunity in COVID-19: a neglected but critical aspect of SARS-CoV-2 infection. Front Immunol November 30, 2020;11:611337. https://doi.org/10.3389/fimmu.2020.611337. PMID: 33329607; PMCID: PMC7733922.

[86] Alkhatib A. Antiviral functional foods and exercise lifestyle prevention of coronavirus. Nutrients August 28, 2020;12(9):2633. https://doi.org/10.3390/nu12092633. PMID: 32872374; PMCID: PMC7551447.

[87] Verruck S, Balthazar CF, Rocha RS, Silva R, Esmerino EA, Pimentel TC, Freitas MQ, Silva MC, da Cruz AG, Prudencio ES. Dairy foods and positive impact on the consumer's health. Adv Food Nutr Res 2019;89:95–164. https://doi.org/10.1016/bs.afnr.2019.03.002. Epub 2019 Apr 17. PMID: 31351531.

[88] Rosa DD, Dias MMS, Grześkowiak ŁM, Reis SA, Conceição LL, Peluzio MDCG. Milk kefir: nutritional, microbiological and health benefits. Nutr Res Rev June 2017;30(1):82–96. https://doi.org/10.1017/S0954422416000275. Epub 2017 Feb 22. PMID: 28222814.

[89] Carasi P, Díaz M, Racedo SM, De Antoni G, Urdaci MC, Serradell Mde L. Safety characterization and antimicrobial properties of kefir-isolated Lactobacillus kefiri. BioMed Res Int 2014:208974. https://doi.org/10.1155/2014/208974. Epub 2014 May 13. PMID: 24955346; PMCID: PMC4052788.

[90] Kim DH, Jeong D, Kang IB, Kim H, Song KY, Seo KH. Dual function of lactobacillus kefiri dh5 in preventing high-fat-diet-induced obesity: direct reduction of cholesterol and upregulation of ppar-alpha in adipose tissue. Mol Nutr Food Res 2017;61. https://doi.org/10.1002/mnfr.201700252.

[91] Carasi P, Racedo SM, Jacquot C, Romanin DE, Serradell MA, Urdaci MC. Impact of kefir derived Lactobacillus kefiri on the mucosal immune response and gut microbiota. J Immunol Res 2015:361604. https://doi.org/10.1155/2015/361604. Epub 2015 Feb 24. PMID: 25811034; PMCID: PMC4355334.

[92] Hong WS, Chen YP, Chen MJ. The antiallergic effect of kefir Lactobacilli. J Food Sci October 2010;75(8):H244–53. https://doi.org/10.1111/j.1750-3841.2010.01787.x. Epub 2010 Sep 20. PMID: 21535502.

[93] Gury-BenAri M, Thaiss CA, Serafini N, Winter DR, Giladi A, Lara-Astiaso D, Levy M, Salame TM, Weiner A, David E, Shapiro H, Dori-Bachash M, Pevsner-Fischer M, Lorenzo-Vivas E, Keren-Shaul H, Paul F, Harmelin A, Eberl G, Itzkovitz S, Tanay A, Di Santo JP, Elinav E, Amit I. The spectrum and regulatory landscape of intestinal innate lymphoid cells are shaped by the microbiome. Cell August 25, 2016;166(5):1231–46. https://doi.org/10.1016/j.cell.2016.07.043. e13. Epub 2016 Aug 18. PMID: 27545347.

[94] Villena J, Chiba E, Tomosada Y, Salva S, Marranzino G, Kitazawa H, Alvarez S. Orally administered Lactobacillus rhamnosus modulates the respiratory immune response triggered by the viral pathogen-associated molecular pattern poly(I:C). BMC Immunol September 18, 2012;13:53. https://doi.org/10.1186/1471-2172-13-53. PMID: 22989047; PMCID: PMC3460727.

[95] Seddik HA, Bendali F, Gancel F, Fliss I, Spano G, Drider D. Lactobacillus plantarum and its probiotic and food potentialities. Probiotics Antimicrob Proteins June 2017;9(2):111–22. https://doi.org/10.1007/s12602-017-9264-z. PMID: 28271469.

[96] Paparo L, Aitoro R, Nocerino R, Fierro C, Bruno C, Canani RB. Direct effects of fermented cow's milk product with Lactobacillus paracasei CBA L74 on human enterocytes. Benef Microbes January 29, 2018;9(1):165–72. https://doi.org/10.3920/BM2017.0038. Epub 2017 Oct 25. PMID: 29065709.

[97] Sindi A, Badsha MB, Ünlü G. Bacterial populations in international artisanal kefirs. Microorganisms August 29, 2020;8(9):1318. https://doi.org/10.3390/microorganisms8091318. PMID: 32872546; PMCID: PMC7565184.

[98] Колмакова ТС, Белик СН, цистяков ВА, Моргуль ЕВ, цистякова ИБ. Характеристика кефира как ценного пробиотического продукта и его биологических свойств. Медицинский вестник Юга России 2014:35–42. – №. 3. – С.

[99] Hamida RS, Shami A, Ali MA, Almohawes ZN, Mohammed AE, Bin-Meferij MM. Kefir: a protective dietary supplementation against viral infection. Biomed Pharmacother January 2021;133:110974. https://doi.org/10.1016/j.biopha.2020.110974. Epub 2020 Nov 11. PMID: 33186795; PMCID: PMC7655491.

[100] Turroni F, Taverniti V, Ruas-Madiedo P, Duranti S, Guglielmetti S, Lugli GA, Gioiosa L, Palanza P, Margolles A, van Sinderen D, Ventura M. Bifidobacterium bifidum PRL2010 modulates the host innate immune response. Appl Environ Microbiol January 2014;80(2):730–40. https://doi.org/10.1128/AEM.03313-13. Epub 2013 Nov 15. PMID: 24242237; PMCID: PMC3911076.

[101] Duranti S, Ruiz L, Lugli GA, Tames H, Milani C, Mancabelli L, Mancino W, Longhi G, Carnevali L, Sgoifo A, Margolles A, Ventura M, Ruas-Madiedo P, Turroni F. Bifidobacterium adolescentis as a key member of the human gut microbiota in the production of GABA. Sci Rep August 24, 2020;10(1):14112. https://doi.org/10.1038/s41598-020-70986-z. PMID: 32839473; PMCID: PMC7445748.

[102] Sankova MV, Kytko OV, Meylanova RD, Vasil'ev YL, Nelipa MV. Possible prospects for using modern magnesium preparations for increasing stress resistance during COVID-19 pandemic. Res Results Pharmacol 2020;6(4):65–76. https://doi.org/10.3897/rrpharmacology.6.59407.

[103] Ricci L, Mackie J, Lenardon MD, Jukes C, Hegazy AN, Brown AJ, Walker AW. Bifidobacterium adolescentis shows potential to strengthen host defence against gastrointestinal infection via inhibition of the opportunistic pathogen Candida albicans and stimulation of human-isolated macrophages killing capacity in vitro. Acc Microbiol 2020:857. – T. 2. – №. 7A. – C.

[104] Wang M, Gong S, Du S, Zhu Y, Rong F, Pan R, Di Y, Li C, Ren D, Jin N. The effect of immunoregulation of Streptococcus lactis L16 strain upon *Staphylococcus aureus* infection. BMC Microbiol June 2, 2017;17(1):130. https://doi.org/10.1186/s12866-017-1038-y. PMID: 28577529; PMCID: PMC5457572.

[105] Yamamoto Y, Saruta J, Takahashi T, To M, Shimizu T, Hayashi T, Morozumi T, Kubota N, Kamata Y, Makino S, Kano H, Hemmi J, Asami Y, Nagai T, Misawa K, Kato S, Tsukinoki K. Effect of ingesting yogurt fermented with Lactobacillus delbrueckii ssp. bulgaricus OLL1073R-1 on influenza virus-bound salivary IgA in elderly residents of nursing homes: a randomized controlled trial. Acta Odontol Scand October 2019;77(7):517–24. https://doi.org/10.1080/00016357.2019.1609697. Epub 2019 May 16. PMID: 31094267.

[106] Клопова АВ. Молоко и молочно-кислые продукты. Фундаментальные и прикладные научные исследования: актуальные вопросы, достижения и инновации 2020:72–4. – С.

[107] Гоголева ОА. Ряженка–высокоценный кисломолочный продукт. Научные труды студентов Ижевской ГСЧА 2020:865–8. – С.

[108] Michalickova DM, Kostic-Vucicevic MM, Vukasinovic-Vesic MD, Stojmenovic TB, Dikic NV, Andjelkovic MS, Djordjevic BI, Tanaskovic BP, Minic RD. Lactobacillus helveticus lafti L10 supplementation modulates mucosal and humoral immunity in elite athletes: a randomized, double-blind, placebo-controlled trial. J Strength Condit Res January 2017;31(1):62–70. https://doi.org/10.1519/JSC.0000000000001456. PMID: 27100317.

[109] Dargahi N, Johnson J, Apostolopoulos V. Streptococcus thermophilus alters the expression of genes associated with innate and adaptive immunity in human peripheral blood mononuclear cells. PLoS One February 11, 2020;15(2):e0228531. https://doi.org/10.1371/journal.pone.0228531. PMID: 32045425; PMCID: PMC7012395.

[110] Farag MA, El Hawary EA, Elmassry MM. Rediscovering acidophilus milk, its quality characteristics, manufacturing methods, flavor chemistry and nutritional value. Crit Rev Food Sci Nutr 2020;60(18):3024–41. https://doi.org/10.1080/10408398.2019.1675584. Epub 2019 Oct 16. PMID: 31617740.

[111] Yan F, Li N, Shi J, Li H, Yue Y, Jiao W, Wang N, Song Y, Huo G, Li B. Lactobacillus acidophilus alleviates type 2 diabetes by regulating hepatic glucose, lipid metabolism and gut microbiota in mice. Food Funct September 1, 2019;10(9):5804–15. https://doi.org/10.1039/c9fo01062a. Epub 2019 Aug 28. PMID: 31461095.

[112] Артемова ЕН, Владимирова ОГ, Флерко ЕС. Исследование потребительских предпочтений при выборе продукции детской молочной кухни. Технология и товароведение инновационных пищевых продуктов 2020:110–6. – №. 2. – С.

[113] Kabeerdoss J, Devi RS, Mary RR, Prabhavathi D, Vidya R, Mechenro J, Mahendri NV, Pugazhendhi S, Ramakrishna BS. Effect of yoghurt containing Bifidobacterium lactis Bb12® on faecal excretion of secretory immunoglobulin A and human beta-defensin 2 in healthy adult volunteers. Nutr J December 23, 2011;10:138. https://doi.org/10.1186/1475-2891-10-138. PMID: 22196482; PMCID: PMC3265429.

[114] Ejtahed HS, Mohtadi-Nia J, Homayouni-Rad A, Niafar M, Asghari-Jafarabadi M, Mofid V, Akbarian-Moghari A. Effect of probiotic yogurt containing lactobacillus acidophilus and Bifidobacterium lactis on lipid profile in individuals with type 2 diabetes mellitus. J Dairy Sci July 2011;94(7):3288–94. https://doi.org/10.3168/jds.2010-4128. PMID: 21700013.

[115] Azevedo RB, Botelho BG, Hollanda JVG, Ferreira LVL, Junqueira de Andrade LZ, Oei SSML, Mello TS, Muxfeldt ES. Covid-19 and the cardiovascular system: a comprehensive review. J Hum Hypertens January 2021;35(1):4–11. https://doi.org/10.1038/s41371-020-0387-4. Epub 2020 Jul 27. PMID: 32719447; PMCID: PMC7384729.

[116] Плоскирева АА, Усенко ДВ. Роль пробиотиков и пробиотических продуктов в лечении и профилактике инфекционных болезней. Инфекционные болезни 2010:58–64. т. 8, №3, с.

[117] Олескин АВ, Шендеров БА. Пробиотики, психобиотики и метабиотики: проблемы и перспективы. Физическая и реабилитационная медицина, медицинская реабилитация 2020:233–43. https://doi.org/10.36425/rehab25811. – Т. 2. – №. 3. – С.

[118] Wang G, Li X, Zhao J, Zhang H, Chen W. Lactobacillus casei CCFM419 attenuates type 2 diabetes via a gut microbiota dependent mechanism. Food Funct September 20, 2017;8(9):3155–64. https://doi.org/10.1039/c7fo00593h. Erratum in: Food Funct. 2017 Oct 18;8(10):3814. PMID: 28782784.

[119] Shida K, Sato T, Iizuka R, Hoshi R, Watanabe O, Igarashi T, Miyazaki K, Nanno M, Ishikawa F. Daily intake of fermented milk with Lactobacillus casei strain Shirota reduces the incidence and duration of upper respiratory tract infections in healthy middle-aged office workers. Eur J Nutr February 2017;56(1):45–53. https://doi.org/10.1007/s00394-015-1056-1. Epub 2015 Sep 29. PMID: 26419583; PMCID: PMC5290054.

[120] Kok CR, Hutkins R. Yogurt and other fermented foods as sources of health-promoting bacteria. Nutr Rev December 1, 2018;76(Suppl. 1):4–15. https://doi.org/10.1093/nutrit/nuy056. PMID: 30452699.

[121] Meng H, Lee Y, Ba Z, Peng J, Lin J, Boyer AS, Fleming JA, Furumoto EJ, Roberts RF, Kris-Etherton PM, Rogers CJ. Consumption of Bifidobacterium animalis subsp. lactis BB-12 impacts upper respiratory tract infection and the function of NK and T cells in healthy adults. Mol Nutr Food Res May 2016;60(5):1161–71. https://doi.org/10.1002/mnfr.201500665. Epub 2016 Mar 1. PMID: 26821116.

[122] Sadrzadeh-Yeganeh H, Elmadfa I, Djazayery A, Jalali M, Heshmat R, Chamary M. The effects of probiotic and conventional yoghurt on lipid profile in women. Br J Nutr June 2010;103(12):1778–83. https://doi.org/10.1017/S0007114509993801. Epub 2010 Jan 26. PMID: 20100374.

[123] Sayon-Orea C, Martínez-González MA, Ruiz-Canela M, Bes-Rastrollo M. Associations between yogurt consumption and weight gain and risk of obesity and metabolic syndrome: a systematic review. Adv Nutr January 17, 2017;8(1):146S–54S. https://doi.org/10.3945/an.115.011536. PMID: 28096138; PMCID: PMC5227971.

[124] Yu J, Mo L, Pan L, Yao C, Ren D, An X, Tsogtgerel T, Zhang H, Liu W. Bacterial microbiota and metabolic character of traditional sour cream and butter in buryatia, Russia. Front Microbiol October 22, 2018;9:2496. https://doi.org/10.3389/fmicb.2018.02496. PMID: 30459729; PMCID: PMC6232932.

[125] Jounai K, Ikado K, Sugimura T, Ano Y, Braun J, Fujiwara D. Spherical lactic acid bacteria activate plasmacytoid dendritic cells immunomodulatory function via TLR9-dependent crosstalk with myeloid dendritic cells. PLoS One 2012;7(4):e32588. https://doi.org/10.1371/journal.pone.0032588. Epub 2012 Apr 10. PMID: 22505996; PMCID: PMC3323594.

[126] Гетманец ВН. Производство сметаны и сметанного продукта. Вестник Алтайского государственного аграрного университета 2017:167–71. – №. 2 (148). – С.

[127] Lin L, Zhang J. Role of intestinal microbiota and metabolites on gut homeostasis and human diseases. BMC Immunol January 6, 2017;18(1):2. https://doi.org/10.1186/s12865-016-0187-3. PMID: 28061847; PMCID: PMC5219689.

[128] Фомина МЮ. Бактериальные закваски для производства творога. вестник магистратуры 2019:18–20. – С.

[129] Poonam PSD, Tomar SK, De S, Singh R. Multifaceted attributes of dairy propionibacteria: a review. World J Microbiol Biotechnol November 2012;28(11):3081–95. https://doi.org/10.1007/s11274-012-1117-z. Epub 2012 Jul 5. PMID: 22806746.

[130] Nam JH, Cho YS, Rackerby B, Goddik L, Park SH. Shifts of microbiota during cheese production: impact on production and quality. Appl Microbiol Biotechnol March 2021;105(6):2307–18. https://doi.org/10.1007/s00253-021-11201-5. Epub 2021 Mar 4. PMID: 33661344.

[131] Das R, Pandey H, Das B, Sarkar S. Fermentation and its application in vegetable preservation: a review. Int J Food Ferment Technol 2016;6(2):207–17. https://doi.org/10.5958/2277-9396.2016.00044.1.

[132] Yang X, Hu W, Xiu Z, Jiang A, Yang X, Sarengaowa, Ji Y, Guan Y, Feng K. Comparison of northeast sauerkraut fermentation between single lactic acid bacteria strains and traditional fermentation. Food Res Int November 2020;137:109553. https://doi.org/10.1016/j.foodres.2020.109553. Epub 2020 Jul 18. PMID: 33233175.

[133] Pham MT, Yang JJ, Balasubramaniam A, Rahim AR, Adi P, Do TTM, Herr DR, Huang CM. Leuconostoc mesenteroides mediates an electrogenic pathway to attenuate the accumulation of abdominal fat mass induced by high fat diet. Sci Rep December 14, 2020;10(1):21916. https://doi.org/10.1038/s41598-020-78835-9. PMID: 33318546; PMCID: PMC7736347.

[134] Traisaeng S, Batsukh A, Chuang TH, Herr DR, Huang YF, Chimeddorj B, Huang CM. Leuconostoc mesenteroides fermentation produces butyric acid and mediates Ffar2 to regulate blood glucose and insulin in type 1 diabetic mice. Sci Rep May 13, 2020;10(1):7928. https://doi.org/10.1038/s41598-020-64916-2. PMID: 32404878; PMCID: PMC7220903.

[135] Le B, Yang SH. Effect of potential probiotic Leuconostoc mesenteroides FB111 in prevention of cholesterol absorption by modulating NPC1L1/PPARα/SREBP-2 pathways in epithelial Caco-2 cells. Int Microbiol June 2019;22(2):279–87. https://doi.org/10.1007/s10123-018-00047-z. Epub 2018 Dec 5. PMID: 30810991.

[136] Patra JK, Das G, Paramithiotis S, Shin HS. Kimchi and other widely consumed traditional fermented foods of Korea: a review. Front Microbiol September 28, 2016;7:1493. https://doi.org/10.3389/fmicb.2016.01493. PMID: 27733844; PMCID: PMC5039233.

[137] Park KY, Jeong JK, Lee YE, Daily 3rd JW. Health benefits of kimchi (Korean fermented vegetables) as a probiotic food. J Med Food January 2014;17(1):6–20. https://doi.org/10.1089/jmf.2013.3083. PMID: 24456350.

[138] Takahashi M, Nagata M, Kaneko T, Suzuki T. Miso soup consumption enhances the bioavailability of the reduced form of supplemental coenzyme Q10. J Nutr Metab January 7, 2020:5349086. https://doi.org/10.1155/2020/5349086. PMID: 31998536; PMCID: PMC6969983.

[139] Kovács ÁT. Bacillus subtilis. Trends Microbiol 2019;27(8):724–5. https://doi.org/10.1016/j.tim.2019.03.008. Epub 15 апреля 2019 г. PMID: 31000489.

[140] Sulistyaningsih I, Afifah DN, Juniarto AZ, Anjani G, Rustanti N. The effect of tempe gembus on high-sensitivity C-reactive protein and adiponectine levels in rats with metabolic syndrome. J Nutr Sci Vitaminol 2020;66(Suppl. ment):S51–5. https://doi.org/10.3177/jnsv.66.S51. PMID: 33612648.

[141] Колесниченко МН, Каменская ЕП. Перспективы использования плодов жимолости в производстве хлебного кваса. Ползуновский вестник 2020:13–20. – №. 1. – С.

[142] Belda I, Ruiz J, Santos A, Van Wyk N, Pretorius IS. Saccharomyces cerevisiae. Trends Genet December 2019;35(12):956–7. https://doi.org/10.1016/j.tig.2019.08.009. Epub 2019 Oct 17. PMID: 31630852.

[143] Lavefve L, Marasini D, Carbonero F. Microbial ecology of fermented vegetables and non-alcoholic drinks and current knowledge on their impact on human health. Adv Food Nutr Res 2019;87:147–85. https://doi.org/10.1016/bs.afnr.2018.09.001. Epub 2018 Dec 7. PMID: 30678814.

[144] Stiemsma LT, Nakamura RE, Nguyen JG, Michels KB. Does consumption of fermented foods modify the human gut microbiota? J Nutr July 1, 2020;150(7):1680–92. https://doi.org/10.1093/jn/nxaa077. PMID: 32232406; PMCID: PMC7330458.

[145] Geva-Zatorsky N, Sefik E, Kua L, Pasman L, Tan TG, Ortiz-Lopez A, Yanortsang TB, Yang L, Jupp R, Mathis D, Benoist C, Kasper DL. Mining the human gut microbiota for immunomodulatory organisms. Cell February 23,

2017;168(5):928–43. https://doi.org/10.1016/j.cell.2017.01.022. e11. Epub 2017 Feb 16. PMID: 28215708; PMCID: PMC7774263.

[146] Haarman M, Knol J. Quantitative real-time PCR assays to identify and quantify fecal Bifidobacterium species in infants receiving a prebiotic infant formula. Appl Environ Microbiol 2005:2318–24. – T. 71. – №. 5. – C.

[147] Odamaki T, Bottacini F, Kato K, Mitsuyama E, Yoshida K, Horigome A, Xiao JZ, van Sinderen D. Genomic diversity and distribution of Bifidobacterium longum subsp. longum across the human lifespan. Sci Rep January 8, 2018;8(1):85. https://doi.org/10.1038/s41598-017-18391-x. PMID: 29311585; PMCID: PMC5758520.

[148] Peirotén A, Arqués JL, Medina M, Rodríguez-Mínguez E. Bifidobacterial strains shared by mother and child as source of probiotics. Benef Microbes February 27, 2018;9(2):231–8. https://doi.org/10.3920/BM2017.0133. PMID: 29488411.

[149] Seppo AE, Bu K, Jumabaeva M, Thakar J, Choudhury RA, Yonemitsu C, Bode L, Martina CA, Allen M, Tamburini S, Piras E, Wallach DS, Looney RJ, Clemente JC, Järvinen KM. Infant gut microbiome is enriched with Bifidobacterium longum ssp. infantis in Old Order Mennonites with traditional farming lifestyle. Allergy November 2021;76(11):3489–503. https://doi.org/10.1111/all.14877. Epub 2021 May 14. PMID: 33905556.

[150] Chichlowski M, Shah N, Wampler JL, Wu SS, Vanderhoof JA. Bifidobacterium longum subspecies infantis (B. Infantis) in pediatric nutrition: current state of knowledge. Nutrients May 28, 2020;12(6):1581. https://doi.org/10.3390/nu12061581. PMID: 32481558; PMCID: PMC7352178.

[151] Escribano J, Ferré N, Gispert-Llaurado M, Luque V, Rubio-Torrents C, Zaragoza-Jordana M, Polanco I, Codoñer FM, Chenoll E, Morera M, Moreno-Muñoz JA, Rivero M, Closa-Monasterolo R. Bifidobacterium longum subsp infantis CECT7210-supplemented formula reduces diarrhea in healthy infants: a randomized controlled trial. Pediatr Res June 2018;83(6):1120–8. https://doi.org/10.1038/pr.2018.34. Epub 2018 May 2. PMID: 29538368.

[152] D'Amico F, Baumgart DC, Danese S, Peyrin-Biroulet L. Diarrhea during COVID-19 infection: pathogenesis, epidemiology, prevention, and management. Clin Gastroenterol Hepatol July 2020;18(8):1663–72. https://doi.org/10.1016/j.cgh.2020.04.001. Epub 2020 Apr 8. PMID: 32278065; PMCID: PMC7141637.

[153] Xiao L, Gong C, Ding Y, Ding G, Xu X, Deng C, Ze X, Malard P, Ben X. Probiotics maintain intestinal secretory immunoglobulin A levels in healthy formula-fed infants: a randomised, double-blind, placebo-controlled study. Benef Microbes October 14, 2019;10(7):729–39. https://doi.org/10.3920/BM2019.0025. Epub 2019 Jul 24. PMID: 31965842.

[154] Huang W, Cho KY, Meng D, Walker WA. The impact of indole-3-lactic acid on immature intestinal innate immunity and development: a transcriptomic analysis. Sci Rep April 13, 2021;11(1):8088. https://doi.org/10.1038/s41598-021-87353-1. PMID: 33850185; PMCID: PMC8044159.

[155] Zimmermann P, Curtis N. COVID-19 in children, pregnancy and neonates: a review of epidemiologic and clinical features. Pediatr Infect Dis J June 2020;39(6):469–77. https://doi.org/10.1097/INF.0000000000002700. PMID: 32398569; PMCID: PMC7363381.

[156] Henrick BM, Chew S, Casaburi G, Brown HK, Frese SA, Zhou Y, Underwood MA, Smilowitz JT. Colonization by B. infantis EVC001 modulates enteric inflammation in exclusively breastfed infants. Pediatr Res December 2019;86(6):749–57. https://doi.org/10.1038/s41390-019-0533-2. Epub 2019 Aug 23. PMID: 31443102; PMCID: PMC6887859.

[157] Turroni F, Serafini F, Foroni E, Duranti S, O'Connell Motherway M, Taverniti V, Mangifesta M, Milani C, Viappiani A, Roversi T, Sánchez B, Santoni A, Gioiosa L, Ferrarini A, Delledonne M, Margolles A, Piazza L, Palanza P, Bolchi A, Guglielmetti S, van Sinderen D, Ventura M. Role of sortase-dependent pili of Bifidobacterium bifidum PRL2010 in modulating bacterium-host interactions. Proc Natl Acad Sci U S A July 2, 2013;110(27):11151–6. https://doi.org/10.1073/pnas.1303897110. Epub 2013 Jun 17. PMID: 23776216; PMCID: PMC3703987.

[158] González-Rodríguez I, Sánchez B, Ruiz L, Turroni F, Ventura M, Ruas-Madiedo P, Gueimonde M, Margolles A. Role of extracellular transaldolase from Bifidobacterium bifidum in mucin adhesion and aggregation. Appl Environ Microbiol June 2012;78(11):3992–8. https://doi.org/10.1128/AEM.08024-11. Epub 2012 Mar 23. PMID: 22447584; PMCID: PMC3346390.

[159] Turroni F, Duranti S, Bottacini F, Guglielmetti S, Van Sinderen D, Ventura M. Bifidobacterium bifidum as an example of a specialized human gut commensal. Front Microbiol 2014;5:437. https://doi.org/10.3389/fmicb.2014.00437.

[160] Lopez P, Gonzalez-Rodriguez I, Gueimonde M, Margolles A, Suarez A. Immune response to Bifidobacterium bifidum strains support Treg/Th17 plasticity. PLoS One 2011;6(9):e24776. https://doi.org/10.1371/journal.pone.0024776.

[161] Tanaka K, Tsukahara T, Yanagi T, Nakahara S, Furukawa O, Tsutsui H, Koshida S. Bifidobacterium bifidum OLB6378 simultaneously enhances systemic and mucosal humoral immunity in low birth weight infants: a non-randomized study. Nutrients February 26, 2017;9(3):195. https://doi.org/10.3390/nu9030195. PMID: 28245626; PMCID: PMC5372858.

[162] Caballero-Franco C, Keller K, De Simone C, Chadee K. The VSL#3 probiotic formula induces mucin gene expression and secretion in colonic epithelial cells. Am J Physiol Gastrointest Liver Physiol 2007;292(1):G315–22. https://doi.org/10.1152/ajpgi.00265.2006.

[163] Jing W, Liu Q, Wang W. Bifidobacterium bifidum TMC3115 ameliorates milk protein allergy in by affecting gut microbiota: a randomized double-blind control trial. J Food Biochem November 2020;44(11):e13489. https://doi.org/10.1111/jfbc.13489. Epub 2020 Sep 29. Erratum in: J Food Biochem. 2021 Nov;45(11):e13591. PMID: 32996156.

[164] Gotoh A, Katoh T, Sakanaka M, Ling Y, Yamada C, Asakuma S, Urashima T, Tomabechi Y, Katayama-Ikegami A, Kurihara S, Yamamoto K, Harata G, He F, Hirose J, Kitaoka M, Okuda S, Katayama T. Sharing of human milk oligosaccharides degradants within bifidobacterial communities in faecal cultures supplemented with Bifidobacterium bifidum. Sci Rep September 18, 2018;8(1):13958. https://doi.org/10.1038/s41598-018-32080-3. PMID: 30228375; PMCID: PMC6143587.

[165] Duranti S, Lugli GA, Milani C, James K, Mancabelli L, Turroni F, Alessandri G, Mangifesta M, Mancino W, Ossiprandi MC, Iori A, Rota C, Gargano G, Bernasconi S, Di Pierro F, van Sinderen D, Ventura M. Bifidobacterium bifidum and the infant gut microbiota: an intriguing case of microbe-host co-evolution. Environ Microbiol October 2019;21(10):3683–95. https://doi.org/10.1111/1462-2920.14705. Epub 2019 Jun 20. PMID: 31172651.

[166] Turroni F, Milani C, Duranti S, Lugli GA, Bernasconi S, Margolles A, Di Pierro F, van Sinderen D, Ventura M. The infant gut microbiome as a microbial organ influencing host well-being. Ital J Pediatr February 5, 2020;46(1):16. https://doi.org/10.1186/s13052-020-0781-0. PMID: 32024556; PMCID: PMC7003403.

[167] Мескина ЕР, Целипанова ЕЕ, Чадисова МК, Галкина ЛА, Сташко ТВ. Лффективность применения сорбированных пробиотиков в комплексной терапии пневмонии, вызванной SARS-COV-2. часть 1. Период разгара клинических проявлений. Терапевтический архив 2021:456–64. – Т. 93. – №. 4. – С.

[168] Duranti S, Lugli GA, Mancabelli L, Armanini F, Turroni F, James K, et al. Maternal inheritance of bifidobacterial communities and bifidophages in infants through vertical transmission. Microbiome 2017;5(1):66. https://doi.org/10.1186/s40168-017-0282-6.

[169] Underwood MA, Davis JCC, Kalanetra KM, Gehlot S, Patole S, Tancredi DJ, Mills DA, Lebrilla CB, Simmer K. Digestion of human milk oligosaccharides by Bifidobacterium breve in the premature infant. J Pediatr Gastroenterol Nutr October 2017;65(4):449–55. https://doi.org/10.1097/MPG.0000000000001590. PMID: 28945208; PMCID: PMC6349036.

[170] James K, O'Connell Motherway M, Penno C, O'Brien RL, van Sinderen D. Bifidobacterium breve UCC2003 employs multiple transcriptional regulators to control metabolism of particular human milk oligosaccharides. Appl Environ Microbiol April 16, 2018;84(9):e02774–17. https://doi.org/10.1128/AEM.02774-17. PMID: 29500268; PMCID: PMC5930313.

[171] Patole SK, Keil AD, Nathan E, Doherty D, Esvaran M, Simmer KN, Conway P. Effect of Bifidobacterium breve M-16V supplementation on faecal bifidobacteria in growth restricted very preterm infants - analysis from a randomised trial. J Matern Fetal Neonatal Med December 2016;29(23):3751–5. https://doi.org/10.3109/14767058.2016.1147554. Epub 2016 Feb 26. PMID: 26821074.

[172] Bozzi Cionci N, Baffoni L, Gaggìa F, Di Gioia D. Therapeutic microbiology: the role of Bifidobacterium breve as food supplement for the prevention/treatment of paediatric diseases. Nutrients November 10, 2018;10(11):1723. https://doi.org/10.3390/nu10111723. PMID: 30423810; PMCID: PMC6265827.

[173] Maldonado-Lobón JA, Blanco-Rojo R, Maldonado J, Ali MA, Almazán MV, Suanes-Cabello A, Callejón E, Jaldo R, Benavídes MR, Negrillo AM, Sañudo A, Rodríguez C, Bañuelos O, Fonollá J, Olivares M, PROBI-COLIC group. Efficacy of Bifidobacterium breve CECT7263 for infantile colic treatment: an open-label, parallel, randomised, controlled trial. Benef Microbes February 24, 2021;12(1):55–67. https://doi.org/10.3920/BM2020.0105. Epub 2020 Dec 22. PMID: 33350361.

[174] Mancabelli L, Mancino W, Lugli GA, Argentini C, Longhi G, Milani C, Viappiani A, Anzalone R, Bernasconi S, van Sinderen D, Ventura M, Turroni F. Amoxicillin-clavulanic acid resistance in the genus Bifidobacterium. Appl Environ Microbiol March 11, 2021;87(7):e03137–20. https://doi.org/10.1128/AEM.03137-20. PMID: 33483308; PMCID: PMC8091617.

[175] Martínez N, Luque R, Milani C, Ventura M, Bañuelos O, Margolles A. A gene homologous to rRNA methylase genes confers erythromycin and clindamycin resistance in Bifidobacterium breve. Appl Environ Microbiol May 1, 2018;84(10):e02888–17. https://doi.org/10.1128/AEM.02888-17. PMID: 29500262; PMCID: PMC5930361.

[176] Arboleya S, Bottacini F, O'Connell-Motherway M, Ryan CA, Ross RP, van Sinderen D, Stanton C. Gene-trait matching across the Bifidobacterium longum pan-genome reveals considerable diversity in carbohydrate catabolism among human infant strains. BMC Genom January 8, 2018;19(1):33. https://doi.org/10.1186/s12864-017-4388-9. PMID: 29310579; PMCID: PMC5759876.

[177] Sakanaka M, Nakakawaji S, Nakajima S, Fukiya S, Abe A, Saburi W, Mori H, Yokota A. A transposon mutagenesis system for Bifidobacterium longum subsp. longum based on an IS3 family insertion sequence, ISBlo11. Appl Environ Microbiol August 17, 2018;84(17):e00824–18. https://doi.org/10.1128/AEM.00824-18. PMID: 29934330; PMCID: PMC6102999.

[178] Oki K, Akiyama T, Matsuda K, Gawad A, Makino H, Ishikawa E, Oishi K, Kushiro A, Fujimoto J. Long-term colonization exceeding six years from early infancy of Bifidobacterium longum subsp. longum in human gut. BMC Microbiol December 12, 2018;18(1):209. https://doi.org/10.1186/s12866-018-1358-6. PMID: 30541439; PMCID: PMC6292050.

[179] Nam YW, Nishimoto M, Arakawa T, Kitaoka M, Fushinobu S. Structural basis for broad substrate specificity of UDP-glucose 4-epimerase in the human milk oligosaccharide catabolic pathway of Bifidobacterium longum. Sci Rep July 31, 2019;9(1):11081. https://doi.org/10.1038/s41598-019-47591-w. PMID: 31366978; PMCID: PMC6668579.

[180] Sundararaman A, Bansal K, Sidhic J, Patil P, Halami PM. Genome of Bifidobacterium longum NCIM 5672 provides insights into its acid-tolerance mechanism and probiotic properties. Arch Microbiol December 2021;203(10):6109–18. https://doi.org/10.1007/s00203-021-02573-3. Epub 2021 Sep 22. PMID: 34553262.

[181] Yamada C, Gotoh A, Sakanaka M, Hattie M, Stubbs KA, Katayama-Ikegami A, Hirose J, Kurihara S, Arakawa T, Kitaoka M, Okuda S, Katayama T, Fushinobu S. Molecular insight into evolution of symbiosis between breast-fed infants and a member of the human gut microbiome Bifidobacterium longum. Cell Chem Biol April 20, 2017;24(4):515–24. https://doi.org/10.1016/j.chembiol.2017.03.012. e5. Epub 2017 Apr 6. PMID: 28392148.

[182] Jakobsen LMA, Sundekilde UK, Andersen HJ, Nielsen DS, Bertram HC. Lactose and bovine milk oligosaccharides synergistically stimulate B. Longum subsp. longum growth in a simplified model of the infant gut microbiome. J Proteome Res August 2, 2019;18(8):3086–98. https://doi.org/10.1021/acs.jproteome.9b00211. Epub 2019 Jul 10. PMID: 31264424.

[183] Mennini M, Reddel S, Del Chierico F, Gardini S, Quagliariello A, Vernocchi P, Valluzzi RL, Fierro V, Riccardi C, Napolitano T, Fiocchi AG, Putignani L. Gut microbiota profile in children with IgE-mediated cow's milk allergy and cow's milk sensitization and probiotic intestinal persistence evaluation. Int J Mol Sci February 6, 2021;22(4):1649. https://doi.org/10.3390/ijms22041649. PMID: 33562104; PMCID: PMC7915344.

[184] Успенский ЮП, Фоминых ЮА, Наджафова КН, Полюшкин СВ. Пробиотики и их место в современном мире. Российский журнал гастроэнтерологии, гепатологии, колопроктологии 2020:24–35. – Т. 30. – №. 3. – С.

[185] Nocerino R, De Filippis F, Cecere G, Marino A, Micillo M, Di Scala C, de Caro C, Calignano A, Bruno C, Paparo L, Iannicelli AM, Cosenza L, Maddalena Y, Della Gatta G, Coppola S, Carucci L, Ercolini D, Berni Canani R. The therapeutic efficacy of Bifidobacterium animalis subsp. lactis BB-12® in infant colic: a randomised, double blind, placebo-controlled trial. Aliment Pharmacol Ther January 2020;51(1):110–20. https://doi.org/10.1111/apt.15561. Epub 2019 Dec 3. PMID: 31797399; PMCID: PMC6973258.

[186] Marsaux B, Van den Abbeele P, Ghyselinck J, Prioult G, Marzorati M, Bogićević B. Synbiotic effect of Bifidobacterium lactis CNCM I-3446 and bovine milk-derived oligosaccharides on infant gut microbiota. Nutrients July 29, 2020;12(8):2268. https://doi.org/10.3390/nu12082268. PMID: 32751149; PMCID: PMC7468906.

[187] Chi C, Xue Y, Liu R, Wang Y, Lv N, Zeng H, Buys N, Zhu B, Sun J, Yin C. Effects of a formula with a probiotic Bifidobacterium lactis Supplement on the gut microbiota of low birth weight infants. Eur J Nutr June 2020;59(4):1493–503. https://doi.org/10.1007/s00394-019-02006-4. Epub 2019 Jun 13. PMID: 31197506.

[188] Holscher HD, Czerkies LA, Cekola P, Litov R, Benbow M, Santema S, Alexander DD, Perez V, Sun S, Saavedra JM, Tappenden KA. Bifidobacterium lactis Bb12 enhances intestinal antibody response in formula-fed infants: a randomized, double-blind, controlled trial. JPEN – J Parenter Enter Nutr January 2012;36(1 Suppl. l):106S–7S. https://doi.org/10.1177/0148607111430817. PMID: 22237870.

[189] Li A, Yang J, Zhang C, Chi H, Zhang C, Li T, Zhang J, Du P. Lactobacillus acidophilus KLDS 1.0738 inhibits TLR4/NF-κB inflammatory pathway in β-lactoglobulin-induced macrophages via modulating miR-146a. J Food Biochem October 2021;45(10):e13662. https://doi.org/10.1111/jfbc.13662. Epub 2021 May 14. PMID: 33990976.

[190] Della Volpe A, Ricci G, Ralli M, Gambacorta V, De Lucia A, Minni A, Pirozzi C, Paccone M, Pastore V, Di Stadio A. The effects of oral supplements with Sambucus nigra, Zinc, Tyndallized Lactobacillus acidophilus (HA122), Arabinogalactans, vitamin D, vitamin E and vitamin C in otitis media with effusion in children: a randomized controlled trial. Eur Rev Med Pharmacol Sci July 2019;23(14):6360–70. https://doi.org/10.26355/eurrev_201907_18460. PMID: 31364144.

[191] Schmidt RM, Pilmann Laursen R, Bruun S, Larnkjaer A, Mølgaard C, Michaelsen KF, Høst A. Probiotics in late infancy reduce the incidence of eczema: a randomized controlled trial. Pediatr Allergy Immunol May 2019;30(3):335–40. https://doi.org/10.1111/pai.13018. Epub 2019 Feb 21. PMID: 30790361.

[192] Castro-Mejía JL, O'Ferrall S, Krych Ł, O'Mahony E, Namusoke H, Lanyero B, Kot W, Nabukeera-Barungi N, Michaelsen KF, Mølgaard C, Friis H, Grenov B, Nielsen DS. Restitution of gut microbiota in Ugandan children administered with probiotics (Lactobacillus rhamnosus GG and Bifidobacterium animalis subsp. lactis BB-12) during treatment for severe acute malnutrition. Gut Microb July 3, 2020;11(4):855–67. https://doi.org/10.1080/19490976.2020.1712982. Epub 2020 Jan 20. Erratum in: Gut Microbes. 2020 Jan 29;:1. PMID: 31959047; PMCID: PMC7524335.

[193] Park MS, Kwon B, Ku S, Ji GE. The efficacy of Bifidobacterium longum BORI and lactobacillus acidophilus AD031 probiotic treatment in infants with rotavirus infection. Nutrients August 16, 2017;9(8):887. https://doi.org/10.3390/nu9080887. PMID: 28813007; PMCID: PMC5579680.

[194] Chen K, Xin J, Zhang G, Xie H, Luo L, Yuan S, Bu Y, Yang X, Ge Y, Liu C. A combination of three probiotic strains for treatment of acute diarrhoea in hospitalised children: an open label, randomised controlled trial. Benef Microbes August 12, 2020;11(4):339–46. https://doi.org/10.3920/BM2020.0046. Epub 2020 Jul 28. PMID: 32720832.

[195] Tremblay A, Xu X, Colee J, Tompkins TA. Efficacy of a multi-strain probiotic formulation in pediatric populations: a comprehensive review of clinical studies. Nutrients June 1, 2021;13(6):1908. https://doi.org/10.3390/nu13061908. PMID: 34206098; PMCID: PMC8226750.

[196] Marißen J, Haiß A, Meyer C, Van Rossum T, Bünte LM, Frommhold D, Gille C, Goedicke-Fritz S, Göpel W, Hudalla H, Pagel J, Pirr S, Siller B, Viemann D, Vens M, König I, Herting E, Zemlin M, Gehring S, Bork P, Henneke P, Härtel C. PRIMAL consortium. Efficacy of Bifidobacterium longum, B. infantis and Lactobacillus acidophilus probiotics to prevent gut dysbiosis in preterm infants of 28+0-32+6 weeks of gestation: a randomised, placebo-controlled, double-blind, multicentre trial: the PRIMAL Clinical Study protocol. BMJ Open November 21, 2019;9(11):e032617. https://doi.org/10.1136/bmjopen-2019-032617. Erratum in: BMJ Open. 2020 Sep 18;10(9):e032617corr1. PMID: 31753895; PMCID: PMC6886923.

[197] DeMuri GP, Lehtoranta LM, Eickhoff JC, Lehtinen MJ, Wald ER. Ex vivo peripheral blood mononuclear cell response to R848 in children after supplementation with the probiotic Lactobacillus acidophilus NCFM/Bifidobacterium lactis Bi-07. Benef Microbes February 24, 2021;12(1):85–93. https://doi.org/10.3920/BM2020.0068. Epub 2021 Feb 8. PMID: 33550937.

[198] Uberos J, Aguilera-Rodríguez E, Jerez-Calero A, Molina-Oya M, Molina-Carballo A, Narbona-López E. Probiotics to prevent necrotising enterocolitis and nosocomial infection in very low birth weight preterm infants. Br J Nutr April 2017;117(7):994–1000. https://doi.org/10.1017/S0007114517000769. Epub 2017 Apr 26. PMID: 28443531.

[199] Meyer MP, Chow SSW, Alsweiler J, Bourchier D, Broadbent R, Knight D, Lynn AM, Patel H. Probiotics for prevention of severe necrotizing enterocolitis: experience of New Zealand neonatal intensive care units. Front Pediatr April 7, 2020;8:119. https://doi.org/10.3389/fped.2020.00119. PMID: 32318522; PMCID: PMC7154127.

[200] Beghetti I, Panizza D, Lenzi J, Gori D, Martini S, Corvaglia L, Aceti A. Probiotics for preventing necrotizing enterocolitis in preterm infants: a network meta-analysis. Nutrients January 9, 2021;13(1):192. https://doi.org/10.3390/nu13010192. PMID: 33435456; PMCID: PMC7827781.

[201] Di Pierro F, Basile I, Danza ML, Venturelli L, Contini R, Risso P, Colombo M. Use of a probiotic mixture containing Bifidobacterium animalis subsp. lactis BB12 and Enterococcus faecium L3 in atopic children. Minerva Pediatr October 2018;70(5):418–24. https://doi.org/10.23736/S0026-4946.18.05203-9. Epub 2018 Apr 12. PMID: 29651835.

[202] Старовойтова СА. Кобиотики – новая концепция пробиотиков. вестник Южно-Казахстанской медицинской академии 2018:38. – 4 (84) Т.1. – С.

[203] Kaiser KA, Arpaia N. Glycans for good. Sci Immunol October 19, 2018;3(28):eaav1041. https://doi.org/10.1126/sciimmunol.aav1041. PMID: 30341146; PMCID: PMC7257804.

[204] Verma R, Lee C, Jeun EJ, Yi J, Kim KS, Ghosh A, Byun S, Lee CG, Kang HJ, Kim GC, Jun CD, Jan G, Suh CH, Jung JY, Sprent J, Rudra D, De Castro C, Molinaro A, Surh CD, Im SH. Cell surface polysaccharides of Bifidobacterium bifidum induce the generation of Foxp3+ regulatory T cells. Sci Immunol October 19, 2018;3(28):eaat6975. https://doi.org/10.1126/sciimmunol.aat6975. PMID: 30341145.

[205] Mahooti M, Abdolalipour E, Salehzadeh A, Mohebbi SR, Gorji A, Ghaemi A. Immunomodulatory and prophylactic effects of Bifidobacterium bifidum probiotic strain on influenza infection in mice. World J Microbiol Biotechnol June 3, 2019;35(6):91. https://doi.org/10.1007/s11274-019-2667-0. PMID: 31161259.

[206] Speciale I, Verma R, Di Lorenzo F, Molinaro A, Im SH, De Castro C. Bifidobacterium bifidum presents on the cell surface a complex mixture of glucans and galactans with different immunological properties. Carbohydr Polym August 15, 2019;218:269–78. https://doi.org/10.1016/j.carbpol.2019.05.006. Epub 2019 May 3. PMID: 31221330.

[207] Hong N, Ku S, Yuk K, Johnston TV, Ji GE, Park MS. Production of biologically active human interleukin-10 by Bifidobacterium bifidum BGN4. Microb Cell Factories January 19, 2021;20(1):16. https://doi.org/10.1186/s12934-020-01505-y. PMID: 33468130; PMCID: PMC7814708.

[208] Chowdhury AH, Cámara M, Verma C, Eremin O, Kulkarni AD, Lobo DN. Modulation of T Regulatory and dendritic cell phenotypes following ingestion of Bifidobacterium longum, AHCC® and azithromycin in healthy individuals. Nutrients October 15, 2019;11(10):2470. https://doi.org/10.3390/nu11102470. PMID: 31618905; PMCID: PMC6835407.

[209] Choi M, Lee Y, Lee NK, Bae CH, Park DC, Paik HD, Park E. Immunomodulatory effects by Bifidobacterium longum KACC 91563 in mouse splenocytes and macrophages. J Microbiol Biotechnol November 28, 2019;29(11):1739–44. https://doi.org/10.4014/jmb.1812.12002. PMID: 31546293.

[210] Groeger D, Schiavi E, Grant R, Kurnik-Łucka M, Michalovich D, Williamson R, Beinke S, Kiely B, Akdis CA, Hessel EM, Shanahan F, O' Mahony L. Intranasal Bifidobacterium longum protects against viral-induced lung inflammation and injury in a murine model of lethal influenza infection. EBioMedicine October 2020;60:102981. https://doi.org/10.1016/j.ebiom.2020.102981. Epub 2020 Sep 11. PMID: 32927273; PMCID: PMC7495089.

[211] Miller LE, Lehtoranta L, Lehtinen MJ. The effect of Bifidobacterium animalis ssp. lactis HN019 on cellular immune function in healthy elderly subjects: systematic review and meta-analysis. Nutrients February 24, 2017;9(3):191. https://doi.org/10.3390/nu9030191. PMID: 28245559; PMCID: PMC5372854.

[212] Shoaib A, Xin L, Xin Y. Oral administration of Lactobacillus acidophilus alleviates exacerbations in *Pseudomonas aeruginosa* and *Staphylococcus aureus* pulmonary infections. Pak J Pharm Sci July 2019;32(4):1621–30. PMID: 31608882.

[213] Mizuno H, Arce L, Tomotsune K, Albarracin L, Funabashi R, Vera D, Islam MA, Vizoso-Pinto MG, Takahashi H, Sasaki Y, Kitazawa H, Villena J. Lipoteichoic acid is involved in the ability of the immunobiotic strain lactobacillus plantarum CRL1506 to modulate the intestinal antiviral innate immunity triggered by TLR3 activation. Front Immunol April 9, 2020;11:571. https://doi.org/10.3389/fimmu.2020.00571. PMID: 32328062; PMCID: PMC7161159.

[214] Finamore A, Roselli M, Donini L, Brasili DE, Rami R, Carnevali P, Mistura L, Pinto A, Giusti A, Mengheri E. Supplementation with Bifidobacterium longum Bar33 and Lactobacillus helveticus Bar13 mixture improves immunity in elderly humans (over 75 years) and aged mice. Nutrition 2019 ;63–64:184–92. https://doi.org/10.1016/j.nut.2019.02.005. Epub 2019 Feb 18. PMID: 31029046.

[215] Garcia-Castillo V, Komatsu R, Clua P, Indo Y, Takagi M, Salva S, Islam MA, Alvarez S, Takahashi H, Garcia-Cancino A, Kitazawa H, Villena J. Evaluation of the immunomodulatory activities of the probiotic strain lactobacillus fermentum UCO-979C. Front Immunol June 13, 2019;10:1376. https://doi.org/10.3389/fimmu.2019.01376. PMID: 31263467; PMCID: PMC6585165.

[216] Guo S, Chen S, Ma J, Ma Y, Zhu J, Ma Y, Liu Y, Wang P, Pan Y. *Escherichia coli* nissle 1917 protects intestinal barrier function by inhibiting NF-κB-Mediated activation of the MLCK-P-MLC signaling pathway. Mediat Inflamm July 3, 2019;2019:5796491. https://doi.org/10.1155/2019/5796491. PMID: 31354386; PMCID: PMC6636522.

[217] Bednorz C, Guenther S, Oelgeschläger K, Kinnemann B, Pieper R, Hartmann S, Tedin K, Semmler T, Neumann K, Schierack P, Bethe A, Wieler LH. Feeding the probiotic Enterococcus faecium strain NCIMB 10415 to piglets specifically reduces the number of *Escherichia coli* pathotypes that adhere to the gut mucosa. Appl Environ Microbiol December 2013;79(24):7896–904. https://doi.org/10.1128/AEM.03138-13. Epub 2013 Oct 11. PMID: 24123741; PMCID: PMC3837809.

[218] Белкина ТВ, Аверина ОВ, Савенкова ЕВ, Даниленко ВН. Микробиом кишечника человека и иммунная система: роль пробиотиков в формировании иммунобиологического потенциала, препятствующего развитию инфекции COVID-19. Успехи современной биологии 2020:523–39. – Т. 140. – №. 6. – С.

[219] Pavlova AS, Ozhegov GD, Arapidi GP, Butenko IO, Fomin ES, Alemasov NA, Afonnikov DA, Yarullina DR, Ivanov VT, Govorun VM, Kayumov AR. Identification of antimicrobial peptides from novel lactobacillus fermentum strain. Protein J February 2020;39(1):73–84. https://doi.org/10.1007/s10930-019-09879-8. PMID: 31933011.

[220] Wang M, Fu T, Hao J, Li L, Tian M, Jin N, Ren L, Li C. A recombinant Lactobacillus plantarum strain expressing the spike protein of SARS-CoV-2. Int J Biol Macromol October 1, 2020;160:736–40. https://doi.org/10.1016/j.ijbiomac.2020.05.239. Epub 2020 May 30. PMID: 32485251; PMCID: PMC7260514.

[221] Li L, Wang M, Hao J, Han J, Fu T, Bai J, Tian M, Jin N, Zhu G, Li C. Mucosal IgA response elicited by intranasal immunization of Lactobacillus plantarum expressing surface-displayed RBD protein of SARS-CoV-2. Int J Biol Macromol November 1, 2021;190:409–16. https://doi.org/10.1016/j.ijbiomac.2021.08.232. Epub 2021 Sep 7. PMID: 34499954; PMCID: PMC8421092.

[222] Keikha R, Hashemi-Shahri SM, Jebali A. The evaluation of novel oral vaccines based on self-amplifying RNA lipid nanparticles (saRNA LNPs), saRNA transfected Lactobacillus plantarum LNPs, and saRNA transfected Lactobacillus plantarum to neutralize SARS-CoV-2 variants alpha and delta. Sci Rep October 29, 2021;11(1):21308. https://doi.org/10.1038/s41598-021-00830-5. PMID: 34716391; PMCID: PMC8556360.

[223] Evans PC, Rainger GE, Mason JC, Guzik TJ, Osto E, Stamataki Z, Neil D, Hoefer IE, Fragiadaki M, Waltenberger J, Weber C, Bochaton-Piallat ML, Bäck M. Endothelial dysfunction in COVID-19: a position paper of the ESC working group for atherosclerosis and vascular biology, and the ESC council of basic cardiovascular science. Cardiovasc Res December 1, 2020;116(14):2177–84. https://doi.org/10.1093/cvr/cvaa230. PMID: 32750108; PMCID: PMC7454368.

[224] Patti G, Lio V, Cavallari I, Gragnano F, Riva L, Calabrò P, Di Pasquale G, Pengo V, Rubboli A. Terapie antitrombotiche in pazienti con infezione da SARS-CoV-2: dalle attuali evidenze alle ragionevoli raccomandazioni – position paper del Gruppo di Studio Aterosclerosi, Trombosi e Biologia Vascolare [Antithrombotic treatments in patients with SARS-CoV-2 infection: from current evidence to reasonable recommendations – a position paper from the Italian Working Group on Atherosclerosis, Thrombosis and Vascular Biology]. G Ital Cardiol July 2020;21(7):489–501. https://doi.org/10.1714/3386.33634. Italian. PMID: 32555564.

[225] Nägele MP, Haubner B, Tanner FC, Ruschitzka F, Flammer AJ. Endothelial dysfunction in COVID-19: current findings and therapeutic implications. Atherosclerosis December 2020;314:58–62. https://doi.org/10.1016/j.atherosclerosis.2020.10.014. Epub 2020 Oct 14. PMID: 33161318; PMCID: PMC7554490.

[226] Chiappetta S, Sharma AM, Bottino V, Stier C. COVID-19 and the role of chronic inflammation in patients with obesity. Int J Obes August 2020;44(8):1790–2. https://doi.org/10.1038/s41366-020-0597-4. Epub 2020 May 14. PMID: 32409680; PMCID: PMC7224343.

[227] Simonnet A, Chetboun M, Poissy J, Raverdy V, Noulette J, Duhamel A, Labreuche J, Mathieu D, Pattou F, Jourdain M. LICORN and the lille COVID-19 and obesity study group. High prevalence of obesity in severe acute respiratory syndrome coronavirus-2 (SARS-CoV-2) requiring invasive mechanical ventilation. Obesity July 2020;28(7):1195–9. https://doi.org/10.1002/oby.22831. Epub 2020 Jun 10. Erratum in: Obesity (Silver Spring). 2020 Oct;28(10):1994. PMID: 32271993; PMCID: PMC7262326.

[228] Michalakis K, Ilias I. SARS-CoV-2 infection and obesity: common inflammatory and metabolic aspects. Diabetes Metabol Syndr July–August 2020;14(4):469–71. https://doi.org/10.1016/j.dsx.2020.04.033. Epub 2020 Apr 29. PMID: 32387864; PMCID: PMC7189186.

[229] Hussain A, Mahawar K, Xia Z, Yang W, El-Hasani S. Obesity and mortality of COVID-19. Meta-analysis. Obes Res Clin Pract July−August 2020;14(4):295−300. https://doi.org/10.1016/j.orcp.2020.07.002. Epub 2020 Jul 9. Retraction in: Obes Res Clin Pract. 2021 Jan-Feb;15(1):100. PMID: 32660813; PMCID: PMC7346803.

[230] Wu J, Zhang J, Sun X, Wang L, Xu Y, Zhang Y, Liu X, Dong C. Influence of diabetes mellitus on the severity and fatality of SARS-CoV-2 (COVID-19) infection. Diabetes Obes Metabol October 2020;22(10):1907−14. https://doi.org/10.1111/dom.14105. Epub 2020 Jul 7. PMID: 32496012; PMCID: PMC7300679.

[231] Fadini GP, Morieri ML, Longato E, Avogaro A. Prevalence and impact of diabetes among people infected with SARS-CoV-2. J Endocrinol Invest June 2020;43(6):867−9. https://doi.org/10.1007/s40618-020-01236-2. Epub 2020 Mar 28. PMID: 32222956; PMCID: PMC7103097.

[232] Zhou Y, Chi J, Lv W, Wang Y. Obesity and diabetes as high-risk factors for severe coronavirus disease 2019 (Covid-19). Diabetes Metab Res Rev February 2021;37(2):e3377. https://doi.org/10.1002/dmrr.3377. Epub 2020 Jul 20. PMID: 32588943; PMCID: PMC7361201.

[233] Lima-Martínez MM, Carrera Boada C, Madera-Silva MD, Marín W, Contreras M. COVID-19 and diabetes: a bidirectional relationship. Clín Invest Arterioscler May−June 2021;33(3):151−7. https://doi.org/10.1016/j.arteri.2020.10.001. English, Spanish. Epub 2020 Oct 28. PMID: 33303218; PMCID: PMC7598432.

[234] Malik M, Suboc TM, Tyagi S, Salzman N, Wang J, Ying R, Tanner MJ, Kakarla M, Baker JE, Widlansky ME. Lactobacillus plantarum 299v supplementation improves vascular endothelial function and reduces inflammatory biomarkers in men with stable coronary artery disease. Circ Res October 12, 2018;123(9):1091−102. https://doi.org/10.1161/CIRCRESAHA.118.313565. PMID: 30355158; PMCID: PMC6205737.

[235] Fuentes MC, Lajo T, Carrión JM, Cuñé J. Cholesterol-lowering efficacy of Lactobacillus plantarum CECT 7527, 7528 and 7529 in hypercholesterolaemic adults. Br J Nutr May 28, 2013;109(10):1866−72. https://doi.org/10.1017/S000711451200373X. Epub 2012 Sep 28. PMID: 23017585.

[236] Макарова СГ, Намазова-Баранова ЛС. Кишечная микробиота и использование пробиотиков в практике педиатра. что нового? Педиатрическая фармакология 2015:38−45. − Т. 12. − №. 1. С.

[237] Tian P, O'Riordan KJ, Lee Y, Wang G, Zhao J, Zhang H, Cryan JF, Chen W. Towards a psychobiotic therapy for depression: bifidobacterium breve CCFM1025 reverses chronic stress-induced depressive symptoms and gut microbial abnormalities in mice. Neurobiology of Stress 2020;12:100216. https://doi.org/10.1016/j.ynstr.2020.100216. ISSN 2352-2895.

[238] Baloch S, Baloch MA, Zheng T, Pei X. The coronavirus disease 2019 (COVID-19) pandemic. Tohoku J Exp Med 2020;250(4):271−8. https://doi.org/10.1620/tjem.250.271.

[239] Stein MB. EDITORIAL: COVID-19 and anxiety and depression in 2020. Depress Anxiety April 2020;37(4):302. https://doi.org/10.1002/da.23014. PMID: 32266767; PMCID: PMC7262238.

[240] Javed B, Sarwer A, Soto EB, Mashwani ZU. Impact of SARS-CoV-2 (coronavirus) pandemic on public mental health. Front Public Health June 23, 2020;8:292. https://doi.org/10.3389/fpubh.2020.00292. PMID: 32656175; PMCID: PMC7324781.

[241] Мосолов СН. Проблемы психического здоровья в условиях пандемии COVID-19. Журнал неврологии и психиатрии им. СС Корсакова 2020:7−15. https://doi.org/10.17116/jnevro20201200517. Т. 120. №. 5. С.

[242] Shigemura J, Ursano RJ, Morganstein JC, Kurosawa M, Benedek DM. Public responses to the novel 2019 coronavirus (2019-nCoV) in Japan: mental health consequences and target populations. Psychiatr Clin Neurosci 2020;74(4):281−2. https://doi.org/10.1111/pcn.12988. Epub 2020 Feb 23. PMID: 32034840; PMCID: PMC7168047.

[243] Xiang YT, Yang Y, Li W, Zhang L, Zhang Q, Cheung T, Ng CH. Timely mental health care for the 2019 novel coronavirus outbreak is urgently needed. Lancet Psychiatr March 2020;7(3):228−9. https://doi.org/10.1016/S2215-0366(20)30046-8. Epub 2020 Feb 4. PMID: 32032543; PMCID: PMC7128153.

[244] Wang C, Pan R, Wan X, Tan Y, Xu L, Ho CS, Ho RC. Immediate psychological responses and associated factors during the initial stage of the 2019 coronavirus disease (COVID-19) epidemic among the general population in China. Int J Environ Res Publ Health 2020;17(5):1729.

[245] Ozamiz-Etxebarria N, Dosil-Santamaria M, Picaza-Gorrochategui M, Idoiaga-Mondragon N. Stress, anxiety, and depression levels in the initial stage of the COVID-19 outbreak in a population sample in the northern Spain. Cad Saúde Pública April 30, 2020;36(4):e00054020. https://doi.org/10.1590/0102-311X00054020. English, Spanish. PMID: 32374806.

[246] Schwartz BJ. New poll: COVID-19 impacting mental well-being: Americans feeling anxious, especially for loved ones. APA News Releases March 25, 2020. https://www.psychiatry.org/newsroom/news-releases/

new-poll-covid-19-impacting-mental-well-being-americans-feeling-anxious-especially-for-loved-ones-older-adults-are-less-anxious.

[247] Taylor S, Landry CA, Paluszek MM, Fergus TA, McKay D, Asmundson GJG. COVID stress syndrome: concept, structure, and correlates. Depress Anxiety 2020;37(8):706–14. https://doi.org/10.1002/da.23071.

[248] Nagaraja AS, Sadaoui NC, Dorniak PL, Lutgendorf SK, Sood AK. SnapShot: stress and disease. Cell Metabol 2016;23(2). https://doi.org/10.1016/j.cmet.2016.01.015. 388-388.e1.

[249] Mazza MG, De Lorenzo R, Conte C, Poletti S, Vai B, Bollettini I, Melloni EMT, Furlan R, Ciceri F, Rovere-Querini P, , COVID-19 BioB Outpatient Clinic Study group, Benedetti F. Anxiety and depression in COVID-19 survivors: role of inflammatory and clinical predictors. Brain Behav Immun October 2020;89:594–600. https://doi.org/10.1016/j.bbi.2020.07.037. Epub 2020 Jul 30. PMID: 32738287; PMCID: PMC7390748.

[250] Demeco A, Marotta N, Barletta M, Pino I, Marinaro C, Petraroli A, Moggio L, Ammendolia A. Rehabilitation of patients post-COVID-19 infection: a literature review. J Int Med Res August 2020;48(8). https://doi.org/10.1177/0300060520948382. 300060520948382. PMID: 32840156; PMCID: PMC7450453.

[251] Yunes RA, Poluektova EU, Dyachkova MS, Klimina KM, Kovtun AS, Averina OV, Orlova VS, Danilenko VN. GABA production and structure of gadB/gadC genes in Lactobacillus and Bifidobacterium strains from human microbiota. Anaerobe December 2016;42:197–204. https://doi.org/10.1016/j.anaerobe.2016.10.011. Epub 2016 Oct 26. PMID: 27794467.

[252] Allen AP, Hutch W, Borre YE, Kennedy PJ, Temko A, Boylan G, Murphy E, Cryan JF, Dinan TG, Clarke G. Bifidobacterium longum 1714 as a translational psychobiotic: modulation of stress, electrophysiology and neurocognition in healthy volunteers. Transl Psychiatry November 1, 2016;6(11):e939. https://doi.org/10.1038/tp.2016.191. PMID: 27801892; PMCID: PMC5314114.

[253] Yang JM, Koh HY, Moon SY, Yoo IK, Ha EK, You S, Kim SY, Yon DK, Lee SW. Allergic disorders and susceptibility to and severity of COVID-19: a nationwide cohort study. J Allergy Clin Immunol October 2020;146(4):790–8. https://doi.org/10.1016/j.jaci.2020.08.008. Epub 2020 Aug 15. PMID: 32810517; PMCID: PMC7428784.

[254] Ovsyannikova IG, Haralambieva IH, Crooke SN, Poland GA, Kennedy RB. The role of host genetics in the immune response to SARS-CoV-2 and COVID-19 susceptibility and severity. Immunol Rev July 2020;296(1):205–19. https://doi.org/10.1111/imr.12897. Epub 2020 Jul 13. PMID: 32658335; PMCID: PMC7404857.

[255] Tavasolian F, Rashidi M, Hatam GR, Jeddi M, Hosseini AZ, Mosawi SH, Abdollahi E, Inman RD. HLA, immune response, and susceptibility to COVID-19. Front Immunol January 8, 2021;11:601886. https://doi.org/10.3389/fimmu.2020.601886. PMID: 33488597; PMCID: PMC7820778.

[256] Galli SJ, Tsai M, Piliponsky AM. The development of allergic inflammation. Nature 2008;454:445–54.

[257] Edwards MR, Strong K, Cameron A, Walton RP, Jackson DJ, Johnston SL. Viral infections in allergy and immunology: how allergic inflammation influences viral infections and illness. J Allergy Clin Immunol 2017;140:909–20.

[258] Guan W-J, Liang W-H, Zhao Y, Liang H-R, Chen Z-S, Li Y-M. Comorbidity and its impact on 1590 patients with Covid-19 in China: a nationwide analysis. Eur Respir J 2020;55.

[259] Reynolds HR, Adhikari S, Pulgarin C, Troxel AB, Iturrate E, Johnson SB. Renin-angiotensin-aldosterone system inhibitors and risk of Covid-19. N Engl J Med 2020;382:2441–8.

[260] Fujimura KE, Lynch SV. Microbiota in allergy and asthma and the emerging relationship with the gut microbiome. Cell Host Microbe May 13, 2015;17(5):592–602. https://doi.org/10.1016/j.chom.2015.04.007. PMID: 25974301; PMCID: PMC4443817.

[261] Aitoro R, Paparo L, Amoroso A, Di Costanzo M, Cosenza L, Granata V, Di Scala C, Nocerino R, Trinchese G, Montella M, Ercolini D, Berni Canani R. Gut microbiota as a target for preventive and therapeutic intervention against food allergy. Nutrients June 28, 2017;9(7):672. https://doi.org/10.3390/nu9070672. PMID: 28657607; PMCID: PMC5537787.

[262] Shu SA, Yuen AWT, Woo E, Chu KH, Kwan HS, Yang GX, Yang Y, Leung PSC. Microbiota and food allergy. Clin Rev Allergy Immunol August 2019;57(1):83–97. https://doi.org/10.1007/s12016-018-8723-y. PMID: 30564985.

[263] Butel MJ. Probiotics, gut microbiota and health. Med Maladies Infect January 2014;44(1):1–8. https://doi.org/10.1016/j.medmal.2013.10.002. Epub 2013 Nov 28. PMID: 24290962.

[264] De Martinis M, Sirufo MM, Suppa M, Ginaldi L. New perspectives in food allergy. Int J Mol Sci February 21, 2020;21(4):1474. https://doi.org/10.3390/ijms21041474. PMID: 32098244; PMCID: PMC7073187.

[265] Cukrowska B, Bierła JB, Zakrzewska M, Klukowski M, Maciorkowska E. The relationship between the infant gut microbiota and allergy. The role of Bifidobacterium breve and prebiotic oligosaccharides in the activation of anti-allergic mechanisms in early life. Nutrients March 29, 2020;12(4):946. https://doi.org/10.3390/nu12040946. PMID: 32235348; PMCID: PMC7230322.

[266] Li N, Yu Y, Chen X, Gao S, Zhang Q, Xu C. Bifidobacterium breve M-16V alters the gut microbiota to alleviate OVA-induced food allergy through IL-33/ST2 signal pathway. J Cell Physiol December 2020;235(12):9464–73. https://doi.org/10.1002/jcp.29751. Epub 2020 May 11. PMID: 32394447.

[267] Terada-Ikeda C, Kitabatake M, Hiraku A, Kato K, Yasui S, Imakita N, Ouji-Sageshima N, Iwabuchi N, Hamada K, Ito T. Maternal supplementation with Bifidobacterium breve M-16V prevents their offspring from allergic airway inflammation accelerated by the prenatal exposure to an air pollutant aerosol. PLoS One September 11, 2020;15(9):e0238923. https://doi.org/10.1371/journal.pone.0238923. PMID: 32915886; PMCID: PMC7485856.

[268] Yamashita M, Miyoshi M, Iwai M, Takeda R, Ono T, Kabuki T. Lactobacillus helveticus SBT2171 alleviates perennial allergic rhinitis in Japanese adults by suppressing eosinophils: a randomized, double-blind, placebo-controlled study. Nutrients November 25, 2020;12(12):3620. https://doi.org/10.3390/nu12123620. PMID: 33255731; PMCID: PMC7760906.

[269] Guan WJ, Ni ZY, Hu Y, Liang WH, Ou CQ, He JX, Liu L, Shan H, Lei CL, Hui DSC, Du B, Li LJ, Zeng G, Yuen KY, Chen RC, Tang CL, Wang T, Chen PY, Xiang J, Li SY, Wang JL, Liang ZJ, Peng YX, Wei L, Liu Y, Hu YH, Peng P, Wang JM, Liu JY, Chen Z, Li G, Zheng ZJ, Qiu SQ, Luo J, Ye CJ, Zhu SY, Zhong NS. China medical treatment expert group for covid-19. Clinical characteristics of coronavirus disease 2019 in China. N Engl J Med April 30, 2020;382(18):1708–20. https://doi.org/10.1056/NEJMoa2002032. Epub 2020 Feb 28. PMID: 32109013; PMCID: PMC7092819.

[270] Забозлаев ФГ, Кравченко ЛВ, Галлямова АР, Летуновский НН. Патологическая анатомия легких при новой коронавирусной инфекции (COVID-19). Предварительный анализ аутопсийных исследований. Клиническая практика 2020:21–37. – Т. 11. – №. 2. – С.

[271] Chinese Research Hospital Association; Respiratory Council. [Expert recommendations for the diagnosis and treatment of interstitial lung disease caused by novel coronavirus pneumonia. Zhonghua Jie He He Hu Xi Za Zhi October 12, 2020;43(10):827–33. https://doi.org/10.3760/cma.j.cn112147-20200326-00419. Chinese. PMID: 32992435.

[272] Mareev VY, Begrambekova YL, Mareev YV. How evaluate results of treatment in patients with COVID-19? Symptomatic hospital and outpatient clinical scale for COVID-19 (SHOCS-COVID). Kardiologiia December 5, 2020;60(11):35–41. https://doi.org/10.18087/cardio.2020.11.n1439. Russian. PMID: 33487148.

[273] He LH, Ren LF, Li JF, Wu YN, Li X, Zhang L. Intestinal flora as a potential strategy to fight SARS-CoV-2 infection. Front Microbiol June 9, 2020;11:1388. https://doi.org/10.3389/fmicb.2020.01388. PMID: 32582138; PMCID: PMC7295895.

[274] Baud D, Dimopoulou Agri V, Gibson GR, Reid G, Giannoni E. Using probiotics to flatten the curve of coronavirus disease COVID-2019 pandemic. Front Public Health May 8, 2020;8:186. https://doi.org/10.3389/fpubh.2020.00186. PMID: 32574290; PMCID: PMC7227397.

[275] Din AU, Mazhar M, Waseem M, Ahmad W, Bibi A, Hassan A, Ali N, Gang W, Qian G, Ullah R, Shah T, Ullah M, Khan I, Nisar MF, Wu J. SARS-CoV-2 microbiome dysbiosis linked disorders and possible probiotics role. Biomed Pharmacother January 2021;133:110947. https://doi.org/10.1016/j.biopha.2020.110947. Epub 2020 Nov 11. PMID: 33197765; PMCID: PMC7657099.

[276] Liong MT. Lactobacillus plantarum DR7 improved upper respiratory tract infections via enhancing immune and inflammatory parameters: a randomized, double-blind, placebo-controlled study. J Dairy Sci June 2019;102(6):4783–97. https://doi.org/10.3168/jds.2018-16103. Epub 2019 Apr 4. PMID: 30954261.

[277] Rather IA, Choi SB, Kamli MR, Hakeem KR, Sabir JSM, Park YH, Hor YY. Potential adjuvant therapeutic effect of lactobacillus plantarum probio-88 postbiotics against SARS-COV-2. Vaccines September 24, 2021;9(10):1067. https://doi.org/10.3390/vaccines9101067. PMID: 34696175; PMCID: PMC8537773.

[278] Ahmadi S, Ghollasi M, Hosseini HM. The apoptotic impact of nisin as a potent bacteriocin on the colon cancer cells. Microb Pathog October 2017;111:193–7. https://doi.org/10.1016/j.micpath.2017.08.037. Epub 2017 Sep 1. PMID: 28867631.

[279] Manna S, Chowdhury T, Chakraborty R, Mandal SM. Probiotics-derived peptides and their immunomodulatory molecules can play a preventive role against viral diseases including COVID-19. Probiotics Antimicrob Proteins June 2021;13(3):611–23. https://doi.org/10.1007/s12602-020-09727-7. Epub 2020 Nov 23. PMID: 33226581; PMCID: PMC7680993.

[280] Balmeh N, Mahmoudi S, Fard NA. Manipulated bio antimicrobial peptides from probiotic bacteria as proposed drugs for COVID-19 disease. Inform Med Unlocked 2021;23:100515. https://doi.org/10.1016/j.imu.2021.100515. Epub 2021 Jan 12. PMID: 33521241; PMCID: PMC7832255.

[281] Artanti D, Sari YES, Azizah F, Puwaningsih NV, Rohmayani V, Nasrullah D. Effect of giving probiotic supplement Lactobacillus acidophilus La-14 as an immunomodulator to maintain a respiratory system in *Mus musculus*. Iran J Microbiol June 2021;13(3):381–8. https://doi.org/10.18502/ijm.v13i3.6401. PMID: 34540177; PMCID: PMC8416592.

[282] Villena J, Kitazawa H. The modulation of mucosal antiviral immunity by immunobiotics: could they offer any benefit in the SARS-CoV-2 pandemic? Front Physiol June 16, 2020;11:699. https://doi.org/10.3389/fphys.2020.00699. PMID: 32670091; PMCID: PMC7326040.

[283] Сарсенбаева АС, Лазебник ЛБ. Диарея при COVID-19 у взрослых. Лкспериментальная и клиническая гастроэнтерология 2020:42–54. – №. 6. – С.

[284] Lin L, Jiang X, Zhang Z, Huang S, Zhang Z, Fang Z, Gu Z, Gao L, Shi H, Mai L, Liu Y, Lin X, Lai R, Yan Z, Li X, Shan H. Gastrointestinal symptoms of 95 cases with SARS-CoV-2 infection. Gut June 2020;69(6):997–1001. https://doi.org/10.1136/gutjnl-2020-321013. Epub 2020 Apr 2. PMID: 32241899; PMCID: PMC7316116.

[285] Lei HY, Ding YH, Nie K, Dong YM, Xu JH, Yang ML, Liu MQ, Wei L, Nasser MI, Xu LY, Zhu P, Zhao MY. Potential effects of SARS-CoV-2 on the gastrointestinal tract and liver. Biomed Pharmacother January 2021;133:111064. https://doi.org/10.1016/j.biopha.2020.111064. Epub 2020 Nov 28. PMID: 33378966; PMCID: PMC7700011.

[286] Gao QY, Chen YX, Fang JY. 2019 Novel Coronavirus infection and gastrointestinal tract. J Dig Dis March 2020;21(3):125–6. https://doi.org/10.1111/1751-2980.12851. Epub 2020 Mar 10. PMID: 32096611; PMCID: PMC7162053.

[287] Ahmed M. Coronavirus disease 2019: a gastroenterologist's perspective in May 2020. Gastroenterol Res June 2020;13(3):89–95. https://doi.org/10.14740/gr1292. Epub 2020 Jun 18. PMID: 32655724; PMCID: PMC7331859.

[288] Ma C, Cong Y, Zhang H. COVID-19 and the digestive system. Am J Gastroenterol July 2020;115(7):1003–6. https://doi.org/10.14309/ajg.0000000000000691. PMID: 32618648; PMCID: PMC7273952.

[289] Hanrahan TP, Lubel JS, Garg M. Lessons from COVID-19, ACE2, and intestinal inflammation: could a virus trigger chronic intestinal inflammation? Clin Gastroenterol Hepatol 2020;19:206. https://doi.org/10.1016/j.cgh.2020.07.036.

[290] Li LY, Wu W, Chen S, Gu JW, Li XL, Song HJ, Du F, Wang G, Zhong CQ, Wang XY, et al. Digestive system involvement of novel coronavirus infection: prevention and control infection from a gastroenterology perspective. J Dig Dis 2020;21:199–204. https://doi.org/10.1111/1751-2980.12862.

[291] Penninger JM, Grant MB, Sung JJY. The role of angiotensin converting enzyme 2 in modulating gut microbiota, intestinal inflammation, and coronavirus infection. Gastroenterology 2020;160. https://doi.org/10.1053/j.gastro.2020.07.067. ahead of print.

[292] Xu J, Chu M, Zhong F, Tan X, Tang G, Mai J, Lai N, Guan C, Liang Y, Liao G. Digestive symptoms of COVID-19 and expression of ACE2 in digestive tract organs. Cell Death Dis 2020;6:76. https://doi.org/10.1038/s41420-020-00307-w.

[293] Vodnar DC, Mitrea L, Teleky BE, Szabo K, Călinoiu LF, Nemes SA, Martău GA. Coronavirus disease (COVID-19) caused by (SARS-CoV-2) infections: a real challenge for human gut microbiota. Front Cell Infect Microbiol December 9, 2020;10:575559. https://doi.org/10.3389/fcimb.2020.575559. PMID: 33363049; PMCID: PMC7756003.

[294] Zuo T, Zhang F, Lui GCY, Yeoh YK, Li AYL, Zhan H, Wan Y, Chung ACK, Cheung CP, Chen N, Lai CKC, Chen Z, Tso EYK, Fung KSC, Chan V, Ling L, Joynt G, Hui DSC, Chan FKL, Chan PKS, Ng SC. Alterations in gut microbiota of patients with COVID-19 during time of hospitalization. Gastroenterology September 2020;159(3):944–55. https://doi.org/10.1053/j.gastro.2020.05.048. e8. Epub 2020 May 20. PMID: 32442562; PMCID: PMC7237927.

[295] Yang B, Huang Z, He Z, Yue Y, Zhou Y, Ross RP, Stanton C, Zhang H, Zhao J, Chen W. Protective effect of Bifidobacterium bifidum FSDJN7O5 and Bifidobacterium breve FHNFQ23M3 on diarrhea caused by enterotoxigenic *Escherichia coli*. Food Funct August 21, 2021;12(16):7271–82. https://doi.org/10.1039/d1fo00504a. Epub 2021 Jun 24. PMID: 34165468.

[296] Kawahara T, Makizaki Y, Oikawa Y, Tanaka Y, Maeda A, Shimakawa M, Komoto S, Moriguchi K, Ohno H, Taniguchi K. Oral administration of Bifidobacterium bifidum G9-1 alleviates rotavirus gastroenteritis through regulation of intestinal homeostasis by inducing mucosal protective factors. PLoS One March 27, 2017;12(3):e0173979. https://doi.org/10.1371/journal.pone.0173979. PMID: 28346473; PMCID: PMC5367788.

[297] Han YO, Jeong Y, You HJ, Ku S, Ji GE, Park MS. The anti-rotaviral activity of low molecular weight and non-proteinaceous substance from Bifidobacterium longum BORI cell extract. Microorganisms April 23, 2019;7(4):108. https://doi.org/10.3390/microorganisms7040108. PMID: 31018530; PMCID: PMC6517874.

[298] Moodley C, Reid SJ, Abratt VR. Molecular characterisation of ABC-type multidrug efflux systems in Bifidobacterium longum. Anaerobe April 2015;32:63–9. https://doi.org/10.1016/j.anaerobe.2014.12.004. Epub 2014 Dec 18. PMID: 25529295.

[299] Chenoll E, Casinos B, Bataller E, Buesa J, Ramón D, Genovés S, Fábrega J, Rivero Urgell M, Moreno Muñoz JA. Identification of a peptide produced by Bifidobacterium longum CECT 7210 with antirotaviral activity. Front Microbiol May 4, 2016;7:655. https://doi.org/10.3389/fmicb.2016.00655. PMID: 27199974; PMCID: PMC4855034.

[300] Fan L, Qi Y, Qu S, Chen X, Li A, Hendi M, Xu C, Wang L, Hou T, Si J, Chen SB. Adolescentis ameliorates chronic colitis by regulating Treg/Th2 response and gut microbiota remodeling. Gut Microb 2021 ;13(1):1–17. https://doi.org/10.1080/19490976.2020.1826746. PMID: 33557671; PMCID: PMC7889144.

[301] María Remes Troche J, Coss Adame E, Ángel Valdovinos Díaz M, Gómez Escudero O, Eugenia Icaza Chávez M, Antonio Chávez-Barrera J, Zárate Mondragón F, Antonio Ruíz Velarde Velasco J, Rafael Aceves Tavares G, Antonio Lira Pedrín M, Cerda Contreras E, Carmona Sánchez RI, Guerra López H, Solana Ortiz R. Lactobacillus acidophilus LB: a useful pharmabiotic for the treatment of digestive disorders. Therap Adv Gastroenterol November 24, 2020;13. https://doi.org/10.1177/1756284820971201. 1756284820971201. PMID: 33281937; PMCID: PMC7692339.

[302] Capurso L. Thirty years of lactobacillus rhamnosus GG: a review. J Clin Gastroenterol March 2019;53(Suppl. 1):S1–41. https://doi.org/10.1097/MCG.0000000000001170. PMID: 30741841.

[303] Aoki-Yoshida A, Saito S, Fukiya S, Aoki R, Takayama Y, Suzuki C, Sonoyama K. Lactobacillus rhamnosus GG increases Toll-like receptor 3 gene expression in murine small intestine ex vivo and in vivo. Benef Microbes June 2016;7(3):421–9. https://doi.org/10.3920/BM2015.0169. Epub 2016 Mar 25. PMID: 27013459.

[304] Ivashkin V, Fomin V, Moiseev S, Brovko M, Maslennikov R, Ulyanin A, Sholomova V, Vasilyeva M, Trush E, Shifrin O, Poluektova E. Efficacy of a probiotic consisting of lacticaseibacillus rhamnosus PDV 1705, Bifidobacterium bifidum PDV 0903, Bifidobacterium longum subsp. infantis PDV 1911, and Bifidobacterium longum subsp. longum PDV 2301 in the treatment of hospitalized patients with COVID-19: a randomized controlled trial. Probiotics Antimicrob Proteins October 2021;13:1–9. https://doi.org/10.1007/s12602-021-09858-5. Epub ahead of print. PMID: 34643888; PMCID: PMC8512595.

[305] Spinler JK, Auchtung J, Brown A, Boonma P, Oezguen N, Ross CL, Luna RA, Runge J, Versalovic J, Peniche A, Dann SM, Britton RA, Haag A, Savidge TC. Next-generation probiotics targeting *Clostridium difficile* through precursor-directed antimicrobial biosynthesis. Infect Immun September 20, 2017;85(10):e00303–17. https://doi.org/10.1128/IAI.00303-17. PMID: 28760934; PMCID: PMC5607411.

[306] Dinleyici EC, Study Group PROBAGE, Vandenplas Y. Lactobacillus reuteri DSM 17938 effectively reduces the duration of acute diarrhoea in hospitalised children. Acta Paediatr July 2014;103(7):e300–5. https://doi.org/10.1111/apa.12617. Epub 2014 Mar 24. PMID: 24579935.

[307] Patman G. Diarrhoea. Lactobacillus reuteri reduces episodes of diarrhoea in healthy children. Nat Rev Gastroenterol Hepatol May 2014;11(5):269. https://doi.org/10.1038/nrgastro.2014.49. Epub 2014 Apr 8. PMID: 24709814.

[308] Urbańska M, Gieruszczak-Białek D, Szajewska H. Systematic review with meta-analysis: lactobacillus reuteri DSM 17938 for diarrhoeal diseases in children. Aliment Pharmacol Ther May 2016;43(10):1025–34. https://doi.org/10.1111/apt.13590. Epub 2016 Mar 16. PMID: 26991503.

[309] Maragkoudaki M, Chouliaras G, Moutafi A, Thomas A, Orfanakou A, Papadopoulou A. Efficacy of an oral rehydration solution enriched with lactobacillus reuteri DSM 17938 and zinc in the management of acute

diarrhoea in infants: a randomized, double-blind, placebo-controlled trial. Nutrients September 1, 2018;10(9):1189. https://doi.org/10.3390/nu10091189. PMID: 30200394; PMCID: PMC6165178.

[310] Patro-Gołab B, Szajewska H. Systematic review with meta-analysis: lactobacillus reuteri DSM 17938 for treating acute gastroenteritis in children. An update. Nutrients November 14, 2019;11(11):2762. https://doi.org/10.3390/nu11112762. PMID: 31739457; PMCID: PMC6893691.

[311] Потапнев МП. Цитокиновый шторм: причины и последствия. Иммунология 2021:175–88. – Т. 42. – №. 2. – С.

[312] Ragab D, Salah Eldin H, Taeimah M, Khattab R, Salem R. The COVID-19 cytokine storm; what we know so far. Front Immunol June 16, 2020;11:1446. https://doi.org/10.3389/fimmu.2020.01446. PMID: 32612617; PMCID: PMC7308649.

[313] Nile SH, Nile A, Qiu J, Li L, Jia X, Kai G. COVID-19: pathogenesis, cytokine storm and therapeutic potential of interferons. Cytokine Growth Factor Rev June 2020;53:66–70. https://doi.org/10.1016/j.cytogfr.2020.05.002. Epub 2020 May 7. PMID: 32418715; PMCID: PMC7204669.

[314] Soy M, Keser G, Atagündüz P, Tabak F, Atagündüz I, Kayhan S. Cytokine storm in COVID-19: pathogenesis and overview of anti-inflammatory agents used in treatment. Clin Rheumatol July 2020;39(7):2085–94. https://doi.org/10.1007/s10067-020-05190-5. Epub 2020 May 30. PMID: 32474885; PMCID: PMC7260446.

[315] Calder PC. Nutrition, immunity and COVID-19. BMJ Nutr Prev Health May 20, 2020;3(1):74–92. https://doi.org/10.1136/bmjnph-2020–000085. PMID:33230497.

[316] Ferreira C, Viana SD, Reis F. Is gut microbiota dysbiosis a predictor of increased susceptibility to poor outcome of COVID-19 patients? An update. Microorganisms December 28, 2020;9(1):53. https://doi.org/10.3390/microorganisms9010053. PMID: 33379162; PMCID: PMC7824665.

[317] Saleh J, Peyssonnaux C, Singh KK, Edeas M. Mitochondria and microbiota dysfunction in COVID-19 pathogenesis. Mitochondrion September 2020;54:1–7. https://doi.org/10.1016/j.mito.2020.06.008. Epub 2020 Jun 20. PMID: 32574708; PMCID: PMC7837003.

[318] Ahlawat S, Asha, Sharma KK. Immunological co-ordination between gut and lungs in SARS-CoV-2 infection. Virus Res September 2020;286:198103. https://doi.org/10.1016/j.virusres.2020.198103. Epub 2020 Jul 24. PMID: 32717345; PMCID: PMC7380259.

[319] Akour A. Probiotics and COVID-19: is there any link? Lett Appl Microbiol September 2020;71(3):229–34. https://doi.org/10.1111/lam.13334. Epub 2020 Jul 16. PMID: 32495940; PMCID: PMC7300613.

[320] Mu Q, Tavella VJ, Luo XM. Role of lactobacillus reuteri in human health and diseases. Front Microbiol April 19, 2018;9:757. https://doi.org/10.3389/fmicb.2018.00757. PMID: 29725324; PMCID: PMC5917019.

[321] Zakharova IN, Berezhnaya IV, Kuchina AE, Dedikova OV. Probiotic Lactobacillus reuteri DSM 17938: what is known about it today? Meditsinskiy sovet Med Council 2019;17:236–42. https://doi.org/10.21518/2079-701X-2019-17-236-242 (In Russ.).

[322] Ratajczak W, Rył A, Mizerski A, Walczakiewicz K, Sipak O, Laszczyńska M. Immunomodulatory potential of gut microbiome-derived short-chain fatty acids (SCFAs). Acta Biochim Pol March 4, 2019;66(1):1–12. https://doi.org/10.18388/abp.2018_2648. PMID: 30831575.

CHAPTER

12

Molecular and immunological evidence for SARS-CoV-2 being the autoimmune virus

Aristo Vojdani[1,2], Avi Rosenberg[3], Elroy Vojdani[4] and Yehuda Shoenfeld[5,6]

[1]Immunosciences Lab, Inc., Los Angeles, CA, United States; [2]Cyrex Laboratories, LLC, Phoenix, AZ, United States; [3]Johns Hopkins Medical Institutions, Baltimore, MD, United States; [4]Regenera Medical, Los Angeles, CA, United States; [5]Zabludowicz Center for Autoimmune Diseases, Sheba Medical Center, Ramat Gan, Israel; [6]Tel Aviv University, Tel Aviv, Israel

Introduction

The most famous or infamous virus at the time of this writing is undoubtedly severe acute respiratory syndrome coronavirus 2 (SARS-CoV-2), the etiological agent for coronavirus disease 2019, the dreaded COVID-19 that has become the pandemic of the new millennium, affecting millions of people all over the world [1,2].

The gathered evidence to date now indicates that SARS-CoV-2 has the ability to hyperstimulate the immune system, leading to the production of multiple autoantibodies, which may potentially trigger preexisting autoimmune diseases. Aside from this ability, this viral agent can also activate autoimmune responses because of the significant molecular resemblance and cross-reactivity between human self-tissues and components of the virus, such as spike and nucleoprotein. The similarity between the SARS-CoV-2 molecular chains and those of many human self-components is so great and so prevalent that it has become known as the autoimmune virus. The virus and its disease, COVID-19, have been linked with many different autoimmune disorders, such as antiphospholipid syndrome, autoimmune hemolytic anemia, Graves' disease, Guillain-Barré syndrome, immune thrombocytopenic purpura, Kawasaki disease, Miller Fisher syndrome, polyneuritis cranialis, postural orthostatic tachycardia syndrome, rheumatoid arthritis, systemic lupus erythematosus, and vasculitis [3,4]. In

Autoimmunity, COVID-19, Post-COVID19 syndrome and COVID-19 vaccination
https://doi.org/10.1016/B978-0-443-18566-3.00036-0

a very recent article, Dotan et al. reviewed the evidence at their time of writing about SARS-CoV-2 being an instrumental trigger of autoimmunity [4].

The involvement of SARS-CoV-2 antigens in human autoimmune diseases is further strengthened by the experimental findings generated from previous studies conducted in our lab with the following criteria:

1. Identification of cross-reactive epitopes that are shared between SARS-CoV-2 and human proteomes that participate in autoimmune diseases
2. Reaction of animal and human monoclonal antibodies made against SARS-CoV-2 antigens with human proteomes
3. Reaction of antibodies made against human tissue with SARS-CoV-2 antigens
4. Detection in sera taken from COVID-19 patients of autoantibodies against human autoantigens that cross-react with SARS-CoV-2

Criteria no. 1: identification of cross-reactive epitopes between SARS-CoV-2 and human tissue

In a very recent study, Dotan et al. [4] showed the homology of the primary sequence between human proteins and components of SARS-CoV-2. The cross-reactivity between these two groups of proteins could very well induce the production of autoantibodies that could result in the onset of an autoimmune disease, marking a possible mechanism in the pathophysiology of autoimmunity. Table 12.1 below shows only 8 of the 34 in Dotan et al.'s study; the homologies involve human proteomes that could lead to severe pathologies if altered, mutated, improperly functioning, deficient or otherwise changed or affected [4,5].

The issue of peptide-sharing between SARS-CoV-2 spike glycoprotein and lung surfactant-related proteins was addressed by Kanduc and Shoenfeld [6]. This peptide sharing consisted of 13 out of 24 pentapeptides. The researchers posited that because of this, the immune response following a SARS-CoV-2 infection might lead to cross-reactivity with pulmonary surfactant proteins, leading to SARS-CoV-2-associated lung disease [6]. Kanduc and

TABLE 12.1 Shortlist (8/34) and description of human proteins and the heptapeptide sequences they share with SARS-CoV-2 [4].

Shared heptapeptide	Human proteins sharing heptapeptides with SARS-CoV-2
SSRSSSR	Corneal antigen
ALALLLL	Ganglioside in peripheral nerve
ALALLLL	Glutamic acid decarboxylase
ALALLLL	Proteolipid protein
IGAGICA	Thyrotropin receptor
TGRLQSL	Leukocyte function-associated antigen
NASVVNI	HLA-B27
AEGSRGG	More than 20 tissue antigens

Shoenfeld have also very recently provided indisputable proof of molecular mimicry as a potential mechanism that contributes toward SARS-CoV-2-associated diseases [7].

Additional evidence for the presence of cross-reactive epitopes between SARS-CoV-2 and human tissue and their contributing role in autoimmunity was presented by Lyons-Weiler when he compared immunogenic epitopes of SARS-CoV-2 to human proteins and found a high degree of similarity with various self-tissues, such as adipose tissue, blood, brain, eye, gastrointestinal tract, heart muscle, kidney, liver, lung, pituitary gland, skeletal muscle, skin, testes, thyroid gland, and many other proteins [8]. With some variations, this was also confirmed in the corresponding author's own study focusing on 55 selected human tissue antigens [9]. While this list unavoidably had some overlap with those used in the Lyons-Weiler study, the corresponding author and his coauthors had made the basis for their study key target human tissue proteins that had been found to be involved not just with common autoimmune diseases but also with extrapulmonary manifestations of COVID-19. The Vojdani-led team investigated the cross-reactivity of SARS-CoV-2 specifically with brain tissue antigens (α-synuclein, amyloid-β, MBP, NFP, synapsin, tTG-6), liver microsomal peptide, M2 protein, PDH peptide, and skin antigens (tTG-3, epithelial cell antigens), while the Lyons-Weiler team studied brain, liver, GI tract and skin.

The Vojdani group also studied many other tissue antigens, such as barrier proteins, that the Lyons-Weiler team did not [9]. We used the Basic Local Alignment Search Tool (BLAST) to do an extensive examination of the degree of identity between SARS-CoV-2 and a carefully selected number of proteins: F-actin, a major component of smooth muscle; thyroid peroxidase (TPO), a target antigen in thyroid autoimmunity; and mitochondria M2. In that study [9], we showed that SARS-CoV-2 shared a significant number of peptide sequences with F-actin (58%–63%), TPO (50%–70%), and mitochondrial M2 protein (50%–78%) as shown in Fig. 12.1.

We also found that some peptide sequences matched with more than one section of a SARS-CoV-2 protein. For example, the F-actin sequence SIL—ASLSTF cross-reacted not only with the SVLYNSASFSTF sequence in chains A, B, C, and E of the SARS-CoV-2 spike

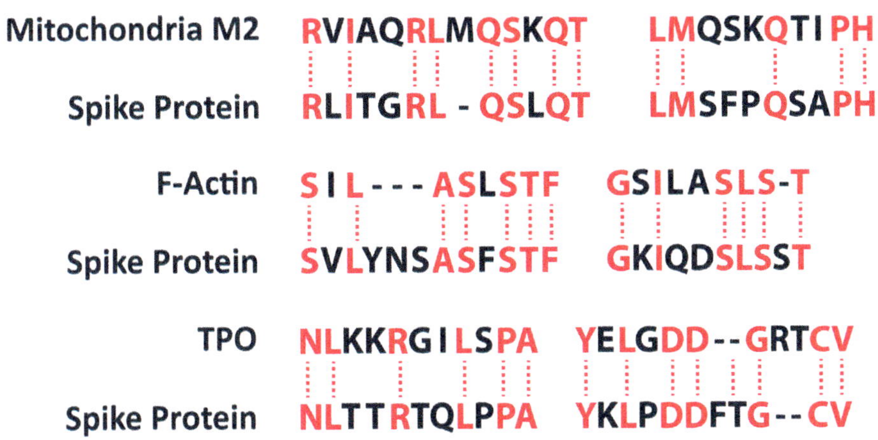
Mitochondria M2
RVIAQRLMQSKQT
LMQSKQTIPH
Spike Protein
RLITGRL - QSLQT
LMSFPQSAPH
F-Actin
SIL---ASLSTF
GSILASLS-T
Spike Protein
SVLYNSASFSTF
GKIQDSLSST
TPO
NLKKRGILSPA
YELGDD--GRTCV
Spike Protein
NLTTRTQLPPA
YKLPDDFTG--CV

FIGURE 12.1 Peptide molecular mimicry between SARS-CoV-2 spike protein and mitochondria M2, F-actin, and thyroid peroxidase (TPO) [9].

protein, it also reacted with chain E of the SARS-CoV-2 spike receptor-binding domain. We detected other peptide sequences with identity percentages ranging from 33% to 49% but they are not shown here.

Additional evidence indicates that SARS-CoV-2 can also target parts of the human reproductive system that express ACE2. In this study, it was shown that SARS-CoV-2 spike protein shared 41 pentapeptides (immune determinants) with 27 human proteins that are related to oogenesis, uterine receptivity, decidualization, and placentation [10]. The authors concluded that the linear sequences shared by SARS-CoV-2 and oogenesis-related proteins might play a role in the production of pathogenic cross-reactive antibodies [10].

This immune cross-reactivity between different antigen groups and SARS-CoV-2 proteins may influence the severity of COVID-19, be involved in the multi-system process of the disease, trigger the onset of autoimmunity in predisposed subgroups, and possibly increase the severity of autoimmunity in subjects that already have preexisting autoimmune disorders.

Criteria no. 2: reaction of animal and human monoclonal antibodies made against SARS-CoV-2 with human tissue antigens

To provide more support for the involvement of SARS-CoV-2 antigens in human autoimmune disorders, our previous study [9] sought to determine whether human monoclonal antibodies that mimic natural antibodies produced against SARS-CoV-2 would react to various human self-antigens. The multi-system disorder found in patients with severe COVID-19 could be a result of such a reaction.

In a different, earlier, limited study [11], we used mouse monoclonal antibodies and rabbit monoclonal antibodies against SARS-CoV-2 proteins to also investigate possible cross-reactivity between SARDS-CoV-2 antigens and human autoantigens. These antibodies showed moderate to strong reactions with 13 different human tissue antigens [11]. When a human monoclonal antibody to SARS-CoV-2 became available, we used this antibody in the previously mentioned study [9], in which we applied the antibody to 55 different human tissue antigens. The SARS-CoV-2 antibody reacted with 24–28 out of the 55 tissue antigens; these 24–28 antigens showed a diversity of tissue groups, including barrier proteins, gastrointestinal, joint, liver, muscle, skin, thyroid, and neural tissues, and various cellular components (ANA, ENA, NCA and more) [9]. The degree of reactivity between SARS-CoV-2 monoclonal antibodies and human autoantigens was classified in Table 12.2 in a scale ranging from "−" for insignificant to "++++" for very strong.

This extensive reactivity of both animal and human monoclonal antibodies to SARS-CoV-2 with so many tissue antigens gives even more support toward a possible role for SARS-CoV-2 spike proteins and nucleoproteins in autoimmune reactivity and autoimmune diseases. These 24–28 tissue antigens are summarized by the groupings shown in Fig. 12.2.

Criteria no. 3: reaction of antibody to human autoantigens with SARS-CoV-2 proteins

In our previous studies [9,11] both animal and human monoclonal antibodies made against spike and nucleoproteins of SARS-CoV-2 reacted strongly with mitochondrial M2 antigens, which shared significant homology with both SARS-CoV-2 proteins. To determine

TABLE 12.2 Optimal density (OD) and % Reactivity of SARS-CoV-2 spike, nucleoprotein, envelope and membrane protein antibodies with the same proteins and different cross-reactive tissue antigens [9].

Antigens	Spike protein OD	% Reactivity	Nucleoprotein OD	% Reactivity
SARS-CoV-2	3.40	100 ++++	3.76	100 ++++
Actin	0.74	17.6 +	1.1	27.1 ++
Mitochondrial antigen (M2)	1.52	41.8 +++	1.94	50.1 +++
ENA	0.85	21.0 +	0.44	9.0 +
NA	1.34	36.2 ++	0.97	23.6 +
Histone	0.65	14.8 +	0.92	22.2 +
S100B	0.46	9.0 +	0.87	20.8 +
MBP	0.53	11.1 +	0.55	12.0 +
NFP	1.98	56 ++++	0.42	8.5 +
Synapsin	0.81	19.8 +	0.95	23.0 +
Beta-amyloid P	0.83	20.4 +	0.82	19.4 +
Tau protein	0.41	7.4 +	0.23	3.3 –
Collagen	0.45	8.6 +	0.65	14.8 +
Alpha-myosin	0.72	17.0 +	0.89	21.3 +
Tropomyosin	0.21	1.2 –	0.25	3.8 –
TPO	0.98	25.1 ++	0.95	23.0 +
Liver microsome	1.00	25.7 ++	1.00	24.4 +
PDH peptide	0.91	22.9 +	0.94	22.7 +
GAD-65	1.35	36.5 ++	1.08	26.5 ++
Insulin	0.25	2.5 –	0.16	0.4 –
Insulin-R	0.72	17.0 +	1.77	45.5 +++
Phospholipid	0.93	23.5 +	0.83	19.7 +

(Continued)

TABLE 12.2 Optimal density (OD) and % Reactivity of SARS-CoV-2 spike, nucleoprotein, envelope and membrane protein antibodies with the same proteins and different cross-reactive tissue antigens [9].—cont'd

Antigens	Spike protein OD	% Reactivity	Nucleoprotein OD	% Reactivity
tTG-6	0.58	12.7 +	0.44	9.0 +
tTG-3	0.42	23.2 +	0.92	22.2 +
tTG-2	0.79	19.2 +	0.72	16.7 +
Int epi cells	0.49	9.9 +	0.46	9.6 +
Beta-catenin	0.95	24.1 +	0.56	12.3 +
Claudin	0.33	4.9 −	0.26	4.1 −
Occludin + zonulin	0.72	17.0 +	1.32	33.0 ++
SCA + NCA[a]	1.10	28.0 ++	1.11	26.0 ++
27 other tissues[b]	0.34	5.2 −	0.36	6.8 −

The percentage of reactivity of tissue antigen(s) with antibody to SARS-CoV-2 spike protein and nucleoprotein was calculated based on the degree of reactivity of the SARS-CoV-2 antibodies with tissue antigens minus background divided by reaction of the same antibody with SARS-CoV-2 antigens minus the background. The antibody reaction percentages were classified according to strength as follows: 0 to percentage based on antibody-specific cutoff point = − or insignificant; above cutoff-based percentage to 25% = + or weak; 25.1%–40% = ++ or moderate; 40.1%–55% = +++ or strong; >55% = ++++ or very strong.

[a]SCA, *Saccharomyces cerevisiae antigen*; NCA, *Neutrophil cytoplasmic antigen.*

[b]*The 27 other tissues are glial fibrillary acidic protein, brain-derived neurotrophic factor, myoglobulin, platelet glycoprotein, alpha-synuclein, acetylcholine receptor, lysosome, elastase, parietal cell antigen, intrinsic factor, laminin, thyroglobulin, myeloperoxidase, neuraminidase, ganglioside* GM_1*, enolase, somatotropin, dipeptidylpeptidase, aquaporin-4, presenilin, fibulin, protein disulfide isomerase, cerebellar, enteric nerve neuronal nuclear antigen, glutamate-R, dopamine-R, dsDNA [9].*

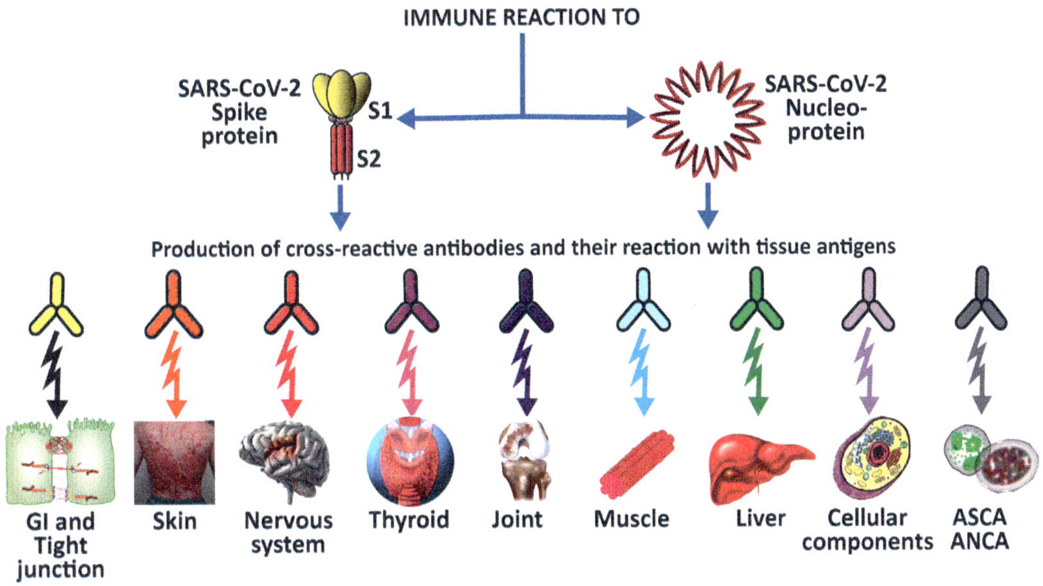

FIGURE 12.2 Diagram of possible relationship between SARS-CoV-2 proteins and autoimmune target proteins.

this, we first used the Trinity Biotech Mitochondrial M2 antibody kit to measure the presence of M2 antibody in four control sera and in the serum of four individuals who tested positive for M2 antibody. We applied the test kit's negative control calibrator, low and high positive controls, the four negative sera, and the four sera positive for M2 antibody to an ELISA plate coated with both SARS-CoV-2 spike proteins and nucleoproteins. The calibrator and positive controls with known levels of M2 antibody reacted moderately with both spike proteins and nucleoproteins. All four sera with elevated M2 antibodies also reacted moderately with these SARS-CoV-2 proteins. There was no reaction to these proteins from the four sera with no detected levels of M2 antibody.

This antibody against mitochondrial M2 is detected in 90%–95% of patients suffering from primary biliary cirrhosis, and occasionally in patients with other liver diseases and scleroderma [12]. Interestingly, a recent study showed that SARS-CoV-2 infection contributes to hepatic impairment in patients with COVID-19 [13].

The results of our previous studies give additional support to molecular mimicry between M2 and SARS-Cov-2 proteins having a role in the production of cross-reactive antibodies. Similar experiments should be performed with other autoantigens that share homology with SARS-CoV-2 proteins to determine the extent of immunological reactivity between the two groups.

Criteria no. 4: detection of autoantibodies against human tissue antigens in COVID-19 patients with different degrees of severity

In our ongoing, 246 adults from Jewish-American communities across five states who had developed symptomatic COVID-19 disease before receiving any vaccine against the disease participated in an online survey that sought to determine the most common symptoms and outcomes of SARS-CoV-2 infection [14,15]. Included in this study were 77 randomly-selected age- and sex-matched healthy controls who had tested SARS-CoV-2 negative and presented no symptoms of COVID-19. The autoantibody data of these controls were compared to data from 169 individuals who had tested SARS-CoV-2 positive by nasopharyngeal swab, and by antibody assay using ELISA kits. The 169 infected individuals were divided into three groups according to the severity of the disease: COVID-19 mild consisted of 74 subjects with fever duration <1 day and a peak fever temperature of 37.8°C; COVID-19 moderate consisted of 63 subjects with fever duration >7 days and a peak fever temperature of 38.8°C; and COVID-19 severe consisted of 32 subjects presenting severe symptoms and requiring supplemental oxygen therapy. This disease severity rating was based on the World Health Organization (WHO) severity classification for COVID-19.

Using these sera, we measured IgG and IgA antibodies against 58 different tissue antigens representing the lungs, heart, muscle, pancreas, liver, brain, skin, tight junction proteins, blood clotting factors, enzymes, and many cellular components, including nuclear and nucleolar antigens, mitochondria, and double-stranded DNA. In comparison to controls, patients with mild symptoms reacted weakly to 14 out of 58 tissue antigens, with the presence of IgG and IgA antibodies being relatively conserved. In severe COVID-19 patients who required oxygen supplementation, these antibodies were detected at much higher levels against 27 tissue antigens for IgG and 29 tissue antigens for IgA (see Figs. 12.3 and 12.4).

Our data indicate that the relationship between autoantibodies targeting so many tissue antigens associated with the clinical severity of COVID-19, especially in those who required oxygen supplementation suggests that this virus contributes to many autoimmune diseases by a variety of novel molecular pathways.

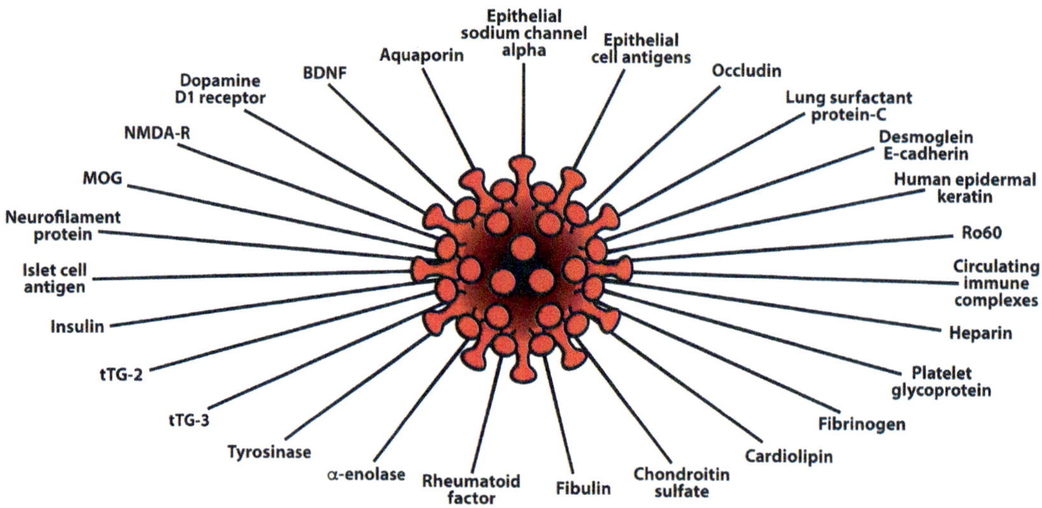

FIGURE 12.3 Detection of IgG antibody against 27 different human tissue antigens in the blood of patients with mild to severe infection with SARS-CoV-2 (positive for PCR and antibody) in comparison to healthy controls ($P < .0001$).

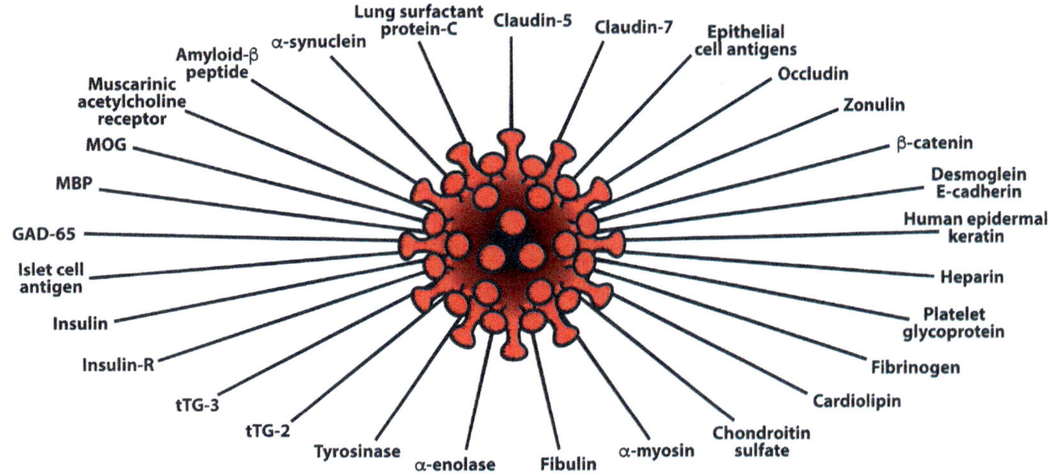

FIGURE 12.4 Detection of IgA antibody against 29 different human tissue antigens in the blood of patients with mild to severe infection with SARS-CoV-2 (positive for PCR and antibody) in comparison to healthy controls ($P < .0001$).

Conclusions

Since the beginning of the SARS-CoV-2 pandemic, a possible rise in autoimmunity has been a subject of interest to many researchers and clinicians [16–28]. In fact, as the number of SARS-CoV-2 infections increased from day to day, scientists learned that the damage caused by the virus extended well beyond the lungs [29]. They learned that the virus could affect the body from head to toe, including the immune, digestive, cardiovascular and nervous systems [30–33]. In our lab, we routinely perform testing for autoimmunity. After the outbreak of SARS-CoV-2, we were surprised to find positivity for ANA, ENA, actin, and mitochondrial antibodies in a significant number of COVID-19 patients to a degree that we had not previously seen in our lab. These results prompted us to investigate possible patterns of cross-reactivity between SARS-CoV-2 and autoantigens that are target proteins for autoimmunity.

A few months later, evidence for epitope sharing between SARS-CoC-2 spike proteins and nucleoproteins began pouring in from different investigators [3,5,7,10,11,17–21]. Furthermore, the association between COVID-19 and the presence of a variety of autoantigens was presented in articles published in different journals [3,4,7–11,17–21,23,24]. Based on this association between SARS-CoV-2 infection and autoimmune reactivity, the virus was named by Gilad and Shoenfeld as the autoimmune virus [3].

However, as we have discussed in this review article, although epitope sharing is a very important factor, it alone is not enough for the production of cross-reactive antibodies that react with autoantigens. This is why, in addition to molecular mimicry we emphasized the importance of the reaction of animal and human monoclonal antibodies made against SARS-CoV-2 spike proteins and nucleoproteins with a variety of human tissue antigens. Additionally, we also emphasized the importance of antibodies made against human tissue

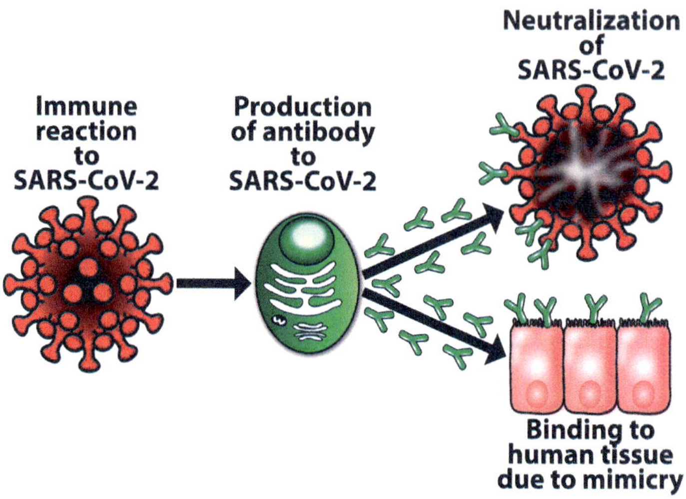

FIGURE 12.5 Exposure to SARS-CoV-2 can induce the production of both beneficial antibodies that work to neutralize SARS-CoV-2 and pathogenic, cross-reactive antibodies that can bind to human tissue antigens because of molecular mimicry, possibly leading to autoimmune reactivity and autoimmunity.

antigens and their reaction with SARS-CoV-2 proteins. Finally, we showed the reaction of sera obtained from COVID patients with different degrees of severity with more than 20 out of about 60 tested human tissue antigens.

Thus, exposure to SARS-CoV-2 results in the production of protective and neutralizing antibodies that bind to the virus, and cross-reactive, pathogenic antibodies that manage to bind to human tissue (see Fig. 12.5).

All the experimental evidence reviewed here lends support to our original findings that molecular mimicry between SARS-CoV-2 and human autoantigens does contribute to autoimmunity, and, thus, the title given to SARS-CoV-2 of "the autoimmune virus" is very well-deserved.

Acknowledgments

The author wishes to thank Joel Bautista for the preparation of this manuscript for publication.

Conflicts of Interest

The author is co-owner, CEO, and technical director of Immunosciences Lab., Inc. in Los Angeles, CA, and is the Chief Scientific Officer of Cyrex Labs LLC in Phoenix, AZ.

References

[1] She J, Jiang J, Ye L, Hu L, Bai C, Song Y. 2019 Novel coronavirus of pneumonia in Wuhan, China: emerging attack and management strategies. Clin Transl Med 2020;9(1):19. https://doi.org/10.1186/s40169-020-00271-z.

[2] Huang C, Wang Y, Li X, Ren L, Zhao J, Hu Y, et al. Clinical features of patients infected with 2019 novel coronavirus in Wuhan, China. Lancet 2020;395:497–506. https://doi.org/10.1016/S0140-6736(20)30183-5.

[3] Halpert G, Shoenfeld Y. SARS-CoV-2, the autoimmune virus. Autoimmun Rev 2020;19(12):102695. https://doi.org/10.1016/j.autrev.2020.102695.

[4] Dotan A, Muller S, Kanduc D, David P, Halpert G, Shoenfeld Y. The SARS-CoV-2 as an instrumental trigger of autoimmunity. Autoimmun Rev 2021;20(4):102792. https://doi.org/10.1016/j.autrev.2021.102792.

[5] Oldstone M. Molecular mimicry and immune-mediated diseases. Faseb J 1998;12(13):1255–65. https://doi.org/10.1096/fasebj.12.13.1255.

[6] Kanduc D, Shoenfeld Y. On the molecular determinants of the SARS-CoV-2 attack. Clin Immunol 2020;215:108426. https://doi.org/10.1016/j.clim.2020.108426.

[7] Kanduc D, Shoenfeld Y. Molecular mimicry between SARS-CoV-2 spike glycoprotein and mammalian proteomes: implication for the vaccine. Immunol Res 2020;68(5):310–3. https://doi.org/10.1007/s12026-020-09152-6.

[8] Lyons-Weiler J. Pathogenic priming likely contributes to serious and critical illness and mortality in COVID-19 via autoimmunity. J Transl Autoimmun 2020;3:100051. https://doi.org/10.1016/j.jtauto.2020.100051.

[9] Vojdani A, Vojdani E, Kharrazian D. Reaction of human monoclonal antibodies to SARS-CoV-2 proteins with tissue antigens: implications for autoimmune diseases. Front Immunol 2021;11:61708919. https://doi.org/10.3389/fimmu.2020.617089.

[10] Dotan A, Kanduc D, Muller S, Makatsariya A, Shoenfeld Y. Molecular mimicry between SARS-CoV-2 and the female reproductive system. J Reprod Immunol 2021;86. https://doi.org/10.1111/aji.13494.

[11] Vojdani A, Kharrazian D. Potential antigenic cross-reactivity between SARSCoV-2 and human tissue with a possible link to an increase in autoimmune disease. Clin Immunol 2020;217:108480. https://doi.org/10.1016/j.clim.2020.108480.

[12] Berg PA, Klein R, Lindenborn-Fotinos J, Klöppel W. ATPase associated antigen (M2): marker antigen for serological diagnosis of primary biliary cirrhosis. Lancet 1982;11:1423–6. https://doi.org/10.1016/S0140-6736(82)91327-7.

[13] Wang Y, Liu S, Liu H, Zhao S, Lu J, Zhao J. SARS-CoV-2 infection of the liver directly contributes to hepatic impairment in patients with COVID-19. J Hepatol 2020;73(4):807–16. https://doi.org/10.1016/j.hep.2020.05.002.

[14] Silverberg JI, Zyskind I, Naiditch H, Zimmerman J, Glatt AE, Printer A, et al. Association of varying clinical manifestations and positive anti-SARS-CoV-2 IgG antibodies: a cross-section of observational study. J Allergy Clin Immunol Pract 2021;9(9):3331–8. https://doi.org/10.1016/j.jaip.2021.06.046. e2.

[15] Zyskind I, Rosenberg AZ, Zimmerman J, Naiditch H, Glatt AE, Printer A, et al. SARS-CoV-2 seroprevalence and symptom onset in culturally linked Orthodox Jewish communities across multipole regions in the United States. JAMA Netw Open 2021;4(3):e212816. https://doi.org/10.1001/jamanetworkopen.2021.2816.

[16] Pascolini S, Vannini A, Deleonardi G, et al. COVID-19 and immunological dysregulation: can autoantibodies be useful? Clin Transl Sci 2021;14(2):502–8. https://doi.org/10.1111/cts.12908.

[17] Lucchese G, Flöel A. Molecular mimicry between SARS-CoV-2 and respiratory pacemaker neurons. Autoimmun Rev 2020;19(7):102556. https://doi.org/10.1016/j.autrev.2020.102556.

[18] Gammazza AM, Légaré S, Lo Bosco G, Fucarino A, Angileri F, de Macario EC, et al. Human molecular chaperones share with SARS-CoV-2 antigenic epitopes potentially capable of eliciting autoimmunity against endothelial cells: possible role of molecular mimicry in COVID-19. Cell Stress Chaperones 2020;25:737–41. https://doi.org/10.1007/s12192-020-01148-3.

[19] Lucchese G, Flöel A. SARS-CoV-2 and Guillain-Barré syndrome: molecular mimicry with human heat shock proteins as potential pathogenic mechanism. Cell Stress Chaperones 2020;25:731–5. https://doi.org/10.1007/s12192-020-01145-6.

[20] Venkatakrishnan A, Kayal N, Anand P, Badley AD, Church GM, Soundararajan V, et al. Benchmarking evolutionary tinkering underlying human-viral molecular mimicry shows multiple host pulmonary-arterial peptides mimicked by SARS-CoV-2. Cell Death Dis 2020;6:96. https://doi.org/10.1038/s41420-020-00321-y.

[21] Kanduc D. From anti-SARS-CoV-2 immune responses to COVID-19 via molecular mimicry. Antibodies 2020;9. https://doi.org/10.3390/antib9030033.

[22] Gil MR, Barouqa M, Szymanski J, Gonzalez-Lugo JD, Rahman S, Billett HH. Assessment of lupus anticoagulant positivity in patients with coronavirus disease 2019 (COVID-19). JAMA Netw Open 2020;3(8):e2017539. https://doi.org/10.1001/jamanetworkopen.2020.17539.

[23] Amezcua-Guerra LM, Rojas-Velasco G, Brianza-Padilla M, Vázquez-Rangel A, Márquez-Velasco R, Baranda-Tovar F, et al. Presence of antiphospholipid antibodies in COVID-19: case series study. Ann Rheum Dis 2020;80(5):e73. https://doi.org/10.1136/annrheumdis-2020-218100.
[24] Pinto AA, Carroll LS, Nar V, Varatharaj A, Galea I. CNS inflammatory vasculopathy with antimyelin oligodendrocyte glycoprotein antibodies in COVID-19. Neurol Neuroimmunol Neuroinflamm 2020;7(5):e813. https://doi.org/10.1212/NXI.0000000000000813.
[25] Gigli G, Vogrig A, Nilo A, Fabris M, Biasotto A, Curcio F, et al. HLA and immunological features of SARS-CoV-2-induced Guillain-Barré syndrome. Neurol Sci 2020;41:3391–4. https://doi.org/10.1007/s10072-020-04787-7.
[26] Finsterer J, Scorza F, Fiorini A. SARS-CoV-2 associated Guillain-Barre syndrome in 62 patients. Eur J Neurol 2021;28(1):e10–2. https://doi.org/10.1111/ene.14544.
[27] Uncini A, Vallat J, Jacobs B. Guillain-Barré syndrome in SARS-CoV-2 infection: an instant systematic review of the first six months of pandemic. J Neurol Neurosurg Psychiatry 2020;91(10):1105–10. https://doi.org/10.1136/jnnp-2020-324491.
[28] Bonometti R, Sacchi M, Stobbione P, Lauritano EC, Tamiazzo S, Marchegiani A, et al. The first case of systemic lupus erythematosus (SLE) triggered by COVID-19 infection. Eur Rev Med Pharmacol Sci 2020;24(18):9695–7. https://doi.org/10.26355/eurrev_202009_23060.
[29] Zhou P, Yang XL, Wang XG, Hu B, Zhang L, Zhang W. A pneumonia outbreak associated with a new coronavirus of probable bat origin. Nature 2020;579(7798):270–3. https://doi.org/10.1038/s41586-020-2012-7.
[30] Nath A. Neurologic complications of coronavirus infections. Neurol 2020;94(19):809–10. https://doi.org/10.1212/WNL.0000000000009455.
[31] Zheng YY, Ma YT, Zhang JY, Xie X. COVID-19 and the cardiovascular system. Nat Rev Cardiol 2020;17(5):259–60. https://doi.org/10.1038/s41569-020-0360-5.
[32] Shi Y, Wang Y, Shao C, Huang J, Gan J, Huang X. COVID-19 infection: the perspectives on immune responses. Cell Death Differ 2020;27:1451–4. https://doi.org/10.1038/s41418-020-0530-3.
[33] Lin L, Jiang X, Zhang Z, Huang S, Zhang Z, Fang Z. Gastrointestinal symptoms of 95 cases with SARS-CoV-2 infection. Gut 2020;69(6):997–1001. https://doi.org/10.1136/gutjnl-2020-321013.

CHAPTER

13

Autoantibodies neutralizing antiinflammatory mediators in the context of SARS-CoV-2 infection and COVID-19

Lorenz Thurner[1] *and Christoph Kessel*[2]

[1]Department of Internal Medicine I, Hematology/Oncology, Clinical Immunology and Rheumatology, and José Carreras Center for Immuno- and Gene Therapy, Saarland University Medical School, Homburg/Saar, Germany; [2]Department of Pediatric Rheumatology and Immunology, Translational Inflammation Research, University Children's Hospital, Münster, Germany

Hyperinflammation initiated by SARS-CoV-2

COVID-19, caused by SARS-CoV-2, shows a very wide spectrum of manifestations and severity ranging from completely asymptomatic courses, to mild cold symptoms or (partial) loss of the sense of taste and smell, to acute respiratory distress syndrome (ARDS) [1–4]. Apart from frequent thromboembolic complications, unconventional hyperinflammatory states belonged to the most striking clinical symptoms in severe and critical COVID-19. Already early in the pandemic those have been proposed to overlap or mimic classic cytokine storm syndromes [5] such as secondary hemophagocytic lymphohistiocytosis (sHLH) or macrophage activation syndrome (MAS), which both reveal strong clinical and immunophenotypic overlap [6,7].

Key molecules or pathways that drive such conditions include IL-1β, IL-6, IL-18, IFN-γ, and JAK/STAT signaling and can be targeted by state-of-the-art therapies. Ever since the proposal regarding an overlap of (critical) COVID-19 with classical cytokine storm conditions has been put forward [5,8] those have been considered as therapeutic targets in COVID-19 with in part mixed results, short-fall of statistical significance (NCT04348071) or still planned trial (NCT04324021) [9–13]. Meanwhile, immunological profiling in critical COVID-19 versus

Autoimmunity, COVID-19, Post-COVID19 syndrome and COVID-19 vaccination
https://doi.org/10.1016/B978-0-443-18566-3.00031-1

classic cytokine storm syndromes rather questions the significance of systemic hyperinflammation following SARS-CoV-2 infection and in part suggests only limited efficacy of specific drugs targeting key molecules and pathways predominantly associated with systemic cytokine storm conditions in COVID-19 [14,15].

Apart from such treatments, other therapeutic approaches involved immunosuppressive drugs like dexamethasone or inhibitors of BCR-signaling pathways as well as immunomodulatory drugs like hydroxychloroquin and azithromycin [16–22]. Of those, however, only dexamethasone and inhibition of IL-1 or IL-6 signaling by anakinra and tocilizumab, respectively, resulted in a reduced 28-day mortality [13,16,23]. Compared to immunosuppressive antiinflammatory drugs, only passive immunization by pools of recombinant monoclonal antibodies have so far resulted in reduced 28-day mortality [24]. Beyond, Remdisivir proofed as the only antiviral resulting in shorter duration of hospitalization [19].

Fortunately, COVID-19 usually does not affect children severely, with the exception of long-COVID and rare but severe hyperinflammatory syndromes, that is, multisystem inflammatory syndrome in children (MIS-C), in Europe frequently called pediatric inflammatory multisystem syndrome (PIMS). This hyperinflammatory syndrome often involves the cardiovascular system and was thus proposed to mimic Kawasaki disease. Ultimately, MIS-C can result in multiorgan failure and shock and therefore requires intensive care treatment [25–30].

Despite the novelty of the hyperinflammatory states in COVID-19 and the rarity of MIS-C, significant insights into specific immunological phenotypes and mechanisms have been gained ever since. Nevertheless, many questions still remain unanswered. At least in MIS-C it has been suggested that the formation of pathophysiologically relevant autoantibodies may accompany hyperinflammation [31,32]. From a clinical perspective, this observation coincides with the frequently noted interval of about two to 6 weeks between SARS-CoV-2 infection [33–35] and manifestation of MIS-C, as well as the fact that most cases of MIS-C respond to glucocorticoids and intravenous immunoglobulins (IVIGs). Of note, the clinical similarity to Kawasaki disease and also the recommendation of the American College of Rheumatology to use anakinra in refractory cases of MIS-C indicates a contribution of a dysregulated IL-1-pathway [36–38].

Autoantibodies in COVID-19

Recent studies have described anti-La antibodies and autoantibody candidates directed against endothelial, gastrointestinal, and immune-cell antigens in MIS-C/PIMS [32]. In adult patients with COVID-19 misdirected, or defective IFN I responses were reported as a key factor for insufficient antiviral immune responses [39–41]. In this context, autoantibodies against IFN I were detected specifically in patients with severe courses of COVID-19 [42]. Moreover, exuberant B-cell responses were regularly found in COVID-19 [43,44], along with a high prevalence of antiphospholipid- [45], anti-Ro/La- [46] or anti-annexin-V-antibodies [47].

A role of proinflammatory acting antibodies has so far not yet been clearly established [48]. Considering the described inflammatory conditions and the observed autoreactivity, the question arose whether proinflammatory acting autoantibodies could be involved in COVID-19 pathology. Potential proinflammatory effects might be mediated by nonneutralizing anti-

SARS-CoV2-antibodies and so-called antibody-enhanced infection and inflammation, by deposition of immunocomplexes, mediated by Fc-domain (afucosylated) [49], or mediated by the reactivity of the Fab-domain itself (Table 13.1).

This latter mechanism may potentially be mediated by binding and activation of proinflammatory-acting receptors like members of the TNF receptor superfamily, by depletion of antiinflammatory-acting receptors like IL-10R, or by neutralization of antiinflammatory secreted mediators like progranulin (PGRN), IL-1-receptor antagonist (IL-1-Ra), IL-10, IL-18 BP, IL-22-BP, IL-36-Ra, IL-38, TGF-β or serpins (Table 13.1).

The break of peripheral immune tolerance in the context of SARS-CoV-2

There are multiple possible mechanisms which may lead to a break of self-tolerance due to an infection with SARS-CoV-2. The most obvious one is molecular mimicry, where the similarity of antigenic determinants of SARS-CoV-2 results in crossreactivity of antiviral immune responses with epitopes of self-proteins.

An in silico search for potential molecular mimicry predicted numerous cross-reactive epitopes [56]. In an effort to further investigate autoimmunity arising from cross-reactive antibody responses targeting the SARS-CoV-2 spike protein in silico screenings identified a set of pentamers regarded as minimal immune determinants with close relation to female germ cells. Yet, neither the existence of such crossreactive antibodies nor eventual functional relevance has not been validated [57].

Further, for vaccine induced thrombotic thrombocytopenia (VITT) upon immunization with vector-based spike protein vaccine, it has been demonstrated, that resulting PF4-specific

TABLE 13.1 Possible proinflammatory antibody-mediated mechanisms in the context of SARS-CoV-2.

Mechanism	(Possible) occurrence associated with SARS-CoV-2.
Fc-domain mediated activation of inflammatory cells	• Afucosylated Fc of IgG1 bind FcγRIIa, FcγRIIIa, and transduce proinflammatory ITAM signaling [49]
Formation of immuno-complexes	• Immune complex mediated [50] • Arthus-reaction • IgA-vasculitis [51] • Antibody enhanced infection and inflammation by nonneutralizing antiviral antibodies [52]
Fab-domain-mediated I. Specific neutralization of secreted antiinflammatory mediators II. ADCC-mediated effects III. Modulation of receptors	• SECONDARY immunodeficiency by antibodies neutralizing type I interferons [42], as reported earlier for IFNy [53] in nontuberculous mycobacterial infection and other opportunistic infections o Autoimmune cytopenia secondary to COVID-19 [54,55] ▪ Direct activation of proinflammatory receptors (potentially possible, e.g., members of TNFRS, or proinflammatory interleukin receptors) ▪ Blockade of antiinflammatory receptors (potentially possible e.g., IL-10R)

antibodies do not cross-reactive to SARS-CoV-2 structural proteins [58,59]. Moreover, in patients with MIS-C, accumulation of T-cell clones with TRBV11-2 or TCR Vbeta 21.3$^+$ outside of the adaptive antiviral immune response against SARS-CoV-2 have been described [60,61].

In general terms, loss of selftolerance can result from defective processes of clonal deletion, induction of anergy or receptor editing and associate with increased maturation of naïve autoreactive B cells. This is attributable to a defect of the early checkpoint of B-cell receptor tolerance [62] and has been described in both SLE and RA as well as other autoimmune conditions [63,64].

Furthermore, peripheral B cells can receive proliferative signals via MHC-II/T-cell receptor and CD40/CD40L-interactions or are depleted via MHCII/T-cell receptor and Fas/FasL-interactions as in the case of highly autoreactive BCRs [65–67]. Both of these tolerance checkpoints can be disturbed during infection as with SARS-CoV-2.

In addition it has been known from before 2019, that altered proinflammatory, B-cell stimulatory signals such as BAFF [67], IL-6 or CpG [68] or decreased, dysbalanced antiinflammatory, immunosuppressive signals such as IL-10 [69], prominent Th17 T cells, or deficiency of CD4$^+$CD25$^+$FoxP3$^+$ and CD4$^+$CD25$^-$FoxP3$^+$ Tregs can influence these peripheral selftolerance checkpoints.

This can be caused by external factors such as a viral infection, especially with a novel virus—as SARS-CoV-2—and a subsequent antiviral response involving both innate (TLR3, TLR7, TLR8, NK cells, macrophages, inflammasome) [70–72] and adaptive immune cells (B-cells, T-cells) [43,73]. Moreover inflammatory environments can result in the activation of normally quiescent autoreactive bystander cells as well as the alteration of selfstructures including exposure of otherwise cryptic determinants, which can now be recognized by immune cells [74,75].

The crucial prerequisite of most autoimmune phenomena is the presence of permissive human leukocyte antigen (HLA) haplotypes [76]. This may influence both the initiation of the cytotoxic antiviral response with the possible desegregation by MHC-I haplotypes as well as the activation and costimulation of B cells depending on permissive MHC-II haplotypes. In adult patients with COVID-19 HLA-C * 04:01 was associated with inflammation and increased mortality [77]. In MIS-C the clonal TRBV11-2 were found shared with following HLA class I alleles A02, B35, and C04 [60].

In addition, there are a large number of polymorphisms within susceptibility genes associated with autoreactivity such as R620W [78,79] or 1858C > T [80] of PTPN22, activity weakening polymorphisms of CTLA4 [81] or A20 [82] or activating SNPs of the TLR9/MYD88 or TLR7/MYD88 [83], CD40/CD40L, ICOS/ICOSL or the BCR pathway [84]. All those have already been described before the advent of SARS-CoV-2 and might contribute to autoreactivity in the course of an infection.

Posttranslational modifications as triggers of neo-epitope formation and autoimmunity

Break of tolerance to selfproteins either by somatic mutations or by secondary modifications has been known for long. In such lines, neoantigens resulting from somatic mutations in the course of cancer have been described, against which humoral immune responses have been detected by SEREX [85]. Also the secondary occurrence of RPC1 autoantibodies and scleroderma in patients with somatically mutated POLR3A gene in precancerous disease can be listed here [86]. In addition to somatically mutated neoantigens, posttranslational modifications (PTMs) can lead to antigen-specific break of tolerance [87]. These immunogenic PTMs are frequently not detected by sequencing-approaches, as in most cases they're not evoked by mutations in the gene with the one exception of the introduction of additional N-glycosylation sites.

The presence of PTM-reactive antibodies such as, that is, anticitrullinated protein antibodies (ACPAs) in RA pin-points toward a weak spot in immune tolerance. PTMs can be introduced either by specialized enzymes or chemical reactions arising from exposure to specific environmental factors or inflammation. Depending on where and when such modifications occur B and T cells may not be adequately tolerized and thus recognize modified antigens as nonself [88]. However, by themselves PTMs frequently do not qualify as full antigen. The resulting molecular mass changes in a protein or peptide can be in the range of less or equivalent to 1 dalton (1Da) and can thus be rather regarded as hapten [89]. Haptens are small structures, which by themselves cannot be recognized as full antigen. However, when in context with a protein or peptide (the carrier) they can induce an immune response [90,91]. Conformational changes induced by these PTMs further benefit the formation of neo-epitopes [92,93].

Following the hapten-carrier model, T cells via their TCR do not just recognize PTMs but rather pick up the modifications in context with the respective peptide back bone once presented by permissive HLA-DR subtypes. Similarly, B cells via their BCR do not recognize just the modification alone, but the altered amino acids in the context of a conformational epitope. This results in some TCR or BCR avidity to go toward the PTM and some to the peptide backbone. As a consequence, such B and T cell clones may then also recognize other similarly modified moieties on self-proteins or the unmodified peptide related to the original priming antigen. This is the basis for the diversification of an immune response via epitope spreading [90,93,94] (Fig. 13.1).

In a proof-of-concept study, we demonstrated the power of the hapten-carrier model in breaking immune tolerance upon even very minor amino acid modifications [94]. By replacing selected natural amino acids located within predicted T-cell epitopes of murine C5a with the unnatural amino acid *p*-nitro-phenylalanine, we showed that the substitution of a hydroxyl-with a nitro-group (a change in three atoms) in a single amino acid can break T-cell tolerance toward the endogenous unmodified antigen and promote a B cellular antibody response toward the modified epitope, which cross-reacts with the unmodified native antigen [94].

Similarly cross-reactive immune responses have also been described in context of atypic phosphorylation and N-glycosylation of antigens as oncogenic stimuli of lymphoproliferative diseases (also Table 13.2) [113,121,122]. For instance, in plasma cell dyscrasia and MGUS T-cells specific for the hyperphosphorylated SLP2 epitope could be characterized in patients [121], who had SLP2-directed paraprotein not differentiating between the native and the hyperphosphorylated isoform [118].

In contrast to non-PTM-specific T cells, PTM-specific T cells are thought to escape central negative selection in the thymus [123]. In this case, break-of-tolerance is not a result of TCR and BCR cross-reactivity with posttranslationally modified epitopes but a consequence of

TABLE 13.2 Immunogenicity by posttranslationally modification of antigens in autoimmune diseases and cancer.

Disease	Antigen	Posttranslational modification
Rheumatoid arthritis	Fibrin/vimentin Synovial tissue Synovial tissue	• Citrullination/Deimination of arginin residue by PADI [95,96] • Homocitrullination/Carbamylation of lysine residue [97] • Malondialdehyde-acetaldehyde (MAA)-modification [98]
Juvenile idiopathic arthritis	DEK protein	Acetylation [99]
Multiple sclerosis	Myelin basic protein MOG	N-terminally acetylated [100] Malondialdehyde-modification [101]
SLE	SR proteins	Phosphorylation [102,103]
ANCA associated vasculitides and several autoimmune diseases	PGRN	Phosphorylation at Ser81 [104]
Celiac disease	Gliadin	Deamidated [105] by transglutaminase
Goodpasture syndrome	Collagen IV	Sulfilimine bonds [106,107]
IgA nephropathy	IgA	Galactose-deficient IgA [108]
Pancreatic adenocarcinoma	Enolase	Phosphorylation [109–111]
Chronic lymphocytic leukemia	LDL	Oxidization [112]
Primary central nervous system lymphoma	SAMD14/neurabin-I	N-glycosylation [113]
Diffuse large B-cell lymphoma of ABC-type	ARS2	Hypo-phosphorylation [114]
Sporadic EBV-negative burkitt lymphoma	HSP40, BYSTIN	SUMOylation and acetylation [115]
Lymphoplasmocytic lymphoma and multiple myeloma	SLP2, ATG HSP90 LGL1, sapC	Phosphorylation [116–118] SUMOylation [119] deficient glucocerebrosidase [120]

specific recognition due to leaky tolerance mechanisms, such has been described for SUMOylation and citrullination of antigens [119].

Proinflammatory autoantibodies in the context of SARS-CoV-2

Given both, the secondary hyperinflammatory states in the course of some SARS-CoV-2 infections, and the association with autoreactivity, we searched for proinflammatory acting autoantibodies using approaches based on published literature, or hypothesis driven approaches and protein-arrays. In these screenings, we found two relevant autoantibodies:

PGRN-antibodies and immunogenic isoform pSer81 PGRN in the context of SARS-CoV-2

PGRN, also called proepithelin, is a secreted precursor protein. Beside several other biological functions [124], a major property of PGRN is its antiinflammatory activity [125,126], which is mediated by direct binding to TNFR1, TNFR2 and DR3 and thus abrogation of responses to TNF-α and TL1-a [127,128]. This has been demonstrated in vivo in several mouse models including collagen and collagen-antibody induced arthritis [127], OXA induced dermatitis [129], and more relevant for COVID-19, also in LPS-induced lung injury/ARDS mouse models [130–132]. Both PGRN and TNF-α bind to cysteine-rich domain two and 3 (CRD2 and 3) of TNFR [133]. Previously, we had identified neutralizing autoantibodies against progranulin (PGRN) in sera from patients with primary small vessel vasculitis [134]. Subsequently we found progranulin-Abs in various rheumatic and other autoimmune diseases, but hardly ever in healthy controls, elderly or obese subjects, patients with sepsis and patients with melanoma [135–137]. The proinflammatory effect of neutralizing PGRN-Abs was characterized in vitro by the analysis of TNF-α-induced cytotoxic effects by MTT-assays and by downmodulation of FoxP3 in $CD4^{+}CD25^{hi}$ Tregs in inflammatory bowel diseases and rheumatic diseases [104,136]. In rheumatologic autoimmune diseases pSer81 isoform had been found exclusively in PGRN-Ab-positive patients and pSer81 isoform preceded the formation of PGRN-Abs. Moreover, the pSer81 isoform was not only immunogenic but also led to a different conversion pattern to mature granulins and to the loss of binding and blockade to TNFR1, TNFR2, and DR3. Of interest, PGRN-Abs are not restricted in their reactivity to the pSer81 PGRN isoform.

In context of hyperinflammation frequently observed in adult patients with COVID-19, those were screened for these antibodies, as we hypothesized defective antiinflammatory mechanisms to contribute to excessive inflammation resulting in poor overall prognosis. Indeed, we found PGRN-Abs in approximately 40% of adult patients with critical COVID-19. These PGRN-Abs were detected at high-titers and belonged to IgM and several IgG subclasses in each patient. In separate cohorts with noncritical COVID-19, PGRN-Abs were detected only in low frequency (i.e., in <5% of patients) and at low titers. Beyond, PGRN-specific Abs were not observed in long-COVID. PGRN-Abs were not found in 40 healthy controls vaccinated against SARS-CoV-2. Importantly, PGRN-Abs were found not to be cross-reactive against SARS-CoV-2 structural proteins [138].

Plasma levels of free PGRN were significantly decreased in autoantibody-positive patients compared to Ab-negative and non-COVID-19 controls [138]. Here we observed discrepancies between different measurement methods. Publications from other groups described increased PGRN levels in acute COVID-19, which had been measured with multiplex cytokine assays [139]. In contrast, we detected significantly suppressed PGRN levels using commercial ELISA. We also validated these ELISAs with dilution curves of rec. PGRN with or without PGRN-Abs, which clearly demonstrated the accuracy of the ELISA in both situations. In subsequent nonreducing native Western blots on plasma, we could show that free PGRN is strongly reduced in PGRN-Ab-positive adult patients with COVID-19, and that immune complexes of PGRN with PGRN-Abs of the IgG and IgM class are detectable [138]. One assumption that could explain the falsely high PGRN levels in antibody-positive patients measured by other groups might be that antibody-bound PGRN might have been measured.

In vitro, PGRN-Abs from patients reduced PGRN-dependent inhibition of TNF-α signaling. The PGRN-Abs as well as the dysfunctional pSer81 isoform of PGRN result in a loss of antagonism to TNF-α and TL-1a, leading to a proinflammatory imbalance in these pathways (Fig. 13.2). The pSer81 hyperphosphorylated PGRN isoform was exclusively detected in patients with PGRN-Abs [138]. In longitudinally collected samples, hyperphosphorylated isoforms of both PGRN emerged transiently and preceded the appearance of autoantibodies [138].

IL-1-Ra-antibodies and the immunogenic pThr111 isoform of IL-1-Ra in the context of SARS-CoV-2

Interleukin-1 receptor antagonist (IL-1-Ra) is the physiologic inhibitor of IL-1α and Il-1β binding to IL-1R1 and is therefore significantly responsible for balancing the IL-1 signaling pathway. Animal models have shown that low IL-1-Ra levels, either due to neutralization after immunization or due to deficiency, induce or exacerbate inflammatory syndromes such as colitis, arthropathy, vasculitis or psoriasis-like manifestations [140–142]. In humans, inherited deficiency of IL-Ra (DIRA) results in a severe inflammatory syndrome [143,144]. Anakinra, a recombinant fragment of IL-1-Ra expressed in *E. coli* is used as an approved drug in the treatment of a number of autoinflammatory and autoimmune diseases [145].

In adult patients with severe to critical COVID-19 autoantibodies against IL-1-Ra (IL-1-Ra-Abs) have been found in approximately 50% of patients [138]. These IL-1-Ra-Abs had high-titers and belonged to IgM and several IgG subclasses in each patient. In patients with noncritical COVID-19, these IL-1-Ra-Abs were detected in low frequency (i.e., in <5% of patients) and at low titers [138]. In contrast, those were not detected in long-COVID or healthy adult controls vaccinated against SARS-CoV-2 or 188 unvaccinated healthy controls [138]. IL-1-Ra-Abs were not cross-reactive against SARS-CoV-2 structural proteins nor against PGRN. Plasma levels of free IL-1-Ra were significantly decreased in autoantibody-positive compared to Ab-negative patients and non-COVID-19 controls [138]. In vitro, IL-1-Ra-Abs from patients reduced IL-1-Ra- or anakinra-dependent inhibition of IL-1β signaling in IL-1-reporter cells [138].

A hyperphosphorylated IL-1-Ra isoform was only found in patients with IL-1-Ra-Abs. Thr111 was identified as the site of hyperphosphorylation for IL-1-Ra. The hyperphosphorylated isoform of IL-1-Ra was transiently and preceded the formation of autoantibodies. Thus, similar to pSer81 PGRN for PGRN-Abs, the concept of transiently occurring immunogenic isoforms also applied to IL-1-Ra-Abs. In a retrospective relatively small analysis of hospitalized adult patients with critical COVID-19, the presence of IL-1-Ra-Abs or IL-1-Ra-Abs in combination with PGRN-Abs was associated with a higher morbidity and mortality [138].

In multisystem inflammatory syndrome in children (MIS-C) antibodies against IL-1-Ra could be detected in approximately 60% of patients, but not in controls [146]. In contrast to critical COVID-19 in adults, IL-1-Ra-antibodies belonged predominantly to IgG1 subclass and PGRN-Abs were infrequently (<5%). Western blots and ELISA showed a concomitant reduction of free IL-1-Ra plasma levels and the presence of IgG-IL-1-Ra immune complexes. Notably, the same additional, hyperphosphorylated, transiently occurring atypical isoform of IL-1-Ra was observed in autoantibody-positive patients as in adult COVID-19.

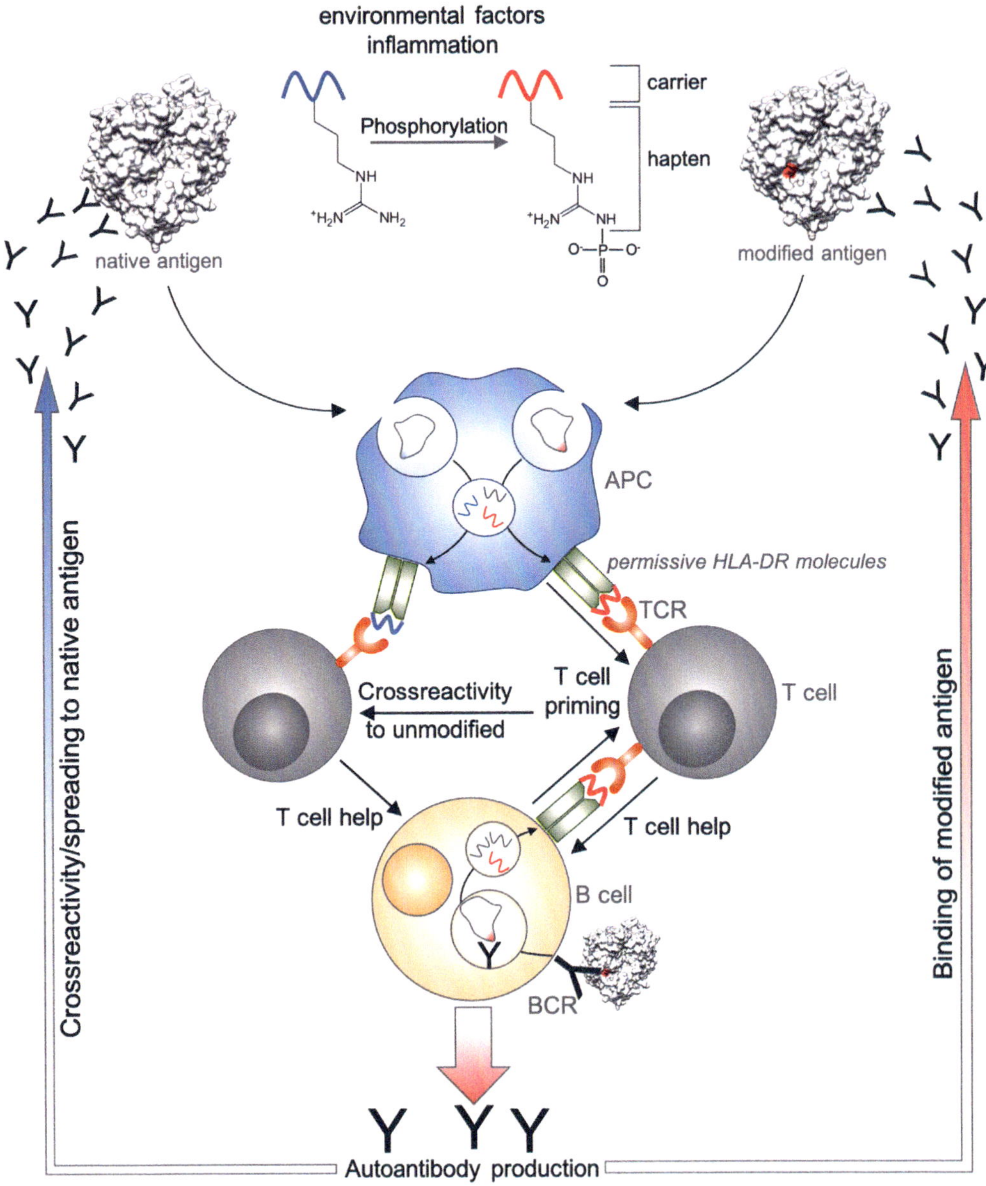

FIGURE 13.1 **The hapten-carrier model and its role in breakdown of peripheral tolerance**. Exposure to environmental noxious agents, infectious triggers and/or (sterile) inflammation can induce posttranslational modifications (as an example: phosphorylation of arginine) to any endogenous protein. By themselves these modifications result in alterations that are too minor to become immunogenic and can thus be regarded as haptens. However, in context of a peptide backbone (the carrier) the modified amino acid side chain may be recognized by T and B cells. Modified as well as unmodified protein can be phagocytosed by APCs and modified and unmodified peptides can be presented via MHCII molecules. As T cells may not recognize the modified peptide as self any longer those can subsequently provide T cell help to antigen presenting B cells. T cells primed by modified antigen may also cross-react to unmodified peptide epitopes and provide further B cell help. B cells mount a local antibody response which is primarily directed against the modified priming antigen but may also cross-react to native protein and may further also spread to other, previously nonimmunogenic sites.

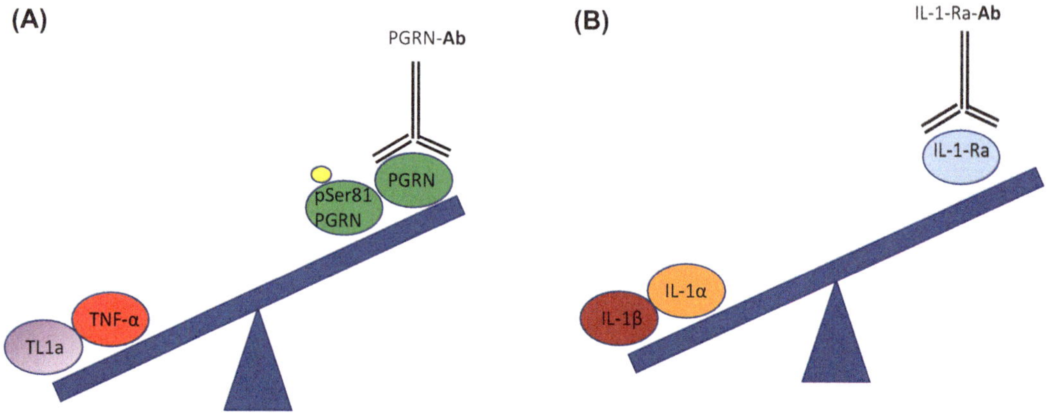

FIGURE 13.2 **Pro-inflammatory Imbalance mediated by autoantibodies.** (A) Inflammatory imbalance in the TNF-α-, TL-1a-pathways evoked by neutralizing PGRN-Abs and the pSer81 isoform of PGRN itself, which lost the ability of inhibitory binding to TNFR1/2 and DR3. (B) Inflammatory imbalance in the IL-1-α- and IL-1β-pathway due to neutralizing IL-1-Ra-Abs. If pThr111 Il-1-Ra is functionally altered due its modification, is not yet clarified.

Concurrent with our publications on IL-1-Ra antibodies in patients with COVID-19, another group published the occurrence of IL-1-Ra-Abs in a subset of IgG4-associated diseases [147] (Table 13.3).

Remaining questions around proinflammatory autoantibodies related to SARS-CoV-2

There are several remnant questions to the described phenomena: (1) Are there other similarly "proinflammatory" antibody responses in context of SARS-CoV2 infection (Table 13.1)? (2) Do autoantibodies as described herein (Table 13.2) also occur in other hyperinflammatory scenarios? (3) What drives introduction of the immunogenic transient modifications and (4) which and (5) why may individuals be susceptible for their development and (6) might there be a prognostic value for disease course and/or predictive value for the response to a specific treatment. Unfortunately, the relevance of the last question is increasing again at the moment while writing this chapter with a frustratingly high incidence during the fourth wave in central Europe and the appearance of the omicron variant. The main cause for the high incidence, and more relevant morbidity and mortality is too low vaccination rates due to insufficient accessibility [152], refusal attitude [153], and due to waning immunity [154]. Not to mention, individuals with preexisting conditions as hematologic neoplasms or immunosuppression [155].

So, possible therapeutic consequences for patients with IL-1-Ra-Abs or PGRN-Abs include immunosuppressive therapies starting from glucocorticoids to B-cell or plasma-cell-depletion, immunomodulation by administration of IVIGs, therapeutic correction of the imbalance of the IL-1α and IL-1-β signaling pathways by either substitution of the decreased IL-1-Ra by the administration of anakinra or by therapeutic neutralization of IL-1β by administration of

TABLE 13.3 Summary of characteristics of IL-1-Ra- and PGRN-autoantibodies.

	IL-1-Ra-abs	PGRN-abs
Prevalence in different diseases	• Critical COVID-19: 50% [138] • Mis-c: 60%–65% [146] • IgG4-related diseases [147]	• Critical COVID-19: 40% [138] • Mis-c: <5% [146] • Various autoimmune diseases including: Aav: 20%–40% [148] • RA: 24% [149] • PsA: 19% [135] • SLE: • CD: 16% and UC: 21% [136]
Neutralizing property	• Shown by ELISA [138,146,147] • Reduction of free IL-1-Ra and occurrence of immune complexes shown in western-blot [138,146] • Neutralizing effect functionally demonstrated in vitro with IL-1 reporter cells. Also neutralizing effect on anakinra [138,146].	• Shown by ELISA [134,138] • Reduction of free PGRN and occurrence of immune complexes shown in western-blot [138] • Neutralizing effect functionally demonstrated in vitro with WEHI-S cells [138,150], and by downmodulation of FOXP3 in $CD4^{+}CD25^{hi}$Tregs [136]
Titer	• Critical COVID-19: 1:400 up to 1:3200 • Mis-c: 1:200 up to 1:800	• Critical COVID-19: 1:400—1:3200 • Autoimmune diseases: 1:400—1:1600 [148]
Ig classes	• Critical COVID-19: IgM and multiple IgG subclasses in each patient • MIS-C: IgG1	• Critical COVID-19: IgM and multiple IgG subclasses in each patient • Autoimmune diseases: Predominantly IgG1 [151], exception of a larger proportion of IgA in CD and UC [136]
Reason of immunogenicity	• Transient pThr111 isoform of IL-1-Ra [138] • No cross reactivity to structural proteins of SARS-cov-2 [138]	• Transient pSer81 isoform of PGRN [104,138] • No cross reactivity to structural proteins of SARS-cov-2 [138]
HLA-restriction	Not known	Not known
Functional effect of modification of the antigen	Not known	• Alternative conversion pattern of pSer81 PGRN [104] • pSer81 PGRN does not bind TNFR1/2 and DR3 [104]

canakinumab. And regarding the imbalance in the TNF-α/TL-1a-pathways, modulation by etanercept, or TNF-α-neutralizing antibodies or indirectly by targeting the related IL-6-pathway. Finally, it remains critical to further elucidate the underlying molecular mechanisms explaining why some patients develop the immunogenic isoforms and whether this can be predicted and or prevented. Ultimately, it needs to be stressed that most efficient control over *any* adverse events associated with SARS-CoV-2 infection is gained by all currently available vaccination strategies and possibly also latest antiviral treatment approaches rushing toward approval [156].

Acknowledgment

The author thanks Natalie Fadle, Evi Regitz, Philipp Klemm, Marina Zaks, Elisabeth Stöger, Jochen Pfeifer, Igor Kos, Frank Langer, Bettina Friesenhahn-Ochs, Gereon Gäbelein, Frank Lammert, Torben Rixecker, Christian Lensch, Philipp Lepper, Marcin Krawczyk, Robert Bals, Michael Böhm, Hashim Abdul-Khaliq, Moritz Bewarder, Dirk Föll, Yvan Fischer, Klaus Roemer, Klaus-Dieter Preuss Michael Pfreundschuh and Bernhard Thurner for their great contributions to the projects, based on which this chapter was written. In particular, we thank Bernhard Thurner for revising this chapter The research of Lorenz Thurner is supported by the NanoBioMed initiative of the University of Saarland. COI: The University of Saarland with Lorenz Thurner, Klaus-Dieter Preuss and Michael Pfreundschuh as investigators had applied for a patent on the role of PGRN as a marker for autoimmunity in 2012. The patent expired in 2017. Christoph Kessel reports consultancy activities for Novartis and Swedish Orphan Biovitrum (SOBI) and receives research support from Novartis.

References

[1] Wölfel R, Corman VM, Guggemos W, et al. Virological assessment of hospitalized patients with COVID-2019. Nature 2020;581(7809):465–9.

[2] Levinson R, Elbaz M, Ben-Ami R, et al. Anosmia and dysgeusia in patients with mild SARS-CoV-2 infection. medRxiv; 2020.

[3] Chen G, Wu D, Guo W, et al. Clinical and immunological features of severe and moderate coronavirus disease 2019. J Clin Invest 2020;130(5):2620–9.

[4] Ackermann M, Verleden SE, Kuehnel M, et al. Pulmonary vascular endothelialitis, thrombosis, and angiogenesis in covid-19. N Engl J Med 2020;383(2):120–8.

[5] Mehta P, McAuley DF, Brown M, Sanchez E, Tattersall RS, Manson JJ. COVID-19: consider cytokine storm syndromes and immunosuppression. Lancet 2020;395(10229).

[6] Crayne C, Cron RQ. Pediatric macrophage activation syndrome, recognizing the tip of the Iceberg. Eur J Rheumatol 2020;7(Suppl 1):1–8.

[7] Kessel C, Vollenberg R, Masjosthusmann K, et al. Discrimination of COVID-19 from inflammation-induced cytokine storm syndromes by disease-related blood biomarkers. Arthritis Rheumatol 2021;73(10):1791–9.

[8] Henderson LA, Canna SW, Schulert GS, et al. On the alert for cytokine storm: immunopathology in COVID-19. Arthritis Rheumatol 2020;72(7).

[9] Mariette X, Hermine O, Resche-Rigon M, et al. Effect of anakinra versus usual care in adults in hospital with COVID-19 and mild-to-moderate pneumonia (CORIMUNO-ANA-1): a randomised controlled trial. Lancet Respir Med 2021;9(3).

[10] Kooistra EJ, Waalders NJB, Grondman I, et al. Anakinra treatment in critically ill COVID-19 patients: a prospective cohort study. Crit Care 2020;24(1).

[11] Cavalli G, De Luca G, Campochiaro C, et al. Interleukin-1 blockade with high-dose anakinra in patients with COVID-19, acute respiratory distress syndrome, and hyperinflammation: a retrospective cohort study. Lancet Rheumatol 2020;2(6):e325–31.

[12] Kaplanski G, Bontemps D, Esnault P, et al. Combined Anakinra and Ruxolitinib treatment to rescue extremely ill COVID-19 patients: a pilot study. Autoimmun Rev 2021;20(2).

[13] Kyriazopoulou E, Poulakou G, Milionis H, et al. Early treatment of COVID-19 with anakinra guided by soluble urokinase plasminogen receptor plasma levels: a double-blind, randomized controlled phase 3 trial. Nat Med 2021;27(10).

[14] Remy KE, Mazer M, Striker DA, et al. Severe immunosuppression and not a cytokine storm characterizes COVID-19 infections. JCI Insight 2020;5(17).

[15] Kessel C, Vollenberg R, Masjosthusmann K, et al. Discrimination of COVID-19 from inflammation-induced cytokine storm syndromes using disease-related blood biomarkers. Arthritis Rheumatol 2021;73(10).

[16] RECOVERY Collaborative Group, Horby P, Lim WS, et al. Dexamethasone in hospitalized patients with covid-19—preliminary report. N Engl J Med 2020;384(8):693–704.

[17] Gupta S, Wang W, Hayek SS, et al. Association between early treatment with tocilizumab and mortality among critically ill patients with COVID-19. JAMA Intern Med 2020;181(1):41–51.

[18] Aomar-Millán IF, Salvatierra J, Torres-Parejo Ú, et al. Anakinra after treatment with corticosteroids alone or with tocilizumab in patients with severe COVID-19 pneumonia and moderate hyperinflammation. A retrospective cohort study. Intern Emerg Med 2021;16(4):843–52.

[19] WHO Solidarity Trial Consortium, Pan H, Peto R, et al. Repurposed antiviral drugs for covid-19—interim WHO solidarity trial results. N Engl J Med 2021;384(6):497–511.

[20] Schlesinger N, Alten RE, Bardin T, et al. Canakinumab for acute gouty arthritis in patients with limited treatment options: results from two randomised, multicentre, active-controlled, double-blind trials and their initial extensions. Ann Rheum Dis 2012;71(11):1839–48.

[21] Lopes MI, Bonjorno LP, Giannini MC, et al. Beneficial effects of colchicine for moderate to severe COVID-19: a randomised, double-blinded, placebo-controlled clinical trial. RMD Open 2021;7(1):e001455.

[22] Treon SP, Castillo JJ, Skarbnik AP, et al. The BTK inhibitor ibrutinib may protect against pulmonary injury in COVID-19 infected patients. Blood 2020;135(21):1912–5.

[23] Abani O, Abbas A, Abbas F, et al. Tocilizumab in patients admitted to hospital with COVID-19 (RECOVERY): a randomised, controlled, open-label, platform trial. Lancet 2021;397(10285).

[24] Group RC, Horby PW, Mafham M, et al. Casirivimab and imdevimab in patients admitted to hospital with COVID-19 (RECOVERY): a randomised, controlled, open-label, platform trial. medRxiv [Internet]. 2021. 2021.06.15.21258542. Available from: http://medrxiv.org/content/early/2021/06/16/2021.06.15.21258542.abstract.

[25] Dufort EM, Koumans EH, Chow EJ, et al. Multisystem inflammatory syndrome in children in New York state. N Engl J Med 2020;383(4):347–58.

[26] Feldstein LR, Rose EB, Horwitz SM, et al. Multisystem inflammatory syndrome in U.S. Children and adolescents. N Engl J Med 2020;383(4):334–46.

[27] Fernández-Sarmiento J, De Souza D, Jabornisky R, Gonzalez GA, Arias López M del P, Palacio G. Paediatric inflammatory multisystem syndrome temporally associated with COVID-19 (PIMS-TS): a narrative review and the viewpoint of the Latin American Society of Pediatric Intensive Care (SLACIP) Sepsis Committee. BMJ Paediatr Open 2021;5:e000894.

[28] Royal College of Paediatrics and Child Health. Paediatric multisystem inflammatory syndrome temporally associated with COVID-19 (PIMS)—guidance for clinicians. 2020.

[29] World Health Organization. Multisystem inflammatory syndrome in children and adolescents temporally related to COVID-19: scientific Brief 15 May 2020. WHO. 2020.

[30] Esteve-Sole A, Anton J, Pino-Ramirez RM, et al. Similarities and differences between the immunopathogenesis of COVID-19-related pediatric multisystem inflammatory syndrome and Kawasaki disease. J Clin Invest 2021;131(6):e144554.

[31] Consiglio CR, Cotugno N, Sardh F, et al. The Immunology of multisystem inflammatory syndrome in children with COVID-19. Cell 2020;183(4):968–981.e7.

[32] Gruber CN, Patel RS, Trachtman R, et al. Mapping systemic inflammation and antibody responses in multisystem inflammatory syndrome in children (MIS-C). Cell 2020;183(4).

[33] Viner RM, Whittaker E. Kawasaki-like disease: emerging complication during the COVID-19 pandemic. Lancet 2020;395(10239):1741–3.

[34] Verdoni L, Mazza A, Gervasoni A, et al. An outbreak of severe Kawasaki-like disease at the Italian epicentre of the SARS-CoV-2 epidemic: an observational cohort study. Lancet 2020;395(10239):1771–8.

[35] Whittaker E, Bamford A, Kenny J, et al. Clinical characteristics of 58 children with a pediatric inflammatory multisystem syndrome temporally associated with SARS-CoV-2. JAMA 2020;324(3):259–69.

[36] Wikén M, Hallén B, Kullenberg T, Koskinen LO. Development and effect of antibodies to anakinra during treatment of severe CAPS: sub-analysis of a long-term safety and efficacy study. Clin Rheumatol 2018;37(12):3381–6.

[37] Henderson LA, Canna SW, Friedman KG, et al. American College of Rheumatology clinical guidance for multisystem inflammatory syndrome in children associated with SARS–CoV-2 and hyperinflammation in pediatric COVID-19: version 1. Arthritis Rheumatol 2020;72(11):1791–805.

[38] Henderson LA, Canna SW, Friedman KG, et al. American College of Rheumatology clinical guidance for multisystem inflammatory syndrome in children associated with SARS–CoV-2 and hyperinflammation in pediatric COVID-19: version 2. Arthritis Rheumatol 2021;73(4):e13–29.

[39] Blanco-Melo D, Nilsson-Payant BE, Liu WC, et al. Imbalanced host response to SARS-CoV-2 drives development of COVID-19. Cell 2020;181(5):1036–1045.e9.

[40] Hadjadj J, Yatim N, Barnabei L, et al. Impaired type I interferon activity and inflammatory responses in severe COVID-19 patients. Science 2020;369(6504):718–24.
[41] Lee JS, Park S, Jeong HW, et al. Immunophenotyping of covid-19 and influenza highlights the role of type i interferons in development of severe covid-19. Sci Immunol 2020;5(49):eabd1554.
[42] Bastard P, Rosen LB, Zhang Q, et al. Autoantibodies against type I IFNs in patients with life-threatening COVID-19. Science 2020;370(6515):eabd4585.
[43] Schultheiß C, Paschold L, Simnica D, et al. Next-generation sequencing of T and B cell receptor repertoires from COVID-19 patients showed signatures associated with severity of disease. Immunity 2020;53(2):442–455.e4.
[44] Halpert G, Shoenfeld Y. SARS-CoV-2, the autoimmune virus. Autoimmun Rev 2020;19(12):102695.
[45] Zhang Y, Cao W, Jiang W, et al. Profile of natural anticoagulant, coagulant factor and anti-phospholipid antibody in critically ill COVID-19 patients. J Thromb Thrombolysis 2020;50(3):580–6.
[46] Fujii H, Tsuji T, Yuba T, et al. High levels of anti-SSA/Ro antibodies in COVID-19 patients with severe respiratory failure: a case-based review: high levels of anti-SSA/Ro antibodies in COVID-19. Clin Rheumatol 2020;39(11):3171–5.
[47] Cristiano A, Fortunati V, Cherubini F, Bernardini S, Nuccetelli M. Anti-phospholipids antibodies and immune complexes in COVID-19 patients: a putative role in disease course for anti-annexin-V antibodies. Clin Rheumatol 2021;40(7):2939–45.
[48] Khamsi R. Rogue antibodies could be driving severe COVID-19. Nature 2021;590(7844):29–31.
[49] Chakraborty S, Gonzalez J, Edwards K, et al. Proinflammatory IgG Fc structures in patients with severe COVID-19. Nat Immunol 2021;22(1):67–73.
[50] Mazzitelli I, Bleichmar L, Ludueña MG, et al. Immunoglobulin G immune complexes may contribute to neutrophil activation in the course of severe coronavirus disease 2019. J Infect Dis 2021;224(4).
[51] Obeid M, Fenwick C, Pantaleo G. Reactivation of IgA vasculitis after COVID-19 vaccination. Lancet Rheumatol 2021;3(9).
[52] Li D, Edwards RJ, Manne K, et al. In vitro and in vivo functions of SARS-CoV-2 infection-enhancing and neutralizing antibodies. Cell 2021;184(16).
[53] Browne SK, Burbelo PD, Chetchotisakd P, et al. Adult-onset immunodeficiency in Thailand and Taiwan. N Engl J Med 2012;367(8):725–34.
[54] Li M, Nguyen CB, Yeung Z, Sanchez K, Rosen D, Bushan S. Evans syndrome in a patient with COVID-19. Br J Haematol 2020;190(2).
[55] Georgy JT, Jayakaran JAJ, Jacob AS, et al. Evans syndrome and immune thrombocytopenia in two patients with COVID-19. J Med Virol 2021;93(5).
[56] Kanduc D, Shoenfeld Y. Molecular mimicry between SARS-CoV-2 spike glycoprotein and mammalian proteomes: implications for the vaccine. Immunol Res 2020;68(5):310–3.
[57] Dotan A, Kanduc D, Muller S, Makatsariya A, Shoenfeld Y. Molecular mimicry between SARS-CoV-2 and the female reproductive system. Am J Reprod Immunol 2021;86(6):e13494.
[58] Greinacher A, Thiele T, Warkentin TE, Weisser K, Kyrle PA, Eichinger S. Thrombotic thrombocytopenia after ChAdOx1 nCov-19 vaccination. N Engl J Med 2021;384(22).
[59] Greinacher A, Selleng K, Mayerle J, et al. Anti–platelet factor 4 antibodies causing VITT do not cross-react with SARS-CoV-2 spike protein. Blood 2021;138(14).
[60] Ramaswamy A, Brodsky NN, Sumida TS, et al. Immune dysregulation and autoreactivity correlate with disease severity in SARS-CoV-2-associated multisystem inflammatory syndrome in children. Immunity 2021;54(5).
[61] Moreews M, Le Gouge K, Khaldi-Plassart S, et al. Polyclonal expansion of TCR Vbeta 21.3+ CD4+ and CD8+ T cells is a hallmark of multisystem inflammatory syndrome in children. Sci Immunol 2021;6(59).
[62] Meffre E, Wardemann H. B-cell tolerance checkpoints in health and autoimmunity. Curr Opin Immunol 2008;20(6):632–8.
[63] Yurasov S, Wardemann H, Hammersen J, et al. Defective B cell tolerance checkpoints in systemic lupus erythematosus. J Exp Med 2005;201(5):703–11.
[64] Samuels J, Ng Y, Coupillaud C, Paget D, Meffre E. Impaired early B cell tolerance in patients with rheumatoid arthritis. J Exp Med 2005;201(10):1659–67.
[65] Rathmell JC, Cooke MP, Ho WY, et al. CD95 (Fas)-dependent elimination of self-reactive B cells upon interaction with CD4+ T cells. Nature [Internet] 1995;376(6536):181–4. Available from: http://www.ncbi.nlm.nih.gov/pubmed/7603571.
[66] Rathmell JC, Townsend SE, Xu JC, Flavell RA, Goodnow CC. Expansion or elimination of B cells in vivo: dual roles for CD40- and Fas (CD95)-ligands modulated by the B cell antigen receptor. Cell 1996;87(2):319–29.

[67] Hervé M, Isnardi I, Ng Y, et al. CD40 ligand and MHC class II expression are essential for human peripheral B cell tolerance. J Exp Med [Internet] 2007;204(7):1583–93. Available from: http://www.pubmedcentral.nih.gov/articlerender.fcgi?artid=2118633&tool=pmcentrez&rendertype=abstract.
[68] Krieg AM, Yi AK, Matson S, et al. CpG motifs in bacterial DNA trigger direct B-cell activation. Nature 1995;374(6522):546–9.
[69] Glocker EO, Kotlarz D, Klein C, Shah N, Grimbacher B. IL-10 and IL-10 receptor defects in humans. Ann N Y Acad Sci 2011;1246(1):102–7.
[70] Van Der Made CI, Simons A, Schuurs-Hoeijmakers J, et al. Presence of genetic variants among young men with severe COVID-19. JAMA, J Am Med Assoc 2020;324(7).
[71] Lesan V, Bewarder M, Metz C, et al. Killer immunoglobulin-like receptor 2DS5 is associated with recovery from coronavirus disease 2019. Intensive Care Med Exp 2021;9(1).
[72] van den Berg DF, te Velde AA. Severe COVID-19: NLRP3 inflammasome dysregulated. Front Immunol 2020:11.
[73] Kos I, Balensiefer B, Lesan V, et al. Increased B-cell activity with consumption of activated monocytes in severe COVID-19 patients. Eur J Immunol 2021;51(6).
[74] Rees JH. Campylobacter jejuni infection and guillain–barré syndrome. NEJM [Internet] 1995;333:1374–9. Available from: http://www.nejm.org/doi/full/10.1056/NEJM199511233332102.
[75] Guilherme L, Kalil J, Cunningham MM. Molecular mimicry in the autoimmune pathogenesis of rheumatic heart disease. Autoimmunity 2006;39(1):31–9.
[76] Fernando MMA, Stevens CR, Walsh EC, et al. Defining the role of the MHC in autoimmunity: a review and pooled analysis. PLoS Genet 2008;4(4).
[77] Weiner J, Suwalski P, Holtgrewe M, et al. Increased risk of severe clinical course of COVID-19 in carriers of HLA-C*04:01. EClinicalMedicine 2021;40:101099.
[78] Bottini N, Musumeci L, Alonso A, et al. A functional variant of lymphoid tyrosine phosphatase is associated with type I diabetes. Nat Genet [Internet] 2004;36(4):337–8. Available from: http://www.ncbi.nlm.nih.gov/pubmed/15004560.
[79] Rieck M, Arechiga A, Onengut-Gumuscu S, Greenbaum C, Concannon P, Buckner JH. Genetic variation in PTPN22 corresponds to altered function of T and B lymphocytes. J Immunol (Baltimore, Md 1950) [Internet] 2007;179(7):4704–10. Available from: http://eutils.ncbi.nlm.nih.gov/entrez/eutils/elink.fcgi?dbfrom=pubmed&id=17878369&retmode=ref&cmd=prlinks%5Cnpapers2://publication/uuid/3553374D-D3C1-4FC7-8A4B-BEC2650EF924.
[80] Stanford SM, Bottini N. PTPN22: the archetypal non-HLA autoimmunity gene. Nat Rev Rheumatol [Internet] 2014;10(10):602–11. Available from: http://www.ncbi.nlm.nih.gov/pubmed/25003765.
[81] Ueda H, Howson JMM, Esposito L, et al. Association of the T-cell regulatory gene CTLA4 with susceptibility to autoimmune disease. Nature 2003;423(May):506–11.
[82] Tavares RM, Turer EE, Liu CL, et al. The ubiquitin modifying enzyme A20 restricts B cell survival and prevents autoimmunity. Immunity 2010;33(2):181–91.
[83] Leadbetter EA, Rifkin IR, Hohlbaum AM, Beaudette BC, Shlomchik MJ, Marshak-Rothstein A. Chromatin-IgG complexes activate B cells by dual engagement of IgM and Toll-like receptors. Nature 2002;416(6881):603–7.
[84] Jackson SW, Kolhatkar NS, Rawlings DJ. B cells take the front seat: dysregulated B cell signals orchestrate loss of tolerance and autoantibody production. Curr Opin Immunol 2015;33:70–7.
[85] Sahin U, Tureci O, Schmitt H, et al. Human neoplasms elicit multiple specific immune responses in the autologous host. ProcNatlAcadSciUSA 1995;92(0027–8424 (Print)):11810–3.
[86] Joseph CG, Darrah E, Shah AA, et al. Association of the autoimmune disease scleroderma with an immunologic response to cancer. Science (80-) 2014;343(1095–9203 (Electronic)):152–7.
[87] Doyle HA, Mamula MJ. Autoantigenesis: the evolution of protein modifications in autoimmune disease. Curr Opin Immunol 2012;24(1):112–8.
[88] Anderton SM. Post-translational modifications of self antigens: implications for autoimmunity. Curr Opin Immunol 2004;16(6).
[89] Tilvawala R, Thompson PR. Peptidyl arginine deiminases: detection and functional analysis of protein citrullination. Curr Opin Struct Biol 2019;59.
[90] Auger I, Balandraud N, Massy E, et al. Peptidylarginine deiminase autoimmunity and the development of anti–citrullinated protein antibody in rheumatoid arthritis: the hapten–carrier model. Arthritis Rheumatol 2020;72(6).

[91] Darrah E, Andrade F. Editorial: citrullination, and carbamylation, and malondialdehyde-acetaldehyde! oh my! entering the forest of autoantigen modifications in rheumatoid arthritis. Arthritis Rheumatol 2015;67(3).
[92] Scally SW, Petersen J, Law SC, et al. A molecular basis for the association of the HLA-DRB1 locus, citrullination, and rheumatoid arthritis. J Exp Med 2013;210(12).
[93] Uysal H, Nandakumar KS, Kessel C, et al. Antibodies to citrullinated proteins: molecular interactions and arthritogenicity. Immunol Rev 2010;233(1).
[94] Kessel C, Nandakumar KS, Peters FB, Gauba V, Schultz PG, Holmdahl R. A single functional group substitution in C5a breaks b cell and t cell tolerance and protects against experimental arthritis. Arthritis Rheumatol 2014;66(3).
[95] Schellekens GA, de Jong BA, van den Hoogen FH, van de Putte LB, van Venrooij WJ. Citrulline is an essential constituent of antigenic determinants recognized by rheumatoid arthritis-specific autoantibodies. J Clin Invest 1998;101(0021–9738 (Print)):273–81.
[96] van Venrooij WJ, Pruijn GJ. Citrullination: a small change for a protein with great consequences for rheumatoid arthritis. Arthritis Res 2000;2(1465–9905 (Print)):249–51.
[97] Mydel P, Wang Z, Brisslert M, et al. Carbamylation-dependent activation of T cells: a novel mechanism in the pathogenesis of autoimmune arthritis. J Immunol 2010;184(12):6882–90.
[98] Thiele GM, Duryee MJ, Anderson DR, et al. Malondialdehyde-acetaldehyde adducts and anti-malondialdehyde-acetaldehyde antibodies in rheumatoid arthritis. Arthritis Rheumatol 2015;67(3).
[99] Mor-Vaknin N, Kappes F, Dick AE, et al. DEK in the synovium of patients with juvenile idiopathic arthritis: characterization of DEK antibodies and posttranslational modification of the DEK autoantigen. Arthritis Rheum 2011;63(2):556–67.
[100] Zamvil SS, Mitchell DJ, Moore AC, Kitamura K, Steinman L, Rothbard JB. T-cell epitope of the autoantigen myelin basic protein that induces encephalomyelitis. Nature 1986;324(0028–0836 (Print)):258–60.
[101] Wållberg M, Bergquist J, Achour A, Breij E, Harris RA. Malondialdehyde modification of myelin oligodendrocyte glycoprotein leads to increased immunogenicity and encephalitogenicity. Eur J Immunol 2007;37(7):1986–95.
[102] Neugebauer KM, Merrill JT, Wener MH, Lahita RG, Roth MB. SR proteins are autoantigens in patients with systemic lupus erythematosus. Importance of phosphoepitopes. Arthritis Rheum 2000;43(0004–3591 (Print)):1768–78.
[103] Utz PJ, Hottelet M, Schur PH, Anderson P. Proteins phosphorylated during stress-induced apoptosis are common targets for autoantibody production in patients with systemic lupus erythematosus. J Exp Med 1997;185(0022–1007 (Print)):843–54.
[104] Thurner L, Fadle N, Regitz E, et al. The molecular basis for development of proinflammatory autoantibodies to progranulin. J Autoimmun 2014;61:17–28.
[105] Arentz-Hansen H, Korner R, Molberg O, et al. The intestinal T cell response to alpha-gliadin in adult celiac disease is focused on a single deamidated glutamine targeted by tissue transglutaminase. J Exp Med 2000;191(0022–1007 (Print)):603–12.
[106] Vanacore RM, Ham AJL, Cartailler JP, et al. A role for collagen IV cross-links in conferring immune privilege to the goodpasture autoantigen: structural basis for the crypticity of B cell epitopes. J Biol Chem 2008;283(33):22737–48.
[107] Vanacore R, Ham AJL, Voehler M, et al. A sulfilimine bond identified in collagen IV. Science 2009;325(5945):1230–4.
[108] Suzuki H, Fan R, Zhang Z, et al. Aberrantly glycosylated IgA1 in IgA nephropathy patients is recognized by IgG antibodies with restricted heterogeneity. J Clin Invest 2009;119(6):1668–77.
[109] Cappello P, Tomaino B, Chiarle R, et al. An integrated humoral and cellular response is elicited in pancreatic cancer by α-enolase, a novel pancreatic ductal adenocarcinoma-associated antigen. Int J Cancer 2009;125(3):639–48.
[110] Tomaino B, Cappello P, Capello M, et al. Circulating autoantibodies to phosphorylated α-enolase are a hallmark of pancreatic cancer. J Proteome Res 2011;10(1):105–12.
[111] Zhou W, Capello M, Fredolini C, et al. Mass spectrometry analysis of the post-translational modifications of alpha-enolase from pancreatic ductal adenocarcinoma cells. J Proteome Res 2010;9(6):2929–36.
[112] Myhrinder AL, Hellqvist E, Sidorova E, et al. A new perspective: molecular motifs on oxidized LDL, apoptotic cells, and bacteria are targets for chronic lymphocytic leukemia antibodies. Blood 2008;111(7):3838–48.
[113] Thurner L, Preuss K-D, Bewarder M, et al. Hyper N-glycosylated SAMD14 and neurabin-I as driver CNS autoantigens of PCNSL. Blood 2018;132(26):2744–53.

[114] Thurner L, Hartmann S, Bewarder M, et al. Identification of the atypically modified autoantigen Ars2 as the target of B-cell receptors from activated B cell-type diffuse large B-cell lymphoma. Haematologica 2020;106(8):2224–32.

[115] Thurner L, Hartmann S, Bock T, et al. Identification of posttranvslationally modified neoantigens as targets of B cell receptors of burkitt lymphoma. Blood 2018;132(Supplement 1):1588.

[116] Grass S, Preuss KD, Wikowicz A, et al. Hyperphosphorylated paratarg-7: a new molecularly defined risk factor for monoclonal gammopathy of undetermined significance of the IgM type and Waldenstrom macroglobulinemia. Blood 2011;117(1528–0020 (Electronic)):2918–23.

[117] Preuss KD, Pfreundschuh M, Fadle N, et al. Hyperphosphorylation of autoantigenic targets of paraproteins is due to inactivation of PP2A. Blood 2011;118(1528–0020 (Electronic)):3340–6.

[118] Grass S, Preuss KD, Pfreundschuh M. Autosomal-dominant inheritance of hyperphosphorylated paratarg-7. Lancet Oncol 2010;11(1474–5488 (Electronic)):12.

[119] Preuss KD, Pfreundschuh M, Fadle N, Regitz E, Kubuschok B. Sumoylated HSP90 is a dominantly inherited plasma cell dyscrasias risk factor. J Clin Invest 2015;125(1558–8238 (Electronic)):316–23.

[120] Nair S, Branagan AR, Liu J, Boddupalli CS, Mistry PK, Dhodapkar MV. Clonal immunoglobulin against lysolipids in the origin of myeloma. N Engl J Med 2016;374(6):555–61.

[121] Neumann F, Pfreundschuh M, Preuss KD, et al. CD4(+) T cells in chronic autoantigenic stimulation in MGUS, multiple myeloma and Waldenstrom's macroglobulinemia. Int J Cancer 2015;137(5):1076–84.

[122] Grass S, Preuss KD, Ahlgrimm M, et al. Association of a dominantly inherited hyperphosphorylated paraprotein target with sporadic and familial multiple myeloma and monoclonal gammopathy of undetermined significance: a case-control study. Lancet Oncol 2009;10(1474–5488 (Electronic)):950–6.

[123] Raposo B, Merky P, Lundqvist C, et al. T cells specific for post-translational modifications escape intrathymic tolerance induction. Nat Commun 2018;9(1):353.

[124] Baker M, Mackenzie IR, Pickering-Brown SM, et al. Mutations in progranulin cause tau-negative frontotemporal dementia linked to chromosome 17. Nature 2006;442(1476–4687 (Electronic)):916–9.

[125] Yin F, Banerjee R, Thomas B, et al. Exaggerated inflammation, impaired host defense, and neuropathology in progranulin-deficient mice. J Exp Med 2010;207(1540–9538 (Electronic)):117–28.

[126] Kessenbrock K, Dau T, Jenne DE. Tailor-made inflammation: how neutrophil serine proteases modulate the inflammatory response. JMolMed(Berl) 2011;89(1432–1440 (Electronic)):23–8.

[127] Tang W, Lu Y, Tian QY, et al. The growth factor progranulin binds to TNF receptors and is therapeutic against inflammatory arthritis in mice. Science (80-) 2011;332(1095–9203 (Electronic)):478–84.

[128] Liu C, Li XX, Gao W, Liu W, Liu DS. Progranulin-derived Atsttrin directly binds to TNFRSF25 (DR3) and inhibits TNF-like ligand 1A (TL1A) activity. PLoS One 2014;9(1932–6203 (Electronic)):e92743.

[129] Zhao YP, Tian QY, Liu CJ. Progranulin deficiency exaggerates, whereas progranulin-derived Atsttrin attenuates, severity of dermatitis in mice. FEBS Lett 2013;587(12):1805–10.

[130] Guo Z, Li Q, Han Y, Liang Y, Xu Z, Ren T. Prevention of lps-induced acute lung injury in mice by progranulin. Mediat Inflamm 2012;2012:540794.

[131] Yu Y, Xu X, Liu L, et al. Progranulin deficiency leads to severe inflammation, lung injury and cell death in a mouse model of endotoxic shock. J Cell Mol Med 2016;20(3):506–17.

[132] Chen YQ, Wang CJ, Xie K, et al. Progranulin improves acute lung injury through regulating the differentiation of regulatory T cells and interleukin-10 immunomodulation to promote macrophage polarization. Mediat Inflamm 2020;2020:9704327.

[133] Jian J, Zhao S, Tian Q, et al. Progranulin directly binds to the CRD2 and CRD3 of TNFR extracellular domains. FEBS Lett 2013:1873–3468 [Electronic)].

[134] Thurner L, Preuss KD, Fadle N, et al. Progranulin antibodies in autoimmune diseases [Internet]. J Autoimmun 2012. https://doi.org/10.1016/j.jaut.2012.10.003 (in press). Available from:.

[135] Thurner L, Zaks M, Preuss KD, et al. Progranulin antibodies entertain a proinflammatory environment in a subgroup of patients with psoriatic arthritis. Arthritis Res Ther 2013;15(1478–6362 (Electronic)):R211.

[136] Thurner L, Stoger E, Fadle N, et al. Proinflammatory progranulin antibodies in inflammatory bowel diseases. Dig Dis Sci 2014:1573–2568 [Electronic)].

[137] Klemm P, Assmann G, Preuss K-D, et al. Progranulin autoantibodies in systemic sclerosis and autoimmune connective tissue disorders: a preliminary study. Immunity, Inflamm Dis 2019;7(4).

[138] L. Thurner, N. Fadle, M. Bewarder, I. Kos, E. Regitz, O. Cetin, B. Thurner, Y. Fischer, T. Rixecker, K.-D. Preuss, C. Schormann, F. Neumann, View ORCID P.S. Hartmann, T. Bock, Dominic Kaddu-Mulind PML.

Autoantibodies against Progranulin and IL-1 receptor antagonist in critically ill COVID-19 (preprint). Homburg/Saar, Germany:

[139] Rieder M, Wirth L, Pollmeier L, et al. Serum protein profiling reveals a specific upregulation of the immunomodulatory protein progranulin in COVID-19. J Infect Dis 2020;223(5):775–84.

[140] Ferretti M, Casini-Raggi V, Pizarro TT, Eisenberg SP, Nast CC, Cominelli F. Neutralization of endogenous IL-1 receptor antagonist exacerbates and prolongs inflammation in rabbit immune colitis. J Clin Invest 1994;94(1):449–53.

[141] Nicklin MJH, Hughes DE, Barton JL, Ure JM, Duff GW. Arterial inflammation in mice lacking the interleukin 1 receptor antagonist gene. J Exp Med 2000;191(2):303–12.

[142] Shepherd J, Little MC, Nicklin MJH. Psoriasis-like cutaneous inflammation in mice lacking interleukin-1 receptor antagonist. J Invest Dermatol 2004;122(3):665–9.

[143] Aksentijevich I, Masters SL, Ferguson PJ, et al. An autoinflammatory disease with deficiency of the interleukin-1–receptor antagonist. N Engl J Med 2009.

[144] Reddy S, Jia S, Geoffrey R, et al. An autoinflammatory disease due to homozygous deletion of the IL1RN locus. N Engl J Med 2009;360(23):2438–44.

[145] Cavalli G, Dinarello CA. Anakinra therapy for non-cancer inflammatory diseases. Front Pharmacol 2018;9(NOV).

[146] Pfeifer J, Thurner B, Kessel C, Fadle N, Kheiroddin P, Regitz E, et al. Autoantibodies against interleukin-1 receptor antagonist in multisystem inflammatory syndrome in children: a multicentre, retrospective, cohort study. Lancet Rheumatol. 2022 May;4(5):e329–37. https://doi.org/10.1016/S2665-9913(22)00064-9. Epub 2022 Mar 29.PMID: 35368387.

[147] Jarrell JA, Baker MC, Perugino CA, et al. Neutralizing anti–IL-1 receptor antagonist autoantibodies induce inflammatory and fibrotic mediators in IgG4-related disease. J Allergy Clin Immunol 2021;149(1):358–68.

[148] Thurner L, Preuss KD, Fadle N, et al. Progranulin antibodies in autoimmune diseases. J Autoimmun 2012:1095–9157 [Electronic))].

[149] Assmann G, Zinke S, Gerling M, Bittenbring JT, Preuss KD, Thurner L. Progranulin-autoantibodies in sera of rheumatoid arthritis patients negative for rheumatoid factor and anti-citrullinated peptide antibodies. Clin Exp Rheumatol 2020;38(1).

[150] Thurner L, Zaks M, Preuss K-D, et al. Progranulin antibodies entertain a proinflammatory environment in a subgroup of patients with psoriatic arthritis. Arthritis Res Ther [Internet] 2013;15(6):R211. Available from: http://www.pubmedcentral.nih.gov/articlerender.fcgi?artid=3978758&tool=pmcentrez&rendertype=abstract.

[151] Thurner L, Preuss KD, Fadle N, et al. Progranulin antibodies in autoimmune diseases. J Autoimmun 2013;42:29–38.

[152] Cardenas NC. 'Europe and United States vaccine hesitancy': leveraging strategic policy for 'Infodemic' on COVID-19 vaccines. J Public Health 2021;44(2):e315–6.

[153] Aborode AT, Olofinsao OA, Osmond E, et al. Equal access of COVID-19 vaccine distribution in Africa: challenges and way forward. J Med Virol 2021;93(9).

[154] Bar-On YM, Goldberg Y, Mandel M, et al. Protection of BNT162b2 vaccine booster against covid-19 in Israel. N Engl J Med 2021;385(15).

[155] Thakkar A, Gonzalez-Lugo JD, Goradia N, et al. Seroconversion rates following COVID-19 vaccination among patients with cancer. Cancer Cell 2021;39(8).

[156] Willyard C. How antiviral pill molnupiravir shot ahead in the COVID drug hunt. Nature 2021. https://doi.org/10.1038/d41586-021-02783-1.

CHAPTER

14

What is common to MDA5 and COVID-19?

Daniela Noa Zohar[1] *and Yehuda Shoenfeld*[2,3]

[1]Department of Neurology, The Chaim Sheba Medical Center, Ramat Gan, Israel; [2]Zabludowicz Center for Autoimmune Diseases, Sheba Medical Center, Ramat Gan, Israel; [3]Tel Aviv University, Tel Aviv, Israel

MDA5 receptor and anti-MDA5 autoantibody

MDA5 is an intracellular protein belonging to the retinoic acid inducible gene-I (RIG-I) like receptors [1]. Acting as an intracellular viral sensor, MDA5 is induced once it interacts with RNA viral nucleic acid, triggering activation of downstream MAVS and NFkB molecules that leads to an intracellular cascade resulting in the production of Type I interferons (Fig. 14.1). Type I interferons play a critical role in immune regulation and provide an innate antiviral response [2]. A defect in MDA5 or its signaling pathway can impact type I interferon production resulting in a reduced innate immune response and high vulnerability to fatal infections [3]. Previously, MDA5 was known for its growth suppressive characteristics in human melanoma cells [4]. In addition, dysregulation of MDA5 contributes to several autoimmune diseases by uncertain mechanism [5]. At the beginning of the 21st century, anti-MDA5 autoantibody was discovered in a group of Asian patients who were diagnosed with clinically amyopathic dermatomyositis (CADM) [6]. CADM is a rare autoimmune disease which is manifested by respiratory symptoms, mild muscular features, and characteristic skin ulcers [7,8]. The presence of anti-MDA5 autoantibody is associated with the development of a rapidly progressive interstitial lung disease (ILD) and hyperferitinemia [7,9]. In spite of aggressive immunosuppressive therapy, CADM patients with rapidly progressive ILD have a poor prognosis [10].

Autoimmunity, COVID-19, Post-COVID19 syndrome and COVID-19 vaccination
https://doi.org/10.1016/B978-0-443-18566-3.00002-5

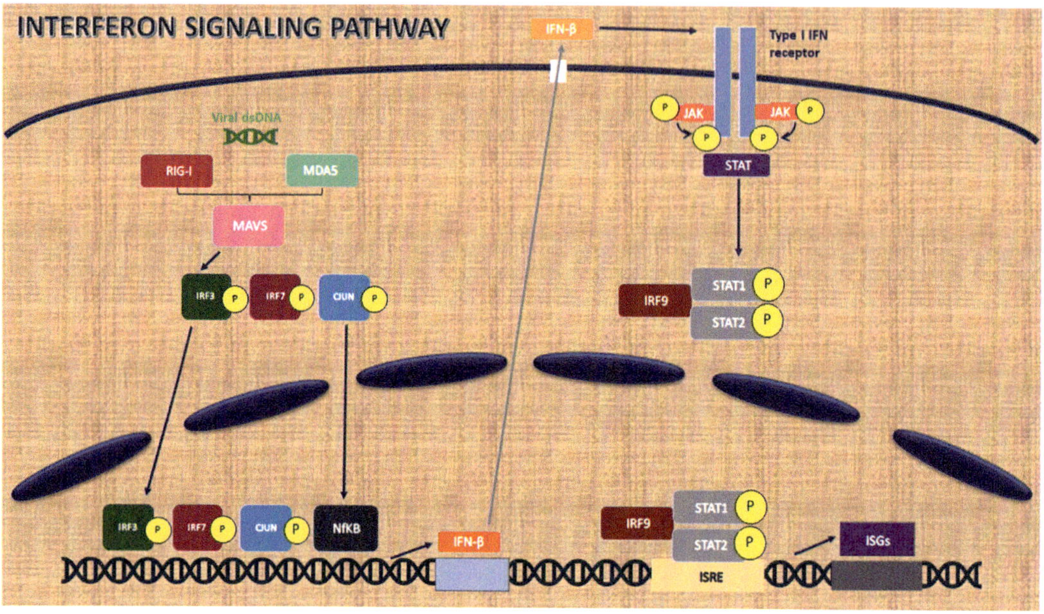

FIGURE 14.1 Interferon signaling pathway.

What are the similarities between COVID-19 disease and anti-MDA5 dermatomyositis?

The COVID-19 respiratory outbreak is extremely contagious and has rapidly distributed all over the world, its clinical presentation is variable, from asymptomatic positive SARS Cov2 patients to severe respiratory disease that may be complicated with acute respiratory distress syndrome (ARDS) [11]. ARDS can lead to respiratory failure and eventually death [12].

The prevalence of anti-MDA5-positive CADM is higher in East Asia predominantly among Chinese compared to the rest of the world [13]. Interestingly, the first cases of COVID-19 occurred in China as well.

On clinical ground, cough, shortness of breath, arthralgia, and general weakness might be an initial clinical presentation of both COVID-19 disease and CADM, representing an interstitial pneumonia which may progress to a respiratory deterioration [7–11]. While the development of ARDS is the main cause of death among COVID-19 patients [12], rapidly progressive ILD is the leading cause of death in CADM patients [9].

In terms of imaging, the hallmark for the diagnosis of COVID-19 is the existence of bilateral ground glass opacities of the lungs with or without peripheral consolidations, other pulmonary radiological findings were described including air bronchogram, reticular or crazy paving patterns airway and pleural changes, fibrosis, nodules, halo sign or reversed halo sign, air bubble sign, vascular enlargement, and pericardial effusion [14]. The diagnosis of rapidly progressive ILD among patients with anti-MDA5-positive CADM is based radiologically mainly on the identification of ground glass opacities and lung consolidations [15,16].

At the laboratory level, similar cytokine profile and hyperferritinemia characterize both COVID-19 disease and anti-MDA5-positive CADM [9,17]. Specifically, elevation in IL6, IL10, IP10 (IFN-γ-induced protein 10), and TNF alpha indicates disease activity both in patients with rapidly progressive ILD dermatomyositis and in severe COVID-19 patients, mainly COVID-19 patients who require treatment in intensive care unit [18–20]. High blood ferritin level is a known marker of inflammation; however, very high ferritin level is correlated with low survival rate in some inflammatory diseases including COVID-19 and anti-MDA5-positive CADM [7,9,17]. Between the proinflammatory markers involving in COVID-19, IL6 is unique because it predicts low survival rate [21].

The pathophysiology of anti-MDA5 dermatomyositis and COVID-19

During the last decades, coronaviruses such as MERS-related coronavirus (MERS-Cov) and SARS-related coronavirus (SARS-Cov) caused severe respiratory disease outbreaks. Previous studies on the pathogenesis of MERS-Cov and SARS-Cov reported the existence of MERS-Cov encoded proteins which inhibit MDA5 and RIG I by dysregulating the production of Type I IFN [22–24].

Equivalently, recent studies showed the importance of IFN signaling in defense against SARS-Cov2 [25]. Specifically, IFN signaling following SARS-Cov2 has been thought to be triggered by MDA5 which is described as the main sensor of SARS-Cov2 [26]. A potential mechanism of evasion of SRAS-Cov2 is by several types of I IFN inhibitory proteins, for example, NSP1 and ORF6 proteins (Fig. 14.1) [27]. This finding may explain the lack of circulating IFN beta among COVID-19 patients regardless of disease severity [25]. Gene analysis demonstrated downregulation of IFN-stimulated genes (ISGs) in severe COVID-19 patients [25]. New data suggest the role of ISG15 in activation of MDA5 for proper induction of an antiviral state. A protein of SARS-cov2 known as papain-like protease is described to play role as an antagonist for the actions of ISG15, and this is another possible mechanism by which SARS-COv2 evades the immune system [28].

Recent studies reveal high levels of follicular T helper cells in severe COVID-19 patients and in positive anti-MDA5-associated idiopathic inflammatory myopathies. This correlation between circulating levels of follicular T helper cells to disease activity and severity is of importance since T helper cells involve in the differentiation of B cells and the production of autoantibodies in autoimmune diseases [29,30]. This may partially explain the fact that 48% of COVID-19 patients in Wuhan (total participants were 274) had anti-MDA5 antibody. Moreover, elevated titer of anti-MDA5 antibody indicated a poor prognosis [31]. A pathological mechanism that may stand behind the production of autoantibodies is molecular mimicry; the immune system may identify accidently selfproteins as viral, since those proteins contain similar peptide sequences as the virus, in such manner autoantibodies are produced and act against self and subsequently lead to a tissue damage and dysregulation of the immune system [32].

The uncontrolled production of inflammatory mediators in COVID19 disease leads to a systemic condition termed cytokine storm which assumed to be triggered by viral infection, this condition has also been described previously in SARS and MERS respiratory outbreaks [33]. It is not surprising to find cytokine storm in patients with anti-MDA5-positive CADM as this disease thought to be linked to viral infection [2]. Eventually cytokine storm reflects the dysregulation of the immune system [33], an excessive immune response is a potential cause of fatality and may explain the high mortality rate in both COVID-19 disease and anti-MDA5-positive CADM.

Immunomodulatory therapies for COVID-19 disease and anti-MDA5-positive CADM

So far, the therapeutic approach for anti-MDA5-positive CADM included the combination of glucocorticoids and calcineurin inhibitors and in some cases with the addition of intravenous cyclophosphamide or mycophenolate mofetil. The mortality rate following these therapies was reported as 40% [34]. For refractory cases with rapid ILD, polymyxin B hemoperfusion, veno-venous extracorporeal membrane oxygenation, and lung transplantation have been suggested as rescue therapies [35]. The benefit from those therapies is uncertain, and only few cases were reported as successful [35].

Since interferon signaling pathway plays essential role in both COVID-19 infection and anti-MDA5-positive CADM-associated IID, some lessons can be learned regarding immunomodulatory therapies for those diseases. The interferon signaling pathway can be modulated by the use of Ineterlukin (IL) six and IL1 receptors antagonists, antitumor necrosis alpha, and Janus kinase (JAK) inhibitors. For example, administration of JAK inhibitors named Tofacitinib and Ruxolitinib led to a lower expression of MDA5 and improvement of six-month survival rate in Japanese patients with anti-MA5-positive CADM-associated ILD [34,36]. The use of JAK inhibitors for COVID-19 disease is still in question because of the development of serious side effects [37]. Following administration of IL1 and IL6 receptors antagonists, pulmonary function of severe COVID-19 patients was improved [37]. Only little evidence exists regarding the use of IL1 antagonist for anti-MDA5-positive CADM, according to it, IL1 antagonist can be helpful for refractory cases [38]. Some studies report the beneficial effects of Interferon beta treatment for COVID-19 patients [37].

The therapeutic effects of intravenous immunoglobulin both for anti-MDA5-positive CADM with ILD and COVID-19 are inconsistent [34,37]. Plasma exchange found to be beneficial in both diseases [35,37].

Conclusion

COVID-19 disease and anti-MDA5 dermatomyositis share similarities on clinical, radiological, and laboratory levels. Those observations together with the identification of anti-MDA5 antibodies in sera of COVID-19-positive patients allude for a common immunogenic basis. The common pathophysiological denominator in both diseases is the cytokine storm. The exact role of anti-MDA5 in COVID-19 disease is uncertain. Still molecular phenomena such as epitope spreading or molecular mimicry may take place in the immunopathology of both diseases. The identification of common immunopathological mechanisms directs us in the way to find potential therapeutic strategies for both COVID-19 disease and anti-MDA5-positive CADM.

References

[1] Goubau D, Deddouche S, Reis e Sousa C. Cytosolic sensing of viruses. Immunity 2013;38(5):855–69. https://doi.org/10.1016/j.immuni.2013.05.007.

[2] Sadler AJ. The role of MDA5 in the development of autoimmune disease. J Leukoc Biol 2017;103(2). https://doi.org/10.1189/jlb.4mr0617-223r. jlb.4MR0617-223R.

[3] Dias Junior AG, Sampaio NG, Rehwinkel J. A balancing act: MDA5 in antiviral immunity and autoinflammation. Trends Microbiol 2019;27(1):75–85. https://doi.org/10.1016/j.tim.2018.08.007.

[4] Kang DC, Gopalkrishnan RV, Wu Q, Jankowsky E, Pyle AM, Fisher PB. mda-5: an interferon-inducible putative RNA helicase with double-stranded RNA-dependent ATPase activity and melanoma growth-suppressive properties. Proc Natl Acad Sci USA 2002;99(2):637–42. https://doi.org/10.1073/pnas.022637199.

[5] Funabiki M, Kato H, Miyachi Y, et al. Autoimmune disorders associated with gain of function of the intracellular sensor MDA5. Immunity 2014;40(2):199–212. https://doi.org/10.1016/j.immuni.2013.12.014.

[6] Sato S, Hirakata M, Kuwana M, et al. Autoantibodies to a 140-kd polypeptide, CADM-140, in Japanese patients with clinically amyopathic dermatomyositis. Arthritis Rheum 2005;52(5):1571–6. https://doi.org/10.1002/ART.21023.

[7] Zohar DN, Seluk L, Yonath H, Shoenfeld Y, Kivity S. Anti-MDA5 positive dermatomyositis associated with rapidly progressive interstitial lung disease and correlation between serum ferritin level and treatment response. Mediterranean J Rheumatol 2020;31(1):75. https://doi.org/10.31138/MJR.31.1.75.

[8] Koga T, Fujikawa K, Horai Y, et al. The diagnostic utility of anti-melanoma differentiation-associated gene 5 antibody testing for predicting the prognosis of Japanese patients with DM. Rheumatology 2012;51(7):1278–84. https://doi.org/10.1093/RHEUMATOLOGY/KER518.

[9] ichiro MS, Sekiguchi A, Toki S, et al. Clinical features and poor prognostic factors of anti-melanoma differentiation-associated gene 5 antibody-positive dermatomyositis with rapid progressive interstitial lung disease. Eur J Dermatol: EJD 2019;29(5):511–7. https://doi.org/10.1684/EJD.2019.3634.

[10] Gupta R, Kumar S, Gow P, Chang L, Yen L. Anti-MDA5-associated dermatomyositis. Intern Med J 2020;50(4):484–7. https://doi.org/10.1111/IMJ.14789.

[11] The WHO-China Joint Mission on Coronavirus Disease 2019, World Health Organization (WHO). Report of the WHO-China joint mission on coronavirus disease 2019 (COVID-19). The WHO-China Joint Mission on Coronavirus Disease 2019 2020;1(16–24 February):1–40.

[12] Li X, Ma X. Acute respiratory failure in COVID-19: is it "typical" ARDS? Crit Care 2020;24(1). https://doi.org/10.1186/S13054-020-02911-9.

[13] Huang K, Vinik O, Shojania K, et al. Clinical spectrum and therapeutics in Canadian patients with anti-melanoma differentiation-associated gene 5 (MDA5)-positive dermatomyositis: a case-based review. Rheumatol Int 2019;39(11):1971–81. https://doi.org/10.1007/S00296-019-04398-2.

[14] Ye Z, Zhang Y, Wang Y, Huang Z, Song B. Chest CT manifestations of new coronavirus disease 2019 (COVID-19): a pictorial review. Eur Radiol 2020;30(8):1. https://doi.org/10.1007/S00330-020-06801-0.

[15] Tanizawa K, Handa T, Nakashima R, et al. HRCT features of interstitial lung disease in dermatomyositis with anti-CADM-140 antibody. Respir Med 2011;105(9):1380–7. https://doi.org/10.1016/J.RMED.2011.05.006.

[16] Xu W, Wu W, Zhang D, et al. A novel CT scoring method predicts the prognosis of interstitial lung disease associated with anti-MDA5 positive dermatomyositis. Sci Rep 2021;11(1). https://doi.org/10.1038/S41598-021-96292-W.

[17] Perricone C, Bartoloni E, Bursi R, et al. COVID-19 as part of the hyperferritinemic syndromes: the role of iron depletion therapy. Immunol Res 2020;68(4):213. https://doi.org/10.1007/S12026-020-09145-5.

[18] Shirakashi M, Nakashima R, Tsuji H, et al. Efficacy of plasma exchange in anti-MDA5-positive dermatomyositis with interstitial lung disease under combined immunosuppressive treatment. Rheumatology 2020;59(11):3284–92. https://doi.org/10.1093/RHEUMATOLOGY/KEAA123.

[19] Gono T, Kaneko H, Kawaguchi Y, et al. Cytokine profiles in polymyositis and dermatomyositis complicated by rapidly progressive or chronic interstitial lung disease. Rheumatology 2014;53(12). https://doi.org/10.1093/RHEUMATOLOGY/KEU258.

[20] Kim JS, Lee JY, Yang JW, et al. Immunopathogenesis and treatment of cytokine storm in COVID-19. Theranostics 2021;11(1):316–29. https://doi.org/10.7150/THNO.49713.

[21] Mandel M, Harari G, Gurevich M, Achiron A. Cytokine prediction of mortality in COVID19 patients. Cytokine 2020;134:155190. https://doi.org/10.1016/J.CYTO.2020.155190.

[22] Lee JY, Bae S, Myoung J. Middle East respiratory syndrome coronavirus-encoded accessory proteins impair MDA5-and TBK1-mediated activation of NF-κB. J Microbiol Biotechnol 2019;29(8):1316–23. https://doi.org/10.4014/JMB.1908.08004.

[23] Lee JY, Bae S, Myoung J. Middle East respiratory syndrome coronavirus-encoded ORF8b strongly antagonizes IFN-β promoter activation: its implication for vaccine design. J Microbiol 2019;57(9):803–11. https://doi.org/10.1007/S12275-019-9272-7.

[24] Kindler E, Thiel V, Weber F. Interaction of SARS and MERS coronaviruses with the antiviral interferon response. Adv Virus Res 2016;96:219. https://doi.org/10.1016/BS.AIVIR.2016.08.006.

[25] Hadjadj J, Yatim N, Barnabei L, et al. Impaired type I interferon activity and inflammatory responses in severe COVID-19 patients. Science (New York, NY) 2020;369(6504):718–24. https://doi.org/10.1126/SCIENCE.ABC6027.

[26] Rebendenne A, Chaves Valadão AL, Tauziet M, et al. SARS-CoV-2 triggers an MDA-5-dependent interferon response which is unable to control replication in lung epithelial cells. J Virol 2021;95(8). https://doi.org/10.1128/JVI.02415-20.

[27] Setaro AC, Gaglia MM. All hands on deck: SARS-CoV-2 proteins that block early anti-viral interferon responses. Current Research in Virological Science 2021;2:100015. https://doi.org/10.1016/J.CRVIRO.2021.100015.

[28] Liu G, Lee JH, Parker ZM, et al. ISG15-dependent activation of the RNA sensor MDA5 and its antagonism by the SARS-CoV-2 papain-like protease. bioRxiv: The Preprint Server for Biology 2020. https://doi.org/10.1101/2020.10.26.356048. Published online October 27.

[29] Circulating TFH cells is correlated with disease activity in anti-MDA5 antibody positive idiopathic inflammatory myopathies—PubMed. 2021. https://pubmed.ncbi.nlm.nih.gov/32896262/. [Accessed 30 November 2021].

[30] Meckiff BJ, Ramírez-Suástegui C, Fajardo V, et al. Imbalance of regulatory and cytotoxic SARS-CoV-2-reactive CD4+ T cells in COVID-19. Cell 2020;183(5):1340. https://doi.org/10.1016/J.CELL.2020.10.001.

[31] Liu C, Wang Q, Wang Y, et al. Analysis of the correlation between anti-MDA5 antibody and the severity of COVID-19: a retrospective study. medRxiv. Published online August 11, 2020:2020.07.29.20164780. 10.1101/2020.07.29.20164780.

[32] Ehrenfeld M, Tincani A, Andreoli L, et al. Covid-19 and autoimmunity. Autoimmun Rev 2020;19(8):102597. https://doi.org/10.1016/J.AUTREV.2020.102597.

[33] Ryabkova VA, Churilov LP, Shoenfeld Y. Influenza infection, SARS, MERS and COVID-19: cytokine storm—the common denominator and the lessons to be learned. Clin Immunol (San Diego, CA, U S) 2021;223:108652. https://doi.org/10.1016/J.CLIM.2020.108652.

[34] Nombel A, Fabien N, Coutant F. Dermatomyositis with anti-MDA5 antibodies: bioclinical features, pathogenesis and emerging therapies. Front Immunol 2021;12. https://doi.org/10.3389/FIMMU.2021.773352.

[35] Selva-O'Callaghan A, Romero-Bueno F, Trallero-Araguás E, et al. Pharmacologic treatment of anti-MDA5 rapidly progressive interstitial lung disease. Curr Treatment Opt Rheumatol 2021. https://doi.org/10.1007/S40674-021-00186-X. Published online December 28.

[36] Chen Z, Wang X, Ye S. Tofacitinib in amyopathic dermatomyositis-associated interstitial lung disease. N Engl J Med 2019;381(3):291–3. https://doi.org/10.1056/NEJMC1900045.

[37] Rizk JG, Kalantar-Zadeh K, Mehra MR, Lavie CJ, Rizk Y, Forthal DN. Pharmaco-immunomodulatory therapy in COVID-19. Drugs 2020;80(13):1. https://doi.org/10.1007/S40265-020-01367-Z.

[38] Interleukin-1 receptor antagonist for refractory anti-MDA5 clinically amyopathic dermatomyopathy—PubMed. Accessed December 1, 2021. https://pubmed.ncbi.nlm.nih.gov/26343354/.

CHAPTER

15

Humoral immunity and thrombosis in COVID-19

G. Lasagni[1], *M.O. Borghi*[2,3], *M. Cugno*[1,4] *and P.L. Meroni*[2]

[1]Department of Pathophysiology and Transplantation, University of Milan, Milan, Italy; [2]Immunorheumatology Research Laboratory, IRCCS Istituto Auxologico Italiano, Milan, Italy; [3]Department of Clinical Sciences and Community Health, University of Milan, Milan, Italy; [4]Fondazione IRCCS Ca' Granda Ospedale Maggiore Policlinico, Internal Medicine and Angelo Bianchi Bonomi Hemophilia and Thrombosis Center, Milan, Italy

Introduction

Coronavirus disease 2019 (COVID-19) is due to severe acute respiratory syndrome coronavirus 2 (SARS-CoV-2) infection and is characterized by clinical symptoms ranging from minor upper airway manifestations to severe and life-threatening acute respiratory distress syndrome (ARDS) [1–3]. COVID-19 displays heterogeneous clinical manifestations, which can be only in part directly related to the virus and largely due to the hyperinflammatory response. In addition, the patients display increased markers of coagulation activation and frequent thrombotic events affecting both medium/large arterial or venous vessels. Microvascular thrombosis has been also reported, which is mechanistically different from Disseminated Intravascular Coagulation [4–6].

COVID-19 coagulopathy is a model of immunothrombosis sustained by several mechanisms such as endothelial perturbation/activation, complement activation, hyperproduction of proinflammatory cytokines, increased neutrophil extracellular traps (NET) formation, monocyte and platelet activation, synthesis of procoagulant autoantibodies, impairment of the fibrinolysis and reduction of the levels of ADAMTS13 with a relative increase of large von Willebrand Factor (vWF) multimers [7–12].

Consistent with the evidence of increased circulating levels of markers of endothelial perturbation/activation, it has been suggested that the involvement of the endothelium plays a central role in sustaining the thrombophilic state [13–15].

Autoimmunity, COVID-19, Post-COVID19 syndrome and COVID-19 vaccination
https://doi.org/10.1016/B978-0-443-18566-3.00037-2

Although SARS-CoV-2 can infect the endothelium via the ACE2 receptor and Transmembrane serine protease 2 (TMPRSS2) expressed on the cell membrane and induce a prothrombotic phenotype by altering the balance of the angiotensin and bradykinin system [16,17], the evidence for such mechanism is still debated. In fact, whether SARS-CoV-2 directly infects endothelial cells (EC) remains a matter of controversy and discrepancies have been reported between SARS-CoV-2 tropism and cellular distribution of ACE2/TMPRSS2 [18]. So, additional players are thought to be involved. In particular, humoral mediators of innate and adaptive immunity have been suggested to contribute to the so-called COVID-19-associated immunothrombosis.

The present chapter will review the role of three main classes of humoral mediators supporting the thrombophilic state in COVID-19: the synthesis of nonorgan specific procoagulant autoantibodies, the hyper-production of proinflammatory cytokines, and the effect of complement activation products. The interaction among these mediators and their association with the clinical manifestations will be discussed as well.

Autoantibodies and thrombosis

Antiphospholipid antibodies

As stated before the presence of thrombotic microangiopathy and/or thrombotic events affecting medium/large arterial and venous vessels might worsen the morbidity and increase the mortality of COVID-19 [19,20]. Initial studies reported prolonged activated partial thromboplastin times and positivity for antiphospholipid antibody (aPL) assays, in particular Lupus Anticoagulant (LA). Both the clinical manifestations and the laboratory abnormalities are mimicking the picture of the antiphospholipid antibody syndrome (APS). Consistently, the issue of whether common pathogenic mechanisms were shared in common by APS and COVID-19 was raised [21,22].

The similarities between COVID-19, APS, and in particular the catastrophic variant (CAPS) are even more intriguing as summarized in the table. All these disorders are characterized by a proinflammatory environment supported by increased levels of proinflammatory cytokines and by the evidence of an increased activation rate of the complement cascade although at different degrees. Comparable cell types playing a key role in the coagulation cascade, such as platelets, monocytes, and neutrophils have been reported to be activated and associated with the proinflammatory and prothrombotic phenotype [5,23]. In particular, with the term "endothelitis" several authors underlined the presence of an endothelial perturbation responsible for the proadhesive (e.g., pro-inflammatory) and procoagulant endothelial phenotype as the common denominator of these diseases [13–15]. This similarity is more evident between the microangiopathy of the catastrophic APS (CAPS) and of COVID-19 [24,25] (Table 15.1).

The presence of ACE2 for entry and TMRPSS2 for S-protein priming/fusion on the endothelial membrane supported the hypothesis of the SARS-CoV-2 endothelial tropism/infection and its direct responsibility for EC perturbation. In fact, after SARS-CoV-2 binding, ACE2 is internalized, and the lack of ACE2 on EC favors the progression of inflammatory and thrombotic processes triggered by local angiotensin II (Ang II) hyperactivity. In addition, the

TABLE 15.1 The thrombophilic mechanisms described in APS, CAPS, and COVID-19

Thrombophilic mechanisms	APS	CAPS	COVID-19
Thrombotic microangiopathy	+/−	++	++
Endothelial activation	+	++	++
Monocyte activation	+	++	+
Platelet activation	+	++	++
Complement activation	+	+	++
NETosis	+/−	?	++
Pro-inflamm. Cytokines	+/−	++	++
Impaired fibrinolysis [29,30]	+	?	++
aPL	++	++	+/−

reduction of ACE2 levels limits the degradation of des-Arg9 bradykinin into inactive peptides, ultimately leading to increased prothrombotic signaling via the activation of bradykinin receptors [16,26,27]. However, both ACE2 and TMRPSS2 expression and SARS-CoV-2 endothelial tropism have been recently questioned, raising doubts about such a mechanism [18].

Besides the ability of proinflammatory cytokine (e.g., Interleukin [IL]-6) and complement activation products (i.e., C5a and C5b9) in mediating the endothelitis [13–15,28,29], additional potential mediators of endothelial perturbation have been suggested. In particular, aPL has been thought to play a role because of their well-known ability to bind and activate endothelium in the APS [30] (Fig. 15.1).

Antiphospholipid antibodies are identified by functional PL-dependent coagulation test (i.e., LA test) and by solid-phase assays detecting antibodies against beta2 glycoprotein I (β2GPI) (i.e., β2GPI-dependent anticardiolipin [aCL] and anti-β2GPI assays) or against prothrombin (PT) complexed with phosphatidylserine (PS) (i.e., aPS-PT). These two last families of autoantibodies are responsible for the large majority of the positive LA [31]. Several papers reported positive aPL tests in COVID-19 patients, but both the inclusion criteria and the laboratory results are quite heterogeneous, making it very difficult to draw conclusive remarks. Moreover, their clinical association with thrombotic events and their eventual impact on the clinical outcome of COVID-19 did not clearly emerge even in a recent meta-analysis and systematic review [32].

Since several variables can affect the reproducibility of LA, specific recommendations have been made by the International Society of Thrombosis and Hemostasis to avoid misinterpretation. In fact, concomitant anticoagulant therapy (e.g., heparin) and systemic inflammation with high CRP plasma levels are well-known factors responsible for LA's false-positive results [33,34]. Both conditions are very frequently met in the course of COVID-19. This is not the case for the aPL solid-phase tests that are not affected by these variables. Positive LA in the absence of anti-β2GPI and aPS/PT antibodies is widely thought to display a low

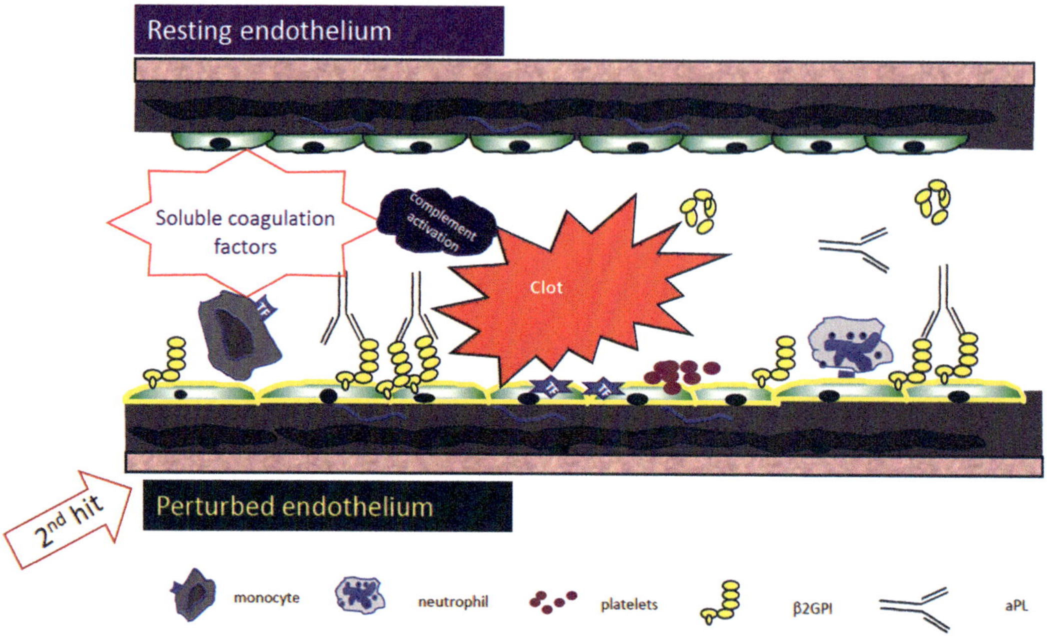

FIGURE 15.1 Antiphospholipid antibody-mediated immunothrombosis. The antibodies are mainly directed against β2GPI in the "open/activated" configuration, which is present at a high density on the endothelium perturbed by the so-called "second hit". Once bound, aPL induces a proadhesive and a procoagulant endothelial phenotype that favors the expression of Tissue Factor (TF) on the endothelium itself and on adhering monocytes, neutrophil adhesion/activation, platelet aggregation, and ultimately clot formation. Complement activation by aPL and proinflammatory cytokine release by activated endothelium and the other involved cells contribute to triggering coagulation [30].

diagnostic and prognostic value in the setting of APS [35,36]. Consistent with this finding, the high frequency of isolated positive LA (and prolonged aPTT) in COVID-19 reduces its predictive value for thrombosis in line with the general assumption that the association between aPL and thrombosis is doubtful [32].

On the other hand, aPL production has been reported in other viral and nonviral infections [37]. So, the occurrence of aPL during SARS-CoV-2 infection is not surprising. However, as in the other infections, the antibodies found are not closely associated with the APS clinical manifestations [38,39].

Moreover, there is evidence that these aPL are transient, usually at medium/low titer, and frequently of the IgM isotype only [31,32]. These are serological characteristics usually associated with low diagnostic and predictive values in the APS setting [31]. Moreover, the β2GPI-dependent aPL was not directed against the domain (D) 1 immune-dominant epitope of the molecule but frequently against D4 [32,39]. While high titer of anti-β2GPI D1 IgG has been associated with the vascular manifestations of the syndrome, found in human tissues from APS patients with thrombosis, and reported to be thrombogenic in animal models, this was not the case for aPL against other domains of the molecule [30,40–42]. Altogether these findings are in line with the lack of an association between aPL and thrombosis in COVID-19 [23,32].

COVID-19 displays an acute form of systemic inflammation with complement activation responsible for endothelial perturbation [15]. It is widely accepted that such a condition increases the density of β2GPI on the activated endothelium, ultimately making the molecule more available to the pathogenic anti-β2GPI antibodies even at a low titer. A condition that has been described in obstetric APS where high quantities of β2GPI are physiologically expressed in the placenta [43,44]. So, the detection of transitory low-titer aPL, usually clinically irrelevant, in a disease with a strong inflammatory phenotype raises the issue of whether or not these antibodies may increase the thrombophilic risk. This point is important to support or not the use of prophylactic or therapeutic heparin therapy during the recovery period or even in the post-COVID-19 follow-up [20]. In fact, if aPL is positive, the patients can theoretically be at higher risk for thrombosis, and prophylactic treatment should be considered. However, we do not have ad hoc clinical studies to support such a therapeutic approach.

In summary, the evidence for the role of aPL in the COVID-19 immunothrombosis is weak but aPL test in these patients should be critically taken into consideration for stratifying the patients at higher thrombophilic profiles.

Finally, the risk of clinical manifestations or the increase in aPL titers in patients suffering from full-blown APS and concomitant SARS-CoV-2 infection should be discussed in line with the hypothesis that immune response against the virus may trigger antibodies toward PL-binding proteins. Besides anecdotal case reports, a recent study showed that both the disease and the COVID-19 vaccination did not affect the aPL titer and were not associated with thrombotic events [45].

Antiplatelet factor 4 antibodies

Heparin-induced thrombocytopenia (HIT) is a severe complication of heparin therapy associated with thrombocytopenia and a high risk of thrombosis. HIT is caused by immune complexes containing antiplatelet factor 4 (PF4) IgG, which trigger platelet aggregation by interacting with the FcγRIIA on the cell membrane. The diagnosis is based on the clinical symptoms (thrombosis, thrombocytopenia), on the demonstration of circulating anti-PF4 immunoglobulins, and the ability of the serum IgG to induce platelet aggregation in vitro [46] (Fig. 15.2).

The thrombotic microangiopathy, the frequent thrombocytopenia, and the large use of heparin anticoagulation have raised the risk of HIT diagnosis during COVID-19. Although some cases of HIT confirmed by platelet aggregation functional test (e.g., serotonin release assay) have been reported, such a mechanism does not seem to play a major role in COVID-19 thrombophilia [47–50].

However, there is evidence of the occurrence of relatively high titers of anti-PF4 immunoglobulins in patients with COVID-19 and clinical signs reminiscent of HIT but without confirmatory positive platelet aggregating tests [51]. The occurrence of immunoglobulins against PF4 but with negative platelet aggregation in vitro assays, no thrombocytopenia or thrombotic events, and no heparin therapy has been reported in other conditions as well. These autoantibodies have been defined as "false-positive tests for HIT" because they are not associated with HIT-related manifestations and do not trigger in vitro platelet activation, despite the fact that most of them display an in vitro heparin-dependent binding activity even in the

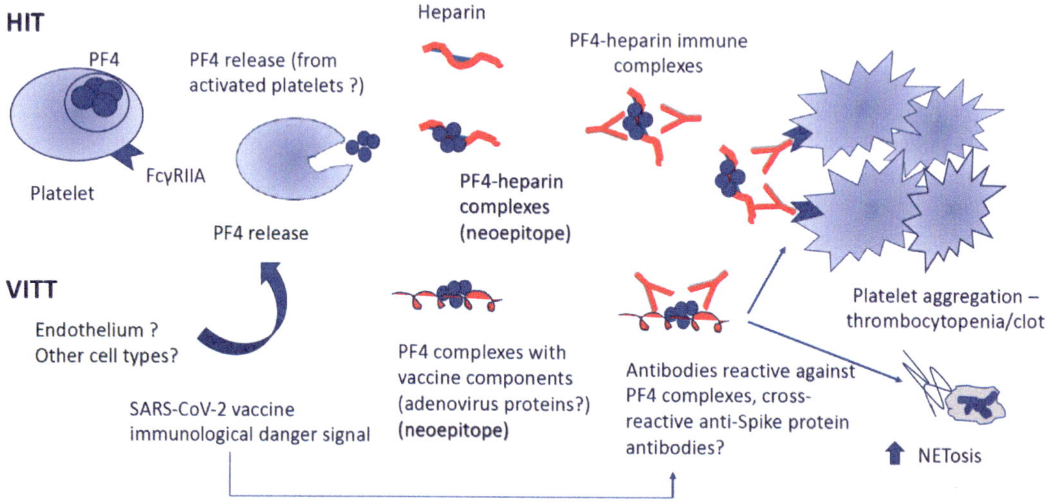

FIGURE 15.2 Heparin-induced thrombocytopenia (HIT) and COVID-19 vaccination-induced immune thrombotic thrombocytopenic syndrome (VITT). The released PF4 from activated platelets might form complexes with heparin in the HIT, ultimately expressing PF4 neo-epitopes that trigger the production of high avidity anti-PF4 immunoglobulins. PF4-heparin-IgG complexes induce platelet aggregation via the engagement of the FcγRIIA. A similar mechanism has been suggested for VITT: PF4 complexes with adenovirus components, in association with the vaccination "danger signal" to the immune system, might trigger the production of high avidity anti-PF4 IgG. The antibodies aggregate platelets and increase neutrophil activation/NETosis, all cooperating in platelet aggregation and clotting [46,63].

absence of heparin treatment [45,52–58]. These so-called "innocent" anti-PF4 immunoglobulins have been described in patients with non-SARS-CoV-2 infectious disorders, in critically ill patients (especially on extracorporeal circuits—ECMO), in systemic autoimmune conditions (e.g., Systemic Lupus Erythematosus [SLE], APS), and even in apparently healthy subjects. Innocent anti-PF4 immunoglobulins are usually at lower titer than those found in full-blown HIT and are always negative in the platelet in vitro activation tests [45,52–58].

The reason why antibodies against PF4 are produced is still a matter of research. Molecular mimicry between self-autoantigens and SARS-CoV-2 spike (S) protein was initially suggested but not completely demonstrated. Alternatively, PF4 released by platelets may form complexes with vaccine components eventually expressing a neo-epitope that can trigger a specific immune response. Ultimately, the formed IgG immune complexes can be responsible for platelet aggregation and clotting [59–63] (Fig. 15.2). This would explain the pathogenesis of the thrombosis with thrombocytopenia after COVID-19 adenovirus-based vaccination (VITT) characterized by the presence of anti-PF4 antibodies active in platelet aggregation assay [64–67]. Accordingly, the issue of a potential thrombophilic danger of COVID-19 vaccination in patients with preexisting anti-PF4 antibodies associated with the underlying disease (such as SLE and APS) was raised. This apparently does not seem to be the case since a recent study showed that vaccination against COVID-19 does not trigger the ex-novo production of anti-PF4 antibodies nor affect the titer of preexisting antibodies in positive SLE/APS patients. More importantly, vaccination does not enable these antibodies to cause platelet activation in vitro. Comparable data were found in a large group of healthcare workers vaccinated with RNA- or adenovirus-based vaccines [45].

In summary, anti-PF4 antibodies mediating a pathogenetic mechanism similar to that described in HIT or in VITT are not usually found in COVID-19 patients. This finding further emphasizes the role of different mechanisms in supporting thrombotic microangiopathy.

Pro-inflammatory cytokines and thrombosis

The cytokine release syndrome

Since the early spread of SARS-Cov-2, patients with severe-to-critical disease display a dysregulated hyperactivation of the immune system characterized by high levels of proinflammatory cytokines, such as IL-6, IL-1β, TNF-α, IL-8, and granulocyte-macrophage colony-stimulating factor (GM–CSF). Such response has been referred to as a cytokine release syndrome rather than "cytokine storm," since recent evidence suggests that the cytokine levels are lower than those reported in patients with the true "cytokine storm" after chimeric antigen receptor (CAR) T-cell therapy [1,68].

SARS-CoV-2 infection induces a prothrombotic state characterized by increased D-dimer, fibrinogen, and vWF levels, and is associated with a relatively modest decrease in platelet count and prolongation of the prothrombin time. Such prothrombotic state is reminiscent of the process known as immunothrombosis, originally defined to describe an innate immune response induced by intravascular thrombi, in particular microvessels, supported by immune cells and by coagulation factors to stop the spread and survival of invading pathogens. If uncontrolled, immunothrombosis can be responsible for organ damage similar to that described in Covid-19 [12,69].

Dysregulated proinflammatory cytokines play an important role in the immunothrombosis process, through the interaction with various components of the coagulation pathway, including EC, platelets, monocytes, and soluble coagulation factors [69].

Cytokines and the endothelium

Vascular EC is actively involved in hemostasis, preserving vascular integrity, controlling coagulation homeostasis by anticoagulant factors, fibrinolysis, and preventing platelet adhesion. However, when stimulated by proinflammatory cytokines or neutrophil extracellular traps, EC may display a proadhesive/inflammatory and procoagulant phenotype, associated with vascular leakage, tissue injury, and immunothrombosis. Proinflammatory cytokines, such as TNF-α and IL-1, modulate the expression of adhesion molecules promoting the endothelial adhesion of activated neutrophils and monocytes and eventually contributing to endothelial injury [70–72].

The same cytokines (IL-1, IL-6, and TNF-α) can stimulate EC to secrete ultralarge vWF (UL-vWF) and P-selectin from the Weibel–Palade (WP) bodies, that in turn are mediating platelet adhesion [9]. Furthermore, IL-6 significantly inhibits the rate of the cleavage of UL-vWF strings by ADAMTS13 leading to the accumulation of hyperreactive ULvWF multimers that aggregate platelets and leukocytes on the endothelium [73]. IL-6 itself also increases vascular permeability and promotes the secretion of proinflammatory cytokines in an autocrine way, thereby amplifying their release [16].

Additionally, proinflammatory cytokines can cause the reduced synthesis of glycosaminoglycans (GAGs), such as heparan sulfate on the endothelial surface. Since glycosaminoglycans act as physiologic heparin-like cofactors promoting the antithrombin (AT) activity, their reduced synthesis may contribute to impaired AT function [74].

Cytokines and their effect on platelets and neutrophils

Besides its role in hemostasis, platelets also act as proinflammatory cells. There is evidence that inflammatory cytokines such as TNF-α, IL-6, and IL-8 can activate platelets. However, activated platelets themselves are also an important source of proinflammatory cytokines, consistent with the cross-talk between inflammation and coagulation [75]. IL-6 has been shown to promote megakaryocyte proliferation and maturation, and it acts also on hepatocytes to increase the production and release of thrombopoietin (TPO), a potent stimulant of platelet production. IL-6 administration results in a significant increase in platelet count and modification of their function (e.g., enhanced thrombin-induced platelet activation) [76,77]. TNF-α induces molecular and metabolic reprogramming associated with platelet's mitochondrial dysfunction and hyperactivity [78]. IL1β, through IL1R1, enhances megakaryocyte maturation and switches the platelet RNA toward a proinflammatory and prothrombotic profile [79].

On the other hand, cytokines such as IL1 β, TNF-α and IL-8 are known to trigger neutrophil extracellular traps (NET) formation. NETosis is emerging as one of the main contributors to the neutrophil-related thromboinflammation in Covid-19. In particular, NET may provide the scaffold for platelet entrapment and subsequent activation through vWF or histones present in NET (especially H3 and H4) [80,81].

Cytokines and the coagulation cascade

Blood coagulation and inflammation closely interact in providing a defense against a variety of potentially injurious stimuli, such as infections and tissue damage [69]. Indeed, proinflammatory cytokines, like IL-1, IL-6, and TNF-α, induce the expression of tissue factor (TF), a potent promoter of thrombin generation through direct activation of factor X by the TF-factor VIIa complex. That complex, in turn, can interact with a protease-activated receptor (PAR) leading to the production of proinflammatory cytokines like TNF-α, IL-1, and IL-6, further emphasizing the link between inflammation and thrombosis [82–84]. IL-6, along with IL-8, has been shown to increase TF production and expression [85]. The effects of IL-6 on TF (including monocyte TF) may also be mediated indirectly through CRP, an acute-phase protein released by hepatocytes after IL-6 stimulation [86,87]. Moreover, other cytokines such as IL-1 and TNF-α as well as complement activation products (see paragraph n. 4) have been shown to contribute to TF upregulation on EC and monocytes.

Proinflammatory cytokines can also downregulate the natural anticoagulants such as AT, protein C (PC), and TF Pathway inhibitor (TFPA). Antithrombin is the main inhibitor of thrombin and its function can be impaired by proinflammatory cytokines through a reduced synthesis of GAGs on the EC surface, as described previously [74]. Protein C is activated by thrombin bound to EC membrane-associated thrombomodulin (TM). Activated protein C (APC) with its cofactor protein S (PS) inactivates FVa and FVIIIa. Moreover, APC displays profibrinolytic activity by neutralizing PAI-1 activity and antiinflammatory effect through the binding to the endothelial protein C receptor (EPCR) [88]. TNF-α and IL-1, down-regulate TM and EPCR on the endothelial surface reducing the capacity of the endothelium to activate protein C. In addition, proinflammatory cytokines down-regulate the mRNA for PC in the liver [89,90]. IL-6 plays a major role in the modulation of the acute-phase proteins, including C4b-binding protein (C4B-BP). Increased plasma levels of C4b binding protein in inflammatory diseases may result in a relative PS deficiency, due to decreased levels of free PS, which further can induce a prothrombotic state [90].

Proinflammatory cytokines, in particular IL-8, can also contribute to the NET formation in COVID-19, which in turn may support immunothrombosis as previously discussed. More specifically, NETs bind to TF leading to TF-mediated thrombin generation through the extrinsic pathway. Neutrophil extracellular traps have also been shown to bind to factor XII (Hageman factor), leading to its activation and prompting the direct activation of the contact pathway of coagulation. On the other hand, neutrophil elastase and serine proteases cleave and inactivate anticoagulants, including TF pathway inhibitor (TFPI) and thrombomodulin [91].

Cytokines and altered fibrinolysis

Plasmin is the active end-enzyme of the fibrinolytic system, able to degrade fibrin clots. As such, the fibrinolytic system can be considered a natural anticoagulant system that seeks to protect the host against excessive clotting. The activation of plasminogen to plasmin is mediated by tissue type and urokinase-type plasminogen activators (t-PA and u-PA). The main inhibitor of both t-PA and u-PA is plasminogen activator inhibitor type 1 (PAI-1). The initial acute fibrinolytic response in inflammation is characterized by an early release of tPA, followed by a rapid increase of PAI-1 levels, leading to an important decline in plasma tPA activity. Proinflammatory cytokines such as TNF-α and IL-1β are the main regulators of PAI-1 activity, stimulating the production of PAI-1 in vascular EC [92]. In vitro stimulation of vascular EC with low amounts of TNF-α suppresses t-PA gene expression, impairing the fibrinolytic system [93].

In summary, the increased production of proinflammatory cytokines plays a critical role in supporting the procoagulant phenotype in COVID-19 by affecting several cell types as well as the soluble factors involved in clotting and fibrinolysis.

Targeting the cytokine pathway

Consistent with the role of proinflammatory cytokines in the pathogenesis of COVID-19, there is evidence that the use of glucocorticoids, in particular dexamethasone, can decrease mortality of patients requiring supplemental oxygen, noninvasive or mechanical ventilation [94,95].

In line with the association between high IL-6 levels and the disease severity, the combination of glucocorticoids and tocilizumab has been shown to reduce disease progression and mortality in severe COVID-19 patients [94,95].

Janus kinase (JAK) inhibitors are drugs modulating immune responses through the inhibition of cytokine production (Fig. 15.3). The combination of glucocorticoids and two JAK inhibitors (baricitinib and tofacitinib) can be also considered in the therapeutic armamentarium since they might decrease disease progression and mortality in patients with COVID-19 requiring oxygen therapy, noninvasive ventilation, or high-flow oxygen [94,95].

Complement activation: endothelial perturbation and interaction with the coagulation cascade

The role of complement

The complement is a biological system that exerts a key role in the innate immune response, representing one of the first lines of the host defense against infectious agents, and it is also involved in the clearance of apoptotic cells [96,97]. The system consists of a large

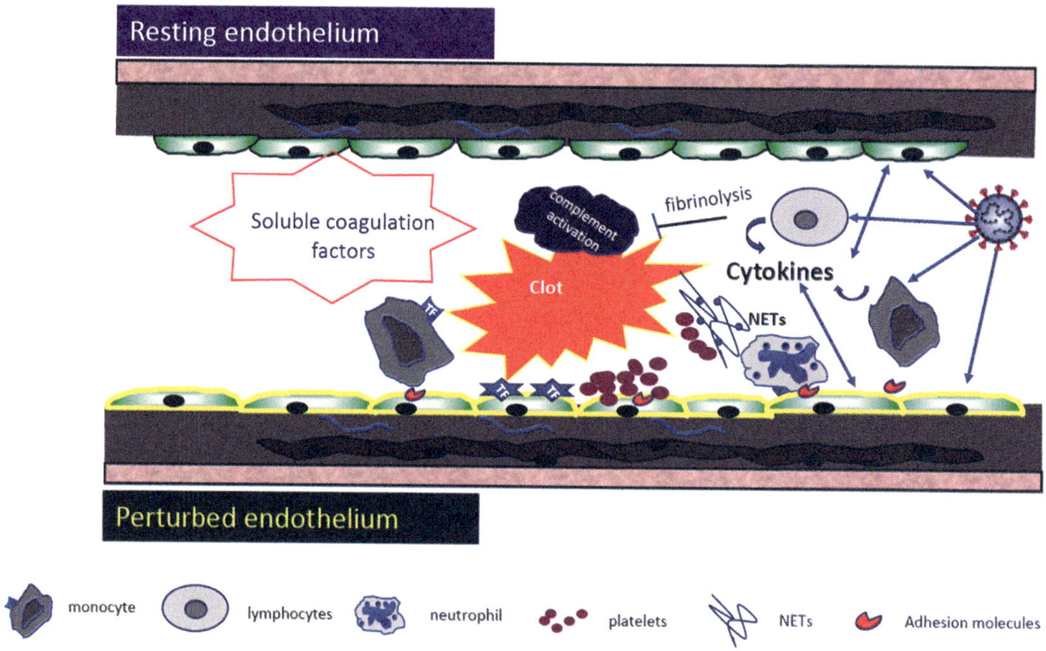

FIGURE 15.3 Cytokine release syndrome and immunothrombosis. SARS-CoV-2 infection might affect EC as well mononuclear cells (lymphocytes, monocytes) triggering the production of proinflammatory cytokines that in turn are responsible for the procoagulant and the proadhesive (inflammatory) phenotype on the EC, the mononuclear cells themselves, and on neutrophils. Activated neutrophils adhere to the endothelium and release extracellular traps (NETs). The proinflammatory milieu induces EC and monocytes tissue factor (TF) expression and favors platelet aggregation/adhesion. Altogether these steps contribute to the activation of the coagulation cascade further supported by complement activation and decreased fibrinolysis pathway.

number of soluble proteins that are present in circulating blood and in tissues. Complement components become activated through proteolytic cascades and work in a coordinated manner toward the activation of three pathways: the classical pathway triggered by antibody-antigen complexes, the alternative pathway by specific surface antigens, and the lectin pathway by binding mannose residues on the pathogen surface. The alternative pathway is constitutively active at a low level (tick-over mechanism) and this allows the system to stay primed for rapid and robust activation. The three pathways converge on the common pathway with the formation of strong inflammatory mediators, such as C3a and C5a, and the formation of the C5b-9 membrane attack complex (MAC) that lyses target cells [96–99].

The activation of the system, which may occur both on cell membranes and in the fluid phase, is controlled by inhibitor proteins synthesized by the liver. In particular, the main inhibitor of both the classical pathway and the lectin pathway is C1-inhibitor whereas the main inhibitors of the alternative pathway are factor I and factor H [99,100].

Complement activation, triggered by pathogen surfaces or immune complexes, elicits local inflammation and clearance mechanisms, including opsonization, chemotaxis, and phagocytosis.

Complement and coagulation cascade

The complement system plays a critical role in the activation of coagulation and the two systems may activate each other [100]. The crosstalk between complement and coagulation represents a defense mechanism but may lead to endothelial injury when the two systems are overactivated, and this condition promotes thrombosis and tissue damage [97,100]. The link between complement and the contact system of blood coagulation has important implications via the renin-angiotensin system in the control of vasodilation and vascular permeability as well [101].

Complement in COVID-19

In patients with COVID-19, from a theoretical point of view, complement activation may be useful in the first phases of viral infection but may become detrimental in the case of overactivation. In the last 2 years of the pandemic, several data from clinicopathological studies have supported the role of complement activation in determining the severity of COVID-19. In 2020, two very early studies showed complement activation in severe cases of COVID-19: the first provided evidence of deposition of the markers of complement activation C4d, C5b-9, and mannose-binding lectin (MBL)-associated serine protease (MASP)2 in the microvasculature of lesional lung tissue in autopsic samples of five patients died for COVID-19 [102]; the second study was from our group, showing increased levels of plasma C5a and soluble C5b-9 (sC5b-9) in 31 patients with moderate and severe COVID-19 (patients requiring continuous positive airway pressure and patients mechanically ventilated, respectively) [103]. Subsequently, the complement involvement in COVID-19 was confirmed by several studies. In particular, Macor et al. showed the deposition of complement components in lung lesions as well as in kidney and liver [104] in 12 patients who died of COVID-19 while the association between complement activation and severity of COVID-19 was confirmed by Holter et al. in 39 patients [105], by Carvelli et al. in 67 patients [106], by Peffault de Latour et al. in 95 patients [107], by de Nooijer et al. in 197 patients [108] and by our further study on 148 patients [15] in which we demonstrated a correlation with endothelial damage.

There is growing evidence that a common pathogenic denominator of the pulmonary and extrapulmonary lesion in COVID-19 is endotheliopathy, as supported by the increased plasma biomarkers of vascular injury [13]. In line with this, we found a significant increase in the plasma levels of vWF in our COVID-19 patients, with higher values observed in those with moderate and severe disease [15]. Interestingly, both humoral markers of complement activation and those of endothelial perturbation paralleled the severity of COVID-19 and normalized or drastically reduced after remission [15]. It has been reported that the terminal complement complex may induce a prothrombotic and proinflammatory endothelium phenotype and mediate vWF release not necessarily as a result of cell death [109]. Although these studies used in vitro models, it is possible to speculate that similar mechanisms take place in vivo, and if so, this would explain the correlation between complement activation and circulating vWF levels. Previous studies had shown that MAC is able to induce the release of vWF from ECs [110], which seems to be accompanied by an increase in procoagulant activity by the expression of tissue factor [111].

The TF is the main initiator of blood coagulation and can be increased also by the action of C5a on EC [112]. Moreover, the two serine proteases that initiate the lectin complement pathway, MASP-1, and MASP-2, can cleave prothrombin to form activated thrombin leading to the conversion of fibrinogen to fibrin [113]. On the other side, thrombin generated from the coagulation system can activate complement C3 and C5 independently [114]. Similarly, it has been reported the cleavage of C3 and C5, with the generation of C3a and C5a, respectively, by the coagulation factors FIXa, FXa, FXIa [115]. In addition, FXIIa has been shown to activate the C1qrs complex [116] and can be inhibited by the inhibitor of the first component of complement, i.e.,. a C1-inhibitor [117] that is also able to inhibit thrombin [118].

The activation of complement, observed in patients with severe acute lung injury during SARS- CoV-2 infection, may be triggered by viral components as shown by Gao et al. [119] who found that the nucleocapsid proteins of SARS- CoV-2 bind to MASP2, thereby activating the lectin pathway of the complement system and by Yu et al. who showed that the viral spike proteins can activate the alternative pathway of complement [120]. Recently, Jarlhert et al. showed that SARS-CoV-2 antibodies might drive significant activation of the classical complement pathway [121]; however, antibodies directed against other tissue molecules may be involved in complement activation, as suggested by immunofluorescence analyses of autopsy tissue specimens [104]. A genetic predisposition to complement activation was observed by our group in 72 patients with COVID-19, showing that the chromosome 3 cluster rs11385942 variant was associated with higher complement activation and more severe disease [122]. The increased C5a levels observed in patients with COVID-19 are consistent with the well-established role of C5a in promoting the lung sequestration of leukocytes and pulmonary dysfunction by causing transendothelial leukocyte migration and vascular leakage [123]. The neutrophils become activated and release neutrophil extracellular traps (NETs) that are networks of extracellular fibers, primarily composed of DNA. NETs can act as a scaffold for thrombus formation during coagulation [124]. Complement and neutrophil activation work in concert to drive severe COVID-19 manifestations by creating a coagulopathic milieu and therein generating microthrombi, a process that leads to acute lung, kidney, and cardiac injury [125].

In conclusion, the complement system may play an important role in the immune response to the infection by SARS- CoV-2 during acute lung injury, contributing to systemic inflammation, endotheliopathy, thrombosis, and multi-organ dysfunction. Preclinical and clinical studies indicate that the complement cascade should be targeted to reduce the pathophysiologic derangements driven by its overactivation. However, further research is necessary to better define the correct time of intervention for blocking the detrimental effects of complement without losing its benefits (Fig. 15.4).

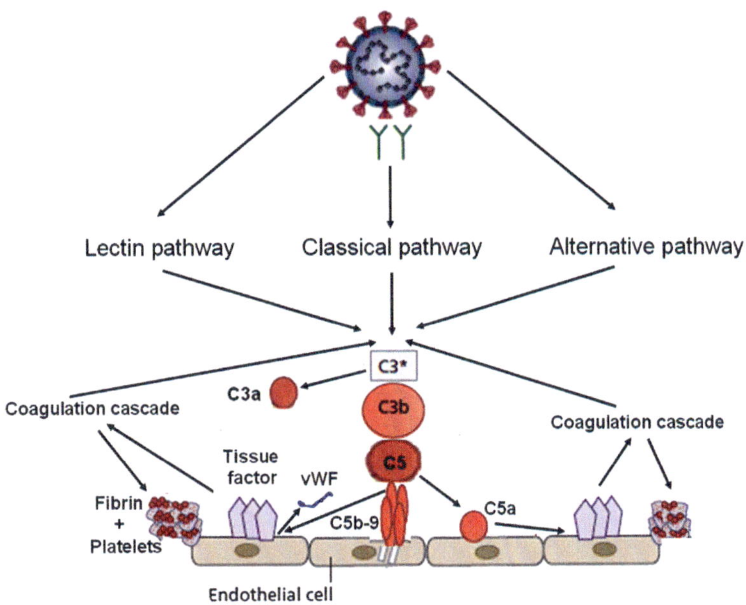

FIGURE 15.4 Complement activation by SARS-CoV-2 and its effect on endothelium and coagulation. The lectin pathway of complement is activated by nucleocapsid proteins of SARS- CoV-2, the alternative pathway is activated by viral spike proteins and the classical pathway by the complex between the spike proteins and the specific antibodies elicited by the viral infection. The three pathways converge on C3 and the subsequent activation leads to the formation of the terminal complex C5b-9 and the release of the anaphylatoxins C3a and C5a. C5b-9 and C5a stimulate the ECs to express tissue factor that is the main initiator of blood coagulation leading to the deposition of fibrin and platelets (i.e., thrombus formation). The coagulation cascade, in turn, can activate C3 and C5.

References

[1] Zhou F, Yu T, Du R, et al. Clinical course and risk factors for mortality of adult inpatients with COVID-19 in Wuhan, China: a retrospective cohort study [published correction appears in. Lancet 2020;395:1038.
[2] Zhu N, Zhang D, Wang W, et al. A novel coronavirus from patients with pneumonia in China, 2019. N Engl J Med 2020;382:727–33.
[3] Guan WJ, Ni ZY, Hu Y, et al. Clinical characteristics of coronavirus disease 2019 in China. N Engl J Med 2020;382:1708–20.
[4] Chen G, Wu D, Guo W, et al. Clinical and immunological features of severe and moderate coronavirus disease 2019. J Clin Invest 2020;130:2620–9.
[5] Tang N, Li D, Wang X, Sun Z. Abnormal coagulation parameters are associated with poor prognosis in patients with novel coronavirus pneumonia. J Thromb Haemostasis 2020;18:844–7.
[6] Tang N, Bai H, Chen X, Gong J, Li D, Sun Z. Anticoagulant treatment is associated with decreased mortality in severe coronavirus disease 2019 patients with coagulopathy. J Thromb Haemostasis 2020;18:1094–9.
[7] Lazzaroni MG, Piantoni S, Masneri S, et al. Coagulation dysfunction in COVID-19: the interplay between inflammation, viral infection and the coagulation system. Blood Rev 2021;46:100745.
[8] Cacciola R, Gentilini Cacciola E, Vecchio V, Cacciola E. Cellular and molecular mechanisms in COVID-19 coagulopathy: role of inflammation and endotheliopathy. J Thromb Thrombolysis 2021;112:1–9.
[9] Gando S, Wada T. Thromboplasminflammation in COVID-19 coagulopathy: three viewpoints for diagnostic and therapeutic strategies. Front Immunol 2021;12:649122.
[10] Portier I, Campbell RA, Denorme F. Mechanisms of immunothrombosis in COVID-19. Curr Opin Hematol 2021;28:445–53.
[11] Al-Gburi S, Beissert S, Günther C. Molecular mechanisms of vasculopathy and coagulopathy in COVID-19. Biol Chem 2021;402:1505–18.
[12] Bonaventura A, Vecchié A, Dagna L, et al. Endothelial dysfunction and immunothrombosis as key pathogenic mechanisms in COVID-19. Nat Rev Immunol 2021;21:319–29.
[13] Goshua G, Pine AB, Meizlish ML, et al. Endotheliopathy in COVID-19-associated coagulopathy: evidence from a single-centre, cross-sectional study. Lancet Haematol 2020;7:e575–82.
[14] Giordo R, Paliogiannis P, Mangoni AA, Pintus G. SARS-CoV-2 and endothelial cell interaction in COVID-19: molecular perspectives. Vasc Biol 2021;3:R15–23.
[15] Cugno M, Meroni PL, Gualtierotti R, et al. Complement activation and endothelial perturbation parallel COVID-19 severity and activity. J Autoimmun 2021;116:102560.
[16] Perico L, Benigni A, Casiraghi F, Ng LFP, Renia L, Remuzzi G. Immunity, endothelial injury and complement-induced coagulopathy in COVID-19. Nat Rev Nephrol 2021;17:46–64.
[17] Legrand M, Bell S, Forni L, et al. Pathophysiology of COVID-19-associated acute kidney injury. Nat Rev Nephrol 2021;17:751–64.
[18] Bernard I, Limonta D, Mahal LK, Hobman TC. Endothelium infection and dysregulation by SARS-CoV-2: evidence and caveats in COVID-19. Viruses 2020;13:29.
[19] Gu SX, Tyagi T, Jain K, et al. Thrombocytopathy and endotheliopathy: crucial contributors to COVID-19 thromboinflammation. Nat Rev Cardiol 2021;18:194–209.
[20] Hadid T, Kafri Z, Al-Katib A. Coagulation and anticoagulation in COVID-19. Blood Rev 2021;47:100761.
[21] Bowles L, Platton S, Yartey N, et al. Lupus anticoagulant and abnormal coagulation tests in patients with covid-19. N Engl J Med 2020;383:288–90.
[22] Zhang Y, Xiao M, Zhang S, et al. Coagulopathy and antiphospholipid antibodies in patients with covid-19. N Engl J Med 2020;382:38.
[23] Meroni PL, Borghi MO. Antiphospholipid antibodies and COVID-19 thrombotic vasculopathy: one swallow does not make a summer. Ann Rheum Dis 2021;80:1105–7.
[24] El Hasbani G, Taher AT, Jawad A, Uthman I. COVID-19, antiphospholipid antibodies, and catastrophic antiphospholipid syndrome: a possible association? Clin Med Insights Arthritis Musculoskelet Disord 2020;13. 1179544120978667.
[25] Previtali G, Seghezzi M, Moioli V, et al. The pathogenesis of thromboembolic disease in covid-19 patients: could be a catastrophic antiphospholipid syndrome? Thromb Res 2020;194:192–4.
[26] Ackermann M, Verleden SE, Kuehnel M, et al. Pulmonary vascular endothelialitis, thrombosis, and angiogenesis in covid-19. N Engl J Med 2020;e 383:120–8.

[27] Varga Z, Flammer AJ, Steiger P, et al. Endothelial cell infection and endotheliitis in COVID-19. Lancet 2020;395:1417–8.
[28] Colling ME, Kanthi Y. COVID-19-associated coagulopathy: an exploration of mechanisms. Vasc Med 2020;25:471–8.
[29] Chauhan AJ, Wiffen LJ, Brown TP. COVID-19: a collision of complement, coagulation and inflammatory pathways. J Thromb Haemostasis 2020;9:2110–7.
[30] Meroni PL, Borghi MO, Raschi E, Tedesco F. Pathogenesis of antiphospholipid syndrome: understanding the antibodies. Nat Rev Rheumatol 2011;7:330–9.
[31] Meroni PL, Borghi MO. Antiphospholipid antibody assays in 2021: looking for a predictive value in addition to a diagnostic one. Front Immunol 2021;12:726820.
[32] Taha M, Samavati L. Antiphospholipid antibodies in COVID-19: a meta-analysis and systematic review. RMD Open 2021;7:e001580.
[33] Martinuzzo ME, Barrera LH, D 'adamo MA, Otaso JC, Gimenez MI, Oyhamburu J. Frequent false-positive results of lupus anticoagulant tests in plasmas of patients receiving the new oral anticoagulants and enoxaparin. Int J Lab Hematol 2014;36:144–50.
[34] Schouwers SM, Delanghe JR, Devreese KM. Lupus Anticoagulant (LAC) testing in patients with inflammatory status: does C-reactive protein interfere with LAC test results? Thromb Res 2010:102–4. e125.
[35] Bertolaccini ML, Amengual O, Andreoli L, et al. 14th international congress on antiphospholipid antibodies task force. Report on antiphospholipid syndrome laboratory diagnostics and trends. Autoimmun Rev 2014;13:917–30.
[36] Pengo V, Bison E, Denas G, Jose SP, Zoppellaro G, Banzato A. Laboratory diagnostics of antiphospholipid syndrome. Semin Thromb Hemost 2018;44:439–44.
[37] Abdel-Wahab N, Talathi S, Lopez-Olivo MA, Suarez-Almazor ME. Risk of developing antiphospholipid antibodies following viral infection: a systematic review and meta-analysis. Lupus 2018:572–83. e27.
[38] Trahtemberg U, Rottapel R, Dos Santos CC, Slutsky AS, Baker A, Fritzler MJ. Anticardiolipin and other antiphospholipid antibodies in critically ill COVID-19 positive and negative patients. Ann Rheum Dis 2021;80:1236–40.
[39] Borghi MO, Beltagy A, Garrafa E, et al. Anti-phospholipid antibodies in COVID-19 are different from those detectable in the anti-phospholipid syndrome. Front Immunol 2020;11:584241.
[40] Meroni PL, Macor P, Durigutto P, et al. Complement activation in antiphospholipid syndrome and its inhibition to prevent rethrombosis after arterial surgery. Blood 2016;127:365–7.
[41] Durigutto P, Grossi C, Borghi MO, et al. New insight into antiphospholipid syndrome: antibodies to β2glycoprotein I-domain 5 fail to induce thrombi in rats. Haematologica 2019;104:819–26.
[42] Agostinis C, Durigutto P, Sblattero D, et al. A non-complement-fixing antibody to β2 glycoprotein I as a novel therapy for antiphospholipid syndrome. Blood 2014;29(123):3478–87.
[43] Agostinis C, Biffi S, Garrovo C, et al. In vivo distribution of β2 glycoprotein I under various pathophysiologic conditions. Blood 2011;118:4231–8.
[44] Pregnolato F, Gerosa M, Raimondo MG, et al. EUREKA algorithm predicts obstetric risk and response to treatment in women with different subsets of anti-phospholipid antibodies. Rheumatology 2021;60:1114–24.
[45] Lonati P, Bodio C, Scavone M, et al. The production of anti-PF4 antibodies in anti-phospholipid antibody-positive patients is not affected by COVID-19 vaccination. RMD Open.
[46] Arepally GM, Cines DB. Pathogenesis of heparin-induced thrombocytopenia. Transl Res 2020:131–40. e225.
[47] Riker RR, May TL, Fraser GL, et al. Heparin-induced thrombocytopenia with thrombosis in COVID-19 adult respiratory distress syndrome. Res Pract Thromb Haemost 2020;4:936–41.
[48] Patell R, Khan AM, Bogue T, et al. Heparin induced thrombocytopenia antibodies in Covid-19. Am J Hematol 2020. https://doi.org/10.1002/ajh.25935.
[49] Daviet F, Guervilly C, Baldesi O, et al. Heparin-induced thrombocytopenia in severe COVID-19. Circulation 2020;142:1875–7.
[50] Delrue M, Siguret V, Neuwirth M, et al. Contrast between prevalence of HIT antibodies and confirmed HIT in hospitalized COVID-19 patients: a prospective study with clinical implications. Thromb Haemostasis 2021;e 121:971–5.
[51] Brodard J, Kremer Hovinga JA, Fontana P, Studt JD, Gruel Y, Greinacher A. COVID-19 patients often show high-titer non-platelet-activating anti-PF4/heparin IgG antibodies. J Thromb Haemostasis 2021;19:1294–8.

[52] Martinuzzo ME, Forastiero RR, Adamczuk Y, Pombo G, Carreras LO. Antiplatelet factor 4–heparin antibodies in patients with antiphospholipid antibodies. Thromb Res 1999:271–9. e95.

[53] Pauzner R, Greinacher A, Selleng K, Althaus K, Shenkman B, Seligsohn U. False-positive tests for heparin-induced thrombocytopenia in patients with antiphospholipid syndrome and systemic lupus erythematosus. J Thromb Haemostasis 2009;7:1070–4.

[54] Alpert D, Mandl LA, Erkan D, Yin W, Peerschke EI, Salmon JE. Anti-heparin platelet factor 4 antibodies in systemic lupus erythematosus are associated with IgM antiphospholipid antibodies and the antiphospholipid syndrome. Ann Rheum Dis 2008:395–401. e67.

[55] Alpert DR, Salmon JE. False-positive tests for heparin-induced thrombocytopenia in patients with antiphospholipid syndrome and systemic lupus erythematosus: a rebuttal. J Thromb Haemostasis 2010;8:1439–41.

[56] Lasne D, Saffroy R, Bachelot C, et al. Tests for heparin-induced thrombocytopenia in primary antiphospholipid syndrome. Br J Haematol 1997:939. e97.

[57] Martin-Toutain I, Piette JC, Diemert MC, Faucher C, Jobic L, Ankri A. High prevalence of antibodies to platelet factor 4 heparin in patients with antiphospholipid antibodies in absence of heparin-induced thrombocytopenia. Lupus 2007;16:79–83.

[58] Satoh T, Tanaka Y, Okazaki Y, Kaburaki J, Ikeda Y, Kuwana M. Heparin-dependent and -independent anti-platelet factor 4 autoantibodies in patients with systemic lupus erythematosus. Rheumatology 2012;51:1721–8.

[59] Vojdani A, Vojdani E, Kharrazian D. Reaction of human monoclonal antibodies to SARS-CoV-2 proteins with tissue antigens: implications for autoimmune diseases. Front Immunol 2021:617089. e11.

[60] Kowarz E, Krutke L, Reis J, et al. Vaccine-Induced Covid-19 Mimicry Syndrome: splice reactions within the SARS-CoV-2 Spike open reading frame result in Spike protein variants that may cause thromboembolic events in patients immunized with vector-bas. Research Square preprint.

[61] Greinacher A, Selleng K, Mayerle J, et al. Anti-platelet factor 4 antibodies causing VITT do not cross-react with SARS-CoV-2 spike protein. Blood 2021;138:1269–77.

[62] Passariello M, Vetrei C, Amato F, De Lorenzo C. Interactions of spike-RBD of SARS-CoV-2 and platelet factor 4: new insights in the etiopathogenesis of thrombosis. Int J Mol Sci 2021;22:8562.

[63] Greinacher A, Selleng K, Palankar R, et al. Insights in ChAdOx1 nCoV-19 vaccine-induced immune thrombotic thrombocytopenia. Blood 2021;138:2256–68.

[64] Scully M, Singh D, Lown R, et al. Pathologic antibodies to platelet factor 4 after ChAdOx1 nCoV-19 vaccination. N Engl J Med 2021;384:2202–11.

[65] Greinacher A, Thiele T, Warkentin TE, Weisser K, Kyrle PA, Eichinger S. Thrombotic thrombocytopenia after ChAdOx1 nCov-19 vaccination. N Engl J Med 2021;384:2092–101.

[66] Schultz NH, Sørvoll IH, Michelsen AE, et al. Thrombosis and thrombocytopenia after ChAdOx1 nCoV-19 vaccination. N Engl J Med 2021;384:2124–30.

[67] Cattaneo M. Thrombosis with Thrombocytopenia Syndrome associated with viral vector COVID-19 vaccines. Eur J Intern 2021;89:22–4.

[68] Hay KA, Hanafi LA, Li D, et al. Kinetics and biomarkers of severe cytokine release syndrome after CD19 chimeric antigen receptor-modified T-cell therapy. Blood 2017;130:2295–306.

[69] Engelmann B, Massberg S. Thrombosis as an intravascular effector of innate immunity. Nat Rev Immunol 2013;e 13:34–45.

[70] Wang J, Doran J. The many faces of cytokine release syndrome-related coagulopathy. Clin Hematol Int 2021;3:3–12.

[71] Teuwen LA, Geldhof V, Pasut A, Carmeliet P. COVID-19: the vasculature unleashed. Nat Rev Immunol 2020;20:389–91.

[72] Libby P, Lüscher T. COVID-19 is, in the end, an endothelial disease. Eur Heart J 2020:3038–44. e41.

[73] Bernardo A, Ball C, Nolasco L, Moake JF, Dong JF. Effects of inflammatory cytokines on the release and cleavage of the endothelial cell-derived ultralarge von Willebrand factor multimers under flow. Blood 2004;104:100–6.

[74] Bourin MC, Lindahl U. Glycosaminoglycans and the regulation of blood coagulation. Biochem J 1993;289:313–30. Pt 2.

[75] Singh A, Bisht P, Bhattacharya S, Guchhait P. Role of platelet cytokines in dengue virus infection. Front Cell Infect Microbiol 2020;10:561366.

[76] Kerr R, Stirling D, Ludlam CA. Interleukin 6 and haemostasis. Br J Haematol 2001;115:3–12.

[77] Kulnigg-Dabsch S, Evstatiev R, Dejaco C, Gasche C. Effect of iron therapy on platelet counts in patients with inflammatory bowel disease-associated anemia. PLoS One 2012;7:e34520.

[78] Davizon-Castillo P, McMahon B, Aguila S, et al. TNF-α-driven inflammation and mitochondrial dysfunction define the platelet hyperreactivity of aging. Blood 2019;134:727–40.

[79] Beaulieu LM, Lin E, Mick E, et al. Interleukin 1 receptor 1 and interleukin 1β regulate megakaryocyte maturation, platelet activation, and transcript profile during inflammation in mice and humans. Arterioscler Thromb Vasc Biol 2014;34:552–64.

[80] Iliadi V, Konstantinidou I, Aftzoglou K, Iliadis S, Konstantinidis TG, Tsigalou C. The emerging role of neutrophils in the pathogenesis of thrombosis in COVID-19. Int J Mol Sci 2021;22:5368.

[81] Fuchs TA, Brill A, Duerschmied D, et al. Extracellular DNA traps promote thrombosis. Proc Natl Acad Sci USA 2010;107:15880–5.

[82] Osterud B, Rapaport SI. Activation of factor IX by the reaction product of tissue factor and factor VII: additional pathway for initiating blood coagulation. Proc Natl Acad Sci USA 1977;e 74:5260–4.

[83] Cugno M, Asero R, Tedeschi A, Lazzari R, Marzano AV. Inflammation and coagulation in urticaria and angioedema. Curr Vasc Pharmacol 2012;10:653–8.

[84] Witkowski M, Landmesser U, Rauch U. Tissue factor as a link between inflammation and coagulation. Trends Cardiovasc Med 2016;26:297–303.

[85] Neumann FJ, Ott I, Marx N, et al. Effect of human recombinant interleukin-6 and interleukin-8 on monocyte procoagulant activity. Arterioscler Thromb Vasc Biol 1997;17:3399–405.

[86] Ogasawara S, Daddona JL, Trimpert J, Stokol T. Effect of recombinant canine interleukin-6 and interleukin-8 on tissue factor procoagulant activity in canine peripheral blood mononuclear cells and purified canine monocytes. Vet Clin Pathol 2012;41:325–35.

[87] Cai H, Song C, Lim IG, Krilis SA, Geczy CL, McNeil HP. Importance of C-reactive protein in regulating monocyte tissue factor expression in patients with inflammatory rheumatic diseases. J. Rheumatol 2005;32:1224–31.

[88] Moore KL, Andreoli SP, Esmon NL, Esmon CT, Bang NU. Endotoxin enhances tissue factor and suppresses thrombomodulin expression of human vascular endothelium in vitro. J Clin Invest 1987;79:124–30.

[89] Yamamoto K, Shimokawa T, Kojima T, Loskutoff DJ, Saito H. Regulation of murine protein C gene expression in vivo: effects of tumor necrosis factor-alpha, interleukin-1, and transforming growth factor-beta. Thromb Haemostasis 1999;82:1297–301.

[90] Phillips DJ, Novinger MS, Evatt BL, Hooper WC. TNF-alpha suppresses IL-1 alpha and IL-6 upregulation of C4b-binding protein in HepG-2 hepatoma cells. Thromb Res 1996;81:307–14.

[91] Jayarangaiah A, Kariyanna PT, Chen X, Jayarangaiah A, Kumar A. COVID-19-Associated coagulopathy: an exacerbated immunothrombosis response. Clin Appl Thromb Hemost 2020;26. 1076029620943293.

[92] van der Poll T, de Jonge E, Levi M. Regulatory role of cytokines in disseminated intravascular coagulation. Semin Thromb Hemost 2001;27:639–51.

[93] Ulfhammer E, Larsson P, Karlsson L, et al. TNF-alpha mediated suppression of tissue type plasminogen activator expression in vascular endothelial cells is NF-kappaB- and p38 MAPK-dependent. J Thromb Haemostasis 2006;4:1781–9.

[94] Alunno A, Najm A, Machado PM, Bertheussen H, Burmester GR, Carubbi F, et al. EULAR points to consider on pathophysiology and use of immunomodulatory therapies in COVID-19. Ann Rheum Dis 2021;80:698–706.

[95] Alunno A, Najm A, Machado PM, et al. 21 more authors) (2021) EULAR points to consider on pathophysiology and use of immunomodulatory therapies in COVID-19. Ann Rheum Dis 2021;7. annrheumdis-2021-221366.

[96] Reis ES, Mastellos DC, Hajishengallis G, Lambris JD. New insights into the immune functions of complement. Nat Rev Immunol 2019;e 19:503–16.

[97] Holers VM. Complement and its receptors: new insights into human disease. Annu Rev Immunol 2014;32:433–59.

[98] Kaplan AP Ghebrehiwet B. The plasma bradykinin-forming pathways and its interrelationships with complement. Mol Immunol 2010;47:2161–9.

[99] Lachmann PJ. The story of complement factor. Immunobiology 2019;224:511–7.

[100] Foley JH. Examining coagulation-complement crosstalk: complement activation and thrombosis. Thromb Res 2016;2:S50–4.

[101] Bekassy Z, Lopatko Fagerström I, Bader M, Karpman D. Crosstalk between the renin-angiotensin, complement and kallikrein-kinin systems in inflammation. Nat Rev Immunol 2021;10:1–18 [Online ahead of print].

[102] Magro C, Mulvey JJ, Berlin D, et al. Complement associated microvascular injury and thrombosis in the pathogenesis of severe COVID-19 infection: a report of five cases. Transl Res 2020:1–13. e220.

[103] Cugno M, Meroni PL, Gualtierotti R, et al. Complement activation in patients with COVID-19: a novel therapeutic target. J Allergy Clin Immunol 2020;146:215–7.

[104] Macor P, Durigutto P, Mangogna A, et al. Multiple-organ complement deposition on vascular endothelium in COVID-19 patients. Biomedicines 2021;9:1003.

[105] Holter JC, Pischke SE, de Boer E, et al. Systemic complement activation is associated with respiratory failure in COVID-19 hospitalized patients. Proc Natl Acad Sci USA 2020;117:25018–25.

[106] Carvelli J, Demaria O, Vély F, et al. Association of COVID-19 inflammation with activation of the C5a-C5aR1 axis. Nature 2020;588:146–50.

[107] Peffault de Latour R, Bergeron A, Lengline E, et al. Complement C5 inhibition in patients with COVID-19 - a promising target? Haematologica 2020;105:2847–50.

[108] de Nooijer AH, Grondman I, Janssen NAF, et al. Complement activation in the disease course of coronavirus disease 2019 and its effects on clinical outcomes. J Infect Dis 2021;223:214–24.

[109] Riedl Khursigara M, Schlam D, Noone DG, et al. Vascular endothelial cells evade complement-mediated membrane injury via Weibel-Palade body mobilization. J Thromb Haemostasis 2020;18:1484–94.

[110] Hattori R, Hamilton KK, McEver RP, Sims PJ. Complement proteins C5b-9 induce secretion of high molecular weight multimers of endothelial von Willebrand factor and translocation of granule membrane protein GMP-140 to the cell surface. J Biol Chem 1989;264:9053–60.

[111] Tedesco F, Pausa M, Nardon E, Introna M, Mantovani A, Dobrina A. The cytolytically inactive terminal complement complex activates endothelial cells to express adhesion molecules and tissue factor procoagulant activity. J Exp Med 1997;185:1619–27.

[112] Ikeda K, Nagasawa K, Horiuchi T, Tsuru T, Nishizaka H, Niho Y. C5a induces tissue factor activity on endothelial cells. Thromb Haemostasis 1997;77:394–8.

[113] Krarup A, Wallis R, Presanis JS, Gál P, Sim RB. Simultaneous activation of complement and coagulation by MBL-associated serine protease 2. PLoS One 2007;2:e623.

[114] Huber-Lang M, Sarma JV, Zetoune FS, et al. Generation of C5a in the absence of C3: a new complement activation pathway. Nat Med 2006;12:682–7.

[115] Amara U, Flierl MA, Rittirsch D, et al. Molecular intercommunication between the complement and coagulation systems. J Immunol 2010;185:5628–36.

[116] Ghebrehiwet B, Silverberg M, Kaplan AP. Activation of the classical pathway of complement by Hageman factor fragment. J Exp Med 1981;153:665–76.

[117] de Agostini A, Lijnen HR, Pixley RA, Colman RW, Schapira M. Inactivation of factor XII active fragment in normal plasma. Predominant role of C-1-inhibitor. J Clin Invest 1984;73:1542–9.

[118] Cugno M, Bos I, Lubbers Y, Hack CE, Agostoni A. In vitro interaction of C1-inhibitor with thrombin. Blood Coagul Fibrinolysis 2001;12:253–60.

[119] Gao T, Hu M, Zhang X, et al. Highly pathogenic coronavirus N protein aggravates lung injury by MASP-2-mediated complement over-activation. medRxiv 2020. 2020.03.29.20041962.

[120] Yu J, Gerber GF, Chen H, Yuan X, Chaturvedi S, Braunstein EM, et al. Complement dysregulation is associated with severe COVID-19 illness. Haematologica May 1 2022;107(5):1095–105. https://doi.org/10.3324/haematol.2021.279155.

[121] Jarlhelt I, Nielsen SK, Jahn CXH, et al. SARS-CoV-2 antibodies mediate complement and cellular driven inflammation. Front Immunol 2021;12:767981.

[122] Valenti L, Griffini S, Lamorte G, et al. Chromosome 3 cluster rs11385942 variant links complement activation with severe COVID-19. J Autoimmun 2011;117:102595.

[123] Bosmann M, Ward PA. Role of C3, C5 and anaphylatoxin receptors in acute lung injury and in sepsis. Adv Exp Med Biol 2012;946:147–59.

[124] de Bont CM, Boelens WC, Pruijn GJM. NETosis, complement, and coagulation: a triangular relationship. Cell Mol Immunol 2019;16:19–27.

[125] Java A, Apicelli AJ, Liszewski MK, et al. The complement system in COVID-19: friend and foe? JCI Insight 2020;5:e140711.

CHAPTER

16

Peripheral nervous system manifestations associated with COVID-19

Tal Davidy and Ofir Zmira

Department of Neurology, Sheba Medical Center, Ramat Gan, Tel Hashomer, Israel affiliated to Sackler Faculty of Medicine, Tel Aviv University, Tel Aviv, Israel

Introduction

Severe acute respiratory syndrome coronavirus 2 (SARS-CoV-2) was first identified in Wuhan, China, in December 2019 and rapidly spread throughout the world [1]. The disease was named COVID-19 The World Health Organization declared it as a pandemic on the 11th of March 2020 [2].

Nowadays, data on different aspects of the disease manifestations, pathology, transmission, prevention, and management strategies have started to emerge.

Although the virus affects the respiratory system [3], a large number of COVID-19 patients also have neurological symptoms which include headache, dizziness, hypogeusia, and neuralgia, encephalopathy, impaired consciousness, and complications such as acute cerebrovascular diseases, encephalitis, myelitis, neuropathy, and skeletal muscular injury [4].

In a retrospective review of 214 patients with COVID-19 in Wuhan, China, 36.5% had neurological symptoms, which were more common in patients with severe disease [5].

This review aimed to discusses the peripheral nervous system (PNS) manifestations and complications in COVID-19. The main purpose is to update the physicians about the possible neurological presentations and complications resulting from this novel virus infection, so that they can better prepared to treat them and improve patient outcomes.

Invasion of SARS-CoV-2 to the nervous system

The exact mechanism of SARS-CoV-2 neuroinvasion is not yet understood. However, there are several hypotheses that suggest routes of entry of the virus into the nervous system.

Autoimmunity, COVID-19, Post-COVID19 syndrome and COVID-19 vaccination
https://doi.org/10.1016/B978-0-443-18566-3.00018-9

Firstly, during the viremia phase of the illness, disruption of the blood–brain barrier may cause the virus to enter the brain directly [6]. Moreover, leukocytes may be infected and serve as a vector to transport the virus to the central nervous system (CNS). The lymphatic route is also considered to be a possible pathway for the virus to enter the CNS(6). Once the virus invades to the CNS, the first line of defense is the activation of microglia; the phagocytes of the brain [7].

Another mechanism of entry is related to the angiotensin converting enzyme-2 receptor.

Structurally, coronaviruses consist a single-stranded RNA within an envelope. Several glycoprotein projections are attached to the envelope. The envelope glycoproteins are crucial for viral entry into the host cell. The spike protein has an avid affinity for angiotensin converting enzyme-2 receptor (ACE-2) on human cells [8]. The ACE-2 receptor is widely distributed in the body [9]. The primary target is the ACE-2 receptor in respiratory epithelium. It is also presented on neural cells. SARS-CoV-2 particles may bind to ACE2 receptors expressed on neural cells, allowing for viral replication and destruction of neuronal tissue [10]. Hence, SARS-CoV-2 can attach multiply and damage neuronal tissue [11]. There is an evidence from animal studies conducted on mice that coronavirus infecting the neuron receptor in the nasal olfactory epithelium to reach the brain via axonal transport along the olfactory nerve or through the cribriform bone. It has been suggested that SARS-CoV-2 behaves in a similar manner [10,12]. Additionally, another possible transsynaptic route from the nasal respiratory epithelium to the brain via the trigeminal nerve branch has recently been hypothesized. A fast-axonal transport mechanism of vesicle transport moving the virus along microtubules back to neuronal cell bodies [13].

Neuropathology of SARS-CoV-2

Damage within the nervous system by SARS-CoV-2 might be caused directly by the virus or by the innate and adaptive immune responses to infection.

Severe COVID-19 induced pneumonia may result in systemic hypoxia, leading to brain damage. The contributory factors to this process include peripheral vasodilatation, hypercarbia, hypoxia, and anaerobic metabolism with accumulation of toxic compounds. These processes may result in neuronal swelling and brain edema which ultimately leads to neurological damage [14].

Furthermore, by attaching to ACE-2 receptors, the virus downregulates ACE-2 in targeted cells leads to the excess production of angiotensin II that promotes the inflammation, vasoconstriction, cell proliferation, and vascular leakage and pulmonary injury [15]. This situation also contributes to the hypoxic state. The virus can infect the PNS or CNS either by direct infection of nerve endings in the tissues and using axonal transport machinery to gain access to the CNS.

Immune-mediated injury associated with COVID-19 infection is mainly due to the cytokine storm that characterized by hyperactivation of the innate immune system with overproduction of inflammatory mediators such as cytokines, chemokines, as well as macrophages. The severe inflammation may cause damage to vital organs [16].

The virus can bind to toll-like receptors, enabling interleukin (IL)-1 synthesis and release. Activation of this receptor leads to a biochemical cascade which is followed by inflammasome activation. In addition, further release of IL-6 causes vascular leak, activation of both the complement and coagulation cascade and disseminated intravascular hyper coagulation [17].

Overproduction of cytokines by macrophages may enhance the inflammatory process and trigger large concentration of ferritin in the blood ("hyperferricemia") [16]. In addition, high levels of D-dimer and ferritin are markedly elevated and associated with poor prognosis [17], also indicated that activated microglia cells in the brain start the neuroinflammatory events [7].

Recently, autoantibodies have been reported in COVID-19 patients [18]. It has been suggested that molecular mimicry exists between COVID-19 and human components [19] and that COVID-19 patients tend to develop autoantibodies and autoimmune diseases [3,16,18].

Peripheral nervous system manifestations of SARS-CoV-2

Guillain–Barré syndrome

Guillain–Barré syndrome (GBS) is an autoimmune process that affects peripheral nerves and manifests with progressive motor weakness, sensory changes, dysautonomia, and areflexia, and facial weakness. Viral infections (e.g., influenza, H1N1, Zika, Epstein–Barr virus) may increase the risk for GBS. Though the exact etiology and pathophysiology have been poorly identified, the syndrome is commonly preceded by a respiratory or gastrointestinal infection [20]. There have evidences of an association between GBS and COVID-19. GBS is one of the frequently manifested PNS complications in SARS-CoV-2 infection.

One review and several case reports described 83 GBS cases associated with COVID-19 [21–28]. The mean age at onset the patients is 60 years old (27 female and 56 male patients). Most of the patients had the typical GBS clinical presentation with a predominantly demyelinating subtype on electrophysiological studies. Preceeding respiratory and/or systemic symptoms were developed in a mean of 12 days after their COVID-19 symptomatology began. GBS manifestations developed after those of COVID-19. Clinically, all patients were presented with paraparesis or tetraparesis. Sensory symptoms were shown in 72% of the patients, either seen in isolation or in combination with paraparesis. Cranial nerve involvement was less frequently described at onset (18%). Miller Fisher syndrome is a variant of GBS and is characterized by ophthalmoplegia, ataxia, and areflexia. It has also been described in patients with COVID-19. Nearly all cases showed lower limb or generalized areflexia. Respiratory failure was seen in 28% of patients.

Albuminocytological dissociation was present in 70% of CSF results, and pleocytosis was noted in 10%. Evidence of SARS-CoV-2 in the CSF was absent in all the reported cases.

Seventy-four percent of the nerve conduction tests of affected patients showed a pattern compatible with demyelinating polyradiculoneuropathy, while axonal damage was prominent in 26%.

Ninety-seven percent of the patients were treated with IVIG, and 19% were treated with plasma exchange therapy. Two patients were given no medical therapy. Seventy-two percent of the patients demonstrated clinical improvement with partial or complete remission while 11.5% showed poor or no improvement and 8% of patients died.

In conclusion, GBS is one of the frequently manifested PNS complications in SARS-CoV-2 infection.

GBS seems to rise as a postinfectious complication of COVID-19. In most reported cases, findings were consistent with demyelinative polyneuropathy. Patients generally had a good prognosis, with more positive outcomes associated with treatment with IVIG. Older patients and patients with respiratory failure had a worse prognosis [21].

Cranial abnormalities

Recent evidence indicates that COVID-19 may also be associated with cranial neuropathies. Anosmia and dysgeusia are the most common reported symptoms [29]. These symptoms were mostly reported in asymptomatic individuals or as the initial stage of SARS-CoV-2 infection with no other symptoms [30] Isolated cranial neuropathies may be associated with COVID-19. Codeluppi et al. found that 21% of patients presenting with facial palsy had active or recent symptoms consistent with SARS-CoV-2 infection, suggesting an excess risk of facial palsy during or after COVID-19 [31].

Wei et al. noted a case of acute unilateral isolated oculomotor nerve palsy in a severely ill patient [32].

Another publication presented a healthy patient diagnosed with COVID-19 presenting with a cranial nerve III palsy [33]. Few cases of abducens nerve palsy have been noted in SARS-CoV-2-infected patients [34].

The inflammatory reaction against the SARS-CoV-2 virus and inflammation of vessels supplying to nerve trunk was a possible reason for cranial nerve damage.

One report of a patient with ipsilateral fifth and seventh cranial nerve involvement that started within 5 days of respiratory symptoms and resolved in 3 weeks suggests that multiple cranial neuropathies may be a manifestation of COVID-19 [35]. As such, cranial neuropathies may be related to immune-mediated injury from pro-inflammatory cytokines rather than direct viral neutrophism.

Myasthenia gravis

Myasthenia gravis (MG) is an autoimmune disease that affects the neuromuscular junction and causes fatigable ocular, limb, and bulbar weakness. Treatment can lead to a remission. A myasthenic exacerbation with worsening of symptoms is called a myasthenic crisis and is characterized by restrictive respiratory failure. Exacerbation can be induced by multiple different bodily stressors, but mostly appears with concurrent infection [36]. Three case reports and two case series described 20 adults (mean age of 60) diagnosed with COVID-19 and also suffered from MG [37–39]. The majority of patients had a known history of MG and manifested with exacerbation. Four patients without previous neurologic or autoimmune disorders were diagnosed with MG after the onset of COVID-19 disease [39,40]. Nine patients showed ocular symptoms (including ptosis, diplopia) and 11 patients had general muscular fatigability. Serum antiacetylcholine receptor (AChR) antibody level were elevated in 11 patients, antimuscle specific tyrosine kinase (MuSk) were elevated in one patient, and four patients were without serological definition.

Regarding treatment, five patients were treated with plasma exchange, and the rest of the patients received varying immunosuppressive therapies (the majority received at least two agents, including pyridostigmine). Most patients (73%) who were hospitalized due to MG exacerbation developed severe respiratory failure and required intubation, while 26% required oxygen nasal canula. Four patients died.

In conclusion, there are very few reports of *de novo* development of MG secondary to COVID-19. However, patients with a past medical history of MG may be considered to be more prone to develop severe complications of COVID-19 including severe respiratory failure. Infections such as viral upper respiratory infection are the most common cause of respiratory failure related to myasthenic crisis [41]. MG patients also have elevated levels of proinflammatory cytokines. Common elevation of IL-6 is seen in both COVID-19 and MG, and it is associated with increased mortality. Thus, preventive approach is essential for these patients.

Myopathy and myositis

Myalgia is reported extensively in the literature as a common musculoskeletal manifestation of COVID-19 infection, presenting in nearly half of all COVID-19-infected patients. COVID-19-related myositis and consequently rhabdomyolysis are other reported manifestations.

Skeletal muscle injury is defined by muscle pain or fatigue associated with elevated serum creatine kinase (CK) level above 200 U/L.

By July 2020, a single case of COVID-19-related myositis had been reported in the literature. Since then, several case reports and series reporting a virus-induced myositis attributed to COVID-19 disease have been published.

In a series of patients from Wuhan, 23 COVID-19 patients (11%) of 214 patients had a muscle injury associated with an increased serum CK [5].

De rosa et al. described 88 patients diagnosed with COVID-19 who had muscular manifestations. 81 complained with fatigue. The mean value of CPK was 262 U/L.

Patients with muscle injury had higher neutrophil counts, lower lymphocyte counts, higher CRP levels, and higher D-dimer levels. Most patients with muscle injury had a multiorgan damage, and high CPK levels were significantly associated with respiratory involvement and a fatal outcome [42].

Conclusion

SARS-CoV-2 may potentially be associated with nervous system complications [43]. We reviewed the peripheral neurological profile of the COVID-19 patient; our review detailed the neurological manifestations of COVID-19 known to date. PNS involvement in the infection include neuropathy of cranial nerves, neuropathy of peripheral nerves, GBS with all its MG and myositis.

Several mechanisms have been theorized, including direct viral involvement, inflammatory response, immune mechanisms, and microvascular disease.

In most cases, the neurological manifestations were observed a few days or even weeks after initial presentation of the viral infection. This time course may indicate either an infectious or postinfectious etiology.

The ability of SARS-CoV-2 to induce hyper-stimulation of the immune system has been recently evidenced [3,18].

And the finding of immune-mediated neurological sequelae following infection with COVID-19 is becoming increasingly evident. All of the complications could be immune mediated in origin [44]. We suggest that the ability of SARS-CoV-2 to produce hyperstimulation of the immune system is the leading mechanism for the development of neurological complications in COVID-19 patients. Additionally, the prevalence of neurological signs and symptoms is higher in patients with severe COVID-19 infection.

Thus, it is important that physician will be better familiarized with the spectrum of clinical, laboratory, and radiologic findings, as well as the proper treatment of those patients.

References

[1] Zhu N, Zhang D, Wang W, Li X, Yang B, Song J, et al. A novel coronavirus from patients with pneumonia in China, 2019. N Engl J Med 2020;382(8):727–33.
[2] Kim J, Zhang J, Cha Y, Kolitz S, Funt J, Chong RE, et al. Coronavirus disease–2019 (COVID-19). ChemRxiv; 2020. 2019(March).
[3] Ehrenfeld M, Tincani A, Andreoli L, Cattalini M, Greenbaum A, Kanduc D, et al. Covid-19 and autoimmunity. Autoimmun Rev 2020:102597.
[4] Berger JR. COVID-19 and the nervous system. 2020. p. 143–8.
[5] Mao L, Jin H, Wang M, Hu Y, Chen S, He Q, et al. Neurologic manifestations of hospitalized patients with coronavirus disease 2019 in Wuhan, China. JAMA Neurol 2020;77(6):683–90.
[6] Koyuncu OO, Hogue IB, Enquist LW. Virus infections in the nervous system. Cell Host Microbe 2013;13(4):379–93.
[7] Streit WJ, Mrak RE, Griffin WST. Microglia and neuroinflammation: a pathological perspective. J Neuroinflammation 2004;1:1–4.
[8] Lu R, Zhao X, Li J, Niu P, Yang B, Wu H, et al. Genomic characterisation and epidemiology of 2019 novel coronavirus: implications for virus origins and receptor binding. Lancet 2020;395(10224):565–74.
[9] Letko M, Marzi A, Munster V. Functional assessment of cell entry and receptor usage for SARS-CoV-2 and other lineage B betacoronaviruses. Nat Microbiol 2020;5(4):562–9.
[10] Li YC, Bai WZ, Hashikawa T. The neuroinvasive potential of SARS-CoV2 may play a role in the respiratory failure of COVID-19 patients. J Med Virol 2020;92(6):552–5.
[11] Yan R, Zhang Y, Li Y, Xia L, Guo Y, Zhou Q. Structural basis for the recognition of SARS-CoV-2 by full-length human ACE2. Science 2020;367(6485):1444–8.
[12] Netland J, Meyerholz DK, Moore S, Cassell M, Perlman S. Severe acute respiratory syndrome coronavirus infection causes neuronal death in the absence of encephalitis in mice transgenic for human ACE2. J Virol 2008;82(15):7264–75.
[13] Ferreira ACA de F, Romão TT, Macedo YS, Pupe C, Nascimento OJM. COVID-19 and herpes zoster co-infection presenting with trigeminal neuropathy. Eur J Neurol September 1, 2020;27(9):1748–50.
[14] Zubair AS, McAlpine LS, Gardin T, Farhadian S, Kuruvilla DE, Spudich S. Neuropathogenesis and neurologic manifestations of the coronaviruses in the age of coronavirus disease 2019: a review. JAMA Neurol 2020;77(8):1018–27.
[15] Rossi GP, Sanga V, Barton M. Potential harmful effects of discontinuing ace-inhibitors and ARBs in covid-19 patients. Elife 2020;9:1–8.
[16] Halpert G, Shoenfeld Y. SARS-CoV-2, the autoimmune virus. Autoimmun Rev 2020;19(12):1–4.
[17] Perricone C, Bartoloni E, Bursi R, Cafaro G, Guidelli GM, Shoenfeld Y, et al. COVID-19 as part of the hyperferritinemic syndromes: the role of iron depletion therapy. Immunol Res 2020;68(4):213–24.
[18] Dotan A, Muller S, Kanduc D, David P, Halpert G, Shoenfeld Y. The SARS-CoV-2 as an instrumental trigger of autoimmunity. Autoimmun Rev 2021:102792.
[19] Kanduc D, Shoenfeld Y. Molecular mimicry between SARS-CoV-2 spike glycoprotein and mammalian proteomes: implications for the vaccine. Immunol Res 2020;68(5):310–3.

[20] Leonhard SE, Mandarakas MR, Gondim FAA, Bateman K, Ferreira MLB, Cornblath DR, et al. Diagnosis and management of Guillain–Barré syndrome in ten steps. Nat Rev Neurol November 1, 2019;15(11):671–83.
[21] Abu-Rumeileh S, Abdelhak A, Foschi M, Tumani H, Otto M. Guillain–Barré syndrome spectrum associated with COVID-19: an up-to-date systematic review of 73 cases. J Neurol 2020;268:1133–70.
[22] Abrams RMC, Kim BD, Markantone DM, Reilly K, Paniz-Mondolfi AE, Gitman MR, et al. Severe rapidly progressive Guillain-Barré syndrome in the setting of acute COVID-19 disease. J Neurovirol 2020;26(5):797–9.
[23] Zito A, Alfonsi E, Franciotta D, Todisco M, Gastaldi M, Cotta Ramusino M, et al. COVID-19 and Guillain–Barré syndrome: a case report and review of literature. Front Neurol 2020;11:1–7.
[24] Pelea T, Reuter U, Schmidt C, Laubinger R, Siegmund R, Walther BW. SARS-CoV-2 associated Guillain–Barré syndrome. J Neurol 2020:2–5. 0123456789.
[25] Rajdev K, Victor N, Buckholtz ES, Hariharan P, Saeed MA, Hershberger DM, et al. A case of Guillain-Barré syndrome associated with COVID-19. J Investig Med High Impact Case Rep 2020;8.
[26] Gale A, Sabaretnam S, Lewinsohn A. Guillain-Barré syndrome and COVID-19: association or coincidence. BMJ Case Rep 2020;13(11):10–4.
[27] Abolmaali M, Heidari M, Zeinali M, Moghaddam P, Ramezani Ghamsari M, Jamshidi Makiani M, et al. Guillain–Barré syndrome as a parainfectious manifestation of SARS-CoV-2 infection: a case series. J Clin Neurosci 2020;83(April 2020):119–22.
[28] Korem S, Gandhi H, Dayag DB. Guillain-Barré syndrome associated with COVID-19 disease. BMJ Case Rep 2020;13(9).
[29] Carrillo-Larco RM, Altez-Fernandez C. Anosmia and dysgeusia in COVID-19: a systematic review, vol 5. Wellcome Open Research. F1000 Research Ltd; 2020.
[30] Gane SBC, Kelly C, Hopkins C. Isolated Sudden onset anosmia in COVID-19 infection. A novel syndrome? Rhinology 2020;58:299–301.
[31] Codeluppi L, Venturelli F, Rossi J, Fasano A, Toschi G, Pacillo F, et al. Facial palsy during the COVID-19 pandemic. Brain Behav January 1, 2021;(1):11.
[32] Wei H, Yin H, Huang M, Guo Z. The 2019 novel cornoavirus pneumonia with onset of oculomotor nerve palsy: a case study. J Neurol 2020;267:1550–3. Springer.
[33] Fitzpatrick JC, Comstock JM, Longmuir RA, Donahue SP, Fitzpatrick JM, Bond III JB. Cranial nerve III palsy in the setting of COVID-19 infection. Neuro-Ophthalmol 2021;41:e286.
[34] Dinkin M, Gao V, Kahan J, Bobker S, Simonetto M, Wechsler P, et al. COVID-19 presenting with ophthalmoparesis from cranial nerve palsy. Neurology August 4, 2020;95(5):221–3.
[35] Gogia B, Gil Guevara A, Rai PK, Fang X. A case of COVID-19 with multiple cranial neuropathies. Int J Neurosci 2020;11:909.
[36] Conti-fine BM, Milani M, Kaminski HJ. Science in medicine Myasthenia gravis: past, present, and future. Sci Med 2006;116(11):2843–54.
[37] Camelo-Filho AE, Silva AMS, Estephan EP, Zambon AA, Mendonça RH, Souza PVS, et al. Myasthenia gravis and COVID-19: clinical characteristics and outcomes. Front Neurol 2020;11(September).
[38] Sriwastava S, Tandon M, Kataria S, Daimee M, Sultan S. New onset of ocular myasthenia gravis in a patient with COVID-19: a novel case report and literature review. J Neurol 2020;268:2690–6.
[39] Restivo DA, Centonze D, Alesina A, Marchese-Ragona R. Myasthenia gravis associated with SARS-CoV-2 infection. Ann Intern Med 2020;173(12):1027–8.
[40] Huber M, Rogozinski S, Puppe W, Framme C, Höglinger G, Hufendiek K, et al. Postinfectious onset of myasthenia gravis in a COVID-19 patient. Front Neurol October 2020;6:11.
[41] Wendell LC, Levine JM. Myasthenic crisis. Neurohospitalist January 2011;1(1):16–22.
[42] De Rosa A. Muscle manifestations and CK levels in COVID infection : results of a large cohort of patients inside a pandemic COVID-19 Area. Acta Myol 2021:1–12.
[43] Saad M, Omrani AS, Baig K, Bahloul A, Elzein F, Matin MA, et al. Clinical aspects and outcomes of 70 patients with Middle East respiratory syndrome coronavirus infection: a single-center experience in Saudi Arabia. Int J Infect Dis 2014;29:301–6.
[44] Manjili RH, Zarei M, Habibi M, Manjili MH. COVID-19 as an acute inflammatory disease. J Immunol 2020;205(1):12–9.

CHAPTER

17

Central nervous system impairments in COVID-19

Polina Sobolevskaia[1], *Andrei Kolobov*[2] and *Leonid P. Churilov*[1,2,3]

[1]Laboratory of the Mosaic of Autoimmunity, Saint Petersburg State University, Saint Petersburg, Russia; [2]Department of Pathology, Saint Petersburg State University, Saint Petersburg, Russia; [3]Saint Petersburg Research Institute of Phthisiopulmonology, Saint Petersburg, Russia

Pathogenesis of central nervous system (CNS) impairments in SARS-CoV-2 infection are still not clear, but the most likely mechanisms are direct neurotropism, the role of aberrant immune response, local circulatory dysfunction and/or hypoxia, inflammatory cytokines in the cerebrospinal fluid (CSF), infected monocytes/macrophages migration across the blood–brain barrier (BBB) [1–3].

Another important aspect of neuropsychiatric impairments in SARS-CoV-2 infection is how does the virus spread to the CNS? The potential tracts of viral spreading can be:

1) from peripheral nervous system (PNS) to CNS via retrograde/anterograde axonal transport, neuron-to-neuron or neuron-to-nonneuronal propagation, through the cranial nerves (olfactory, facial, glossopharyngeal, vagus) [1,4];
2) hematogenous path—is associated with the interrelationship between the COVID-19 and ACE2 receptor in endothelial cells, with straight BBB penetration [1];
3) immunological tract—COVID-19 affects resident mucosal immune cells that spread to other organs [1];
4) CSF and fenestrated blood vessels virus can be spreaded to meningeal structures, choroid plexus, etc. [1,3].
5) pathogenic transmission through the enterocytes, enteric plexus, sympathetic nerves, dendritic cells, as well as in cases of Herpes virus, influenza, and enteroviral entities [1,5].

Neurovirulence is not the only reason of the neuroinflammation in SARS-CoV-2. However, not only SARS-CoV-2 infection itself can cause CNS damage to the CNS, but also its

Autoimmunity, COVID-19, Post-COVID19 syndrome and COVID-19 vaccination
https://doi.org/10.1016/B978-0-443-18566-3.00020-7

consequences. The cytokine storm, which is observed in some severe cases of SARS-CoV-2 infection, can cause BBB injury, astrocytes disruption, and activation of microglia. A complex of such violations can lead to acute encephalopathy, hypoperfusion, hypoxia and coagulation disturbances, demyelination, aberrant neuronal signaling, cell damage, and even death [1,2,6–8].

SARS-CoV-2 infection affects both central and peripheral nervous systems. It is quite effectually to divide manifestations of COVID-19 to: 1. Neurological COVID-19 manifestations (which cover both CNS and PNS) such as olfactory and gustatory disturbances, headaches, acute cerebrovascular disease in ischemic and hemorrhagic form, seizures, encephalitis, myelopathies, Guillain–Barré syndrome, neuropathies, viral or autoimmune myositis (myalgia, hyperCKemia and rhabdomyolysis cases) [1,9,10]; 2. Psychiatric COVID-19 manifestations (which are associated with CNS) such as encephalopathy, psychosis, delirium, cognitive dysfunction, memory dysfunction, insomnia, fatigue, depression, anxiety, agitation, brain fog, impaired consciousness, and confusion [1,4].

SARS-CoV-2 infection and meningoencephalitis: In 2020, a group of Japanese scientists have described a case of a patient with generalized seizures and presence of the SARS-CoV-2 RNA in the CSF [11].

Another one case report of meningoencephalitis associated with SARS-CoV-2 infection was described later, but it was not a result of direct SARS-CoV-2 invasion into the brain, rather it could be the consequenses of a cytokine storm. It was a case of 58-year-old female with cough, fever, and altered mental status, who was positive for SARS-CoV-2 [12].

At the same time in the literature, we see publications, describing autoimmune encephalitis as a complication of SARS-CoV-2 infection. A group of scientists from Singapore published a meta-analysis of incidence, outcomes, and predictors of encephalitis as a neurological complication of COVID-19 [13]. They have analyzed 23 original studies with a combined population of 129,008 patients, including 138 patients with encephalitis. This analysis revealed that the incidence of encephalitis was about 0.215%, the mortality rate among the patients with encephalitis as a complication of COVID-19 was 13.4%. The supposed pathogenetic mechanisms of encephalitis as a complication of COVID-19 suggested in this paper were direct invasion of the nervous system, systemic inflammation, and molecular mimicry [13]. We also have noticed the signs of brain injury in postmortem studies. We have revealed that with a new coronavirus infection, the brain is affected with the development of encephalitis—the signs of fibrous and cellular gliosis, diffuse mononuclear infiltration are detected (Fig. 17.1A–D).

One of the autoimmune encephalitides—an encephalitis with positive autoantibodies to glutamate receptor type.

N-methyl-D-aspartate (anti-NMDAR encephalitis) was described in COVID-19 adult patients [14,15] as well as in pediatric patients [16]. That means that COVID-19 infection can provoke an anti-brain autoimmunity.

SARS-CoV-2 infection and olfactory/gustatory disturbances

A group of scientists from London, UK have shown that patients with SARS-CoV-2 antibodies with an acute loss of smell and taste sense were significantly less likely to recover their

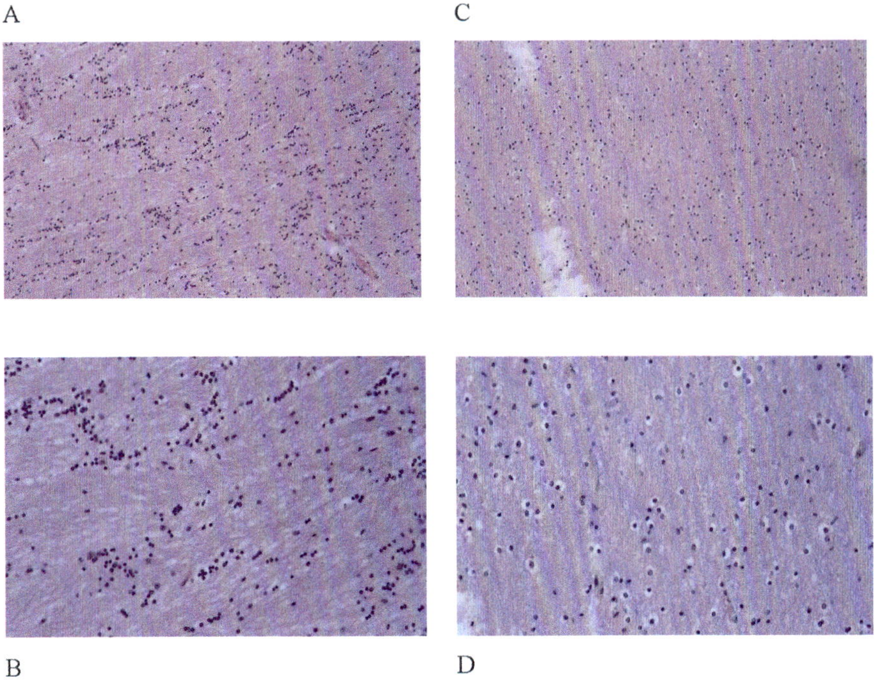

FIGURE 17.1 Representative microphotographs illustrating pathological parameters. Hematoxylin and eosin staining (H&E). A—mononuclear infiltrates in the white matter of the brain, x100; B—mononuclear infiltrates in the white matter of the brain, x200; C—white matter of the brain without signs of viral damage, x100; D—white matter of the brain without signs of viral damage, x200.

sense of smell/taste than people who were seronegative [17]. Another group of scientists from Iran demonstrated the increased TNF-α levels in the olfactory epithelium of the COVID-19 patients compared to the uninfected control subjects at the same time no differences in IL-1β levels were observed [18].

We still can't exactly say what is the mechanism of CNS impairments in SARS-CoV-2 infection, is it a result of a direct effect of a virus to the CNS or is it a result of secondary injury. Possible hypothesis needs to be checked in clinical and experimental trials. But at the same time, we see that SARS-CoV-2 infection can strike the CNS and it is important to notice these complications and start the therapy in time.

Acknowledgment

The work was supported by the grant of Russian Science Foundation, No. 22-15-00113, agreement of 13.05.2022, https://rscf.ru/project/22-15-00113/.

References

[1] Sieracka J, Sieracki P, Kozera G, Szurowska E, Gulczyński J, Sobolewski P, et al. COVID-19 - neuropathological point of view, pathobiology, and dilemmas after the first year of the pandemic struggle. Folia Neuropathol 2021;59:1–6. https://doi.org/10.5114/fn.2021.105128.

[2] Al-Sarraj S, Troakes C, Hanley B, Osborn M, Richardson MP, Hotopf M, et al. Invited Review: the spectrum of neuropathology in COVID-19. Neuropathol Appl Neurobiol 2021;47:3–16. https://doi.org/10.1111/nan.12667.

[3] Altable M, Moisés de la Serna J. Neuropathogenesis in COVID-19. J Neuropathol Exp Neurol 2020;79:1247–9. https://doi.org/10.1093/jnen/nlaa116.

[4] Han Y, Yuan K, Wang Z, Liu W-J, Lu Z-A, Liu L, et al. Neuropsychiatric manifestations of COVID-19, potential neurotropic mechanisms, and therapeutic interventions. Transl Psychiatry 2021;11:1–20. https://doi.org/10.1038/s41398-021-01629-8.

[5] Deffner F, Scharr M, Klingenstein S, Klingenstein M, Milazzo A, Scherer S, et al. Histological evidence for the enteric nervous system and the choroid plexus as alternative routes of neuroinvasion by SARS-CoV2. Front Neuroanat 2020;14:596439. https://doi.org/10.3389/fnana.2020.596439.

[6] Al-Dalahmah O, Thakur KT, Nordvig AS, Prust ML, Roth W, Lignelli A, et al. Neuronophagia and microglial nodules in a SARS-CoV-2 patient with cerebellar hemorrhage. Acta Neuropathol Commun 2020;8:147. https://doi.org/10.1186/s40478-020-01024-2.

[7] Franca RA, Ugga L, Guadagno E, Russo D, Del Basso De Caro M. Neuroinvasive potential of SARS-CoV2 with neuroradiological and neuropathological findings: is the brain a target or a victim? APMIS 2021;129:37–54. https://doi.org/10.1111/apm.13092.

[8] Jaunmuktane Z, Mahadeva U, Green A, Sekhawat V, Barrett NA, Childs L, et al. Microvascular injury and hypoxic damage: emerging neuropathological signatures in COVID-19. Acta Neuropathol 2020;140:397–400. https://doi.org/10.1007/s00401-020-02190-2.

[9] Delamarre L, Gollion C, Grouteau G, Rousset D, Jimena G, Roustan J, et al. COVID-19-associated acute necrotising encephalopathy successfully treated with steroids and polyvalent immunoglobulin with unusual IgG targeting the cerebral fibre network. J Neurol Neurosurg Psychiatry 2020;91:1004–6. https://doi.org/10.1136/jnnp-2020-323678.

[10] Josephson SA, Kamel H. Neurology and COVID-19. JAMA 2020;324:1139–40. https://doi.org/10.1001/jama.2020.14254.

[11] Moriguchi T, Harii N, Goto J, Harada D, Sugawara H, Takamino J, et al. A first case of meningitis/encephalitis associated with SARS-Coronavirus-2. Int J Infect Dis 2020;94:55–8. https://doi.org/10.1016/j.ijid.2020.03.062.

[12] Poyiadji N, Shahin G, Noujaim D, Stone M, Patel S, Griffith B. COVID-19-associated acute hemorrhagic necrotizing encephalopathy: imaging features. Radiology 2020;296:E119–20. https://doi.org/10.1148/radiol.2020201187.

[13] Siow I, Lee KS, Zhang JJY, Saffari SE, Ng A. Encephalitis as a neurological complication of COVID-19: a systematic review and meta-analysis of incidence, outcomes, and predictors. Eur J Neurol 2021;28:3491–502. https://doi.org/10.1111/ene.14913.

[14] Panariello A, Bassetti R, Radice A, Rossotti R, Puoti M, Corradin M, et al. Anti-NMDA receptor encephalitis in a psychiatric Covid-19 patient: a case report. Brain Behav Immun 2020;87:179–81. https://doi.org/10.1016/j.bbi.2020.05.054.

[15] Monti G, Giovannini G, Marudi A, Bedin R, Melegari A, Simone AM, et al. Anti-NMDA receptor encephalitis presenting as new onset refractory status epilepticus in COVID-19. Seizure 2020;81:18–20. https://doi.org/10.1016/j.seizure.2020.07.006.

[16] Sarigecili E, Arslan I, Ucar HK, Celik U. Pediatric anti-NMDA receptor encephalitis associated with COVID-19. Childs Nerv Syst 2021;37:3919–22. https://doi.org/10.1007/s00381-021-05155-2.

[17] Makaronidis J, Firman C, Magee CG, Mok J, Balogun N, Lechner M, et al. Distorted chemosensory perception and female sex associate with persistent smell and/or taste loss in people with SARS-CoV-2 antibodies: a community based cohort study investigating clinical course and resolution of acute smell and/or taste loss in people with and without SARS-CoV-2 antibodies in London, UK. BMC Infect Dis 2021;21:221. https://doi.org/10.1186/s12879-021-05927-w.

[18] Torabi A, Mohammadbagheri E, Akbari Dilmaghani N, Bayat A-H, Fathi M, Vakili K, et al. Proinflammatory cytokines in the olfactory mucosa result in COVID-19 induced anosmia. ACS Chem Neurosci 2020;11:1909–13. https://doi.org/10.1021/acschemneuro.0c00249.

CHAPTER

18

Neuropsychiatric side of the COVID-19

Margarita A. Mayorova[1], *Leonid P. Churilov*[1,2,3], *Natalia N. Petrova*[4] *and Yehuda Shoenfeld*[5,6]

[1]Laboratory of the Mosaic of Autoimmunity, Saint Petersburg State University, Saint Petersburg, Russia; [2]Department of Pathology, Department of Pathology, Saint Petersburg State University, Saint Petersburg, Russia; [3]Saint Petersburg Research Institute of Phthisiopulmonology, Saint Petersburg, Russia; [4]Department of Psychiatry and Addiction, Saint Petersburg State University, Saint Petersburg, Russia; [5]Zabludowicz Center for Autoimmune Diseases, Sheba Medical Center, Ramat Gan, Israel; [6]Tel Aviv University, Tel Aviv, Israel

Introduction

COVID-19 as an acute infection may be characterized in general by its respiratory symptoms. However, the latest data shows that neurological and neuropsychiatric symptoms are common in new coronavirus infections as well. In that case, symptoms may be nonspecific, such as muscle soreness, headache, dizziness, anxiety, sleep and mood disturbances, fatigue, or more specific ones: stroke, seizures, encephalitis, ataxia, and myelitis; with peripheral nervous system (PNS) disorders including loss of smell and taste (anosmia/hyposmia and ageusia/dysgeusia), Guillain-Barré syndrome and Miller Fisher syndrome; or psychiatric and neuropsychiatric syndromes including major depressive disorder, bipolar disorder, obsessive-compulsive disorder and posttraumatic stress disorder [1].

Mirfazeli et al. [2] proposed to divide neuropsychiatric symptoms in COVID-19 into three distinct groups: olfactory symptoms (anosmia, hypogeusia), general constitutional-like neuropsychiatric symptoms (dizziness, headache, limb force reduction), and specific neuropsychiatric symptoms (photophobia, mental state change, hallucination, vision and speech problems, seizure, delirium, stroke, and balance disturbance) [2].

In turn, patients with verified psychiatric diseases may also be at high risk for contacting the viral infection due to a huge spectrum of various factors including the dysregulated

https://doi.org/10.1016/B978-0-443-18566-3.00007-4

innate immune system, altered/impaired cognitive and motor functioning, and sometimes, complications with personal hygiene [3].

Pathogenesis

Proof of the COVID-19 invasion into the CNS

Human coronaviruses are characterized by neuroinvasive and neurotropic potential. It was also recently hypothesized that the SARS-CoV-2 virus may be able to render a direct effect on the central nervous system (CNS) [4,5].

According to the recent data SARS-CoV-2 may be detected *via* reverse-transcription polymerase chain reaction (RT-PCR) assay in CSF of most of the COVID-19 infected patients with active neuropsychiatric symptoms [1,6]. Furthermore, later studies have shown that the presence of COVID-19 RNA may be detected not only in CSF of patients (especially those with viral encephalitis) but also in hypothalamic and cortical neurons [4,7,8].

Postmortem studies have detected the presence of SARS-CoV-2 spike protein in cortical neurons and endothelium in line with hypoxic-ischemic damages in the brain [1,9]. Other neuropathological studies have shown evidence of demyelination, vascular disturbances, development of encephalitis, and meningitis in patients, infected with COVID-19 [1,10].

Despite the growing number of postmortem evidence of COVID-19 influence on CNS, there is a significant lack of such data on survivors [1].

Fortunately, the rapidly evolving technology based on stem cell culture has allowed for the generation of human-induced pluripotent stem cells (iPSCs) that can be differentiated into virtually any cell lineage [11].

Another interesting perspective in this direction is three-dimensional tissue cultures known as organoids, which contain multiple cell types and recapitulate tissue structures and development. Cerebral organoids (COs) accurately resemble the molecular, cellular, and structural features of the developing brain and may be derived from human iPSCs and be infected with COVID-19 [1,11].

As early as 2008, after the first epidemic of SARS, Netland et al. have traced in detail the pathways and steps of SARS-CoV-1 intracerebral spreading. They used transgenic mice with human ACE2R. It appeared that virus within the first 4 days after inoculation spreads from the nasal epithelium through the structures related to the olfactory analyzer: piriform cortex, basal ganglia, midbrain, and hypothalamus. Later it involves substantia nigra, amygdala, hippocampus, and cerebellum, causing the death of neurons and hyperproduction of proinflammatory cytokines, thus brain changes in these experiments were more tightly related to mice perish than lung involvement [12]. SARS-CoV-1 and SARS-CoV-2 are close phylogenetically.

The latest data of similar SARS-CoV-2 studies on CO models have shown that the virus of COVID-19 can actively infect CO models and replicate within them—particles of the virus were detected in neurons by electron microscopy [13,14]. Interestingly, Ramani et al. described that COVID-19 infected COs' cells on Day 60 much quicker than on Day 15, suggesting that the virus prefers infecting more mature neural cells [13]. However, these studies do not explain the details of the COVID-19 pathway through the blood-brain barrier (BBB). However, some studies showed that SARS-CoV-2 may spread through peripheral lymphatic vessels connected to the brain glymphatic system [15].

In addition, a recent study has shown that patients after COVID-19 infection may have within neuron-enriched extracellular vesicles (nEV) increased levels of amyloid-beta, total tau, and p-T181 proteins, neurogranin, and neurofilament light protein indicating an association with neuroinflammation and neurodegeneration [16].

Mechanisms of SARS-CoV-2 impact on CNS

Precise mechanisms of COVID-19 infection influence on CNS are not yet fully understood and seem to result from a combination of direct viral infection, indirect systemic disease complication, and post-COVID neuroinflammation [1].

Morgun et al. emphasize the role of impaired intercellular interactions (neuron-astrocytic and astrocyte-endothelial), "local neuroinflammation, increased permeability of the BBB, and failed neuroplasticity; the above mechanisms include the so-called vascular component (for example, neurogenesis in neurogenic niches of the brain)" [17]. Dinein and kinesin are two proteins that can help in the anterograde and retrograde transmission of the virus in neurons. Recent postmortem animal studies have shown that the nucleus of the solitary fascicle in the brainstem could be one of the important regions of viral load [18].

According to the latest data, potential receptors, required for the entrance of COVID-19 into the host cells are angiotensin-converting enzyme-2 (ACE2), neuropilin-1, CD147, CD26, CD133, CD209, furin, and cadherin-17 [19–22].

It was recently discovered that infection by SARS-CoV-2 could occur *via* the binding of its spike (S) protein to the ACE2 receptor (ACE2R), decreasing its availability for ACE. ACE acting in the CNS can mediate neuroinflammation, neurodegeneration, and neurotoxicity. Thus, SARS-CoV-2 may render a negative effect on neuroprotective mechanisms in the brain [23].

ACE2R is a widespread receptor among a spectrum of tissues, including CNS, heart, kidneys, lungs, small intestine, thyroid, adrenals, gonads, pituitary, and blood vessels. Various types of cells in the central nervous system have differences in ACE2R expression, thus, in susceptibility to COVID-19, and also may vary with physiological and pathological conditions [1,24,25].

For example, the ACE2R expressing neural cells were found in subfornical organs, paraventricular nucleus, solitary tract, and rostral ventrolateral medulla. The aforementioned regions have weak protection of BBB and are important for cardiovascular and respiratory regulation. Thus, these CNS sites are more vulnerable to the neuroinflammatory process and invasion of various pathogens [24,26].

A recent study has shown that ACE2R in the brain blood vessels is highly expressed in pericytes instead of endothelium cells [27,28].

However, despite the lack of ACE2R in the endothelium, SARS-CoV-2 particles have been detected in the vascular endothelial cells in line with clinical cases of endothelialitis [29]. Interestingly, the iPSC-derived endothelial cells are also susceptible to SARS-CoV-2 [11]. In line with that, direct evidence for COVID-19 infection in brain pericytes is still lacking, although there are some strains of coronaviruses displaying considerable tropism to endotheliocytes of primate and human cerebral blood vessels [30].

Pericytes are located around the vascular endothelium and maintain vascular integrity, being an essential element of so-called neurovascular units of the brain, the key structures of brain protection and intracerebral transportation of molecules [17]. Although isolated damage to this pool of cells is not enough for SARS-CoV-2 passage across the BBB and first of all, it requires more significant disturbances in the structure of the endothelial barrier (or combination with pericytes' damage). It may result from preexisting conditions, direct viral influence, and immune response against infection. In clinical practice, it leads to massive cerebrovascular complications in infected patients such as ischemic infarcts in small and large arteries, ischemic strokes, and intracranial hemorrhages [4,31]. Moreover, the severity of vasculopathy may correlate with the severity of neurological symptoms within COVID-19 infection (stroke, mental alterations) [1].

On the other hand, some cells with weak expression of ACE2 can have strong expression of other types of potentially valid penetration receptors. For example, this phenomenon occurs in human brain cortical neurons, which have a high level of CD147 and neuropilin-1 and low expression of ACE2 receptor [1].

CD147 is a transmembrane glycosylated protein, the receptor of cyclophilins, and an inducer of metalloproteinases, important instrument of alteration in the inflammatory process. It is expressed on cerebral endothelium and intracerebral leukocytes and controls the integrity of BBB *via* local metalloproteinase activity. This is a target molecule for penetration of several viruses and Plasmodium falciparum, the lack of CD147 causes severe learning and memorizing disorders in knockout animals. Moreover, in the lungs (and hypothetically in the brain also) interaction of CD147 with SARS-CoV-2 may damage the stem and progenitor cells, thus jeopardizing postnatal organogenesis [17].

The low expression of CD147 is associated with the activation of lactate receptors on vessels endothelium (in vitro). Alzheimer's disease mice model has shown a significant decrease in CD147 expression in the hippocampus region. It correlates with data that a low level of CD147 is associated with the overproduction of amyloid-beta [17].

Cyclophilin A (a ligand of CD147), is also associated with chronic neurodegeneration. For example, an increase in its expression and proinflammatory effects combined with MMP-9 metalloproteinase activation may result in high BBB permeability in patients with Alzheimer's disease [32].

Another interesting question includes the role of olfactory bulbs and cranial nerves in the pathway of COVID-19 to CNS. It was recently shown that olfactory neurons have low expression of ACE2R, unlike epithelial and stem cells (for example, horizontal basal cells, involved in the regeneration of olfactory epithelium) [17].

The S protein-immunoreactivity was recently detected in brain neurons of K18-hACE2 mice after SARS-CoV-2 infection by intranasal delivery, suggesting the possibility that the SARS-CoV-2 live virus can infect brain neurons via the intranasal route [33].

Authors suggest that the virus may attach to ACE2 on the brain vessels endothelium or on the olfactory epithelium. It might result in the virus penetration into the brain tissue via a palatine plate [17]. It is especially relevant to know about the virus's prolonged presence in the respiratory tract. On average about 30% of patients may have this viral RNA present in the respiratory tract for 20 or more days [24].

CD147 (including cyclophilin A) and ACE2 could mediate the SARS-CoV-2-induced damage of stem and progenitor cells in the CNS suppressing neurogenesis and causing neurodegeneration. It also could be an additional cause of anosmia, associated with chronic neurodegeneration, which ultimately leads to dysfunction of the olfactory epithelium [17].

However, the findings on this issue still are quite contradictory and it was not yet been fully proven that this way of passing through the BBB is crucially significant for COVID-19 as a neuroinfection.

For example, a recent study of patients who died of COVID-19 identified structural brain abnormalities on postmortem brain imaging, with 21% of subjects having asymmetric olfactory bulbs [5]. In addition, Bulfamante et al. described the presence of virus particles in the olfactory nerve and gyrus rectus in the patient's brainstem with signs of severe damage of all tissue cell elements [34]. Brain imaging in COVID-19 regularly reveals predominant involvement of the olfactory system extended to the corpus callosum, cingulate cortex, and insula [35].

On the other hand, a magnetic resonance imaging (MRI) case study on a patient with COVID-19 with acute onset of anosmia described a nasal mucosa with no signs of congestion, as well as a normal volume in the bilateral olfactory bulbs [4,36]. It was also recently suggested that the COVID-19 virus could be able to invade the brain through other cranial nerves, such as the trigeminal nerve and sensory fibers of the vagus. The gustatory pathways implicating intermediate and glossopharingeal nerves could be also involved. However, the data is still scarce [8,24].

Microglia is well known for its activation during many psychiatric diseases (for example, it takes part in the pathogenesis of depression and schizophrenia) and for its association with the neuroinflammatory process *via* overproduction of a spectrum of proinflammatory cytokines [37].

It was recently described that patients with SARS-CoV-2 infection also have microglial activation, especially in the brainstem and olfactory bulb [38]. Although it remains unknown whether SARS-CoV-2 can directly infect microglial cells. The overproduction of cytokines in cytokine storm represents the basis for the indirect mechanism of neuronal damage (both directly and *via* cerebral hypoxia in hemodynamic shock), which may itself lead to a spectrum of neuropsychiatric symptoms [1].

In a late study, SARS-CoV-2 particles were detected in human macrophages from lymph nodes and lungs. Thus, whether infected macrophages infiltrate the brain, serving as a hijacking mechanism for SARS-CoV-2, remains to be determined [1,39]. Astrocytes play an important role in the functioning and structure of BBB. However, COVID-19 viral influence is very low or absent in this pool of cells. It may be explained by the high astrocyte cell subsets heterogeneity and low expression of ACE2 receptors [40].

Another interesting question is whether COVID-19 can pass through the blood–CSF–barrier (BCSFB), including passage through the choroid plexus with its complex network of epithelial cells surrounding capillaries. It is especially relevant knowing that choroid plexus cells express high rates of ACE2R and TMPRSS2 [41]. Recent studies have shown that choroid plexus epithelial cells, expressed in hippocampal COs are severely susceptible to SARS-CoV-2 invasion, unlike other neural cells subtypes. Further analysis of choroid plexus COs has revealed very high rates of infection even at low viral titer and leakage of BCSFB due to viral choroid plexus epithelial damage [41,42]. Thus, SARS-CoV-2 may be strongly able to use this pathway to enter CNS [42]. Approximately 1.28% of those COVID-19 patients who were tested for SARS-CoV-2 presence in CSF appeared to be positive, although the percentage of CNS infection with SARS-CoV-2 according to the postmortem data is much higher [8].

We already cited above the article suggested that SARS-CoV-2 also may enter and spread in the lymphatic system of the brain, regardless of the ACE2 receptor system [15].

Peripheral myeloid cells may be also infected by SARS-CoV-2 and subsequently recruited or transmigrate to the CNS in line with BBB structure impairment causing neuroinflammation via microglia activation. It is also noteworthy, that infected immune cells can maintain the neuroinflammatory process long after the initial infection when acute symptoms faded out [43].

A new study has identified auto-reactive lymphocytes that can cross-react with SARS-CoV-2 epitopes and human myelin. Thus, molecular mimicry could be a potential mechanism by which COVID-19 infection could potentiate the development of autoimmune brain involvement and corresponding neuropsychiatric manifestations [43].

COVID-19 may be a cause of limbic encephalitides. Molecular mimicry of COVID-19 and NMDA receptors was recently suggested as one of the mechanisms of autoimmune damage to neural tissue. One of the latest studies has identified 8 cases of COVID-19-associated anti-NMDAR encephalitis with the presence of a full clinical picture of encephalitis and high titer of NMDAR autoantibodies in CSF even after 3 weeks of infection. All patients had psychiatric and neurological symptoms (disturbance of consciousness, delirium, psychosis, catatonia, motor failures, dysarthria) and 75% of patients had seizures during the course of the disease [44].

Vojdani and Kharazian [45] identified significant immunological cross-reaction between monoclonal antibodies against SARS-CoV-2 S-protein and several human CNS antigens, like myelin basic protein (MBP), protein S100B and a key element of BBB molecular structure—claudin 5. Monoclonal antibodies against SARS-CoV-2 nucleoprotein cross-reacted with universally expressed human nuclear and mitochondrial antigens as well as with MBP. Both types of anti-SARS-CoV-2 monoclonal immunoglobulins cross-reacted with thyroid antigens, which are expressed in CNS also [45].

Several postmortem studies revealed lymphocytic infiltration in brain tissue of COVID-19 victims (as well as in many other organs) suggesting immunopathological/autoimmune links to pathogenesis [46].

In several studies development of autoimmune Guillain-Barré and Miller−Fisher syndromes was also described in patients, infected with SARS-CoV-2 [1,47,48]. Another possible mechanism of COVID-induced neuropsychiatric symptoms is an association with gut-brain axis alterations. ACE2R is widely expressed in gut epithelium and about 40% of patients with COVID-19 suffer from gastrointestinal symptoms [43]. Gut organs on postmortem investigation are infiltrated with lymphocytes and demonstrate the signs of viral damage [46]. In gut involvement, SARS-CoV-2 could be able to alter the microbiota diversity and composition, causing neuropsychiatric symptoms *via* the gut-immune system-brain axis. This mechanism is largely speculative but still is mechanistically feasible [49]. Moreover, key autoantigens of celiac disease, namely transglutaminases, showed the greatest immunological cross-reaction against anti-SARS-CoV-2 monoclonal antibodies among 50 tested human antigens [45]. In view of the known association of gut-brain axis disorders with some mental diseases, these findings should not be ignored.

COVID-19-associated neuropsychiatric manifestations

Neuropsychiatric manifestations of COVID-19 infection

Up to 36% of patients with COVID-19 may suffer from various neurological complications. Nonspecific and the most frequent central neurological symptoms are dizziness, headache, and cognitive impairment, sleep disturbances whereas the peripheral nervous system (PNS) manifestations mainly include polyneuropathy, muscle pain, alterations in smell and taste (hyposmia, anosmia, hypogeusia) [48,50]. Some authors also suggest that in up to 60% of cases anosmia and ageusia may appear before other overt symptoms of the disease [51]. A Spanish survey-based study showed that smell disorders can persist for several weeks in about 1/3 of patients [52]. In addition, consciousness disturbances also take place in COVID-19 neuropsychiatric picture, especially in cases of severe infection [48].

Headache mostly may be precipitated by hypoxia and impaired cerebral blood circulation [50].

Rogers et al. described that up to 41.7% of patients with acute COVID-19 infection suffer from sleep disturbances, anxiety, irritability, fatigue, depression symptoms, cognitive impairment, and sometimes, even hallucinations [53].

Many patients in the acute phase of the disease had complaints of memory difficulties, attention impairment, asthenia, and "brain fog" [54].

In a recent big study (with 40,469 patients) polyneuropathy along with nerve root and plexus, disorders have been registered in about 1% ($n = 392$) of patients. Authors suggested that this kind of symptom could develop due to demyelination caused by direct viral invasion or immune-mediated damage *via* cytokine storm [50].

Encephalopathy, myalgia, and chronic pain could be met in up to 2% of patients and possibly are caused by severe metabolic disturbances resulting from multiorgan involvement, with possible direct viral neuronal damage [50]. In the latest study authors have described the neurological status of patients with COVID-19-induced encephalopathy during hospitalization and 6 months after disease onset. The clinical picture included seizures, delirium, sleep disturbances, depression, anxiety, cognitive impairments, apathy, and behavior impairments varying in different patients. A pattern of PET/CT hypometabolism in a cerebral network including the prefrontal cortex, anterior cingulate, insula, and caudate nucleus was observed in patients with COVID-19-induced encephalopathy. Interestingly, a case of Hashimoto encephalopathy provocation during and after COVID-19 infection in female autoimmune thyroiditis patient have been reported recently [55].

A long row of studies showed that patients with COVID-19 are at a considerable risk of developing encephalitis with positive neurological signs, ischemic and hemorrhagic stroke, and cerebral sinus thrombosis [7,48,56]. A significant proportion of patients also may have an ischemic stroke or transient ischemic attack (TIA) [50]. This is especially dangerous in the elderly and immune-compromised group of patients [57]. Cascade of viral binding to ACE2 inhibitors, triggering the massive cytokine release and impaired coagulation cascade was proposed as a possible mechanism for stroke-like symptoms [50]. Risk for cerebrovascular complications correlated with higher levels of D-dimer and C-reactive protein in these patients.

Furthermore, the indirect influence of COVID-19 on CNS may result from cytokine storm, which in turn causes hemodynamic shock, accompanied by disseminated intravascular coagulation, multiple tromboembolism, and finally severe hypoxic organ damage, including the cerebral one [48,58].

The skeletal muscle injuries that have been documented in COVID-19 patients might concur with the development of respiratory failure. Moreover, it is well known that severe hypoxia, which often presents in patients with COVID-19, results in brain damage with cerebral vasodilation and interstitial edema. These effects might indeed be precipitated or worsened by an overlapping respiratory failure [48]. It was also recently described that patients with CNS-associated (dizziness, headache, ataxia) and muscular (myalgia) manifestations had low total blood lymphocyte counts in line with a high level of sera C-reactive protein (CRP) levels [43]. In addition, the neurological symptoms correlated with the severity of the disease and serum antiviral antibody titer [57].

About 1% of COVID-19 patients are susceptible to seizures. Decreased seizure threshold from cytokine surge and severe psychological stress could be the underlying mechanism for COVID-19-associated seizures [50]. A recent study has shown the presence of seizure-triggering metabolic changes such as electrolyte imbalance in 27% of patients with COVID-19 [59]. Encephalopathy or cerebral edema also may lead to new-onset seizures or even to activation of latent epilepsy [18]. Although, the direct epileptogenic potential of SARS-CoV-2 is not yet established. It is important to remember that certain antiviral drugs such as remdesavir or lopinavir can have cytochrome-based interactions with antiepileptics [57].

It is not surprising that patients with a history of psychiatric diseases (especially with psychotic, affective, and anxiety spectrum of diseases) in COVID-19 are more susceptible to worsening their mental state with exacerbation or even with the development of additional neuropsychiatric comorbidities [60]. For example, a recent study described exacerbation of schizophrenia following COVID-19 infection. In addition, the courses of dementia and Parkinson's disease also seems to be negatively influenced by an infection with SARS-CoV-2 [61].

Delirium

COVID-19 is well known for its negative effect on the neuropsychiatric status of patients (even in long-term periods), which effects are associated with significant morbidity and mortality. For example, about 20% of patients during their hospitalization suffered from a confusion state [4].

Delirium is usually described as an acutely disturbed state of mind characterized by restlessness, illusions, and incoherence, defined by other authors as confusion, altered mental status, acute onset of psychotic symptoms, disorientation, and decreased level of consciousness, cognitive dysfunction, and encephalopathy [4,15].

Development of delirium, as a severe disturbance of consciousness with acute onset and fluctuating course, was also described among many other symptoms of COVID-19 in patients with moderate and severe course of the disease. The inflammatory process in the CNS, prodromal hypoxia, acute pain, impaired attention, and cognitive-communication deficits due to coronavirus infection may contribute to delirium pathogenesis [62]. It is especially dangerous in elderly patients with premorbid evidence of cognitive decline and neuropsychiatric comorbidity [5,63,64]. According to a late study, delirium may represent a marker of a severe disease course in this group of patients [64]. In addition, in patients with dementia delirium may represent a prodromal phase of COVID-19 [62].

Delirium may play a role as a predictor of low patient survival, especially in prolonged hospitalizations. The severity of coronavirus infection makes the greatest contribution to the poor outcome: the risk of death increases by 33.17 times. The severity of the mental disorder had a greater impact on the risk of death compared with age, increasing it by 4.55 times [54].

The clinical appearance of impaired consciousness and/or delirium in most cases of SARS-CoV-2 infection may suggest that the virus penetrates the brain and spreads to the neocortex [4,53]. Altered consciousness can be met in up to 70% of patients with severe COVID-19 infection. It was also described in patients without typical symptoms and may be the only presenting symptom [63,65].

The highest occurrence of delirium was found in patients with severe COVID-19 infection in the intensive care unit (ICU) (ranging from 65% to 79.5%). Studies in adult and elderly patients have shown that delirium is often associated with frailty, senile age, history of epilepsy, presence of dementia, schizophrenia, depressive disorder, use of vasodilators and antipsychotics, higher serum urea, and increased lactate-dehydrogenase levels [5,64,66]. Other authors suggest that tissue hypoxia, oxygen desaturation, cytokine overproduction, and the use of hydroxychloroquine could be associated with the prolonged form of delirium [18].

Patients in intensive care units (ICU) may suffer from various subtypes of delirium. For example, the authors describe the presence of motor subtype delirium, agitation, or specifically, hyper- and hypoactive delirium. Khan *et al.* found that on the first assessment, most ICU patients (86.8%) had hypoactive delirium [67].

Possible mechanisms of delirium

On the one hand, pneumonia and acute respiratory distress syndrome (ARDS) are well-known risk factors for delirium development, established long before the current pandemic started. For example, hypoxia, respiratory acidosis, respiratory failure, disseminated intravascular coagulation, and systemic organ dysfunction associated with ARDS may contribute to delirium [68]. In addition, a long-term admission to the ICU ventilation support and sedation are also deliriogenic. Hypercoagulation state within COVID-19 infection may also predispose patients to ischemic brain injury [5,68].

Cuperlovic-Culf et al. hypothesized a relationship between delirium and SARS-CoV-2 infection *via* a possible binding of SARS-CoV-2 spike protein to monoamine oxidase B (MAO-B) enzymes, which influences the enzyme activity and possibly leads to many of the observed neurological and platelet-based complications of SARS-CoV-2 infection [4,69].

On the other hand, systemic inflammation with CNS involvement (independently from direct virus CNS infection) and overproduction of a spectrum of proinflammatory cytokines, such as IL-1, IL-6, and TNF-α, can also render a negative effect on the consciousness state. It is known, that such an inflammatory state in different kinds of shock and shock-like syndromes with excessive systemic action of inflammatory mediators - equally may lead to an impairment of the blood-brain barrier causing further neuronal damage and secondary encephalopathy [63]. Moreover, this condition is thought to involve an intracranial wave of cytokine storm mediated by BBB disturbances rather than direct viral neuronal damage [5].

Very essential results were brought in by the experiments of Frank et al. [70] published just a few days ago. They demonstrated that SARS-CoV-2 spike S1 subunit is a ligand of TLR4 receptors expressed in CNS. After intracerebrocysternal injection, this viral protein directly induces neuroinflammatory, microglial, and behavioral sickness responses. In vitro series of experiments with microglial cells also confirmed that this subunit of S-protein *per se* acts as a classical pathogen-associated molecular pattern (PAMP) and induces the expression of several proinflammatory cytokines by the target glial cells [70].

Taking into account the possible direct effect of SARS-CoV-2 on glial and neuronal cell subsets, delirium also could manifest either directly due to neuronal damage within the brain or indirectly due to hypoxia caused by disruptions in the function of the medullary respiratory centers [5]. Ultimately, further investigation is required before any conclusions can be drawn regarding deliriogenic pathobiology and whether direct neuroinvasion by SARS-CoV-2 plays a role.

Delayed and long-term COVID-19-induced neuropsychiatric complications

Despite many patients meeting discharge criteria, up to 19.9% of COVID-19 survivors still suffer from sleep disturbances, anxiety, irritability, fatigue, depression symptoms, cognitive impairment, hallucinations, and other psychotic symptoms [53].

Cognitive impairment may be present in 38%–50% of patients and includes impairments of psychomotor and processing speed, attention (inability to concentrate and hold attention for a long time), memory (short-term, working), executive functioning (cognitive tasks solving, planning), and abstract thinking. These changes are especially significant and dangerous in elderly patients and positively correlate with the severity of the infection [53,71].

Brain PET 6 months follow-up has shown the presence of prefrontal hypermetabolism in half of the patients. In the other half of the patients, the metabolism has returned to almost normal. Thus, longitudinal data suggest that this network may remain mildly to severely impaired even 6 months after disease onset [72].

In the latest 1-year follow-up study, COVID-19 survivors had greatly increased amplitude of low-frequency fluctuation (ALFF) values in the left frontal lobe, and parietal and temporal lobe within the left hemisphere. This might indicate that COVID-19 damages the function of multiple brain lobes to varying degrees. As the study was conducted 1 year after discharge, the authors suggest that the cause of this finding could be related to the compensatory repair of brain tissue after hypoxia and inflammation, which results in increased spontaneous activity of neurons and ALFF [73].

Mood and anxiety disorders

The development of depressive disorder is one of the most frequent consequences of COVID-19 infection. It is also well known that depression is often associated with the neuroinflammatory process (more exactly, with overproduction of a spectrum of proinflammatory cytokines and activated microglia). This picture can be also frequently met during the SARS-CoV-2 infection course, especially during severe infection and characterized by very high levels of proinflammatory cytokines (especially IL-6), high suicidal risk, and unfavorable outcomes of the disease [24].

Systemic infection can itself trigger major depression, especially in elderly patients due to age-dependent immune homeostasis alterations [24]. It was also recently described that levels of some proinflammatory cytokines may correlate with severity of apathy, motor inhibition, anhedonia, treatment resistance, and suicidal risk [74]. COVID-19 may critically impact psychosocial wellbeing and influence suicidal attempts among the affected individuals, which may also aggravate if the patient has other comorbid diseases [75].

About 31%–38% of COVID-19 survivors may suffer from depression, 22%–42% - have problems with anxiety, and 20% - with obsessive-compulsive symptoms. The aforementioned symptoms can be met during hospitalization in up to 36% of cases [76,77]. The latest meta-analysis revealed even higher rates of depression, anxiety, and sleep disorders occurrence in patients with COVID-19—45%, 47%, and 34%, respectively [78].

It is noteworthy, that patients with and after SARS-CoV-2 infection usually suffer from separate psychiatric symptoms, however, a quite voluminous proportion meet the diagnostic criteria for a psychiatric disorder. For example, the onset of anxiety and depressive spectrum disorders following SARS-CoV-2 infection was described in 12.8% and 9.9% of patients respectively [77,79].

Frequency of COVID-induced depression and anxiety positively correlated with the presence of infected family members, postinfection physical complications, the severity of the infection, level of proinflammatory markers, and psychiatric comorbidity [77]. It is also noteworthy, that patients of younger age (up to 40 years old) were more susceptible to the development of generalized anxiety and depression. The female gender was also reported as a common risk factor for depression and anxiety disorders [75]. SARS-CoV-2 may be associated with high suicidal risk in this group of patients.

One of the studies showed that even 1 month after infection about 38% of patients reported symptoms of depression [80]. Moreover, some patients suffered from suicidal ideation even at 1-month postdischarge [76].

The 3 months follow-up study of patients with COVID-19-related depression has shown that about 35% of patients had residual depressive symptoms. There was also a tendency to intensify depressive symptoms, especially in patients with a history of mental disorders. Executive functioning and motor speed were significantly impaired in 78% of patients with post-COVID depression [81].

Depression as a syndrome may have various etiology. But in the case of COVID-19 probably it is essential to emphasize the following aspect. Many COVID-19 patients have early debuted and long-lasting anosmia. Anosmia and depression are intimately interrelated. For the early mammal ancestors of humans, good olfaction was a key pillar of vitality and chance for survival in the struggle for existence. And archetypes of reactivity still are with us, although nowadays olfaction loss for humans is significance [82]. That's why disorders of olfaction are frequently associated with hopeless moods and depressive thoughts. Olfaction is often damaged during autoimmune diseases, as a rule in their initial phase, and aromatherapy renders some positive effects [83]. This is true for example for lupus and especially for lupus encephalitis, associated with depression, which was first demonstrated by Shoenfeld et al. who obtained the experimental model of olfactory and depressive disorders on animals treated with IgG of lupus patients binding ribosomal P-antigen. Moreover, it was shown that such autoantibodies may penetrate into CNS affecting the limbic system [84].

Hence, the observations about the depressive symptoms in COVID-19 and post-COVID health disturbances may stand in line with the characteristic of SARS-CoV-2 as the "virus of autoimmunity" [85].

Recently, a case report showed that patients with COVID-19 and no history of psychiatric disease may suffer from manic-like symptoms. It was suggested as a delayed response to neuroinfection by SARS-CoV-2 [86]. The latest study also described that COVID-19 survivors may also suffer from mania and hypomania even after an asymptomatic type of infection. The risk for mania positively correlated with psychosocial stress, history of mania/bipolar disorder or psychosis, and high level of proinflammatory markers. It is also noteworthy, that only 40% of patients with COVID-induced mania had bipolar disorder history. It means that about 60% of patients had an onset of bipolar disorder after surviving the infection [87].

Posttraumatic stress disorder (PTSD)

Severe COVID-19 has many common mechanistic links with other possible reasons for shock and shock-like states, including traumatic shock, which is accompanied by excessive systemic action of inflammatory mediators and multiorganic hypoxic failure [58]. That's why it is not surprising that posttraumatic stress disorder appeared to be one of the most common neuropsychiatric complications of SARS and MERS infections even at a 6-month postdischarge. The frequency of PTSD symptoms among COVID-19 infected patients is high as well—about 20%–30% of patients have become diagnosed with PTSD following the infection and a much higher rate of patients is suffering from various separate posttraumatic symptoms (from 31% to 96.2%). Moreover, these symptoms could be met even after 2–2.5 months after discharge [77,88,89].

Risk of COVID-19 following PTSD associated with younger age, female gender, obesity, diabetes, presence of autoimmune and psychiatric comorbidity [77].

Delirium and ICU-level care, both common complications of COVID-19, also represent the risk factors for PTSD/PTSS, with approximately 20% of critical care survivors experiencing PTSS 12 month after discharge [77,90].

COVID-induced psychosis and catatonia

It is known that the active neuroinflammatory process with overproduction of the whole spectrum of proinflammatory markers may lead to a significantly higher risk for the onset of psychosis and schizophrenia. This picture is also a frequent characteristic of ongoing exacerbation of schizophrenia and may persist for a long time after state stabilization [91]. COVID-19, in turn, is strongly associated with the massive inflammatory response that can lead to further indirect neuronal damage even after the acute phase of the disease.

The CoroNerve surveillance study identified new-onset psychosis in at least 6.5% of patients with COVID-19 and neuropsychiatric manifestations [92]. Recent studies also identified several separate cases of first-episode psychosis in COVID-19 infected patients including ones without a history of psychiatric diseases [93–95].

The clinical picture of COVID-19-induced psychosis may be characterized by disorganization, paranoia, confusional and delusional symptoms with the subacute onset, and a good response to antipsychotic therapy [77,95,96]. However, these patients should be carefully treated due to the high risk of suicidal behavior [97].

In addition, the medicines used in COVID-19 treatment (chloroquine, hydroxychloroquine, lopinavir, ritonavir, and high-dose corticosteroids) also may increase the risk for hallucinations and other psychotic symptoms, especially in elderly patients [77,98].

It is also noteworthy, that COVID-19 is associated not only with the debut of the psychosis but also may lead to exacerbation in patients with a history of psychotic symptoms. For example, Yao et al. describe that many of their patients with schizophrenia have had post-COVID exacerbations even despite receiving adequate therapy [99].

Zain et al. described a case of a sudden onset of excited catatonia, developed after COVID-19 infection. The patient was seropositive for COVID-19 and displayed at least three of the signs needed to diagnose catatonia—agitation, rigidity, and echolalia—and had a therapeutic response to lorazepam, confirming suspicions of excited catatonia [100].

Thus, apart from the main significant COVID-19-induced problems with mental health, in close future we may expect a growth in the frequency of psychotic disorders, including schizophrenia.

Post-COVID syndrome

Symptoms following COVID-19 infection may persist for up to several weeks after an acute infection and can be met in up to one-third of the survivors, even if the acute disease was not severe. When these symptoms persist more than 3 weeks after diagnosis it means that patient has post-COVID syndrome [101].

The syndrome has been suggested to result from prolonged inflammation following a SARS-CoV-2 infection, and contribution from autoimmune mechanisms is suspected, although the pathogenesis is still under investigation and is not entirely clear [102].

Characteristic symptoms of this syndrome include dizziness, headache, dyspnea, chronic pain, cough, myalgia, chronic fatigue without relief after sleep/rest, and taste and smell disturbances, as well as mental status disorders such as depression, anxiety, sleep disorders, PTSD, and cognitive impairment (Fig. 18.1) [104,105].

Seizures also may occur in a clinical picture during this syndrome [103]. Anosmia and ageusia persist at least for several weeks after COVID-19 infection. A recent study has shown hypometabolism in the olfactory/rectus gyrus with 4 weeks of prolonged anosmia. Additional regions of hypometabolism were also discovered in the amygdala, hippocampus, parahippocampus, cingulate cortex, pre-/postcentral gyrus, thalamus/hypothalamus, cerebellum, pons, and medulla in the other patient with chronic pain [106].

Up to 20.2% of patients with post-COVID have severe problems with cognitive functioning. A recent UK study has shown that many COVID-19 survivors have significant impairment in learning and gnosis. Moreover, a general picture of their cognition shows that their intellect aged for about 10 years [107].

Moreover, it was recently noted that even 4 months after discharge 51% of patients have at least one persisting symptom of the post-COVID syndrome. The most frequent symptoms were fatigue (31% of patients), cognitive impairment (21%), and dyspnea. Cognitive impairment includes disturbances in learning, executive functioning, neuromotor sphere, attention, processing speed, immediate and delayed verbal memory, verbal fluency, and working

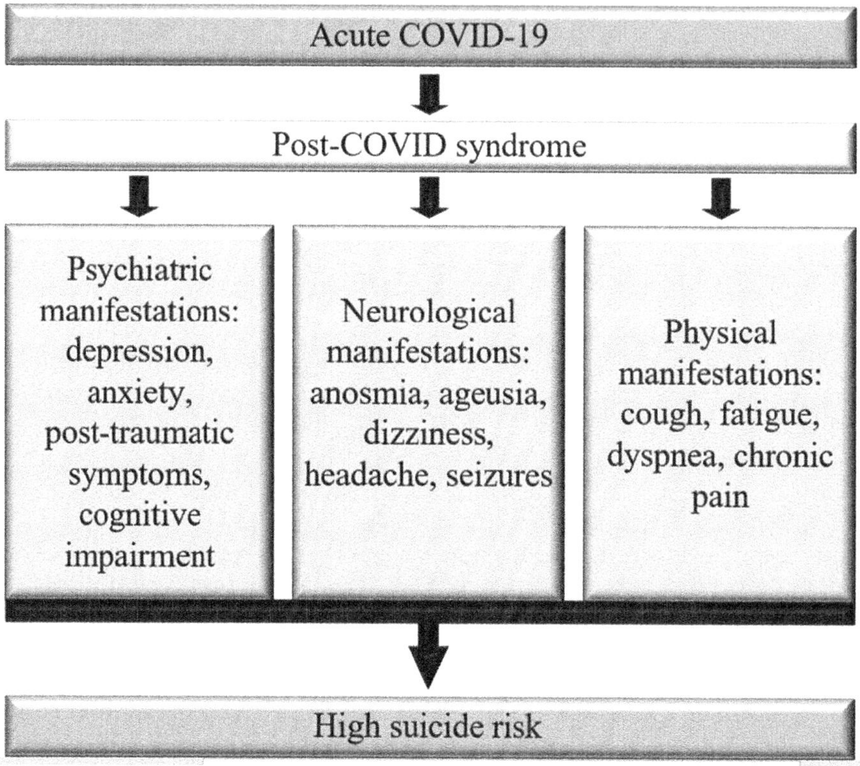

FIGURE 18.1 Suicide risk in patients with the post-COVID [103].

memory [108,109]. Patients who required ICU stay demonstrated greater breadth and severity of cognitive impairment than those requiring less intensive treatment [110].

Posttraumatic associated manifestations of post-COVID also seemed to persist for several months after discharge [111]. Moreover, the authors suggest that these symptoms in COVID-19 survivors may even worsen over time [105].

In addition, it all seems to be associated with COVID-19 severity and psychiatric comorbidity. For example, about 80% of patients who survived a severe form of the disease and patients as well as patients with Parkinson's disease also had severe post-COVID syndrome [16].

It was recently noted that symptoms may persist even 6 months after COVID-19 infection. In this case, brain MRI can show hyper-intensive areas in white matter and semi-left areas, which indicates neurodegeneration and microvascular impairment [112]. Picture of an increased level of proinflammatory cytokines (in particular, IL-4, IL-6, CRP) even after a long time postdischarge also indicates the presence of ongoing neuroinflammation [16]. Psychiatric manifestations, including depressive disorder, may affect up to 40% of patients even 6 months after the onset of symptoms [113].

In a 1-year follow-up study authors described significantly increased ALFF values in the left brain of COVID-19 survivors suggesting it is a consequence of compensatory repair of the brain after hypoxia and neuroinflammation [73].

Post-COVID syndrome and suicidality

It was recently described that anxiety and sleep disorders, PTSD, depression, and cognitive impairment are strongly interrelated with a high risk of suicidality. For example, patients with depression have a 25 times greater risk for suicide, especially when untreated [103]. Neurological manifestations (for example, chronic pain and seizures) are also associated with high rates of suicide attempts [103,114] (Fig. 18.1).

It is highly possible that a combination of psychiatric, neurological, and physical manifestations of the post-COVID syndrome in line with inflammatory neuronal damage may lead to a significant increase in the occurrence of suicidal ideation and behavior in these patients (Fig. 18.1). Moreover, it was recently noted that patients still may have a suicide risk even without severe symptoms of post-COVID [103,115].

Thus, studies of suicidality in COVID-19 survivors are urgently needed and could represent a new area of suicide research. It is also important to keep in mind that appropriate treatment of neuropsychiatric and physical conditions may reduce suicide risk among virus survivors with or without post-COVID syndrome [103].

Conclusion

Apart from the main respiratory and other somatic negative effects of COVID-19 one also can see the wide spectrum of various neuropsychiatric manifestations in this illness, often persisting after its acute phase. Neuropsychiatric complications of COVID-19 vary from nonspecific neural impairments to the development of a full clinical picture of psychiatric diseases (especially of psychotic, anxiety, and affective spectrum). The complex symptoms, persisting after several weeks of infection were called a post-COVID syndrome and a huge proportion of patients suffer from its various symptoms, including psychoneurological ones, as long as a year after discharge. It has a devastating effect on health-related quality of life and is associated with a high risk of suicidal behavior, which additionally increases summary mortality of COVID-19. Clinicians need to be aware of these manifestations in COVID-19 infected patients, especially because of known high rates of morbidity and mortality. Early recognition, prompt management, and long-term follow-up are warranted to provide better and more efficient patient care.

The exact pathways of the SARS-CoV-2 effect on the CNS remain not fully understood and require further research. At this moment we just have a collection of hypotheses about its indirect (via cytokine storm and further prolonged overproduction, hypoxia, ARDS, neuroinflammation, immune system dysregulation, including postinfection autoimmunity and immune cell transmigration) and possible direct COVID-19-related neuronal damage/CNS infiltration in the spectrum of neural tissues and vascular system of the brain. The direct PAMP-like effect of SARS-CoV-2 components on Toll-like receptors of glia was proven. Autoimmune and immunopathological links of COVID-19 pathogenesis, most probably, play an essential mechanistic role in its neuropsychiatric complications.

Further research is required to expand the knowledge on the impact of SARS-CoV-2 infection on the development of psychotic, affective, anxiety, and neurocognitive spectrum of disorders. Of course, the nature of humans is dual, bio-social, hence sociopathogenic effect of a prolonged pandemic (with all its social limitations and stressful atmosphere of hysteria around the COVID-19 problem facilitating phobic ideas) also has a negative influence on the psychic health of the population. But first of all, it is biomedical research, which could broaden our awareness of the long-term neuropsychiatric COVID-related consequences. At the same time, the studies will help to identify risk groups in terms of difficulties in treating psychiatric disorders and also could help to find new therapeutic methods in the future. In particular, it could provide the identification of new markers and targets for therapy.

References

[1] Bodnar B, Patel K, Ho W, Luo JJ, Hu W. Cellular mechanisms underlying neurological/neuropsychiatric manifestations of COVID-19. J Med Virol 2021;93(4):1983–98. https://doi.org/10.1002/jmv.26720.

[2] Mirfazeli FS, Sarabi-Jamab A, Jahanbakhshi A, Kordi A, Javadnia P, Shariat SV, et al. Neuropsychiatric manifestations of COVID-19 can be clustered in three distinct symptom categories. Sci Rep 2020;10:20957. https://doi.org/10.1038/s41598-020-78050-6.

[3] Jansen van Vuren E, Steyn SF, Brink CB, Möller M, Viljoen FP, Harvey BH. The neuropsychiatric manifestations of COVID-19: interactions with psychiatric illness and pharmacological treatment. Biomed Pharmacother 2021;135:111200. https://doi.org/10.1016/j.biopha.2020.111200.

[4] Fabrazzo M, Russo A, Camerlengo A, Tucci C, Luciano M, De Santis V, et al. Delirium and cognitive impairment as predisposing factors of COVID-19 infection in neuropsychiatric patients: a narrative review. Medicina 2021;57(11):1244. https://doi.org/10.3390/medicina57111244.

[5] Hawkins M, Sockalingam S, Bonato S, Rajaratnam T, Ravindran M, Gosse P, Sheehan KA. A rapid review of the pathoetiology, presentation, and management of delirium in adults with COVID-19. J Psychosom Res 2021;141:110350. https://doi.org/10.1016/j.jpsychores.2020.110350.

[6] Bellon M, Schweblin C, Lambeng N, Cherpillod P, Vasquez J, Lalive PH, et al. Cerebrospinal fluid features in SARS-CoV-2 RT-PCR positive patients. Clin Infect Dis 2021;73(9):e3102–5. https://doi.org/10.1093/cid/ciaa1165.

[7] Moriguchi T, Harii N, Goto J, Harada D, Sugawara H, Takamino J, et al. A first case of meningitis/encephalitis associated with SARS-coronavirus-2. Int J Infect Dis 2020;94:55–8. https://doi.org/10.1016/j.ijid.2020.03.062.

[8] Liu JM, Tan BH, Wu S, Gui Y, Suo JL, Li YC. Evidence of central nervous system infection and neuroinvasive routes, as well as neurological involvement, in the lethality of SARSCoV2 infection. J Med Virol 2021;93:1304–13. https://doi.org/10.1002/jmv.26570.

[9] Song E, Zhang C, Israelow B, Lu-Culligan A, Prado AV, Skriabine S, et al. Neuroinvasion of SARS-CoV-2 in human and mouse brain. bioRxiv 2020;218. https://doi.org/10.1101/2020.06.25.169946.

[10] Reichard RR, Kashani KB, Boire NA, Constantopoulos E, Guo Y, Lucchinetti CF. Neuropathology of COVID-19: a spectrum of vascular and acute disseminated encephalomyelitis (ADEM)-like pathology. Acta Neuropathol 2020;140:1–6. https://doi.org/10.1007/s00401-020-02166-2.

[11] Yang L, Han Y, Nilsson-Payant BE, Gupta V, Wang P, Duan X, et al. A human pluripotent stem cell-based platform to study SARS-CoV-2 tropism and model virus infection in human cells and organoids. Cell Stem Cell 2020;27(1):125–36. https://doi.org/10.1016/j.stem.2020.06.015. e7.

[12] Netland J, Meyerholz DK, Moore S, Cassell M, Perlman S. Severe acute respiratory syndrome coronavirus infection causes neuronal death in the absence of encephalitis in mice transgenic for human ACE2. J Virol 2008;82(15):7264–75. https://doi.org/10.1128/jvi.00737-08.

[13] Ramani A, Müller L, Ostermann PN, Gabriel E, Abida-Islam P, Müller-Schiffmann A, et al. SARS-CoV-2 targets neurons of 3D human brain organoids. EMBO J 2020;39:e106230. https://doi.org/10.15252/embj.2020106230.

[14] Yi SA, Nam KH, Yun J, Gim D, Joe D, Kim YH, et al. Infection of brain organoids and 2D cortical neurons with SARS-CoV-2 pseudovirus. Viruses 2020;12(9):1004. https://doi.org/10.3390/v12091004.

[15] Bostancıklıoğlu M. SARS-CoV2 entry and spread in the lymphatic drainage system of the brain. Brain Behav Immun 2020;87:122–3. https://doi.org/10.1016/j.bbi.2020.04.080.

[16] Dabrowska E, Galińska-Skok B, Waszkiewicz N. Depressive and neurocognitive disorders in the context of the inflammatory background of COVID-19. Life 2021;11(10):1056. https://doi.org/10.3390/life11101056.
[17] Morgun AV, Salmin VV, Boytsova EB, Lopatina OL, Salmina AB. Molecular mechanisms of proteins - targets for SARS-CoV-2 (review). Sovrem Tekhnologii Med 2021;12(6):98–108. https://doi.org/10.17691/stm2020.12.6.11.
[18] Wu Z, McGoogan JM. Characteristics of and important lessons from the coronavirus disease 2019 (COVID-19) outbreak in China: summary of a report of 72 314 cases from the Chinese center for disease control and prevention. JAMA 2020;323(13):1239–42. https://doi.org/10.1001/jama.2020.2648.
[19] Latini A, Agolini E, Novelli A, Borgiani P, Giannini R, Gravina P, et al. COVID-19 and genetic variants of protein involved in the SARS-CoV-2 entry into the host cells. Genes 2020;11(9). https://doi.org/10.3390/genes11091010.
[20] Kotani N, Nakano T. Candidate screening of host cell membrane proteins involved in SARS-CoV-2 entry. bioRxiv 2020. https://doi.org/10.1101/2020.09.09.289488.
[21] Amraei R, Napoleon M, Yin W, Suder EL, Berrigan J, Zhao Q, et al. CD209L/L-SIGN and CD209/DC-SIGN act as receptors for SARS-CoV-2 and are differentially expressed in lung and kidney epithelial and endothelial cells. bioRxiv 2020. https://doi.org/10.1101/2020.06.22.165803.
[22] Cantuti-Castelvetri L, Ojha R, Pedro LD, Djannatian M, Franz J, Kuivanen S, et al. Neuropilin-1 facilitates SARS-CoV-2 cell entry and infectivity. Science 2020;370:856–60. https://doi.org/10.1126/science.abd2985.
[23] Chiappelli F. Towards neuro-CoViD-19. Bioinformation 2020;16(4):288–92. https://doi.org/10.6026/97320630016288.
[24] Steardo L, Steardo Jr L, Verkhratsky A. Psychiatric face of COVID-19. Transl Psychiatry 2020;10(1):261. https://doi.org/10.1038/s41398-020-00949-5.
[25] Soldevila B, Puig-Domingo M, Marazuela M. Basic mechanisms of SARS-CoV-2 infection. What endocrine systems could be implicated? Rev Endocr Metab Disord July 2021;31:1–14. https://doi.org/10.1007/s11154-021-09678-6.
[26] Panariello F, Cellini L, Speciani M, De Ronchi D, Atti AR. How does SARS-CoV-2 affect the central nervous system? A working hypothesis. Front Psychiatry 2020;16(11):582345. https://doi.org/10.3389/fpsyt.2020.582345.
[27] He L, Mäe MA, Muhl L, Sun Y, Pietilä R, Nahar K, et al. Pericyte-specific vascular expression of SARS-CoV-2 receptor ACE2- implications for microvascular inflammation and hypercoagulopathy in COVID-19 patients. bioRxiv 2020. https://doi.org/10.1101/2020.05.11.088500.
[28] Ziegler CGK, Allon SJ, Nyquist SK, Mbano IM, Miao VN, Tzouanas CN, et al. SARS-CoV-2 receptor ACE2 is an interferon-stimulated gene in human airway epithelial cells and is detected in specific cell subsets across tissues. Cell 2020;181(5):1016–35. https://doi.org/10.1016/j.cell.2020.04.035. e19.
[29] Varga Z, Flammer AJ, Steiger P, Haberecker M, Andermatt R, Zinkernagel AS, et al. Endothelial cell infection and endotheliitis in COVID-19. Lancet 2020;395:1417–8. https://doi.org/10.1016/S0140-6736(20)30937-5.
[30] Cabirac GF, Murray RS, McLaughlin LB, Skolnick DM, Hogue B, Dorovini-Zis K, Didier PJ. In vitro interaction of coronaviruses with primate and human brain microvascular endothelial cells. Adv Exp Med Biol 1995;380:79–88. https://doi.org/10.1007/978-1-4615-1899-0_11.
[31] Li Y, Li M, Wang M, Zhou Y, Chang J, Xian Y, et al. Acute cerebrovascular disease following COVID19: a single center, retrospective, observational study. Stroke Vasc Neurol 2020;5:279–84. https://doi.org/10.1136/svn-2020-000431.
[32] Halliday MR, Rege SV, Ma Q, Zhao Z, Miller CA, Winkler EA, Zlokovic BV. Accelerated pericyte degeneration and blood-brain barrier breakdown in apolipoprotein E4 carriers with Alzheimer's disease. J Cerebr Blood Flow Metabol 2016;36(1):216–27. https://doi.org/10.1038/jcbfm. 2015.44.
[33] Golden JW, Cline CR, Zeng X, Garrison AR, Carey BD, Mucker EM, et al. Human angiotensin-converting enzyme 2 transgenic mice infected with SARS-CoV-2 develop severe and fatal respiratory disease. JCI Insight 2020;5(19):e142032. https://doi.org/10.1172/jci.insight.142032.
[34] Bulfamante G, Chiumello D, Canevini MP, Priori A, Mazzanti M, Centanni S, Felisati G. First ultrastructural autoptic findings of SARS-Cov-2 in olfactory pathways and brainstem. Minerva Anestesiol 2020;86(6):678–9. https://doi.org/10.23736/S0375-9393.20.14772-2.
[35] Najt P, Richards HL, Fortune DG. Brain imaging in patients with COVID-19: a systematic review. Brain Behav Immun Health 2021;16:100290. https://doi.org/10.1016/j.bbih.2021.100290.

[36] Galougahi MK, Ghorbani J, Bakhshayeshkaram M, Naeini AS, Haseli S. Olfactory bulb magnetic resonance imaging in SARS-CoV-2-induced anosmia: the first report. Acad Radiol 2020;27:892–3. https://doi.org/10.1016/j.acra.2020.04.002.
[37] Mayorova MA, Butoma BG, Churilov LP, Gilburd B, Petrova NN, Shoenfeld Y. Autoimmune concept of schizophrenia: historical roots and current facets. Psychiatr Danub 2021;33(1):3–17. https://doi.org/10.24869/psyd.2021.3. Spring.
[38] Deigendesch N, Sironi L, Kutza M, Wischnewski S, Fuchs V, Hench J, et al. Correlates of critical illness-related encephalopathy predominate postmortem COVID-19 neuropathology. Acta Neuropathol 2020;140:583–6. https://doi.org/10.1007/s00401-020-02213-y.
[39] Martines RB, Ritter JM, Matkovic E, Gary J, Bollweg BC, Bullock H, et al. Pathology and pathogenesis of SARS-CoV-2 associated with fatal coronavirus disease, United States. Emerg Infect Dis 2020;26:2005–15. https://doi.org/10.3201/eid2609.202095.
[40] Murta V, Villarreal A, Ramos AJ. Severe acute respiratory syndrome coronavirus 2 impact on the central nervous system: are astrocytes and microglia main players or merely bystanders? ASN Neuro 2020;12. https://doi.org/10.1177/1759091420954960.
[41] Pellegrini L, Albecka A, Mallery DL, Kellner MJ, Paul D, Carter AP, et al. SARS-CoV-2 infects the brain choroid plexus and disrupts the blood-CSF barrier in human brain organoids. Cell Stem Cell 2020;27:951–61. https://doi.org/10.1016/j.stem.2020.10.001. e5.
[42] Jacob F, Pather SR, Huang WK, Zhang F, Wong SZH, Zhou H, et al. Human pluripotent stem cell-derived neural cells and brain organoids reveal SARS-CoV-2 neurotropism predominates in choroid plexus epithelium. Cell Stem Cell 2020;27(6):937–50. https://doi.org/10.1016/j.stem.2020.09.016.
[43] Troyer EA, Kohn JN, Hong S. Are we facing a crashing wave of neuropsychiatric sequelae of COVID-19? Neuropsychiatric symptoms and potential immunologic mechanisms. Brain Behav Immun 2020;87:34–9. https://doi.org/10.1016/j.bbi.2020.04.027.
[44] Vasilevska V, Guest PC, Bernstein HG, Schroeter ML, Geis C, Steiner J. Molecular mimicry of NMDA receptors may contribute to neuropsychiatric symptoms in severe COVID-19 cases. J Neuroinflammation 2021;18(1):245. https://doi.org/10.1186/s12974-021-02293-x.
[45] Vojdani A, Kharrazian D. Potential antigenic cross-reactivity between SARS-CoV-2 and human tissue with a possible link to an increase in autoimmune diseases. Clin Immunol 2020;217:108480. https://doi.org/10.1016/j.clim.2020.108480.
[46] Zinserling VA, Vashukova MA, Vasilyeva MV, Isakov AN, Lugovskaya NA, Narkevich TA, Sukhanova YV, Semenova NY, Gusev DA. Issues of pathology of a new coronavirus infection COVID-19. J Infect 2020;12(2):5–11. https://doi.org/10.22625/2072-6732-2020-12-2-5-11 (In Russ.).
[47] Ehrenfeld M, Tincani A, Andreoli L, Cattalini M, Greenbaum A, Kanduc D, Alijotas-Reig J, Zinserling V, Semenova N, Amital H, Shoenfeld Y. COVID-19 and autoimmunity. Autoimmun Rev 2020;19(8):102597. https://doi.org/10.1016/j.autrev.2020.102597.
[48] Orsini A, Corsi M, Santangelo A, Riva A, Peroni D, Foiadelli T, et al. Challenges and management of neurological and psychiatric manifestations in SARS-CoV-2 (COVID-19) patients. Neurol Sci 2020;41(9):2353–66. https://doi.org/10.1007/s10072-020-04544-w.
[49] Li N, Ma WT, Pang M, Fan QL, Hua JL. The commensal microbiota and viral infection: a comprehensive review. Front Immunol 2019;10:1–16. https://doi.org/10.3389/fimmu.2019.01551.
[50] Nalleballe K, Reddy Onteddu S, Sharma R, Dandu V, Brown A, Jasti M, et al. Spectrum of neuropsychiatric manifestations in COVID-19. Brain Behav Immun August 2020;88:71–4. https://doi.org/10.1016/j.bbi.2020.06.020.
[51] Almqvist J, Granberg T, Tzortzakakis A, Klironomos S, Kollia E, Öhberg C, et al. Neurological manifestations of coronavirus infections—a systematic review. Ann Clin Transl Neurol October 2020;7(10):2057–71. https://doi.org/10.1002/acn3.51166.
[52] Chiesa-Estomba CM, Lechien JR, Radulesco T, Michel J, Sowerby LJ, Hopkins C, Saussez S. Patterns of smell recovery in 751 patients affected by the COVID-19 outbreak. Eur J Neurol 2020;27(11):2318–21. https://doi.org/10.1111/ene.14440.
[53] Rogers JP, Chesney E, Oliver D, Pollak TA, McGuire P, Fusar-Poli P, et al. Psychiatric and neuropsychiatric presentations associated with severe coronavirus infections: a systematic review and meta-analysis with comparison to the COVID-19 pandemic. Lancet Psychiatr 2020;7(7):611–27. https://doi.org/10.1016/S2215-0366(20)30203-0.

[54] Petrova NN, Pashkovskiy VE, Sivashova MS, Gvozdetskiy AN, Prokopovich GA. Impact of mental disorders on COVID-19 outcomes. Neurol Neuropsychiatr Psychosom 2021;13(5):40–7 [In Russian].

[55] Vermeersch G, Maes J. Encephalopathy associated with autoimmune thyroid disease: a rare but frequently missed neuropsychiatric syndrome. Acta Neurol Belg 2021;121(3):821–2. https://doi.org/10.1007/s13760-021-01682-6.

[56] Xiang P, Xu XM, Gao LL, Wang HZ, Xiong HF, Li RH. First case of 2019 novel coronavirus disease with encephalitis. China 2020:00015. 202003.

[57] Banerjee D, Viswanath B. Neuropsychiatric manifestations of COVID-19 and possible pathogenic mechanisms: insights from other coronaviruses. Asian J Psychiatr 2020;54:102350. https://doi.org/10.1016/j.ajp.2020.102350.

[58] Ryabkova VA, Churilov LP, Shoenfeld Y. Influenza infection, SARS, MERS and COVID-19: cytokine storm–the common denominator and the lessons to be learned. Clin Immunol 2021a;223:108652. https://doi.org/10.1016/j.clim.2020.108652.

[59] Lu L, Xiong W, Liu D, Liu J, Yang D, Li N, et al. New onset acute symptomatic seizure and risk factors in coronavirus disease 2019: a retrospective multicenter study. Epilepsia 2020;61(6):e49–53. https://doi.org/10.1111/epi.16524.

[60] Robinson-Agramonte MA, Gonçalves CA, Noris-García E, Préndes Rivero N, Brigida AL, Schultz S, et al. Impact of SARS-CoV-2 on neuropsychiatric disorders. World J Psychiatr 2021;11(7):347–54. https://doi.org/10.5498/wjp.v11.i7.347.

[61] Rittmannsberger H, Barth M, Malik P, Yazdi K. Neuropsychiatrische Aspekte von COVID-19 – eine narrative Übersicht [Neuropsychiatric Aspects of COVID-19 - a Narrative Overview]. Fortschr Neurol Psychiatr 2021. https://doi.org/10.1055/a-1523-3850. German.

[62] Wang H. Delirium: a suggestive sign of COVID-19 in dementia. EClinicalMedicine 2020;26:100524. https://doi.org/10.1016/j.eclinm.2020.100524.

[63] Beach SR, Praschan NC, Hogan C, Dotson S, Merideth F, Kontos N, et al. Delirium in COVID-19: a case series and exploration of potential mechanisms for central nervous system involvement. Gen Hosp Psychiatr 2020;65:47–53. https://doi.org/10.1016/j.genhosppsych.2020.05.008.

[64] Ticinesi A, Cerundolo N, Parise A, Nouvenne A, Prati B, Guerra A, et al. Delirium in COVID-19: epidemiology and clinical correlations in a large group of patients admitted to an academic hospital. Aging Clin Exp Res 2020;32:2159–66. https://doi.org/10.1007/s40520-020-01699-6.

[65] O'Hanlon S, Inouye SK. Delirium: a missing piece in the COVID-19 pandemic puzzle. Age Ageing 2020;49(4):497–8. https://doi.org/10.1093/ageing/afaa094.

[66] Anmella G, Arbelo N, Fico G, Murru A, Llach CD, Madero S, et al. COVID-19 inpatients with psychiatric disorders: real-world clinical recommendations from an expert team in consultation-liaison psychiatry. J Affect Disord 2020;274:1062–7. https://doi.org/10.1016/j.jad.2020.05.149.

[67] Khan SH, Lindroth H, Perkins AJ, Jamil Y, Wang S, Roberts S, et al. Delirium incidence, duration and severity in critically ill patients with COVID-19. Crit Care Explor 2020;2(12):e0290. https://doi.org/10.1097/CCE.0000000000000290.

[68] Kim H-C, Yoo S-Y, Lee B-H, Lee SH, Shin H-S. Psychiatric findings in suspected and confirmed Middle East respiratory syndrome patients quarantined in hospital: a retrospective chart analysis. Psychiatry Investig 2018;15:355–60. https://doi.org/10.30773/pi.2017.10.25.1.

[69] Cuperlovic-Culf M, Cunningham EL, Teimoorinia H, Surendra A, Pan X, Bennett SAL, et al. Metabolomics and computational analysis of the role of monoamine oxidase activity in delirium and SARS-CoV-2 infection. Sci Rep 2021;11:10629. https://doi.org/10.1038/s41598-021-90243-1.

[70] Frank MG, Nguyen KH, Ball JB, Hopkins S, Kelley T, Baratta MV, Fleshner M, Maier SF. SARS-CoV-2 spike S1 subunit induces neuroinflammatory, microglial and behavioral sickness responses: evidence of PAMP-like properties. Brain Behav Immun 2022;100:267–77. https://doi.org/10.1016/j.bbi.2021.12.007.

[71] Beaud V, Crottaz-Herbette S, Dunet V, Vaucher J, Bernard-Valnet R, Du Pasquier R, Bart PA, Clarke S. Pattern of cognitive deficits in severe COVID-19. J Neurol Neurosurg Psychiatry 2021;92(5):567–8. https://doi.org/10.1136/jnnp-2020-325173.

[72] Kas A, Soret M, Pyatigoskaya N, Habert MO, Hesters A, Le Guennec L, et al. The cerebral network of COVID-19-related encephalopathy: a longitudinal voxel-based 18F-FDG-PET study. Eur J Nucl Med Mol Imag 2021;48(8):2543–57. https://doi.org/10.1007/s00259-020-05178-y.

[73] Du YY, Zhao W, Zhou XL, Zeng M, Yang DH, Xie XZ, et al. Survivors of COVID-19 exhibit altered amplitudes of low frequency fluctuation in the brain: a resting-state functional magnetic resonance imaging study at 1-year follow-up. Neural Regen Res 2022;17(7):1576–81. https://doi.org/10.4103/1673-5374.327361.

[74] Schmidt FM, Schröder T, Kirkby KC, Sander C, Suslow T, Holdt LM, et al. Pro- and anti-inflammatory cytokines, but not CRP, are inversely correlated with severity and symptoms of major depression. Psychiatr Res 2016;239:85–91. https://doi.org/10.1016/j.psychres.2016.02.052.

[75] Hossain MM, Tasnim S, Sultana A, Faizah F, Mazumder H, Zou L, et al. Epidemiology of mental health problems in COVID-19: a review. F1000Res 2020;9:636. https://doi.org/10.12688/f1000research.24457.1.

[76] Mazza MG, De Lorenzo R, Conte C, Poletti S, Vai B, Bollettini I, et al. Anxiety and depression in COVID-19 survivors: role of inflammatory and clinical predictors. Brain Behav Immun 2020;89:594–600. https://doi.org/10.1016/j.bbi.2020.07.037.

[77] Nakamura ZM, Nash RP, Laughon SL, Rosenstein DL. Neuropsychiatric complications of COVID-19. Curr Psychiatr Rep 2021;23(5):25. https://doi.org/10.1007/s11920-021-01237-9.

[78] Deng J, Zhou F, Hou W, Silver Z, Wong CY, Chang O, et al. The prevalence of depression, anxiety, and sleep disturbances in COVID-19 patients: a meta-analysis. Ann N Y Acad Sci 2021;1486(1):90–111. https://doi.org/10.1111/nyas.14506.

[79] Taquet M, Luciano S, Geddes JR, Harrison PJ. Bidirectional associations between COVID-19 and psychiatric disorder: a study of 62,354 COVID-19 cases. Lancet Psychiatr 2020:30462–4. https://doi.org/10.1016/S2215-0366(20)30462-4. S2215–0366.

[80] Cai X, Hu X, Ekumi IO, Wang J, An Y, Li Z, Yuan B. Psychological distress and its correlates among COVID-19 survivors during early convalescence across age groups. Am J Geriatr Psychiatr 2020;28:1030–9. https://doi.org/10.1016/j.jagp.2020.07.003.

[81] Gennaro MM, Mariagrazia P, De Lorenzo R, Cristiano M, Sara P, Roberto F, et al. Persistent psychopathology and neurocognitive impairment in COVID-19 survivors: effect of inflammatory biomarkers at three-month follow-up. Brain Behav Immun 2021;94:138–47. https://doi.org/10.1016/j.bbi.2021.02.021.

[82] Kivity S, Ortega-Hernandez OD, Shoenfeld Y. Olfaction–a window to the mind. Isr Med Assoc J 2009;11(4):238–43.

[83] Perricone C, Shoenfeld N, Agmon-Levin N, de Carolis C, Perricone R, Shoenfeld Y. Smell and autoimmunity: a comprehensive review. Clin Rev Allergy Immunol 2013;45(1):87–96. https://doi.org/10.1007/s12016-012-8343-x.

[84] Katzav A, Solodeev I, Brodsky O, Chapman J, Pick CG, Blank M, Zhang W, Reichlin M, Shoenfeld Y. Induction of autoimmune depression in mice by anti–ribosomal P antibodies via the limbic system. Arthritis Rheum 2007;56:938–48.

[85] Dotan A, Muller S, Kanduc D, David P, Halpert G, Shoenfeld Y. The SARS-CoV-2 as an instrumental trigger of autoimmunity. Autoimmun Rev 2021;20(4):102792. https://doi.org/10.1016/j.autrev.2021.102792.

[86] Lu S, Wei N, Jiang J, Wu L, Sheng J, Zhou J, et al. First report of manic-like symptoms in a COVID-19 patient with no previous history of a psychiatric disorder. J Affect Disord 2020;277:337–40. https://doi.org/10.1016/j.jad.2020.08.031.

[87] Iqbal Y, Alabdulla M, Latoo J, Kumar R, Albrahim S, Wadoo OM, Haddad P. Mania and hypomania associated with COVID-19: a series of 15 cases seen by the consultation-liaison psychiatry service in Qatar. Qatar Med J 2021;2021(3):65. https://doi.org/10.5339/qmj.2021.65.

[88] Bo HX, Li W, Yang Y, Wang Y, Zhang Q, Cheung T, et al. Posttraumatic stress symptoms and attitude toward crisis mental health services among clinically stable patients with COVID-19 in China. Psychol Med 2020;51(6):1052–3. https://doi.org/10.1017/S0033291720000999. Cambridge University Press.

[89] Halpin SJ, McIvor C, Whyatt G, Adams A, Harvey O, McLean L, et al. Postdischarge symptoms and rehabilitation needs in survivors of COVID-19 infection: a cross-sectional evaluation. J Med Virol 2021;93(2):1013–22. https://doi.org/10.1002/jmv.26368.

[90] Righy C, Rosa RG, Da Silva RTA, Kochhann R, Migliavaca CB, Robinson CC, et al. Prevalence of post-traumatic stress disorder symptoms in adult critical care survivors: a systematic review and meta-analysis. Crit Care 2019;23:1–13. https://doi.org/10.1186/s13054-019-2489-3.

[91] Dadkhah M, Talei S, Doostkamel D, Molaei S, Rezaei N. The impact of COVID-19 on diagnostic biomarkers in neuropsychiatric and neuroimmunological diseases: a review. Rev Neurosci 2021;33(1):79–92. https://doi.org/10.1515/revneuro-2020-0154.

[92] Varatharaj A, Thomas N, Ellul MA, NWS D, Pollak TA, Tenorio EL, et al. Neurological and neuropsychiatric complications of COVID-19 in 153 patients: a UK-wide surveillance study. Lancet Psychiatr 2020;7:875–82. https://doi.org/10.1016/S2215-0366(20)30287-X.

[93] Rentero D, Juanes A, Losada CP, Álvarez S, Parra A, Santana V, et al. New-onset psychosis in COVID-19 pandemic: a case series in Madrid. Psychiatr Res 2020;290:113097. https://doi.org/10.1016/j.psychres.2020.113097.

[94] Tariku M, Hajure M. Available evidence and ongoing hypothesis on corona virus (COVID-19) and psychosis: is corona virus and psychosis related? A narrative review. Psychol Res Behav Manag 2020;13:701–4. https://doi.org/10.2147/PRBM.S264235.

[95] Smith CM, Komisar JR, Mourad A, Kincaid BR. COVID-19-associated brief psychotic disorder. BMJ Case Rep 2020;13(8):e236940. https://doi.org/10.1136/bcr-2020-236940.

[96] Parra A, Juanes A, Losada CP, Álvarez-Sesmero S, Santana VD, Martí I, et al. Psychotic symptoms in COVID-19 patients. A retrospective descriptive study. Psychiatr Res 2020;291:113254. https://doi.org/10.1016/j.psychres.2020.113254.

[97] Chacko M, Job A, Caston 3rd F, George P, Yacoub A, Cáceda R. COVID-19-Induced psychosis and suicidal behavior: case report. SN Compr Clin Med 2020;26:1–5. https://doi.org/10.1007/s42399-020-00530-7.

[98] Mascolo A, Berrino PM, Gareri P, Castagna A, Capuano A, Manzo C, et al. Neuropsychiatric clinical manifestations in elderly patients treated with hydroxychloroquine: a review article. Inflammopharmacology 2018;26:1141–9. https://doi.org/10.1007/s10787-018-0498-5.

[99] Yao H, Chen JH, Xu YF. Patients with mental health disorders in the COVID-19 epidemic. Lancet Psychiatr 2020;7(4):e21. https://doi.org/10.1016/S2215-0366(20)30090-0.

[100] Zain SM, Muthukanagaraj P, Rahman N. Excited catatonia—a delayed neuropsychiatric complication of COVID-19 infection. Cureus 2021;13(3):e13891. https://doi.org/10.7759/cureus.13891.

[101] Amenta EM, Spallone A, Rodriguez-Barradas MC, El Sahly HM, Atmar RL, Kulkarni PA. Postacute COVID-19: an overview and approach to classification. Open Forum Infect Dis 2020;7. https://doi.org/10.1093/ofid/ofaa509. ofaa509.

[102] Ryabkova VA, Gavrilova NY, Kanduc D, Churilov LP, Shoenfeld Y. Post-COVID syndrome and its immunopathological mechanisms. The role of autoimmunity. Russ Biomed Res 2021b;6(3):7–11.

[103] Sher L. Post-COVID syndrome and suicide risk. QJM 2021;114(2):95–8. https://doi.org/10.1093/qjmed/hcab007.

[104] Havervall S, Rosell A, Phillipson M, Mangsbo SM, Nilsson P, Hober S, Thålin C. Symptoms and functional impairment assessed 8 Months after mild COVID-19 among health care workers. JAMA 2021;325:2015–6. https://doi.org/10.1001/jama.2021.5612.

[105] Kyzar EJ, Purpura LJ, Shah J, Cantos A, Nordvig AS, Yin MT. Anxiety, depression, insomnia, and trauma-related symptoms following COVID-19 infection at long-term follow-up. Brain Behav Immun Health 2021;16:100315. https://doi.org/10.1016/j.bbih.2021.100315.

[106] Guedj E, Million M, Dudouet P, Tissot-Dupont H, Bregeon F, Cammilleri S. Raoult D. ^{18}F-FDG brain PET hypometabolism in post-SARS-CoV-2 infection: substrate for persistent/delayed disorders? Eur J Nucl Med Mol Imag 2021;48(2):592–5. https://doi.org/10.1007/s00259-020-04973-x.

[107] Hampshire A, Trender W, Chamberlain SR, et al. Cognitive deficits in people who have recovered from COVID-19. EClinicalMedicine 2021;39. https://doi.org/10.1016/j.eclinm.2021.101044.

[108] Kumar S, Veldhuis A, Malhotra T. Neuropsychiatric and cognitive sequelae of COVID-19. Front Psychol 2021;12:577529. https://doi.org/10.3389/fpsyg.2021.577529.

[109] Méndez R, Balanzá-Martínez V, Luperdi SC, Estrada I, Latorre A, González-Jiménez P, et al. Short-term neuropsychiatric outcomes and quality of life in COVID-19 survivors. J Intern Med 2021;290(3):621–31. https://doi.org/10.1111/joim.13262.

[110] Vannorsdall TD, Brigham E, Fawzy A, Raju S, Gorgone A, Pletnikova A, et al. Rates of cognitive dysfunction, psychiatric distress, and functional decline after COVID-19. JACLP 2021. https://doi.org/10.1016/j.jaclp.2021.10.006. S2667-2960(21)00185-3.

[111] Van Helvoort MA, Pop-Purceleanu M, Tendolkar I, Everaerd DS. Neuropsychiatrisch herstel na COVID-19; een observationeel cohortonderzoek [Neuropsychiatric recovery after COVID-19—an observational cohort-study]. Tijdschr Psychiatr 2021;63(7):514–21.

[112] Nuzzo D, Cambula G, Bacile I, Rizzo M, Galia M, Mangiapane P, et al. Long-term brain disorders in post COVID-19 neurological syndrome (PCNS) patient. Brain Sci 2021;11:454. https://doi.org/10.3390/brainsci11040454.

[113] Huang C, Huang L, Wang Y, Li X, Ren L, Gu X, et al. 6-month consequences of COVID-19 in patients discharged from hospital: a cohort study. Lancet 2021;397:220–32. https://doi.org/10.1016/S0140-6736(20)32656-8.

[114] Coughlin SS, Sher L. Suicidal behavior and neurological illnesses. J Depress Anxiety 2013;02:12443. https://doi.org/10.4172/2167-1044.S9-001.

[115] Wilson N, Kvalsvig A, Barnard LT, Baker MG. Case-fatality risk estimates for COVID-19 calculated by using a lag time for fatality. Emerg Infect Dis 2020;26(6):1339–441. https://doi.org/10.3201/eid2606.200320.

CHAPTER

19

Myocarditis following vaccination with Pfizer-BioNTech BNT162b2 against coronavirus infection (COVID-19)

Dror Mevorach

Department of Medicine B, and Division of Rheumatology-Immunology-Allergology and the Wohl Institute for Translational Medicine, Department of Medicine, Hadassah Medical Center and the Faculty of Medicine, Hebrew University, Jerusalem, Israel

Background

Postvaccination myocarditis was reported as early as 1957, in association with smallpox vaccination [1–5]. Vaccine-associated myocarditis received further attention when several cases were reported among healthcare workers (HCW) and military personnel who received the smallpox vaccine [2]. Among over 25,000 HCWs who received the smallpox vaccine in the first quarter of 2003, seven cases of adverse cardiac events were recorded among civilians and 10 cases of myocarditis among military personnel. Rare reports of vaccine-associated myocarditis were not limited to the smallpox vaccine; Makaryus et al. described myocarditis associated with pneumococcal vaccination [3]. Cheng et al. described an association with seasonal inactivated influenza vaccine [4], and several other reports of myocarditis associated with different vaccines have been suggested [5].

Myocarditis following adult vaccination with two doses of Pfizer-BioNTech BNT162b2

Following Emergency Use Authorization (EUA) of the Pfizer-BioNTech BNT162b2 vaccine by the FDA on December 11, 2020 [6], approval was granted in Israel on December 20, 2020. A national vaccination campaign for novel coronavirus infection (COVID-19)

Autoimmunity, COVID-19, Post-COVID19 syndrome and COVID-19 vaccination
https://doi.org/10.1016/B978-0-443-18566-3.00019-0

using the Pfizer vaccine ensued in Israel. The vaccination campaign was based on a 2-dose regimen administered with a 21-day interval. The campaign initially targeted at-risk populations of HCW and citizens aged 60 and over, but eligibility criteria rapidly expanded to include all eligible adults aged 16 years and above. By May 31, 2021 over 5.45 million individuals were vaccinated.

The first known patient in the world with postvaccination myocarditis was hospitalized on January 10, 2020 in the Department of Medicine B, Hadassah Ein Karem Medical Center in Jerusalem, Israel. The case was reported to the Israeli Ministry of Health (MoH) and the World Health Organization (WHO), and in a personal twitter (Profesor Dror Mevorach), as possibly related to the vaccination. Passive surveillance was conducted during the campaign, with adverse events following immunization (AEFI) within 30 days of vaccination reported to the MoH by healthcare providers. Upon receipt of several myocarditis reports, the MoH initiated active surveillance, requesting all 28 medical centers in Israel to report myocarditis cases, with or without pericardial effusion (i.e., perimyocarditis), regardless of vaccination status. Cases of suspected myocarditis are almost always hospitalized in Israel, and therefore these data represent a complete set of myocarditis patients on the national level. A preliminary report in April 2021 identified this association [7] as required by Israeli law.

The U.S. Centers for Disease Control (CDC) [8] and the European Medicines Agency (EMA) of the European Union [9] also reported a small number of cases of myocarditis following the COVID-19 mRNA vaccination with Comirnaty (Pfizer) and Spikevax (Moderna). Case reports, surveillance data and other reports from the United States, Israel, and Canada indicated an increased risk of myocarditis after vaccination with SARS-CoV2 mRNA vaccines, higher after the second dose, especially in younger men [10–16]. Data from Canada and France indicated more cases of myocarditis after Moderna's mRNA-1273 than after Pfizer's BNT162b2 [17,18]. However, these reports were all based on passive surveillance, and it was difficult to draw a clear conclusion prior to publication of three reports based on active surveillance for cases of myocarditis across the whole country of Israel that evaluated risk based on observed cases in relation to expected. The initial clinical and epidemiological active studies performed in Israel included patient characteristics, treatment, and outcomes. The analyses focused on risk following the first and second vaccine in adults [19] and in adolescents [12], as well as risk in adults following the third (booster) vaccine [20].

The Israeli studies are based on patients admitted to hospital with a primary or secondary discharge diagnosis of myocarditis or diagnostic codes (*International Classification of Diseases, 10th Revision*, 422.0-9*x* and 429.0*x*) that have been shown to have 85% positive predictive value for myocarditis in patients below the age of 60 [21]. Cases were included after review of clinical and laboratory data and discharge summaries associated with the active surveillance reports by cardiologists and a rheumatologist (all board certified) for classification as myocarditis based on Brighton criteria [22] or criteria for adverse events after smallpox vaccination [23–25]. Verification of vaccination status and date was obtained from a national database and intensive statistical risk analysis was based on national historical data for myocarditis incidence. The observed-to-expected ratio (standardized incidence ratio, SIR) with approximate 95% confidence intervals for all myocarditis cases was also computed based on a national pre-COVID-19 reference (2017–2019). A diagnosis within 21 days following receipt of the first vaccine dose (the interval between the two doses) or within 30 days after the second dose was deemed possibly related to vaccination.

The first study [19] included the period from December 2020 when the vaccination campaign began through May 2021, at which point approximately 5.1 million Israelis had received both doses of the Pfizer vaccine. We found higher incidence of myocarditis in Israeli adults aged >16 years, mainly in young males, who had received Pfizer-BioNTech BNT162b2 vaccinations compared to historical controls and unvaccinated individuals. Among 304 persons with symptoms of myocarditis, 21 received an alternative diagnosis. Of the remaining 283 cases, 142 occurred after receipt of the BNT162b2 vaccine and 136 diagnoses of the 142 were definitive or probable. The clinical presentation was judged to be mild in 129 recipients (95%), but one fulminant case was fatal. The overall risk difference between the first and second doses was 1.76 per 100,000 persons (95% confidence interval [CI], 1.33 to 2.19), with the largest difference among male recipients between the ages of 16 and 19 years (difference, 13.73 per 100,000 persons; 95% CI, 8.11 to 19.46). As compared to the expected incidence based on historical data, the standardized incidence ratio was 5.34 (95% CI, 4.48 to 6.40) and was highest after the second dose in male recipients between the ages of 16 and 19 years (13.60; 95% CI, 9.30 to 19.20). The rate ratio 30 days after the second vaccine dose in fully vaccinated recipients, as compared to unvaccinated persons, was 2.35 (95% CI, 1.10 to 5.02); the rate ratio was again highest in male recipients between the ages of 16 and 19 years (8.96; 95% CI, 4.50 to 17.83), with a ratio of 1 in 6637.

Myocarditis in adolescents following vaccination with two doses of Pfizer-BioNTech BNT162b2

Given the elevated risk we had found in young men, the second study focused on risk of myocarditis in individuals aged 12–15 years following vaccination with Pfizer-BioNTech BNT162b2 [12]. Again, using the active nationwide surveillance system administered by the Israeli MoH, we reported he incidence of hospitalization for myocarditis between June 2 and October 20, 2021 in this age group, within 21 days after receipt of the first vaccine dose and within 30 days after receipt of the second dose. Clinical data were reviewed by a cardiologist and a rheumatologist, and the severity of disease was classified according to the Brighton Collaboration Case Definition [22]. During the period under study, 404,407 adolescents (195,579 of whom were male) received the first dose of vaccine and 326,463 adolescents (157,153 of whom were male) received the second dose. There were 18 cases of myocarditis leading to hospitalization reported. Two cases of myocarditis were excluded from the study owing to reasonable alternative diagnoses. Of the remaining 16 cases, one occurred in an unvaccinated adolescent and 15 occurred in vaccinated adolescents, one case within 21 days after receipt of the first vaccine dose, 12 cases within 1 week after receipt of the second dose, and two later cases (1 each at 46 and 70 days after receipt of the second dose). The two later cases were considered by the investigators as unlikely to be related to the vaccine. The demographic characteristics of the 13 adolescents with myocarditis occurring within 21 days after receipt of the first vaccine dose or within 30 days after receipt of the second dose. These 13 cases were classified as probable or definitive myocarditis according to the case definition. All the cases were clinically mild, involving a mean duration of hospitalization of 3.1 days (range, 1 to 6) and no readmissions during 30 days of follow-up. The risk estimates of myocarditis among male recipients in the 21 days after the first and second doses were 0.56 cases per 100,000 after the first dose and 8.09 cases per 100,000 after the second dose; the risk estimates among female recipients were 0 cases per 100,000 after the first dose and 0.69 cases per 100,000 after the second dose. The risk of myocarditis after receipt of the second vaccine dose among male adolescents 12-to-15 years of age was estimated to be 1 case per 12,361; the corresponding risk among female adolescents was estimated to be 1 case per 144,439. The risk estimates per person in this study were lower than the previously reported risks among male recipients 16–24 years of age [19], but they were slightly higher than the Centers for Disease Control and Prevention estimate of approximately 1 case per 16,129 male recipients 12-to-17 years of age after receipt of the second dose [26]. These differences may be explained by the active surveillance in our population. In a phase three trial of the BNT162b2 vaccine, the relatively small number of vaccinated adolescents 12-to-15 years of age (1131), of whom 567 were male, is a possible explanation for the absence of reported cases of myocarditis during the trial [27].

Myocarditis following adult vaccination with a third (booster) dose of Pfizer-BioNTech BNT162b2

Although the efficacy of the vaccine was demonstrated in both in clinical trials and post-vaccination observational studies [28–30], there has been uncertainty about the duration of protection, particularly in whom an adequate antibody response to the vaccines was not detected. In the follow-up phase of trials conducted with Pfizer-BioNTech COVID-19 vaccine, overall clinical effectiveness of over 95% for severe disease and around 65% for asymptomatic disease was reported; however, follow-up was limited to 2 months [31]. In real life, the efficacy data found in clinical trials by studies in large populations has been confirmed [28,29], but, as observation time increased, differences related to age groups and in some cases to disease progression and concerns of waning vaccine-induced immunity were found. Waning of spike protein antibody levels was observed over time following the administration of a second dose of SARS-CoV-2 vaccines [32,33], and the need for a booster was considered. Indeed, FDA emergency authorization of the vaccine expanded the EAU for the Pfizer and Moderna Covid-19 vaccine boosters on November 17, 2021 [34], indicating that the shots can be given to anyone aged 18 or older at least 6 months after completion of the primary vaccine series.

Based on evidence of waning protection, vaccine boosters were authorized and given earlier in Israel than in the United States, with the vaccination campaign for the booster vaccination beginning on July 30, 2021. Since the incidence of myocarditis had been increased in association with the original 2-dose regimen, particularly at a younger age, it was important to evaluate and compare the risk for development of myocarditis following the booster. In our third study [20], we therefore evaluated the risk of the third (booster) vaccination. All cases of myocarditis from July 31, 2021, when booster shots were first administered, through November 5, 2021, regardless of vaccination status, were reported to the MOH by all hospitals in Israel. Clinical data were again reviewed by a cardiologist and a rheumatologist and classified based on the Brighton Collaboration Myocarditis Case Definition. Descriptive statistics were used to describe the clinical picture of patients, including age and sex analysis. Myocarditis risk for definite/probable cases was computed with 95% confidence interval (95%CI) and compared to previous vaccinations, and SIRs were calculated. Analyses were repeated for a follow up of 90 days to cover myocarditis cases occurring later.

During the surveillance period, 3,610,023 individuals (1,766,617 males, 48.9%) received the Pfizer booster dose and 91 cases of myocarditis were reported, including 35 cases reported within 30 days of booster vaccination. Among them, 29 were probable or confirmed myocarditis; 18/29 occurred during the first week after the booster. All 29 cases were clinically mild and the patients recovered following an average hospitalization of 3.5 days (range 1–6), with no readmissions after discharge. Risk estimates in the 30 days following the booster were 6.44/100,000 and 5.21/100,000 for males aged 16–19 and 20–24, respectively. Compared to vaccine dose 1 and 2, for males the overall risk differences per 100,000 were 0.69 (95%CI, 0.08 to 1.34) and −2.66 (95%CI 3.62 to −1.67), respectively, mainly driven by younger males. For females, the corresponding differences were 0.09 (95%CI −0.12 to 0.34) and −0.48 (95%CI −0.83 to −0.09). Observed-to-expected myocarditis incidence in the 30 days following the booster vaccine dose was SIR = 2.29 (95% CI 1.56 to 3.23) and SIR = 1.03 (95% CI 0.21 to 3.00) in males and females, respectively, with significantly elevated ratios for males aged 16–19 (SIR = 5.45, 95%CI 1.99–11.87), 20–24 (SIR = 4.68, 95%CI 2.01–9.22) and 40+ (SIR = 2.59, 95%CI 1.29 to 4.63) years. To summarize, there was increased risk of myocarditis following the third vaccine dose, mainly in males ages 16–24, with estimated prevalence as 1:17,498. This risk was lower compared to the risk following the second vaccine dose, which could be because susceptible individuals who had previously developed myocarditis following vaccination did not receive the booster, or due to the longer interval length between the second and third vaccinations.

Limitations of the three studies described [12,19,20] are that myocarditis was not validated by myocardial biopsy, misclassification, and reporting bias may have taken place, and we acquired only hospitalized cases. On the other hand, these were the only studies based on active nationwide surveillance that verified all diagnoses, whereas most other studies were based on a case series, passive data collection, or facilitated passive data collection. Therefore, despite having the limitation of some ethnicity variation, these three studies provide the more accurate estimates of risk for postvaccination myocarditis.

mRNA-1273 (Moderna)

The second mRNA vaccine is mRNA-1273 and was not included in the studies in Israel due to limited use. On December 18, 2020, the Food and Drug Administration (FDA) issued an EUA for the Moderna COVID-19 (mRNA-1273) vaccine [35]. Like the Pfizer vaccine, the Moderna vaccine is a lipid nanoparticle-encapsulated, nucleoside-modified mRNA vaccine encoding the stabilized prefusion spike glycoprotein of SARS-CoV-2, the virus that causes coronavirus disease 2019 (COVID-19) [36]. Vaccination with the Moderna COVID-19 vaccine consists of two doses (100 μg, 0.5 mL each) administered intramuscularly, 1 month (4 weeks) apart. On December 19, 2020, the Advisory Committee on Immunization Practices (ACIP) issued an interim recommendation for use of the Moderna COVID-19 vaccine in persons aged ≥18 years for the prevention of COVID-19. To guide its deliberations regarding the vaccine, the ACIP employed the Evidence to Recommendation (EtR) Framework [37], using the Grading of Recommendations Assessment, Development and Evaluation (GRADE) approach. The Moderna COVID-19 vaccine received U.S. Food and Drug Administration (FDA) approval on January 31, 2022, for individuals ages 18 years and older. Once vaccines are approved by the FDA, companies can market the vaccines under brand names. Spikevax is the brand name for the Moderna COVID-19 vaccine. The FDA-authorized Moderna COVID-19 vaccine for individual ages 18 years and older will now be marketed as Spikevax. No change has been made to the vaccine's formula with the name change.

Mechanism of action of post-mRNA myocarditis

The mechanism of vaccine-induced myocarditis is not known but may be directly related to the active component of the vaccine. [36], the mRNA sequence that codes for the spike [S] protein of SARS-CoV-2, and/or to the immune response that follows vaccination. mRNA vaccines tend to act as their own adjuvant and stimulate a further immune response that improves their efficacy [38]. RNA is encapsulated in liposomes to avoid degradation by RNases, and the molecule is delivered inside target cells following a process of endocytosis [39]. mRNA is then translated into immunogenic proteins by cell ribosomal processing. Prior to translation, mRNA may bind pattern recognition receptors (PRRs) in endosomes or cytosol. Toll-like receptors (TLR)3, TLR7, and TLR8 are able to recognize chains of double-stranded RNA (dsRNA) or single-stranded RNA (ssRNA) in endosomes, while retinoic acid-inducible gene-I (RIG-I) and melanoma differentiation-associated protein 5 (MDA5) may detect short and long filaments of dsRNA in the cytosol. In any of these scenarios, the result would be activation of several pro-inflammatory cascades, including inducing expression of complement components [40], assembly of inflammasome platforms, type I interferon (IFN) response, and nuclear activation of nuclear factor (NF)-kB [41]. This suggests that the possible explanation for lower risk in the current study may indeed be related to the 3-week interval between the first and second vaccine doses and proximity to already stimulated PRRs, compared to the 20–24 week interval between the second and third vaccine doses where the response to PRRs may already have subsided.

Myocarditis associated with additional vaccines

As mentioned above, postvaccination myocarditis was reported in association with smallpox vaccination.

The FDA has approved three vaccines against SARS-CoV-2, the Pfizer–BioNTech BNT162b2 (Comirnaty), Moderna mRNA-1273 (Spikevax), and Johnson and Johnson Ad26.COV2.S (Janssen). The EMA of the European Commission has approved four vaccines against SARS-CoV-2, from Pfizer–BioNTech, Moderna, AstraZeneca AZD1222 (Vaxzevria), and Johnson and Johnson. In Israel the two mRNA vaccines (Pfizer-BioNTech and Moderna) along with AZD1222, are available, but most of the population received the Pfizer vaccine. These vaccines have proven to be efficient and safe, although it is noteworthy that the small number of cases of myocarditis or pericarditis during the first weeks after vaccination have been reported mainly in individuals who received mRNA vaccines. Data from Canada and France indicate that may be more cases of myocarditis after mRNA-1273 than after BNT162b2 [42,43] but this remains to be elucidated.

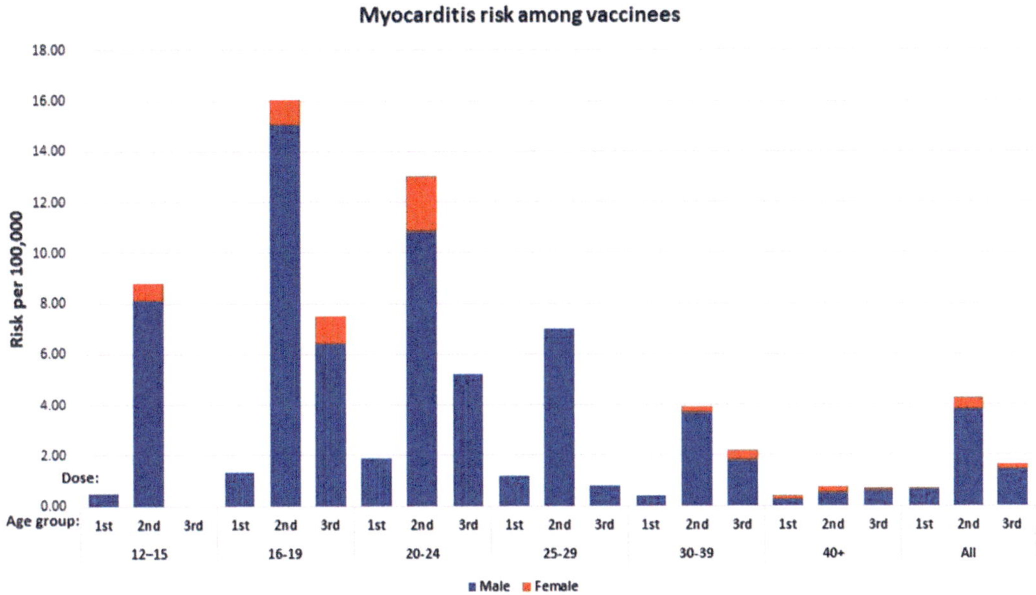

FIGURE 19.1 Sex- and age-dependent risks for myocarditis among individuals who have received the BNT162b2 vaccine.

Summary

Myocarditis is associated with mRNA vaccines. The relative risk according to gender and age are presented in Fig. 19.1. The data received form Pfizer-BioNTech BNT162b2 mRNA vaccination was from an active nationwide surveillance, and hence, the most solid data of myocarditis associated with vaccines and correlate the natural occurrence of myocarditis in general which is predominant in young males.

References

[1] Dalgaard JB. Fatal myocarditis following smallpox vaccination. Am Heart J 1957;54(1):156–7. https://doi.org/10.1016/0002-8703(57)90090-x. pmid:13435214.

[2] Cardiac adverse events following smallpox vaccination—United States. MMWR Morbid Mortal Wkly Rep. Washington, DC., U.S.A: U.S. Department of Health and Human Services (HHS), Centers for Disease Control (CDC) 2003; 2003. Available from: https://www.ncbi.nlm.nih.gov/pubmed/12680519. Accessed July 22, 2021.

[3] Makaryus AN, Revere DJ, Steinberg B. Recurrent reversible dilated cardiomyopathy secondary to viral and streptococcal pneumonia vaccine-associated myocarditis. Cardiol Rev 2006;14(4). https://doi.org/10.1097/01.crd.0000174803.68564.65. pmid:16788323.

[4] Cheng MP, Kozoriz MG, Ahmadi AA, Kelsall J, et al. Post-vaccination myositis and myocarditis in a previously healthy male. Allergy Asthma Clin Immunol 2016;12:6. https://doi.org/10.1186/s13223-016-0114-4. pmid:26877725.

[5] Miller ER, Moro PL, Cano M, Shimabukuro TT. Deaths following vaccination: what does the evidence show? Vaccine 2015;33(29):3288–92. https://doi.org/10.1016/j.vaccine.2015.05.023. pmid:26004568.

[6] FDA takes key action in fighting against COVID-19 by issuing Emergency Use Authorization for first COVID-19 vaccination. Washington, DC, USA: Food and Drug Administration (FDA), U.S. Department of Health and Human Services (HHS) 2020 Available from: https://www.fda.gov/news-events/press-announcements/fda-takes-key-action-fight-against-covid-19-issuing-emergency-use-authorization-first-covid-19/Accessed February 13, 2022.

[7] Israel examining heart inflammation cases in people who received Pfizer COVID shot. Jerusalem, Israel: Reuters; 2021. Available from: https://www.reuters.com/world/middle-east/israel-examining-heart-inflammation-cases-people-who-received-pfizer-covid-shot-2021-04-25//. Accessed February 13, 2022.

[8] Clinical considerations: myocarditis and pericarditis after receipt of mRNA COVID-10 vaccines among adolescents and young adults. Washington, DC, USA: Centers for Disease Control (CDC), U.S. Department of Health and Human Services (HHS) 2021 Available from: https://www.cdc.gov/vaccines/covid-19/clinical-considerations/myocarditis.html/Accessed February 13, 2022.

[9] Comirnaty and Spikevax: possible link to very rare cases of myocarditis and pericarditis. Amsterdam, The Netherlands: European Medicines Agency (EMA) of the European Union (EU); 2021. Available from: https://www.ema.europa.eu/en/news/comirnaty-spikevax-possible-link-very-rare-cases-myocarditis-pericarditis/. Accessed February 13, 2022.

[10] Klein NP, Donahue JG, Weintraub E, Co-Investigators V. Rapid cycle analysis (RCA) to monitor the safety of COVID-19 vaccines in near real-time within the vaccine safety datalink (VSD). Atlanta, GA, USA: Vaccine Safety Datalink Investigators in cooperation with the US Centers for Disease Control (CDC); 2021. Available from: https://www.cdc.gov/vaccines/acip/meetings/downloads/slides-2021-10-20-21/08-COVID-Klein-508.pdf/. Accessed February 13, 2022.

[11] Klein NP, Lewis N, Goddard K, Fireman B, et al. Surveillance for adverse events after COVID-19 mRNA vaccination. JAMA 2021;326(14):1390–9. https://doi.org/10.1001/jama.2021.15072. pmid:34477808.

[12] Mevorach D, Anis E, Cedar N, Hasin T, et al. Myocarditis after BNT162b2 vaccination in Israeli adolescents. N Engl J Med 2022. https://doi.org/10.1056/NEJMc2116999.

[13] Montgomery J, Ryan M, Engler R, Hoffman D, et al. Myocarditis following immunization with mRNA COVID-19 vaccines in members of the US military. JAMA Cardiol 2021;6(10):1202–6. https://doi.org/10.1001/jamacardio.2021.2833. pmid:34185045.

[14] Witberg G, Barda N, Hoss S, Richter I, et al. Myocarditis after Covid-19 vaccination in a large health care organization. N Engl J Med 2021;385(23):2132–9. https://doi.org/10.1056/NEJMoa2110737. pmid:34614329.

[15] Wong H-L. Surveillance updates of myocarditis/pericarditis and mRNA COVID-10 vaccination in the FDA BEST System. Washington, DC, USA: Food and Drug Administration (FDA), U.S. Department of Health and Human Services 2021 Available from: https://www.fda.gov/media/153090/download/Accessed February 13, 2022.

[16] Su JR. Myopericarditis following COVID-19 vaccination: updates from the vaccine adverse event reporting system (VAERS). Washington, DC, USA: Vaccine Safety Team of the Centers for Disease Control (CDC) COVID-19 Vaccine Task Force, U.S. Department of Health and Human Services (HHS); 2021. Available from: https://www.cdc.gov/vaccines/acip/meetings/downloads/slides-2021-10-20-21/07-COVID-Su-508.pdf/. Accessed February 13, 2022.

[17] Le risque de myocardite et péricardite après la vaccination Covid-19 est confirmé mais peu fréquent et d'évolution favorable [in French]. Paris, France: Agence Nationale de Sécurité du Médicament et des produits de santé (ANSM), French Ministry of Health; 2021. Available from: https://ansm.sante.fr/actualites/le-risque-de-myocardite-et-pericardite-apres-la-vaccination-covid-19-est-confirme-mais-peu-frequent-et-devolution-favorable/. Accessed February 13, 2022.

[18] Myocarditis and pericarditis following vaccination with COVID-19 mRNA vaccines in Ontario: December 13, 2020 to November 21, 2021. Ontario, Canada: Ontarior Department of Public Health; 2022. Available from: https://www.publichealthontario.ca/-/media/documents/ncov/epi/covid-19-myocarditis-pericarditis-vaccines-epi.pdf?sc_lang=en/. Accessed February 13, 2022.

[19] Mevorach D, Anis E, Cedar N, Bromberg M, et al. Myocarditis after BNT162b2 mRNA vaccine against Covid-19 in Israel. N Engl J Med 2021;385(23):2140–9. https://doi.org/10.1056/NEJMoa2109730. pmid:34614328.

[20] Mevorach D, et al. Myocarditis after the third BNT162b2 COVID-19 vaccine in Israel. N Engl J Med 2021;385:2140–9.

[21] Sundboll J, Adelborg K, Munch T, Froslev T, et al. Positive predictive value of cardiovascular diagnoses in the Danish National Patient Registry: a validation study. BMJ Open 2016;6(11):e012832. https://doi.org/10.1136/bmjopen-2016-012832. pmid:27864249.

[22] Brighton Collaboration. Myocarditis/pericarditis case definition. Decatur, GA, USA: Brighton Collaboration of the Task Force for Global Health; 2021. Available from: https://brightoncollaboration.us/myocarditis-case-definition-update/. Accessed December 26, 2021.

[23] Update: cardiac-related events during the civilian smallpox vaccination program - United States. MMWR Morb Mortal Wkly Rep 2003;52(21):492–6. Washington, DC, USA: U.S. Department of Health and Human Services (HHS), Centers for Disease Control (CDC) 2003 Available from: https://pubmed.ncbi.nlm.nih.gov/12809110/. Accessed December 12, 2021.

[24] Casey C, Vellozzi C, Mootrey GT, et al. Surveillance guidelines for smallpox vaccine (vaccinia) adverse reactions. MMWR Morb Mortal Wkly Rep 2006;55(RR-1):1–16. Washington, DC, USA: U.S. Department of Health and Human Services (HHS), Centers for Disease Control (CDC) 2006 Available from: https://www.cdc.gov/mmwr/preview/mmwrhtml/rr5501a1.htm#top. Accessed July 22, 2021.

[25] Mei R, Raschi E, Forcesi E, Diemberger I, et al. Myocarditis and pericarditis after immunization: gaining insights through the vaccine adverse event reporting system. Int J Cardiol 2018;273:183–6. https://doi.org/10.1016/j.ijcard.2018.09.054. pmid:30236504.

[26] Wallace M, Oliver S. COVID-19 mRNA vaccines in adolescents and young adults: benefit-risk discussion. Meeting of the advisory committee on immunization Practices (ACIP), centers for disease control (CDC). Atlanta, GA, USA: Centers for Disease Control (CDC); 2021. U.S. Department of Health and Human Services (HHS) 2021 Available from: https://www.cdc.gov/vaccines/acip/meetings/downloads/slides-2021-06/05-COVID-Wallace-508.pdf/. Accessed February 13, 2022.

[27] Frenck RW, Klein NP, Kitchin N, Gurtman A, et al. Safety, immunogenicity, and efficacy of the BNT162b2 Covid-19 vaccine in adolescents. N Engl J Med 2021;385(3):239–50. https://doi.org/10.1056/NEJMoa2107456.

[28] Glatman-Freedman A, Bromberg M, Dichtiar R, Hershkovitz Y, et al. The BNT162b2 vaccine effectiveness against new COVID-19 cases and complications of breakthrough cases: a nation-wide retrospective longitudinal multiple cohort analysis using individualised data. EBioMedicine 2021;72:103574. https://doi.org/10.1016/j.ebiom.2021.103574. pmid:34537449.

[29] Glatman-Freedman A, Hershkovitz Y, Kaufman Z, Dichtiar R, et al. Effectiveness of BNT162b2 vaccine in adolescents during outbreak of SARS-CoV-2 delta variant infection, Israel, 2021. Emerg Infect Dis 2021;27(11):2919–22. https://doi.org/10.3201/eid2711.211886. pmid:34570694.

[30] Haas EJ, Angulo FJ, McLaughlin JM, Anis E, et al. Impact and effectiveness of mRNA BNT162b2 vaccine against SARS-CoV-2 infections and COVID-19 cases, hospitalisations, and deaths following a nationwide vaccination campaign in Israel: an observational study using national surveillance data. Lancet 2021;397(10287):1819–29. https://doi.org/10.1016/S0140-6736(21)00947-8. pmid:33964222.

[31] Thomas SJ, Moreira Jr ED, Kitchin N, Absalon J, et al. Safety and efficacy of the BNT162b2 mRNA Covid-19 vaccine through 6 months. N Engl J Med 2021;385(19):1761–73. https://doi.org/10.1056/NEJMoa2110345. pmid:34525277.

[32] Levin EG, Lustig Y, Cohen C, Fluss R, et al. Waning immune humoral response to BNT162b2 Covid-19 vaccine over 6 months. N Engl J Med 2021. https://doi.org/10.1056/NEJMoa2114583. pmid:34614326.

[33] Shrotri M, Navaratnam AMD, Nguyen V, Byrne T, et al. Spike-antibody waning after second dose of BNT162b2 or ChAdOx1. Lancet 2021;398(10298):385–7. https://doi.org/10.1016/S0140-6736(21)01642-1. pmid:34274038.

[34] Coronavirus (CORONA-19) update: FDA expands eligibility for COVID-19 vaccine boosters. Washington, D.C., U.S.A: U.S. Department of Health and Human Services (HHS), Food and Drug Administration (FDA); 2021. Available from: https://www.fda.gov/news-events/press-announcements/coronavirus-covid-19-update-fda-expands-eligibility-covid-19-vaccine-boosters. Accessed February 13, 2022.

[35] FDA takes additional action in fight against COVID-19 by issuing Emergency Use Authorization for second COVID-19 vaccine (issued December 18, 2020). Washington, DC, USA: Food and Drug Administration (FDA), U.S. Department of Health and Human Services (HHS); 2021. Available from: https://www.fda.gov/news-events/press-announcements/fda-takes-additional-action-fight-against-covid-19-issuing-emergency-use-authorization-second-covid/. Accessed February 13, 2022.

[36] Dolgin E. The tangled history of mRNA vaccines. Nature 2021;597:318–24.

[37] Advisory committee on immunization Practices (ACIP) evidence to recommendation for use of Moderna COVID-19 vaccine under an emergency use authorization. Washington, DC, USA: Centers for Disease Control (CDC), U.S. Department of Health and Human Services (HHS) 2020. Available from: https://www.cdc.gov/vaccines/acip/recs/grade/covid-19-moderna-etr.html/Accessed February 13, 2022.

[38] Zhang C, Maruggi G, Shan H, Li J. Advances in mRNA vaccines for infectious diseases. Front Immunol 2019;10:594. https://doi.org/10.3389/fimmu.2019.00594. pmid:30972078.

[39] Marć MA, Dominguez-Alvarez E, Gamazo C. Nucleic acid vaccination strategies against infectious diseases. Expert Opin Drug Deliv 2015;12(12):1851–65. https://doi.org/10.1517/17425247.2015.1077559. pmid:26365499.

[40] Caskey M, Lefebvre F, Filali-Mouhim A, Cameron MJ, et al. Synthetic double-stranded RNA induces innate immune responses similar to a live viral vaccine in humans. J Exp Med 2011;208(12):2357–66. https://doi.org/10.1084/jem.20111171. pmid:22065672.

[41] Reikine S, Nguyen JB, Modis Y. Pattern recognition and signaling mechanisms of RIG-I and MDA5. Front Immunol 2014;5:342. https://doi.org/10.3389/fimmu.2014.00342. pmid:25101084.

[42] Myocardite et péricardite après la vaccination Covid-19 [in French]. Paris, France: EPI-PHARE: Agence Nationale de Sécurité du Médicament et des produits de santé (ANSM), French Ministry of Health 2021; 8 Novembre 2021. Available from: https://www.epi-phare.fr/rapports-detudes-et-publications/myocardite-pericardite-vaccination-covid19/#:~:text=Depuis%20juillet%202021%2C%20les%20myocardites,notamment%20chez%20-les%20hommes%20jeunes./. Accessed February 14, 2022.

[43] Ontario recommends the use of Pfizer-BioNTech COVID-19 vaccine for individuals aged 18-24 years old (September 29, 2021). Toronto, Ontario: Canada: Government of Ontario; 2021. Available from: https://news.ontario.ca/en/statement/1000907/ontario-recommends-the-use-of-pfizer-biontech-covid-19-vaccine-for-individuals-aged-18-24-years-old/. Accessed February 14, 2022.

CHAPTER

20

Rheumatic manifestations and autoimmunity associated with COVID-19

Danielle Zemer Lev[1], *Arad Dotan*[2,3] *and Michael Ehrenfeld*[2,3]

[1]Faculty of Medicine, Ben-Gurion University of the Negev, Beersheba, Israel; [2]Zabludowicz Center for Autoimmune Diseases, Sheba Medical Center, Ramat Gan, Israel; [3]Sackler Faculty of Medicine, Tel Aviv University, Tel Aviv, Israel

Introduction

As the number of patients infected by coronavirus disease, 2019 (COVID-19) globally rises many case studies, reviews, and clinical trials have been published regarding the relationship between COVID-19 and the generation of autoantibodies that may cause rheumatic diseases [4]. In adults, a broad spectrum of complications following COVID-19 has been documented including the new onset of autoimmune manifestations and rheumatic diseases. Some of the immune dysregulations that will be described in this chapter appeared in the acute stage of COVID-19 [3]. Yet, the clinical presentation of autoimmunity can also be expressed years after an infection that acts as a trigger. Thus, in the future, we may witness a rise of such disorders in SARS-CoV-2-infected individuals. Importantly, recent reports imply that the range of autoimmune and auto-inflammatory disorders in individuals infected with severe acute respiratory syndrome coronavirus 2 (SARS-CoV-2) should respond to immunosuppressive and immunomodulatory treatments, as well as intravenous immunoglobulin (IVIG) therapy and corticosteroids [1].

Pathophysiology of COVID-19 as a trigger of autoimmune disease

The pathophysiology of viral infections as the cause of rheumatic diseases has been long known and studied by the scientific community. The two main mechanisms are molecular mimicry and immune hyperstimulation.

Autoimmunity, COVID-19, Post-COVID19 syndrome and COVID-19 vaccination
https://doi.org/10.1016/B978-0-443-18566-3.00028-1

The theory behind molecular mimicry suggests that similarities between viral peptides and self-peptides may facilitate the activation of autoreactive T or B cells [2]. It seems that autoreactive T is a dominant feature of molecular mimicry as a cause of autoimmune disease. The development of autoimmunity is related to the activation of T cells that were previously autoreactive, which may occur in response to hidden antigens [2].

Hyperstimulation of the immune system may be triggered by viral diseases. This may cause dysregulation of the immune system that may result in autoreactivity [3]. Hyperstimulation may be a result of environmental factors, such as robust exposure to reactive antigens. Hyperstimulation can also be a result of genetic tendencies that may cause the familial nature of autoimmune diseases.

Rheumatic diseases

Axial SPA

A couple of case reports of axial and peripheral spondylarthritis following a SARS-CoV-2 infection have been published. One such report describes two patients [4]:

A 25-year-old Lebanese male presented with severe pain, swelling and redness on the left ankle, severe back pain, and morning stiffness. An RT-PCR confirmed - symptomatic COVID-19 disease. His ANA, anti-CCP, and RF were negative, and he was found to be HLA-B27 positive.

A 57-year-old Lebanese male presented with pain and swelling of his left wrist that was worst in the morning and associated with large joint arthralgia all occurring 1 month after an RT-PCR confirmed him as a case of symptomatic COVID-19 disease. His ANA, anti-CCP, and RF were negative, and he was found to be HLA-B27 positive.

Another case report describes a 21-year-old female that suffered diffuse joint pain mainly in her hips, knees, and back pain that was worst in the mornings. She also presented with low-grade fever and mild diarrhea. She had not been tested for COVID-19 at the time of the investigation, but a later serologic test revealed she had been in fact infected. Further follow-up revealed ANA and RF to be negative. Imaging showed grade 2 sclerosis of the sacroiliac joint. She improved under treatment with Certolizumab within a week [6].

Reactive arthritis and psoriatic arthritis

Approximately 36% of COVID-19-affected patients, described arthralgia but had no notable evidence of inflammation on physical examination [7]. Several anecdotal case reports of reactive arthritis were published. Four out of 5 cases reported, began anywhere from 3 days to 1 month following COVID-19 resolution. HLA-B27 was found to be positive in a couple of them. RF, ANA as well as anti-CCP were negative in all of them [8–12].

Another case report published was of a 53-year-old male presenting with new-onset inflammatory back pain in the lumbar, thoracic, and cervical regions. Additionally, he described anterior chest wall pain. These symptoms followed an episode of self-limiting systematic symptoms suggestive of COVID-19; however, a nasopharyngeal swab for PCR was not obtained at the time of the disease. A later SARS-CoV-2 antibody test was found to be positive. Reactive arthritis often presents as oligoarthritis but in some cases can cause axial arthritis. In the case of this patient, there was a definite temporal association between the suspected COVID-19 infection and the axial disease, in a timeframe that is appropriate for reactive arthritis. HLA-B27 was also found to be positive in this case [13].

It is essential to mention that besides the pathophysiology of SARS-CoV-2 itself, there are numerous factors related to the pandemic scale of COVID-19 that could contribute to that. Such factors include psychological distress, socioeconomic factors, poor sleep, and reduced physical activity. All the above factors may contribute to the development of chronic pain that may mimic a rheumatic disease [14].

Rheumatoid arthritis and Still's disease

Anti-CCP (cyclic citrullinated peptide) is an antibody known to have a major role in RA (rheumatoid arthritis). A study performed to determine the seroprevalence of anti-CPA following COVID-19 infection, studied 61 patients with moderate to severe COVID-19 in a post-COVID-19 outpatient clinic, 5 weeks after hospitalization. None of the patients tested positive for anti-CPA, except two with a previous diagnosis of anti-CPA-positive RA. However, there were five patients who suffered from polyarthritis consistent with RA. The average onset of symptoms was 6.6 weeks after the infection, though two patients reported symptoms before infection. Four of the five patients fulfilled the 2010 American College of Rheumatology criteria for RA. Three patients resembled clinically typical new-onset RA [5].

Still's disease is an uncommon inflammatory disorder that often presents with fever, rash, joint involvement, lymphadenopathy, and serositis. It is in fact a range of disorders that vary from systemic juvenile idiopathic arthritis (SJIA) to the adult-onset Still's a disease (AOSD) [15]. A 29-year-old woman with no past medical history presented with signs suggestive of COVID-19, including sore throat, headache, anosmia, ageusia, generalized weakness, shortness of breath, and diarrhea. The patient had a positive RT-PCR nasopharyngeal swab for SARS-CoV-2. Her initial symptoms did not require hospitalization. After 15 days, her RT-PCR nasopharyngeal swab for SARS-CoV-2 became negative. Six months following her infection, the patient developed persistent fatigue, resting tachycardia, dyspnea, and recurrent macular rashes. A TTE (transthoracic echocardiogram) did not show any irregularities. The patient suffered from a sore throat, but RT-PCR for SARS-CoV-2 was again found to be negative. During the following days, her condition had deteriorated, suffering from myalgia, arthralgia, fever of up to 41·0°C, lymphadenopathy, and a "salmon colored" rash. Her liver enzymes were elevated, (AST levels of 123 U/L and ALT levels of 165 U/L), NT-pro-BNP was significantly increased (3856 pg/mL) and troponin T was found to be elevated (463 pg/mL). Laboratory tests for ANA, RF (rheumatoid factor), and various infectious agents were all negative. The patient underwent a cardiac MRI that revealed mild pericarditis with a small amount of pericardial and pleural effusions. During her hospitalization, she fulfilled all major and minor criteria of the Yamaguchi classification and was diagnosed with Still's disease. She was initially treated with IV prednisolone (50 mg/day) that didn't lead to any improvement. The dose was thus increased to 100 mg/day, again without any sufficient improvement. The third line of treatment was initiated with the IL-1 receptor antagonist Anakinra (SC, 100 mg/day), which led to a significant improvement in symptoms [16].

Viral arthralgia

A single-center retrospective cohort study found that among hospitalized COVID-19 patients 30% reported musculoskeletal complaints. Of those patients 37.5% suffered from myalgia, 5.7% suffered from arthralgia, 6.8% suffered from new-onset back pain, and 50%

from generalized body ache. COVID-19 arthralgia was often more severe than the respiratory symptoms and had a variable temporal relationship with COVID-19 diagnosis. In order to avoid missing a COVID-19 diagnosis, one should be aware of its variability and have a high index of suspicion when diagnosing arthralgia and musculoskeletal pain [17].

Sjogren's disease

Only one small study reported that about 25% of patients mentioned suffered from symptoms associated with sicca syndrome, mainly during the acute phase of the disease, and some reported during the follow-up period [7].

Lofgren's syndrome

Lofgren's syndrome is an acute clinical phenotype of sarcoidosis. It typically presents with fever, erythema nodosum, bilateral hilar lymphadenopathy, and migratory polyarthritis. It seldom presents with uveitis [18].

One case report from Slovakia described a 30-year-old male patient in generally good health who presented with a 10-day history of low-grade fever, pain in both ankles, wrists, and right elbow, dry cough, dull chest pain, and difficulty breathing for 4 days. Upon physical examination, several erythematous and warm plaques with palpable subcutaneous nodules in the malleolar and pretibial areas were noted bilaterally. A nasopharyngeal swab for SARS-CoV-2 was negative, however, ELISA for SARS-CoV-2 antibodies was found to be positive. Once diagnosed, the patient was treated with corticosteroids (40 mg of prednisone daily) and following 2 days of treatment, the fever and joint pain had resolved [19].

Myositis

Roughly 24% of COVID-19 patients reported suffering from myalgia, in large study populations and the rate of elevated creatine kinase (CK) levels was about 11%. A chronic form of this myalgia was noted in approximately 10%–20% of cases of acute COVID-19 [20].

To date, only two studies have assessed the rate of myositis in hospitalized COVID-19 patients. These studies approximated myositis in 3%–11% of patients [21]. In both studies, most patients with suspected myositis did not complete tests that provide definitive diagnoses such as EMG, imaging, or histopathological tests. Anecdotal reports suggest that most cases occurred in adult males with symptoms consistent with myalgia, occurring primarily in the first week of COVID-19, with CK levels higher than 10,000 U/L in most of them [22].

A recent review of the muscular presentations of COVID-19 revealed COVID-19-associated myositis has a variety of presentations that may range from muscle weakness to dermatomyositis accompanied by classic rashes or back pain with muscle disease on imaging. About 23 cases of myositis considered to be induced by COVID-19 have been described thus far. Most patients tested positive for COVID-19 upon initial clinical presentation. The vast majority of these patients were males, with an age range from 33 to 87. This presentation may or may not be associated with elevated enzyme markers such as CK, and muscle enzyme elevation does not necessarily indicate the prognosis [23].

Systemic sclerosis

A case report of a 47-year-old man with no history of any autoimmune diseases has been published. The patient was in generally good health until he started to develop mild systemic flu-like disease: fatigue, fever, cough, and sore throat. Oropharyngeal swab for SARS-CoV-2 PCR tested positive. This disease was self-limiting, and most of the symptoms subsided after 3 weeks. At the same time, he started to feel extremely tired and experienced abdominal discomfort and redness of the skin. Two months after his COVID-19 disease subsided, he required emergency care due to abdominal pain, vomiting, generalized skin rash with diffuse erythema, and burning skin sensation. He also presented with swollen eyelids and conjunctivitis, followed by a heliotropic skin rash. Other additional new symptoms included Raynaud's phenomenon, swollen fingers, pain at the fingertip, myalgia, muscular weakness, and dysphagia. ANA was strongly positive and raised suspicions of systemic sclerosis. Anti-PM/Scl 75 and anti-PM/Scl 100 tested positive. Anti-Scl-70, anti-Jo 1, and anti-RNA-polymerase III tested negative. The patient was diagnosed with systemic sclerosis or scleroderma/polymyositis overlap. He was treated with calcium channel blockers for 6 months, improving some of his symptoms [24].

Chilblains

Chilblains (also known as pernio) are a rare inflammatory vasculitis of the small vessels of the limbs, causing painful or itchy erythematous or violaceous lesions after exposure to cold temperature [25].

The association between COVID-19 and chilblains was initially noticed due to several case reports from southern Europe during the first wave of the pandemic. One case series followed 505 patients who presented with cutaneous manifestations associated with a COVID-19 infection. Sixty-three percent of the patients presented with Perino-like symptoms, of these patients 7% were laboratory-confirmed COVID-19 positive, and 6% were in close contact with confirmed patients. The rest were suspected of COVID-19 or had never been tested. Therefore, current data supports only a weak link between Chilblains and a COVID-19 infection [26].

Another smaller case series evaluated the condition of 31 referred patients who had recently developed chilblains or Perino-like symptoms. This study performed RT-PCR to detect SARS-CoV-2 RNA from a nasopharyngeal swab for all patients and a skin biopsy specimen of 22 of the patients. This study also found that Chilblains did not appear to be directly associated with COVID-19 [27].

SLE—systemic lupus erythematosus

SLE is a disease characterized by immune dysregulation that causes multisystem inflammation. Diagnosis of systemic lupus erythematosus (SLE) is often made when a patient fits several clinical criteria [28]. Patients recovering from COVID-19 can present with similar related features, including lymphopenia, thrombocytopenia, hemolytic anemia, arthralgia, serositis, chilblain lesions, or antiphospholipid antibodies [21]. The suggested mechanism of COVID-19 as a trigger involves the dysregulation of the immune response to the infection: high expression of proinflammatory cytokines (IL-1, IL-6, and TNF-alpha) that could be worsened by the shift from Th1 to Th2 response that is typical SLE.

A review that collected data from several case studies reported that all patients responded well to immunosuppression except for one patient in this series that had passed away [8–14]. This patient was an 18-year-old Hispanic female with a medical history of ASD (autistic spectrum disorder) and panic disorder. She had suffered a cardiac tamponade and went into PEA (pulseless electrical activity) arrest on the 17th day of hospitalization [30]. One of the cases mentioned above is a 39-year-old man that presented with fever, rash, and proteinuria 2 months after a confirmed COVID-19 infection. Blood works revealed ANA, dsDNA, anti-Ro, and anti-La antibodies. Renal biopsy showed class 1 lupus nephritis [29].

To date, it remains unknown whether these cases present a transient phenomenon or develop into a full-blown chronic disease, as well as the long-term outcome and prognosis [31].

Hematological diseases

Evan's syndrome

Evan's syndrome is an autoimmune condition characterized by autoantibodies that attack platelets and red blood cells and cause immune thrombocytopenia (ITP) and autoimmune hemolytic anemia (AIHA). In some cases, it may also attack neutrophils and cause autoimmune neutropenia (AIN) [32]. Up to half of Evan's syndrome cases may be secondary and attributed to various etiologies, including infections [33].

Two case reports describing COVID-19 patients were reported detailing their condition and disease progression:

A 22-year-old, previously healthy male patient presented to the Emergency Department with jaundice, fatigue, dyspnea, and fever. His blood counts showed severe anemia with a hemoglobin of 3.9 g/dL and marked alterations in markers of hemolysis. Thoracic CT findings were suggestive of COVID-19 pneumonia, though RT-PCR for SARS-CoV-2 was negative twice. Nonetheless, provided the clinical presentation and CT findings, the patient was treated with hydroxychloroquine, moxifloxacin, and favipiravir for 5 days as though he was a COVID-19 patient. His Evan's syndrome was treated with 1 mg/kg of methylprednisolone, folic acid, vitamin B12, and a PPI. On the fifth day of treatment, the hemoglobin level had increased to 7.4 g/dL [34].

Another case of a 39-year-old man that presented to the Emergency hemoptysis and epistaxis with and history of sore throat, productive cough, fevers, chills, and dyspnea for 1 week. Blood counts demonstrated a leukocyte count of 11,000 cells/μL, hemoglobin of 15.6 g/dL, and platelet count of 3000 cells/μL. Neutrophil count was 8700 cells/μL, and lymphocyte count was 1700 cells/μL. A rapid nasopharyngeal PCR swab for COVID-19 was positive. While hospitalized, the patient suffered from worsening bleeding with hematemesis, melena, and hematochezia, associated with a hemoglobin decrease to 6.4 g/dL. He was treated with PPI. His platelet count recovered to 52 cells/μL with the resolution of the bleeding. When his platelet count was 308 cells/μL and hemoglobin was stable at 7.6 g/dL, the patient was discharged. Four days following his discharge, he returned to the Emergency Department with extreme weakness, intermittent fever, and cough without bleeding. Hemoglobin was 6.0 g/dL with a normal platelet count. When the diagnosis of Evan's syndrome was made, he was treated with two rounds of IVIG [16].

The two cases described above suggest that in the case of Evan's syndrome related to acute infections such as COVID-19, the treating physicians should balance the aggressive course of immunosuppression and the potential for bone marrow stimulation in patients with inadequate hematopoiesis. IVIG and plasmapheresis are treatments to be considered on an individual patient level. The severity of AIHA at onset (specifically Hb < 6 g/dL) is the primary determinant of relapse and risk of mortality [33].

Antiphospholipid antibodies

Some patients with COVID-19 suffer from different coagulopathy disorders, especially patients who are severely ill and admitted to an ICU [35]. Though the virus itself does not appear to have coagulation-promoting effects, and the abnormal results of coagulation tests often found in patients with COVID-19 appear to be primarily associated with the systemic inflammatory response [36], yet, as the autoimmune mechanism has shown to also play a major role in the coagulopathy disorders, a study has reported more than 90% of COVID-19 patients were positive for Lupus anticoagulants [37].

Several studies reported antiphospholipid (aPL) antibodies in patients with COVID-19. Thirteen studies included patients with COVID-19 admitted to the ICU. Lupus anticoagulants were positive in more than half of the patients, although the rate of positive results had a vast range among the studies, ranging from 3% to 91% [21].

Lastly, it is essential to note that Lupus anticoagulants may be detected in different settings, particularly infections and inflammations, which might cause the exposure of cell phospholipids that are not typically exposed to the immune system. Thus, a positive result is not necessarily due to the antiphospholipid syndrome [38].

ITP

Viral infection as a trigger to ITP (immune thrombocytopenic purpura) is a widely known and studied phenomenon. The suggested mechanism is that antibodies targeted at the viral glycoproteins might cross-react with platelet surface integrins like glycoprotein IIb/IIIa (GPIIb/IIIa) or GPIb-IX-V [39].

Mild thrombocytopenia has been detected in roughly 5%–10% of patients with symptomatic COVID-19 [40]. Some COVID-19 patients may display signs and symptoms of ITP. About 75% of the patients presenting with COVID-19-related ITP are above the age of 50, and nearly half started presenting with purpura and mucosal bleeding at least 2 weeks after contracting COVID-19 [41]. One example of such a case series is a French study in which all patients, but one had an initial platelet count of $<20 \times 109/L$, and 79% of patients had a platelet count of $\leq 10 \times 109/L$. For all patients, either a previous normal platelet count was obtained or no report of a prior history of bleeding was mentioned. Hemorrhagic manifestations were diverse: 29% of the patients suffered from severe bleeding (i.e., intracranial hemorrhage, gastrointestinal, severe metrorrhagia, and gross hematuria) and 21% of patients had mucosal bleeding. The first-line treatment was prednisone (1 mg/kg/day) alone, resulting in an initial response in 29% of patients after a median of 10 days (ranging between 5 and 15). One patient who received 40 mg of dexamethasone for 4 days also achieved a complete response on the fifth day. This study concluded that COVID-19-associated ITP appears predominantly in the second phase (after 1 week) of SARS-CoV-2 infection, with considerable bleeding and a favorable prognosis [42].

Aortic thrombosis

One of the most noteworthy extrapulmonary manifestations of COVID-19 is hypercoagulability. It may lead to severe complications, including aortic thrombosis [43].

An 80-year-old male with a substantial cardiac and vascular medical history presented with cough and dyspnea for 2 weeks and tested positive for COVID-19 infection. He was hospitalized and later began to suffer from acute left ankle pain and coolness, with discoloration of his fifth toe. A duplex test revealed a blocked left lower extremity artery, with a partial blockage to the level of the external iliac artery and complete blockage of the common femoral artery. He was treated with continuous heparin anticoagulation, and vascular surgery was considered. A review of his thoracic CT in a PE (pulmonary embolus) protocol demonstrated a focal 6.2 cm intraluminal thrombus was narrowing 40% of the aorta at the diaphragmatic hiatus level. The patient underwent a thrombectomy, femoral-popliteal bypass via groin cutdown, femoral endarterectomy, dorsalis pedis, and posterior tibial exploration, and medial and lateral fasciotomy. Yet the persistent ischemia of the left lower extremity resulted in a left above-knee amputation [44].

Endocrine diseases

Thyroid

A retrospective study evaluated thyroid function in hospitalized COVID-19 patients under the assumption that cytokine storm associated with COVID-19 may cause thyroid dysfunction. The study found that 20.2% were experienced thyrotoxicosis, 5.2% had been diagnosed with hypothyroidism, and 74.6% with normal thyroid function [45].

Another retrospective study evaluated thyroid function in patients with COVID-19 with no previous history of thyroid disease. This study found that TSH levels, lower than the normal range were present in 56% of the patients. Additionally, TSH and serum total triiodothyronine (TT3) of the patients with COVID-19 were significantly lower than those of the control group [46].

Overall, most patients with thyroid dysfunction were tested for the presence of antithyroid antibodies and the vast majority had negative results [21].

Diabetes mellitus

The expression of the SARS coronavirus receptor—ACE2 (angiotensin-converting enzyme 2) in the endocrine part of the pancreas, may contribute to the pathogenesis of COVID-19 as a cause of damage to the Langerhans islets and acute diabetes [47].

An 8-year-old boy with no past medical history of note was hospitalized for a week due to increased polyuria. He was diagnosed with type I diabetes mellitus with autoantibodies against glutamic acid decarboxylase, tyrosine phosphatase, and insulin. His Hba1C value was 11.6%. When hospitalized, he was tested for COVID-19 and found to be positive. As he was asymptomatic the duration of the infection was not established. Initially, he had no antibodies and when he was tested again, he had significantly elevated antibodies against COVID-19 15 days later [48].

Neurological diseases

Encephalitis and anti-NMDA receptor encephalitis

Several patients with COVID-19 presented with neurological symptoms consistent with encephalitis following the infection. In one-third of those patients, the symptoms began 2 weeks after COVID-19 diagnosis or disease onset. The incidence was similar between males and females with a mean age at diagnosis of 55 years old and a range of 11–84 [21].

Even though most cases were diagnosed generally as encephalitis caused by a viral infection, some were diagnosed with a specific condition—autoimmune encephalitis associated with anti-NMDA receptor autoantibodies [45].

The exact pathogenesis that causes COVID-19 infection to induce encephalitis remains mostly unclear. Though, a study now suspects that patients with COVID-19 may present with neurological features that share prominent resemblances with CAR-T cell-related encephalopathy. Such similarities include similar pathophysiological features such as CRS (cytokine release syndrome), endothelial activation, blood-brain barrier dysfunction, and immune-related injury [46].

Guillain Barre syndrome

Guillain Barre syndrome (GBS) is described as a neuropathic condition characterized by progressive muscle weakness and reduced or missing myotatic reflexes following an infectious disease [47].

The incidence of COVID-19-related GBS remains largely unknown. To date, only one large study estimated post-COVID-19 GBS to be about 0.1% among hospitalized patients [48]. Thus far, 90% of the reported cases were of men above the age of 50. In 75% of the cases, diagnosis occurred at least 2 weeks after the onset of COVID-19 symptoms and diagnosis. The clinical features mostly resembled typical "non-COVID-19" features [49]. Anti-ganglioside antibodies were negative in most patients. Serum and CSF were negative for SARS-CoV-2. Over 70% of the patients experienced a favorable prognosis, particularly after IVIG (intravenous immunoglobulin) treatment. Older age was often associated with a worse prognosis [50].

Movement disorders

Ninety-three recorded cases of movement disorders triggered by or temporally linked to SARS-CoV-2 infection, or its treatments were assessed, and the following results were observed:

Myoclonus presented in 63.4%, ataxia in 38.7%, action/postural tremor in 10.8%, parkinsonism (rigid-akinetic syndrome) in 5.38%, oculomotor abnormalities in 20.4%, catatonia in 2.1%, dystonia in 1.1%, chorea in 1.1%, functional (psychogenic) movement disorders in 3.2%. Encephalopathy was a common association found in 39.8% of cases, and stroke was identified in a small fraction of cases—5.4% of cases.

Most cases of patients that suffered from myoclonus were accompanied by either encephalopathy or delirium.

Imaging studies that supported the clinical findings were present in 82.8% of cases. Treatment options ranged from corticosteroids (that targeted either the COVID-19 infection movement disorder itself) to IVIG, plasmapheresis, antiepileptic drugs, and benzodiazepines [51].

Myasthenia gravis

A 61-year-old male with a medical history of bronchial asthma and diabetes mellitus was diagnosed with a mild case of COVID-19. He was treated with noninvasive ventilation, corticosteroids, and antiviral agents. Two months later, the patient presented with an acute episode of shortness of breath, dysphagia, and fatigue. He was diagnosed with myasthenia gravis and treated with IVIG, corticosteroids, and pyridostigmine. He was aided by intermittent noninvasive ventilation. Thoracic CT demonstrated an anterior mediastinal mass, which was suggestive of a thymoma. Thus, the patient was diagnosed with thymomatous myasthenia gravis and was referred to surgery. The patient underwent a thymomectomy, had an uneventful postoperative course, and was discharged 3 days after his surgery with a maintenance treatment of prednisone 30 mg daily. When myasthenic symptoms improved, he began tapering down on his treatment from 30 mg once daily to 15 mg on alternate days now. By the sixth week of follow-up, the patient was asymptomatic [52].

Other nonrheumatic autoimmune diseases

Autoimmune hepatitis

The first case reported of autoimmune hepatitis—primary biliary cholangitis overlap syndrome was published. The patient is a 57-year-old male with a past medical history of prediabetes, essential hypertension, and beta thalassemia minor. He presented with sore throat, cough, fatigue, and arthralgia and was diagnosed by nasopharyngeal swab RT-PCR with COVID-19. His blood tests revealed hyperferritinemia, elevated liver enzymes (AST/ALT/GGT), hypergammaglobulinemia, ASMA (antismooth muscle antibody), AMA (antimitochondrial antibody), and antidsDNA (double-stranded DNA antibodies). Subsequently, the patient was diagnosed with autoimmune hepatitis—primary biliary cholangitis overlap syndrome that was determined to be triggered by COVID-19. The patient was treated with ursodeoxycholic acid [53].

The specific mechanism that causes autoimmune hepatitis—primary biliary cholangitis overlap syndrome is not completely understood to date. Genetic predispositions, viral infections, and drugs were suggested as provoking agents for the autoimmune disease [54].

Possible mechanisms in this particular case may be immune dysregulation or excessive immune response to COVID-19 that in turn caused a cytokine storm and hyperferritinemia, ultimately leading to molecular mimicry between pathogenic viruses and human proteins, and the production of autoantibodies [55].

Pemphigus vulgaris

Pemphigus vulgaris is a dermatological autoimmune disorder that causes the formation of bullae on the skin. It may be triggered by several causes, including viral infections [56]. A 43-year-old, with a history of resistant mediastinal stage II Hodgkin's lymphoma, without current treatment, presented with monomorphic flaccid bullae over his trunk 40 days after testing positive COVID-19. Even though he had risk factors for IgA and paraneoplastic pemphigus, there was no evidence for these diseases. The patient responded well to treatment with prednisolone 1 mg/kg per day and methotrexate 15 mg subcutaneously, which was added after a week. He was later discharged with oral methotrexate and prednisolone at the same dose. Prednisolone was tapered down to 20 mg per day during the follow-up [57].

References

[1] Rojas M, Restrepo-Jiménez P, Monsalve DM, Pacheco Y, Acosta-Ampudia Y, Ramírez-Santana C, et al. Molecular mimicry and autoimmunity. J Autoimmun December 2018;95:100–23.

[2] Sercarz EE, Lehmann PV, Ametani A, Benichou G, Miller A, Moudgil K. Dominance and crypticity of T cell antigenic determinants. Annu Rev Immunol April 1993;11(1):729–66.

[3] Ryabkova VA, Churilov LP, Shoenfeld Y. Hyperstimulation of the immune system as a cause of autoimmune diseases. Annal Russ Acad Med Sci August 31, 2020;75(3).

[4] Dotan A, Muller S, Kanduc D, David P, Halpert G, Shoenfeld Y. The SARS-CoV-2 as an instrumental trigger of autoimmunity. Autoimmun Rev April 2021;20(4).

[5] el Hasbani G, Jawad A, Uthman I. Axial and peripheral spondyloarthritis triggered by sars-cov-2 infection: a report of two cases. Reumatismo April 19, 2021;(1):73.

[6] Saikali W, Gharib S. The first non-radiographic axial spondyloarthrits with COVID-19. Immun Inflamm Dis September 12, 2021;9(3).

[7] Carfì A, Bernabei R, Landi F. Persistent symptoms in patients after acute COVID-19. JAMA August 11, 2020;(6):324.

[8] de Stefano L, Rossi S, Montecucco C, Bugatti S. Transient monoarthritis and psoriatic skin lesions following COVID-19. Ann Rheum Dis August 4, 2020:1–2.

[9] Yokogawa N, Minematsu N, Katano H, Suzuki T. Case of acute arthritis following SARS-CoV-2 infection. Ann Rheum Dis June 2021;80(6).

[10] Danssaert Z, Raum G, Hemtasilpa S. Reactive arthritis in a 37-year-old female with SARS-CoV2 infection. Cureus August 12, 2020;12.

[11] Hønge BL, Hermansen M-LF, Storgaard M. Reactive arthritis after COVID-19. BMJ Case Rep March 2021;14(3).

[12] Saricaoglu EM, Hasanoglu I, Guner R. The first reactive arthritis case associated with COVID-19. J Med Virol January 19, 2021;93(1).

[13] Coath FL, Mackay J, Gaffney JK. Axial presentation of reactive arthritis secondary to COVID-19 infection. Rheumatology July 1, 2021;60(7).

[14] Clauw DJ, Häuser W, Cohen SP, Fitzcharles M-A. Considering the potential for an increase in chronic pain after the COVID-19 pandemic. Pain August 2020;161(8).

[15] Föll D, Wittkowski H, Hinze C. Das still-syndrom als biphasische Erkrankung. Z Rheumatol September 6, 2020;79(7).

[16] Bamidis AD, Koehler P, di Cristanziano V, Rasche K, Demirel B, Bacher P, et al. First manifestation of adult-onset Still's disease after COVID-19. Lancet Rheumatol May 2021;3(5).

[17] Hoong CWS, Amin MNME, Tan TC, Lee JE. Viral arthralgia a new manifestation of COVID-19 infection? A cohort study of COVID-19-associated musculoskeletal symptoms. Int J Infect Dis March 2021;104.

[18] Karakaya B, Kaiser Y, van Moorsel C, Grunewald J. Löfgren's syndrome: diagnosis, management, and disease pathogenesis. Semin Respir Crit Care Med August 27, 2017;38(04).

[19] Mihalov P, Krajčovičová E, Káčerová H, Sabaka P. Lofgren syndrome in close temporal association with mild COVID-19 – case report. IDCases 2021;26.

[20] Carvalho-Schneider C, Laurent E, Lemaignen A, Beaufils E, Bourbao-Tournois C, Laribi S, et al. Follow-up of adults with noncritical COVID-19 two months after symptom onset. Clin Microbiol Infect February 2021;27(2).

[21] Ramos-Casals M, Brito-Zerón P, Mariette X. Systemic and organ-specific immune-related manifestations of COVID-19. Nat Rev Rheumatol June 26, 2021;17(6).

[22] Romero-Sánchez CM, Díaz-Maroto I, Fernández-Díaz E, Sánchez-Larsen A, Layos-Romero A, García-García J, et al. Neurologic manifestations in hospitalized patients with COVID-19. Neurology August 25, 2020;95(8).

[23] Saud A, Naveen R, Aggarwal R, Gupta L. COVID-19 and myositis: what we know so far. Curr Rheumatol Rep August 3, 2021;23(8).

[24] Fineschi S. Case report: systemic sclerosis after covid-19 infection. Front Immunol June 2021;28:12.

[25] Crowson AN, Magro CM. Idiopathic perniosis and its mimics: a clinical and histological study of 38 cases. Hum Pathol April 1997;28(4).

[26] Freeman EE, McMahon DE, Lipoff JB, Rosenbach M, Kovarik C, Takeshita J, et al. Pernio-like skin lesions associated with COVID-19: a case series of 318 patients from 8 countries. J Am Acad Dermatol August 2020;83(2).

[27] Herman A, Peeters C, Verroken A, Tromme I, Tennstedt D, Marot L, et al. Evaluation of chilblains as a manifestation of the COVID-19 pandemic. JAMA Dermatol September 1, 2020;156(9).

[28] Aringer M, Leuchten N, Johnson SR. New criteria for lupus. Curr Rheumatol Rep June 13, 2020;22(6).

[29] Zamani B, Moeini Taba S-M, Shayestehpour M. Systemic lupus erythematosus manifestation following COVID-19: a case report. J Med Case Rep December 25, 2021;15(1).

[30] Mantovani Cardoso E, Hundal J, Feterman D, Magaldi J. Concomitant new diagnosis of systemic lupus erythematosus and COVID-19 with possible antiphospholipid syndrome. Just a coincidence? A case report and review of intertwining pathophysiology. Clin Rheumatol September 28, 2020;39(9).
[31] Zacharias H, Dubey S, Koduri G, D'Cruz D. Rheumatological complications of covid 19. Autoimmun Rev September 2021;20(9).
[32] Audia S, Grienay N, Mounier M, Michel M, Bonnotte B. Evans' syndrome: from diagnosis to treatment. J Clin Med November 27, 2020;9(12).
[33] Fattizzo B. Evans syndrome and infections: a dangerous cocktail to manage with caution. Blood Transfus 2021;19:5–8. Edizioni SIMTI.
[34] Demir NA, Basturk A, Ural O, Sumer S, Erdogdu B, Kiratli HE, et al. A case of Evans syndrome secondary to COVID-19. Blood Transfus January 1, 2021;19(1):85–8.
[35] Levi M, Thachil J, Iba T, Levy JH. Coagulation abnormalities and thrombosis in patients with COVID-19. Lancet Haematol June 2020;7(6).
[36] Connors JM, Levy JH. COVID-19 and its implications for thrombosis and anticoagulation. Blood June 4, 2020;135(23).
[37] Bowles L, Platton S, Yartey N, Dave M, Lee K, Hart DP, et al. Lupus anticoagulant and abnormal coagulation tests in patients with covid-19. N Engl J Med July 16, 2020;383(3).
[38] Helms J, Tacquard C, Severac F, Leonard-Lorant I, Ohana M, Delabranche X, et al. High risk of thrombosis in patients with severe SARS-CoV-2 infection: a multicenter prospective cohort study. Intensive Care Med June 4, 2020;46(6).
[39] Assinger A. Platelets and infection–an emerging role of platelets in viral infection. Front Immunol December 2014;18:5.
[40] Chen N, Zhou M, Dong X, Qu J, Gong F, Han Y, et al. Epidemiological and clinical characteristics of 99 cases of 2019 novel coronavirus pneumonia in Wuhan, China: a descriptive study. Lancet February 2020;395(10223).
[41] Terpos E, Ntanasis-Stathopoulos I, Elalamy I, Kastritis E, Sergentanis TN, Politou M, et al. Hematological findings and complications of COVID-19. Am J Hematol July 23, 2020;95(7).
[42] Mahévas M, Moulis G, Andres E, Riviere E, Garzaro M, Crickx E, et al. Clinical characteristics, management and outcome of COVID-19-associated immune thrombocytopenia: a French multicentre series. Br J Haematol August 4, 2020;190(4).
[43] Abou-Ismail MY, Diamond A, Kapoor S, Arafah Y, Nayak L. The hypercoagulable state in COVID-19: incidence, pathophysiology, and management. Thromb Res October 2020;194.
[44] Burley NB, Dy PS, Kalantri S, Razzaq K. Aortic thrombosis and acute limb ischemia secondary to COVID hypercoagulability. Cureus July 4, 2021;13.
[45] Lania A, Sandri MT, Cellini M, Mirani M, Lavezzi E, Mazziotti G. Thyrotoxicosis in patients with COVID-19: the THYRCOV study. Eur J Endocrinol October 2020;183(4).
[46] Chen M, Zhou W, Xu W. Thyroid function analysis in 50 patients with COVID-19: a retrospective study. Thyroid January 1, 2021;31(1).
[47] Yang J-K, Lin S-S, Ji X-J, Guo L-M. Binding of SARS coronavirus to its receptor damages islets and causes acute diabetes. Acta Diabetol September 31, 2010;47(3).
[48] Robert Kästner gor AH. COVID-19 infection as a trigger for new-onset type 1 diabetes in a susceptible individual – or just coincidence? GMS Hyg Infect Control April 22, 2021;16.
[49] Ellul MA, Benjamin L, Singh B, Lant S, Michael BD, Easton A, et al. Neurological associations of COVID-19. Lancet Neurol September 2020;19(9).
[50] Perrin P, Collongues N, Baloglu S, Bedo D, Bassand X, Lavaux T, et al. Cytokine release syndrome-associated encephalopathy in patients with COVID-19. Eur J Neurol January 5, 2021;28(1).
[51] Brandão PRP, Grippe TC, Pereira DA, Munhoz RP, Cardoso F. New-onset movement disorders associated with COVID-19. Tremor Other Hyperkinet Mov July 8, 2021;11(1).
[52] Bhandarwar A, Jadhav S, Tandur A, Dhimole N, Wagh A, Bhondve S. Management of thymomatous myasthenia gravis – case report of a rare Covid19 infection sequelae. Int J Surg Case Rep April 2021;81.
[53] Singh B, Kaur P, Maroules M. Autoimmune hepatitis–primary biliary cholangitis overlap syndrome triggered by COVID-19. Eur J Case Rep Intern Med February 4, 2021;8 [LATEST ONLINE)].
[54] Rahim MN, Miquel R, Heneghan MA. Approach to the patient with acute severe autoimmune hepatitis. JHEP Rep December 2020;2(6).

[55] Halpert G, Shoenfeld Y. SARS-CoV-2, the autoimmune virus. Autoimmun Rev December 2020;19(12).
[56] Porro AM, Seque CA, Ferreira MCC, Enokihara MMS e S. Pemphigus vulgaris. An Bras Dermatol May 2019;94(3).
[57] de Medeiros VLS, Monteiro-Neto AU, França DDT, Castelo Branco R, de Miranda Coelho ÉO, Takano DM. Pemphigus vulgaris after COVID-19: a case of induced autoimmunity. SN Compr Clin Med August 27, 2021;3(8).

Further reading

Abu-Rumeileh S, Abdelhak A, Foschi M, Tumani H, Otto M. Guillain–Barré syndrome spectrum associated with COVID-19: an up-to-date systematic review of 73 cases. J Neurol April 25, 2021;268(4).

Bonometti R, Sacchi MC, Stobbione P, Lauritano EC, Tamiazzo S, Marchegiani A, et al. The first case of systemic lupus erythematosus (SLE) triggered by COVID-19 infection. Eur Rev Med Pharmacol Sci September 2020;24(18).

Caress JB, Castoro RJ, Simmons Z, Scelsa SN, Lewis RA, Ahlawat A, et al. COVID-19–associated Guillain-Barré syndrome: the early pandemic experience. Muscle Nerve October 11, 2020;62(4).

Derksen VFAM, Kissel T, Lamers-Karnebeek FBG, van der Bijl AE, Venhuizen AC, Huizinga TWJ, et al. Onset of rheumatoid arthritis after COVID-19: coincidence or connected? Ann Rheum Dis August 2021;80(8).

El Aoud S, Morin C, Lorriaux P, Obert J, Sorial D, Chaabouni T, et al. COVID-19 presenting as lupus erythematosus-like syndrome. Disaster Med Public Health Prep August 10, 2021;15(4).

Galeotti C, Bayry J. Autoimmune and inflammatory diseases following COVID-19. Nat Rev Rheumatol August 4, 2020;(8):16.

Gracia-Ramos AE, Saavedra-Salinas MÁ. Can the SARS-CoV-2 infection trigger systemic lupus erythematosus? A case-based review. Rheumatol Int April 4, 2021;41(4).

Hali F, Jabri H, Chiheb S, Hafiani Y, Nsiri A. A concomitant diagnosis of COVID-19 infection and systemic lupus erythematosus complicated by a macrophage activation syndrome: a new case report. Int J Dermatol August 17, 2021;60(8).

Slimani Y, Abbassi R, el Fatoiki F, Barrou L, Chiheb S. Systemic lupus erythematosus and varicella-like rash following COVID-19 in a previously healthy patient. J Med Virol February 28, 2021;93(2).

Walling AD, Dickson G. Guillain-Barré syndrome. Am Fam Physician February 1, 2013;87(3).

CHAPTER

21

SARS-CoV-2 induction and COVID-19 manifestations related to autoimmune gastrointestinal diseases

Aaron Lerner[1,2] *and Carina Benzvi*[1]

[1]Chaim Sheba Medical Center, Zabludowicz Research Center for Autoimmune Diseases, Ramat Gan, Israel; [2]Ariel University, Ariel, Israel

The COVID -19 pandemic: a short update

Following the severe acute respiratory syndrome (SARS) and the middle east respiratory syndrome (MERS), our globus is currently facing the third member of the coronavirus family, where the SARS-CoV-2 is the most contagious and pathogenic of them.

It originated in the mega-metropolis of Wuhan in the Chinese province of Hubei in December 2019 and spread worldwide with incredible speed in quite a short time [1]. We are facing an ongoing Pandemic that teaches us totally new aspects of viral behavior, genetic adaptation, human-to-human transmission, geo-epidemiologic, clinical presentations, morbidity, and mortality [2–4]. Due to its devastating short and long-term outcomes, Coronavirus disease 2019 (COVID-19) represents a medical and a scientific challenge, hence brainstorming many health communities and pharmaceutical industries to treat the affected patients and, not less important, to prevent the disease individually and globally. In fact, according to the WHO, as of November 5, 2021 there are 248,467,363 confirmed cases, 5,027,183 deaths, and a total of 7,027,377,238 vaccine doses were administered [5]. Common presenting symptoms include dry cough, fever, and fatigue. Less common are dizziness, headache, abdominal pain, nausea, and vomiting. Some present with dysgeusia (distortion/loss of taste) and anosmia (loss of smell); however, many infected individuals are asymptomatic. Unfortunately, those presentations are not specific to COVID-19 and extensively overlap with a plethora of other microbial and viral infections [6], including the influenza ones [7]. No doubt that the respiratory tract and the lungs are the main target organs representing the primary indicator for disease activity, morbidity, and mortality.

Autoimmunity, COVID-19, Post-COVID19 syndrome and COVID-19 vaccination
https://doi.org/10.1016/B978-0-443-18566-3.00009-8

The disease usually starts with respiratory and pulmonary signs and symptoms, but extrapulmonary presentations are continuously reported [8]. The wide range of nonpulmonary affected organs' manifestations includes the heart, central and peripheral nervous systems, ears, olfactory system, muscles, skin, the coagulation network and vessels, and the list is not final [8,9]. Intriguingly, the human gut occupies a significant part of the list (Fig. 21.1). In fact, more and more publications continuously appear on the SARS-CoV-2 and gut association [10]. Applying COVID-19 and intestine words on PubMed, the number of publications between January 2019 and November 2021 increased substantially from 19 to 602, meaning a 32-fold surge (updated for 6, November 2021). The present review will expand on the epidemiology, symptoms and signs, pathology, morbidity, infectivity, and the pathophysiology of the gastrointestinal (GI) involvement in COVID -19 disease.

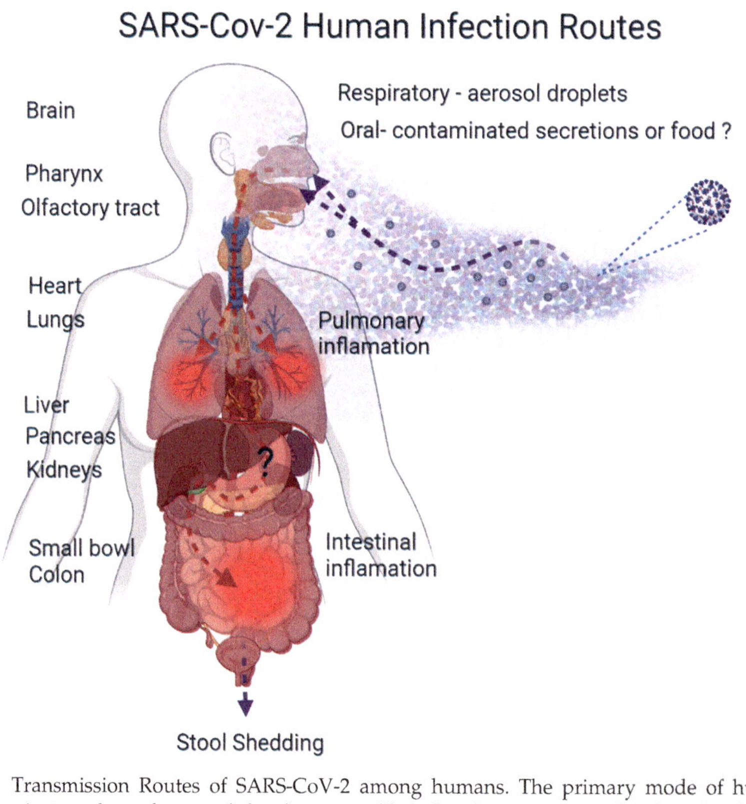

FIGURE 21.1 Transmission Routes of SARS-CoV-2 among humans. The primary mode of human-to-human transmission is respiratory through aerosol droplets, most likely by close contact with infected individuals, mainly when they exhibit active coughing or by urine. Vomiting and diarrheal routes are debatable. The inhaled viruses usually infect the respiratory tract first, inducing pulmonary symptoms. SARS-CoV-2 affects a wide range of nonpulmonary organs, including the intestine, esophagus, pancreas, liver, biliary tract and the vascular network. It infects the digestive system epithelium, either indirectly via circulation or directly through oral routes. Infected secretions (saliva) or contaminated foods could potentially carry the virus and spread the disease.

The human intestine is a target organ for SARS-CoV-2

To enter target cells, the surface spike protein of the SARS-CoV-2 virus binds to the angiotensin one converting enzyme 2 (ACE2) [11]. Still, it needs the type II transmembrane serine protease, TMPRSS2, for the viral spike membrane fusion in order to penetrate the host cell. Both receptors are highly expressed along the enteric tract and its associated organs (Fig. 21.2). In fact, esophageal, small bowel, and colonic epitheliums are rich in ACE2s, but other GI-associated organs like the liver, cholangiocytes in the biliary tract, and pancreas, also express the receptor [12–15]. The cell ACE2 expression of various organs was recently provided by the genotype-tissue expression (GTEx) project [16]. Zooming on the intestinal and other GI-associated organs, the small bowel terminal ileum had the highest expression,

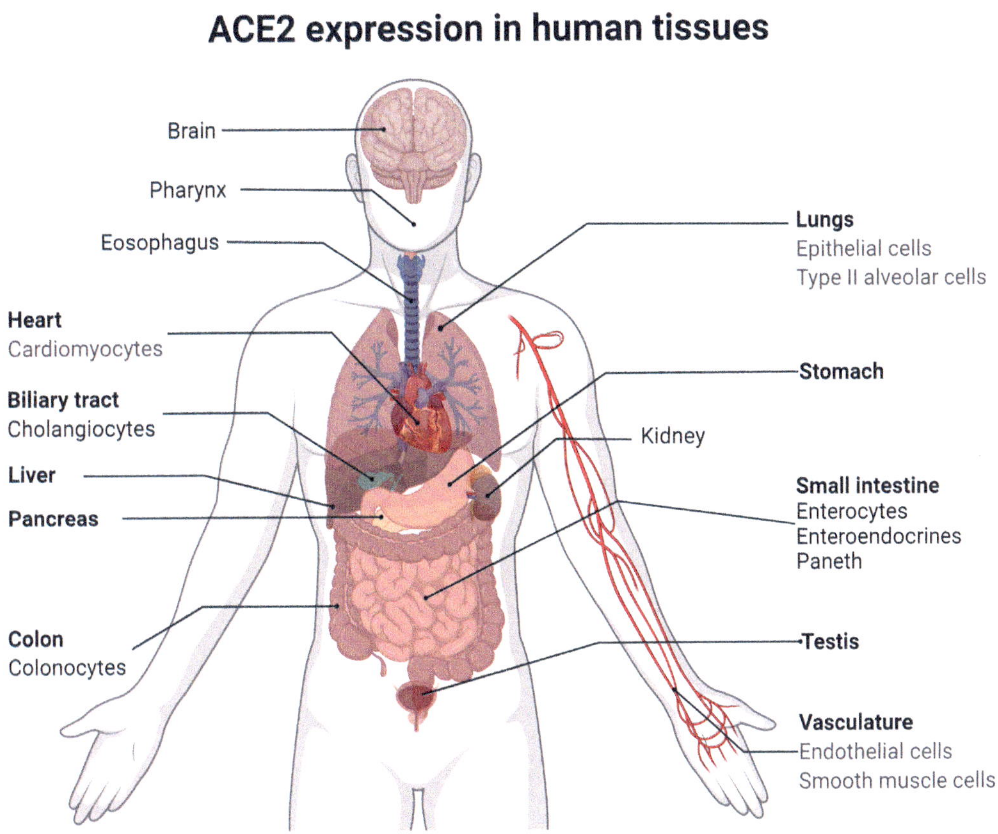

FIGURE 21.2 ACE2 expression in human organs. SARS-CoV-2 requires both ACE2 receptor and TMPRSS2 to penetrate the host cell. Those receptors are expressed in various organs, enabling the virus to target cells throughout the human body. The expression in the respiratory system is relatively low, whereas, in the GI tract, it is highly present, especially in the small intestine, colon, duodenum, biliary tract (cholangiocytes), and, to a lesser extent, in the pancreas, esophagus, and liver. The kidney, pharynx, testis, heart, vascular endothelial cells, and smooth muscle cells are additional sites.

followed by the esophageal mucosa and the pancreas. Intriguingly, all of them surpassed the lung expression. The esophageal muscularis, the gastro-esophageal junction, and the liver had less expression, while the stomach had the lowest [16]. The virus can impair patients' taste. Ageusia is present in half of the COVID-19 patients, and one-seventh of them had gustatory abnormalities as their initial symptoms [17].

The close proximity between the SARS-CoV-2 virus particles to its GI ACE2 receptor strongly suggests the presence, infectivity and pathologic injury induced by the virus in the human GI tract [12,18–24].

Pathologically wise, COVID -19 pathology affects all along the GI tract. Starting from the esophagus up to the recto-sigmoid. The esophagus squamous epithelium is infiltrated with lymphocytes, the stomach with plasma cells, lymphocytic infiltration, and edema. Screening the entire enteric mucosa, necrosis, degeneration, edema, and shedding of the epithelium can be detected [19,25]. The SARS-CoV-2 tropism to its intestinal ACE2 receptors was reported in China and other centers. The virus itself and some of its components, like the nucleocapsid proteins, were detected in the cytoplasm of colonic, duodenal, and gastric epithelial cells, as well excreted in the patients' stools [19,26,27]. It can be summarized that those numerous publications can point to the fact that the virus resides, penetrates, induces GI damage, and the human mucosal immune systems are activated against the aggressive intruder. Interestingly, ACE2 is known for its pivotal role in maintaining intestinal homeostasis; however, its mRNA expression is strongly reduced in cells infected by SARS-CoV-2, thus compromising its physiological functions [28].

Gastrointestinal manifestations of COVID-19

Gastrointestinal symptoms are common in infected patients. They may occur in the absence of any respiratory complaints. Patients with enteric symptoms present higher morbidity, worse clinical outcomes, and higher mortality when compared with those with respiratory presentations [29,30]. Others reported no correlation between GI symptoms and the COVID-19 severity [31].

The incidence of GI manifestations is quite broad, depending on inclusion and exclusion criteria and the experimental designs of the publications. Anorexia, nausea, or vomiting incidences range between 1% and 83.8%, diarrhea between 1.3% and 29.3%, and abnormal liver transglutaminases between 3.75% and 53.1% [29]. Recent data from outside of Wuhan, China, showed that overall GI symptoms, such as loss of appetite, nausea, vomiting, diarrhea, abdominal pain and even GI bleeding were presented in up to 79% of the infected patients [32]. Anorexia was the most prevalent GI complaint in adults (39.9%–50.2%), while diarrhea was the most common one in adults and children combined (2%–49.5%). Vomiting was more common in the pediatric age compared to adults (6.5%–66.7%, 3.6%–15.9%, respectively) [32]. Other GI manifestations include bloody diarrhea, constipation hemorrhagic colitis, multiple round herpetic erosions and ulcers, ulcerative and ischemic changes in recto sigmoidoscopy, and several other Intestinal Ischemic Manifestations [33,34]. Most recently, GI manifestations of the SARS-CoV-2 -Related Multisystem Inflammatory Syndrome in Children were described [35]. Having predominant intestinal symptoms is associated with a significant delay in diagnosis and later hospitalization compared to those with respiratory ones (9 vs. 7.3 d16 and 16 vs. 11.6 d15) [33]. Overall, the reported incidences of COVID-GI-related manifestations are variable, might be underestimated, and should be taken with reservation [36]. Table 21.1 summarizes the manifestations of GI and gut-associated organs in COVID-19 patients.

TABLE 21.1 Gastrointestinal and gut-associated organs' manifestations in COVID-19 patients.

Organs	Manifestations
Gastrointestinal	Abdominal pains
	Diarrhea
	Nausea
	Vomiting
	Hematochezia
	Bloody diarrhea
	Hemorrhagic colitis
	Constipation
	A/hypogeusia
Hepatobiliary	Transaminasemia-hepatitis
	Cholestasis-Jaundice
	Cholecystitis
	Hepatic failure
	Drug-induced hepatic damage
Pancreatic	Pancreatitis
	Acute diabetes
	Drug-induced pancreatic damage

Lee IC, Huo TI Huang, Y.H. Gastrointestinal and liver manifestations in patients with COVID-19. J Chin Med Assoc June 1, 2020;83(6):521–523; Patel KP, Patel PA, Vunnam RR, Hewlett AT, Jain R, Jing R. et al. Gastrointestinal, hepatobiliary, and pancreatic manifestations of COVID-19. J Clin Virol [Internet] July 1, 2020 [cited 2021 Nov 28];128. Available from: https://pubmed.ncbi.nlm.nih.gov/32388469/; Wan Y, Li J, Shen L, Zou Y, Hou L, Zhu L, et al. Enteric involvement in hospitalised patients with COVID-19 outside Wuhan. Lancet Gastroenterol Hepatol [Internet] June 1, 2020 [cited 2021 Nov 28];5(6):534–535. Available from: https://pubmed.ncbi.nlm.nih.gov/32304638/; Kariyawasam JC, Jayarajah U, Riza R, Abeysuriya V, Seneviratne SL. Gastrointestinal manifestations in COVID-19. Trans R Soc Trop Med Hyg [Internet] March 16, 2021 [cited 2021 Nov 29]; Available from: https://academic.oup.com/trstmh/advance-article/doi/10.1093/trstmh/trab042/6174402; Ponzetto A, Holton J, Porta M. Intestinal ischemic manifestations of COVID-19. Gastroenterology [Internet] May 1, 2021 [cited 2021 Nov 29];160(6):2191. Available from: https://pubmed.ncbi.nlm.nih.gov/33385437/; Sahn B, Eze OP, Edelman MC, Chougar CE, Thomas RM, Schleien CL, et al. Features of intestinal disease associated with COVID-related Multisystem inflammatory syndrome in children. J Pediatr Gastroenterol Nutr [Internet] March 1, 2021 [cited 2021 Nov 29];72(3):384–387. Available from: https://pubmed.ncbi.nlm.nih.gov/32969960/; Liang W, Feng Z, Rao S, Xiao C, Xue X, Lin Z, et al. Diarrhoea may be underestimated: a missing link in 2019 novel coronavirus. Gut June 1, 2020;69(6):1141–1143; Yang L, Tu L. Implications of gastrointestinal manifestations of COVID-19. Lancet Gastroenterol Hepatol [Internet] July 1, 2020 [cited 2021 Nov 29];5(7):629–630. Available from: https://pubmed.ncbi.nlm.nih.gov/32405602/.

The topic of the viral RNA or the virus itself shedding in stools and fecal-oral transmission is crucial for the contemporary pandemic spreading. Since viral RNA can be detected in a patient's stool, and viral constituents are detected in human feces, major questions arise: are stools infective, and does fecal-oral transmission occur? In addition to the respiratory and nasal secretion, the potency of stool infectivity was reported [37,38]. Interestingly, even when the SARS-CoV-2 was cleared from the respiratory tract, the virus continued to replicate in the enteric lumen, hence, Spilled through the feces [37,39]. The mean duration of the virus stool shading was 17.2 days, while the maximal duration was 126 days [40]. Stool RT-PCR positive rate from the time of diagnosis was 25% in week 1% and 37.5% in week 2 [41]. Stool viral loads in CT values were 31.65 in week 1 and 26.5 in week 2 [38]. SARS-CoV-2 RNA can persist for a prolonged time in several non-respiratory fluid samples. For example, the RNA was detected in bile even 75 days postinfections [42]. Finally, SARS-CoV-2 Infection in a Nonhuman Primate Model was most recently described [43]. It should be stressed that, as far as today, the fecal-oral transmission of the COVID-19 was not yet fully established. Unlike the well-established aerosol droplet transmission, fecal transmission and the degree of stool infectivity are still debatable. When the topic is discussed in the literature, the words like potential, possible, questionable, and debatable are frequently used [12,19,23,44–47].

A new route of transmission of the virus has recently been described. It is well known that contaminating pathogens can be carried by water-generated toilet flushing aerosols [48]. The flushed bio-aerosols are small and light enough to be air-born infective messengers [49]. In fact, the index case in the Hong Kong SARS epidemic presented with diarrhea, suggesting a local flashed aerosol spreading [50]. More recently, numerous publications reported bio-aerosol transmission of the virus via high-rise housing drainage stacks [51,52] and through ambient urban waters and raw wastewaters [53,54].

The fact that fecal shedding is longer compared to the respiratory droplet pouring and the fact that COVID-19 GI manifestation might predict a severe disease course, important consequences can be deducted [24,39,47]. The suggested fecal-oral environmental spreading should alert the public health authorities to direct efforts to fecal environmental COVID-19 control and build future therapeutic strategies to limit and stop the actual Pandemic. On the other side, one has to take into account that viral RNA presence in stools does not point to transmissibility and infectivity. Indeed, nucleic acid detection does not distinguish between infective from noninfective SARS-CoV-2 virus [33,55].

Pathophysiological aspects for SARS-CoV-2-Associated Gastrointestinal Illness

The pathophysiology of the COVID-19 related GI manifestations, complications, and fecal shedding is complicated and enrolls multiple aspects and pathways. Fig. 21.3 schematically presents some of them, and they are detailed below:

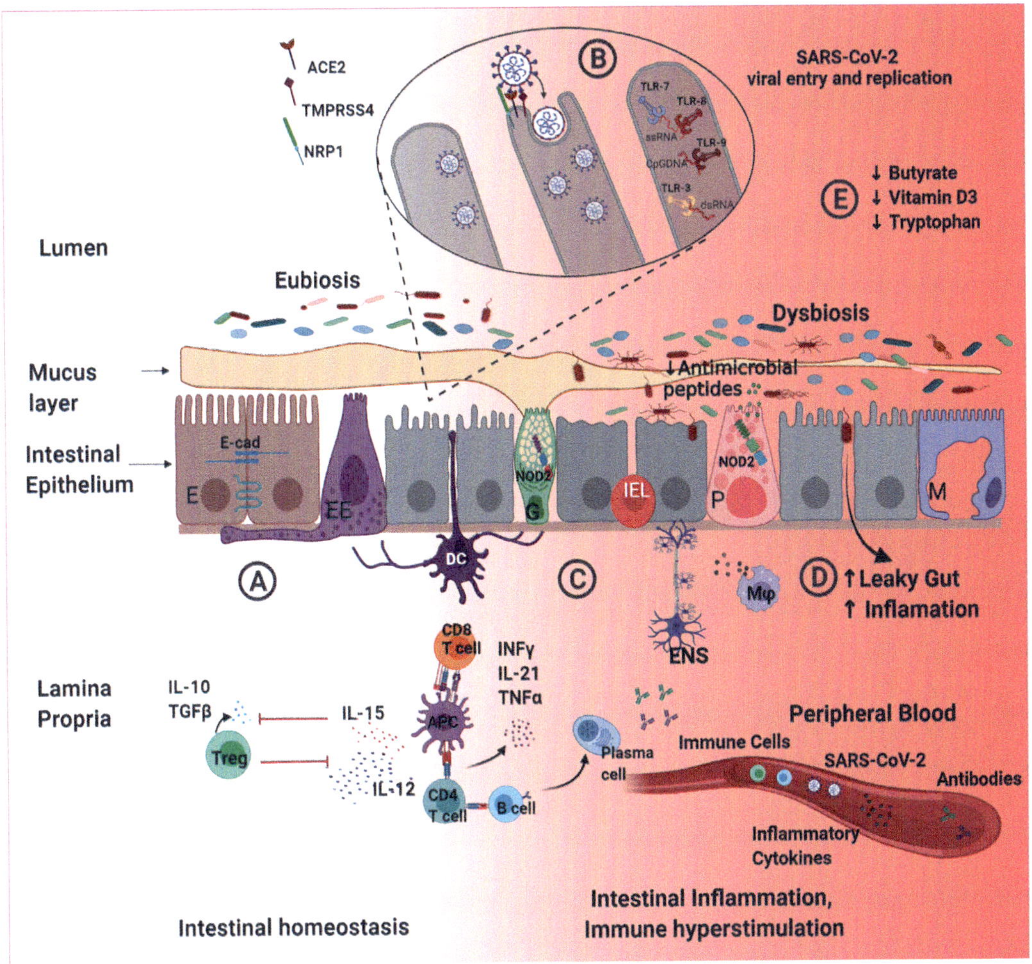

FIGURE 21.3 A schematic presentation of the pathophysiological aspects for SARS-CoV-2-Associated Gastrointestinal Illness. (A) During homeostasis, the epithelial cells interact together and maintain tight junction functional integrity. Goblet cells secrete mucins which act as a mucosal barrier against microbiota in the lumen while enabling enterocytes to uptake nutrients. Paneth cells express antimicrobial peptides upon sensing microbial infection. ACE2 is highly expressed on enterocytes; it plays a role in the expression and secretion of antimicrobial peptides, maintains local amino acid homeostasis, and modulates innate immunity. (B) Epithelial cells that express ACE2 are exposed to SARS-CoV-2 infection. Upon cellular penetration, the level of ACE2 expression is strongly reduced, affecting intestinal homeostasis and luminal microbiome integrity. The intruders are sensed by TLR3, TLR7, TLR8, and TLR9 receptors, which release stress signals enhancing gut inflammation. (C) Viral constituents are detected and processed by M cells, dendritic cells, and macrophages. APCs deliver them to lymphoid tissues, such as mesenteric lymph nodes (MLNs) and gut-associated lymphoid tissues (GALT). When those antigens activate immune cells, they proliferate and migrate to the site of infection, trying to eliminate the invasive pathogen. (D) The release of antimicrobial peptides and maintenance of a protective mucus layer is compromised, leading to a decrease in microbiota diversity resulting in enteric dysbiosis. The damaged epithelium enhances intestinal permeability and increases local and systemic inflammation, resulting in hyperstimulation of the immune responses. (E) SARS-CoV-2 infection leads to a decrease in butyrate, tryptophan, and vitamin D3 levels. These three have an essential role in maintaining intestinal homeostasis, and their deficiencies contribute to the inflammatory state of this viral infection.

Compromising the beneficial functions of the ACE2 receptors

The virus enters the enteric monolayer epithelial cells through the ACE2 receptors [28,33]. Subsequently to SARS-CoV-2 binding to its ACE2 receptor, both are endocytosed, reducing cell surface ACE2 levels' expression. The reduced ACE2 levels have major consequences since it plays a pivotal role in intestinal luminal microbiome integrity, antimicrobial peptides expression and secretion, maintain local amino acid homeostasis, and modulate innate immunity. Suppressing enteric ACE2 levels' expression perturbates those events and enhances gut inflammation [28,33].

The saliva adds to the virus intestinal inoculation

In addition to the naso-oral and respiratory viral load, the continuously swallowed saliva adds SARS-CoV-2 particles to the gut lumen, thus increasing the viral cargo [56].

The gut microbiome/dysbiome ratio is decreased

The SARS-CoV-2 decreases the gut commensal microbe diversity and composition, resulting in enteric dysbiosis. The dysbiome causes increased proinflammatory cytokines' levels, induces local and systemic inflammation, gut leakage, and hyperstimulates the immune system responses [33,57,58].

Intestinal self-defense and protective barriers are compromised

The ACE2 loss of enteric functions, the reduction of antimicrobial peptides produced by the cryptic Paneth's cells and other gut epithelial cells, the dysbiotic and the pathobiotic detrimental effects, the thinning and disruption of the overlining mucus layer, the dysfunctional local innate immunity, the damaged epithelial layer and finally, the resulting leaky gut, join forces to damage the intestinal system during the SARS-CoV-2 infection [28,33,57–60]. In addition, some second-line protective mechanisms can be suppressed. The failure of the homotypic interaction of enter-enterocytic E-cad in trans might increase the trans-epithelial intruder's transmigration and systemic invasion [28,61].

In parallel, the cryptic paneth cells' protective functions are suppressed. In response to luminal bacterial stimuli, the secretion of α-defensins, human α-defensin 5 (HD-5), and human α-defensin 6 (HD-6) might be less effective upon SARS-CoV-2 intestinal damage. The lack of those microbicides might compromise microbial control and the enteric homeostasis [28,62].

Tissue-specific patterns of SARS-CoV-2 variants and toll-like receptors (TLR)

Out of 13 TLRsrelated to the SARS-CoV-2 virus and the mucosal innate immunity, TLR-3 recognizes double-stranded RNA, TLR-7 and TLR-8 recognize single-stranded RNA, and TLR-9 is activated by unmethylated CpGDNA [63]. While those receptors were not thoroughly explored in humans, TLRs/TLR4-deficient mice are more susceptible to the virus infection [64], and the associated lymphopenia is a known marker of the human disease activity [65].

The host ACE2, TMPRSS4, and NRP-1 receptors facilitate SARS-CoV-2 infectivity in the GI tract

Neuropilin 1(NRP1) is a coreceptor that facilitates SARS-CoV-2 entry to the host cell, and it is present in the human intestine. Thus, all three receptors: ACE2, TMPRSS4, and NRP-1, might join together to potentiate SARS-CoV-2 infectivity [66,67].

The nucleotide-binding oligomerization domain 2 (NOD2)

The cytosolic innate receptor, NOD2, is able to sense peptidoglycan conserved motifs, muramyl dipeptide from Gram-positive and -negative bacteria. Thus, it triggers RIP2- and NF-κB-mediated pro-inflammatory and antibacterial responses and protects the body against bacterial invasiveness [68]. It appears that the NOD2 has some anti-viral functions, also against the SARS-CoV-2. Most recently, nodosome Inhibition was suggested as a novel broad-spectrum antiviral therapeutic strategy against SARS-CoV-2 [69].

Induction of a leaky gut

Intestinal permeability depends on the tight junction functional integrity. It is tightly regulated and evolutionary conserved, hence, avoiding foreign antigen's entry inside the body [70]. Predisposing individual conditions for COVID-19 severity are the elderly and certain underlying diseases like high blood pressure, diabetes, obesity, immune deficiencies, malnutrition, and other dysbiotic states. In many of those, increased intestinal permeability was reported [58]. Fecal calprotectin is a well-established marker for intestinal inflammation. Its abnormal high levels, were detected in COVID-19 patient's stool samples [71]. Thus, the hypothesis that SARS-CoV-2 induces bowel inflammation, potentially associated with the "leaky gut" syndrome, is supported.

Inadequacy of butyrate, tryptophan, and vitamin D3 levels in COVID-19

All three play a pivotal role in many gut functions and intestinal homeostasis [72–74]. Their local and systemic deficiencies were suggested to induce and maintain the enteric inflammatory state in COVID-19 [28,73,74]. More so, promoting oral butyrate, L-tryptophan, and vitamin D3 intake was suggested as a supplemental therapy for the patients [28,73–76].

Coronaviruses egress the host cells by lysosomal exocytosis and disrupt lysosomal and phagocytic functions

Most recently, it was shown that the b-coronaviruses don't use the conventional synthetic pathways but rather egress the host cell by the Arl8b-dependent lysosomal exocytosis in small secretory vesicles. In their intracellular way, they suppress the lysosomal proteolytic enzymes and compromise antigen processing and presentation [77,78]. Nevertheless, the studies were not performed on gut epithelial cells; this mode of non-lytic viral release may represent a new mode of epithelial shading to the human enteric lumen.

Post-COVID-19 gut manifestations

Months after recovery from acute COVID-19, people continue to suffer, and this represents a new entity termed long COVID-19 [79]. Gastrointestinal complaints and sequela are part of this new, still undefined condition. Nausea, vomiting, dysgeusia, loss of appetite, abdominal pain, hematemesis/melena, dysphagia, gastroesophageal reflux disease, constipation, and fatigue are some of the list. In a recent study, 6 months post-COVID diagnosis, 29% of the patients reported COVID-related GI symptoms. 9.6% had diarrhea, 11% constipation, 9.4% abdominal pain, 7.1% nausea or vomiting, and 16% with heartburn. GI symptoms were the most self-reported bothersome current symptom in 11% [80]. Interestingly, the presence of post-COVID mental health symptoms was significantly related to post-COVID GI symptoms.

SARS-CoV-2 impact on gastrointestinal diseases

Since the SARS-CoV-2 infects the human GI tract, induces inflammation and histological abnormalities, provokes clinical gut manifestation and is shaded in the stools, it is interesting to study the relations between COVID-19 and various GI diseases.

Inflammatory bowel disease (IBD)

The pathogenesis, molecular pathways, and implications of innate and adaptive immune responses following infection with SARS-CoV-2 in patients with IBD were recently summarized [81]. The COVID-19 Pandemic brought dramatic challenges for the patients, as well as for the healthcare teams of IBD. Those challenges provoked many questions about the virus-gut cross-talks in IBD and changed patients' habits and care centers' protocols [82].

Age, inflammatory state, and anatomic location were found to be key players of ACE2 and TMPRSS2 expression in IBD patients [83]. The inflammation-induced surge in colonic ACE2 expression in the colon may elude the proinflammatory cytokine effects, as demonstrated at the respiratory level. It was suggested that patients with high disease activity are at higher risk for the SARS-CoV-2 uptake and proliferation, hence, aggravating the colitis [83]. In opposite, others reported on lack of higher expression of ACE2 upon inflammation [84]. On the other hand, the reduction of the ACE2 in Crohn's disease active ileitis may suggest a better outcome. Interestingly, pharmaceutical therapy was associated with reduced levels of ACE2, Thus, reassuring the IBD community [84]. Staying on the optimistic plan, recent observational studies concluded that neither IBD nor immunosuppressants represent a risk factor for severe COVID-19 during a 1-year follow-up [85,86]. However, IBD patients had a higher hospitalization rate due to COVID-19 [87].

The outcome of IBD patients is highly variable and debatable. Comorbidity, increasing age, and systemic corticosteroid therapy were associated with severe COVID-19; hence, no causality could be established. Of note, antitumor necrosis factor therapy was not associated with severe SARS-CoV-2 infection in IBD-affected patients [88]. However, in younger patients, clinically active IBD may be a risk factor for severe COVID-19 [89].

As for the treating teams and the IBD centers, various guidelines were recently reported recommending the reorganization of endoscopy and gastroenterology services for patients, healthcare providers, and public health safety. Using telemedicine is increasingly recommended and addressing mental health aspects and stress management are highlighted during the COVID-19 era [90].

Finally, as of October 6, 2021, as reported by the SECURE-IBD database (https://covidibd.org), the number of registered cases of COVID-19 in patients with IBD mounted to 6635. Reported from 71 countries [91]. 57% had Crohn's disease, 40% had ulcerative colitis, and 3% had unspecified IBD. The results suggest that biologicals, mesalamine or sulfasalazine, are not associated with severe SARS-CoV-2 infection outcomes. On the contrary, the combination of anti-TNF with methotrexate might confer some protection from COVID-19 adverse effects compared to the combination with thiopurines. However, corticosteroids appear to increase the risk of severe COVID-19 outcomes. It is recommended to lower the doze or to wean off corticosteroids when possible. Since the number of IBD patients infected with SARS-CoV-2 is continuously increasing daily, further research is needed to explore the pathophysiology, the dominant molecular pathways, and short- and long-term consequences of SARS-CoV-2 infection in IBD patients.

Celiac disease (CD)

At the COVID-19 pandemic onset, there were some concerns that celiac patients might be at a higher risk for the SARS-CoV-2 infection [92]. Their occasional associations with immune dysregulation [93], IgA deficiency [94], immune deficiency conditions [95], Immune suppressive therapy in refractory celiac [96], obesity [97], and pulmonary diseases [98–101] could have played against them. Fortunately, this is not the case. They don't have any additional risk of attracting COVID-19, if they follow a gluten-free diet [102–104]. In screening Brazilian CD patients for the quality of life, GI aspects were more affected than emotional, social, or worrisome ones [105]. The authors reported lower quality of life and a greater burden in the non-adhering to gluten withdrawal patients. The elderly [106], women and those CD patients with other comorbidities [107–109] were more impacted by the pandemic, and large-scale remote consultation, practicing telemedicine, became a more popular means of CD healthcare [110,111]. At least in Italy, the lockdown improved adherence to a gluten-free diet in one-third of the survey participants, mainly non-adherent ones [112]. When studying the levels of risk perceptions in the CD population, the level was highly associated with higher self-COVID-19-related stress, and negative mental health consequences [113]. Based on CD referral center experience, recommendations were suggested to manage CD patients and their gluten-restricted diet, paying attention to social and psychological aspects [110,114–116].

As for the CD patient's anti-SARS-CoV-2 serological profile, a similar immunoglobulins profile was reported compared to non-CD controls, except for the anti-N IgA [117]. Concerning the hesitations and concerns about the various COVID-19 vaccinations, it is recommended that they should be vaccinated, and specific strategies should be developed and implemented to address the hesitant and wary patients [118,119].

In summary, CD patients are not at high risk for the COVID-19, except when comorbidity, nonadherence, and complicated situations occur. Despite that, SARS-CoV-2 is a new runner in the GI tracts [24], compared to other more severe autoimmune conditions [120–124], CD patients are relatively safe [92,102–104,119,125]. Several viruses were associated with CD induction [126], but it seems that the SARS-CoV-2 virus is not involved in CD autoimmunogenesis.

Conclusions

The scientific and medical communities should be aware of the wide range of GI symptoms and signs in the ongoing Pandemic of COVID-19. The healthcare givers should develop a high degree of suspicion in those individuals presented with the above-mentioned gut symptoms. The GI clinical symptoms can present the only indicator of COVID-19. This high awareness may predict the progression to more severe disease, complications, and long COVID complaints, along the road [28,33,125]. SARS-CoV-2 might impact autoimmune GI diseases like IBD and CD, but no cause-and-effect relations were depicted concerning their induction or initiation. On the contrary, at least in children with functional abdominal pains, the COVID-19 quarantine showed the satisfactory quality of life and anxiety scores [127]. The authors alluded to the positive effects of school closure and enhanced parental attention. The COVID-19 Pandemic changed protocols and recommendations in order to keep GI healthcare teams and the affected patient's health safety as a prime goal.

Conflicts of Interest: The authors declare that the research was conducted in the absence of any commercial or financial relationships that could be construed as a potential conflict of interest.

Author Contributions: Conceptualization, Formal Analysis, Writing – Original Draft Preparation, Supervision A.L.; Methodology, Software, Visualization, designing the figure using BioRender.com. C.B.; Validation, Data Curation, Writing – Review & Editing A.L. and C.B.;Visualization, C.B.; designing the figure using BioRender.com. C.B.; Supervision, A.L.
The authors agreed to the published version of the manuscript.

Abbreviations: ACE2—angiotensin 1 converting enzyme 2; CD—celiac disease; GALT—gut-associated lymphoid tissues; GI—gastrointestinal; IBD—Inflammatory bowel disease; MLNs—mesenteric lymph nodes; TLR—Toll-like receptors; TMPRSS2—type II transmembrane serine protease.

References

[1] Boni MF, Lemey P, Jiang X, Lam TTY, Perry BW, Castoe TA, et al. Evolutionary origins of the SARS-CoV-2 sarbecovirus lineage responsible for the COVID-19 pandemic. Nat Microbiol November 1, 2020;5(11):1408–17.

[2] Salimi-Jeda A, Abbassi S, Mousavizadeh A, Esghaie M, Bokharaei-Salim F, Jeddi F, et al. SARS-CoV-2: current trends in emerging variants, pathogenesis, immune responses, potential therapeutic, and vaccine development strategies. Int Immunopharm December 2021;101:108232.

[3] Wang C, Wang Z, Wang G, Lau JYN, Zhang K, Li W. COVID-19 in early 2021: current status and looking forward. Signal Transduct Targeted Ther December 1, 2021;6(1).

[4] Rana R, Tripathi A, Kumar N, Ganguly NK. A comprehensive overview on COVID-19: future perspectives. Front Cell Infect Microbiol September 2021;14:11.

[5] WHO coronavirus (COVID-19) dashboard | WHO coronavirus (COVID-19) dashboard with vaccination data. 2021 [cited 2021 Nov 28]. Available from: https://covid19.who.int/.
[6] Gallo Marin B, Aghagoli G, Lavine K, Yang L, Siff EJ, Chiang SS, et al. Predictors of COVID-19 severity: a literature review. Rev Med Virol January 1, 2021;31(1):1–10.
[7] Deng LS, Yuan J, Ding L, Chen YL, Zhao CH, Chen GQ, et al. Comparison of patients hospitalized with COVID-19, H7N9 and H1N1. Infect Dis Poverty December 1, 2020;9(1).
[8] Finsterer J, Scorza FA, Scorza CA, Fiorini AC. Extrapulmonary onset manifestations of COVID-19. Clinics 2021:76.
[9] Pousa PA, Mendonça TSC, Oliveira EA, Simões-e-Silva AC. Extrapulmonary manifestations of COVID-19 in children: a comprehensive review and pathophysiological considerations [cited 2021 Nov 29] J Pediatr March 1, 2021;97(2):116–39. Available from: https://pubmed.ncbi.nlm.nih.gov/32980319/.
[10] Perisetti A, Gajendran M, Mann R, Elhanafi S, Goyal H. COVID-19 extrapulmonary illness – special gastrointestinal and hepatic considerations. Dis Mon September 1, 2020;66(9).
[11] Yan R, Zhang Y, Li Y, Xia L, Guo Y, Zhou Q. Structural basis for the recognition of SARS-CoV-2 by full-length human ACE2. Science March 27, 2020;367(6485):1444–8. 80-.
[12] Zhang H, Kang Z, Gong H, Xu D, Wang J, Li Z, et al. The digestive system is a potential route of 2019-nCov infection: a bioinformatics analysis based on single-cell transcriptomes. bioRxiv January 31, 2020 [cited 2021 Nov 28];2020.01.30.927806. Available from: https://www.biorxiv.org/content/10.1101/2020.01.30.927806v1.
[13] Debes JD. COVID-19 and the liver: the perils of non–peer-reviewed science in times of a pandemic. Gastroenterology October 1, 2020;159(4):1620.
[14] Liu F, Long X, Zhang B, Zhang W, Chen X, Zhang Z. ACE2 expression in pancreas may cause pancreatic damage after SARS-CoV-2 infection. Clin Gastroenterol Hepatol August 1, 2020;18(9):2128–30. e2.
[15] Kumar A, Faiq MA, Pareek V, Raza K, Narayan RK, Prasoon P, et al. Relevance of SARS-CoV-2 related factors ACE2 and TMPRSS2 expressions in gastrointestinal tissue with pathogenesis of digestive symptoms, diabetes-associated mortality, and disease recurrence in COVID-19 patients. Med Hypotheses November 2020;1:144.
[16] Sarkesh A, Sorkhabi AD, Sheykhsaran E, Alinezhad F, Mohammadzadeh N, Hemmat N, et al. Extrapulmonary clinical manifestations in COVID-19 patients. Am J Trop Med Hyg November 1, 2020;103(5):1783–96.
[17] Chi H, Chiu NC, Peng CC, Lin CH, Tai YL, Lee MD, et al. One-seventh of patients with covid-19 had olfactory and gustatory abnormalities as their initial symptoms: a systematic review and meta-analysis. Life September 1, 2020;10(9):1–8.
[18] Rothan HA, Byrareddy SN. The epidemiology and pathogenesis of coronavirus disease (COVID-19) outbreak. J Autoimmun May 2020;1:109.
[19] Fang D, Ma J, Guan J, Wang M, Song Y, Tian D, et al. Manifestations of Digestive system in hospitalized patients with novel coronavirus pneumonia in Wuhan, China: a single-center, descriptive study. Chinese J Dig 2020. https://doi.org/10.3760/cma.j.issn.0254-1432.2020.0005 [cited 2021 Nov 28];E005–E005. Available from:.
[20] Tian Y, Rong L, Nian W, He Y. Review article: gastrointestinal features in COVID-19 and the possibility of faecal transmission [cited 2021 Nov 28] Aliment Pharmacol Ther May 1, 2020;51(9):843–51. Available from: https://pubmed.ncbi.nlm.nih.gov/32222988/.
[21] Wei XS, Wang X, Niu YR, Ye LL, Peng WB, Wang ZH, et al. Diarrhea is associated with prolonged symptoms and viral carriage in corona virus disease 2019. Clin Gastroenterol Hepatol July 1, 2020;18(8):1753–9. e2.
[22] Kam KQ, Yung CF, Cui L, Pin Lin RT, Mak TM, Maiwald M, et al. A well infant with coronavirus disease 2019 with high viral load [cited 2021 Nov 28] Clin Infect Dis August 1, 2020;71(15):847–9. Available from: https://pubmed.ncbi.nlm.nih.gov/32112082/.
[23] Wong SH, Lui RNS, Sung JJY. Covid-19 and the digestive system [cited 2021 Nov 28] J Gastroenterol Hepatol May 1, 2020;35(5):744–8. Available from: https://pubmed.ncbi.nlm.nih.gov/32215956/.
[24] Lerner A. Covid-19 and the human gut: a new runner on the tract [cited 2021 Nov 28] Int J Celiac Dis June 25, 2020;8(2):64–7. Available from: http://www.sciepub.com/IJCD/abstract/11998.
[25] Liu Q, Wang RS, Qu GQ. Gross examination report of a COVID-19 death autopsy. J Forensic Med February 25, 2020;36(1):21–3.
[26] YANG Z, LI G, DAI X, LIU G, LI G, JIE Y. Three cases of novel coronavirus pneumonia with viral nucleic acids still positive in stool after throat swab detection turned negative. Chinese J Dig 2020. https://doi.org/10.3760/cma.j.issn.0254-1432.2020.0002 [cited 2021 Nov 28];E002–E002. Available from:.

[27] Zhang JC, Wang SB, Xue YD. Fecal specimen diagnosis 2019 novel coronavirus–infected pneumonia. J Med Virol June 1, 2020;92(6):680–2.
[28] Devaux CA, Lagier JC, Raoult D. New insights into the physiopathology of COVID-19: SARS-CoV-2-Associated gastrointestinal illness [cited 2021 Nov 28] Front Med February 18, 2021;8. Available from: https://pubmed.ncbi.nlm.nih.gov/33681266/.
[29] Lee IC, Huo TI, Huang YH. Gastrointestinal and liver manifestations in patients with COVID-19. J Chin Med Assoc June 1, 2020;83(6):521–3.
[30] Patel KP, Patel PA, Vunnam RR, Hewlett AT, Jain R, Jing R, et al. Gastrointestinal, hepatobiliary, and pancreatic manifestations of COVID-19 [cited 2021 Nov 28] J Clin Virol July 1, 2020;128. Available from: https://pubmed.ncbi.nlm.nih.gov/32388469/.
[31] Guan W, Ni Z, Hu Y, Liang W, Ou C, He J, et al. Clinical characteristics of coronavirus disease 2019 in China [cited 2021 Nov 28] N Engl J Med April 30, 2020;382(18):1708–20. Available from: https://www.nejm.org/doi/full/10.1056/nejmoa2002032.
[32] Wan Y, Li J, Shen L, Zou Y, Hou L, Zhu L, et al. Enteric involvement in hospitalised patients with COVID-19 outside Wuhan [cited 2021 Nov 28] Lancet Gastroenterol Hepatol June 1, 2020;5(6):534–5. Available from: https://pubmed.ncbi.nlm.nih.gov/32304638/.
[33] Kariyawasam JC, Jayarajah U, Riza R, Abeysuriya V, Seneviratne SL. Gastrointestinal manifestations in COVID-19. Trans R Soc Trop Med Hyg March 16, 2021 [cited 2021 Nov 29]; Available from: https://academic.oup.com/trstmh/advance-article/doi/10.1093/trstmh/trab042/6174402.
[34] Ponzetto A, Holton J, Porta M. Intestinal ischemic manifestations of COVID-19 [cited 2021 Nov 29] Gastroenterology May 1, 2021;160(6):2191. Available from: https://pubmed.ncbi.nlm.nih.gov/33385437/.
[35] Sahn B, Eze OP, Edelman MC, Chougar CE, Thomas RM, Schleien CL, et al. Features of intestinal disease associated with COVID-related Multisystem inflammatory syndrome in children [cited 2021 Nov 29] J Pediatr Gastroenterol Nutr March 1, 2021;72(3):384–7. Available from: https://pubmed.ncbi.nlm.nih.gov/32969960/.
[36] Liang W, Feng Z, Rao S, Xiao C, Xue X, Lin Z, et al. Diarrhoea may be underestimated: a missing link in 2019 novel coronavirus. Gut June 1, 2020;69(6):1141–3.
[37] Yang L, Tu L. Implications of gastrointestinal manifestations of COVID-19 [cited 2021 Nov 29] Lancet Gastroenterol Hepatol July 1, 2020;5(7):629–30. Available from: https://pubmed.ncbi.nlm.nih.gov/32405602/.
[38] Wu Y, Guo C, Tang L, Hong Z, Zhou J, Dong X, et al. Prolonged presence of SARS-CoV-2 viral RNA in faecal samples. Lancet Gastroenterol Hepatol May 1, 2020;5(5):434–5.
[39] Santos VS, Gurgel RQ, Cuevas LE, Martins-Filho PR. Prolonged fecal shedding of SARS-CoV-2 in pediatric patients: a quantitative evidence synthesis [cited 2021 Nov 29] J Pediatr Gastroenterol Nutr August 1, 2020;71(2):150–2. Available from: https://pubmed.ncbi.nlm.nih.gov/32452978/.
[40] Cevik M, Tate M, Lloyd O, Maraolo AE, Schafers J, Ho A. SARS-CoV-2, SARS-CoV, and MERS-CoV viral load dynamics, duration of viral shedding, and infectiousness: a systematic review and meta-analysis. The Lancet Microbe January 1, 2021;2(1):e13–22.
[41] Yan Y, Chang L, Wang L. Laboratory testing of SARS-CoV, MERS-CoV, and SARS-CoV-2 (2019-nCoV): current status, challenges, and countermeasures [cited 2021 Nov 29] Rev Med Virol May 1, 2020;30(3). Available from: https://pubmed.ncbi.nlm.nih.gov/32302058/.
[42] Scutari R, Piermatteo L, Manuelli MC, Iannetta M, Salpini R, Bertoli A, et al. Long-term sars-cov-2 infection associated with viral dissemination in different body fluids including bile in two patients with acute cholecystitis. Life November 1, 2020;10(11):1–9.
[43] Jiao L, Li H, Xu J, Yang M, Ma C, Li J, et al. The gastrointestinal tract is an alternative route for SARS-CoV-2 infection in a nonhuman primate Model [cited 2021 Nov 29] Gastroenterology April 1, 2021;160(5):1647–61. Available from: https://pubmed.ncbi.nlm.nih.gov/33307034/.
[44] Gu J, Han B, Wang J. COVID-19: gastrointestinal manifestations and potential fecal-oral transmission [cited 2021 Nov 29] Gastroenterology May 1, 2020;158(6):1518–9. Available from: https://pubmed.ncbi.nlm.nih.gov/32142785/.
[45] Hindson J. COVID-19: faecal-oral transmission? [cited 2021 Nov 29] Nat Rev Gastroenterol Hepatol May 1, 2020;17(5):259. Available from: https://pubmed.ncbi.nlm.nih.gov/32214231/.
[46] McDermott CV, Alicic RZ, Harden N, Cox EJ, Scanlan JM. Put a lid on it: are faecal bio-aerosols a route of transmission for SARS-CoV-2? [cited 2021 Nov 29] J Hosp Infect July 1, 2020;105(3):397–8. Available from: https://pubmed.ncbi.nlm.nih.gov/32315667/.

[47] Xu Y, Li X, Zhu B, Liang H, Fang C, Gong Y, et al. Characteristics of pediatric SARS-CoV-2 infection and potential evidence for persistent fecal viral shedding [cited 2021 Nov 29] Nat Med April 1, 2020;26(4):502–5. Available from: https://pubmed.ncbi.nlm.nih.gov/32284613/.

[48] Knowlton SD, Boles CL, Perencevich EN, Diekema DJ, Nonnenmann MW. Bioaerosol concentrations generated from toilet flushing in a hospital-based patient care setting [cited 2021 Nov 29] Antimicrob Resist Infect Control January 26, 2018;7(1). Available from: https://pubmed.ncbi.nlm.nih.gov/29423191/.

[49] Johnson D, Lynch R, Marshall C, Mead K, Hirst D. Aerosol generation by modern flush toilets. Aerosol Sci Technol 2013;47(9):1047–57.

[50] Yu ITS, Li Y, Wong TW, Tam W, Chan AT, Lee JHW, et al. Evidence of airborne transmission of the severe acute respiratory syndrome virus [cited 2021 Nov 29] N Engl J Med April 22, 2004;350(17):1731–9. Available from: https://pubmed.ncbi.nlm.nih.gov/15102999/.

[51] Wang Q, Li Y, Lung DC, Chan PT, Dung CH, Jia W, et al. Aerosol transmission of SARS-CoV-2 due to the chimney effect in two high-rise housing drainage stacks [cited 2021 Nov 29] J Hazard Mater January 5, 2022;421. Available from: https://pubmed.ncbi.nlm.nih.gov/34396958/.

[52] Kang M, Wei J, Yuan J, Guo J, Zhang Y, Hang J, et al. Probable evidence of fecal aerosol transmission of SARS-CoV-2 in a high-rise building [cited 2021 Nov 29] Ann Intern Med December 15, 2020;173(12):974–80. Available from: https://pubmed.ncbi.nlm.nih.gov/32870707/.

[53] Kumar M, Srivastava V, Mazumder P, Deka JP, Gupta S, Goswami R, et al. Spectre of SARS-CoV-2 RNA in the ambient urban waters of Ahmedabad and Guwahati: a tale of two Indian cities [cited 2021 Nov 29] Environ Res March 1, 2021;204(Pt B). Available from: https://pubmed.ncbi.nlm.nih.gov/34543636/.

[54] Gwenzi W. Leaving no stone unturned in light of the COVID-19 faecal-oral hypothesis? A water, sanitation and hygiene (WASH) perspective targeting low-income countries. Sci Total Environ January 2021;20:753.

[55] Joynt GM, Wu WK. Understanding COVID-19: what does viral RNA load really mean? [cited 2021 Nov 29] Lancet Infect Dis June 1, 2020;20(6):635–6. Available from: https://pubmed.ncbi.nlm.nih.gov/32224308/.

[56] To KKW, Tsang OTY, Yip CCY, Chan KH, Wu TC, Chan JMC, et al. Consistent detection of 2019 novel coronavirus in saliva [cited 2021 Nov 29] Clin Infect Dis August 1, 2020;71(15):841–3. Available from: https://pubmed.ncbi.nlm.nih.gov/32047895/.

[57] Villapol S. Gastrointestinal symptoms associated with COVID-19: impact on the gut microbiome. Transl Res December 1, 2020;226:57–69.

[58] Kim HS. Do an altered gut microbiota and an associated leaky gut affect COVID-19 severity? [cited 2021 Nov 29] mBio 2021;12(1):1–9. Available from: https://pubmed.ncbi.nlm.nih.gov/33436436/.

[59] Dhar D, Mohanty A. Gut microbiota and Covid-19- possible link and implications. Virus Res August 2020;1:285.

[60] Vanella G, Capurso G, Burti C, Fanti L, Ricciardiello L, Souza Lino A, et al. Gastrointestinal mucosal damage in patients with COVID-19 undergoing endoscopy: an international multicentre study [cited 2021 Nov 29] BMJ Open Gastroenterol February 24, 2021;8(1). Available from: https://pubmed.ncbi.nlm.nih.gov/33627313/.

[61] Devaux CA, Mezouar S, Mege J-L. The E-cadherin cleavage associated to pathogenic bacteria infections can favor bacterial invasion and transmigration, dysregulation of the immune response and cancer induction in humans [cited 2021 Nov 29] Front Microbiol November 8, 2019;10:2598. Available from: http://www.ncbi.nlm.nih.gov/pubmed/31781079.

[62] Yang E, Shen J. The roles and functions of Paneth cells in Crohn's disease: a critical review [cited 2021 Nov 29] Cell Prolif January 1, 2021;54(1). Available from: https://pubmed.ncbi.nlm.nih.gov/33174662/.

[63] Lester SN, Li K. Toll-like receptors in antiviral innate immunity [cited 2021 Nov 29] J Mol Biol March 20, 2014;426(6):1246–64. Available from: https://pubmed.ncbi.nlm.nih.gov/24316048/.

[64] Totura AL, Whitmore A, Agnihothram S, Schäfer A, Katze MG, Heise MT, et al. Toll-like receptor 3 signaling via TRIF contributes to a protective innate immune response to severe acute respiratory syndrome coronavirus infection. mBio May 26, 2015;6(3):1–14.

[65] Huang G, Kovalic AJ, Graber CJ. Prognostic value of leukocytosis and lymphopenia for coronavirus disease severity. Emerg Infect Dis August 1, 2020;26(8):1839–41.

[66] Cantuti-Castelvetri L, Ojha R, Pedro LD, Djannatian M, Franz J, Kuivanen S, et al. Neuropilin-1 facilitates SARS-CoV-2 cell entry and infectivity. Science 2020;370. 6518, https://pubmed.ncbi.nlm.nih.gov/33082293/.

[67] Chekol Abebe E, Mengie Ayele T, Tilahun Muche Z, Asmamaw Dejenie T. Neuropilin 1: a novel entry factor for SARS-CoV-2 infection and a potential therapeutic target [cited 2021 Nov 29] Biol Targets Ther May

2021;15:143–52. Available from: https://www.dovepress.com/neuropilin-1-a-novel-entry-factor-for-sars-cov-2-infection-and-a-poten-peer-reviewed-fulltext-article-BTT.

[68] Negroni A, Pierdomenico M, Cucchiara S, Stronati L. NOD2 and inflammation: current insights [cited 2021 Nov 29] J Inflamm Res 2018:11–49. https://doi.org/10.2147/JIR.S137606. Available from:.

[69] Limonta D, Dyna-Dagman L, Branton W, Mancinelli V, Makio T, Wozniak RW, et al. Nodosome inhibition as a novel broad-spectrum antiviral strategy against arboviruses, enteroviruses, and SARS-CoV-2 [cited 2021 Nov 29] Antimicrob Agents Chemother July 16, 2021;65(8). Available from: https://journals.asm.org/doi/10.1128/AAC.00491-21.

[70] Lerner A, McCarty MF. The aging bowel dysfunction and elderly vulnerability towards COVID-19 infection [cited 2021 Nov 29] Life January 28, 2021;11(2):97. Available from: https://www.mdpi.com/2075-1729/11/2/97.

[71] Zerbato V, Di Bella S, Giuffrè M, Jaracz AW, Gobbo Y, Luppino D, et al. High fecal calprotectin levels are associated with SARS-CoV-2 intestinal shedding in COVID-19 patients: a proof-of-concept study [cited 2021 Nov 29] World J Gastroenterol June 14, 2021;27(22):3130–7. Available from: https://www.wjgnet.com/1007-9327/full/v27/i22/3130.htm.

[72] Lerner A, Patricia J, Matthias T. Nutrients, bugs and us: the short-chain fatty acids story in celiac disease [cited 2021 Nov 29] Int J Celiac Dis October 11, 2016;4(3):92–4. Available from: http://pubs.sciepub.com/ijcd/4/3/12/index.html.

[73] Eroğlu İ, Eroğlu BÇ, Güven GS. Altered tryptophan absorption and metabolism could underlie long-term symptoms in survivors of coronavirus disease 2019 (COVID-19) [cited 2021 Nov 29] Nutrition October 2021;90:111308. Available from: https://linkinghub.elsevier.com/retrieve/pii/S0899900721001702.

[74] Mercola J, Grant WB, Wagner CL. Evidence regarding vitamin D and risk of COVID-19 and its severity [cited 2021 Nov 29] Nutrients October 31, 2020;12(11):3361. Available from: https://www.mdpi.com/2072-6643/12/11/3361.

[75] Jardou M, Lawson R. Supportive therapy during COVID-19: the proposed mechanism of short-chain fatty acids to prevent cytokine storm and multi-organ failure [cited 2021 Nov 29] Med Hypotheses September 2021;154:110661. Available from: https://linkinghub.elsevier.com/retrieve/pii/S0306987721001808.

[76] Patil P, Bhandary SK, Haridas V, Sarth Kumar E, et al. Is butyrate a natural alternative to dexamethasone in the management of CoVID-19? [cited 2021 Nov 29] F1000Research April 6, 2021;10:273. Available from: https://f1000research.com/articles/10-273/v1.

[77] Ghosh S, Dellibovi-Ragheb TA, Kerviel A, Pak E, Qiu Q, Fisher M, et al. β-Coronaviruses use lysosomes for egress instead of the biosynthetic secretory pathway [cited 2021 Nov 29] Cell December 2020;183(6):1520–35. e14, https://linkinghub.elsevier.com/retrieve/pii/S009286742031446X.

[78] Eymieux S, Uzbekov R, Rouillé Y, Blanchard E, Hourioux C, Dubuisson J, et al. Secretory vesicles are the principal means of SARS-CoV-2 egress [cited 2021 Nov 29] Cells August 10, 2021;10(8):2047. Available from: https://www.mdpi.com/2073-4409/10/8/2047.

[79] Yelin D, Wirtheim E, Vetter P, Kalil AC, Bruchfeld J, Runold M, et al. Long-term consequences of COVID-19: research needs [cited 2021 Nov 29] Lancet Infect Dis October 2020;20(10):1115–7. Available from: https://linkinghub.elsevier.com/retrieve/pii/S1473309920307015.

[80] Blackett JW, Wainberg M, Elkind MSV, Freedberg DE. Potential long COVID-19 gastrointestinal symptoms 6 months after coronavirus infection are associated with mental health symptoms [cited 2021 Nov 29]; Available from: Gastroenterology October 2021. https://linkinghub.elsevier.com/retrieve/pii/S0016508521037124.

[81] Dvornikova KA, Bystrova EY, Churilov LP, Lerner A. Pathogenesis of the inflammatory bowel disease in context of SARS-COV-2 infection [cited 2021 Nov 29] Mol Biol Rep July 22, 2021;48(7):5745–58. Available from: https://link.springer.com/10.1007/s11033-021-06565-w.

[82] Danese S, Cecconi M, Spinelli A. Management of IBD during the COVID-19 outbreak: resetting clinical priorities [cited 2021 Nov 29] Nat Rev Gastroenterol Hepatol May 15, 2020;17(5):253–5. Available from: http://www.nature.com/articles/s41575-020-0294-8.

[83] Nowak JK, Lindstrøm JC, Kalla R, Ricanek P, Halfvarson J, Satsangi J. Age, inflammation, and disease location are critical determinants of intestinal expression of SARS-CoV-2 receptor ACE2 and TMPRSS2 in inflammatory bowel disease [cited 2021 Nov 29] Gastroenterology September 2020;159(3):1151–4. e2, https://linkinghub.elsevier.com/retrieve/pii/S0016508520306533.

[84] Burgueño JF, Reich A, Hazime H, Quintero MA, Fernandez I, Fritsch J, et al. Expression of SARS-CoV-2 entry molecules ACE2 and TMPRSS2 in the gut of patients with IBD [cited 2021 Nov 29] Inflamm Bowel Dis May 12, 2020;26(6):797–808. Available from: https://academic.oup.com/ibdjournal/article/26/6/797/5825063.

[85] Gilissen LPL, Heinen SGH, Rijpma-Jacobs L, Schoon E, Schreuder R-M, Wensing A-M, et al. Neither inflammatory bowel disease nor immunosuppressants are associated with an increased risk of severe COVID-19: an observational Dutch cohort study. Clin Exp Med September 20, 2021 [cited 2021 Nov 29]; Available from: https://link.springer.com/10.1007/s10238-021-00755-3.

[86] Ludvigsson JF, Axelrad J, Halfvarson J, Khalili H, Larsson E, Lochhead P, et al. Inflammatory bowel disease and risk of severe COVID-19: a nationwide population-based cohort study in Sweden [cited 2021 Nov 29] United Eur Gastroenterol J March 11, 2021;9(2):177–92. Available from: https://onlinelibrary.wiley.com/doi/10.1002/ueg2.12049.

[87] Creemers RH, Rezazadeh Ardabili A, Jonkers DM, Leers MPG, Romberg-Camps MJ, Pierik MJ, et al. Severe COVID-19 in inflammatory bowel disease patients in a population-based setting. In: Pittet V, editor. PLoS One; October 5, 2021 [cited 2021 Nov 29];16(10):e0258271. Available from: https://dx.plos.org/10.1371/journal.pone.0258271.

[88] Brenner EJ, Ungaro RC, Gearry RB, Kaplan GG, Kissous-Hunt M, Lewis JD, et al. Corticosteroids, but not TNF antagonists, are associated with adverse COVID-19 outcomes in patients with inflammatory bowel diseases: results from an international registry [cited 2021 Nov 29] Gastroenterology August 2020;159(2):481–91. e3, https://linkinghub.elsevier.com/retrieve/pii/S0016508520306557.

[89] Ricciuto A, Lamb CA, Benchimol EI, Walker GJ, Kennedy NA, Kuenzig ME, et al. Inflammatory bowel disease clinical activity is associated with COVID-19 severity especially in younger patients. J Crohn's Colitis September 27, 2021 [cited 2021 Nov 29]; Available from: https://academic.oup.com/ecco-jcc/advance-article/doi/10.1093/ecco-jcc/jjab172/6376474.

[90] Chebli JMF, Queiroz NSF, Damião AOMC, Chebli LA, Costa MH de M, Parra RS. How to manage inflammatory bowel disease during the COVID-19 pandemic: a guide for the practicing clinician [cited 2021 Nov 29] World J Gastroenterol March 21, 2021;27(11):1022–42. Available from: https://www.wjgnet.com/1007-9327/full/v27/i11/1022.htm.

[91] Ungaro RC, Brenner EJ, Agrawal M, Zhang X, Kappelman MD, Colombel J-F. Impact of medications on COVID-19 outcomes in inflammatory bowel disease: analysis of more than 6000 patients from an international registry. Gastroenterology September 2021 [cited 2021 Nov 29]; Available from: https://linkinghub.elsevier.com/retrieve/pii/S0016508521034909.

[92] lerner aaron. Are my patients with celiac disease at higher risk of COVID-19 virus [cited 2021 Nov 29] Int J Celiac Dis February 18, 2020;8(1):35–8. Available from: https://www.academia.edu/43329691/Are_My_Patients_with_Celiac_Disease_at_Higher_Risk_of_COVID_19_Virus.

[93] Levy J, Bernstein L, Silber N. Celiac disease: an immune dysregulation syndrome. Curr Probl Pediatr Adolesc Health Care December 1, 2014;44(11):324–7.

[94] Lerner A, Neidhöfer S, Matthias T. The gut-gut axis: cohabitation of celiac, Crohn's disease and IgA deficiency. Int J Celiac Dis 2016;4(2):68–70.

[95] Uzzan M, Ko HM, Mehandru S, Cunningham-Rundles C. Gastrointestinal disorders associated with common variable immune deficiency (CVID) and chronic granulomatous disease (CGD) [cited 2021 Nov 29] Curr Gastroenterol Rep April 1, 2016;18(4). Available from: https://pubmed.ncbi.nlm.nih.gov/26951230/.

[96] Woodward J. Improving outcomes of refractory celiac disease - current and emerging treatment strategies [cited 2021 Nov 29] Clin Exp Gastroenterol August 3, 2016;9:225–36. Available from: https://pubmed.ncbi.nlm.nih.gov/27536154/.

[97] Livshits OE, Shauol R, Reifen R, Matthias T, Lerner A. Can celiac disease present along with childhood obesity? [cited 2022 Feb 2] Int J Celiac Dis March 2, 2017;5(1):19–23. Available from: http://pubs.sciepub.com/ijcd/5/1/7/index.html.

[98] Yaqoob Z, Al-Kindi SG, Zein J. Association between celiac disease and asthma. Dig Dis Sci December 1, 2016;61(12):3636–7.

[99] Pichardo C, Muinos W, Brathwaite C, Hernandez E. Pulmonary hemosiderosis associated with celiac disease: lane Hamilton syndrome. J Pediatr Gastroenterol Nutr May 1, 2017;64(5):e133.

[100] Lerner A. Balanced polymorphism: a survival advantage in celiac disease [cited 2022 Feb 2] Med Hypotheses July 2011;77(1):1–2. Available from: https://pubmed.ncbi.nlm.nih.gov/21601992/.

[101] Lerner A. The last two millennias echo-catastrophes are the driving forces for the potential genetic advantage mechanisms in celiac disease [cited 2021 Nov 29] Med Hypotheses November 2011;77(5):773–6. Available from: https://pubmed.ncbi.nlm.nih.gov/21856087/.

[102] Gokden Y, Hot S, Adas M, Ogutmen Koc D, Atak S, Hot AB. Celiac disease and COVID-19 pandemic: should we worry? Acta Gastroenterol Belg October 1, 2020;83(4):517–25.

[103] Zhen J, Stefanolo JP, Temprano M, Tedesco S, Seiler C, Caminero AF, et al. The risk of contracting COVID-19 is not increased in patients with celiac disease [cited 2021 Nov 29] Clin Gastroenterol Hepatol February 2021;19(2):391–3. Available from: https://linkinghub.elsevier.com/retrieve/pii/S1542356520313987.

[104] Lionetti E, Fabbrizi A, Catassi C. Prevalence of COVID-19 in Italian children with celiac disease: a cross-sectional study [cited 2021 Nov 29] Clin Gastroenterol Hepatol May 2021;19(5):1075. Available from: https://linkinghub.elsevier.com/retrieve/pii/S1542356520316256.

[105] Falcomer AL, Farage P, Pratesi CB, Pratesi R, Gandolfi L, Nakano EY, et al. Health-related quality of life and experiences of Brazilian celiac individuals over the course of the sars-cov-2 pandemic [cited 2021 Nov 29] Nutrients [Internet] May 9, 2021;13(5):1582. Available from: https://www.mdpi.com/2072-6643/13/5/1582.

[106] Lerner A, Matthias T. Increased knowledge and awareness of celiac disease will benefit the elderly. Int J Celiac Dis 2015;3(3):112–4.

[107] Lerner A, Matthias T. Extra intestinal manifestations of CD: common pathways in the gut- remote organs' axes [cited 2021 Nov 29] Int J Celiac Dis 2017;5(1):24–7.

[108] Lerner A, Matthias T, Wusterhausen P. Autoimmunity in celiac disease: extra-intestinal manifestations [cited 2021 Feb 16] Autoimmun Rev March 1, 2019;18(3):241–6. Available from: https://pubmed.ncbi.nlm.nih.gov/30639642/.

[109] Samasca G, Ajay R, Sur D, Aldea C, Sur L, Floca E, et al. Polyautoimmunity-the missing ingredient [cited 2022 Feb 3] Autoimmun Rev August 1, 2018;17(8):840–1. Available from: https://pubmed.ncbi.nlm.nih.gov/29885545/.

[110] Siniscalchi M, Zingone F, Savarino EV, D'Odorico A, Ciacci C. COVID-19 pandemic perception in adults with celiac disease: an impulse to implement the use of telemedicine [cited 2021 Nov 29] Dig Liver Dis October 2020;52(10):1071–5. Available from: https://linkinghub.elsevier.com/retrieve/pii/S1590865820302206.

[111] Muhammad H, Reeves S, Ishaq S, Jeanes Y. Experiences of outpatient clinics and opinions of telehealth by caucasian and south asian patients' with celiac disease [cited 2021 Nov 29] J Patient Exp January 1, 2021;(8). 237437352110180, http://journals.sagepub.com/doi/10.1177/23743735211018083.

[112] Monzani A, Lionetti E, Felici E, Fransos L, Azzolina D, Rabbone I, et al. Adherence to the gluten-free diet during the lockdown for COVID-19 pandemic: a web-based survey of Italian subjects with celiac disease [cited 2021 Nov 29] Nutrients November 12, 2020;12(11):3467. Available from: https://www.mdpi.com/2072-6643/12/11/3467.

[113] Zhen J, Stefanolo JP, de la Paz Temprano M, Seiler CL, Caminero A, de-Madaria E, et al. Risk perception and knowledge of COVID-19 in patients with celiac disease. World J Gastroenterol March 28, 2021;27(12):1213–25.

[114] Elli L, Barisani D, Vaira V, Bardella MT, Topa M, Vecchi M, et al. How to manage celiac disease and gluten-free diet during the COVID-19 era: proposals from a tertiary referral center in a high-incidence scenario [cited 2021 Nov 29] BMC Gastroenterol December 19, 2020;20(1):387. Available from: https://bmcgastroenterol.biomedcentral.com/articles/10.1186/s12876-020-01524-4.

[115] Galli G, Esposito G, Dilaghi E, Annibale B, Lahner E, Conti L. Successful coping with SARS-CoV-2 infection of adult celiac patients assessed by telemedicine [cited 2021 Nov 29] Dig Liver Dis April 2021;53(4):391–3. Available from: https://linkinghub.elsevier.com/retrieve/pii/S159086582100013X.

[116] Dipasquale V, Passanisi S, Cucinotta U, Cascio A, Romano C. Implications of SARS-COV-2 infection in the diagnosis and management of the pediatric gastrointestinal disease [cited 2021 Nov 29] Ital J Pediatr December 24, 2021;47(1):71. Available from: https://ijponline.biomedcentral.com/articles/10.1186/s13052-021-01020-9.

[117] Elli L, Facciotti F, Lombardo V, Scricciolo A, Sanders DS, Vaira V, et al. Anti-SARS-CoV-2 immunoglobulin profile in patients with celiac disease living in a high incidence area. Dig Liver Dis September 2021 [cited 2021 Nov 29]; Available from: https://linkinghub.elsevier.com/retrieve/pii/S1590865821007696.

[118] Costantino A, Topa M, Roncoroni L, Doneda L, Lombardo V, Stocco D, et al. COVID-19 vaccine: a survey of hesitancy in patients with celiac disease [cited 2021 Nov 29] Vaccines May 16, 2021;9(5):511. Available from: https://www.mdpi.com/2076-393X/9/5/511.

[119] Lerner A. The COVID-19 vaccination debate: CoV-2 in celiac disease: a pathogen or just along for the ride? [cited 2021 Nov 29] Int J Celiac Dis January 18, 2021;9(1):6–9. Available from: http://pubs.sciepub.com/ijcd/9/1/8.

[120] Halpert G, Shoenfeld Y. SARS-CoV-2, the autoimmune virus. Autoimmun Rev December 1, 2020;19(12):102695.

[121] Vojdani A, Kharrazian D. Potential antigenic cross-reactivity between SARS-CoV-2 and human tissue with a possible link to an increase in autoimmune diseases [cited 2021 Nov 29] Clin Immunol August 1, 2020;217. Available from: https://pubmed.ncbi.nlm.nih.gov/32461193/.

[122] Sacchi MC, Tamiazzo S, Stobbione P, Agatea L, De Gaspari P, Stecca A, et al. SARS-CoV-2 infection as a trigger of autoimmune response [cited 2021 Nov 29] Clin Transl Sci May 21, 2021;14(3):898–907. Available from: https://onlinelibrary.wiley.com/doi/10.1111/cts.12953.

[123] Ehrenfeld M, Tincani A, Andreoli L, Cattalini M, Greenbaum A, Kanduc D, et al. Covid-19 and autoimmunity [cited 2021 Nov 29] Autoimmun Rev 2020;19(8). Available from: https://pubmed.ncbi.nlm.nih.gov/32535093/.

[124] Kanduc D, Shoenfeld Y. Molecular mimicry between SARS-CoV-2 spike glycoprotein and mammalian proteomes: implications for the vaccine [cited 2021 Nov 29] Immunol Res October 1, 2020;68(5):310–3. Available from: https://pubmed.ncbi.nlm.nih.gov/32946016/.

[125] Samasca G, Lerner A. Celiac disease in the COVID-19 pandemic [cited 2021 Nov 29] J Transl Autoimmun 2021;4:100120. Available from: https://linkinghub.elsevier.com/retrieve/pii/S258990902100040X.

[126] Lerner A, Ramesh A, Matthias T. The revival of the battle between David and Goliath in the enteric viruses and microbiota struggle: potential implication for celiac disease [cited 2021 Nov 29] Microorganisms June 14, 2019;7(6):173. Available from: https://www.mdpi.com/2076-2607/7/6/173.

[127] Strisciuglio C, Martinelli M, Lu P, Bar Lev MR, Beinvogl B, Benninga MA, et al. Overall impact of coronavirus disease 2019 outbreak in children with functional abdominal pain disorders: results from the first pandemic phase [cited 2021 Nov 29] J Pediatr Gastroenterol Nutr December 2021;73(6):689–94. Available from: https://journals.lww.com/10.1097/MPG.0000000000003286.

CHAPTER

22

Multisystem inflammatory syndrome in children

Nina Emeršič[1] *and Tadej Avčin*[1,2]

[1]Department of Allergology, Rheumatology and Clinical Immunology, University Children's Hospital, University Medical Center Ljubljana, Ljubljana, Slovenia; [2]Faculty of Medicine, University of Ljubljana, Ljubljana, Slovenia

Introduction

The infection with severe acute respiratory syndrome coronavirus 2 (SARS-CoV-2) is usually mild or even asymptomatic in pediatric population. In rare cases, children may be severely affected, and the SARS-CoV-2 infection is now recognized as an infection with a significant risk for serious complications [1]. In late April 2020, the first reports from Italy and the United Kingdom described a new clinical syndrome with severe heart disease and shock in children after exposure to SARS-CoV-2 virus, which was similar to incomplete Kawasaki disease (KD) and toxic shock syndrome [2]. The condition has been termed multisystem inflammatory syndrome in children (MIS-C), which is also known as pediatric inflammatory multisystem syndrome (PIMS).

Epidemiology

MIS-C is a rare life-threatening hyperinflammatory complication of usually mild or even asymptomatic COVID-19, that occurs in less than 1% of patients with SARS-CoV-2 infection. The incidence in the USA was estimated at 0.2 to 11.4 cases per 100,000 persons younger than 21 years [1,3,4]. In a prospective nationwide cohort study in Denmark the estimated incidence of MIS-C among SARS-CoV-2-infected children and adolescents during the first year of the pandemic was two per 100,000 individuals under 18 years of age, which is one in 4100 infected children [5]. An Italian study reported an incidence of MIS-C at 10.3/100,000 persons under 19 years of age [6]. The incidence is mostly related to the movement of the epidemic, with the peak of cases occurring 2–4 weeks after the peak in the number of cases of laboratory-confirmed SARS-CoV-2 infections.

Autoimmunity, COVID-19, Post-COVID19 syndrome and COVID-19 vaccination
https://doi.org/10.1016/B978-0-443-18566-3.00015-3

The syndrome most commonly affects children aged 8–11 years but occurs in the entire pediatric population including infants and adolescents [2,3,7–9]. In the adult population, the disease is rare and has been termed the multisystem inflammatory syndrome in adults (MIS-A). The male:female ratio is close to 1:1 for patients aged 0–4 years and progressively increases for subsequent age categories to 2:1 for patients aged 18–20 years [1]. It usually affects previously completely healthy children. It is more prevalent in patients of African and Hispanic descent, less common in Caucasians, and very rare in Asians [2,3,8,9].

Pathophysiology

Given the delay of a few weeks after an acute infection, it is hypothesized that MIS-C is a postinfectious immunologically mediated hyperinflammatory syndrome. It is clearly distinguished from the early, infectious phase of SARS-CoV-2 virus infection (COVID-19) [10]. Patients with MIS-C usually have a negative nasopharyngeal swab for the presence of SARS-CoV-2 virus.

The pathophysiological mechanism of disease is unclear. It seems to be a complex intertwining of immune dysregulation of natural and acquired immunity. The acute phase is characterized by an activated innate immune system with highly activated neutrophils and macrophages [11], increased levels of cytokines, including interleukin (IL)-1β and IL-6, tumor necrosis factor-α, interferon-γ (IFN-γ) and raised CRP. The two proposed immunopathogenic drivers of MIS-C are either altered IFN responses or antibody-dependent enhancement of disease (ADE), however, these may differ between patients. The first hypothesis for the marked cytokine storm experienced by children with MIS-C derives from the well-known ability of coronaviruses to block type I and type III interferon responses, with the potential outcome of delayed cytokine storm in patients with immune responses that cannot control viral replication well due to genetic factors or in those with initially high SARS-CoV-2 viral load [12]. On the other hand, ADE is a phenomenon by which the complex consisting of the antigen and nonneutralizing virus-specific antibodies enhance virus entry. The second might be supported by several reports showing that most of the individuals presenting with MIS-C have significant levels of SARS-CoV-2 antibodies in their sera, but they are negative for SARS-CoV-2 by real-time polymerase chain reaction (RT-PCR) testing [13].

The reason why only some SARS-CoV-2 infected children develop MIS-C, but most do not, suggest a possible role of host genetic susceptibility [14]. The relatively rare occurrence of life-threatening acute MIS-C in healthy children indeed suggests the presence of rare, single-gene mutations or noncoding variation. Patients with MIS-C usually have T and B cell lymphopenia, which resolves with recovery [15].

Diagnostic approach

American College of Rheumatology (ACR) issued clinical guidance on the management and treatment of children with suspected MIS-C [16]. Any child with suspected MIS-C should have a thorough clinical examination with special attention to monitoring basic life functions that may deteriorate rapidly. Clinical evaluation should include assessment of the involvement of various organ systems (heart, gastrointestinal tract, kidneys, liver), confirmation of SARS-CoV-2 infection or exposure, and exclusion of other causes.

The suggested initial laboratory tests are complete blood count with differential, inflammatory markers (C-reactive protein (CRP), erythrocyte sedimentation rate (ESR), ferritin, procalcitonin (PCT)), liver enzymes (aspartate aminotransferase (AST), alanine transaminase (ALT), lactate dehydrogenase (LDH)), electrolytes, urea, creatinine, urine analysis, troponin, N-terminal pro-B-type natriuretic peptide (NT-proBNP), D-dimer, coagulation tests. Investigations need to be repeated during the acute phase to monitor the dynamics of the results.

Other causes of fever, especially infections, must be excluded with blood and urine culture, stool tests for bacterial and viral pathogens of intestinal infections, throat swabs for Streptococcus, nasopharyngeal swabs for respiratory viruses and quantitative PCR test for *Epstein–*Barr virus (EBV), *cytomegalovirus* (CMV), adenoviruses and enteroviruses as required.

The assessment of cardiac involvement in addition to the determination of laboratory indicators includes regular recording of 12-channel electrocardiogram (ECG) and echocardiogram. Additional investigations in patients with more severe cardiac involvement include a 24-hour ECG and *magnetic resonance imaging* (MRI) of the heart.

X-rays of the chest and abdominal and pleural ultrasound are performed to determine the involvement of other internal organ systems.

Clinical picture

MIS-C occurs 2–6 weeks after the acute infection with SARS-CoV-2. The disease starts with high fever and chills, which last for at least 3–5 days. Patients are usually admitted to hospital approximately 4 days after the onset of symptoms [3]. Various organ systems may be affected, and the presenting symptoms may be varied. The most common manifestations are presented in Table 22.1 [1–3,7–9,17]. Among the leading symptoms are gastrointestinal problems, such as nausea, abdominal pain, vomiting and diarrhea. These can be so pronounced as to resemble acute appendicitis or bacterial intestinal infection. Patients may present also with muco-cutaneous symptoms (skin rash (Fig. 22.1), bilateral conjunctivitis (Fig. 22.2), swelling, cracking or redness of the lips, edema of the palms (Fig. 22.3) and soles of the feet, strawberry tongue). The rash can be varied, from maculopapular, reticular, purpuric to urticarial. Prominent cardiac involvement (myocarditis, cardiac dysfunction, or coronary artery dilatations) has been reported in a proportion of MIS-C patients in many studies [2,3,7,8,17,18]. The cardiac involvement can be asymptomatic, only occasionally, there is chest pain, but it is less pronounced than in non-MIS-C myocarditis. Heart disease can lead to rapidly progressing cardiogenic shock.

It has been observed that age may impact the clinical phenotype of MIS-C. Younger children are more likely to present with KD-like features, while older children are more likely to develop myocarditis and shock [3,9].

Respiratory symptoms may also occur. Dry cough is common in early stages, most likely due to pleural effusion. Rarely, breathing problems may occur in the later stages of shock or cardiogenic pulmonary edema. Non-specific pain in the neck and muscles occurs several times. Patients often complain of neurologic symptoms such as headache, meningismus

TABLE 22.1 Clinical manifestations.

	Frequency (%)
Fever	**100**
GIT symptoms (abdominal pain, nausea, vomiting, diarrhea)	60–100
Muco-cutaneous symptoms:	
- Skin rash - Bilateral conjunctivitis - Strawberry tongue, swelling, cracking or redness of the lips - Edema of the palms and soles of the feet–	45–75 30–80 25–75 10–15
Cardiac involvement (myocarditis, cardiac dysfunction, or coronary artery dilatations)	50–90
Serositis	25–60
Respiratory symptoms	20–60
Neurologic symptoms (headache, meningismus, lethargy, seizures, altered mental status)	30–55
Acute kidney failure	8–50
Pain in the neck and muscles	5–20
Hepatitis/hepatomegaly	5–20
Lymphadenopathy	5–15

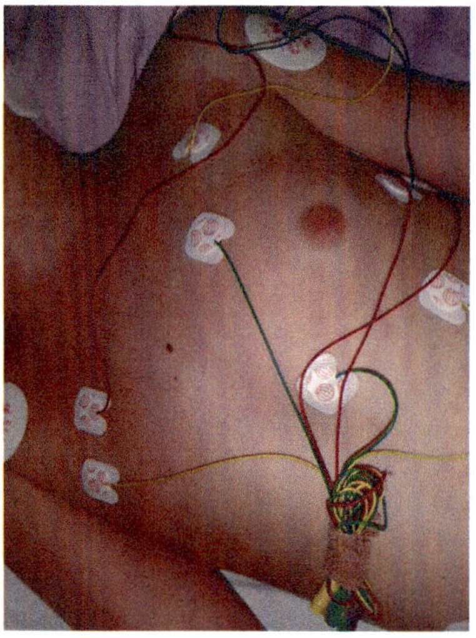

FIGURE 22.1 Maculopapular skin rash in a patient with MIS-C.

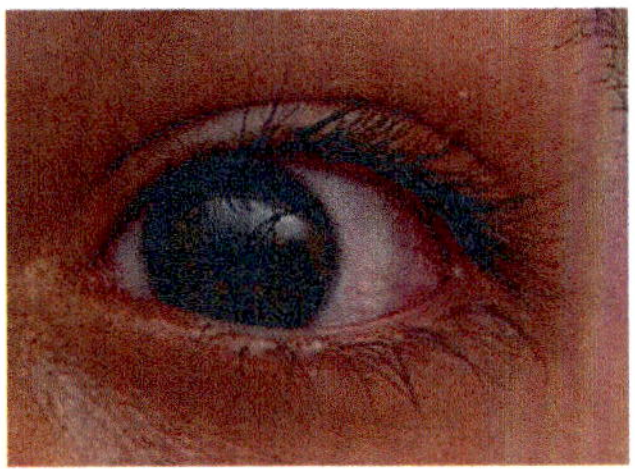

FIGURE 22.2 Conjunctivitis in a patient with MIS-C.

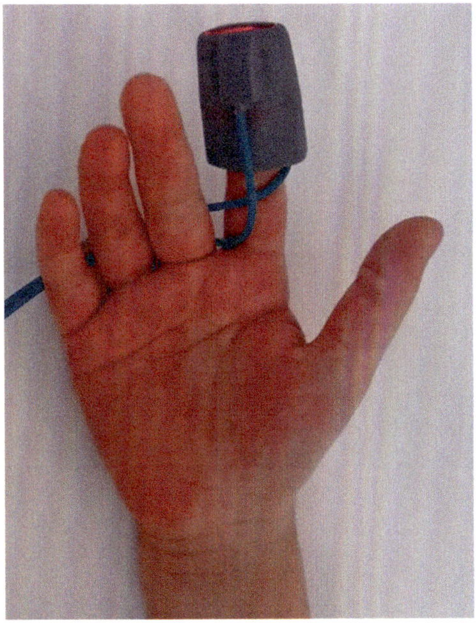

FIGURE 22.3 Palmar erythema with slight edema in a patient with MIS-C.

and lethargy. Seizures or altered mental status are also possible. Acute kidney failure may also develop.

Examination reveals fever, tachycardia and decreased blood pressure. In the first published cases, a state of shock was reported, which is still as high as 30%–75% in larger cohorts. Thrombosis also occurs in 7% of patients, and in 19% of patients over 12 years of age [19].

Laboratory results

All patients with MIS-C have significantly elevated levels of inflammatory markers, particularly CRP, but also ESR, PCT, ferritin, fibrinogen, IL-6. The value of inflammatory markers is related to the severity of the disease [8]. The complete blood cell count is characterized by a combination of lymphopenia, neutrophilia and thrombocytopenia. Thrombocytopenia can range from mild to moderate and usually progresses to thrombocytosis in the second week of illness. Mild anemia may also occur.

Elevated cardiac laboratory values (levels of troponin T and NT-proBNP) may help identify patients with cardiac sequelae [7,8], which are present in the vast majority of cases. Because there are few cardiac symptoms, cardiac involvement should be actively sought and sequential measurements of troponin T and NT-proBNP should be performed whenever MIS-C is suspected. Troponin increases with a lag of a few days relative to fever and an increase in CRP value. It is important to note that mild and transient elevations in NT-proBNP are nonspecific, as BNP is an acute-phase reactant, and can be elevated in inflammatory conditions without cardiac involvement [8].

Hyponatremia, hypoalbuminemia, increased liver transaminases and LDH levels have been observed in biochemical studies. Pancreatic enzyme levels may be elevated [20] and coagulation is also impaired, D-dimer values are very high. Urea and creatinine are elevated in the event of acute renal impairment.

Microbiology

Case definition for MIS-C requires evidence of recent infection with SARS-CoV-2. Due to the delay in the occurrence of MIS-C relative to the infection, the majority of patients are already negative for the presence of the virus itself in the nasopharyngeal space (RT-PCR testing). If there is no information on the primary acute infection with SARS-CoV-2, the infection needs to be demonstrated with serological testing for virus-specific antibodies [3,7,21]. If a nasopharyngeal swab and serology do not show SARS-CoV-2 virus infection, a clear exposure to the infection is required in the appropriate time window to make a diagnosis [22,23]. The use of serological testing may complicate with evolving COVID-19 pandemic, as seropositivity for SARS–CoV-2 IgG may not be any more indicative of a recent infection [16].

Radiologic examinations

If MIS-C is suspected, an echocardiography should be performed by an experienced pediatric cardiologist. Echocardiography may reveal myocardial edema, segmental contractility disorders and left ventricular dysfunction with reduced ejection fraction. Left ventricular global longitudinal strain (GLS), which measures the maximal shortening of myocardial longitudinal length during systole compared to the resting length in diastole, is typically lowered in patients with MIS-C. Less often dilatation or aneurysms of coronary vessels, mitral regurgitation or pericardial effusion is seen [24]. Nonspecific repolarization disorders are most often present on ECG recordings. In hospitalized patients, ECG should be obtained at a minimum of every 48 h [8,24]. If electrical conduction abnormalities are present, the patient should be placed on telemetry while in the hospital [16].

Ultrasound of the abdomen may show hepatosplenomegaly, ascites, pleural effusion, mesenterial lymphadenopathy, inflammation of the intestinal wall, especially the terminal ileum, and cholecystitis [20]. Parenchymal thickenings and pleural effusion are occasionally present on chest X-ray.

Diagnosis

The diagnosis of MIS-C is based on the case definition for MIS-C according to World Health Organization (WHO) and the Centers for Disease Control and Prevention (CDC). The case definitions overlap in most of the criteria and are shown in Table 22.2. CDC lists only cases that require hospitalization, while WHO does not have this criterion [22,23].

Differential diagnosis

MIS-C often overlaps with KD, a vasculitis affecting medium-sized arteries, while 25%–50% patients meet the criteria for both diseases [3,7–9,24]. Children with KD who develop KD shock syndrome (less than 10% of KD patients) with cardiovascular involvement are most similar to those with MIS-C. The incidence of KD is highest in Japan, where MIS-C is not so common. The main trigger of KD is probably infectious agents, although no unique specific microorganism has been identified yet. The most important features that distinguish MIS-C from KD are older age (most children with KD present with symptoms before the age of 5 years [7,8]), frequency of gastrointestinal and myocardial involvement, and the frequent need for intensive care. Neurologic symptoms are also more frequently encountered in the MIS-C population [16]. Changes in the coronary arteries occur in up to 20% of MIS-C patients and close to one-quarter of untreated KD patients develop coronary artery aneurysms (CAAs) [2,3,7–9,24]. The values of inflammatory indicators are higher in MIS-C, but platelet count is lower, as well as absolute lymphocyte count [7,8,25]. Inflammatory response in MIS-C shares several features with Kawasaki disease, but also differs from this condition in terms of T cell subsets, IL-17A, and biomarkers associated with arterial damage [10]. The treatment of both is similar in the initial phase [2,3,8,9,17].

In the severe acute form of COVID-19, the values of inflammatory indicators are slightly lower, with respiratory involvement in the foreground (pneumonia and/or ARDS). Injury to other organ systems is secondary. RT-PCR examination of the nasopharyngeal swab for SARS-CoV-2 is positive and antibody titer of SARS-CoV-2 is still low.

Many infections can occur with high fever, high values of inflammatory parameters and rash. Bacterial sepsis can quickly lead to a progressive state of shock, and in clinical practice, patients could first start empirical antibiotic treatment while awaiting the results of the microbiological investigations. Streptococcal and staphylococcal shock syndrome, in addition to fever, high inflammation and rash, can affect many other organ systems, including the gastrointestinal tract and eyes (conjunctivitis). Gastrointestinal infections, especially bacterial infections, are ruled out by microbiological examination of the feces. Intensive gastrointestinal symptoms may be similar to acute appendicitis.

TABLE 22.2 Case definition for MIS-C according to WHO and CDC.

CDC case definition	WHO case definition
All 4 criteria must be met:	All 6 criteria must be met:
1. Age <21 years	1. Age 0–19 years
2. Clinical presentation consistent with MIS-C, including all of the following:	2. Fever for ≥3 days
- Fever • Documented fever >38.0°C for ≥24 h or • Report of subjective fever lasting ≥24 h	
- Laboratory evidence of inflammation • including, but not limited to, **any** of the following: • Elevated CRP • Elevated ESR • Elevated fibrinogen • Elevated procalcitonin • Elevated D-dimer • Elevated ferritin • Elevated LDH • Elevated IL-6 level • Neutrophilia • Lymphocytopenia • Hypoalbuminemia - Multisystem involvement • **2 or more** organ systems involved: • Cardiovascular (e.g., shock, elevated troponin, elevated NT-proBNP, abnormal echocardiogram, arrhythmia) • Respiratory (e.g., pneumonia, ARDS, pulmonary embolism) • Renal (e.g., AKI, kidney failure) • Neurologic (e.g., seizure, stroke, aseptic meningitis) • Hematologic (e.g., coagulopathy) • Gastrointestinal (e.g., abdominal pain, vomiting, diarrhea, elevated liver enzymes, ileus, gastrointestinal bleeding) • Dermatologic (e.g., erythroderma, mucositis, other rash)	3. Clinical signs of multisystem involvement (**at least 2** of the following): • Rash, bilateral nonpurulent conjunctivitis, or mucocutaneous inflammation signs (oral, hands, or feet) • Hypotension or shock • Cardiac dysfunction, pericarditis, valvulitis, or coronary abnormalities (including echocardiographic findings or elevated troponin/NT-proBNP) • Evidence of coagulopathy (prolonged PT or PTT; elevated D-dimer) • Acute gastrointestinal symptoms (diarrhea, vomiting, or abdominal pain)
3. Severe illness requiring hospitalization 4. No alternative plausible diagnoses	4. Elevated markers of inflammation (e.g., ESR, CRP, or procalcitonin)
5. Recent or current SARS-CoV-2 infection or exposure	5. No other obvious microbial cause of inflammation, including bacterial sepsis and staphylococcal/streptococcal toxic shock syndromes
• **Any** of the following: • Positive SARS-CoV-2 RT-PCR	6. Evidence of SARS-CoV-2 infection

TABLE 22.2 Case definition for MIS-C according to WHO and CDC.—cont'd

CDC case definition	WHO case definition
• Positive serology • Positive antigen test • COVID-19 exposure within the 4 weeks prior to the onset of symptoms	• **Any** of the following: • Positive SARS-CoV-2 RT-PCR • Positive serology • Positive antigen test • Contact with an individual with COVID-19

AKI: acute kidney injury, ARDS: acute respiratory distress syndrome, CDC: Centers for Disease Control and Prevention, COVID-19: coronavirus disease 2019, CRP: C-reactive protein, ESR: erythrocyte sedimentation rate, IL-6: interleukin 6, LDH: lactate dehydrogenase, MIS-C: Multisystem inflammatory syndrome in children, MIS-C: multisystem inflammatory syndrome in children, NT-proBNP: N-terminal pro-B-type natriuretic peptide, PT: prothrombin time, PTT: partial prothrombin time, RT-PCR: real-time polymerase chain reaction, SARS-CoV-2: severe acute respiratory syndrome coronavirus 2, WHO: World Health Organization.

Viral infections must also be ruled out, as well as viral myocarditis if heart is affected. Primary EBV infection can occur with high fever, sore throat or neck, lymphadenopathy, rash and high inflammatory parameters, mild hepatitis and elevated lymphocyte counts. In acute COVID-19 patients with septic shock, viremia with CMV or EBV is common, but not the cause of the disease. EBV and CMV are also known triggers of hemphagocytic lymphohistiocytosis.

Hemphagocytic lymphohistiocytosis is characterized by a cytokine storm with high fever, high values of inflammatory indicators, cytopenia, hyperferritinemia, pathological values of liver tests, and multiorgan involvement. Genetic forms are most often expressed very early in childhood. Macrophage activation syndrome is a similar syndrome that occurs in patients with rheumatic diseases and may also be the first manifestation of the disease.

Systemic inflammation is also present in systemic connective tissue diseases, systemic vasculitis, systemic forms of juvenile idiopathic arthritis, and autoinflammatory disease.

Treatment

The approach to treatment depends on the child's clinical condition. If the patient is in a life-threatening condition, the first goal is to stabilize the patient. Immunomodulatory treatment, which is started as soon as possible after the diagnosis, is crucial to stop the inflammation. Early initiation of intravenous immunoglobulin (IVIG) and systemic glucocorticosteroid (GC) reduces admissions to intensive care unit (ICU) and length of hospitalization. In addition, patients require introduction of supportive symptomatic treatment depending on the involvement of organ systems. Management of patients with MIS-C includes also prevention of long-term sequelae, especially sequelae on the heart, such as CAAs, myocardial fibrosis/scarring and conduction abnormalities. A multidisciplinary approach is important.

Immunomodulatory treatment

First-line drugs are IVIG, systemic GC, or a combination [9,26].

Immune globulin (IVIG)

IVIG has been used for a long time in similar immune-mediated diseases such as KD and fulminant myocarditis. They have an antiinflammatory effect on monocytes/macrophages and consequently on the amount of circulating inflammatory molecules [24]. IVIG is given as soon as possible after the diagnosis at a dose of 2 g/kg body weight. To avoid overloading the heart, especially with left ventricular dysfunction, IVIG is usually divided into two separate doses and given at a slow infusion rate [16]. To avoid volume overload, diuretics may also be considered. Blood must be taken for serological tests before IVIG injection, as the results are not valid after application, nor is the measured ESR.

If the disease is refractory (persistent fevers, significant end-organ involvement despite initial therapy), a second dose of IVIG is not recommended (as opposed to KD). Instead, systemic GC is recommended.

Among children with MIS-C, treatment with IVIG and GC versus IVIG alone was associated with a more favorable fever course [26]. The combination therapy was also associated with less severe acute complications, including acute left ventricular dysfunction and hemodynamic support requirement.

Systemic glucocorticoids (GC)

Systemic GC is added to patients in shock from the onset, if the disease threatens a vital organ, or if the patient looks ill and has severely elevated troponin, NT-proBNP, or tachycardia. In refractory patients who have already received GC at low/moderate doses, treatment is escalated to high-dose pulse therapy [16].

GC are initially prescribed at high dose (methylprednisolone in total doses of 1–2 mg/kg body weight (BW) divided into three daily doses, intravenous or orally). In severely ill or refractory patients, intravenous pulse therapy with methylprednisolone at a dose of 10–30 mg/kg BW is used for 3–5 days [16]. Doses are gradually tapered and finally discontinued within about 6 weeks. In addition to GC treatment, patients require close monitoring and introduction of supportive therapy with proton pump inhibitors, calcium and vitamin D supplementation.

A French observational study compared the outcome of the disease in more than 100 children with MIS-C after treatment with IVIG alone and combination therapy with IVIG and GC. The combination of drugs was associated with greater treatment success, less hemodynamic support, and shorter time in the intensive care unit [26]. Licciardi et al. developed a treatment protocol that avoids IVIG as first-line therapy. They retrospectively analyzed a cohort of 31 patients and reported that timely start of GC therapy and careful fluid management might improve the outcomes of MIS-C patients [27].

Biologics—anakinra

High-dose anakinra is used to treat MIS-C patients with refractory disease, who do not respond to IVIG and GC treatment, or as a steroid-sparing agent. It is given at a dose of 4 mg/kg BW daily and can be even increased in selected cases [16]. Anakinra is tapered in 2 weeks [27].

There are various reports of individual cases of treatment with other biologics, such as tocilizumab, infliximab, and canakinumab, but there is insufficient evidence for their routine use.

Anticoagulant and antiplatelet therapy

Disorders of blood clotting and platelet count are common in patients with MIS-C. The risk of thrombosis in the natural course of the disease among patients ages 13–20 years is estimated at 7% [19]. In KD, the risk of thrombosis in affected coronaries is lower with acetylsalicylic acid (ASA).

Antiplatelet therapy with ASA at a dose of 3–5 mg/kg BW is administered daily to all MIS-C patients who are without active bleeding or significant bleeding risk for at least 4–6 weeks [16,28]. If patients meet the criteria for KD or have affected coronary arteries, the guidelines for KD treatment should be followed including a high dose of ASA.

In MIS-C, there are many factors that may contribute to the procoagulant state [29]. These are widespread endothelial injury, increased platelet–vessel wall interaction, and activation of coagulation. The risk of thromboembolic events in MIS-C may further be increased by the systemic inflammatory disease itself, immobility, and central catheterization. According to the ACR recommendations, anticoagulation therapy is advised only in patients with major coronary aneurysms and should be considered in patients with more than mild LV dysfunction [16]. ISTH recommendations and some other centers advice prophylactic anticoagulant therapy with enoxaparin in all patients with clinical risk factors for venous thromboembolism or markedly elevated plasma D-dimer levels in the absence of contraindications for the treatment [30,31]. Prophylactic anticoagulation therapy with LMWH is used and the target antifactor Xa level is 0.2–0.3 IU/mL. If D-dimer is extremely elevated or is rising, prophylactic anticoagulation therapy should be intensified at a target antifactor Xa level of 0.4–0.5 IU/mL. In the published cohorts, approximately 60% of patients received anticoagulant treatment with enoxaparin [19].

Treatment targeting the affected organ system

The treatment is highly multidisciplinary.

With heart disease, patients often receive angiotensin-converting enzyme (ACE) inhibitors, beta-blockers, and diuretics. They often need fluid and ionotropic support. Physical activity is not recommended 6 months after suffering from MIS-C with involvement of the heart.

Antibiotic treatment has no place in the treatment of MIS-C, but it is often introduced at the onset of the disease until the results of microbiological tests are received, and the diagnosis is confirmed.

Disease outcome

The disease course is characteristically monophasic. Most patients exhibit rapid clinical improvement with therapy including resolution of left ventricular systolic dysfunction and other symptoms, concomitantly with a decline in the inflammatory markers. More than half of the patients in the larger published cohorts required intensive care [3]. Mortality is about 1% [1,5,9]. Patients who survive the acute phase and are treated promptly, have a good prognosis of disease outcome. Children are usually hospitalized for a median of 8 days. After the acute phase, no severe long-term damage to the organ systems is seen, and cardiac function is usually normalized [9], although electrical conduction abnormalities may develop.

Reinfection and Mis-C

So far, we do not know, whether MIS-C recurs after reinfection with SARS-CoV-2. There is only one published case report of reinfection with SARS-CoV-2 13 months after the diagnosis of MIS-C. There was no recurrence of MIS-C within 2 months after reinfection in this patient [32]. It seems that, with increasingly high numbers of infected and reinfected children with SARS-CoV-2 and no reports of recurrence of MIS-C, that recurrence is not very likely.

Vaccinations and Mis-C

COVID-19 vaccines are well-tolerated and safe in adults and children after the age of 5 [33]. Nevertheless, case reports have been published on the occurrence of MIS-C following SARS-CoV-2 vaccination. An 18-year-old and a 12-year-old boy developed MIS-C 10 and 5 weeks after second vaccination with Pfizer/BioNTech and Moderna vaccine, respectively. Anti-N antibodies were not determined [34,35]. There are also two reports of a 12 and 17 year old boy who were diagnosed with MIS-C 27 and 5 days after receiving the first and second dose of Pfizer/BioNTech vaccine, respectively. Both had negative anti-N antibodies and high levels of anti-S antibodies against SARS-CoV-2, indicating a vaccine-induced rather than a SARS-CoV-2 infection-induced antibody response [36,37].

On the other side, there is growing evidence demonstrating that vaccination against SARS-CoV-2 is protective against developing MIS-C. Recently, Levy et al. estimated the risk of MIS-C among adolescents by COVID-19 vaccination status [21]. They observed 107 patients with MIS-C. Seven patients had received a single dose of COVID-19 mRNA vaccine and all others were unvaccinated against SARS-CoV-2. Their results suggest that COVID-19 mRNA vaccination was associated with a lower incidence of MIS-C. Yet it is important to be alert on possible myocarditis occurring in adolescents after COVID-19 mRNA vaccine.

Similarly, the report from Zambrano et al. evaluated the effectiveness of two doses of Pfizer/BioNTech vaccine against MIS-C in adolescents aged 12–18 years, which was estimated to 91% (Zambrano et al. no date). 97 of 102 hospitalized children with MIS-C were unvaccinated and 39% of unvaccinated MIS-C patients required respiratory or cardiovascular life support, while none of the fully vaccinated patients did.

The association between mRNA vaccination and MIS-C in younger children has not yet been evaluated as vaccines for this age group have been approved only recently.

Conclusion

MIS-C is a rare but potentially life-threatening complication of childhood SARS-CoV-2 infection that occurs 2–6 weeks after primary infection. It is an aggressive systemic inflammatory response that can attack many organs. It starts with high, unremitting fever, which is most often accompanied by gastrointestinal symptoms, skin and mucous membrane manifestations, and headache. In most cases, the heart is affected. Antiinflammatory treatment suppresses inflammation and achieves a favorable treatment outcome.

References

[1] Belay ED, Abrams J, Oster ME, et al. Trends in geographic and temporal distribution of US children with multisystem inflammatory syndrome during the COVID-19 pandemic. JAMA Pediatr 2021;175(8):837–45. https://doi.org/10.1001/jamapediatrics.2021.0630.

[2] Riphagen S, Gomez X, Gonzalez-Martinez C, Wilkinson N, Theocharis P. Hyperinflammatory shock in children during COVID-19 pandemic. Lancet 2020;395(10237):1607–8. https://doi.org/10.1016/S0140-6736(20)31094-1.

[3] Dufort EM, Koumans EH, Chow EJ, et al. Multisystem inflammatory syndrome in children in New York state. N Engl J Med 2020;383(4):347–58. https://doi.org/10.1056/nejmoa2021756.

[4] Payne AB, Gilani Z, Godfred-Cato S, et al. Incidence of multisystem inflammatory syndrome in children among US persons infected with SARS-CoV-2. JAMA Netw Open 2021;4(6). https://doi.org/10.1001/jamanetworkopen.2021.16420.

[5] Holm M, Hartling UB, Schmidt LS, et al. Multisystem inflammatory syndrome in children occurred in one of four thousand children with severe acute respiratory syndrome coronavirus 2. Acta Paediatr Int J Paediatr 2021;110(9):2581–3. https://doi.org/10.1111/apa.15985.

[6] Castagnola E, Mariani M, Sticchi C, et al. Incidence rate of MIS-C in paediatrics: a good reason to vaccinate children against SARS-CoV-2. Acta Paediatr Int J Paediatr 2022;111(1):123–4. https://doi.org/10.1111/apa.16081.

[7] Verdoni L, et al. An outbreak of severe kawasaki-like disease at the Italian epicentre of the SARS-CoV-2 epidemic: an observational cohort study. Pediatrics 2021;148(Suppl. 3). https://doi.org/10.1542/peds.2021-053843ddddd. S74-S74.

[8] Whittaker E, Bamford A, Kenny J, et al. Clinical characteristics of 58 children with a pediatric inflammatory multisystem syndrome temporally associated with SARS-CoV-2 group information: the PIMS-TS study group and EUCLIDS and PERFORM consortia members are listed in supplement 1. JAMA 2020;324(3):259–69. https://doi.org/10.1001/jama.2020.10369.

[9] Feldstein LR, Tenforde MW, Friedman KG, et al. Characteristics and outcomes of US children and adolescents with multisystem inflammatory syndrome in children (MIS-C) compared with severe acute COVID-19. JAMA J Am Med Assoc 2021;325(11):1074–87. https://doi.org/10.1001/jama.2021.2091.

[10] Consiglio CR, Cotugno N, Sardh F, et al. The immunology of multisystem inflammatory syndrome in children with COVID-19. medRxiv 2020;(January. https://doi.org/10.1101/2020.07.08.20148353.

[11] Syrimi E, Fennell E, Richter A, et al. The immune landscape of SARS-CoV-2-associated Multisystem Inflammatory Syndrome in Children (MIS-C) from acute disease to recovery. iScience 2021;24(11):103215. https://doi.org/10.1016/j.isci.2021.103215.

[12] Rowley AH. Understanding SARS-CoV-2-related multisystem inflammatory syndrome in children. Nat Rev Immunol 2020;20(8):453–4. https://doi.org/10.1038/s41577-020-0367-5.

[13] Rothan HA, et al. The potential threat of multisystem inflammatory syndrome in children during the COVID-19 pandemic. Pediatr Allergy Immunol 2021;32(1):17–22. https://doi.org/10.1111/pai.13361.

[14] Zhang SY, Zhang Q, Casanova JL, et al. Severe COVID-19 in the young and healthy: monogenic inborn errors of immunity? Nat Rev Immunol 2020;20(8):455–6. https://doi.org/10.1038/s41577-020-0373-7.

[15] Carter MJ, Fish M, Jennings A, et al. Peripheral immunophenotypes in children with multisystem inflammatory syndrome associated with SARS-CoV-2 infection. Nat Med 2020;26:1701–7. https://doi.org/10.1038/s41591-020-1054-6.

[16] Henderson LA, Canna SW, Friedman KG, et al. American College of Rheumatology clinical guidance for multisystem inflammatory syndrome in children associated with SARS–CoV-2 and hyperinflammation in pediatric COVID-19: version 2. Arthritis Rheumatol 2021;73(4):e13–29. https://doi.org/10.1002/art.41616.

[17] Capone CA, Subramony A, Sweberg T, et al. Characteristics, cardiac involvement, and outcomes of multisystem inflammatory syndrome of childhood associated with severe acute respiratory syndrome coronavirus 2 infection. J Pediatr 2020;224:141–5. https://doi.org/10.1016/j.jpeds.2020.06.044.

[18] Grimaud M, Starck J, Levy M, et al. Acute myocarditis and multisystem inflammatory emerging disease following SARS-CoV-2 infection in critically ill children. Ann Intensive Care 2020;10:69. https://doi.org/10.1186/s13613-020-00690-8.

[19] Whitworth H, Sartain SE, Kumar R, et al. Rate of thrombosis in children and adolescents hospitalized with COVID-19 or MIS-C 2021;138:190–8. https://doi.org/10.1182/blood.2019000962.

[20] Zajc Avramovic M, Vincek K, Mlakar G, et al. POS1318 a nationwide cohort study on clinical and laboratory manifestations in children with multisystem inflammatory syndrome (MIS-C). Ann Rheum Dis 2021;80(Suppl. 1):941–2. https://doi.org/10.1136/ANNRHEUMDIS-2021-EULAR.3022.

[21] Levy M, Recher M, Hubert H, et al. Multisystem inflammatory syndrome in children by COVID-19 vaccination status of adolescents in France. JAMA 2022;327:281–3. https://doi.org/10.1001/jama.2021.23262.

[22] CDC. Multisystem Inflammatory Syndrome in Children (MIS-C) Associated with Cor "Centers for Disease Control and Prevention. Multisystem Inflammatory Syndrome in Children (MIS-C) Associated with Coronavirus Disease 2019 (COVID-19). 2020 March 27, 2020." n.d. Htt. https://emergency.cdc.gov/han/2020/han00432.asp.

[23] WHO. Multisystem inflammatory syndrome in children and adolescents temporally related to COVID-19. Accessed January 29, 2022. https://www.who.int/news-room/commentaries/detail/multisystem-inflammatory-syndrome-in-children-and-adolescents-with-covid-19.

[24] Belhadjer Z, et al. Acute heart failure in multisystem inflammatory syndrome in children in the context of global SARS-CoV-2 pandemic. Circulation 2020;142:429–36. https://doi.org/10.1161/CIRCULATIONAHA.120.048360.

[25] Pouletty M, Borocco C, Ouldali N, et al. Paediatric multisystem inflammatory syndrome temporally associated with SARS- CoV-2 mimicking Kawasaki disease (Kawa- COVID-19): a multicentre cohort. Ann Rheum Dis :999-1006. doi:10.1136/annrheumdis-2020-217960.

[26] Ouldali N, Toubiana J, Antona D, et al. Association of intravenous immunoglobulins plus methylprednisolone vs immunoglobulins alone with course of fever in multisystem inflammatory syndrome in children. JAMA 2021;325:854–64. https://doi.org/10.1001/jama.2021.0694.

[27] Licciardi F, Baldini L, Dellepiane M, et al. MIS-C treatment: is IVIG always necessary? Front Pediatr 2021;9(November):1–6. https://doi.org/10.3389/fped.2021.753123.

[28] Harwood R, Allin B, Jones CE, et al. A national consensus management pathway for paediatric inflammatory multisystem syndrome temporally associated with COVID-19 (PIMS-TS): results of a national Delphi process Rachel. Lancet Child Adolesc Heal 2021;5:133–41.

[29] Borrello GD, Giraudo I, Bondone C, et al. SARS-COV-2-associated coagulopathy and thromboembolism prophylaxis in children: a single-center observational study. Thromb Haemost 2021;19(2):522–30. https://doi.org/10.1111/jth.15216.

[30] Goldenberg NA, Sochet A, Albisetti M, et al. Consensus-based clinical recommendations and research priorities for anticoagulant thromboprophylaxis in children hospitalized for COVID-19–related illness. J Thromb Haemost 2020;18(11):3099–105. https://doi.org/10.1111/jth.15073.

[31] Faganel Kotnik B, Zajc Avramovič M, Kitanovski L, Avčin T. Prophylactic Anticoagulation Therapy: comment on the Article by Henderson et al. Arthritis Rheumatol 2021;73(7):1341–2. https://doi.org/10.1002/ART.41690.

[32] Buddingh EP, Vossen ACTM, Lamb HJ, van der Palen RLF, Brinkman DMC. Reinfection with severe acute respiratory syndrome coronavirus 2 without recurrence of multisystem inflammatory syndrome in children. Pediatr Infect Dis J 2021;40(12):e491–2. https://doi.org/10.1097/inf.0000000000003280.

[33] Castells MC, Phillips EJ. Maintaining safety with SARS-CoV-2 vaccines. N Engl J Med 2021;384(7):643–9. https://doi.org/10.1056/nejmra2035343.

[34] Buchhorn R, Meyer C, Schulze-Forster K, Junker J, Heidecke H. Autoantibody release in children after corona virus mRNA vaccination: a risk factor of multisystem inflammatory syndrome? Vaccines 2021;9:1353. https://doi.org/10.3390/vaccines9111353.

[35] Abdelgalil AA, Saeedi FA. Multisystem inflammatory syndrome in a 12-Year-old boy after mRNA-SARS-CoV-2 vaccination. J Nerv Ment Dis 1995;183(5):337–9. https://doi.org/10.1097/00005053-199505000-00011.

[36] Chai Q, Nygaard U, Schmidt RC, Zaremba T, Møller AM, Thorvig CM. Multisystem inflammatory syndrome in a male adolescent after his second Pfizer-BioNTech COVID-19 vaccine. Acta Paediatr Int J Paediatr 2022;111(1):125–7. https://doi.org/10.1111/apa.16141.

[37] Yalçinkaya R, Öz FN, Polat M, et al. A case of multisystem inflammatory syndrome in a 12-year-old male after COVID-19 mRNA vaccine. Pediatr Infect Dis J 2021;(Xx):9–11. https://doi.org/10.1097/inf.0000000000003432.

CHAPTER

23

Anosmia in COVID-19 and post-COVID syndrome

Paula David[1,2] *and Anna Malkova*[3,4]

[1]Internal Medicine B, Sheba Medical Center, Ramat Gan, Israel; [2]Zabludowicz Center for Autoimmune Diseases, Sheba Medical Center, Ramat Gan, Israel; [3]Ariel University, Ariel, Israel; [4]Saint Petersburg State University, Saint Petersburg, Russia

Introduction

Since the beginning of the COVID-19 pandemics, *anosmia*—or the loss of smell—have been reported as one of the disease's most common symptom [1], occurring on an average of 41%–62% of the patients [2,3]. It can be the first and/or only sign of the infection, usually appears within 3 days of the disease's onset and is recovered in up to a month [4–6]. However, sometimes patients experience disturbances in the sense of smell for a longer period: among post-COVID syndrome (PCS) patients, an anosmia/hyposmia incidence of 21%–23% is described, being it a sequelae of previous illness [7], or a de novo symptom with late-onset of more than a month after the acute infection [8].

Ano/parosmia has a high specificity and low sensitivity for the COVID-19 infection diagnosis, and had no statistically significant association with the prognosis for the disease course [4,9,10], thus, for now, it is difficult to determine its clinical significance. However, it has been proposed as a predictor factor for the development of PCS, in particular fatigue [11].

In this chapter, we will discuss what is known to date in respect to anosmia in COVID-19 and PCS, its potential pathogenesis pathways, and its implication in clinical practice.

Epidemiology of anosmia in COVID-19 and PCS

The high prevalence of loss of smell in COVID-19 patients is undeniable. It is hard to obtain a reliable number, since there is a wide range of prevalence rates among the studies. This discrepancy is probably due to the fact that the earlier studies, in which lower anosmia rates were found [12], were mostly based on retrospective data and self-report

Autoimmunity, COVID-19, Post-COVID19 syndrome and COVID-19 vaccination
https://doi.org/10.1016/B978-0-443-18566-3.00010-4

questionnaires, since anosmia was then not well established as a COVID-19 symptom. On the other hand, most recent studies found a higher prevalence, possibly because they could access patients with these specific symptoms [13]. A big meta-analysis published in 2021 found an overall anosmia incidence of 51% in COVID-19 patients [14]; however, we should consider that this number is probably underestimated for the reasons mentioned above.

In the University of Pennsylvania, a quantitative smell testing was applied to 60 confirmed COVID-19 and to 60 controls matched for gender and age, showing that COVID-19 infected patients had a higher incidence, with 98% of them having a level of olfactory dysfunction and more than half being either completely anosmic or with severe hyposmia [13].

The current literature suggest that around 10%–17% of COVID-19 patients that present with anosmia will not spontaneously recover their smell function [14,15]. It is clear that smell dysfunction is one of the symptoms of PCS, but is still not clear its prevalence among PCS patients.

Pathogenesis

To understand the possible pathways through which the SARS-Cov-2 could lead to the loss it is important to review how our olfactory system works.

The structure of the olfactory organ

The olfactory organ is represented in Fig. 23.1. It can be divided un [1] peripheral, comprised by the nasal/olfactory epithelium (OE) and the olfactory bulb (OB), and [2] central, by the piriform olfactory cortex, the thalamus, and the frontal lobes.

The OE consists in around 50 million olfactory sensory neurons (OSN) [16]. Every OSN has a specific type of olfactory receptors (OR), which are in the cilia membrane. Each OSN dendrite has around 5–10 immotile cilia that forms the apical part of the OE [17]. One OR may respond to multiple odorous molecules, as well as one odorant may activate more than one OR, resulting in a unique combination of ORs for each odorant.

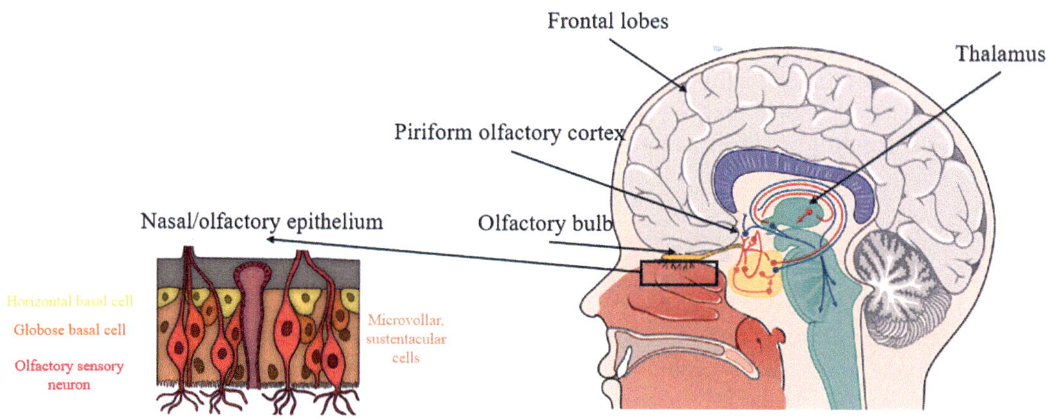

FIGURE 23.1 The structure of the olfactory organ.

The OB contains the axons of the neurons, represented in Fig. 23.1 above the cribriform plate, the glomerulus and the mitral or tufted cells. After an odorant stimulus, all activated OSN fire an action potential to a specific glomerulus. An olfactory glomerulus is a structure consisting primarily of neutrophils, that receives OSN synapses and transfer them to the mitral cell, that in turn, are responsible to send neuronal signals to the primary olfactory cortex [18].

Olfactory receptors (OR)

The ORs are classic G-protein-coupled surface receptors (GPCRs), with seven transmembrane helical domains, three putative extracellular loops (EL) and three putative intracellular loops (IL), an extracellular N-terminus, an intracellular C-terminus [19], similar to a beta-adrenergic receptor, for example, except for the fact that in the ORs binding sites, there are hydrophobic interactions between odorants and the receptor, while in β-adrenergic receptor, ionic bonds, including hydrogen bonds and electrostatic interactions, are found [20] (Fig. 23.2).

Interestingly, ORs can also be found outside the olfactory mucosa [21], presenting different functions, such taking part in sperm chemotaxis [22], regulating migration and adhesion of muscle cells [23], and participating in cell positioning during embryogenesis and cell-cell recognition [24].

Pathogenesis of anosmia

The most common cause of anosmia in respiratory disease is mucosa edema with increased mucus production [25]. However, with COVID-19, there are several peculiarities may suggest an alternative pathogenesis of the olfactory disorder.

Anosmia has been reported in COVID-19 patients without signs of nasal congestion [26,27] and after the respiratory symptoms resolution [7]. This, together with the fact that phantosmia and parosmia have also been described in these patients, is consistent with a sensorineural anosmia. Most COVID-19 patients with impaired sense of smell complained had parallel additional neurological symptoms, such as headache, balance impairment, dysphonia, dizziness, mild confusion, sensory disturbances, and visual disturbances [26].

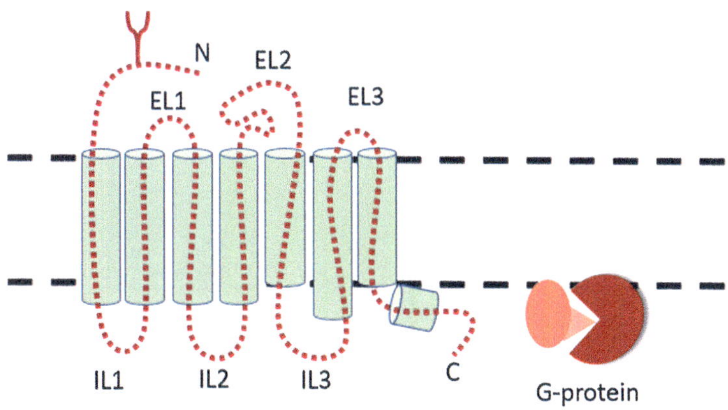

FIGURE 23.2 The Olfactory receptor structure. EL—extracellular loops, IL—intracellular loops.

Table 23.1 resumes some of histological findings that can help us understand the pathogenesis leading to smell dysfunction in COVID patients; those findings suggest that during COVID-19 infection damages both the central and the peripheral olfactory system.

On the one hand, direct viral invasion, that occurs through ACE2 and opioid receptors sigma-1 and sigma-2 receptors, leads to supporting cells, microvillar cells, and pericytes death [1,28,29]. Those opioid receptors are also G-protein-coupled receptors [30,31].

On the other hand, the development of persistent olfactory disorders or in combination with PCS can be explained by the development of autoimmune inflammation with nerve system damage. In fact, other neurologic symptoms, specially autonomic, that are well documented in PCS patients, such as extreme fatigue, attention deficit, tremors, dysautonomia and postorthostatic tachycardia syndrome (POTS), are associated with the presence of autoantibodies against autonomic receptors in these patients [32], such as the β2-adrenoceptor, the α1-adrenoceptor, the angiotensin II AT1-receptor, muscarinic M2-receptor. Those G-protein-couple receptors, as previously mentioned, are very structurally similar to the OR receptors, suggesting that antibodies targeting OR could explain the persistence and the appearance of anosmia and other smell dysfunction long after COVID-19 symptoms had resolved.

Association of anosmia and other autoimmune diseases have been well established, including both neurologic diseases, such as Multiple Sclerosis (high prevalence of 20%–40%), and nonneurologic disorders, including systemic lupus erythematosus (SLE), Sjogren disease, Mikulicz's disease, antiphospholipid antibodies syndrome, among others [33–41].

The fact that impairment of smell has also been described following vaccination validates the hypothesis of an autoimmune response as a pathogenic mechanism [42]. Olfactory and

TABLE 23.1 Histological findings related to anosmia pathogenesis in COVID-19.

Histological findings	References
ACE-2 is not expressed by olfactory sensory neurons and olfactory bulbs mitral cells	[50,51]
ACE-2 is expressed at a significant level by other supporting cells in the olfactory mucosa, including sustentacular and microvillar cells	[50,51]
Significant amounts of SARS-CoV S protein and RNA have been found in the cells of the olfactory mucosa.	[31]
Viral RNA was also detected in central nervous system areas not directly connected with olfactory structures, arguing for a possible SARS-CoV-2 neurotropism. The evidence of the presence of viral RNA in the brain and cerebrospinal fluid (CSF) has been published; however, according to the researchers, it does not indicate a true in-fection with SARS-CoV-2. On the other hand, ACE2 expression was found in neuronal and glial cells of the central nervous system, in the olfactory mucosa	[31,50,52,53]
Magnetic resonance microscopy study found evidence of microvascular injury in the olfactory bulbs of COVID-19 patients	[54]

gustatory disorders were reported following both Pfizer-BioNTech (mRNA vaccine) and AstraZeneca (DNA vector with the viral spike protein—S-protein) vaccination [42]. The patients had negative nasal swabs, were mostly women (around 83%) and the symptoms duration ranged from 4 to 42 days [42]. Since the two vaccines are based on the initiation of the s-protein, a possible mechanism explanation would be molecular mimicry between this protein and human peptides that take part in the olfactory system [43]. Actually, molecular mimicry between the S-protein and several G-couple proteins has been described [44,45]. Matches with other proteins, including some with neuronal function, have also been found, including the plasminogen receptor, previously proposed as a risk factor for COVID-19 and that can be highly found in the microglia cells, that as mentioned before, are part of the olfactory system [46–48].

Conclusion

Smell dysfunction is an important symptom that is found in both COVID-19 disease and in the PCS. The exact pathogenic mechanism of this symptom is still not well established. The mentioned data suggest that the virus enters in nasopharyngeal cavity, where it damages olfactory epithelium and induce acute inflammation with edema and the development of anosmia. In the case of effective immune response after the acute phase, the impairment of olfactory is recovered. However, in genetic predisposed patients to an autoimmune processes, the virus induces autoimmune reaction against OR and similar peptides (G-protein-coupled receptors), migrate to central nervous system through the OB, where induces inflammation with the development of neurological symptoms, including persistent anosmia, fatigue, brain fog, etc, which can prolong in post-COVID syndrome (Fig. 23.3) [49].

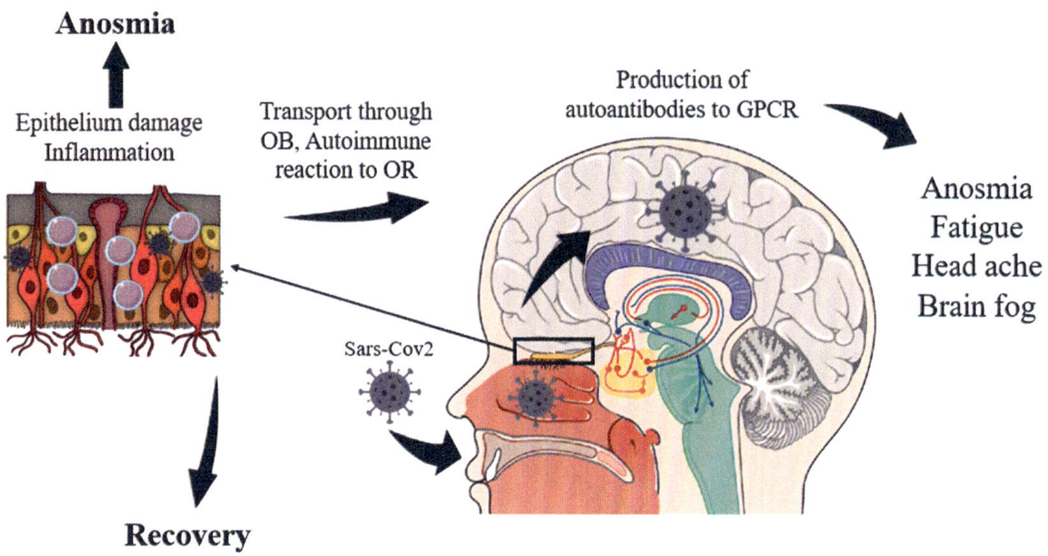

FIGURE 23.3 The hypothesis on anosmia pathogenesis. OR—olfactory receptors, OB—olfactory bulb.

References

[1] Mastrangelo A, Bonato M, Cinque P. Smell and taste disorders in COVID-19: from pathogenesis to clinical features and outcomes. Neurosci Lett March 2021;748:135694.
[2] Rocke J, Hopkins C, Philpott C, Kumar N. Is loss of sense of smell a diagnostic marker in COVID-19: a systematic review and meta-analysis. Clin Otolaryngol 2020;45:914–22.
[3] Agyeman AA, Chin KL, Landersdorfer CB, Liew D, Ofori-Asenso R. Smell and taste dysfunction in patients with COVID-19: a systematic review and meta-analysis. Mayo Clin Proc August 2020;95(8):1621–31.
[4] Brandão Neto D, Fornazieri MA, Dib C, Di Francesco RC, Doty RL, Voegels RL, et al. Chemosensory dysfunction in COVID-19: prevalences, recovery rates, and clinical associations on a large Brazilian sample. Otolaryngol Head Neck Surg March 2021;164(3):512–8.
[5] Speth MM, Singer-Cornelius T, Oberle M, Gengler I, Brockmeier SJ, Sedaghat AR. Olfactory dysfunction and sinonasal symptomatology in COVID-19: prevalence, severity, timing, and associated characteristics. Otolaryngol Head Neck Surg July 2020;163(1):114–20.
[6] Boscolo-Rizzo P, Borsetto D, Fabbris C, Spinato G, Frezza D, Menegaldo A, et al. Evolution of altered sense of smell or taste in patients with mildly symptomatic COVID-19. JAMA Otolaryngol Head Neck Surg August 2020;146(8):1–5.
[7] Chiesa-Estomba CM, Lechien JR, Radulesco T, Michel J, Sowerby LJ, Hopkins C, et al. Patterns of smell recovery in 751 patients affected by the COVID-19 outbreak. Eur J Neurol November 2020;27(11):2318–21.
[8] Carod-Artal FJ. Post-COVID-19 syndrome: epidemiology, diagnostic criteria and pathogenic mechanisms involved. Rev Neurol June 2021;72(11):384–96.
[9] Villerabel C, Makinson A, Jaussent A, Picot MC, Nègre-Pagès L, Rouvière JA, et al. Diagnostic value of patient-reported and clinically tested olfactory dysfunction in a population screened for COVID-19. JAMA Otolaryngol Head Neck Surg March 2021;147(3):271–9.
[10] Wee LE, Chan YFZ, Teo NWY, Cherng BPZ, Thien SY, Wong HM, et al. The role of self-reported olfactory and gustatory dysfunction as a screening criterion for suspected COVID-19. Eur Arch Otorhinolaryngol 2020;277:2389–90.
[11] Wostyn P. Anosmia as a predictor for post-COVID-19 fatigue syndrome. Lancet Reg Heal Eur. August 2021;7:100162.
[12] Mao L, Jin H, Wang M, Hu Y, Chen S, He Q, et al. Neurologic manifestations of hospitalized patients with coronavirus disease 2019 in Wuhan, China. JAMA Neurol April 2020;77:683–90.
[13] Moein ST, Hashemian SMR, Mansourafshar B, Khorram-Tousi A, Tabarsi P, Doty RL. Smell dysfunction: a biomarker for COVID-19. Int Forum Allergy Rhinol April 2020;10(8).
[14] Aziz M, Goyal H, Haghbin H, Lee-Smith WM, Gajendran M, Perisetti A. The association of "loss of smell" to COVID-19: a systematic review and meta-analysis. Am J Med Sci February 2021;361(2):216–25.
[15] Paderno A, Mattavelli D, Rampinelli V, Grammatica A, Raffetti E, Tomasoni M, et al. Olfactory and gustatory outcomes in COVID-19: a prospective evaluation in nonhospitalized subjects. Otolaryngol Head Neck Surg December 2020;163(6):1144–9.
[16] Breer H, Fleischer J, Strotmann J. The sense of smell: multiple olfactory subsystems. Cell Mol Life Sci 2006:1465–75.
[17] Breer H. Olfactory receptors: molecular basis for recognition and discrimination of odors. Anal Bioanal Chem 2003;377:427–33.
[18] Sharma A, Kumar R, Aier I, Semwal R, Tyagi P, Varadwaj P. Sense of smell: structural, functional, mechanistic advancements and challenges in human olfactory research. Curr Neuropharmacol December 2018;17(9):891–911.
[19] Baldwin JM. Structure and function of receptors coupled to G proteins. Curr Opin Cell Biol 1994;6(2):180–90.
[20] Katada S, Hirokawa T, Touhara K. Exploring the odorant binding site of a G-protein-coupled olfactory receptor. Curr Comput Aided Drug Des June 2008;4(2):123–31.
[21] Flegel C, Manteniotis S, Osthold S, Hatt H, Gisselmann G. Expression profile of ectopic olfactory receptors determined by deep sequencing. PLoS One February 2013;8(2).
[22] Fukuda N, Touhara K. Developmental expression patterns of testicular olfactory receptor genes during mouse spermatogenesis. Gene Cell January 2006;11(1):71–81.
[23] Griffin CA, Kafadar KA, Pavlath GK. MOR23 promotes muscle regeneration and regulates cell adhesion and migration. Dev Cell November 2009;17(5):649–61.

[24] Dreyer WJ. The area code hypothesis revisited: olfactory receptors and other related transmembrane receptors may function as the last digits in a cell surface code for assembling embryos. Proc Natl Acad Sci USA 1998;95:9072–7.

[25] Hummel T, Whitcroft KL, Andrews P, Altundag A, Cinghi C, Costanzo RM, et al. Position paper on olfactory dysfunction. Rhinol J June 2017;56(1):1–30.

[26] Cocco A, Amami P, Desai A, Voza A, Ferreli F, Albanese A. Neurological features in SARS-CoV-2-infected patients with smell and taste disorder. J Neurol 2021;268:1570–2.

[27] Beltrán-Corbellini A, Chico-García JL, Martínez-Poles J, Rodríguez-Jorge F, Natera-Villalba E, Gómez-Corral J, et al. Acute-onset smell and taste disorders in the context of COVID-19: a pilot multicentre polymerase chain reaction based case–control study. Eur J Neurol September 2020;27(9):1738–41.

[28] Perrin R, Riste L, Hann M, Walther A, Mukherjee A, Heald A. Into the looking glass: post-viral syndrome post COVID-19. Med Hypotheses 2020;144:110055.

[29] Morbini P, Benazzo M, Verga L, Pagella FG, Mojoli F, Bruno R, et al. Ultrastructural evidence of direct viral damage to the olfactory complex in patients testing positive for SARS-COV-2. JAMA Otolaryngol Head Neck Surg 2020;146:972–3.

[30] Gordon DE, Jang GM, Bouhaddou M, Xu J, Obernier K, White KM, et al. A SARS-CoV-2 protein interaction map reveals targets for drug repurposing. Nature April 2020;583(7816):459–68.

[31] Meinhardt J, Radke J, Dittmayer C, Franz J, Thomas C, Mothes R, et al. Olfactory transmucosal SARS-CoV-2 invasion as a port of central nervous system entry in individuals with COVID-19. Nat Neurosci November 2021;24(2):168–75.

[32] Wallukat G, Hohberger B, Wenzel K, Fürst J, Schulze-Rothe S, Wallukat A, et al. Functional autoantibodies against G-protein coupled receptors in patients with persistent Long-COVID-19 symptoms. J Transl Autoimmun January 2021;4:100100.

[33] Perricone C, Shoenfeld N, Agmon-Levin N, de Carolis C, Perricone R, Shoenfeld Y. Smell and autoimmunity: a comprehensive review. Clin Rev Allergy Immunol December 2012;45(1):87–96.

[34] Fleiner F, Dahlslett SB, Schmidt F, Harms L, Goektas O. Olfactory and gustatory function in patients with multiple sclerosis. Am J Rhinol Allergy September 2010;24(5).

[35] Gatto M, Zen M, Ghirardello A, Bettio S, Bassi N, Iaccarino L, et al. Emerging and critical issues in the pathogenesis of lupus. Autoimmun Rev 2013;12:523–36.

[36] Kamel UF, Maddison P, Whitaker R. Impact of primary Sjögren's syndrome on smell and taste: effect on quality of life. Rheumatology 2009;48(12):1512–4.

[37] Takano K, Yamamoto M, Kondo A, Takahashi H, Himi T. A clinical study of olfactory dysfunction in patients with Mikulicz's disease. Auris Nasus Larynx June 2011;38(3):347–51.

[38] Perricone C, Shoenfeld N, Agmon-Levin N, de Carolis C, Perricone R, Shoenfeld Y. Smell and autoimmunity: a comprehensive review. Clin Rev Allergy Immunol August 2013;45(1):87–96.

[39] Rattazzi L, Cariboni A, Poojara R, Shoenfeld Y, D'Acquisto F. Impaired sense of smell and altered olfactory system in RAG-1(-/-) immunodeficient mice. Front Neurosci 2015;9:318.

[40] Katzav A, Ben-Ziv T, Blank M, Pick CG, Shoenfeld Y, Chapman J. Antibody-specific behavioral effects: intracerebroventricular injection of antiphospholipid antibodies induces hyperactive behavior while anti-ribosomal-P antibodies induces depression and smell deficits in mice. J Neuroimmunol July 2014;272(1–2):10–5.

[41] Shoenfeld Y. Corona (COVID-19) time musings: our involvement in COVID-19 pathogenesis, diagnosis, treatment and vaccine planning. Autoimmun Rev 2020:102538.

[42] Lechien JR, Diallo AO, Dachy B, Le Bon SD, Maniaci A, Vaira LA, et al. COVID-19: post-vaccine smell and taste disorders: report of 6 cases. Ear Nose Throat J September 2021. https://doi.org/10.1177/01455613211033125. 2021:1455613211033125 Epub ahead of print. PMID: 34467793.

[43] Mascellino MT, Di Timoteo F, De Angelis M, Oliva A. Overview of the main anti-sars-cov-2 vaccines: mechanism of action, efficacy and safety. Infect Drug Resist 2021;14:3459–76.

[44] Kanduc D, Shoenfeld Y. On the molecular determinants of the SARS-CoV-2 attack. Clin Immunol 2020;215:108426.

[45] Kanduc D. From anti-SARS-CoV-2 immune response to the cytokine storm via molecular mimicry. Antibodies September 2021;10(4):36.

[46] Adiguzel Y. Molecular mimicry between SARS-CoV-2 and human proteins. Autoimmun Rev 2021;20:102791.

[47] Ji HL, Zhao R, Matalon S, Matthay MA. Elevated plasmin(Ogen) as a common risk factor for COVID-19 susceptibility. Physiol Rev 2020;100(3):1065–75.

[48] Flick MJ, Bugge TH. Plasminogen−receptor KT: plasminogen activation and beyond. J Thromb Haemost 2017;15:150−4.
[49] Malkova A, Kudryavtsev I, Starshinova A, Kudlay D, Zinchenko Y, Glushkova A, et al. Post COVID-19 syndrome in patients with asymptomatic/mild form. Pathogens October 2021;10(11):1408.
[50] Brann DH, Tsukahara T, Weinreb C, Lipovsek M, Van Den Berge K, Gong B, et al. Non-neuronal expression of SARS-CoV-2 entry genes in the olfactory system suggests mechanisms underlying COVID-19-associated anosmia. Sci Adv July 2020;6(31).
[51] Chen M, Shen W, Rowan NR, Kulaga H, Hillel A, Ramanathan M, et al. Elevated ACE2 expression in the olfactory neuroepithelium: implications for anosmia and upper respiratory SARS-CoV-2 entry and replication. Eur Respir J 2020;56(3).
[52] Moriguchi T, Harii N, Goto J, Harada D, Sugawara H, Takamino J, et al. A first case of meningitis/encephalitis associated with SARS-Coronavirus-2. Int J Infect Dis May 2020;94:55−8.
[53] Khan S, Gomes J. Neuropathogenesis of SARS-CoV-2 infection. Elife July 2020;9:1−9.
[54] Lee M-H, Perl DP, Nair G, Li W, Maric D, Murray H, et al. Microvascular injury in the brains of patients with covid-19. N Engl J Med February 2021;384(5):481−3.

CHAPTER

24

The effect of COVID-19 on patients with preexisting autoimmune diseases

Olga Vera-Lastra[1,2], *Alberto Ordinola Navarro*[1,2,3], *Gabriela Medina*[2,4], *María Pilar Cruz-Domínguez*[2,5] and *Luis J. Jara*[6]

[1]Internal Medicine Department, Hospital de Especialidades "Dr. Antonio Fraga Mouret" Centro Médico Nacional La Raza, Instituto Mexicano del Seguro Social, México City, México; [2]Division of Postgraduate Studies, Faculty of Medicine, Universidad Nacional Autónoma de México, México City, México; [3]Infectious Disease Department, Instituto Nacional de Ciencias Médicas y Nutrición Salvador Zubirán, México City, México; [4]Translational Research Unit, Hospital de Especialidades "Dr. Antonio Fraga Mouret" Centro Médico Nacional La Raza, Instituto Mexicano del Seguro Social, México City, México; [5]Direction of Education and Research, Hospital de Especialidades "Dr. Antonio Fraga Mouret" Centro Médico Nacional La Raza, Instituto Mexicano del Seguro Social, México City, México; [6]Rheumatology Division, Instituto Nacional de Rehabilitación "Luis Guillermo Ibarra Ibarra", México City, México

Introduction

Acute viral respiratory infections are mainly infectious diseases in the world, caused by more than 200 viruses. The etiological agents are rhinoviruses, 30%–50%, coronaviruses, 10%–15%, influenza viruses, 5%–15%, respiratory syncytial virus, parainfluenza viruses, 5%, adenoviruses, enteroviruses, <5%, and unknown 20%–30% [1]. In December

Autoimmunity, COVID-19, Post-COVID19 syndrome and COVID-19 vaccination
https://doi.org/10.1016/B978-0-443-18566-3.00001-3

2019, a new Coronavirus, called Severe Acute Respiratory Syndrome Coronavirus-2 (SARS-CoV-2), appeared in China, spreading rapidly globally and becoming a global pandemic. SARS-CoV-2 is the cause of a serious life-threatening disease known as COVID-19 [2].

Since the beginning of the COVID-19 pandemic, we have learned that several groups are at higher risk of developing the SARS-CoV-2 infection and evolving to its most serious form, such as cytokine storm syndrome (CSS) multi-organ disease that endangers the patient's life. The main recognized risk groups are the following: old age (<65 years old), male gender, comorbidities such as hypertension, diabetes, obesity, chronic lung diseases, heart, liver, and kidney diseases, cancer, immunodeficiencies, local immunodeficiency, such as early-type I interferon secretion capacity, and pregnancy [3]. The risk of SARS-CoV-2 infection in patients with systemic autoimmune rheumatic diseases appears to be slightly higher than in the general population, but the clinical course does not appear to be different. However, we must bear in mind that the use of corticosteroids, immunomodulatory drugs, and biological therapy in patients with autoimmune rheumatic diseases can modulate the risk of hospitalization and death [4]. The pandemic of COVID-19 is the cause of high morbidity and mortality in the world. The SARS-CoV-2 virus leads to a picture of severe acute respiratory distress syndrome (ARDS) and pulmonary insufficiency. This clinical picture develops as a consequence of a complex interaction between the virus and the immune system and leads to an immune/inflammatory/coagulation cascade hyper-responsiveness, with the release of cytokines and other proinflammatory proteins by the affected cells, thus rapidly developing a true or perfect CSS and macrophage activation syndrome. Given the severity of these syndromes and the absence of a specific antiviral treatment, various antirheumatic drugs have been used to try to save the lives of our patients, such as corticosteroids, anticoagulants, chloroquine, hydroxychloroquine, JAK, IL-6, IL-1 inhibitors, anti-TNF-α agents, intravenous immunoglobulin (IVIG), and colchicine, with varying degrees of evidence. The alterations in the innate and adaptive immune response found in patients with CSS due to COVID-19 and their high morbidity and mortality indicate that clinicians should identify early and closely monitor patients with risk factors for developing these complications [5–7].

Multiple studies conducted in different countries and continents during the pandemic indicate that COVID-19 infection is a very important cause of stress, with the impact of the SARS-CoV-2 on the CNS and mental health outcomes, which activates the immune-neuro-endocrine system. Suppose the infection progresses and the patient develops a cytokine storm. In that case, the axis of the immune-neuro endocrine system such as the hypothalamic-pituitary-adrenal axis (HPAA), the hypothalamic-pituitary-thyroid axis (HPTA), the hypothalamic-pituitary gonad axis (HPGA), among others, are directly affected by the SARS -CoV-2 virus or by the cytokine storm, causing a significant imbalance in these defense systems against stress. These disorders can occur in patients with risk factors, including patients with autoimmune diseases. In this sense, it has been proposed that the immune response of patients with COVID-19 is very similar to the one of patients with autoimmune diseases through cross-reactivity with host cells [8–10], and probably leads to immuno-neuro-endocrine alterations.

This chapter aims to review the impact of COVID-19 infection, on patients with preexisting autoimmune diseases, with emphasis on autoimmune rheumatic diseases (ARD), autoimmune endocrine diseases (AED), and autoimmune neurological diseases (ANR).

Preexisting autoimmune rheumatic diseases

General aspects

The effect of the therapies used in patients with an autoimmune rheumatic disease (ARD) has led health personnel to question if patients with autoimmune diseases may be more susceptible to acquiring COVID-19 and may have an increased risk of complications and mortality. Patients with ARD are considered more susceptible to infectious diseases, which may be related to the activity of the condition, the damage it has produced, the comorbidities, and its treatment. Thus, in patients with chronic damage caused by (ARD), the risk of severe complications for COVID-19 could be higher than for other patients [11].

Autoimmune diseases are heterogeneous, derived from the presence of autoantibodies that, due to loss of immune tolerance and dysregulation of the immune system, lead to inflammatory reactions to target organ damage. These immune-mediated lesions also exist in COVID-19. The excessive production and release of proinflammatory cytokines and chemokines can cause severe damage to organs in critical cases due to the degree of imbalance of these cytokines and the activation of immune cells. Another change found in autoimmune diseases is that neutrophilia and associated excessive extracellular neutrophil traps (NETs) are also part of the pathophysiology of lung injury in patients with severe COVID-19 [10].

During the COVID-19 pandemic, autoimmune diseases have caused the most significant concern regarding SARS-CoV-2 infection because immunosuppressive drugs used to treat autoimmune diseases can increase the susceptibility to being infected due to COVID-19 causes immune dysfunction [12]. Some of the patients with autoimmune diseases discontinued their medication because they feared that the immunosuppressive effect of the pills would make them more susceptible to infection, which decreased medical visits. Most patients with autoimmune diseases have received or are receiving immunomodulatory drugs or biological agents. However, interrupted continuity of medical care and noncompliance with medication are associated with flare-ups of the rheumatologic disease and worsening disease activity [13].

In an Italian study, they evaluated the association between autoimmune disease and COVID-19 risk in the population of Milan. They found a negative association between autoimmune status and COVID-19 risk, thus proposing that autoimmune disease is not a risk factor for being positive for COVID-19 and that patients with autoimmune diseases do not have a worse prognosis than individuals without the presence of these types of diseases [14]. In contrast, D'Silva et al. [15], in a multicenter study with patients with systemic ARD and diagnosis of COVID-19, evaluated the risks of having a severe illness. They found that patients with ARD had significantly higher chances of hospitalization, admission to the intensive care unit, acute renal failure, and venous thromboembolism than matched comparators but did not have significantly higher risks of mechanical ventilation or death.

Autoimmune rheumatic diseases and factors that influence COVID 19

Patients with ARD have a high frequency of women, elderly patients, and patients with preexisting comorbidities (metabolic syndrome), although these factors do not appear to have a decisive effect on disease severity. In this way, it is important to mention the use of antirheumatic treatments, which have been studied for the efficacy of treating COVID 19, mainly TNF $-\alpha$ and IL-6 receptor antagonists, but they have not provided conclusive information [16].

Age and gender

Aging has been seen as a factor independently related to hospital admission in ARD patients infected with SARS-CoV-2 [17]. In these patients with ARD, age older than 50 and older than 35 years was a risk factor for their hospitalization and death, respectively [18–23].

Male and female patients behave differently in COVID-19 infection. The majority of ARD patients infected with COVID-19 were female, generally exceeding 60%. The overall mortality during COVID-19 development was higher in female ARD patients, which is different from the general population in that males account for a more significant proportion. However, other studies reported that males could be an independent factor associated with the severity of COVID-19, for male ARD patients may have a worse prognosis, higher hospitalization rate, and risk of severe pneumonia [23–25].

Races

Among different races, exists the influence of different factors: genetics, survival environment or lifestyles, and social aspects, among others, it has been observed that African American, Asiatic and Latin races had higher COVID-19 associated hospitalization rates than white patients, and the need for respiratory assistance was more significant, but it did not reach statistical significance [16–26].

Comorbidities

The most common three comorbidities in ARDs patients infected with COVID-19 were cardiovascular diseases (arterial hypertension), endocrine diseases (diabetes), and respiratory diseases (chronic obstructive pulmonary disease and asthma). In the COVID-19 pandemic, the number of comorbidities is strongly associated with patients' general condition, and comprehensive recognition of the complexity of the diseases is of great significance [27,28].

Drugs

Among the most common drugs used in ARD are glucocorticoids, conventional disease-modifying antirheumatic drugs (csDMARDs), antimalarial drugs, and biologic or targeted synthetic disease-modifying antirheumatic drugs (b/tsDMARDs). These drugs act on COVID-19-infected ARD patients based on different pharmacological mechanisms [16].

Glucocorticoids have a crucial role in treating rheumatic diseases, while their role in rheumatic patients with COVID-19 infection is controversial. Compared with nonhospitalized patients, the proportion of SLE and vasculitis was higher in hospitalized patients, while psoriatic arthritis and ankylosing spondylitis were lower [29]. In addition, Nuño et al. [27] found increased mortality after glucocorticoid treatment in ARD patients. It is important to emphasize that the use of glucocorticoids seems to increase the risk of COVID 19. Therefore, it is suggested to reduce glucocorticoids to less than 10 mg/day gradually. The discontinuation of glucocorticoids during the COVID pandemic is not recommended. According to the case reported, improvements in kidney, respiratory, neurological, and liver function in systemic lupus erythematosus (SLE) or SLE-like patients infected with COVID-19 were observed [30,31].

Conventional synthetic disease-modifying antirheumatic drugs

It has been reported that csDMARDs may have clinical results to reduce the risk of COVID, the protective effect of leflunomide on the cytokine storm emerging in severe COVID -19 cases was also recommended [32].

A meta-analysis involving eight studies showed that colchicine reduced the mortality of COVID-19 patients and the number of severe cases, which could be good news for people with gout [33].

However, in the vast majority of cases, the effect of csDMARDs on COVID-19 infection was neutral. Likewise, ARD patients treated with csDMARDs alone (methotrexate or cyclosporine) or in conjunction with biological agents or Janus Kinase inhibitors do not influence the susceptibility to COVID-19 or hospitalization rate was observed [34].

The antimalarials (AM) for the treatment of COVID 19 generated a great expectation. Patients with ARD who took AM were less susceptible to COVID-19 than patients who took other csDMARDs [35]. Other retrospective studies suggested that long-term treatment of HCQ in RADs patients can protect against COVID-19 infection [36]. The American College of Rheumatology's guideline suggested that it was reasonable to adjust HCQ dosing intervals or dosage according to practical situations [37]. Noteworthy, most adverse events (AEs) tend to occur with the first cumulative dose of 1 g. However, its use has been controversial and is not recommended for the prevention or treatment of SARS-COV-2 [38].

Biologic or targeted synthetic disease-modifying antirheumatic drugs

Biologic or targeted synthetic disease-modifying antirheumatic drugs may be potentially helpful in alleviating inflammatory cytokine storm under COVID-19 attack [39]. Compared with ARD patients treated with CD20 monoclonal antibody rituximab or IL-17A antagonist secukinumab, patients receiving tumor necrosis factor (TNF) inhibitors etanercept and adalimumab or IL-6 receptor antagonist tocilizumab may experience a relatively mild course [40]. In addition, the effects of TNF inhibitors and tocilizumab on clinical epidemiology have also been reported. Patients receiving adalimumab or infliximab treatment had a reduced risk of COVID-19 infection [16] and monotherapy of TNF-inhibitor prior to COVID-19 infection may reduce the COVID-19-related hospitalization or severity [41].

Treatment of tocilizumab has been proven to ensure the stability of vascular permeability and myocardial functions in RA patients infected with COVID-19 [42,43] and reduce the COVID-19-associated mortality and inflammatory indicators [44,45]. For the treatment after the infection of COVID-19, in general, most studies have reported that these treatments just have a neutral effect on ARD patients; the mortality or hospitalization rate of patients has not been particularly affected. In contrast to the possible positive effect of maintenance treatment before a diagnosis of COVID-19, the use of biologic agents after the COVID-19 diagnosis did not stop the disease from progressing [16].

COVID-19 in inflammatory arthritis

There are few studies about the course of the disease in patients with immune-mediated inflammatory diseases. A study included 50 cases of inflammatory arthritis: rheumatoid arthritis (RA), psoriatic arthritis (PsA), and ankylosing spondylitis (ASp) diagnosed with COVID-19. They found differences between outpatient and inpatient treatment: most inpatients received biological disease-modifying antirheumatic drugs (bDMARD) or Janus kinase inhibitors (JAK). Furthermore, hospitalized patients most frequently used oral glucocorticoids, hydroxychloroquine, and methotrexate, while biologics (mainly TNF blockers and anti-IL12) were more frequent in outpatients. All this could suggest a possible protective effect of these biologics to prevent the appearance of a cytokine release syndrome in patients with rheumatic diseases. However, this remains controversial [46].

COVID 19 in rheumatoid arthritis

Rheumatoid arthritis is an autoimmune disease that affects the joints and internal organs that significantly impact health systems. The COVID-19 pandemic has made these patients more vulnerable. In patients with RA, risk factors for severe COVID-19 outcomes include older age and comorbidities, similar to those in the general population. Glucocorticoids, but not other classes of disease-modifying antirheumatic drugs (DMARDs), appear to be associated with a higher risk of severe COVID-19 outcomes. RA patients have been affected by changes in access to care, telemedicine, drug shortages, anxiety, and social isolation, contributing to disease flares [47].

Regarding some studies in patients with preexisting RA and COVID 19, the following has been reported.

In a French cohort of 694 patients, it was found that 63% had mild disease, 24% had moderate disease, and severe disease up to 13%. The factors associated with severe COVID were age, being a woman, body mass index, hypertension, and use of corticosteroids, mycophenolate mofetil, and rituximab; these patients were compared with 175 matched hospitalized patients only with COVID, and the OR of mortality associated with hospitalized patients with AID and COVID-19 was 1.45 (95% CI: 0.87–2.42). Regarding RA, the mortality was 20 out of 58 died (34%) [48].

In a study of individuals with rheumatic disease and COVID-19 from the COVID-19 Global Rheumatology Alliance registry [19] of a total of 600 cases from 40 countries, nearly half of the cases were hospitalized (277, 46%), and 55 (9%) died. Prednisone of ≥10 mg/day was associated with a higher odds of hospitalization and anti-TNF with a decreased odds of hospitalization in patients with rheumatic disease. Neither exposure to DMARDs nor NSAIDs were associated with increased odds of hospitalization. In a Brazilian study of 334 participants enrolled, a majority of them were women, with a median age of 45 years;

they found that the age >50 years and immunosuppression with GC and cyclophosphamide were associated with unfavorable outcomes of COVID-19 and treatment with TNF may have been protective [49].

An Italian study of 916 patients comprised 397 SLE, 182 ANCA-Associated Vasculitis, 176 Systemic Sclerosis, 111 Rheumatoid Arthritis, and 50 Inflammatory Myopathy. Of those, 148 patients developed at least one symptom compatible with COVID-19. No deaths occurred. In this study, COVID-19 incidence seems to be similar to the general population [50].

In a Canadian study, regarding comorbidities, RA was associated with a higher risk of COVID-19 mortality and severity among individuals under 50 years old, compared to their effect in older age groups. This study highlights that the number of comorbidities was a strong risk factor for deaths and severe outcomes among younger individuals with COVID-19 [51].

Based on the above, RA is one of the main diseases that have suffered by COVID 19; in general, immunosuppressant use could have prevented a less severe disease.

According to the European League Against Rheumatism, there is no evidence that patients with inflammatory rheumatic disease are at a higher risk of SARS-CoV-2 infection than individuals without an inflammatory disease, and do not have worse prognostic with a diagnosis of COVID. In patients with inflammatory ARD, glucocorticoid at doses >10 mg/day was associated with higher odds of hospitalization rates and antitumor necrosis factor with fewer odds [48].

COVID-19 in spondyloarthropathies

According to data from the Global Rheumatology Alliance physician-reported registry, patients with PsA, axial spondyloarthritis (axSpA), or other spondyloarthritis that required hospitalization for COVID-19 infection had a lower proportion of patients (8% and 6%, respectively) compared with those with these diseases and COVID-19 that were not hospitalized (16% and 10%, respectively). Likewise, PsA and axSpA ranked fifth and sixth place in the number of rheumatic disease patients hospitalized in this registry. In general, factors associated with a higher risk of hospitalization were older age, presence of comorbidities, and higher doses of prednisone (≥10 mg/day) [20]. The BIOBADASER registry, with more than 6600 patients prospectively followed in Spain, identified 41 patients with COVID-19 and rheumatic diseases, treated with biological (bDMARD) or targeted synthetic disease-modifying antirheumatic drug (tsDMAR). Twelve out of 41 patients had SpA, 66.7% required hospitalization, and one patient died. However, the mortality rate and hospitalization did not differ from the general population rate by COVID-19 in Spain [52]. In another cohort of 228 patients with rheumatic diseases and hospitalized for COVID-19 infection, 16% had SpA while 15% had PsA. Of note, neither having a chronic inflammatory rheumatic disease such as SpA and PsA, nor previous immunosuppressive therapies were associated with severe COVID-19 [53].

Regarding reactive arthritis, there is one case report in a male patient without previous rheumatic disease that developed reactive arthritis after severe acute respiratory syndrome due to SARS-CoV-2 infection, with immunologic tests negative, including HLA-B27 and without evidence of bacterial coinfection [54]. Haberman et al. [55] reported the findings in a cohort of 126 adults with inflammatory arthritis including RA, PsA, ankylosing spondylitis, or inflammatory bowel disease (IBD)-associated arthritis), confirmed or highly suspected of

COVID-19 infection. They found that RA patients had a higher hospitalization rate in comparison with SpA groups (38% vs. 16%; $P = .02$). Of great relevance was that the regular use of anticytokine biologic therapies was not associated with worse outcomes of COVID-19 in patients with inflammatory arthritis.

In general, age, comorbidities, and having a systemic autoimmune condition increased the risk of hospital admission, although DMARD was not associated with hospital admission [56]. Therefore, patients with PsA or axSpA seem not to increase the risk of COVID-19 severe infection.

COVID-19 in antiphospholipid syndrome

It is known that COVID-19 infection can predispose to thrombotic events because of endothelial dysfunction, increased levels of von Willebrand factor (VWF), systemic inflammation, activation of Toll-like receptors, and tissue factor pathway activation [57]. Another mechanism is through the formation of antiphospholipid antibodies (aPL) in patients with severe acute respiratory distress syndrome (ARDS), suggesting an antiphospholipid syndrome (APS) like condition. Some patients with SARS-CoV-2 two infection had elevated anticardiolipin (aCL) IgA antibodies and anti-β2-glycoprotein I (anti-β2-GPI) with clinical presentation of multiple cerebral infarctions, as well as LAC (Lupus anticoagulant) [58,59]. However, aCL and anti-β2-GPI antibodies have been found positive in a few patients with venous thrombotic complications [59].

In a big series of 150 COVID-19 patients managed at the ICU by ARDS, up to 64 thrombotic events were registered with several coagulation abnormalities. Regarding the immunological profile, most of the patients had positive LAC, leaving the question of whether COVID 19 can precipitate APS [60]. Borghi et al. [61] found in 122 COVID 19 patients anti-b2GPI in a low percentage of patients without association with thrombosis, possibly due to a different epitope specificity. In another study, aPL Abs were frequent in patients with severe COVID-19. These antibodies appeared after 35–39 days of disease onset, and repeated testing showed medium to high titers of aPL. Antiphospholipid antibodies may be transient and disappear in a few weeks, however in genetically predisposed patients; COVID-19 may trigger an APS-like syndrome [62].

On the other hand, the clinical behavior of COVID-19 infection appears to be different in patients with preexisting autoimmune diseases or patients undergoing immunosuppressive therapy. In this regard, immunosuppressed heart-transplanted patients present a milder form of COVID-19. There is scarce information about the course of COVID-19 in patients with preexisting autoimmune diseases. A man with severe APS, treated with anticoagulation and immunosuppressors with COVID-19 infection, received remdesivir and steroid doses because of suspected diffuse alveolar hemorrhage. He was discharged without supplemental oxygen. Subsequently, the patient had several complications that required hospitalization for persistent SARS-CoV-2 infections, suggesting that the torpid course of the disease was associated with an immunocompromised state [63]. Escher et al. [64] reported a case of a patient with COVID-19 with respiratory and renal failure, elevated anticardiolipin, anti-β2-GP IgM antibodies, and von Willebrand factor (VWF), and factor VIII. The patient was treated with prophylactic LMWH, followed by a therapeutic dose of unfractionated heparin, with clinical improvement, suggesting a role of therapeutic anticoagulation in patients with

COVID-19. Nevertheless, testing of aPL Abs and LA in a larger number of COVID-19 patients, as well as longitudinal follow-up of patients who recovered from COVID-19 infection and that are positive for aPL Abs with thrombotic events are necessary to ascertain whether they disappeared after recovery of the infection or whether they develop definite APS [65].

COVID-19 in systemic lupus erythematosus

Prolonged activated partial-thromboplastin time (aPTT) has been observed in COVID-19 patients, corresponding to LAC in 91% of patients with aberrant results [66]. The presence of LAC, in approximately 50% of SLE patients and SLE, considered a risk factor for both venous and arterial thrombosis, alerts the need to monitor especially patients with both conditions, COVID 19 and SLE [67].

Pascolini et al. [68] determined the presence of antinuclear antibodies (ANA), among other autoantibodies, in patients with COVID-19. Furthermore, cases of SLE triggered by SARS-CoV-2 as well as a concomitant new diagnosis of SLE, APS, and COVID-19 have been reported [69,70]. It is not well known how SLE patients respond to COVID-19 and whether they are at an increased risk of getting infected because of their maladaptive immune system [71]. He F et al. reported a case of recurrence of SARS-CoV-2 infection in an SLE patient possibly due to difficulty removing the virus because of the immunosuppressive treatment. Therefore, patients with SLE and COVID-19 possibly require closer monitoring and testing than the general population with SARS-CoV-2 infection. However, limitations in epidemiologic data available to date do not allow us to ascertain if SLE per se will be a significant risk factor for contracting COVID-19 or developing subsequent poor outcomes [72]. Patients with rheumatic diseases, including SLE, seem to have a slightly increased risk of death from COVID-19 compared to those without these diseases, even though the role of both disease activity and treatment in this risk estimation is not taken into consideration [73].

Several studies have suggested that having SLE does not increase the risk of SARS-CoV-2, which has been the subject of discussion because the prevalence has varied significantly depending on the autoimmune disease studied. For example, Pablos et al. found a 1.32 times higher prevalence of hospitalized for COVID-19 in patients with chronic inflammatory disorders than the reference population (0.76% vs. 0.58%), showing a significant increase, while patients with inflammatory arthritis or SLE did not [14]. However, other studies have found that SLE patients infected with COVID-19 have a high hospitalization rate (59%), but the mortality rate is not different from that of the general population [74]. More information about the behavior of COVID-19 infection in patients with SLE and APS will be treated more extensively in another chapter.

COVID-19 in systemic sclerosis

Systemic sclerosis (SSc) is an autoimmune disease characterized by immune-system alterations, diffuse microangiopathy, and fibrosis involving the skin and internal organs. COVID-19 is due to a direct attack of SARS-CoV-2 on the vascular system as an acute infection; in the same way, SSc is a vasculopathy.

An Italian study found a statistically higher prevalence of COVID-19 in connective tissue diseases than in the chronic arthritis subgroup and in ASD patients with preexisting interstitial lung involvement. Patients treated with either conventional disease-modifying antirheumatic drugs (DMARDs) and/or biological DMARDs showed a significantly lower prevalence of COVID-19 in both) [75].

On the other hand, in other ARD such as systemic sclerosis (SSc), pulmonary and cardiovascular manifestations must be considered when specifying the risk of COVID-19 in these patients. In a cohort study where 110 patients with SSc were studied, 35% had interstitial lung disease, while none had pulmonary arterial hypertension; only 10% had a history of cardiovascular disease. They only reported one case of COVID-19 in this cohort. The patient was a 77-year-old woman with limited cutaneous SSc of 6 years of evolution on treatment with methylprednisolone and methotrexate. She had a history of high blood pressure and interstitial lung disease. This hospitalized patient showed a good prognosis after being treated with methylprednisolone, hydroxychloroquine, azithromycin, and tocilizumab. She had a complete resolution of symptoms [75].

Also, Nicoletta Del Papa et al. [76] studied a cohort of 526 patients with SSc, of which 270 and 256 had limited cutaneous and diffuse cutaneous systemic sclerosis, respectively. They had 45% of the patients with interstitial lung disease, and 68% received immunosuppressive therapy. Eleven patients reported symptoms consistent with a mild form of COVID-19, and only two patients needed hospitalization. They were hospitalized for signs of respiratory failure and treated with antibiotics, hydroxychloroquine, and steroids. The first patient had diffused cutaneous SSc, mild interstitial lung disease, was on weekly methotrexate, and received a cycle of two rituximab infusions 6 months earlier. Unfortunately, this patient remained very feverish, required invasive ventilatory support, and died. The second patient had limited systemic cutaneous sclerosis, and pulmonary hypertension and was on treatment with endothelin receptor antagonists and sildenafil, recovering in 3 weeks. An essential piece of information is that none of these patients modified their therapy during the COVID-19 outbreak. In this study, they conclude that despite the high prevalence of interstitial lung disease and immunosuppressive therapies, which can be considered risk factors for being more susceptible to being infected by COVID-19 and manifesting as a severe disease, in terms of mortality and morbidity rates, it does not seem particularly severe in these con SSc. Ferri et al. [77] reported in SSc patients with preexisting interstitial lung involvement undergoing low-dose aspirin had a significantly lower rate of COVID-19 compared to those without.

Regarding mental symptoms, anxiety, but not depression symptoms, increased dramatically during COVID-19 among people with SS [78].

In our experience on 116 patients with SSc, 13 (11.2%) patients (12 female and one man) have become ill with COVID-19 during follow-up from March to December 2020. Only one of them had minor symptoms of COVID-19 (stage 1 of viral replication) and 11 developed mild to moderate atypical pneumonia, but only seven required supplemental oxygen (stage 2 of invasion). All these patients with pneumonia improved with steroids and anticoagulants and only one evolved to severe atypical pneumonia and died in the Intensive Care Unit. Most of our patients with pulmonary disease continued their immunosuppressive treatment. Our results suggest that the patients with SS and Covid-19 infection become mild atypical pneumonia. In this sense, our results support the hypothesis that patients with interstitial lung disease- SSc with immunosuppressive treatment are susceptible to presenting serious complications from COVID-19 almost similar to the general population (Table 24.1).

TABLE 24.1 Demographics, clinical manifestations, comorbidities and treatment of patients with systemic sclerosis and Covid-19.

Characteristic	Data value
Age, median (IQR) (years)	57 (52, 63)
SSc subtype, no. (%)	
• diffususe cutaneous SSc	9 (69.2)
• limites cutáneos SSc	4 (30.8)
IMC, median (IQR) (Kg/m^2)	25.9 (21.4, 29.8)
SO_2% (FIO_2 21%), median (IQR)	90 (88, 92)
Disease duration, median (IQR) (years)	15 (9, 20)
Treatment for COVID-19, n (%)	
Steroids	9 (69.2)
Anticoagulants	8 (61.5)
Antiplatelet agents	7 (53.8)
Comorbidities, no. (%)	
Diabetes	2 (15.4)
Arterial hypertension	2 (15.4)
PAH	4 (30.8)
Hypothyroidism	3 (23.1)
Treatment for SSc, no. (%)	
Amlodipine	8 (61.5)
Mycophenolate	5 (38.5)
Metothrexate	2 (15.4)
Prednisone	4 (30.8)
Sildenafil citrate	1 (7.7)
Outcomes associated with Covid-19	
Hospitalization, n (%)	2 (15.4)
Home oxygen	7 (53.8)
Deaths, no. (%)	1 (7.7)

IQR, Interquartile range; *PAH*, Pulmonary arterial hypertension; *SSc*, Systemic sclerosis.

COVID 19 in primary Sjogren syndrome

Primary SS (SS) is a systemic autoimmune disease characterized by affecting the exocrine glands and internal organs, predominantly affecting women. The clinical feature of primary SS is the development of dryness symptoms, reported by> 95% of patients, accompanied in a significant number of cases by a wide variety of systemic manifestations, including autoimmune damage to internal organs [79,80].

People with ARD, especially SS, are considered at-risk for severe COVID-19, considering their underlying abnormal immune response and the frequent use of immunosuppressive drugs. So far, no study has evaluated the impact of COVID-19 on primary SS, which has some specific features that could favor an increased risk for developing severe COVID-19 (pulmonary autoimmune damage, use of immunosuppressive agents, among others) [81–83]. Brito-Zeron et al. [84] analyzed the prognosis and outcomes of COVID-19 in patients with primary SS from the Big Data Sjogren Registry, an international, multicentre registry. A total of 51 patients were included in the study; the majority were women. According to the number of patients with primary SS evaluated in the registry (n = 8211), the estimated frequency of SARS-CoV-2 infection was 0.62%. All but two presented with symptoms suggestive of COVID-19, with typical manifestations including fever (82%), cough (57%), dyspnea (39%), among others. Infection was managed at home in 26 (51%) cases, and 25 (49%) required hospitalization (five required admissions to ICU, four died). Compared with patients managed at home, those requiring hospitalization had higher odds of having lymphopenia in a laboratory. Patients with comorbidities had an older age and showed a risk for hospital admission. This study, it was evaluated the outcomes of SARS-CoV-2 infection in patients with primary SS. Primary SS-infected individuals seemed to be similarly affected by SARS-CoV-2 compared with the general population's clinical presentation. Notably, baseline comorbidities were risk factors for a more complicated COVID-19 in this population, especially chronic pulmonary disease, not only interstitial lung disease (closely related to poor outcome in primary SS) [85] but also asthma (recently related to a more complicated outcome in SARS-CoV-2 infection) [86]. Patients with primary SS and comorbidities had higher hospitalization rates and poor outcomes (intensive care admission, death) compared with those without baseline comorbidities. In conclusion, baseline comorbidities were a key risk factor for a more complicated COVID-19 in patients with primary SS, with higher rates of hospitalization and poor outcomes in comparison with patients without comorbidities.

Serban A et al. [87] investigate the perspective of patients with Sjögren syndrome (SS) on various aspects of the disease during the SARS-CoV-2 outbreak, including the impact of COVID-19 on the disease. The study was an online questionnaire-based survey. It received responses from 137 SS patients. Regarding the general emotional status, 33 patients (24.0%) and 47 patients (34.3%) declared to have been sadder/depressive and more agitated/anxious during the SARS-CoV-2 outbreak. In this study, 22.6% of patients with SS reported that they had had COVID-19 versus <1% informed in the study of Brito-Zeron [84]. Only one patient was completely asymptomatic, while the most frequently declared symptom was weakness (84.0%). In 17 patients among the respondents (68%), the symptoms lasted for at least 2 weeks; the most frequent long-lasting symptoms were fatigue (40.0%) and weakness (36.0%).

Notably, baseline comorbidities were risk factors for a more complicated COVID-19 in this population, especially chronic pulmonary disease, not only interstitial lung disease (closely related to poor outcome in primary SS) [85] but also asthma (recently related to a more complicated outcome in SARS-CoV-2 infection) [86].

One Italian study showed a higher frequency of COVID-19 occurrence in patients with systemic autoimmune diseases when compared to the general population, especially in patients without ongoing immunosuppressive [3].

To conclude, the results of an online survey reflect the perception of Romanian patients with SS on the SARS-CoV-2 outbreak, COVID-19 infection, and vaccination. SS does not appear to be a risk factor for severe COVID-19. Moreover, the vaccination against COVID-19 in our group of patients appeared to be safe [87].

COVID 19 in vasculitis

Vasculitis is a large group of disorders that may evolve into systemic diseases; as the name says, it is an inflammation of the blood vessel wall that can occur in any organ, including the skin. Therapy is based on the diameter of the affected vessels (small, medium, or large), the type of lessons, and the systemic affection [88].

Patients with vasculitis diagnosis are usually on cytotoxic, corticosteroids and synthetic disease-modifying antirheumatic drugs (b/tsDMARDs) treatment; this puts these patients at particular risk because it has been reported the capacity of COVID-19 damage into the endothelial cells; SARS-CoV-2 could damage the main functions of the endothelium, which goes from a barrier to thromboregulation and angiogenesis functions. Affecting, the endothelium could release an autoimmune reaction that could last several times, realizing cycling in the reaction, creating antibodies that continue to damage the endothelium [89].

In addition to this well-known affection, COVID-19 may mimic classic vasculitis lesions, such as transient livedo reticularis, Kawasaki-like disease, or some cases of macrophagic activate syndrome, realizing confusion in some cases getting a differential diagnosis and choice of treatment [90].

The affection of COVID-19 could go to the endothelium in the body; for example, there are reports of vasculitis in the brain related to COVID-19 possible due to angiotensin-converting enzyme (ACE2), which primary receptor for SARS-CoV-2 is expressed by endothelial cells and uncomplicated cases like vasculitis leukocytoclastic in the skin [91,92].

In relation to pathogenesis, it is essential to mention that after COVID-19 endothelial cell and diffuse endothelial inflammation have been reported, followed by endothelium, apoptosis, and pyroptosis in autopsies of COVID-19 cases.

An acceptable theory would be that type 2 T-helper immune response to type 3 hypersensitivity is involved in these alterations, with immune complexes inside the vessels. It is causing a severe inflammatory reaction with the help of interleukin-6.

The findings have been mononuclear cell infiltrations into the vascular intima along the lumen of many vessels, suggesting that the SARS CoV-2 can invade the vessels, causing vasculitis [93].

The extensive antigen-antibody immune complexes cannot be quickly cleared. Thus, patients start to create type III hypersensitivity immune response, including protease releases, that can damage the endothelium, inducing inflammation through the body, causing Kawasaki or Kawasaki-like syndrome, but following that, there could be secondary antibodies that could continue damaging the endothelium [94].

According to epidemiological aspects, there are several case reports of patients with vasculitis. However, some Centers have had a follow-up of these, with interesting results. There is a multicentric cohort in the UK and Ireland that was able to follow 65 patients with COVID-19 and vasculitis diagnosis, being the most common vasculitis 55/65 (85%) antineutrophil cytoplasm antibody-associated vasculitis, 24 with granulomatosis with polyangiitis, 25 with microscopic polyangiitis, and 6 with eosinophilic granulomatosis with polyangiitis. Most of these patients were on corticosteroid treatment. Seven of these patients died (28%). However, of interest that 59/65 patients (90.8%) required hospitalization [95].

In addition, the Department of Rheumatology at Istanbul reported 211 cases with vasculitis within 1 year, 49 with systemic vasculitis in their cohort. None of the patients reported symptoms associated with COVID-19.

There was the possibility of follow-up with 103 patients. The main findings were that four patients applied to the hospital with suspicion of COVID-19, but were ruled out, just one patient with granulomatosis with polyangiitis during hospitalization for disease flare was diagnosed with COVID-19, but despite treatment, died in the hospital [96].

There are some reports of cerebral vasculitis, small and medium vessels; these studies, they compare two groups of patients with neurological involvements; of note, patients with vasculitis were found just in the SARS-CoV-2 group, and these patients presented multifocal involvements in the brain and were older than the control group with negative SARS-CoV-2. This reinforces the idea that the ACE2 receptors have a high affinity for endothelial cells event in the brain [97].

Patients with ANCA-associated vasculitis usually have the affection of predominantly small and medium-sized arteries, with similar affection in the kidney histology (necrotizing, pauci-immune glomerulonephritis, these patients are on immunosuppression, that in concept, put them at risk of complications. Besides that, there is a cross-sectional study by Kant et al. [98] who followed up 206 patients; all patients followed personal protective measures, 193 patients were asymptomatic during the follow-up, and there were just three positive COVID-19 patients, two with PR3 positive and one with MPO positive, two requiring hospitalizations but the three recovered in a median of 25 days. Although there were 12 patients with disease relapse, those patients did not have a SARS-CoV-2 infection during the relapse [98].

Regarding Kawasaki disease, there have been reports that suggest that the number of children with multisystem inflammatory symptoms has been increasing, mainly 2 weeks after the COVID-19 epidemic; the sudden exposure to new antigens might trigger a particular uncontrolled immune response in susceptible individuals, of interest, Ouldai et al. [99] found two peaks of Kawasaki disease, one with the influenza A H1NI1 (up to 365% increase) and one in the SARS Cov2 pandemic (up to 6 cases per month) and were available to test 10 patients with SARS-CoV-2 PCR or serology, obtaining a positive result in 80% of the cases, all of the patients were treated with IgG; suggesting a link between these viral infections because of the exposure to a new pathogen without previous immunological memory.

Patients with Behcet's disease are in immunosuppressive and immunomodulatory treatment. Dutson et al. [100] reported a follow-up of 4 months of patients with this disease;

the study included 54 patients with different strategies, seven of them reduced the doses of treatments and three changed in the prescription, none of them developed COVID-19 or life treatment activations. There were just three cases of thrombophlebitis that were not related to COVID-19; the main utilized drugs were colchicine, colchicine + azathioprine; there was home isolation for most patients.

Long COVID. Post-COVID Syndrome, or long haulers, as it has been called, is one of the exciting topics of research; it is true that the persistent symptoms, including neurologic alterations, have been reported even after mild COVID-19 [101].

Nevertheless, of interest, Sollini et al. [102] realized a comparative study in recovered COVID-19 patients with FDG positron emission tomography, and finding a target to blood pool ratio significantly higher in three vascular regions of COVID-19 recovered patients (thoracic aorta, right iliac artery and femoral arteries) suggesting that this vascular inflammation, may be responsible for the persisting symptoms.

In conclusion, patients with vasculitis are constantly on immunosuppressor or immunomodulatory treatments, putting them at risk for complications due to COVID-19. However, due to date, there is no evidence to discontinue treatment or change on prescription. These patients may benefit from protective measures and, if possible, home isolation, mainly when receiving a subsequent therapy, such as rituximab, or cyclophosphamide, or have had a change in medication due to a disease flare. Although there are cohorts with a high number of hospitalizations, the outcomes are favorable for most cases. When hospitalized, they should receive treatment for the life treatment condition, or if not, standard care for COVID-19.

Preexisting endocrine disorders and COVID-19

General aspects

The immune-neuroendocrine system is essential to maintain homeostasis, especially during stressful situations. COVID 19 produces an intense activation and interaction of the immune system and other ways, such as neuroendocrine and hematological. Therefore, COVID-19 infection produces stress and activates different axis of the immune–neuroendocrine system, such as the HPA axis, HPT axis, and HPG axis, among others [103,104].

Several independent risk factors have been described for increased morbidity and mortality in patients with COVID 19. These factors are age ≥65 years, diabetes mellitus, arterial hypertension, overweight/obesity, asthma, chronic obstructive pulmonary disease, immunocompromise chronic systemic disease, immunosuppressive therapies, especially the preexistent cardiometabolic diseases such as diabetes and obesity [105]. Innate and adaptive immune systems are hyperactive with overproduction of IL-1β, IL-6, IL-10, TNF-α, and IFN-γ, among others, leading to CSS respiratory complications [105].

Multiple biomarkers have been associated with more significant mortality: elevated levels of cardiac troponin, C-reactive protein, interleukin-6, D-dimer, creatinine, as well as decreased levels of albumin. Other biomarkers of morbimortality are lymphopenia, increased lactic dehydrogenase (LDH), C-reactive protein, procalcitonin, D-dimer, and ferritin. Patients with underlying cardiometabolic disease, acute inflammation, and end-organ damage are at higher risk of mortality due to COVID-19 infection and should be managed with greater intensity [106].

COVID-19 in pituitary disorders

Coronavirus entry into host cells is mediated by the viral transmembrane spike (S) glycoprotein binding the metallopeptidase ACE2(114–115). ACE2 has been identified as the functional receptor for infection of SARS-CoV-2 and SARS-CoV-2 mediating viral entry in concert with S glycoprotein priming by the host cell transmembrane serine protease 2 (TMPRSS2) [107,108]. SARS-CoV-2 revealed a 10–20-fold higher binding affinity than the SARS-CoV, explaining at least its higher transmissibility and infectivity [109]. ACE2 expression on cerebral vascular endothelium, neurons, and glial cells may play a role in SARS-CoV-2 neural invasion and COVID-19 neurological involvement presenting with headache, confusion, dysgeusia, anosmia, nausea, and vomiting [110,111]. ACE2 mRNA expression was also reported in hypothalamus and pituitary gland cells [112]. Moreover, in a previous study, SARS-CoV was detected in pituitary tissues of patients who died from SARS [113]. Some disorders of the endocrine glands and their main axes will be mentioned below.

Hypothalamic–pituitary–adrenal axis

The Hypothalamic-pituitary-adrenal axis is activated after a viral infection and stress situation. Cytokines are released to stimulate the hypothalamus and release the corticotrophin-releasing hormone (CRH) [113,114], subsequently the anterior pituitary gland and consequently releasing the adrenocorticotropic hormone (ACTH), ending with the release of corticoids by the adrenal glands [115,116]. These corticoids yield negative feedback on immune cells, suppressing the synthesis and release of the cytokines TNF-α, IL-1β, and IL-6 [117]. Another function of glucocorticoids is to change from Th1- to Th2-type immune responses, thus counterbalancing tissue damage [118]. The SARS-CoV-2 virus is neurotropic. COVID-19 infection alters the stress response system, which contributes to the worsening of elderly patients or those with an autoimmune disease. Patients severely infected with COVID-19 exhibited significantly lower cortisol levels than severely infected non-COVID-19 patients [119].

Another study evaluated adrenocortical function in a group of patients with COVID-19, in which the study's findings suggest an inadequate response of the HPA axis [120]. In support of these findings, an autopsy study of COVID-19 patients revealed enlarged hematomas, diffuse bleeding, thrombus, necrosis, and the inflammatory infiltrate of adrenal glands. Taken this evidence together, COVID-19 has a devastating effect on the hypothalamic-pituitary-adrenal axis, that is, the central stress response system [121].

Hypothalamic–pituitary-gonadal axis

The relation between HPGA and the immune response can be sustained by specific facts, such as the gonadotropin-releasing hormone (GnRH) produced by immune cells; estrogens stimulate the immune response, and androgens inhibit this response [122]. It was observed that men present more complications than women due to the levels of androgens, particularly in the expression of a gene, TMPRSS2, whose transcription is regulated by androgen receptors [123]. Concerning ACE2 receptors and SARS-CoV-2 interaction, estrogens and androgens increase their expression [124]. It was evidenced that the hypothalamic-pituitary-gonadal axis can be directly affected by COVID-19, destroying Sertoli cells and Leydig cells, causing a worsening of spermatogenesis and a decrease in testosterone levels [125]. Several investigations have shown the involvement of the COVID-19 infection in the ovarian reserve and can affect the reproductive function of fertile women. Therefore, the latter will be monitored when COVID-19 occurs in women of reproductive age [126]. This evidence indicates the involvement of COVID-19 infection with the HPG axis. The consequence of this damage needs to be studied in the post-COVID-19 stage.

Hypothalamic–pituitary–thyroid axis

The HPT axis has a clear relation with the immune system, and low T3 and T4 were found in some infections [127]. During the cytokine storm for COVID-19, thyrotoxicosis and low free T3 concentrations have been described. Infection by SARS-CoV-2 can destroy thyroid follicular cells and could be the reason for thyrotoxicosis [128]. Affectation of the HPT axis can occur in two ways: by direct interaction between the SARS-CoV-2 and the thyroid glands or using the hyperinflammatory response. In either situation, thyroiditis occurs. This is probably due to the high number of ACE-2 receptors in the thyroid glands [129]. The description is of interest of some cases of Graves' disease and thyroiditis in post-COVID19 vaccinated patients [130,131].

Preexisting pituitary condition, glands disorders, and COVID-19

Several pituitary diseases, that is., hypopituitarism, Cushing disease, adrenal insufficiency, and frequent comorbidities such as diabetes, may be a risk factor for severe COVID 19 in affected patients [132].

Endocrine diseases, especially those of autoimmune origin, play an essential role in COVID 19. An endocrine phenotype has been described for COVID-19 due to the involvement of multiple endocrine organs and tissues and hormonal substances, the alterations that can adversely affect patients with COVID-19 [133,134]. Susceptibility to infections, hypertension, and increased mortality independently of sex and age are specific risk factors for pituitary patients like those affected by Cushing's disease [135]. Cardiovascular disease (heart attack and stroke) is the leading cause of death, consistent with the increased cardiovascular risk profile that this condition entails. However, the mortality excess is also associated with bacterial, viral, and fungal infections, particularly pneumonia, to which patients with hypercortisolism are particularly exposed due to the inhibitory effect of supraphysiological doses of glucocorticoids on the immune system [136,137], such as inhibition of proinflammatory genes [138], stimulation of genes coding for antiinflammatory proteins, inhibition of cytokines, direct action on immune system cells [139,140].

A young woman with Cushing's disease reported moderate to severe COVID-19 despite the lack of known risk factors associated with severe SARS-CoV-2 infection [141]. Recently, in a large Italian series of 61 patients with Cushing disease, it has been reported that 3.2% of them had confirmed COVID-19 as compared to the 0.6% of the general population. Severe clinical presentation was observed, especially in patients with active Cushing disease, suggesting that chronic hypercortisolism may be associated with more SARS-CoV-2 severe infection and confirming that patients with biochemically active Cushing disease may be considered a high-risk population for COVID-19 [142]. This was recently confirmed in another case series of 22 patients with active Cushing's syndrome, in which three cases of COVID-19 were found ranging from very severe to mild depending on the severity of hypercortisolism [144]. Therefore, strict surveillance and early intervention in suspected SARS-CoV-2 infection patients with severe hypercortisolism may be recommended.

Recently, a frequency of COVID 19 of 3.2% has been reported in patients with preexisting Cushing disease, especially in patients with active disease, suggesting that chronic hypercortisolism may be associated with a more severe form of COVID-19, for which these patients are considered at high risk of COVID-19 [141–144]. These results have been observed in other studies.

COVID-19 in hypopituitarism and adrenal insufficiency

In patients with adrenal insufficiency, there is twice the mortality than in the average population, mainly due to cardiovascular disease and infections [145], especially for respiratory causes, and a higher number of hospitalizations due to altered immune responses with reduced cytotoxic function of NK cells [145–147].

Importantly, patients with adrenal insufficiency are at high risk of overtreatment since established glucocorticoid replacement regimens do not wholly reproduce the endogenous hormonal production, and reliable clinical and biochemical markers are lacking [148] with consequent increased risk for Diabetes Mellitus, overweight, hypertension, and chronic inflammatory disease, all conditions currently recognized as risk factors for poor outcomes and death in COVID-19 [136,149].

Importantly, patients with adrenal insufficiency are at high risk of overtreatment since established glucocorticoid replacement regimens do not entirely reproduce the endogenous hormonal production and reliable clinical and biochemical markers are lacking [148] with consequent increased risk for DM, overweight, hypertension, and chronic inflammatory disease, all conditions currently recognized as risk factors for poor outcomes and death in COVID-19 [149,150]. However, there are still few reports regarding the prevalence and clinical outcomes in patients with hypopituitarism and/or adrenal insufficiency infected (Table 24.2).

TABLE 24.2 Characteristics of patients with autoimmune/inflammatory diseases with COVID-19 (n: 113).

Variables	n = 113	Frequency (%)
Diagnostic and type		
Rheumatoid arthritis	30	26.5
Systemic lupus erythematosus	24	21.2
Lupus nephritis	8	7.1
Systemic sclerosis	16	14.2

TABLE 24.2 Characteristics of patients with autoimmune/inflammatory diseases with COVID-19 (n: 113).—cont'd

Variables	n = 113	Frequency (%)
Diffuse	10	8.8
Limited	6	5.3
Primary antiphospholipid syndrome	12	10.6
ANCA vasculitis	8	7.1
Granulomatosis with polyangiitis	6	5.3
Microscopic polyangiitis	1	0.9
Eosinophilic granulomatosis with polyangiitis	1	0.9
Autoimmune encephalitis	6	5.3
Multiple sclerosis	3	2.7
Sjögren's syndrome	2	1.8
Hashimoto's thyroiditis	2	1.8
ASIA	2	1.8
Systemic lupus erythematosus + rheumatoid arthritis	2	1.8
Polymyositis	1	0.9
Gout	1	0.9
Immune thrombocytopenic purpura	1	0.9
Fibromyalgia	1	0.9
Undifferentiated arthritis	1	0.9
Psoriasis	1	0.9
Years of follow-up π	11.87	±9.4
Immunosuppressive therapy prior COVID		
Prednisone	70	61.9
Methotrexate	23	20.3
Mycophenolate mofetil	16	14.2
Chloroquine	15	13.2
Azathioprine	3	2.7
Rituximab	3	2.7
Cyclophosphamide	2	1.8

ANCA, antineutrophil cytoplasmic antibodies; *ASIA*, autoimmune/inflammatory syndrome induced by adjuvants.
π, Mean ± standard deviation.

Three cases of hypopituitarism and adrenal insufficiency have been reported, during their hospitalization, the hydrocortisone dose was increased without observing a greater severity of COVID 19 than the general population, and they were discharged between 3 and 6 days [151].

Noteworthy, recent findings hypothesized possible beneficial effects in severe COVID-19 for dexamethasone and methylprednisolone [152], likely via inhibition of SARS-CoV-2 entry into cells by binding to ACE2 [153]. The use of high-dose potent exogenous glucocorticoids may suppress the hypothalamic-pituitary-adrenal axis and consequent adrenal insufficiency depending on dose, duration of treatment, and individual sensitivity to the drug [154].

Endocrine and diabetes societies have responded to COVID-19 by producing guidance in cortisol-deficient patients (due to primary adrenal failure or hypopituitarism), patients treated with glucocorticoids for underlying inflammatory conditions, and in patients with diabetes [155]. However, patients with thyroid disorders have not been given specific advice.

COVID-19 in autoimmune thyroids diseases

Autoimmune thyroid disease (AITD) is prevalent, and patients with hypothyroidism or hyperthyroidism belong to a high-risk group [156].

To date, there are no reports of preexisting conditions, specifically, thyroid/AITD and COVID-19. Thyroid abnormalities may represent an isolated alteration, but they also may be the herald of a future autoimmune polyglandular syndrome [157]. They may also precede or follow connective tissue diseases or RA. The mechanisms by which AITD may be linked to systemic autoimmune diseases have not yet been fully understood [158,159]. However, it has been suggested that RA patients do not belong to a high-risk group for COVID-19, and since immunological dysfunction has features related to AITD, one may infer that this is likely also to be the case for AITD [160].

Affected patients with AITD such as Graves' disease often experience as consequences of treatment present severe neutropenia over several weeks and up to several months after first drug exposure. Antithyroid drugs are most frequently associated with thiamazole (methimazole) and carbimazole. Patients may experience acute, severe neutropenia or agranulocytosis and develop fever, chills, sore throat, and muscle/joint pain [161]. Diagnosis can be difficult, especially during the COVID-19 pandemic, but timely recognition is critical because, if left untreated, there is an increase in mortality [162].

A study evaluated the thyroid function of a cohort of COVID-19 patients concerning their clinical features, and biochemical, immunological, and inflammatory markers. The main results were that in 191 patients with COVID-19, 13.1% had abnormal thyroid function. Ten patients had isolated low TSH, suggestive of subclinical thyrotoxicosis due to thyroiditis, although the contribution of autoimmunity was likely in two of them. Autoimmune thyroiditis probably also contributed to subclinical hypothyroidism in another patient. Ten patients had isolated low fT3, likely representing nonthyroidal illness syndrome. A decreasing trend of free triiodothyronine 3 (fT3) with increasing COVID-19 severity ($P = .032$) was found. Patients with low fT3 had severe COVID-19-related outcomes.

In conclusion, around 15% of patients with mild to moderate COVID-19 had thyroid dysfunction. There may be a direct effect of SARS-CoV-2 on thyroid function, potentially exacerbating preexisting autoimmune thyroid disease.

Autoimmune neurological disease and COVID-19

COVID-19 in multiple sclerosis

Multiple sclerosis (MS) is an immune-manifested, chronic immune-mediated, and neurodegenerative disorder. These patients are a group of individuals that received disease-modifying therapy (DMT). They indeed have a higher background of infection when compared to the general population.

Due to the previously explained mechanism, it is expected that COVID-19 can trigger and exacerbate the disease by the potential invasion of SARS-CoV-2 in neurological tissue [163].

The Swedish National Board of Health realized a follow of patients with Sclerosis Multiple in an electronic database; they found that as of January 2021, 501 patients reported as COVID-19 positive, 79 were hospitalized, and 20 required intensive care, suggesting a lower proportion of cases of severe COVID-19 than the general population. They did not find any relation that MS confers a higher risk of more severe infection [164].

There is a significant multicentric study in Italy that included 232 MS patients with suspected or confirmed COVID-19 infection. They followed up with these patients to evaluate the outcomes, although there were just 57/232 cases with positive SARS CoV2- two infections; the rest of the sample with respiratory symptoms (222/232) were fully recovered, and there were just 10 cases with severe disease, with fatal outcome in five of them. Concluding that the severity of the disease was similar to the general population [165].

Kataria et al. [1,163] presented three cases of patients with MS who presented to the clinic with an exacerbation of the disease and a COVID-19 positive test. All three patients presented good evolution.

Of interest there Novi et al. [166] described a case of a patient in treatment with ocrelizumab; he mentioned in his manuscript the probability of a protective role due to the immunosuppressive therapy; in addition, Thornton et al. [167] reported two cases with ocrelizumab treatment with mild disease, and finally, Monterol-Escribano et al. [168], reported six patients on ocrelizumab with mild disease, all recovered, the clinical course of these patients could support the hypothesis of a protective role of the immunosuppressive therapy.

Monterol-Escribano also reported the follow-up of his patients on rituximab, finding that those patients were not at risk of severe disease, just one was hospitalized, but with good outcomes; those findings support that the presence of the B cells are not required for recovery from COVID-19 [168].

To summarize the COVID-19 cases, Möhn et al. [169] realized a review of 873 published cases, reporting the outcomes of 700; he reported that up to 317/873 were under anti-CD20 treatment, but of note, the most exciting report is the global mortality rate was 4%. With all these previously reported studies, we can conclude that immunosuppressive therapy itself does not appear to be substantial; the protective role could be due to the mitigation of the cytokine storm. To date, there is no support to change or alter the standard treatment of MS patients; they should continue standard care and self-protective measures.

COVID-19 in autoimmune encephalitis

In patients with preexisting autoimmune neurological diseases, Neurological complications have been observed coexisting or after COVID-19. These complications could go from mild, nonspecific symptoms, such as headache (a common symptom of SARS-CoV-2 infection), from flare-ups to neurological disease, severe neurological diseases, or the manifestation of Guillain Barre Syndrome, Autoimmune encephalitis, among others. The neurological disorder due to COVID-19 has many mechanisms; at the beginning of the pandemic, it was demanded that it was just for metabolic alterations and due to the cytokine storm; however, further information revealed the presence of SARS-CoV-2 in the brain tissue of a patient, and mechanism such as direct viral invasion of the virus, navigation across nerve synapses, the olfactory nerve, or even due to molecular mimicking of created antibodies increase the interest of the neuroimmunology research. Autoimmune encephalitis is a relatively new disorder that could be underdiagnosed due to some centers' limitations to access the diagnosis tools [170–172].

Regarding, preexisting AE there is no information, only cases post-COVID. In addition to that, COVID-19 critically ill patients present neurological alterations that end with a fatal outcome attributed to critically ill COVID-19 disease. The global pathogeny of COVID-19 has been previously reported; however, regarding the Central Nervous system, some theories try to explain the mechanism of affection in the system; one of them is "cytokine-induced sickness behavior."

This has been reported after viral infections or vaccinations, described as "psychiatric symptoms, such as depressive mood, paranoid and hallucinatory symptoms"; this disease has been attributed to the release of cytokines, such as IL1, Il6, IFN, and tumor necrosis factor-alpha. The pathogeny explains that there is a decreased availability of serotonin due to the cytokines [173]. Moreover, TH17 would play an essential role since it is necessary to activate and difference IL-6 (essential to neutrophil granulocyte migration); in addition, the proinflammatory cytokine IL-17 produced by TH17 and CD4 may disrupt the blood–brain barriers and contribute to secondary autoimmune reactions of SARS-CoV2 with other autoimmune diseases [174].

Another theory is that some viruses can change the development of neuronal circuits, which can trigger an autoimmune response due to molecular mimicking; in genetically vulnerable individuals, AE has been related to these, for example.

NMDAR-encephalitis has been reported after infections such as herpes simplex virus due to the production of antineuronal antibodies; this cross-reactivity is explained because some viruses share a ligand with different antibodies; for example, M transmembrane protein of Influenza A and NMDAR share amantadine ligand [171].

COVID-19 has described a mimicry between the NMDAR-NR1 subunit and viral nonstructural protein eight and between NMDAR-NR2 subunit and viral nonstructural protein 9. This mimicry may lead to generating IgG antibodies against NMDAR subunits for other antibodies [173].

Of interest, a study realized by Sanchez-Valencia et al. [175] tested serum samples of COVID-19 consecutive patients in a laboratory cohort, including residual samples of 556 patients evaluated due to neurological alterations for AE neural antibodies. In this laboratory cohort, they tested the patients' samples for antibodies against the SARS- CoV-2 spike glycoprotein using an FDA-authorized assay; they found five patients that met diagnostic criteria for AE; four of them with favorable outcomes, suggesting just occasional cases of the disease, even in patients with neurological alterations.

Unfortunately, to date, no other cohort has described the characteristics or following of AE diagnosticated patients in the context of the pandemic.

In our hospital, for a year of the patients hospitalized with AID, six patients had AE, all of them undergoing treatment with steroids and rituximab, and IGIV. Of these, five had preexisting AE, one was post-COVID, one patient died from complications of pneumonia, and the rest had a good evolution.

Bennussi et al. [176] in Italy reported clinical and laboratory characteristics, treatment, and clinical outcomes of patients admitted for neurologic diseases with and without coronavirus disease 2019 (COVID-19). They studied 173 patients were included in this study, of whom 56 were positive and 117 were negative for COVID-19. Patients with COVID-19 were older (77.0 years), interquartile range [IQR] 67.0–83.8 versus. 70.1 years, IQR 52.9–78.6 years, $P = .006$), had a different distribution regarding admission diagnoses, including cerebrovascular disorders (n = 43, 76.8% vs. n = 68, 58.1%), and had a higher quick Sequential Organ Failure Assessment (qSOFA) score on admission (0.9, IQR 0.7–1.1 vs. 0.5, IQR 0.4–0.6, $P = .006$). In hospital mortality rates (n = 21, 37.5% vs. n = 5, 4.3%, $P < .001$) and incident delirium (n = 15, 26.8% vs. n = 9, 7.7%, $P = .003$) were significantly higher in the COVID-19 group. Patients with COVID-19 and without COVID with stroke had similar baseline characteristics, but patients with COVID-19 had higher modified Rankin Scale scores at discharge (5.0, IQR 2.0–6.0 vs. 2.0, IQR 1.0–3.0, $P < .001$), with a significantly lower number of patients with a good outcome (n = 11, 25.6% vs. n = 48, 70.6%, $P < .001$). In patients with COVID-19, multivariable regressions showed increased odds of in-hospital death associated with higher qSOFA scores (odds ratio [OR] 4.47, 95% [CI] 1.21–16.5, $P = .025$), lower platelet count (OR 0.98, 95% CI 0.97–0.99, $P = .005$), and higher lactate dehydrogenase (OR 1.01, 95% CI 1.00–1.03, $P = .009$) on admission. In conclusion, patients with COVID-19 admitted with neurologic disease, including stroke, have a significantly higher in-hospital mortality and incident delirium and higher disability than patients without COVID-19.

Experience in autoimmune diseases and COVID-19 in a single Mexican center

To conclude this chapter, we will share our center's experience with COVID-19 patients with preexisting AID.

We performed a comparative prospective cohort study in a Tertiary Referral Center between April 2020 and April 2021 in México City. We included ≥18-year-old patients with autoimmune diseases, according to the American College of Rheumatology/European League Against Rheumatism (ACR/EULAR) with COVID-19. We paired patients by age and gender, comparing them with patients without AID. There were 113 AID patients with a median follow-up of 11.87 years; most of them were on immunosuppressive treatment; the autoimmune diseases are reported in Table 24.3. These patients were compared with 113 patients only with COVID-19.

The global mortality of COVID-AID patients was 33/113 (29%), although this seems like a high number compared with worldwide mortality when compared with patients without AID, the latter group has a higher mortality rate 48/113 (43%); this may be due to different

TABLE 24.3 Clinical, biochemical characteristics, comorbidities, and treatment of patients with AID (n: 113) and controls (n: 113) with COVID-19.

Variables	AID, n = 113 (%)	Controls n = 113 (%)	p[a]
Age (years) π	51.15 (±14.3)	53.45 ± (13.3)	0.216[d]
Female gender	81 (71.7)	83 (73.5)	0.766
Obesity	**37 (32.7)**	**98 (86.7)**	**<0.0001[b]**
Arterial hypertension	41 (36.3)	47 (41.6)	0.451
Diabetes mellitus	26 (23.0)	33 (29.2)	0.289
Ischemic heart disease	**7 (6.2)**	**0 (0)**	**0.007[b]**
Neoplasms	**6 (5.3)**	**19 (16.8)**	**0.006**
Hypothyroidism	9 (8.0)	3 (2.7)	0.068[b]
Initial O_2 saturation (%) μ	88.0 (78–92)	85 (77–92)	0.387[c]
CO-RADS Ω			
1	**6 (9.8)**	**0 (0)**	**0.005**
2	3 (4.9)	3 (3.9)	0.782
3	11 (18.0)	12 (15.8)	0.727
4	12 (19.7)	12 (15.8)	0.552
5	**25 (41.0)**	**49 (64.5)**	**0.006**
6	**4 (6.6)**	**0 (0)**	**0.023**
CT severity score Ω			
Mild	31 (50.8)	27 (35.5)	0.071
Moderate	27 (44.2)	34 (44.7)	0.955
Severe	**3 (4.9)**	**15 (19.7)**	**0.010**
Leukocytes (cels/mm3) μ	7100 (46,00–113,50)	8700 (60,00–129,42)	0.067[c]
Lymphocytes (cels/mm3) μ	**1450 (800–3290)**	**860 (570–1332)**	**<0.0001[c]**
Platelets (K/uL) μ	201.70 (150.0–294.1)	229.00 (146.2–314.2)	0.071[c]
Glucose (mg/dL) μ	111.6 (91.2–143.2)	119.1 (100.0–176.7)	0.085[c]
Creatinine (mg/dL) μ	0.80 (0.6–1.1)	0.84 (0.6–1.25)	0.324[c]
LDH (U/L) μ	**398.50 (280.5–574.0)**	**552.00 (409.0–864.0)**	**<0.0001[c]**
ESR (mm/h) μ	36.00 (29.0–40.0)	35.50 (20.0–43.2)	0.738[c]
CRP (mg/L) μ	**21.80 (9.5–59.6)**	**72.35 (19.9–165.0)**	**0.002[c]**
Fibrinogen (g/L) μ	464.00 (398.0–664.5)	500.00 (356.2–632.2)	0.842[c]
D-dimer (ng/mL)	861.0 (315.0–3892.0)	854.0 (443.5–2360.5)	0.907[c]

TABLE 24.3 Clinical, biochemical characteristics, comorbidities, and treatment of patients with AID (n: 113) and controls (n: 113) with COVID-19.—cont'd

Variables	AID, n = 113 (%)	Controls n = 113 (%)	p[a]
Treatment			
Antimalarial	32 (28.3)	24 (21.2)	0.218
Glucocorticoid	**68 (60.2)**	**34 (30.1)**	**<0.0001**
Anticoagulant	**83 (73.5)**	**66 (58.4)**	**0.017**
Outcomes			
LoS μ	7.00 (0.5–10.0)	6.0 (2.0–12.0)	0.633[c]
Days with IMV μ	6.0 (2.0–15.0)	3.0 (1.5–7.5)	0.251[c]
IMV	**19 (16.8)**	**33 (29.2)**	**0.027**
Death	**33 (29.2)**	**48 (42.5)**	**0.037**
Septic shock	22 (19.4)	21 (18.5)	0.960
Respiratory insufficiency	11 (9.7)	13 (11.5)	0.912
Discharge with O_2	**11 (13.6)**	**27 (41.5)**	**<0.0001**

[a]*Chi-square test.*
[b]*Fisher's exact test.*
[c]*Mann–Whitney U test.*
[d]*T student for independent samples.*
AID, autoimmune/inflammatory diseases; *CO-RADS*, COVID-19 Reporting and Data System; *CRP*, C reactive protein; *CT*, computed tomography; *ESR*, erythrocyte sedimentation rate; *IMV*, invasive mechanical ventilation; *LDH*, lactic dehydrogenase; *LoS*, length of stay.
π, Mean ± standard deviation.
μ Median and IQR.
Ω AID n = 61; controls n = 76.

factors: Mexican population has a high proportion of obesity, diabetes, and hypertension, in addition, being our Hospital a Referral Center, there were a high proportion of critically ill patients requiring invasive mechanical ventilation (IMV) and due to limitation of UCI beds, must of the patients, were treated in the general ward, being a challenge for nonintensive care physicians. In this study patients with AID had better outcomes for COVID-19 (less mortality, IMV, and less oxygen on discharge) than patients without AID. Also, the use of anticoagulation was associated with a lower death in patients with AID [177].

Conclusions

Patients with preexisting autoimmune diseases may flare during the SARS-CoV-2 infection.

The SARS-CoV-2 virus penetrates various tissues and organs through ACE- two and leads to endothelial damage that may cause vascular manifestations, including thrombosis. The pathogenesis of COVID 19 is complex and involves a CSS shared by immunoinflammatory disease.

According to studies carried out in patients with inflammatory arthritis, especially RA and seronegative spondyloarthropathies, it has been suggested that the immunosuppressive therapy, older age, male sex, and the presence of comorbidities similar to those in the general population (hypertension, lung disease, diabetes, cardiovascular diseases, and chronic renal insufficiency/end-stage renal disease) could be associated with an increased risk of infections and high rate of hospitalization. On the other hand, it has been shown that lower odds of hospitalization were associated with bDMARD or tsDMARDs monotherapy, mainly driven by anti-TNF therapies.

The risk for critical COVID-19 in patients with systemic inflammatory diseases such as inflammatory arthritis, SLE, SS, SSc, and vasculitis might be increased.

Regarding endocrine diseases, in general, it has been described that there is a dysfunction of the main axis, especially the hypothalamic-pituitary-adrenal axis. It is essential to evaluate thyroid diseases due to the primary injury to this gland may play a key role in the pathogenesis of thyroid disorders in COVID-19 patients.

Patients with preexisting autoimmune neurological diseases may also increase the risk of neurologic manifestations in COVID-19 patients. The clinical spectrum and consequences of neurologic manifestations in COVID-19 patients are broad and heterogeneous.

References

[1] Heikkinen T, Järvinen A. The common cold. Lancet January 4, 2003;361(9351):51–9. https://doi.org/10.1016/S0140-6736(03)12162-9.

[2] Adil MT, Rahman R, Whitelaw D, et al. SARS-CoV-2 and the pandemic of COVID-19. Postgrad Med J February 2021;97(1144):110–6. https://doi.org/10.1136/postgradmedj-2020-138386.

[3] Gao YD, Ding M, Dong X, et al. Risk factors for severe and critically ill COVID-19 patients: a review. Allergy February 2021;76(2):428–55. https://doi.org/10.1111/all.14657.

[4] Lakota K, Perdan-Pirkmajer K, Hočevar A, et al. COVID-19 in association with development, course, and treatment of systemic autoimmune rheumatic diseases. Front Immunol January 26, 2021;11:611318. https://doi.org/10.3389/fimmu.2020.611318.

[5] Kobak S. The perfect storm: a rheumatologist's point of view on COVID-19 infection. Curr Rheumatol Rev 2021;17(2):141–52. https://doi.org/10.2174/1573397116666201029155105.

[6] Soy M, Keser G, Atagündüz P, et al. Cytokine storm in COVID-19: pathogenesis and overview of anti-inflammatory agents used in treatment. Clin Rheumatol July 2020;39(7):2085–94. https://doi.org/10.1007/s10067-020-05190-5.

[7] Hu B, Huang S, Yin L. The cytokine storm and COVID-19. J Med Virol January 2021;93(1):250–6. https://doi.org/10.1002/jmv.26232.

[8] Szcześniak D, Gładka A, Misiak B, et al. The SARS-CoV-2 and mental health: from biological mechanisms to social consequences. Prog Neuro-Psychopharmacol Biol Psychiatry January 10, 2021;104:110046. https://doi.org/10.1016/j.pnpbp.2020.110046.

[9] Jara LJ, López-Zamora B, Ordoñez-González I, et al. The immune-neuroendocrine system in COVID-19, advanced age and rheumatic diseases. Autoimmun Rev November 2021;20(11):102946. https://doi.org/10.1016/j.autrev.2021.102946.

[10] Liu Y, Sawalha AH, Lu Q. COVID-19 and autoimmune diseases. Curr Opin Rheumatol March 1, 2021;33(2):155–62. https://doi.org/10.1097/BOR.0000000000000776.

[11] Stradner MH, Dejaco C, Zwerina J, Fritsch-Stork RD. Rheumatic musculoskeletal diseases and COVID-19 A review of the first 6 Months of the pandemic. Front Med 2020;7:562142. https://doi.org/10.3389/fmed.2020.562142. Published 2020 Oct 9.

[12] Li J, Liu HH, Yin XD, Li CC, Wang J. COVID-19 illness and autoimmune diseases: recent insights. Inflamm Res 2021;70(4):407–28. https://doi.org/10.1007/s00011-021-01446-1.

[13] Khabbazi A, Kavandi H, Paribanaem R, et al. Adherence to medication in patients with rheumatic diseases during COVID-19 pandemic. Ann Rheum Dis September 7, 2020.

[14] Murtas R, Andreano A, Gervasi F, et al. Association between autoimmune diseases and COVID-19 as assessed in both a test-negative case-control and population case-control design. Auto Immun Highlights 2020;11(1):15. https://doi.org/10.1186/s13317-020-00141-1. Published 2020 Oct 6.

[15] D'Silva KM, Jorge A, Cohen A, et al. COVID-19 outcomes in patients with systemic autoimmune rheumatic diseases compared to the general population: a US multicenter, comparative cohort study. Arthritis Rheumatol 2021;73(6):914–20. https://doi.org/10.1002/art.41619.

[16] Zhu Y, Zhong J, Dong L. Epidemiology and clinical management of rheumatic autoimmune diseases in the COVID-19 pandemic: a review. Front Med August 19, 2021;8:725226. https://doi.org/10.3389/fmed.2021.725226.

[17] Vázquez-Díaz M, Freites Nuñez DD, Leon L. Risk factors for hospital admissions related to COVID-19 in patients with autoimmune inflammatory rheumatic diseases. Rheumatol Int 2020;79:1393–9. https://doi.org/10.1136/annrheumdis-2020-217984.

[18] Sarzi-Puttini P, Marotto D, Caporali R, et al. Prevalence of COVID infections in a population of rheumatic patients from Lombardy and Marche treated with biological drugs or small molecules: a multicentre retrospective study. J Autoimmun 2021;116:102545. https://doi.org/10.1016/j.jaut.2020.102545.

[19] Tiendrébéogo WJS, Kaboré F, Ntsiba H, Montero F. Coronavirus disease 2019. (COVID-19) in autoimmune and inflammatory conditions: clinical characteristics of poor outcomes. Clin Rheumatol 2020;40:1593–8. https://doi.org/10.1007/s00296-020-04676-4.

[20] Gianfrancesco M, Hyrich KL, et al. Characteristics associated with hospitalisation for COVID-19 in people with rheumatic disease: data from the COVID-19 global rheumatology alliance physician-reported registry. Rheumatol Int 2020;79:859–66. https://doi.org/10.1136/annrheumdis-2020-217871.

[21] Pablos JL. Clinical outcomes of hospitalised patients with COVID-19 and chronic inflammatory and autoimmune rheumatic diseases: a multicentric matched cohort study. Cells 2020;79:1544–9. https://doi.org/10.1136/annrheumdis-2020-218296.

[22] Ji W, Huh K, Kang M, et al. Effect of underlying comorbidities on the infection and severity of COVID-19 in Korea: a nationwide case-control study. J Korean Med Sci 2020;35:e237. https://doi.org/10.3346/jkms.2020.35.e237.

[23] Peach E, Rutter M, Lanyon P, et al. Risk of death among people with rare autoimmune diseases compared to the general population in England during the 2020. COVID-19 pandemic. Rheumatology 2020:60. https://doi.org/10.1101/2020.10.09.20210237. eaa855.

[24] Scirè CA, Carrara G, Zanetti A, et al. COVID-19 in rheumatic diseases in Italy: first results from the Italian registry of the Italian Society for Rheumatology (CONTROL-19). Clin Exp Rheumatol 2020;38:748–53.

[25] Tan EH, Sena AG, Prats-Uribe A, You SC, Ahmed WU, Kostka K, et al. COVID-19 in patients with autoimmune diseases: characteristics and outcomes in a multinational network of cohorts across three countries. Rheumatology 2021:keab250. https://doi.org/10.1093/rheumatology/keab250.

[26] Haberman RH, Castillo R, Chen A, et al. COVID-19 in patients with inflammatory arthritis: a prospective study on the effects of comorbidities and disease-modifying antirheumatic drugs on clinical outcomes. Arthritis Rheumatol 2020;72:1981–9. https://doi.org/10.1002/art.41456.

[27] Nuño L, Novella Navarro M, et al. Clinical course, severity and mortality in a cohort of patients with COVID-19 with rheumatic diseases. Ann Rheum Dis 2020;79:1659–61. https://doi.org/10.1136/annrheumdis-2020-218054.

[28] Gianfrancesco MA, Leykina LA, et al. Association of race and ethnicity with COVID-19 outcomes in rheumatic disease: data from the COVID-19 global rheumatology alliance physician registry. Arthritis Rheumatol 2020;73:374–80. https://doi.org/10.1002/art.41567.

[29] Arleo T, Tong D, Shabto J, O'Keefe G, Khosroshahi A. Clinical course and outcomes of COVID-19 in rheumatic disease patients: a case cohort study with a diverse population. Clin Rheumatol 2021;40:2633–42. https://doi.org/10.1007/s10067-021-05578-x.

[30] Kichloo A, Aljadah M, Albosta M, Wani F, Singh J, Solanki S. COVID-19 and acute lupus pneumonitis: diagnostic and treatment dilemma. J Investig Med High Impact Case Rep 2020:8. https://doi.org/10.1177/2324709620933438.

[31] Alharthy A, Faqihi F, Nasim N, et al. COVID-19 in a patient with a flare of systemic lupus erythematosus: a rare case-report. Respir Med Case Rep 2020;31:101252. https://doi.org/10.1016/j.rmcr.2020.101252.

[32] Cavagna L, Seminari E, Zanframundo G, et al. Calcineurin inhibitor-based immunosuppression and COVID-19: results from a multidisciplinary cohort of patients in northern Italy. Microorganisms 2020;8:977. https://doi.org/10.3390/microorganisms8070977.

[33] Misra DP, Agarwal V, Gasparyan AY, Zimba O. Rheumatologists' perspective on coronavirus disease 19 (COVID-19) and potential therapeutic targets. Clin Rheumatol 2020;39:2055–62. https://doi.org/10.1007/s10067-020-.

[34] Favalli EG, Bugatti S, Klersy C, et al. Impact of corticosteroids and immunosuppressive therapies on symptomatic SARS-CoV-2 infection in a large cohort of patients with chronic inflammatory arthritis. Arthritis Res Ther 2020;22:290. https://doi.org/10.1186/s13075-020-02395-6.

[35] Ghazawi FM, Lim M, Dutz JP, Kirchhof MG. Infection risk of dermatologic therapeutics during the COVID-19 pandemic: an evidence-based recalibration. Int J Dermatol 2020;59:1043–56. https://doi.org/10.1111/ijd.

[36] Hariyanto TI, Halim DA, Jodhinata C, Yanto TA, Kurniawan A. Colchicine treatment can improve outcomes of coronavirus disease 2019 (COVID-19): a systematic review and meta-analysis. Clin Exp Pharmacol Physiol 2021;48:823–30. https://doi.org/10.1111/1440-1681.13488.

[37] Zhong J, Shen G, Yang H, et al. COVID-19 in patients with rheumatic disease in Hubei province, China: a multicentre retrospective observational study. Lancet Rheumatol 2020;2:e557–64. https://doi.org/10.1016/S2665-9913(20)30227-7.

[38] Teh CL, Cheong YK, Wan M, et al. COVID-19 among Malaysian patients with systemic lupus erythematosus on hydroxychloroquine. Ann Rheum Dis 2020;80:e69. https://doi.org/10.1136/annrheumdis-2020-218154.

[39] Littlejohn E. Keeping lupus patients on hydroxychloroquine during the COVID-19 pandemic. Cleve Clin J Med 2020. https://doi.org/10.3949/ccjm.87a.ccc023.

[40] Nagaraja BS, Ramesh KN, Dhar D, et al. HyPE study: hydroxychloroquine prophylaxis-related adverse events' analysis among healthcare workers during COVID-19 pandemic: a rising public health concern. J Public Health 2020;42:493–503. https://doi.org/10.1093/pubmed/fdaa074.

[41] Ahmadinejad Z, Assari R, Ayoobi, et al. COVID-19 pandemic and biological therapy in rheumatologic disorders: how to deal with? Reumatismo 2020;72:173–7. https://doi.org/10.4081/reumatismo.2020.1289.

[42] Sharmeen S, Elghawy A, Zarlasht F, Yao Q. COVID-19 in rheumatic disease patients on immunosuppressive agents. Semin Arthritis Rheum 2020;50:680–6. https://doi.org/10.1016/j.semarthrit.2020.05.010.

[43] Ikonomidis I, Pavlidis G, Katsimbri P, et al. Tocilizumab improves oxidative stress and endothelial glycocalyx: a mechanism that may explain the effects of biological treatment on COVID-19. Food Chem Toxicol 2020;145:111694. https://doi.org/10.1016/j.fct.2020.111694.

[44] Rossi B, Nguyen LS, Zimmermann P, et al. Effect of tocilizumab in hospitalized patients with severe COVID-19 pneumonia: a case-control cohort study. Pharmaceuticals 2020;13:317. https://doi.org/10.3390/ph13100317.

[45] Hariyanto TI, Hardyson W, Kurniawan A. Efficacy and safety of tocilizumab for coronavirus disease 2019 (COVID-19) patients: a systematic review and meta-analysis. Drug Res 2021;71:265–74. https://doi.org/10.1055/a-1336-2371.

[46] Ti H, Kurniawan A. Tocilizumab administration is associated with the reduction in biomarkers of coronavirus disease 2019 infection. J Med Virol 2021;93:1832–6. https://doi.org/10.1002/jmv.26698.

[47] D'Silvaa KM, Wallacea ZS. COVID-19 and rheumatoid arthritis. Curr Opin Rheumatol 2021;33:255–61. https://doi.org/10.1097/BOR.0000000000000786.

[48] FAI2R/SFR/SNFMI/SOFREMIP/CRI/IMIDIATE consortium and contributors. Severity of COVID-19 and survival in patients with rheumatic and inflammatory diseases: data from the French RMD COVID-19 cohort of 694 patients. Ann Rheum Dis 2020;80:527–38. https://doi.org/10.1136/annrheumdis-2020-218310.

[49] Marques CDL, Kakehasi AM, Pinheiro MM, et al. High levels of immunosuppression are related to unfavourable outcomes in hospitalised patients with rheumatic diseases and COVID-19: first results of ReumaCoV Brasil registry. RMD Open 2021;7:e001461. https://doi.org/10.1136/rmdopen-.

[50] Zen M, Fuzzi E E, Astorri D, et al. SARS-CoV-2 infection in patients with autoimmune rheumatic diseases in northeast Italy: a cross-sectional study on 916 patients. J Autoimm 2020. https://doi.org/10.1016/j.jaut.2020.102502.

[51] Ge E, Li Y, Wu S, et al. Association of pre-existing comorbidities with mortality and disease severity among 167,500 individuals with COVID-19 in Canada: a population-based cohort study. PLoS One 2021;16(10):e0258154. https://doi.org/10.1371/journal.pone.0258154. eCollection 2021.

[52] Sanchez-Piedra C, Diaz-Torne C, Manero J, Pego-Reigosa JM, Rúa-Figueroa Í, Gonzalez-Gay MA, et al. Clinical features and outcomes of COVID-19 in patients with rheumatic diseases treated with biological and synthetic targeted therapies. Ann Rheum Dis 2020;79(7):988–90. https://doi.org/10.1136/annrheumdis-2020-217948.

[53] Pablos JL, Galindo M, Carmona L, et al. Clinical outcomes of hospitalised patients with COVID-19 and chronic inflammatory and autoimmune rheumatic diseases: a multicentric matched cohort study. Ann Rheum Dis 2020;79(12):1544–9. https://doi.org/10.1136/annrheumdis-2020-218296.

[54] Ono K, Kishimoto M, Shimasaki T, Uchida H, Kurai D, Deshpande GA, Komagata Y, Kaname S. Reactive arthritis after COVID-19 infection. RMD Open August 2020;6(2):e001350. https://doi.org/10.1136/rmdopen-2020-001350.

[55] Freites Nuñez DD, Leon L, Mucientes A, et al. Risk factors for hospital admissions related to COVID-19 in patients with autoimmune inflammatory rheumatic diseases. Ann Rheum Dis 2020;79(11):1393–9. https://doi.org/10.1136/annrheumdis-2020-217984.

[56] Ferrara F, Santilli P, D'Aiuto V, Vitiello A. Clinical pharmacology aspects in patients treated with TNF inhibitors during SARS-CoV-2 pandemic. Adv Pharm Bull May 2021;11(3):393–4. https://doi.org/10.34172/apb.2021.045. Epub 2020 Oct 20.

[57] Giannis D, Ziogas IA, Gianni P. Coagulation disorders in coronavirus infected patients: COVID-19, SARS-CoV-1, MERS-CoV and lessons from the past. J Clin Virol 2020;127:104362.

[58] Zhang Y, Xiao M, Zhang S, et al. Coagulopathy and antiphospholipid antibodies in patients with COVID-19. N Engl J Med 2020;382(17):e38.

[59] El Hasbani G, Taher AT, Jawad A, Uthman I. COVID-19, antiphospholipid antibodies, and Catastrophic antiphospholipid syndrome: a possible association? Clin Med Insights Arthritis Musculoskelet Disord 2020;13. https://doi.org/10.1177/1179544120978667. 1179544120978667.

[60] Helms J, Tacquard C, Severac F, et al. High risk of thrombosis in patients with severe SARS-CoV-2 infection: a multicenter prospective cohort study. Intensive Care Med 2020;46(6):1089–98. https://doi.org/10.1007/s00134-020-06062-x.

[61] Borghi MO, Beltagy A, Garrafa E, et al. Anti-phospholipid antibodies in COVID-19 are different from those detectable in the anti-phospholipid syndrome. Front Immunol 2020;11:584241. https://doi.org/10.3389/fimmu.2020.584241.

[62] Xiao M, Zhang Y, Zhang S, et al. Antiphospholipid antibodies in critically ill patients with COVID-19. Arthritis Rheumatol 2020;72(12):1998–2004. https://doi.org/10.1002/art.41425. Epub 2020 Oct 7. PMID: 32602200; PMCID: PMC7361932.

[63] Choi B, Choudhary MC, Regan J, et al. Persistence and evolution of SARS-CoV-2 in an immunocompromised host. N Engl J Med 2020;383(23):2291–3. https://doi.org/10.1056/NEJMc2031364.

[64] Escher R, Breakey N, Lämmle B. Severe COVID-19 infection associated with endothelial activation. Thromb Res 2020;190:62. https://doi.org/10.1016/j.thromres.2020.04.014.

[65] Colafrancesco S, Alessandri C, Conti F, Priori R. COVID-19 gone bad: a new character in the spectrum of the hyperferritinemic syndrome? Autoimmun Rev 2020;19(7):102576. https://doi.org/10.1016/j.autrev.2020.102573.

[66] Harzallah I, Debliquis A, Drénou B. Frequency of lupus anticoagulant in COVID-19 patients. J Thromb Haemost 2020;18:2778. https://doi.org/10.1111/jth.14937.

[67] Spihlman AP, Gadi N, Wu SC, Moulton VR. COVID-19 and systemic lupus erythematosus: focus on immune response and therapeutics. Front Immunol October 30, 2020;11:589474. https://doi.org/10.3389/fimmu.2020.589474.

[68] Pascolini S, Vannini A, Deleonardi G, et al. COVID-19 and immunological dysregulation: can autoantibodies be useful? Clin Transl Sci March 2021;14(2):502–8.

[69] Bonometti R, Sacchi M, Stobbione P, et al. The first case of systemic lupus erythematosus (SLE) triggered by COVID-19 infection. Eur Rev Med Pharmacol Sci 2020;24:9695–7.

[70] Mantovani Cardoso E, Hundal J, Feterman D, Magaldi J. Concomitant new diagnosis of systemic lupus erythematosus and COVID-19 with possible antiphospholipid syndrome. Just a coincidence? A case report and review of intertwining pathophysiology. Clin Rheumatol 2020;39(9):2811–5. https://doi.org/10.1007/s10067-020-05310-1.

[71] Monti S, Balduzzi S, Delvino P, Bellis E, Quadrelli VS, Montecucco C. Clinical course of COVID-19 in a series of patients with chronic arthritis treated with immunosuppressive targeted therapies. Ann Rheum Dis 2020;79:667–8. https://doi.org/10.1136/annrheumdis-2020-217424.

[72] Thanou A, Sawalha AH. SARS-CoV-2 and systemic lupus erythematosus. Curr Rheumatol Rep 2021;23(2):8. https://doi.org/10.1007/s11926-020-00973-w.

[73] Hyrich KL, Machado PM. Rheumatic disease and COVID-19: epidemiology and outcomes. Nat Rev Rheumatol February 2021;17(2):71–2. https://doi.org/10.1038/s41584-020-00562-2.

[74] Fernandez-Ruiz R, Masson M, Kim MY, et al. Leveraging the United States epicenter to provide insights on COVID-19 in patients with systemic lupus erythematosus. Arthritis Rheumatol 2020;72(12):1971–80. https://doi.org/10.1002/art.41450.

[75] Pellegrino G, Mohammad Reza Beigi D, Angelelli C, et al. COVID-19 and systemic sclerosis: analysis of lifestyle changes during the SARS-CoV-2 pandemic in an Italian single-center cohort. Clin Rheumatol 2021;40(4):1393–7. https://doi.org/10.1007/s10067-020-05504-7.

[76] Del Papa N, Sambataro G, Minniti A, et al. Impact of COVID-19 outbreak in an Italian cohort of patients with systemic sclerosis. Ther Adv Musculoskelet Dis 2020;12. https://doi.org/10.1177/1759720X20953356. 1759720X20953356. Published 2020 Sep. 24.

[77] Ferri C, Giuggioli D, Raimondo V, et al. COVID-19 and rheumatic autoimmune systemic diseases: role of pre-existing lung involvement and ongoing treatments. Curr Pharm Des 2021;27(41):4245–52. https://doi.org/10.2174/1381612827666210903103935.

[78] Thombs BD, Kwakkenbos L, Henry RS, et al. Changes in mental health symptoms from pre-COVID-19 to COVID-19 among participants with systemic sclerosis from four countries: a Scleroderma Patient-centered Intervention Network (SPIN) Cohort study. J Psychosom Res December 2020;139:110262. https://doi.org/10.1016/j.jpsychores.2020.110262.

[79] Brito-Zeron P, Acar-Denizli N, Zeher M, et al. Influence of geolocation and ethnicity on the phenotypic expression of primary Sjogren's syndrome at diagnosis in 8310 patients: a cross-sectional study from the Big Data Sjogren Project Consortium. Ann Rheum Dis 2017;76:1042–50.

[80] Mariette X, Criswell LA. Primary Sjogren's syndrome. N Engl J Med 2018;378:931–9.

[81] Brito-Zeron P, Kostov B, Fraile G, et al. Characterization and risk estimate of cancer in patients with primary Sjogren syndrome. J Hematol Oncol 2017;10:90.

[82] Ramos-Casals M, Brito-Zeron P, Bombardieri S, et al. EULAR recommendations for the management of Sjö gren's syndrome with topical and systemic therapies. Ann Rheum Dis 2020;79:3–18.

[83] Sambataro G, Ferro F, Orlandi M, et al. Clinical, morphological features and prognostic factors associated with interstitial lung disease in primary Sjö gren's syndrome: a systematic review from the Italian Society of Rheumatology. Autoimmun Rev 2020;19:102447.

[84] Brito-Zerón P, Melchor S, Seror R. Sjögren Big Data Consortium, Members of the EULAR-SS Task Force Big Data Consortium who contributed to this study. SARS-CoV-2 infection in patients with primary Sjogren syndrome: characterization and outcomes of 51 patients. Rheumatology June 18, 2021;60(6):2946–57. https://doi.org/10.1093/rheumatology/keaa74.

[85] Nannini C, Jebakumar AJ, Crowson CS, et al. Primary Sjogren's syndrome 1976-2005 and associated interstitial lung disease: a population-based study of incidence and mortality. BMJ Open 2013;3:e003569.

[86] Mahdavinia M, Foster KJ, Jauregui E, et al. Asthma prolongs intubation in COVID-19. J Allergy Clin Immunol Pract 2020;8:2388–91.

[87] Serban A, Mihai A, Dima A, Balaban DV, Jinga M, Jurcut C. The impact of the COVID-19 pandemic on patients with primary Sjogren syndrome. Rheumatol Int November 2021;41(11):1933–40. https://doi.org/10.1007/s00296-021-04967-4.

[88] Shavit E, Alavi A, Sibbald RG. Vasculitis-what do we have to know? A review of literature. Int J Low Extrem Wounds 2018;17(4):218–26. https://doi.org/10.1177/1534734618804982.

[89] Becker RC. COVID-19-associated vasculitis and vasculopathy. J Thromb Thrombolysis 2020;50(3):499–511. https://doi.org/10.1007/s11239-020-02230-4.

[90] Iba T, Connors JM, Levy JH. The coagulopathy, endotheliopathy, and vasculitis of COVID-19. Inflamm Res 2020;69(12):1181–9. https://doi.org/10.1007/s00011-020-01401-6.

[91] Camprodon Gómez M, González-Cruz C, Ferrer B, Barberá MJ. Leucocytoclastic vasculitis in a patient with COVID-19 with positive SARS-CoV-2 PCR in skin biopsy. BMJ Case Rep 2020;13(10):e238039. https://doi.org/10.1136/bcr-2020-238039. Published 2020 Oct 29.

[92] Lersy F, Anaheim M, Willaume T, et al. Cerebral vasculitis of medium-sized vessels as a possible mechanism of brain damage in COVID-19 patients. J Neuroradiol 2021;48(3):141–6. https://doi.org/10.1016/j.neurad.2020.11.004.

[93] Dourmishev L, Guleva D, Pozharashka J, et al. Autoimmune connective tissue diseases in the COVID-19 pandemic. Clin Dermatol 2021;39(1):56–63. https://doi.org/10.1016/j.clindermatol.2020.12.013.

[94] Bukulmez H. Current understanding of multisystem inflammatory syndrome (MIS-C) following COVID-19 and its distinction from Kawasaki disease. Curr Rheumatol Rep 2021;23(8):58. https://doi.org/10.1007/s11926-021-01028-4. Published 2021 Jul 3.

[95] Rutherford MA, Scott J, Karabayas M, et al. Risk factors for severe outcomes in patients with systemic vasculitis and COVID-19: a binational, registry-based cohort study. Arthritis Rheumatol 2021;73(9):1713–9. https://doi.org/10.1002/art.41728.

[96] Ince B, Bektas M, Koca N, et al. A single center survey study of systemic vasculitis and COVID-19 during the first months of pandemic. Turk J Med Sci 2021;51(5):2243–7. https://doi.org/10.3906/sag-2010-267. Published 2021 Oct 21.

[97] Vahedi A, Apap Mangion S, Silber E, Sibtain N, Chandra J. COVID-19 leukoencephalopathy with subacute magnetic resonance imaging findings of vasculitis and demyelination. J Neurovirol 2021;27(4):656–61. https://doi.org/10.1007/s13365-021-00990-0.

[98] Kant S, Morris A, Ravi S, et al. The impact of COVID-19 pandemic on patients with ANCA associated vasculitis. J Nephrol 2021;34(1):185–90. https://doi.org/10.1007/s40620-020-00881-3.

[99] Ouldali N, Pouletty M, Mariani P, et al. Emergence of Kawasaki disease related to SARS-CoV-2 infection in an epicentre of the French COVID-19 epidemic: a time-series analysis. Lancet Child Adolesc Health 2020;4(9):662–8. https://doi.org/10.1016/S2352-4642(20)30175-9.

[100] Dursun R, Temiz SA, Özer İ, Daye M, Ataseven A. Management of patients with Behçet's disease during the COVID-19 pandemic. Dermatol Ther 2020;33(6):e14063. https://doi.org/10.1111/dth.14063.

[101] Ordinola Navarro A, Cervantes-Bojalil J, Cobos Quevedo OJ, et al. Decreased quality of life and spirometric alterations even after mild-moderate COVID-19. Respir Med 2021;181:106391. https://doi.org/10.1016/j.rmed.2021.106391.

[102] Sollini M, Ciccarelli M, Cecconi M, et al. Vasculitis changes in COVID-19 survivors with persistent symptoms: an [18F]FDG-PET/CT study. Eur J Nucl Med Mol Imaging 2021;48(5):1460–6. https://doi.org/10.1007/s00259-020-05084-3.

[103] Jara LJ, López-Zamora B, et al. The immune-neuroendocrine system in COVID-19, advanced age and rheumatic diseases. Autoimmun Rev November 2021;20(11):102946. https://doi.org/10.1016/j.autrev.2021.102946.

[104] Pérez-Aguilar MC, Rondon-Mercado R. Neuroimmunoendocrine system in health and disease. EC Microbiol 2018;14(1):02–6.

[105] Li X, Xu S, Yu M, et al. Risk factors for severity and mortality in adult COVID-19 inpatients in Wuhan. J Allergy Clin Immunol July 2020;146(1):110–8. https://doi.org/10.1016/j.jaci.2020.04.006. doi: 10.1016/j.jaci.2020.04.006.

[106] Tian W, Jiang W, Yao J, et al. Predictors of mortality in hospitalized COVID-19 patients: a systematic review and meta-analysis. J Med Virol October 2020;92(10):1875–83. https://doi.org/10.1002/jmv.26050. DOI: 10.1002/jmv.26050.

[107] Li W, Moore MJ, Vasilieva N, et al. Angiotensin-converting enzyme 2 is a functional receptor for the SARS coronavirus. Nature 2003;426(6965):450–4.

[108] Walls AC, Park YJ, Tortorici MA, Wall A, McGuire AT, Veesler D. Structure, function, and antigenicity of the SARSCoV-2 spike glycoprotein. Cell 2020;183(6):1735.

[109] Hofmann M, Kleine-Weber H, et al. SARS-CoV-2 cell entry depends on ACE2 and TMPRSS2 and is blocked by a clinically proven protease inhibitor. Cell 2020;181(2):271–280 e278.

[110] Mao L, Jin H, Wang M, et al. Neurologic manifestations of hospitalized patients with coronavirus disease 2019 in Wuhan, China. JAMA Neurol 2020;77(6):683–90. https://doi.org/10.1001/jamaneurol.2020.1127.

[111] Conde Cardona G, Quintana Pajaro LD, et al. Neurotropism of SARS-CoV 2: mechanisms and manifestations. J Neurol Sci 2020;412:116824.

[112] Han T, Kang J, Li G, Ge J, Gu J. Analysis of 2019-nCoV receptor ACE2 expression in diferent tissues and its signifcance study. Ann Transl Med 2020;8(17):1077. https://doi.org/10.21037/atm-20-4281.

[113] Ding Y, He L, Zhang Q, Huang Z, Che X, Hou J, Wang H, Shen H, Qiu L, Li Z, Geng J, Cai J, Han H, Li X, Kang W, Weng D, Liang P, Jiang S. Organ distribution of severe acute respiratory syndrome (SARS) associated coronavirus (SARSCoV) in SARS patients: implications for pathogenesis and virus transmission pathways. J Pathol 2004;203(2):622–30. https://doi.org/10.1002/path.1560.

[114] Jara LJ, Navarro C, Medina G, Vera-Lastra O, Blanco F. Immune-neuroendocrine interactions and autoimmune diseases. Clin Dev Immunol 2006;13(2–4):109–23.
[115] Tsigos C, Chrousos GP. Hypothalamic-pituitary-adrenal axis, neuroendocrine factors and stress. J Psychosom Res 2002;53:865–71.
[116] Perez AR, Bottasso O, Savino W. The impact of infectious diseases upon neuroendocrine circuits. Neuroimmunomodulation 2009;16:96–105.
[117] Silverman M, Pearce B, Biron C, Miller A. Immune modulation of the hypothalamic-pituitary-adrenal (HPA) axis during viral infection. Viral Immunol 2005;18(1):41–78.
[118] Jara LJ, Izquierdo E, Medina G. Is the immune neuroendocrine system the connection between epipharyngitis and chronic fatigue syndrome induced by HPV vaccine? Editorial Immunol Res 2017;65(1):5–7.
[119] Mao Y, Xu B, Guan W, Xu D, Li F, Ren R, et al. The adrenal cortex, an underestimated site of SARS-CoV-2 infection. Front Endocrinol 2021;11:593179.
[120] Alzahrani AS, Mukhtar N, Aljomaiah A, et al. The impact of COVID-19 viral infection on the hypothalamic-pituitary-adrenal axis. Endocr Pract 2021;27(2):83–9.
[121] Freire Santana M, Borba MGS, Baía-da-Silva DC, Val F, Alexandre MAA, BritoSousa JD, et al. Case report: adrenal pathology findings in severe COVID-19: an autopsy study. Am J Trop Med Hyg 2020;103(4):1604–7.
[122] 20OTanriverdi F, Silveira LF, MacColl GS, Bouloux PM. The hypothalamic-pituitarygonadal axis: immune function and autoimmunity. J Endocrinol 2003;176(3):293–304.
[123] Moradi F, Enjezab B, Ghadiri-Anari A. The role of androgens in COVID-19. Diabetes Metab Syndr 2020;14(6):2003–6.
[124] Chen J, Jiang Q, Xia X, Liu K, Yu Z, Tao W, et al. Individual variation of the SARSCoV-2 receptor ACE2 gene expression and regulation. Aging Cell 2020;19(7):e13168.
[125] Khalili MA, Leisegang K, Majzoub A, et al. Male fertility and the COVID-19 pandemic: systematic review of the literature. World J Mens Health 2020;38(4):506–20.
[126] Ding T, Wang T, Zhang J, et al. Analysis of ovarian injury associated with COVID-19 disease in reproductive-aged women in Wuhan, China: an observational Study. Front Med 2021;8:635255.
[127] Fekete C, Lechan RM. Central regulation of hypothalamic-pituitary-thyroid axis under physiological and pathophysiological conditions. Endocr Rev 2014;35(2):159–94.
[128] Caron P. Thyroid disorders and SARS-CoV-2 infection: from pathophysiological mechanism to patient management. Ann Endocrinol 2020;81(5):507–10.
[129] Scappaticcio L, Pitoia F, Esposito K, et al. Impact of COVID-19 on the thyroid gland: an update. Rev Endocr Metab Disord 2020;25:1–13.
[130] Vera-Lastra O, Ordinola Navarro A, et al. Two cases of Graves' disease following SARS-CoV-2 vaccination: an autoimmune/inflammatory syndrome induced by adjuvants. Thyroid 2021. https://doi.org/10.1089/thy.2021.0142.
[131] Iremli BG, Ş endur SN, Ünlütürk U. Three cases of subacute thyroiditis following SARS-CoV-2 vaccine: post-vaccination ASIA syndrome. J Clin Endocrinol Metab August 18, 2021;106(9):2600–5.
[132] Frara S, Allora A, Castellino L, di Filippo L, Loli P, Giustina A. COVID-19 and the pituitary. Pituitary June 2021;24(3):465–81. https://doi.org/10.1007/s11102-021-01148-1. Epub 2021 May 3.
[133] Ackermann M, Verleden SE, et al. Pulmonary vascular endothelialitis, thrombosis, and angiogenesis in COVID-19. N Engl J Med 2020;383(2):120–8. https://doi.org/10.1056/NEJMoa2015432.
[134] Bilezikian JP, Bikle D, Hewison M, et al. Mechanisms in endocrinology: vitamin D and COVID-19. Eur J Endocrinol 2020;183(5):R133–47. https://doi.org/10.1530/EJE-20-0665.
[135] Brandi ML. Giustina A Sexual Dimorphism of coronavirus 19 morbidity and lethality. Trends Endocrinol Metab 2020;31(12):918–27.
[136] Marazuela M, Giustina A, Puig-Domingo M. Endocrine and metabolic aspects of the COVID-19 pandemic. Rev Endocr Metab Disord 2020;21(4):495–507. https://doi.org/10.1007/s11154-020-09569-2.
[137] Arnaldi G, Angeli A, Atkinson AB. Bertagna XDiagnosis and complications of Cushing's syndrome: a consensus statement. J Clin Endocrinol Metab 2003;88(12):5593–602. https://doi.org/10.1210/jc.2003-030871.
[138] Tatsi C, Boden R, Sinaii N, Keil M, et al. Decreased lymphocytes and increased risk for infection are common in endogenous pediatric Cushing syndrome. Pediatr Res 2018;83(2):431–7.
[139] Yang M, Chen J, Wei W. Dimerization of glucocorticoid receptors and its role in infammation and immune responses. Pharmacol Res April 2021;166:105334.

[140] Bruno NE, Nwachukwu JC, Srinivasan S, et al. Chemical systems biology reveals mechanisms of glucocorticoid receptor signaling. Nat Chem Biol 2021;17(3):307–16. https://doi.org/10.1038/s41589-020-00719-w.

[141] Hasenmajer V, Sbardella E, Sciarra F, et al. The immune system in Cushing's syndrome. Trends Endocrinol Metab 2020;31(9):655–69. https://doi.org/10.1016/j.tem.2020.04.004.

[142] Serban AL, Ferrante E, Carosi G, et al. COVID-19 in Cushing disease: experience of a single tertiary centre in Lombardy. J Endocrinol Invest June 2021;44(6):1335–6. https://doi.org/10.1007/s40618-020-01419-x.

[143] Yuno A, Kenmotsu Y, Takahashi Y, et al. Successful management of a patient with active Cushing's disease complicated with coronavirus disease 2019 (COVID-19) pneumonia. Endocr J April 28, 2021;68(4):477–84. https://doi.org/10.1507/endocrj.EJ20-0613.

[144] Belaya Z, Golounina O, Melnichenko G, et al. Clinical course and outcome of patients with ACTH-dependent Cushing's syndrome infected with novel coronavirus disease-19 (COVID-19): case presentations. Endocrine April 2021;72(1):12–9. https://doi.org/10.1007/s12020-021-02674-5.

[145] Quinkler M, Ekman B, Zhang P, et al. Mortality data from the European adrenal insufciency registry-patient characterization and associations. Clin Endocrinol 2018;89(1):30–5. https://doi.org/10.1111/cen.13609.

[146] Stewart PM, Biller BM. Exploring inpatient hospitalizations and morbidity in patients with adrenal insufciency. J Clin Endocrinol Metab 2016;101(12):4843–50. https://doi.org/10.1210/jc.2016-2221.

[147] Bancos I, Hazeldine J, Chortis V, et al. Primary adrenal insufciency is associated with impaired natural killer cell function: a potential link to increased mortality. Eur J Endocrinol 2017;176(4):471–80. https://doi.org/10.1530/EJE-16-0969.

[148] Mazziotti G, Formenti AM, et al. Management of endocrine disease: risk of overtreatment in patients with adrenal insufciency: current and emerging aspects. Eur J Endocrinol 2017;177(5):R231–48. https://doi.org/10.1530/EJE-17-0154.

[149] Puig-Domingo M, Marazuela M, Giustina A. COVID-19 and endocrine diseases. A statement from the European Society of Endocrinology. Endocrine 2020;68(1):2–5. https://doi.org/10.1007/s12020-020-02294-5-.

[150] Loli P, Frara S, Pasquali R, Di Filippo L, Rovere-Querini P, Giustina A. COVID-19 and hypopituitarism. Experience from an endocrine center in a high-impact area. Endocrine Abstract 2020;70:AEP1075.

[151] Carosi G, Morelli V, Del Sindaco G, Serban AL, Cremaschi A, Frigerio S, Rodari G, Profka E, Indirli R, Mungari R, Resi V, Orsi E, Ferrante E, Dolci A, Giavoli C, Arosio M, Mantovani G. Adrenal insufciency at the time of COVID-19: a retrospective study in patients referring to a tertiary center. J Clin Endocrinol Metab 2021;106(3):e1354–61.

[152] Ko JJ, Wu C, Mehta N, et al. A comparison of methylprednisolone and dexamethasone in intensive care patients with COVID-19. J Intensive Care Med June 2021;36(6):673–80. https://doi.org/10.1177/0885066621994057.

[153] Zhang Y, Hu S, Wang J, Xue Z, Wang C, Wang N. Dexamethasone inhibits SARS-CoV-2 spike pseudotyped virus viropexis by binding to ACE2. Virology 2021;554:83–8. https://doi.org/10.1016/j.virol.2020.12.001.

[154] Ilias I, Zabuliene L. Hyperglycemia and the novel COVID-19 infection: possible pathophysiologic mechanisms. Med Hypotheses 2020;139:109699.

[155] Kaiser UB, Mirmira RG, Stewart PM. Our response to COVID-19 as endocrinologists and diabetologists. JCEM 2020;105(5):dgaa148.

[156] Dworakowska D, Grossman AB. Thyroid disease in the time of COVID-19. Endocrine June 2020;68(3):471–4. https://doi.org/10.1007/s12020-020-02364-8.

[157] Pham-Dobor G, Hanak L, Hegyi P, et al. Prevalence of other autoimmune diseases in polyglandular autoimmune syndromes type II and III. J Endocrinol Invest September 2020;43(9):1–9.

[158] Bourji K, Gatto M, Cozzi F, Doria A, Punzi L. Rheumatic and autoimmune thyroid disorders: a causal or casual relationship? Autoimmun Rev 2015;14:57–63.

[159] Conigliaro P, D'Antonio A, Pinto S, et al. Autoimmune thyroid disorders and rheumatoid arthritis: a bidirectional interplay. Autoimmun Rev 2020;19(6):102529.

[160] Figueroa-Parra G, Aguirre-Garcia GM, Gamboa-Alonso CM, et al. Are my patients with rheumatic diseases at higher risk of COVID-19? Ann Rheum Dis 2020;79(6):839–40. https://doi.org/10.1136/annrheumdis-2020-217322.

[161] Curtis BR. Non-chemotherapy drug-induced neutropenia: key points to manage the challenges. Hematology Am Soc Hematol. 2017 Educ. Program 2017:187–93.

[162] Lui DTW, Lee CH, Chow WS, et al. Thyroid dysfunction in relation to immune profile, disease status, and outcome in 191 patients with COVID-19. J Clin Endocrinol Metab January 23, 2021;106(2):e926–35. https://doi.org/10.1210/clinem/dgaa813.

[163] Kataria S, Tandon M, Melnic V, Sriwastava S. A case series and literature review of multiple sclerosis and COVID-19: clinical characteristics, outcomes and a brief review of immunotherapies. eNeurologicalSci 2020;21:100287. https://doi.org/10.1016/j.ensci.2020.100287.

[164] Landtblom AM, Berntsson SG, Boström I, Iacobaeus E. Multiple sclerosis and COVID-19: the Swedish experience. Acta Neurol Scand 2021;144(3):229–35. https://doi.org/10.1111/ane.13453.

[165] Sormani MP. Italian Study Group on COVID-19 infection in multiple sclerosis. An Italian programme for COVID-19 infection in multiple sclerosis [published correction appears in Lancet Neurol. 2020 May 28. Lancet Neurol 2020;19(6):481–2. https://doi.org/10.1016/S1474-4422(20)30147-2.

[166] Novi G, Mikulska M, Briano F, et al. COVID-19 in a MS patient treated with ocrelizumab: does immunosuppression have a protective role? Mult Scler Relat Disord 2020;42:102120. https://doi.org/10.1016/j.msard.2020.102120.

[167] Thornton JR, Harel A. Negative SARS-CoV-2 antibody testing following COVID-19 infection in Two MS patients treated with ocrelizumab. Mult Scler Relat Disord 2020;44:102341. https://doi.org/10.1016/j.msard.2020.102341.

[168] Montero-Escribano P, Matías-Guiu J, Gómez-Iglesias P, Porta-Etessam J, Pytel V, Matias-Guiu JA. Anti-CD20 and COVID-19 in multiple sclerosis and related disorders: a case series of 60 patients from Madrid, Spain. Mult Scler Relat Disord 2020;42:102185. https://doi.org/10.1016/j.msard.2020.102185.

[169] Möhn N, Konen FF, Pul R, et al. Experience in multiple sclerosis patients with COVID-19 and disease-modifying therapies: a review of 873 published cases. J Clin Med 2020;9(12):4067. https://doi.org/10.3390/jcm9124067. Published 2020 Dec 16.

[170] Berger JR. COVID-19 and the nervous system. J Neurovirol 2020;26(2):143–8. https://doi.org/10.1007/s13365-020-00840-5.

[171] Scoppettuolo P, Borrelli S, Naeije G. Neurological involvement in SARS-CoV-2 infection: a clinical systematic review. Brain Behav Immun Health 2020;5:100094. https://doi.org/10.1016/j.bbih.2020.100094.

[172] Valadez-Calderon J, Ordinola Navarro A, Rodriguez-Chavez E, Vera-Lastra O. Co-expression of anti-NMDAR and anti-GAD65 antibodies. A case of autoimmune encephalitis in a post-COVID-19 patient [published online ahead of print, 2021 Oct 13]. Neurologia 2021. https://doi.org/10.1016/j.nrl.2021.09.003. 10.1016/j.nrl.2021.09.003.

[173] Vasilevska V, Guest PC, Schlaaff K, Incesoy EI, Prüss H, Steiner J. Potential cross-links of inflammation with Schizophreniform and affective symptoms: a review and outlook on autoimmune encephalitis and COVID-19. Front Psychiatry 2021;12:729868. https://doi.org/10.3389/fpsyt.2021.729868. Published 2021 Sep. 16.

[174] Vasilevska V, Guest PC, Bernstein HG, Schroeter ML, Geis C, Steiner J. Molecular mimicry of NMDA receptors may contribute to neuropsychiatric symptoms in severe COVID-19 cases. J Neuroinflammation 2021;18(1):245. https://doi.org/10.1186/s12974-021-02293-x. Published 2021 Oct 28.

[175] Valencia Sanchez C, Theel E, Binnicker M, Toledano M, McKeon A. Autoimmune encephalitis post-SARS-CoV-2 infection: case frequency, findings, and outcomes [published online ahead of print, 2021 oct 11]. Neurology 2021. https://doi.org/10.1212/WNL.0000000000012931. 10.1212/WNL.0000000000012931.

[176] Benussi A, Pilotto A, Premi E, et al. Clinical characteristics and outcomes of inpatients with neurologic disease and COVID-19 in Brescia, Lombardy, Italy. Neurology August 18, 2020;95(7):e910–20. https://doi.org/10.1212/WNL.0000000000009848.

[177] Vera-Lastra O Cimé-Aké ES, Ordinola Navarro A, et al. Risk factors and outcomes for COVID-19 in autoimmune/inflammatory diseases during sars-cov-2 pandemic. a comparative study. IMAJ submitted to publication; 2021.

Further reading

He F, Luo Q, Lei M, et al. Successful recovery of recurrence of positive SARS-CoV-2 RNA in COVID-19 patient with systemic lupus erythematosus: a case report and review. Clin Rheumatol 2020;39(9):2803–10. https://doi.org/10.1007/s10067-020-05230-0.

Pablos JL, Abasolo L, Alvaro-Gracia JM, et al. Prevalence of hospital PCR-confirmed COVID-19 cases in patients with chronic inflammatory and autoimmune rheumatic diseases. Ann Rheum Dis 2020;79(9):1170–3. https://doi.org/10.1136/annrheumdis-2020-217763.

Rodríguez Y, Novelli L, Rojas M, et al. Autoinflammatory and autoimmune conditions at the crossroad of COVID-19. J Autoimmun 2020;114:102506. https://doi.org/10.1016/j.jaut.2020.102506.

CHAPTER

25

COVID-19 in patients with Systemic Lupus Erythematosus and the antiphospholipid syndrome

Francesca Crisafulli[1], *Silvia-Ebe-Lucia Della-Pina*[1], *Giulia Fontana*[1], *Jorge-Manuel Rodrigues-Fernandes*[2], *Franco Franceschini*[1], *Laura Andreoli*[1] *and Angela Tincani*[1,3]

[1]Rheumatology and Clinical Immunology Unit, ASST Spedali Civili and Department of Clinical and Experimental Sciences, University of Brescia, Brescia, Italy; [2]Internal Medicine/ Autoimmune Diseases Unit, Curry Cabral Hospital, Central Lisbon University Hospital Centre, Lisbon, Portugal; [3]I.M. Sechenov First Moscow State Medical University of the Ministry of Health of the Russian Federation (Sechenov University), Moscow, Russia

Introduction

The emergence of SARS-CoV-2 infection raised concerns about patients with established rheumatic diseases such as Systemic Lupus Erythematosus (SLE) and the antiphospholipid syndrome (APS).

SLE is a chronic, multisystem autoimmune disease with heterogeneous manifestations and a remitting-relapsing clinical course [1]. The dysregulation of the innate, adaptive, and cytokine mediated immune response along with the use of immunosuppressive medications may confer an increased susceptibility to SARS-CoV-2 infection and lead to a prolonged viral shedding or predispose to more severe disease [2–4].

The use of immunosuppressive therapy may also rise some concerns about the efficacy of anti-SARS-CoV-2 vaccines, which nevertheless can be beneficial in patients to reduce the risk of infection or severe disease [5,6].

Moreover, hyperstimulation of the immune system with production of autoantibodies, bystander activation of T-cells, and molecular mimicry, are mechanisms that may stimulate autoimmunity by SARS-CoV-2 infection [6–8]. Whether this can impact patients with already

Autoimmunity, COVID-19, Post-COVID19 syndrome and COVID-19 vaccination
https://doi.org/10.1016/B978-0-443-18566-3.00003-7

established autoimmune disease causing serological modifications or flares is not clearly established.

Both SARS-CoV-2 infection and SLE interact with the host immune system. The pathogenic pathways common to both diseases are: disturbances in B-cell and T-cell responses, dysregulation of Type I interferon (IFN) response, and dysregulation of the apoptosis mechanisms. These pathogenic pathways may ultimately promote a proinflammatory environment that includes activation of the complement system, excessive neutrophil extracellular traps (NETs) formation (NETosis) with neutrophil-associated cytokine responses and endothelial damage [6,9,10].

Common clinical and laboratory features in SLE and COVID-19 patients may be explained by these mechanisms but the extent of how this correlates with COVID-19 expression and outcomes in SLE patients is not well defined [2,11].

Moreover, the contribution of COVID-19 or SLE for the outcomes of infected patients is difficult to determine since both diseases may have similar phenotypical expression, including the occurrence of antiphospholipid (aPL) autoantibodies positivity, antiphospholipid syndrome, or thrombotic phenomena [10]. Antiphospholipid antibodies are antibodies directed against proteins that bind to anionic phospholipids on plasma membranes, such as β-2-glycoprotein I (β2GPI) or annexin A5. They can be found in 5% of healthy population and in at least 20%–30% of patients with SLE with or without APS [12,13]. APS can occur also in otherwise healthy subjects and it is characterized by an hypercoagulable state that cause thrombosis in both arteries and veins and pregnancy-related complications such as miscarriage, stillbirth, preterm delivery, and severe pre-eclampsia [14].

The presence of aPL is detected by three serological tests: lupus anticoagulant (LA) coagulation test, anti-cardiolipin (aCL, IgG and IgM), and anti-β2-glycoprotein-I (aβ2GPI, IgG and IgM) immunoassays. Although these are the laboratory tests included in the classification criteria for APS, it's been suggested that other "non-criteria" antibodies, such as IgG and IgM phosphatidiylserine/prothrombin complex (aPS/PT), IgA aβ2GPI and/or aCL, may play a role in APS pathogenesis [15].

Common pathogenic mechanisms and clinical features of APS, SLE, and COVID-19 include thrombotic microangiopathy, endothelium damage, complement activation, NETosis, and proinflammatory cytokines. The association between SLE and APS is well known but the presence of aPL autoantibodies in COVID-19 without established autoimmune diseases raised the question about the role of SARS-CoV-2 infection in the emergence of aPL, and of their responsibility in endothelial damage, and the occurrence of thrombotic phenomena [10].

In fact, inflammation and coagulation are strongly related and abnormal coagulation tests or coagulopathy may occur in SLE and COVID-19 patients due to the inflammatory state by itself, independently of the presence of aPL [9,16,17].

Finally, the common immune phenotypical expression of SLE with or without aPL/APS and COVID-19 may also explain the beneficial role of some medications, normally used to treat SLE or APS patients, when they are prescribed in COVID-19 patients [2,18].

Another concern regarding COVID-19 relies on the persistence of debilitating symptoms for weeks or even months after the acute phase, which has been defined as "post-COVID syndrome" [19,20].

The World Health Organization (WHO) developed a clinical case definition of post-COVID-19 condition by Delphi methodology: "*Post COVID-19 condition occurs in individuals with a history of probable or confirmed SARS-CoV-2 infection, usually 3 months from the onset of COVID-19 with symptoms and that last for at least 2 months and cannot be explained by an alternative diagnosis. Common symptoms include fatigue, shortness of breath, cognitive dysfunction but also others and generally have an impact on everyday functioning. Symptoms may be new onset following initial recovery from an acute COVID-19 episode or persist from the initial illness. Symptoms may also fluctuate or relapse over time. A separate definition may be applicable for children.*" [21]

The clinical picture of post-COVID syndrome can include, among others, long-term organ dysfunction as consequence of thrombotic events, and chronic fatigue syndrome, which is one of its most common expression [22,23]. The etiology and pathogenesis of post-COVID syndrome remain unknown but seems to be multifactorial and partially overlapping with that of SLE and APS [20]. Certainly, some common symptoms and laboratory findings in post-COVID syndrome are also found in rheumatic diseases. Therefore, it is important to differentiate these conditions.

In this chapter, we will focus on COVID-19, anti-COVID vaccinations, and the post-COVID syndrome in patients with SLE and APS.

COVID-19: the disease in SLE patients with or without APS/aPL

COVID-19 & SLE

As previously reported, COVID-19 and SLE patients share some common features.

On the clinical side, fever, asthenia, myalgia, arthralgia, lung involvement, hepatitis, general neurological involvement, general renal involvement, and thrombosis are common in both diseases so that, in some cases, a differential diagnosis between these two conditions had to be considered [24–26].

On the immunological side, some of the abnormalities in patients with SLE were found also in patients with COVID-19 infection [27]. As an example, lymphopenia is frequently found in SLE patients and it can occur either because of disease-mediated mechanisms (active inflammation with increased apoptosis of immune cells, complement-mediated or antibody-dependent cytotoxicity and decreased lymphopoiesis) or it can occur as a side effect of immunosuppressants [2,3]. Similarly, reversible low lymphocyte count has been also observed in patients with COVID-19, especially those with severe disease due to infection of lymphocytes by SARS-CoV-2, exhaustion, and induction of apoptosis by cell hyperactivation and/or increase in proinflammatory cytokines and proapoptotic signals [28].

Both in COVID-19 and in SLE CD8 T cell responses are impaired, including defects in phagocytosis, cytotoxic capacity, degranulation, and chemotaxis [29].

Proinflammatory mediators, like Tumor Necrosis Factor α (TNF-α) and Interleukin-6 (IL-6), play an important role in the occurrence and development of SLE and compromise the Th1 type of response, which is involved in antiviral-defense. Similarly, proinflammatory cytokines are increased also in plasma of patients with COVID-19, likely due to a combination of rapid virus replication, delayed IFN response, macrophage and neutrophil accumulation, and infection of alveolar epithelial cells. This condition is typical of severe COVID-19 infection: an uncontrolled proinflammatory cytokine response can lead to cytokine storm, which causes multi-organ damage, characterized by significant morbidity and mortality [30].

On the other hand, most patients with SLE show elevated circulating type I IFN, which has antiviral proprieties and could be protective to COVID-19 infection [31]. In fact, a recent study found that patients with severe COVID-19 infection present low type I IFN activity and the importance of IFN response is also sustained by the evidence that patients treated with IFN-a2b present a shorter duration of detectable virus [32].

As it has been postulated for other viruses, infections lead to the activation of innate and acquired immune response in genetically predisposed patients, inducing a lupus-like syndrome by transient positive autoantibodies synthesis, characterized by symptoms such as malar rash, arthralgia, nephritis and hepatitis [33]. This condition can be characterized by the presence of transient autoantibodies typical of SLE like ANA, dsDNA, and aPL. As shown by some reports, COVID-19 infection could shortly precede de novo diagnosis of SLE or could occur concomitantly, suggesting the possibility of SARS-CoV-2 being a trigger of autoimmunity [24,34], but the development of SLE, following the COVID-19 infection is not currently confirmed by the available data [35]. In fact, despite the presence of some clinical similarities, in infected patients these findings seem to be related to high expression of pro-inflammatory cytokines, such as IL-1, IL-6, and TNF-α [36].

It's also unclear whether COVID-19 can cause a disease flare in SLE patients, indeed various reports have indicated that it may worsen SLE manifestations [37,38].

However, attributing SLE flares only to a SARS-CoV-2 infection is challenging because during the pandemic period many of these patients might had greater difficulty accessing health care. Therefore, the lack of medical care, the difficulty continuing SLE medications and psychosocial stressors of the pandemic could cause worsening of the disease even without the infection [27].

Although patients with SLE are more susceptible to infections because of the impaired immune response, the damage from comorbidity and the use of immunosuppressive therapies [39,40], studies seem to suggest that most patients may not be at increased risk of developing COVID-19 [41–43].

Regarding COVID-19, patients with SLE were more frequently hospitalized [44], but it seems that comorbidities like obesity, diabetes, and hypertension, more than SLE itself, were responsible for a more severe course of the infection [45].

Infected SLE patients displayed also a higher risk of admission to the intensive care unit (ICU), mechanical ventilation, stroke, venous thromboembolism (VTE), and sepsis as compared to the general population [43].

In the general population, male gender is a risk factor for poor outcome of COVID-19, especially in men over the age of 60 years and with comorbidities. Conversely, SLE affects mostly women in young age: in this case, female gender may represent a protective factor because biological factors, which protect men from autoimmunity, may cause worse clinical outcomes of COVID-19 in males [2].

Ethnic minority communities, like Afro-Americans and Hispanics, are at increased risk of both COVID-19 infection and SLE development and they present worse outcomes: this association is likely multifactorial, involving both biological aspects and socioeconomic disparities [46].

Further studies shown that worse COVID-19 outcomes in SLE patients are associated with moderate or high rheumatic disease activity, flare preceding the COVID-19 diagnosis, renal lupus, and glucocorticoids use (>5 mg/day of prednisone) [47].

It is interesting to note that in SLE patients renal involvement reflects more aggressive disease requiring higher doses of immunosuppressants and corticosteroids compared to joint or cutaneous manifestations [48] and the presence of a compromised renal function due to lupus may be an important predictor of acute kidney injury during COVID-19 infection [43].

Data about COVID-19 mortality in SLE patients are unclear. An observational cohort study shown that patients with rheumatologic diseases have a slightly higher risk of mortality from COVID-19, especially those affected with SLE [49]. At the same time, a retrospective study displayed that the risk of death due to COVID among SLE was comparable to that in the general population [43].

Fig. 25.1 summarizes the characteristics involved in the interplay between SLE and COVID-19.

COVID-19 & APS

Both COVID-19 and APS could be characterized by the presence of thrombotic microangiopathy, arterial and venous thrombosis, and pulmonary embolisms [10]. The risk of venous thromboembolism in patients with COVID-19 was estimated at about 16%, while risk of arterial thrombosis was 11% [50].

Also, from the pathogenic point of view these two diseases had some common features, in particular considering the pathogenesis of particular conditions such as the catastrophic APS (CAPS). CAPS is a rare condition, often triggered by infections, and characterized by increased circulating levels of proinflammatory cytokine and systemic thrombotic microangiopathy. This condition causes rapid organ failure and is associated with an high risk of death [14,51]. In the early observations, it was noticed a certain similarities between COVID-19 acute phase and CAPS: in fact both diseases present cytokine storm and coagulation

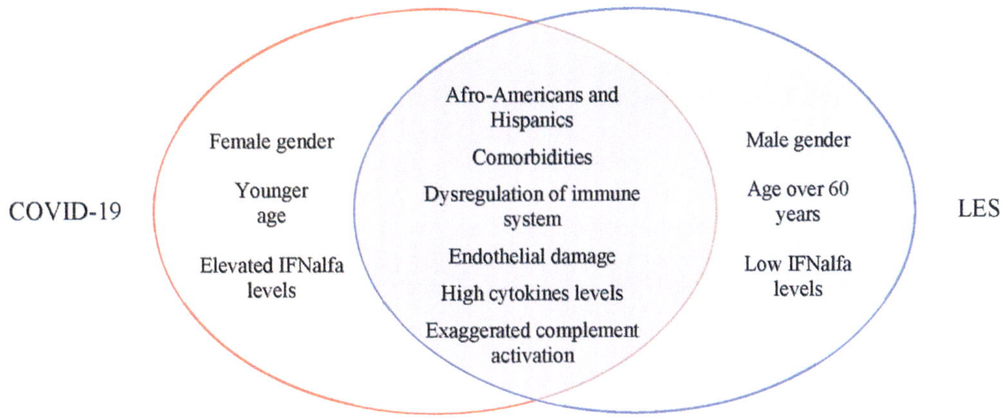

FIGURE 25.1 The interplay between SLE and COVID-19. *Modified from Spihlman AP, Gadi N, Wu SC, Moulton VR. COVID-19 and systemic lupus erythematosus: focus on immune response and therapeutics. Front Immunol. Published online 2020. https://doi.org/10.3389/fimmu.2020.589474.*

abnormalities like prolonged aPTT, as well as similar clinical manifestations characterizes by thrombosis and mycroangiopathy [51,52].

The common pathogenic pathways between APS, CAPS, and COVID-19 include endothelial damage and the release of NETs [10,53].

Endothelial damage can be due to a complex systemic inflammatory caused by proinflammatory cytokines, like IL-6, TNF-α, and IL-1β, released after virus infection [54]. As an example large quantities of IL-6 can induce endothelial cells to activate and express factors such as von Willebrand factor, factor VIII and tissue factor, resulting in a hypercoagulability state. IL-6 can also induce neutrophil infiltration and nitric oxide (NO)-mediated increase in vascular permeability [54].

Another cause of endothelial dysregulation is due to complement activation. COVID-19 is able to activate complement system by the lectin and alternative pathways, although the classical complement pathway could also be activated in this setting by immune complexes [55].

This common pathogenic mechanism between CAPS and severe COVID-19 represent possible targets of intervention: eculizumab, an antibody that binds to the terminal complement component 5, can be an effective therapy for both COVID-19 and CAPS [56].

Instead, NETs are web-like chromatin fibers with microbicidal proteins and granule enzymes released by neutrophils as a host defense mechanism against microbes. NETs can enhance inflammation and type I IFN responses. Dysregulated NETs can also potentiate thrombosis in APS [57] and several studies suggested their key role in COVID-19 pathogenesis [58].

The presence of aPL, the marker of APS, might be another pathogenic pathway shared by the two conditions. In fact, it is known that some infectious agents are able to trigger the in vivo production of aPL through a molecular mimicry mechanism between viruses and β2GPI, especially in genetically susceptible patients [59]. Given that thrombosis can occur in patients with COVID-19, various studies aimed to identify the presence of aPL in patients with COVID-19 trying to define if SARS-CoV-2 itself could be responsible for aPL production and if these antibodies could have a pathogenic or prognostic value [10,50].

aPL were detected in nearly half of in -patients with COVID-19,; however, their true prevalence is unknown. LA is the most frequent positive test reported, with a pooled prevalence rate of 50.7%, followed by aCL (13.9%) and aβ2GPI (6.7%) [50].

Trahtemberg et al. have studied longitudinally 42 hospitalized patients (22 COVID-19+ and 20 COVID-19-) with respiratory failure admitted to ICU: aPL were found in both groups, with a tendency toward higher frequency among the COVID-19+ (predominantly IgG aCL (48%), followed by IgM (21%) in all patients) [60]. Positive aPL serology seems to be associated with worse disease severity in both COVID-19+ and COVID-19- patients, so aPL status has an independent association with disease severity and doesn't modulate the outcomes differentially based on COVID status [60]. Similarly there's no association between aPL positivity and COVID-19 mortality or invasive ventilation [50].

Increased titer of non-criteria aPL test, such as IgG and IgM phosphatidiylserine/prothrombin complex (aPS/PT), IgA aβ2GPI, and aCL were also shown in COVID-19 patients [61,62].

Another recent report, however, clearly showed that prolonged aPTT and positive LA results represent nonspecific findings in patients admitted to ICU with or without COVID-19 [63].

Although the presence of aPL in COVID-19 patients is established, the pathological significance of aPL in COVID-19 patients is still unclear.

In patients with established diagnosis of APS or with aPL positivity, SARS-CoV-2 may trigger thrombosis through a "two-hit hypothesis": in fact, thanks to its special tropism to the endothelium, SARS-CoV-2 may favor the pathogenic effects of aPL by causing endothelial cells damage and proinflammatory states, determining a disease flare that could be precipitated in CAPS [64].

However, additional findings are supporting the idea that aPL in COVID-19 are not associated with thrombosis [50].

First at all, the lack of longitudinal studies assessing the persistence of aPL in COVID-19 infected patients does not allow to know if these antibodies are comparable to those linked to clinical and biological effects in APS [65].

Furthermore, there is evidence that in COVID-19 aPL are transient, usually at medium/low titer, with a high rate of isolated positivity and frequently of the IgM isotype only [10,50].

However, the low titer of aPL in COVID-19 does not exclude pathogenicity: the systemic inflammation with complement system activation and release of cytokines typical of COVID-19 causes endothelial injury and there is evidence that β2GPI can accumulate on the activated endothelium at high density, being much more available to the aβ2GPI antibodies and ultimately favoring their pathogenic effect [66]. A comparable condition in which low titers of aPL can cause substantial damage was reported in obstetric APS, where high quantities of β2GPI are physiologically expressed in the placenta [67].

Despite these considerations, Borghi et al. reported sound evidence that COVID-19 aβ2GPI were not directed against the Domain (D)-1 of β2GPI molecule, which are typical of the syndrome with the vascular manifestations, but frequently against D4/-5, that is the target of "innocent" antibodies [68,69].

In conclusion, a recent meta-analysis and literature review highlighted that the presence of aPL autoantibodies in COVID-19 patients appeared not to be associated with disease outcomes such as venous thrombosis, invasive ventilation and mortality [50]. Overall, the occurrence of aPL in COVID-19 patients is possible, but their prevalence, specific isotypes, and titers may not be the primary cause of thrombosis in the acute stage of disease [70]: the coagulopathy may be due to the inflammatory state by itself, independently of the presence of aPL autoantibodies, that represent markers of endothelial damage [16,71,72].

The last report from EULAR COVID-19 Registry (on October 1, 2021) shows that APS is reported in 1% of rheumatological patients with COVID-19 (60/10,350); however, data on COVID-19 outcomes in patients with aPL (with or without APS) are limited and heterogenous. Some case reports described the course of COVID-19 infection in patients with APS or aPL-positivity: an SLE patient with triple aPL-positivity but no APS developed VTE [73]; a patient with SLE and APS developed severe thrombocytopenia (in this case authors suggested that SARS-CoV-2 infection was more likely a trigger for clinical exacerbation of APS rather than the direct cause of thrombocytopenia) [74]; a patient with primary APS on therapeutic anticoagulation developed bilateral adrenal gland hemorrhage and limb arterial ischemia [64]; another APS patient developed recurrent diffuse alveolar hemorrhage complicated by fungal pneumonia [75].

Zhang et al. reported multiple cerebral infarctions in three COVID-19 patients with aPL (aCL IgA, aβ2GPI IgA, and IgG): patients with higher and persistent levels of aPL or multiple aPL positivity may be more at risk of cerebral infarction during COVID-19 [52].

A survey described that none of 18 patients with SARS-CoV-2 infection and APS with triple positive aPL profile suffer thromboembolic events, although at high risk of thrombosis [76].

More clinical data are needed to clarify COVID-19 outcomes in patients with APS.

COVID-19 & SLE/APS treatment

Due to shared pathogenic and clinical manifestations of SLE and COVID-19, some strategies used for SLE may be also used as therapeutic options for COVID-19 [77].

SLE management involves the use of multiple therapeutic strategies to treat the specific manifestations, to lower disease activity, and to prevent irreversible organ damage [78]. General standard treatment strategies include the use of antimalarials, nonbiologic and biologic agents, glucocorticoids (sGC), and nonsteroidal antiinflammatory drugs (NSAIDs) [27].

Because of their antiinflammatory activity, many of the standard treatments for SLE were studied as potential treatments for COVID-19 infection, especially in patients who developed the abnormal immune response that characterize the cytokine storm syndrome [2]. In addition, some antirheumatic drugs, such as hydroxychloroquine (HCQ), have also shown an antiviral action [79].

Some management strategies have been provided by COVID-19 Global Rheumatology Alliance (C19-GRA), an international database aiming to capture detailed data from rheumatology providers on COVID-19 outcomes in patients with rheumatic diseases in order to address the knowledge gap regarding factors associated with severe disease [44].

Table 25.1. describes some examples of SLE drugs with possible application in COVID-19 treatment.

In conclusion, the immune response is important not only in the antiviral defense, but also in the disease progression, severity, and clinical outcomes of COVID-19 because an uncontrolled proinflammatory cytokine response can lead to cytokine storm [30].

According to the today available data, SLE treatments are not associated with an increased rate of COVID-19 diagnosis or mortality, except patients treated with B-cell depletion therapy or high dose sGC at baseline that present higher risk of more severe COVID-19 outcomes if infected [5].

The management of COVID-19 in SLE patients should find the right balance between the risk of immunosuppression due to treatment and the risk of flare of SLE due to drugs removal.

Better understanding of the underlying immune response and therapeutic strategies in SLE and COVID-19 is important to guide management of this infectious disease in the context of SLE and vice-versa [77].

The treatment of aPL-positive COVID-19 patients can be also challenging, hence recommendations were recently proposed, taking into consideration the required level of care (inpatient/outpatient), additional thrombosis risk factors, and the presence of contraindications to anticoagulation [53].

Generally, aPL-positive outpatients not on anticoagulation should receive a prophylactic dose with low-molecular weight heparin (LMWH), especially in the setting of additional venous thromboembolism risk factors, such as reduced mobility or malignancy. Instead,

TABLE 25.1 SLE drugs with possible application in COVID-19 treatment.

Drug	Role in SLE treatment	Possible antiviral mechanisms	Use in SLE and COVID-19
NSAIDs	Used to relieve symptoms in patients with SLE [77].	Possible prevention of the cascade of proinflammatory cytokines caused by COX-2 upregulation induced by SARS-CoV-2 [80].	NSAIDs can be safely used to relieve the symptoms of COVID-19. SLE patients should continue to take NSAIDs as needed [77].
sGC	First-line treatment in the management of organ- and life-threatening manifestations of SLE [46].	– Inhibition of the infiltration of excessive macrophages, neutrophils and T-lymphocytes, and reduction of cytokine storm risk [81]. – Induction of the production of NO, that can inhibit the SARS-CoV replication cycle [82].	– Higher odds of hospitalization in patients with rheumatic diseases taking sGC at doses >10 mg/day [44] – Use of sGC as a COVID-19 treatment may increase the risk of death in patients with mild infection [83]. – SLE patients who do not have COVID-19 should continue to take low dose sGC to maintain the stability of their disease. – SLE patients with mild COVID-19 complications should continue to use low dose sGC to maintain a stable condition and use antiviral drugs to reduce the side effects of sGC, -SLE patients with severe disease can be treated with high dose sGC to prevent the development of cytokine storm, as the general population [77].
Hydroxychloroquine (HCQ)	Recommended in most patients with SLE, owing to multiple health benefits and overall safety [84].	– Increase of lysosomal pH and prevention of posttranslational modification of synthesized proteins that are crucial for replication and dissemination of viruses [84]. Randomized controlled trials proved that HCQ has no clinical benefit in inhibiting SARS-CoV-2 infection [85,86].	SLE patients should continue taking HCQ even they suffer from COVID-19 [77].

(*Continued*)

TABLE 25.1 SLE drugs with possible application in COVID-19 treatment.—cont'd

Drug	Role in SLE treatment	Possible antiviral mechanisms	Use in SLE and COVID-19
Methotrexate (MTX)	Commonly used to manage moderate to severe manifestations [27].	– Could be able to inhibit SARS-CoV-2 replication by purine biosynthesis inhibition (In vitro studies) [87]. – Antagonize IL-6 production by JAK-STAT pathway inhibition, preventing hypercoagulable state and lung injury [88].	Clinical studies do not support an increased risk of SARS-CoV-2 infection in SLE patients on MTX, MMF, and cyclophosphamide. Based on these evidences, patients with SLE should continue taking these drugs to maintain stable disease, while patients with severe COVID-19 and SLE should receive DMARDs to avoid multi-organ complications [77].
Mycophenolate mofetil (MMF)	Commonly used to manage moderate to severe manifestations [27].	Possible inhibition of SARS-CoV-2 replication by purine biosynthesis inhibition [77]	
Cyclophosphamide	Used to manage severe, organ-threatening manifestations	Inhibition of B lymphocyte proliferation and antibody production [89].	
Calcineurin inhibitors (CNI)	– Inhibition of abnormal T cell and B cell hyperactivity – Inhibition of the release of proinflammatory cytokines by blocking NF-κB [90].	Can inhibit the replication of a variety of coronaviruses at low concentrations without cytotoxicity [91].	There is clinical evidence that CNI are beneficial for COVID-19 patients. It's important to monitor blood pressure in the treated patients because both COVID-19 and CNI are associated with hypertension and hypercoagulable state [77].
Belimumab	Can prevent naïve B cells from producing antibody secreting cells [92].	Down-regulation of the excessive inflammatory response in patients with severe COVID-19 by displaying activation of extrafollicular B cell responses and antibody secreting cells expansions [27].	Based on data from randomized controlled trials, there is no suggestion of a significantly increased risk of severe respiratory viral infections with belimumab use [27].
Rituximab	Used in SLE patients who are refractory or intolerant to conventional therapies [93].	Could have antiviral effect by avoid antibody secreting cells expansions [27].	2 small studies reported high rates of severe COVID-19 and mortality in patients on rituximab for various indications [94,95]. However, larger studies and longer follow-up are needed to confirm these observations [27].

not-hospitalized patients with COVID-19 and aPL on anticoagulation should keep their treatment.

Inpatients not on anticoagulation should receive prophylactic dose with LMWH or unfractionated heparin (UFH), while inpatients on oral anticoagulation, should be transitioned to therapeutic dose LMWH or UFH. LMWH is preferable to UFH because requires once daily injections and less heparin-induced thrombocytopenia (HIT), and it's also preferred to vitamin K antagonists because of potential variability of the INR due to acute illness-related factors and for its shorter half-life.

After hospital discharge thromboprophylaxis is generally recommended for at least 14 days for patients at high thrombotic risk.

LMWH on therapeutic dose should be given in COVID-19 and APS pregnant patients because pregnancy is an independent risk factor for severe COVID-19 and for thrombosis. Pregnant women with COVID-19 infection and APS on anticoagulation should not increase the prophylactic dose to therapeutic dose anticoagulation because there's no evidence that this change improves outcomes.

Pregnancy

SLE commonly occur in reproductive-aged women and population-based cohorts have demonstrated that women with this disease have fewer live births because of maternal and fetal complications (lupus flare, diabetes, pre-eclampsia, miscarriage, intrauterine fetal death, preterm birth, intrauterine growth restriction, and congenital heart block) [96]. Obviously maternal treatments have to be tailored according to the patient's pregnancy desire taking into account the disease control and the fetal safety, that requires the avoidance of teratogenic drugs (i.e., MTX, MMF and cyclophosphamide) [97].

An additional challenge in the management of this disease in pregnancy is represented by COVID-19 infection. It seems that healthy pregnant women are not thought to be more susceptible to the infection than the general population. However, changes to the immune system determine that they may be more vulnerable to severe infection. In fact it's known in scientific literature that pregnant women with COVID-19 are significantly more likely to be admitted to an ICU, receive invasive ventilation and extracorporeal membrane oxygenation and die compared to nonpregnant women [98].

A recent study has valuated 39 women affected by rheumatic disease: nine of them present SLE (23%), six APS (15%) and, among them, two patients present SLE with coexisting APS. In this small patient series, the presence of both a systemic rheumatic disease and pregnancy did not portend worse outcomes from COVID-19 infection than what has been observed in the general population of pregnant women [98]. Worse outcomes were increased in ethnic minorities, older age women and with the presence of high disease activity, comorbidities, and higher doses of prednisone [98,99].

Furthermore, evidence suggests that there is a low risk of vertical transmission or fetal distress [44,100].

Currently there is no information on how to manage COVID-19 during pregnancy in patients diagnosed with rheumatic diseases, so an individualized and multidisciplinary therapeutic approach in pregnant SLE patients diagnosed with COVID-19 is recommended [101].

Existing information on the safety of breastfeeding of COVID-19 patients is reassuring; however, since few studies have investigated this matter, larger studies are needed to clarify this issue [102].

COVID-19: vaccination SLE patients with or without APS/aPL

Since the start of the COVID-19 pandemic in March 2020, scientists and researchers have made enormous efforts to develop safe and effective vaccines against SARS-CoV-2. There are several COVID-19 vaccines validated for use by WHO (given Emergency Use Listing) detailed elsewhere in this book.

Among these vaccines, two mRNA vaccines (BNT162b2 and mRNA-1273) and one adenovirus-based vaccine (Johnson & Johnson) have been widely used both in Europe and the USA. Another adenovirus-based vaccine (ChAdOx1nCoV-19) has been dispensed in Europe while still awaiting emergency use authorization (EUA) from the Food and Drug Administration (FDA) to enter the USA [103].

Patients with SLE are, at least theoretically, among the most vulnerable population in terms of SARS-CoV-2 infection, so they have been among the first to receive the vaccines [103]. On the other hand, there is still a paucity of data regarding the safety of COVID-19 vaccines in patients with autoimmune rheumatic diseases such as SLE and APS, because these patients have largely been excluded from vaccine trials [83,104–106]. Furthermore, the use of mRNA vaccines has raised substantial concerns about the tolerance of these new vaccine technologies in patients with SLE, as Toll-like receptor stimulation by nucleic acids might increase the risk of flare [104,107]. These uncertainties have been shown to be major determinants of reduced vaccination willingness in patients with SLE and in general musculoskeletal and rheumatic diseases [83,104].

Immunogenicity and effectiveness of Covid-19 vaccines in SLE patients

Given the dysregulation of the immune system which characterize SLE patients, with a lower ability to generate adequate immune responses, these patients have been reported to have poor immune responses to vaccines against several pathogens [107] and these data were also confirmed for COVID-19 vaccines [103,107]. This is probably driven by immunosuppressants commonly used to treat SLE, including sGC, MTX, MMF, and RTX that may delay or further impair vaccine responses [103].

Some studies evaluated COVID-19 vaccine efficacy in patients with autoimmune inflammatory rheumatic diseases that included SLE, also considering the effect of different immunosuppressive regimens [103,108–111].

Taken together, these studies suggest that immunosuppressive treatments, rather than underlying autoimmune diseases, may be the main factor limiting immune responses against COVID-19 vaccines [103,108,111]. Treatments that mostly affected the humoral response were B-cell depletion therapies (BCDT), particularly RTX and GCs, followed by JAK inhibitors, and antimetabolites including MTX. Other risk factors for reduced immunogenicity of BNT162b2 vaccine are treatment with Abatacept and MMF [103,108–111].

B cell depletion following RTX treatment was significantly associated with nonseroconversion, although the majority of these patients developed T-cell responses to SARS-CoV-2 [112]. The time between the vaccination and the last exposure to RTX is an important element in maximizing the chances of a serological response: confirmation of B-cell reconstitution prior to vaccination may increase the likelihood of a positive serological response. Indeed, it was found that patients who had even low levels of B-cell reconstitution had higher rates of seropositive responses to vaccines, while patients depleted of B cells invariably demonstrated a negative serological response to vaccination [112,113].

Experimental data suggest that CD8+T cell responses may play a protective role in the presence of transient or subprotective antibody titers. It is reassuring that vaccine-induced T-cell responses were detected in the majority of patients, including those who were depleted of B cells at the time of vaccination and those who failed to seroconvert [109,112]. The use of Tacrolimus has been associated with a reduced T-cell response and further studies are needed to investigate the impact of calcineurin inhibitors and other T-cell directed therapies on vaccine both humoral and cellular responses in more detail [109].

The use of MTX as monotherapy or in combination with other treatments has mainly been associated with reduced seropositivity rate and the development of lower levels of antibodies [110] as well as a reduction in activated CD8+T cell induction which could further impair efficacy of COVID-19 vaccines [114].

In what concerns the inhibitor of B-Lymphocyte stimulating (BLyS) protein, belimumab, there are few data evaluating the specific effect on COVID-19 vaccines [115]. Spiera et al. described the serological response to COVID-19 vaccines in a series of patients with rheumatic diseases; two patients were on treatment with belimumab and one had a serological response while the other did not [116].

Although immunosuppressive therapies are the main determinants of a reduced humoral and cellular response to the vaccine, there would also seem to be a role of the immune alterations typical of the disease: in fact, in the study by *Simon* et al. in which the humoral responses to at least one dose of BNT162b2 vaccine were compared between untreated patients, patients with autoimmune rheumatic diseases (including SLE) treated with conventional or biologic DMARDs, and healthy controls, the immune response against SARS-CoV-2 was delayed and reduced in patients with rheumatic diseases and this effect seems to be based on the disease itself rather than concomitant treatment as it was also present in patients not taking any type of therapy [113]. It was, however, highlighted that following the administration of the second dose of the BNT162b2, the vast majority of patients with autoimmune rheumatic diseases developed a significant humoral response [108,113]; therefore, repeat vaccine doses may be necessary to optimize the immunological responses of these patients.

Concern has recently been raised about the effectiveness of the vaccine in the general population and also in SLE patients by the emergence of the Delta variant and even more recently of Omicron variant; in fact, the efficacy of the BNT162b2 and ChAdOx1nCoV-19 vaccines against this variant was initially unclear. Currently available data highlight only modest differences in the efficacy of the vaccines with the Delta variant compared to the Alpha variant after the administration of two doses of vaccine [117]. As regards the Omicron variant, an early estimation of vaccine effectiveness (VE) against symptomatic infection finds a significantly lower VE for Omicron infection compared to Delta infection. Nevertheless, a moderate to high vaccine effectiveness of 70%–75% is seen in the early period after a booster dose [118].

It remains to be urgently studied in greater detail whether Omicron spreads faster makes vaccines and drugs less effective or leads to more serious illnesses and deaths.

Unfortunately, there are currently no data that fully vaccinated SLE patients are at an increased risk of becoming infected with emerging variants, whether they would benefit from a booster dose and, if so, when is the optimal time to administer the booster and how to adjust the immunosuppressive regimen to optimize the effects of booster but the current recommendations of the American College of Rheumatology are the same as for the healthy population and the booster dose is recommended in any case [103,119].

Another interesting aspect that has recently been taken into consideration is the use of a heterologous vaccination booster program (ChAd/BNT) compared to a homologous one (BNT/BNT-ChAd/ChAd). The data that emerged in this regard were that the antispike IgG concentrations SARS-CoV-2 of both heterologous programs were higher than those of the homologous authorized vaccination program (ChAd/ChAd) with proven efficacy against the COVID-19 disease. Together with the higher immunogenicity of ChAd/BNT compared to ChAD/ChAd, these data support flexibility in the use of heterologous prime-boost vaccination using the ChAd and BNT COVID-19 vaccines [120].

Safety of Covid-19 vaccines in patients with SLE

The pathogenesis of SLE and COVID-19 rely on the activation of similar molecular networks, including Type I interferon and proinflammatory cytokine pathways. The nucleic acid-based vaccines used for COVID-19 can activate these pathways by signaling through endosomal Toll-like receptors (TLRs) and cytosolic RNA and DNA sensors (such as MDA5, RIG-I, and cGAS) that trigger inflammasome activation and Type I interferon production, raising initial concern that such approaches could induce disease flares [103]. In addition, it has been speculated that the mRNA vaccines may interact with cytoplasmic RNA-binding proteins involved in the posttranslational regulation of inflammatory mediators, thus triggering autoimmune disease activity [103].

Despite all the theoretical concerns above, current data on the safety of COVID19 vaccines in SLE patients have been reassuring even if scarce: in the study by *Izmirly* et al., 90 SLE patients were assessed for pre- and postvaccination disease activities by clinical and serological parameters. SLEDAI scores, percentages of patients with anti-dsDNA antibodies positivity and/or complement reduction, and levels of C3 and C4 remained similar pre- and postvaccination. Nine (11.4%) patients had postvaccination flares, of which only one was severe and characterized by arthritis requiring MTX treatment [103,121]. Furthermore *Watad* et al. presented a series of 27 cases including 17 disease flares and 10 de novo onsets of autoimmune inflammatory rheumatic diseases following administration of SARS-CoV-2 vaccines. Among them, two SLE flares and one case of discoid SLE that converted to pleuropericarditis were recorded [103]. Another study described local and systemic reactogenicity after completion of vaccination with the BNT162b2 in patients with SLE and RA compared to health controls and the data showed that patients experienced reactions following vaccination more frequently; however, these reactions were no more severe than controls. Particularly for patients with SLE and RA, pain at the injection site, fatigue, and headache were the most common events. Regarding systemic events, it has been found that patients with SLE and RA suffered more frequently from fatigue, fever, headache, chills, muscle pain, and joint pain.

No patients were hospitalized or died [105]. To date, only a single report has been made in the literature of a case of SLE arising following COVID-19 vaccination with ChAdOx1nCoV-19 in a 22-year-old woman [122]. In the International Vaccination against COVID in Systemic Lupus (VACOLUP) study, Felten et al. surveyed a group of 696 patients with SLE focusing on the tolerance, including the risk of incident flare. The results did not show a significant association between vaccination and particular side effects or the onset of SLE exacerbation. The side effects after COVID-19 vaccination in patients with SLE were common (around 50%) but did not impair daily functioning in most cases. No difference was found in the occurrence of side effects after receipt of mRNA vaccines compared with vaccines with other modes of action, which is an important and reassuring finding. Finally, the number of medically confirmed flares reported after COVID-19 vaccination was low. In conclusion, the VACOLUP study suggests that COVID-19 vaccination appears well tolerated in patients with SLE, with only a minimal risk of flare, if any, including after the mRNA vaccines, without any difference among different vaccines [104].

The results of the VACOLUP study were confirmed by the Covid-19 Global Rheumatology Alliance (C19-GRA) Vaccine Survey, the largest international survey of patients outcomes related to COVID-19 vaccines among vaccinated people with autoimmune rheumatic diseases, included SLE and APS who received BNT162b2 (53.2%), ChAdOx1nCoV-19 (22.6%), mRNA-1273 (21.3%), Ad26.COV2.S (1.7%). In fact, similarly to the data reported in the general population, only a minority of patients suffered systemic reactions to vaccination, which including fatigue, fever and pain. Systemic rheumatics disease flare-ups that require a change in medication were very rare [106].

Therefore, recent studies argue that COVID-19 vaccines are safe in SLE patients [105].

Covid-19 vaccines & aPL

Some concerns have been raised regarding the safety of the vaccines in patients with antiphospholipid antibodies, as these antibodies have been reported to appear following both infection and vaccination and have been identified in patients with COVID-19. Furthermore, several cases of Vaccine-Induced Immune Thrombocytopenia (VITT), Cerebral Venous Sinus Thrombosis (CVST), and others thrombotic events with clinical features resembling antiphospholipid syndrome have been reported in recipients of either adenoviral vector-based or mRNA-based COVID-19 vaccines, raising more concerns about the risks associated in vaccinating patients with aPL.

Regarding VITT, it clinically resembles spontaneous autoimmune HIT caused by platelet-activating IgG antibodies against platelet factor 4 (PF4) complexed with heparin. This complex then binds to the platelet FcRγIIA receptors and causes platelet activation and formation of platelet microparticles. These microparticles initiate the formation of blood clots and inducing a prothrombotic cascade, which consequently decreases platelet count and causes thrombocytopenia. Moreover, the reticuloendothelial system, particularly the spleen, removes the antibody-coated platelets and aggravates thrombocytopenia. Furthermore, PF4 is regarded as the main β2-glycoprotein I-interacting factor and, according to in vitro and in silico studies, anti-β2-glycoprotein I antibodies selectively bind β2-glycoprotein I that is complexed to PF4. The formation of such immunocomplexes can give rise to platelet activation through p38MAPK phosphorylation and release of thromboxane B2. It may be hypothesized that the binding of anti-β2-glycoprotein I antibodies to their ligand unmasks epitope domains of PF4, inducing the subsequent generation of antiplatelet PF4 antibodies. As a consequence, the dual action of both anti-β2-glycoprotein I and anti-PF4 autoantibodies would greatly increase the risk of disseminated thrombosis [123].

But despite these observations regarding VITT, a pathogenic link and, more critically, the clinical relevance of aPL in these clinical settings are yet to be fully elucidated [124]. The hypothetical immunothrombotic pathways triggered by COVID-19 vaccines are:

1. The administration of adenoviral vector-based vaccine can cause platelet aggregation and their sequestration in the reticulo-endothelial system, thus leading to thrombocytopenia and platelet activation. Furthermore, adenoviral epitopes may cross-react with epitopes within selfcomplexes of proteins and anionic lipids, generating aPLs. Anti-Spike antibodies may induce after several weeks the generation of antiidiotype antibodies, able to support platelet activation through the interaction with platelet ACE2 [125];
2. With the mRNA-based vaccine formulations, minimal amounts of mRNA released from liposomal capsules may activate Toll-like receptors in plasmacytoid dendritic cells and concur to the synthesis of Type I IFN-related cytokines. These may encourage the production of aPLs from plasma cells and NETosis. Moreover, mRNA may promote the initiation of the coagulation cascade by activating the coagulation factors VII, XI, and XII. At last, liposomal formulations may interfere with the physiological cross-talk occurring between platelets and endothelial cells and promote the activation of the inflammasome platforms into endothelial cells and thus the secretion of proinflammatory cytokines [125].

The safety and tolerability of COVID-19 vaccines have been studied in a large-scale survey study by Pengo et al. [=18] on 161 high-risk thrombotic APS patients with triple positive antiphospholipid tests (LA, aCL, and aβ2GPI) confirmed 12 weeks apart with a previous arterial or venous thromboembolic event or catastrophic variant of the syndrome. The type of vaccines administered were BNT162b2, ChAdOx1nCoV-19, and mRNA-1273. The results showed that vaccination side effects were minimal and, in most cases, limited to injection site pain. No serious safety problems were reported and no patient was hospitalized. In particular, the two patients with previous CAPS and the five patients receiving the ChAdOx1nCoV-19 vaccine did not report thrombotic complications or Vaccine-induced Immune Thrombotic Thrombocytopenia (VITT) (indeed, this complication was observed in young individuals, likewise the participants in this survey, and particularly in those having the ChAdOx1nCoV-19 vaccine) [76]. These results should reassure patients and caregivers on the safety of COVID-19 vaccination. Moreover, the results of this survey can also be translated to lower risk APS patients with incomplete positive aPL profile (double and single positivity) [76]. In another study by *Sciascia* et al., 102 vaccinated patients were studied, 52 of which had a diagnosis of antiphospholipid syndrome and 50 have antiphospholipid antibodies without clinical features of the syndrome. The 66% of the 102 patients received BNT162b2 and the 34% receive mRNA-1273 vaccine. The data showed that 76% of 102 patients had at least one side effect: 44% reported pain at the injection site, 36% fatigue, and 28% headache. Symptoms were transient and selflimiting within 10 days. There were no differences in frequencies of systemic side-effects between the two mRNA vaccines. Symptoms were reported as mild in 71% patients and moderate in 29%. No symptoms compatible with new thrombotic events were reported. The rate of reactions was not different when comparing those after the first and second doses. Only one patient with thrombotic antiphospholipid syndrome and a known history of mild thrombocytopenia (110,000/mm^3), who was on long-term vitamin K antagonist therapy, reported the occurrence of self-limiting purpuric lesions on her calves 10 days after the second dose [124]. The C19-GRA Vaccine Survey data, which included 68 patients with APS, also agree with those of these two studies [106], so, although more data are needed, including from long-term follow-up, immunogenicity data from these surveys show that mRNA COVID-19 vaccines seem to have an acceptable safety and tolerability profile in patients with antiphospholipid antibodies. No major adverse effects nor thrombotic events were reported. Side effects seem frequent, but mild and transient in nature.

Covid-19 vaccines and pregnancy

Pregnant women were excluded from preauthorization clinical studies and only limited human data on safety during pregnancy were available at the time of EUA. However, as previously treated, people who are pregnant with COVID-19 are at greater risk of serious illness (hospitalization in an intensive care unit, extracorporeal membrane oxygenation, or mechanical ventilation) and death, compared to nonpregnant people at reproductive age. Additionally, pregnant women with COVID-19 may be at increased risk of adverse pregnancy outcomes, such as preterm birth [126].

The Centers for Disease Control and Prevention (CDC) and Advisory Committee on Immunization Practices (ACIP), in partnership with the American College of Obstetricians and Gynecologists (ACOG) and the American Academy of Pediatrics (AAP), have issued guidance indicating that Covid-19 vaccines should not be withheld from pregnant person but rather actively offered regardless of age and working condition: in fact, with regards to effectiveness, there are limited data available on the efficacy of COVID-19 vaccines in pregnancy, but so far, the vaccines appear to be equally effective in pregnant individuals and nonpregnant individuals. Regarding safety the first data do not indicate any obvious risk associated with vaccination against COVID-19 in the third trimester for the safety of pregnancy and neonatal outcomes, Local and systemic solicited reactions were similar between pregnant and nonpregnant women and the proportions of adverse pregnancies and neonatal outcomes appear not significantly different from that published in the pregnancy populations studied before the COVID-19 pandemic. Emerging evidence also showed transplacental transfer of antibodies to SARS-CoV-2 after maternal vaccination during the third trimester, suggesting that maternal vaccination could provide some level of protection to the newborn [126]. Current ACOG guidelines recommend the vaccine in any trimester and that the pregnant woman be given the booster dose following the completion of their initial COVID-19 vaccine series [119].

The safety of the vaccine in pregnant women with rheumatic diseases (in particular SLE and APS) and taking immunosuppressive regimens is unclear as this patient group was not included in clinical trials and the data present in the literature on the subject are absent. Among pregnant women, mother and fetal safety and efficacy emerged as the main concerns. The risk of flare and other potential side effects, particularly in those with autoimmune conditions, is another widely voiced concern. Vaccination among breastfeeding women is another gray area, with recommendations largely based on understanding the pharmacodynamics of vaccines and antibodies [127]. However, the possible infection related damage in SLE/APS patients during pregnancy should be considered. Until there is more data in the literature, SLE/APS future mothers need to follow ACOG guidelines. Recommendations are not only that pregnant women can be vaccinated in any trimester, but also that moderately to severely immunocompromised individuals should receive an additional dose (a third dose) of an mRNA COVID-19 vaccine at least 28 days after a second dose of BNT162b2 and mRna-1273 vaccines.

Continuous monitoring is needed to further assess maternal, pregnancy, neonatal, and infant outcomes associated with maternal vaccination against Covid-19, including in the early stages of pregnancy and during the preconception period. Meanwhile, current data can help make informed vaccination decisions for pregnant people and their healthcare professionals.

Current recommendations by the American College of Rheumatology

In conclusion, the data currently available demonstrate that patients with SLE and APS with a selection of immunosuppressive therapies for inflammatory autoimmune diseases are able to develop an effective immune response after vaccination with SARS-CoV-2 mRNA without significant side effects or exacerbations. Therefore, the current recommendations of the American College of Rheumatology are to vaccinate patients with systemic autoimmune diseases because they are considered to be at greater risk because of disease itself and related treatment [128]. There is a theoretical risk of flare-up or worsening of the disease following vaccination against COVID-19; however, the benefit of COVID-19 vaccination for these patients outweighs the potential risk of developing new autoimmunity [128].

More recently, other recommendations are those concerning the type of vaccine in this category of patients, in fact: for patients not yet vaccinated, one of the mRNA vaccines is preferred over the single dose of adenovirus vaccine. There is no recommendation for one mRNA vaccine over another [128].

Patients receiving any immunosuppressant or immunomodulatory therapy other than hydroxychloroquine monotherapy and have previously completed the 2-dose vaccine series, an additional (booster) vaccine dose is recommended at least 28 days after completion of the series. Finally for booster dose mRNA vaccines of both types (BNT162b2 and mRna-1273) are preferred [128].

ACR guidelines regarding dosage and timing of immunomodulatory therapy in relation to COVID-19 vaccination are summarized in Table 25.2 [128].

Post-COVID and SLE/APS: similar manifestations

Post-COVID syndrome refers to the long-term consequences of the acute infection by SARS-CoV-2 and includes a lot of clinical manifestations, many of which could resemble those of SLE. The clinical picture of post-COVID syndrome can include, among others, long-term organ dysfunction as consequence of thrombotic events, and chronic fatigue

TABLE 25.2 Recommendations regarding dosage and timing of immunomodulatory therapy with regard to COVID-19 vaccination.

Medication	Timing consideration for immunomodulatory therapy and vaccination
Rituximab or other anti-CD20 B-cell depleting agents	Provide the booster 2–4 weeks before next anticipated rituximab dose.
Belimumab S.Q	Discontinue for 1–2 weeks after each COVID vaccine dose (depending on disease activity).
Intravenous cyclophosphamide	Administer the drug about a week after the vaccine.
Hydroxychloroquine	No changes are required.
All other conventional and targeted immunomodulatory or immunosuppressive medications including: Azathioprine, calcineurin inhibitors, cyclophosphamide (oral), methotrexate, Janus Kinase inhibitors, Mychophenolate Mofetile	Discontinue for 1–2 weeks after each COVID vaccine dose (depending on disease activity).
Acetaminophen, NSAIDs	If the disease is stable, stop for 24 h prior to vaccination. No restrictions on use postvaccination to treat symptoms.
Glucocorticoids	The suspension is not necessary in case of dosage <10 mg/day, in case of higher dosages it is useful to evaluate the disease activity with the physician.

Modified from the ACR guidelines.

syndrome, which is one of the most common expression of post-COVID syndrome [22,23]. Other common manifestations in the general population include dyspnea, nervous system involvement with associated olfactory and gustatory dysfunction, chest pain, myalgia, sleep, and mental disorders [22,23]. Although these manifestations are common in patients with rheumatic diseases (and also in SLE patients), some features can help the physicians in distinguishing these conditions. For example, myalgia in rheumatic disease is frequently associated with other signs or symptoms such as Raynaud phenomenon, skin rashes, and specific autoantibodies positivity, which occurred less frequently in post-COVID syndrome [129]. Data from the international registry for COVID-19 dermatological manifestation (promoted by the International League of Dermatological Societies and the American Academy of Dermatology) showed that one patient developed livedo reticularis (a frequent skin manifestation in patients with APS) and a lupus pernio 1 month after the exposure to a Sars-CoV-2 positive family member and that the patient tested positive for SARS-CoV-2 serum IgG 1 month after the appearance of skin lesions; his cutaneous manifestations persisted for over 150 days [130]. Moreover, in literature are reported some cases of chilblain acral lesions which resembled those of connective tissue diseases [131]. In the majority of cases, these lesions resolved spontaneously but in other cases they could be persistent [130,131]. Finally, other symptoms such as fatigue, arthralgia, and breathlessness could be frequent findings in both post-COVID syndrome and in SLE and should be deepened.

On the laboratory side, two cases of post-COVID syndrome with positivity for aPL were reported [132,133]. One, described the case of a patient with postural orthostatic tachycardia (POTS) and mast cell activation syndrome, developed after COVID-19 infection, with persistent positivity of aPL (anti-beta2GPI IgM; anti-phosphatidylethanolamine IgM, anti-phosphatidylserine IgG) [132]. The other, reported a case of a patient with post-COVID syndrome characterized by neurologic symptoms and persistent aCL IgG positivity and low eosinophils count 1 year after COVID-19 infection [133]. Since aCL autoantibodies and eosinopenia were recognized as independent factors associated with COVID-19 severity, the authors suggested that they could be predictors of post-COVID syndrome [133] but more data are needed to better understand these findings.

References

[1] Thanou A, Sawalha AH. SARS-CoV-2 and systemic lupus erythematosus. Curr Rheumatol Rep 2021. https://doi.org/10.1007/s11926-020-00973-w. Published online.

[2] Spihlman AP, Gadi N, Wu SC, Moulton VR. COVID-19 and systemic lupus erythematosus: focus on immune response and therapeutics. Front Immunol 2020;11(October):1–12. https://doi.org/10.3389/fimmu.2020.589474.

[3] Danza A, Ruiz-Irastorza G. Infection risk in systemic lupus erythematosus patients: susceptibility factors and preventive strategies. Lupus 2013. https://doi.org/10.1177/0961203313493032. Published online.

[4] Felsenstein S, Herbert JA, McNamara PS, Hedrich CM. COVID-19: immunology and treatment options. Clin Immunol 2020. https://doi.org/10.1016/j.clim.2020.108448. Published online.

[5] Winthrop KL, Whitley RJ, Aletaha D. CoV-2 and the rheumatology patient: the last 12 months and a boost in the future 1249–1251. https://doi.org/10.1136/annrheumdis-2021-221251.

[6] Dotan A, Muller S, Kanduc D, David P, Halpert G, Shoenfeld Y. The SARS-CoV-2 as an instrumental trigger of autoimmunity. Autoimmun Rev 2021. https://doi.org/10.1016/j.autrev.2021.102792. Published online.

[7] Moody R, Wilson K, Flanagan KL, Jaworowski A, Plebanski M. Adaptive immunity and the risk of autoreactivity in covid-19. Int J Mol Sci 2021. https://doi.org/10.3390/ijms22168965. Published online.

[8] Smatti MK, Cyprian FS, Nasrallah GK, Al Thani AA, Almishal RO, Yassine HM. Viruses and autoimmunity: a review on the potential interaction and molecular mechanisms. Viruses 2019. https://doi.org/10.3390/v11080762. Published online.

[9] Najafi S, Rajaei E, Moallemian R, Nokhostin F. The potential similarities of COVID-19 and autoimmune disease pathogenesis and therapeutic options: new insights approach. Clin Rheumatol November 2020;39(11):3223–35. https://doi.org/10.1007/s10067-020-05376-x. Published online 2020.

[10] Meroni PL, Borghi MO. Antiphospholipid antibodies and COVID-19 thrombotic vasculopathy: one swallow does not make a summer 2021;80(9):1105–7. https://doi.org/10.1136/annrheumdis-2021-220520.

[11] Misra DP, Agarwal V, Gasparyan AY, Zimba O. Rheumatologists' perspective on coronavirus disease 19 (COVID-19) and potential therapeutic targets. Clin Rheumatol 2020;39(7):2055–62. https://doi.org/10.1007/s10067-020-05073-9.

[12] Pons-Estel GJ, Andreoli L, Scanzi F, Cervera R, Tincani A. The antiphospholipid syndrome in patients with systemic lupus erythematosus. J Autoimmun 2017. https://doi.org/10.1016/j.jaut.2016.10.004. Published online.

[13] Linnemann B. Antiphospholipid syndrome - an update. Vasa Eur J Vasc Med 2018. https://doi.org/10.1024/0301-1526/a000723. Published online.

[14] Tung ML, Tan B, Cherian R, Chandra B. Anti-phospholipid syndrome and COVID-19 thrombosis: connecting the dots. Rheumatol Adv Pract 2021. https://doi.org/10.1093/rap/rkaa081. Published online.

[15] Khamashta M, Taraborelli M, Sciascia S, Tincani A. Antiphospholipid syndrome. Best Pract Res Clin Rheumatol 2016. https://doi.org/10.1016/j.berh.2016.04.002. Published online.

[16] Jackson SP, Darbousset R, Schoenwaelder SM. Thromboinflammation: challenges of therapeutically targeting coagulation and other host defense mechanisms. Blood 2019. https://doi.org/10.1182/blood-2018-11-882993. Published online.

[17] Abou-Ismail MY, Diamond A, Kapoor S, Arafah Y, Nayak L. The hypercoagulable state in COVID-19: incidence, pathophysiology, and management. Thromb Res 2020. https://doi.org/10.1016/j.thromres.2020.06.029. Published online.

[18] Fredi M, Cavazzana I, Moschetti L, et al. COVID-19 in patients with rheumatic diseases in northern Italy: a single-centre observational and case–control study. Lancet Rheumatol 2020. https://doi.org/10.1016/S2665-9913(20)30169-7. Published online.

[19] Kabi A, Mohanty A, Mohanty AP, Kumar S. Post COVID-19 syndrome: a literature review. J Adv Med Med Res 2020. https://doi.org/10.9734/jammr/2020/v32i2430781. Published online.

[20] Amenta EM, Spallone A, Rodriguez-Barradas MC, Sahly HME, Atmar RL, Kulkarni PA. Postacute covid-19: an overview and approach to classification. Open Forum Infect Dis 2020. https://doi.org/10.1093/ofid/ofaa509. Published online.

[21] WHO/2019-nCoV/Post_COVID-19_condition/Clinical_case_definition/2021.1.

[22] Sengupta R, Sisodia M, Kumar A, Verma G, Banerjee S. Challenges of post covid syndrome-A. New Menace 2021;4(9).

[23] Maltezou HC, Pavli A, Tsakris A. Post-COVID syndrome: an insight on its pathogenesis. Vaccines 2021. https://doi.org/10.3390/vaccines9050497. Published online.

[24] El Aoud S, Morin C, Lorriaux P, et al. COVID-19 presenting as lupus erythematosus-like syndrome. Disaster Med Public Health Prep 2021. https://doi.org/10.1017/dmp.2020.358. Published online.

[25] Kouhsari E, Azizian K, Sholeh M, et al. Clinical, epidemiological, laboratory, and radiological characteristics of novel Coronavirus (2019-nCoV) in retrospective studies: a systemic review and meta-analysis. Indian J Med Microbiol 2021. https://doi.org/10.1016/j.ijmmb.2020.10.004. Published online.

[26] Cojocaru M, Cojocaru IM, Silosi I, Vrabie CD. Manifestations of systemic lupus erythematosus. Mædica J Clin Med 2011;6(4):330–6.

[27] Fernandez-Ruiz R, Paredes JL, Niewold TB. COVID-19 in patients with systemic lupus erythematosus: lessons learned from the inflammatory disease. Transl Res 2021. https://doi.org/10.1016/j.trsl.2020.12.007. Published online.

[28] Tan L, Wang Q, Zhang D, et al. Lymphopenia predicts disease severity of COVID-19: a descriptive and predictive study. Signal Transduct Targeted Ther 2020. https://doi.org/10.1038/s41392-020-0148-4. Published online.

[29] Katsuyama E, Suarez-Fueyo A, Bradley SJ, et al. The CD38/NAD/SIRTUIN1/EZH2 Axis mitigates cytotoxic CD8 T cell function and identifies patients with SLE prone to infections. Cell Rep 2020. https://doi.org/10.1016/j.celrep.2019.12.014. Published online.

[30] Hadjadj J, Yatim N, Barnabei L, et al. Impaired type I interferon activity and inflammatory responses in severe COVID-19 patients. Science 2020;80. https://doi.org/10.1126/science.abc6027. Published online.

[31] Niewold TB. Interferon alpha as a primary pathogenic factor in human lupus. J Interferon Cytokine Res 2011. https://doi.org/10.1089/jir.2011.0071. Published online.

[32] Zhou Q, Chen V, Shannon CP, et al. Interferon-α2b treatment for COVID-19. Front Immunol 2020. https://doi.org/10.3389/fimmu.2020.01061. Published online.

[33] Georges E, Rihova Z, Cmejla R, Decleire PY, Langen C. Parvovirus B19 induced lupus-like syndrome with nephritis. Acta Clin Belgica Int J Clin Lab Med 2016. https://doi.org/10.1080/17843286.2015.1111673. Published online.

[34] Cardoso EM. Concomitant new diagnosis of systemic lupus erythematosus and COVID-19 with possible antiphospholipid syndrome. Just a coincidence ? A case report and review of intertwining pathophysiology. Clin Rheumatol 2020:6–10. Published online.

[35] Bonometti R, Sacchi MC, Stobbione P, et al. The first case of systemic lupus erythematosus (SLE) triggered by COVID-19 infection. Eur Rev Med Pharmacol Sci 2020. https://doi.org/10.26355/eurrev_202009_23060. Published online.

[36] Najafi S, Rajaei E, Moallemian R, Nokhostin F. The potential similarities of COVID-19 and autoimmune disease pathogenesis and therapeutic options: new insights approach. Clin Rheumatol 2020. https://doi.org/10.1007/s10067-020-05376-x. Published online.

[37] Raghavan S, Gonakoti S, Asemota IR, Mba B. A case of systemic lupus erythematosus flare triggered by severe coronavirus disease 2019. J Clin Rheumatol. Published online 2020. https://doi.org/10.1097/RHU.0000000000001531.

[38] Kondo Y, Kaneko Y, Oshige T, et al. Exacerbation of immune thrombocytopenia triggered by COVID-19 in patients with systemic lupus erythematosus. Ann Rheum Dis 2021. https://doi.org/10.1136/annrheumdis-2020-218157. Published online.

[39] Doria A, Canova M, Tonon M, et al. Infections as triggers and complications of systemic lupus erythematosus. Autoimmun Rev 2008. https://doi.org/10.1016/j.autrev.2008.07.019. Published online.

[40] Bruce IN, O'Keeffe AG, Farewell V, et al. Factors associated with damage accrual in patients with systemic lupus erythematosus: results from the systemic lupus international collaborating clinics (SLICC) inception cohort. Ann Rheum Dis 2015. https://doi.org/10.1136/annrheumdis-2013-205171. Published online.

[41] Ramirez GA, Gerosa M, Beretta L, et al. COVID-19 in systemic lupus erythematosus: data from a survey on 417 patients. Semin Arthritis Rheum 2020. https://doi.org/10.1016/j.semarthrit.2020.06.012. Published online.

[42] Murtas R, Andreano A, Gervasi F, et al. Association between autoimmune diseases and COVID-19 as assessed in both a test-negative case-control and population case-control design. Autoimmun Highlights 2020. https://doi.org/10.1186/s13317-020-00141-1. Published online.

[43] Raiker R, Pakhchanian H, DeYoung C, et al. Short term outcomes of COVID-19 in lupus: propensity score matched analysis from a nationwide multi-centric research network. J Autoimmun 2021. https://doi.org/10.1016/j.jaut.2021.102730. Published online.

[44] Gianfrancesco M, Hyrich KL, Hyrich KL, et al. Characteristics associated with hospitalisation for COVID-19 in people with rheumatic disease: data from the COVID-19 Global Rheumatology Alliance physician-reported registry. Ann Rheum Dis 2020. https://doi.org/10.1136/annrheumdis-2020-217871. Published online.

[45] Akiyama S, Hamdeh S, Micic D, Sakuraba A. Prevalence and clinical outcomes of COVID-19 in patients with autoimmune diseases: a systematic review and meta-analysis. Ann Rheum Dis 2021. https://doi.org/10.1136/annrheumdis-2020-218946. Published online.

[46] Spihlman AP, Gadi N, Wu SC, Moulton VR. COVID-19 and systemic lupus erythematosus: focus on immune response and therapeutics. Front Immunol 2020. https://doi.org/10.3389/fimmu.2020.589474. Published online.

[47] Sakthiswary R, Chuah HY, Chiang KS, Liew YS, Muhammad Aizat NA. COVID-19 in systemic lupus erythematosus: a pooled analysis and systematic review of case reports and series. Lupus 2021. https://doi.org/10.1177/09612033211045057. Published online.

[48] Alarcón GS. Multiethnic lupus cohorts: what have they taught us? Reumatol Clínica 2011. https://doi.org/10.1016/j.reuma.2010.11.001. Published online.

[49] Williamson EJ, Walker AJ, Bhaskaran K, et al. OpenSAFELY: factors associated with COVID-19 death in 17 million patients. Nature 2020. https://doi.org/10.1038/s41586-020-2521-4. Published online.

[50] Taha M, Samavati L. Antiphospholipid antibodies in COVID-19: a meta-analysis and systematic review. RMD Open 2021. https://doi.org/10.1136/rmdopen-2021-001580. Published online.

[51] El Hasbani G, Taher AT, Jawad A, Uthman I. COVID-19, antiphospholipid antibodies, and catastrophic antiphospholipid syndrome: a possible association? Clin Med Insights Arthritis Musculoskelet Disord 2020. https://doi.org/10.1177/1179544120978667. Published online.

[52] Zhang Y, Xiao M, Zhang S, et al. Coagulopathy and antiphospholipid antibodies in patients with covid-19. N Engl J Med 2020. https://doi.org/10.1056/nejmc2007575. Published online.

[53] Wang X, Gkrouzman E, Castro Oliveira Andrade D, Andreoli L, Barbhaiya M, Belmont HM, Ware Branch D, de Jesús GR, Efthymiou M, Ríos-Garcés R, Gerosa M, Georges El Hasb AA. COVID-19 and antiphospholipid antibodies: a position statement and management guidance from AntiPhospholipid syndrome alliance for clinical trials and international networking (APS ACTION). Lupus 2021;(Dec). https://doi.org/10.1177/09612033211062523.

[54] Pearce L, Davidson SM, Yellon DM. The cytokine storm of COVID-19: a spotlight on prevention and protection. Expert Opin Ther Targets August 2020;24(8):723–30. https://doi.org/10.1080/14728222.2020.1783243. Epub 2020 Jun 27. PMID: 32594778.

[55] Skendros P, Mitsios A, Chrysanthopoulou A, et al. Complement and tissue factor–enriched neutrophil extracellular traps are key drivers in COVID-19 immunothrombosis. J Clin Invest 2020. https://doi.org/10.1172/JCI141374. Published online.

[56] Diurno F, Numis FG, Porta G, et al. Eculizumab treatment in patients with COVID-19: preliminary results from real life ASL Napoli 2 Nord experience. Eur Rev Med Pharmacol Sci 2020. https://doi.org/10.26355/EUR-REV_202004_20875. Published online.

[57] Meng H, Yalavarthi S, Kanthi Y, et al. In vivo role of neutrophil extracellular traps in antiphospholipid antibody–mediated venous thrombosis. Arthritis Rheumatol 2017. https://doi.org/10.1002/art.39938. Published online.
[58] Middleton EA, He XY, Denorme F, et al. Neutrophil extracellular traps contribute to immunothrombosis in COVID-19 acute respiratory distress syndrome. Blood 2020. https://doi.org/10.1182/blood.2020007008. Published online.
[59] Willis R, Pierangeli SS. Pathophysiology of the antiphospholipid antibody syndrome. Autoimmun Highlights 2011. https://doi.org/10.1007/s13317-011-0017-9. Published online.
[60] Trahtemberg U, Rottapel R, Santos CCD, Slutsky AS, Baker A, Fritzler MJ. Anticardiolipin and other antiphospholipid antibodies in critically ill COVID-19 positive and negative patients. 2021. p. 1236–40. https://doi.org/10.1136/annrheumdis-2021-220206. Published online.
[61] Devreese KMJ, Linskens EA, Benoit D, Peperstraete H. Antiphospholipid antibodies in patients with COVID-19: a relevant observation? J Thromb Haemostasis 2020. https://doi.org/10.1111/jth.14994. Published online.
[62] Zhang Y, Cao W, Jiang W, et al. Profile of natural anticoagulant, coagulant factor and anti-phospholipid antibody in critically ill COVID-19 patients. J Thromb Thrombolysis 2020. https://doi.org/10.1007/s11239-020-02182-9. Published online.
[63] Harzallah I, Debliquis A, Drénou B. Frequency of lupus anticoagulant in COVID-19 patients. J Thromb Haemostasis 2020. https://doi.org/10.1111/jth.14937. Published online.
[64] Maria ATJ, Diaz-Cau I, Benejean J-M, et al. Flare of antiphospholipid syndrome in the course of COVID-19. TH Open 2020. https://doi.org/10.1055/s-0040-1716735. Published online.
[65] Gkrouzman E, Barbhaiya M, Erkan D, Lockshin MD. Reality check on antiphospholipid antibodies in COVID-19–associated coagulopathy. Arthritis Rheumatol 2021. https://doi.org/10.1002/art.41472. Published online.
[66] Agostinis C, Biffi S, Garrovo C, et al. In vivo distribution of β2 glycoprotein I under various pathophysiologic conditions. Blood 2011. https://doi.org/10.1182/blood-2011-01-333617. Published online.
[67] Pregnolato F, Gerosa M, Raimondo MG, et al. EUREKA algorithm predicts obstetric risk and response to treatment in women with different subsets of anti-phospholipid antibodies. Rheumatol (United Kingdom) . Published online 2021. doi:10.1093/rheumatology/keaa203
[68] Borghi MO, Beltagy A, Garrafa E, et al. Anti-phospholipid antibodies in COVID-19 are different from those detectable in the anti-phospholipid syndrome. Front Immunol 2020. https://doi.org/10.3389/fimmu.2020.584241. Published online.
[69] Andreoli L, Chighizola CB, Nalli C, et al. Clinical characterization of antiphospholipid syndrome by detection of IgG antibodies against β2-glycoprotein i domain 1 and domain 4/5: ratio of anti-domain 1 to anti-domain 4/5 as a useful new biomarker for antiphospholipid syndrome. Arthritis Rheumatol 2015. https://doi.org/10.1002/art.39187. Published online.
[70] Meroni PL, Borghi MO, Raschi E, Tedesco F. Pathogenesis of antiphospholipid syndrome: understanding the antibodies. Nat Rev Rheumatol 2011. https://doi.org/10.1038/nrrheum.2011.52. Published online.
[71] Sène D, Piette JC, Cacoub P. Antiphospholipid antibodies, antiphospholipid syndrome and infections. Autoimmun Rev 2008. https://doi.org/10.1016/j.autrev.2007.10.001. Published online.
[72] Lazzaroni MG, Piantoni S, Masneri S, Garrafa E, Martini G, Tincani A, Andreoli L, Franceschini F. Coagulation dysfunction in COVID-19: the interplay between inflammation, viral infection and the coagulation system. Blood Rev March 2021;46:100745. https://doi.org/10.1016/j.blre.2020.100745. Epub 2020 Aug 24. PMID: 32868115; PMCID: PMC7444609.
[73] Aguirre-Alastuey ME, Suárez-Díaz S, Rodríguez-Jerez F, Coto-Hernández R, Caminal-Montero L. Venous thrombosis in a systemic lupus erythematosus patient with antiphospholipid antibodies coinciding with mild Covid-19. Lupus 2021. https://doi.org/10.1177/0961203320967407. Published online.
[74] Hayden A, Vyas-Lahar A, Rella V, Rudinskaya A. Severe refractory thrombocytopenia in a woman positive for coronavirus disease 2019 with lupus and antiphospholipid syndrome. Lupus 2020. https://doi.org/10.1177/0961203320940389. Published online.
[75] Choi B, Choudhary MC, Regan J, et al. Persistence and evolution of SARS-CoV-2 in an immunocompromised host. N Engl J Med 2020. https://doi.org/10.1056/nejmc2031364. Published online.
[76] Pengo V, Del Ross T, Tonello M, Andreoli L, Tincani A, Gresele P, Silvestri E, Simioni P, Campello E, Hoxha A, Anna F, Ghirarduzzi A, Denas G. COVID-19 APS collaborators. Impact of COVID-19 and COVID-19 vaccination on high-risk patients with Antiphospholipid Syndrome. [Submitted].

[77] Zhou B, Li S, Ye J, et al. Immunopathological events surrounding IL-6 and IFN-α: a bridge for anti-lupus erythematosus drugs used to treat COVID-19. Int Immunopharm. Published online 2021. https://doi.org/10.1016/j.intimp.2021.108254.

[78] Durcan L, O'Dwyer T, Petri M. Management strategies and future directions for systemic lupus erythematosus in adults. Lancet 2019. https://doi.org/10.1016/S0140-6736(19)30237-5. Published online.

[79] Zhong J, Shen G, Yang H, et al. COVID-19 in patients with rheumatic disease in Hubei province, China: a multicentre retrospective observational study. Lancet Rheumatol 2020. https://doi.org/10.1016/S2665-9913(20)30227-7. Published online.

[80] Chen JS, Alfajaro MM, Chow RD, et al. Nonsteroidal anti-inflammatory drugs dampen the cytokine and antibody response to SARS-CoV-2 infection. J Virol 2021;95(7):1–16. https://doi.org/10.1128/jvi.00014-21.

[81] García LF. Immune response, inflammation, and the clinical spectrum of COVID-19. Front Immunol 2020;11:1441. https://doi.org/10.3389/fimmu.2020.01441. Published 2020 Jun 16.

[82] Åkerström S, Mousavi-Jazi M, Klingström J, Leijon M, Å L, Mirazimi A. Nitric oxide inhibits the replication cycle of severe acute respiratory syndrome coronavirus. J Virol 2005. https://doi.org/10.1128/jvi.79.3.1966-1969.2005. Published online.

[83] Lu S, Zhou Q, Huang L, et al. Effectiveness and safety of glucocorticoids to treat COVID-19: a rapid review and meta-analysis. Ann Transl Med 2020. https://doi.org/10.1101/2020.04.17.20064469. Published online.

[84] Bansal P, Goyal A, Cusick A, Lahan S, Dhaliwal HS. Hydroxychloroquine: a comprehensive review and its controversial role in coronavirus disease 2019. Ann Med 2021;53(1):117–34. https://doi.org/10.1080/07853890.2020.1839959.

[85] Mitjà O, Corbacho-Monné M, Ubals M, et al. A cluster-randomized trial of hydroxychloroquine for prevention of covid-19. N Engl J Med. Published online 2021. doi:10.1056/nejmoa2021801

[86] Konig MF, Kim AHJ, Scheetz MH, et al. Baseline use of hydroxychloroquine in systemic lupus erythematosus does not preclude SARS-CoV-2 infection and severe COVID-19. Ann Rheum Dis 2020. https://doi.org/10.1136/annrheumdis-2020-217690. Published online.

[87] Stegmann KM, Dickmanns A, Gerber S, Nikolova V, Klemke L, Manzini V, Schlösser D, Bierwirth C, Freund J, Sitte M, Lugert R, Salinas G, Meister TL, Pfaender S, Görlich D, Wollnik B, Groß U, Dobbelstein M. The folate antagonist methotrexate diminishes replication of the coronavirus SARS-CoV-2 and enhances the antiviral efficacy of remdesivir in cell culture models. Virus Res September 2021;302:198469. https://doi.org/10.1016/j.virusres.2021.198469. Epub 2021 Jun 6.

[88] Meletiadis J, Tsiodras S, Tsirigotis P. Interleukin-6 blocking vs. JAK-STAT inhibition for prevention of lung injury in patients with COVID-19. Infect Dis Ther 2020;9:707–13. https://doi.org/10.1007/s40121-020-00326-1.

[89] Moeinzadeh F, et al. Newly diagnosed glomerulonephritis during COVID-19 infection undergoing immunosuppression therapy, a case report. Iran J Kidney Dis 2020;14(3):239–42.

[90] McHugh J. Targeted delivery of immunosuppressant in SLE. Nat Rev Rheumatol 2020. https://doi.org/10.1038/s41584-020-0462-9. Published online.

[91] de Wilde AH, Raj VS, Oudshoorn D, Bestebroer TM, van Nieuwkoop S, Limpens RWAL, Posthuma CC, van der Meer Y, arcena MB, Haagmans BL, Snijder EJ, van den Hoogen BG. MERS-coronavirus replication induces severe in vitro cytopathology and is strongly inhibited by cyclosporin A or interferon-α treatment. J Gen Virol August 2013;94(Pt 8):1749–60. https://doi.org/10.1099/vir.0.052910-0. Epub 2013 Apr 25. PMID: 23620378; PMCID: PMC3749523.

[92] Blair HA, Duggan ST. Belimumab: a review in systemic lupus erythematosus. Drugs March 2018;78(3):355–66. https://doi.org/10.1007/s40265-018-0872-z. PMID: 29396833.

[93] Mok CC. Current role of rituximab in systemic lupus erythematosus. Int J Rheum Dis 2015. https://doi.org/10.1111/1756-185X.12463. Published online.

[94] Notz Q, Meybohm P, Kranke P, Weismann D, Lotz C, Schmalzing M. Antirheumatic drugs, B cell depletion and critical COVID-19: correspondence on 'Clinical course of corona- virus disease 2019 (COVID-19) in a series of 17 patients with systemic lupus erythematosus. Ann Rheum Dis August 2020;28. https://doi.org/10.1136/annrheumdis-2020-218778. annrheumdis-2020-218778.

[95] Loarce-Martos J, Garcıa-Fernandez A, Lopez-Gutierrez F, et al. High rates of severe disease and death due to SARS-CoV-2 infection in rheumatic disease patients treated with rituximab: a descriptive study. Rheumatol Int 2020;1–7. https://doi.org/10.1007/s00296-020-04699-x. Epub 2020 Sep 18. PMID: 32945944; PMCID: PMC7499013.

[96] Andreoli L, Bertsias GK, Agmon-Levin N, et al. EULAR recommendations for women's health and the management of family planning, assisted reproduction, pregnancy and menopause in patients with systemic lupus erythematosus and/or antiphospholipid syndrome. Ann Rheum Dis 2017;76(3):476–85. https://doi.org/10.1136/annrheumdis-2016-209770.

[97] Peart E, Clowse MEB. Systemic lupus erythematosus and pregnancy outcomes: an update and review of the literature. Curr Opin Rheumatol 2014. https://doi.org/10.1097/BOR.0000000000000030. Published online.

[98] Bermas BL, Gianfrancesco M, Tanner HL, et al. COVID-19 in pregnant women with rheumatic disease: data from the COVID-19 global rheumatology alliance. Published online 2021:1-5. https://doi.org/10.3899/jrheum.210480.

[99] Zambrano LD, Ellington S, Strid P, et al. Update: characteristics of symptomatic women of reproductive age with laboratory-confirmed SARS-CoV-2 infection by pregnancy status — United States, January 22–October 3, 2020. MMWR Morb Mortal Wkly Rep 2020. https://doi.org/10.15585/mmwr.mm6944e3. Published online.

[100] Fenizia C, Biasin M, Cetin I, et al. Analysis of SARS-CoV-2 vertical transmission during pregnancy. Nat Commun 2020;11(1). https://doi.org/10.1038/s41467-020-18933-4.

[101] Smeele HTW, Perez-garcia LF, Grimminck K, Schoenmakers S, Mulders AG, Dolhain RJEM. Systemic lupus erythematosus and COVID-19 during pregnancy. 2021. https://doi.org/10.1177/09612033211002270. Published online.

[102] Raschetti R, Vivanti AJ, Vauloup-Fellous C, Loi B, Benachi A, De Luca D. Synthesis and systematic review of reported neonatal SARS-CoV-2 infections. Nat Commun 2020. https://doi.org/10.1038/s41467-020-18982-9. Published online.

[103] Tang W, Gartshteyn Y, Ricker E, et al. The use of COVID-19 vaccines in patients with SLE. Curr Rheumatol Rep 2021;23:79. https://doi.org/10.1007/s11926-021-01046-2. PMID: 34767100; PMCID: PMC8586600.

[104] Felten R, Kawka L, Dubois M, Ugarte-Gil MF, Fuentes-Silva Y, Piga M, Arnaud L. Tolerance of COVID-19 vaccination in patients with systemic lupus erythematosus: the international VACOLUP study. Lancet Rheumatol September 2021;3(9):e613–5. https://doi.org/10.1016/S2665-9913(21)00221-6. Epub 2021 Jul 21. PMID: 34312612; PMCID: PMC8294805.

[105] Bartels LE, Ammitzbøll C, Andersen JB, Vils SR, Mistegaard CE, Johannsen AD, Hermansen MF, Thomsen MK, Erikstrup C, Hauge EM, Troldborg A. Local and systemic reactogenicity of COVID-19 vaccine BNT162b2 in patients with systemic lupus erythematosus and rheumatoid arthritis. Rheumatol Int November 2021;41(11):1925–31. https://doi.org/10.1007/s00296-021-04972-7. Epub 2021 Sep. 2.

[106] Sattui SE, Liew JW, Kennedy K, Sirotich E, Putman M, Moni TT, Akpabio A, Alpízar-Rodríguez D, Berenbaum F, Bulina I, Conway R, Singh AD, Duff E, Durrant KL, Gheita TA, Hill CL, Howard RA, Hoyer BF, Hsieh E, El Kibbi L, Kilian A, Kim AH, Liew DFL, Lo C, Miller B, Mingolla S, Nudel M, Palmerlee CA, Singh JA, Singh N, Ugarte-Gil MF, Wallace J, Young KJ, Bhana S, Costello W, Grainger R, Machado PM, Robinson PC, Paul S, Wallace ZS, Yazdany J, Harrison C, Larché M, Levine M, Foster G, Thabane L, Rider LG, Hausmann JS, Simard JF, Sparks JA. Early experience of COVID-19 vaccination in adults with systemic rheumatic diseases: results from the COVID-19 Global Rheumatology Alliance Vaccine Survey. RMD Open September 2021;7(3):e001814. https://doi.org/10.1136/rmdopen-2021-001814.

[107] Mason A, Anver H, Lwin M, Holroyd C, Faust SN, Edwards CJ. Lupus, vaccinations and COVID-19: what we know now. Lupus September 2021;30(10):1541–52. https://doi.org/10.1177/09612033211024355. Epub 2021 Jun 17. PMID: 34134555.

[108] Braun-Moscovici Y, Kaplan M, Braun M, Markovits D, Giryes S, Toledano K, Tavor Y, Dolnikov K, Balbir-Gurman A. Disease activity and humoral response in patients with inflammatory rheumatic diseases after two doses of the Pfizer mRNA vaccine against SARS-CoV-2. Ann Rheum Dis October 2021;80(10):1317–21. https://doi.org/10.1136/annrheumdis-2021-220503. Epub 2021 Jun 18.

[109] Prendecki M, Clarke C, Edwards H, McIntyre S, Mortimer P, Gleeson S, Martin P, Thomson T, Randell P, Shah A, Singanayagam A, Lightstone L, Cox A, Kelleher P, Willicombe M, McAdoo SP. Humoral and T-cell responses to SARS-CoV-2 vaccination in patients receiving immunosuppression. Ann Rheum Dis October 2021;80(10):1322–9. https://doi.org/10.1136/annrheumdis-2021-220626. Epub 2021 Aug 6.

[110] Furer V, Eviatar T, Zisman D, Peleg H, Paran D, Levartovsky D, Zisapel M, Elalouf O, Kaufman I, Meidan R, Broyde A, Polachek A, Wollman J, Litinsky I, Meridor K, Nochomovitz H, Silberman A, Rosenberg D, Feld J, Haddad A, Gazzit T, Elias M, Higazi N, Kharouf F, Shefer G, Sharon O, Pel S, Nevo S, Elkayam O. Immunogenicity and safety of the BNT162b2 mRNA COVID-19 vaccine in adult patients with autoimmune

inflammatory rheumatic diseases and in the general population: a multicentre study. Ann Rheum Dis October 2021;80(10):1330–8. https://doi.org/10.1136/annrheumdis-2021-220647. Epub 2021 Jun 14.

[111] Friedman MA, Curtis JR, Winthrop KL. Impact of disease-modifying antirheumatic drugs on vaccine immunogenicity in patients with inflammatory rheumatic and musculoskeletal diseases. Ann Rheum Dis October 2021;80(10):1255–65. https://doi.org/10.1136/annrheumdis-2021-22.

[112] Mrak D, Tobudic S, Koblischke M, Graninger M, Radner H, Sieghart D, Hofer P, Perkmann T, Haslacher H, Thalhammer R, Winkler S, Blüml S, Stiasny K, Aberle JH, Smolen JS, Heinz LX, Aletaha D, Bonelli M. SARS-CoV-2 vaccination in rituximab-treated patients: B cells promote humoral immune responses in the presence of T-cell-mediated immunity. Ann Rheum Dis October 2021;80(10):1345–50. https://doi.org/10.1136/annrheumdis-2021-220781. Epub 2021 Jul 20.

[113] Simon D, Tascilar K, Fagni F, Krönke G, Kleyer A, Meder C, Atreya R, Leppkes M, Kremer AE, Ramming A, Pachowsky ML, Schuch F, Ronneberger M, Kleinert S, Hueber AJ, Manger K, Manger B, Berking C, Sticherling M, Neurath MF, Schett G. SARS-CoV-2 vaccination responses in untreated, conventionally treated and anticytokine-treated patients with immune-mediated inflammatory diseases. Ann Rheum Dis October 2021;80(10):1312–6. https://doi.org/10.1136/annrheumdis-2021-220461. Epub 2021 May 6.

[114] Haberman RH, Herati R, Simon D, Samanovic M, Blank RB, Tuen M, Koralov SB, Atreya R, Tascilar K, Allen JR, Castillo R, Cornelius AR, Rackoff P, Solomon G, Adhikari S, Azar N, Rosenthal P, Izmirly P, Samuels J, Golden B, Reddy SM, Neurath MF, Abramson SB, Schett G, Mulligan MJ, Scher JU. Methotrexate hampers immunogenicity to BNT162b2 mRNA COVID-19 vaccine in immune-mediated inflammatory disease. Ann Rheum Dis October 2021;80(10):1339–44. https://doi.org/10.1136/annrheumdis-2021-220597. Epub 2021 May 25.

[115] Wack S, Patton TFL. COVID-19 vaccine safety and efficacy in patients with immune-mediated inflammatory disease: review of available evidence. J Am Acad Dermatol November 2021;85(5):1274–84. https://doi.org/10.1016/j.jaad.2021.07.054. Epub 2021 Aug 4. PMID: 34363909; PMCID: PMC8336973.

[116] Spiera R, Jinich SJ-KD. Rituximab, but not other antirheumatic therapies, is associated with impaired serological response to SARS- CoV-2 vaccination in patients with rheumatic diseases. Ann Rheum Dis October 2021;80(10):1357–9. https://doi.org/10.1136/annrheumdis-2021-220604. Epub 2021 May 11. PMID: 33975857.

[117] Harder T, Külper-Schiek W, Reda S, Treskova-Schwarzbach M, Koch J, Vygen-Bonnet S, Wichmann O. Effectiveness of COVID-19 vaccines against SARS-CoV-2 infection with the Delta (B.1.617.2) variant: second interim results of a living systematic review and meta-analysis, 1 January to 25 August 2021. Euro Surveill October 2021;26(41):2100920.

[118] SARS-CoV-2 variants of concern and variants under investigation in England. UK Health Security Agency; December 10 , 2021. Technical Briefing 31.

[119] COVID-19 vaccines and pregnancy: conversation guide. Am Coll Obstetr Gynecol December 2021. https://www.acog.org/covid-19/covid-19-vaccines-and-pregnancy-conversation-guide-for-clinicians.

[120] Liu X, Shaw RH, Stuart ASV, Greenland M, Aley PK, Andrews NJ, Cameron JC, Charlton S, Clutterbuck EA, Collins AM, Dinesh T, England A, Faust SN, Ferreira DM, Finn A, Green CA, Hallis B, Heath PT, Hill H, Lambe T, Lazarus R, Libri V, Long F, Mujadidi YF, Plested EL, Provstgaard-Morys S, Ramasamy MN, Ramsay M, Read RC, Robinson H, Singh N, Turner DPJ, Turner PJ, Walker LL, White R, Nguyen-Van-Tam JS, Snape MD, Study Group C-COV. Safety and immunogenicity of heterologous versus homologous prime-boost schedules with an adenoviral vectored and mRNA COVID-19 vaccine (Com-COV): a single-blind, randomised, non-inferiority trial. Lancet September 4, 2021;398(10303):856–69. https://doi.org/10.1016/S0140-6736(21)01694-9. Epub 2021 Aug 6. PMID: 34370971; PMCID: PMC8346248.

[121] Izmirly PM, Kim MY, Samanovic M, Fernandez-Ruiz R, Ohana S, Deonaraine KK, Engel AJ, Masson M, Xie X, Cornelius AR, Herati RS, Haberman RH, Scher JU, Guttmann A, Blank RB, Plotz B, Haj-Ali M, Banbury B, Stream S, Hasan G, Ho G, Rackoff P, Blazer AD, Tseng. Evaluation of immune response and disease status in SLE patients following SARS-CoV-2 vaccination. Arthritis Rheumatol August 4, 2021. https://doi.org/10.1002/art.41937. https://doi.org/10.1002/art.41937.

[122] Patil S, Patil A. Systemic lupus erythematosus after COVID-19 vaccination: a case report. J Cosmet Dermatol October 2021;20(10):3103–4. https://doi.org/10.1111/jocd.14386. Epub 2021 Aug 21. PMID: 34418261; PMCID: PMC8661983.

[123] Sharifian-Dorche M, Bahmanyar M, Sharifian-Dorche A, Mohammadi P, Nomovi MMA. Vaccine-induced immune thrombotic thrombocytopenia and cerebral venous sinus thrombosis post COVID-19 vaccination; a

systematic review. J Neurol Sci 2021;Sep;15:428. https://doi.org/10.1016/j.jns.2021.117607. Epub 2021 Aug 3. PMID: 34365148; PMCID: PMC8330139.

[124] Sciascia S, Costanzo P, Radin M, Schreiber K, Pini M, Vaccarino A, Cecchi I, Baldovino S, Roccatello D. Safety and tolerability of mRNA COVID-19 vaccines in people with antiphospholipid antibodies. Lancet Rheumatol December 2021;3(12):e832. https://doi.org/10.1016/S2665-9913(21)00320-9. Epub 2021 Oct 20. PMID: 34697607; PMCID: PMC8528471.

[125] Talotta R, Robertson ES. Antiphospholipid antibodies and risk of post-COVID-19 vaccination thrombophilia: the straw that breaks the camel's back? Cytokine Growth Factor Rev August 2021;60:52–60. https://doi.org/10.1016/j.cytogfr.2021.05.001. Epub 2021 May 28. PMID: 34090785; PMCID: PMC8159713.

[126] Shimabukuro TT, Kim SY, Myers TR, Moro PL, Oduyebo T, Panagiotakopoulos L, Marquez PL, Olson CK, Liu R, Chang KT, Ellington SR, Burkel VK, Smoots AN, Green CJ, Licata C, Zhang BC, Alimchandani M, Mba-Jonas A, Martin SW, Gee JM, Meaney-Delman DM. CDCv-safe COVID-19 pregnancy registry team. Preliminary findings of mRNA covid-19 vaccine safety in pregnant persons. N Engl J Med June 17, 2021;384(24):2273–82. https://doi.org/10.1056/NEJMoa2104983. Epub 2021 Apr 21. Erratum in: N Engl J Med. 2021 Oct 14;385(16):1536. PMID: 33882218; PMCID: PMC8117969.

[127] Tariq J, Gupta L. Safety and efficacy of COVID-19 vaccines in pregnant women with rheumatic diseases: an immunologic perspective. Rheumatol Int August 2021;41(8):1545–7. https://doi.org/10.1007/s00296-021-04918-z. Epub 2021 Jun 10. PMID: 34110465; PMCID: PMC8190165.

[128] Covid-19 vaccine clinical guidance summary for patients with rheumatic and musculoskeletal diseases. Am Coll Rheumatol Version4 October 27, 2021. https://www.rheumatology.org/Portals/0/Files/COVID-19-Vaccine-Clinical-Guidance-Rheumatic-Dis.

[129] Sapkota HR, Nune A. Long COVID from rheumatology perspective - a narrative review. Clin Rheumatol November 2021;30:1–12. https://doi.org/10.1007/s10067-021-06001-1. Epub ahead of print. PMID: 34845562; PMCID: PMC8629735.

[130] McMahon DE, Gallman AE, Hruza GJ, Rosenbach M, Lipoff JB, Desai SR, French LE, Lim H, Cyster JG, Fox LP, Fassett MS, Freeman EE. Long COVID in the skin: a registry analysis of COVID-19 dermatological duration. Lancet Infect Dis March 2021;21(3):313–4. https://doi.org/10.1016/S1473-3099(20)30986-5. Epub 2021 Jan 15. PMID: 33460566; PMCID: PMC7836995.

[131] Mehta P, Bunker CB, Ciurtin C, Porter JC, Chambers RC, Papdopoulou C, Garthwaite H, Hillman T, Heightman M, Howell KJ, Eleftheriou D, Denton CP. Chilblain-like acral lesions in long COVID-19: management and implications for understanding microangiopathy. Lancet Infect Dis July 2021;21(7):912. https://doi.org/10.1016/S1473-3099(21)00133-X. Epub 2021 Mar 8. PMID: 33705725; PMCID: PMC8221732.

[132] Schofield JR. Persistent antiphospholipid antibodies, mast cell activation syndrome, postural orthostatic tachycardia syndrome and post-COVID syndrome: 1 Year on. Eur J Case Rep Intern Med March 22, 2021;8(3):002378. https://doi.org/10.12890/2021_002378. PMID: 3386909.

[133] Bertin D, Kaphan E, Weber S, Babacci B, Arcani R, Faucher B, Ménard A, Brodovitch A, Mege JL, Bardin N. Persistent IgG anticardiolipin autoantibodies are associated with post-COVID syndrome. Int J Infect Dis December 2021;113:23–5. https://doi.org/10.1016/j.ijid.2021.0.

CHAPTER

26

Psoriatic arthritis and psoriasis in the era of COVID-19

Panagiotis Athanassiou[1], Lambros Athanassiou[2] and Ifigenia Kostoglou-Athanassiou[3]

[1]Department of Rheumatology, St. Paul's Hospital, Thessaloniki, Greece; [2]Department of Rheumatology, Asclepeion Hospital, Athens, Greece; [3]Department of Endocrinology, Asclepeion Hospital, Athens, Greece

Introduction

Psoriatic arthritis is a seronegative oligoarthritis. It is a spondyloarthropathy [1]. It can occur simultaneously with psoriasis. Psoriatic arthritis may present before, simultaneously or after psoriasis. Psoriatic arthritis is an inflammatory arthritis with ocular, intestinal, metabolic, and cardiovascular manifestations. It is characterized by arthritis, enthesitis, dactylitis, spondylitis, psoriasis, and nail disease. Psoriatic arthritis and psoriasis are autoimmune diseases. The management of psoriatic arthritis and psoriasis depends on traditional immune modulating agents and biologic agents. Various biologics have entered the field of the management of psoriatic arthritis and psoriasis and have improved patient quality of life. The SARS-CoV-2 virus is a coronavirus and has caused the recent pandemic [2]. The disease may run as a mild disease or may cause severe pneumonia which may be lethal [3]. The discussion in the scientific community on risk factors for the development of COVID-19 disease and risk factors for severe disease and death has been in the focus of world-wide interest [4–6]. The question has arisen as to whether patients with psoriatic arthritis and psoriasis on treatment with immune modulating biologic agents may be at increased risk of infection by the SARS-CoV-2 virus. It is also discussed whether patients with psoriasis and psoriatic arthritis on treatment with biologic agents are at increased risk for severe disease or death from COVID-19. The problem of psoriatic arthritis and psoriasis management during the COVID-19 pandemic has also attracted interest. The therapeutic management of patients with psoriatic arthritis or psoriasis on treatment with biologics who get infected with the SARS-CoV-2 virus is also of great interest and is currently discussed.

Autoimmunity, COVID-19, Post-COVID19 syndrome and COVID-19 vaccination
https://doi.org/10.1016/B978-0-443-18566-3.00038-4

Psoriatic arthritis and psoriasis

Pathophysiology

Cutaneous psoriasis and psoriatic arthritis are complex heterogeneous diseases with similar pathophysiology [1,7]. Various efforts have tried to elucidate the soluble and cellular mediators implicated in the pathogenesis of psoriatic arthritis and psoriasis through genetic approaches such as genome-wide association studies, as well as by using molecular models [8–10]. New therapeutic agents which target mediators of the immune response such as IL-12, IL-23, IL-17, IL-17 receptor, and TNFa have proven to be effective in the treatment of both skin and joint disease and have shown that both diseases are immune mediated [11].

Comorbidities

Psoriatic arthritis and psoriasis are associated with comorbidities such as the metabolic syndrome, diabetes mellitus type 2, and obesity [12–14].

Metabolic syndrome

Psoriatic arthritis and psoriasis are known to be associated with the metabolic syndrome. It has been observed that the occurrence of metabolic syndrome and hyperuricemia is higher in patients with psoriasis [14]. It thus appears that cutaneous involvement is greater in psoriatic arthritis with evidence of metabolic syndrome and hyperuricemia.

Diabetes mellitus type 2

Psoriatic arthritis and psoriasis are known to be associated with the presence of diabetes mellitus type 2 [13,15–17]. The possible presence of diabetes mellitus type 2 and its associated cardiometabolic factors should be taken into account when management of psoriatic arthritis and psoriasis is planned.

Obesity

Obesity is known to accompany psoriatic arthritis and psoriasis [18,19]. Obesity is a common comorbidity in patients with psoriatic arthritis and psoriasis [20–22]. It should be taken into account when planning treatment for the disease [15]. Dietary intervention with main aim weight loss seems to be a significant factor in the treatment of both psoriatic arthritis and psoriasis [21,22].

Treatment of psoriatic arthritis

The current treatment of psoriatic arthritis involves a step-up approach. Initially analgesic agents and nonsteroidal antiinflammatory agents are applied [23]. If large joints are involved local steroid injections may be used. Next step is the application of conventional DMARDs (disease modifying antirheumatic drugs) such as methotrexate [24]. When conventional DMARDs fail to induce disease remission biologics are considered. Various classes of biologics are available [25]. TNFa inhibitors, interleukin 12/23 inhibitors (IL12/23i), interleukin-17 inhibitors, interleukin-23 inhibitors, CTLA4-Ig (abatacept), and a JAK inhibitor (tofacitinib) are a choice for the management of psoriatic arthritis. Ustekinumab, an interleukin 12/23 inhibitor, has efficacy in psoriatic arthritis [26]. Secukinumab, an interleukin-17 inhibitor is also used effectively in psoriatic arthritis [27,28]. Guselkumab, an IL-23 inhibitor is also applied in psoriatic arthritis treatment successfully [29]. TNFa inhibitors are used quite frequently as they have efficacy across all domains of psoriatic arthritis, namely arthritis, enthesitis, dactylitis, skin, and nail disease [30]. TNFa inhibitors often show efficacy in the treatment of psoriatic arthritis related conditions, such as inflammatory bowel disease [29], Crohn's disease and ulcerative colitis and in some cases uveitis. Additionally, TNFa inhibitors are used quite frequently, as this treatment has been available for a long time and they are available as biosimilars for a considerably lower cost. Tofacitinib, a JAK inhibitor, used orally has also efficacy in psoriatic arthritis [31].

Treatment of psoriasis

Psoriasis may be associated with psoriatic arthritis, or may not be accompanied by it. The treatment of psoriasis attains great significance as it relates to the skin and the appearance of the patient. Many treatment options exist for psoriasis [32] and all of them are discussed with the patient as psoriasis greatly affects quality of life. Local agents may be applied for mild disease such as topical corticosteroids. Vitamin D analogs may also be used [33]. Calcineurin inhibitors, pipecrolimus, and tacrolimus may be applied in the form of ointments and creams [34]. Phototherapy, ultraviolet B phototherapy may also be used and it is very helpful in controlling psoriasis [35].

Nonbiological DMARDs such as methotrexate may be applied [36]. Acitretin has also been used successfully in the past before the advent of biologics. Cyclosporine is also an option [37]. If these steps do not control psoriasis then biologic drugs may be used. Apremilast, a phosphodiesterase inhibitor, which is an orally administered agent may be applied [38]. As far as biologic drugs, TNFa inhibitors, interleukin 12/23 inhibitors, interleukin-17 inhibitor, and interleukin-23 inhibitor may be used [39,40]. It is important to individualize treatment, that is, to apply the use of biologic agents to the needs of each patient.

The SARS-CoV-2 virus

The SARS-CoV-2 pandemic

The SARS-CoV-2 virus belongs to the family of Coronaviridae and has caused the recent pandemic. Coronaviruses are responsible for various epidemics over the years. In particular, coronaviruses have caused the severe acute respiratory syndrome (SARS-CoV) in 2002 and a decade later the Middle East respiratory syndrome (MERS-CoV) [41]. The SARS-CoV-2 virus may cause a mild or even asymptomatic disease, but may also lead to severe pneumonia, which may be lethal [42,43]. Various comorbidities seem to make patients susceptible to the virus and to severe disease and/or death. Such comorbidities are the metabolic syndrome, arterial hypertension, diabetes mellitus type 2, and obesity [4,5].

Risk factors for severe SARS-CoV-2 infection

Diabetes mellitus type 2 and SARS-CoV-2 infection

The presence of diabetes mellitus has been described as a risk factor for severe or fatal disease in Covid-19 infection [44]. In Mexico and other Latin America countries, diabetes mellitus type 2 may have an early onset, before the age of 40, and even at this rather young age it confers a high risk for severe COVID-19 disease [45]. Arterial hypertension and obesity are other risk factors for severe or fatal disease course in COVID-19 infection [46].

Obesity and SARS-CoV-2 infection

Obesity and impaired metabolic health increase complications and mortality in COVID-19 [47]. Obesity and in particular severe obesity is a strong and independent risk factor for severe COVID-19 disease [47]. Obesity is also a risk factor for death from COVID-19 disease, although this appears to be true especially for younger patients [6,48]. Visceral obesity increases the risk of complications of COVID-19 disease [49].

Psoriatic disease and SARS-CoV-2

Psoriatic arthritis and psoriasis are interrelated autoimmune diseases [39]. They are treated with immune modulating agents, such as biologics which alter the immune response [50–52]. In addition, both are related with metabolic syndrome, hyperuricemia, obesity, and diabetes mellitus type 2 [53–55]. Obesity and diabetes mellitus type 2 seem to be related with severe or even fatal COVID-19 disease [6,56,57]. Therefore, the question has arisen as to the prevalence and incidence of COVID-19 infection in psoriatic arthritis and psoriasis patients. The question has also arisen as to the effect of immunomodulatory treatment administered to COVID-19 patients on the severity of COVID-19 disease. It is also important to know if there is a need for psoriatic arthritis and psoriasis treatment modification in the presence of COVID-19 disease.

Psoriatic arthritis, psoriasis, and SARS-CoV-2 infection

Patients with psoriasis are at increased risk for thrombosis and comorbidities related to worse COVID-19 outcomes and may be more susceptible to infection. Despite that, patients with psoriasis appear to have the same risk of infection from SARS-CoV-2 and similar COVID-19 outcomes as the general population [58–60]. Studies in patients with psoriatic arthritis also show that they have similar rates of infection with SARS-CoV-2 and similar rates of COVID-19 outcome [61,62]. The severity of COVID-19 is driven by risk factors such as smoking, male sex, older age, and comorbidities [63,64]. Cardiovascular disease is a risk factor for severe COVID-19 infection. Cardiovascular disease accompanies psoriatic arthritis and psoriasis. According to a British study methotrexate, etanercept, adalimumab, and ustekinumab decrease cardiovascular risk in psoriasis patients [65].

Psoriatic arthritis, psoriasis treatment, and SARS-CoV-2

In a paper, Wollina et al. [66] addressed the question whether the COVID-19 pandemic should modify immunosuppressive treatment of psoriasis. They concluded that in the absence of active infection there seems to be no need to stop immune modulating treatment in psoriasis patients. Research so far has found that treatment for psoriatic arthritis and psoriasis does not alter the risk of getting SARS-CoV-2 infection or having worse Covid-19 outcome. In a group of psoriasis patients in Italy on biologics, the rate of confirmed SARS-CoV-2 infection was similar to that in the general Italian population [59]. In a group of patients with psoriasis on biologics in northern Italy, hospitalization and death was similar to that of the general population [60]. Chronic systemic corticosteroid treatment should be avoided, if possible, for patients with psoriatic arthritis and psoriasis as it is associated with worse COVID-19 outcome [67]. It has been observed that hospitalization for COVID-19 was more frequent in patients using nonbiologic systemic therapy than in those using biologic treatment [68]. In a global study, no evidence for increased COVID-19 hospitalization was observed in patients on tumor necrosis factor inhibitors or methotrexate or both [69]. It thus appears that patients with psoriatic arthritis or psoriasis who are not infected with SARS-CoV-2 should continue their biologic or oral treatment for either psoriatic arthritis and/or psoriasis.

Psoriatic arthritis, psoriasis management in the COVID-19 pandemic

The COVID-19 pandemic has attacked all the world and changed many aspects of life. Various activities, which have always taken place with person-to-person contact have changed and are taking place online. In the medical world, the management of other diseases than the COVID-19 disease has taken a second role. However, the needs of the patients remain unaltered [70]. Therefore, various methods have been proposed to tackle the problem. One of these methods is telemedicine, which is appropriate for some psoriatic arthritis and psoriasis patients [71]. However, if the appropriate safety measures are taken, such as the use of masking among the medical personnel, distancing, restrictions in visits, and the use of PCR testing for COVID-19 as needed medical care may be administered safely.

Protection from COVID-19 infection in psoriatic patients

The pandemic from the SARS-CoV-2 infection, a highly contagious disease has made the development of vaccines against the disease necessary. Thus, novel vaccines have been developed using the mRNA technology [72] or the more traditional adenovirus vectored [73] technology for COVID-19 infection. It has been discussed whether psoriatic arthritis and psoriasis patients should modify their treatment for the disease before or after vaccination against COVID-19. The literature so far agrees that patients with psoriatic arthritis or psoriasis on treatment with biologics and/or methotrexate should continue their treatment before and after vaccination against the SARS-CoV-2 virus.

Treatment of SARS-CoV-2 infection in psoriatic patients

For outpatients with psoriatic disease in the presence of COVID-19 infection at high risk for progressing to severe COVID-19, the use of monoclonal antibodies directed against the spike protein of SARS-CoV-2 is recommended [74,75]. For hospitalized patients, in addition to remdesivir and dexamethasone, baricitinib in combination with remdesivir may be applied [76–78]. Convalescent plasma may be used in the setting of clinical trials [79]. It is necessary to inform patients with psoriatic disease that infection with COVID-19 may cause a flare of psoriasis, even pustular flare [80,81]. It is suggested that treatment which targets the immune system should be withheld in the setting of suspected or confirmed SARS-CoV-2 infection in psoriatic arthritis and psoriasis patients [71] and reinstituted upon recovery.

Conclusion

Psoriatic arthritis and psoriasis are interrelated autoimmune diseases. They are associated with metabolic syndrome, obesity, and diabetes mellitus type 2. Patients are treated with immune modulating agents. The SARS-CoV-2 infection appears to have a worse outcome in patients with obesity and diabetes mellitus type 2. Despite that, patients with psoriatic arthritis and psoriasis have the same risk of infection and the same outcome to that of the general population. They should be vaccinated against COVID-19 to be protected from the disease. Immune modulating treatment in psoriatic disease should not be modified during the SARS-CoV-2 pandemic. If infected with the SARS-CoV-2 virus psoriatic disease patients may be treated with the various agents available today for the infection, such as monoclonal antibodies, remdesivir, dexamethasone, and baricitinib. Immune modulating treatment should be withheld in the presence or suspicion of SARS-CoV-2 infection and should be reintroduced upon recovery.

References

[1] Napolitano M, Caso F, Scarpa R, et al. Psoriatic arthritis and psoriasis: differential diagnosis. Clin Rheumatol 2016;35(8):1893–901.
[2] Chams N, Chams S, Badran R, et al. COVID-19: a multidisciplinary review. Front Public Health 2020;8:383.
[3] Parasher A. COVID-19: current understanding of its pathophysiology, clinical presentation and treatment. Postgrad Med May 2021;97(1147):312–20.
[4] Gao YD, Ding M, Dong X, et al. Risk factors for severe and critically ill COVID-19 patients: a review. Allergy 2021;76(2):428–55.
[5] Jordan RE, Adab P, Cheng KK. Covid-19: risk factors for severe disease and death. BMJ March 26, 2020;368. m1198.
[6] Zhou Y, Chi J, Lv W, Wang Y. Obesity and diabetes as high-risk factors for severe coronavirus disease 2019 (Covid-19). Diabetes Metab Res Rev 2021;37(2):e3377.
[7] Menter A. Psoriasis and psoriatic arthritis overview. Am J Manag Care 2016;22(8 Suppl. l):s216–24.
[8] Mathieu A, Cauli A, Vacca A, et al. Genetics of psoriasis and psoriatic arthritis. Reumatismo 2007;59(Suppl.1):25–7.
[9] Coates LC, FitzGerald O, Helliwell PS, Paul C. Psoriasis, psoriatic arthritis, and rheumatoid arthritis: is all inflammation the same? Semin Arthritis Rheum 2016;46(3):291–304.
[10] Veale DJ, Fearon U. The pathogenesis of psoriatic arthritis. Lancet June 2, 2018;391(10136):2273–84.
[11] Sukhov A, Adamopoulos IE, Maverakis E. Interactions of the immune system with skin and bone tissue in psoriatic arthritis: a comprehensive review. Clin Rev Allergy Immunol 2016;51(1):87–99.
[12] Puig L. Cardiometabolic comorbidities in psoriasis and psoriatic arthritis. Int J Mol Sci December 25, 2017;19(1).
[13] Takeshita J, Grewal S, Langan SM, et al. Psoriasis and comorbid diseases: Epidemiology. J Am Acad Dermatol 2017;76(3):377–90.
[14] Caso F, Del Puente A, Oliviero F, et al. Metabolic syndrome in psoriatic arthritis: the interplay with cutaneous involvement. Evidences from literature and a recent cross-sectional study. Clin Rheumatol 2018;37(3):579–86.
[15] Takeshita J, Grewal S, Langan SM, et al. Psoriasis and comorbid diseases: implications for management. J Am Acad Dermatol 2017;76(3):393–403.
[16] Coto-Segura P, Eiris-Salvado N, González-Lara L, et al. Psoriasis, psoriatic arthritis and type 2 diabetes mellitus: a systematic review and meta-analysis. Br J Dermatol 2013;169(4):783–93.

[17] Queiro R, Lorenzo A, Pardo E, Brandy A, Coto P, Ballina J. Prevalence and type II diabetes-associated factors in psoriatic arthritis. Clin Rheumatol 2018;37(4):1059–64.
[18] Ogdie A, Eder L. The need for strategies to address obesity and psoriatic arthritis prevention in psoriasis. Br J Dermatol 2020;182(3):523–4.
[19] Zafiriou E, Daponte AI, Siokas V, Tsigalou C, Dardiotis E, Bogdanos DP. Depression and obesity in patients with psoriasis and psoriatic arthritis: is IL-17-mediated immune dysregulation the connecting link? Front Immunol 2021;12: 699848.
[20] Jensen P, Skov L. Psoriasis and obesity. Dermatology 2016;232(6):633–9.
[21] Ford AR, Siegel M, Bagel J, et al. Dietary recommendations for adults with psoriasis or psoriatic arthritis from the medical board of the national psoriasis foundation: a systematic review. JAMA Dermatol August 1, 2018;154(8):934–50.
[22] Debbaneh M, Millsop JW, Bhatia BK, Koo J, Liao W. Diet and psoriasis, part I: impact of weight loss interventions. J Am Acad Dermatol 2014;71(1):133–40.
[23] Ungprasert P, Thongprayoon C, Davis 3rd JM. Indirect comparisons of the efficacy of biological agents inpatients with psoriatic arthritis with an inadequate response to traditional disease-modifying anti-rheumatic drugs or to non-steroidal anti-inflammatory drugs: a meta-analysis. Semin Arthritis Rheum 2016;45(4):428–38.
[24] Vieira-Sousa E, Alves P, Rodrigues AM, et al. GO-DACT: a phase 3b randomised, double-blind, placebo-controlled trial of GOlimumab plus methotrexate (MTX) versus placebo plus MTX in improving DACTylitis in MTX-naive patients with psoriatic arthritis. Ann Rheum Dis 2020;79(4):490–8.
[25] Singh JA, Guyatt G, Ogdie A, et al. Special article: 2018 American college of rheumatology/national psoriasis foundation guideline for the treatment of psoriatic arthritis. Arthritis Rheumatol 2019;71(1):5–32.
[26] Ghosh S, Gensler LS, Yang Z, et al. Ustekinumab safety in psoriasis, psoriatic arthritis, and Crohn's disease: an integrated analysis of phase II/III clinical development programs. Drug Saf 2019;42(6):751–68.
[27] Abrouk M, Gandy J, Nakamura M, et al. Secukinumab in the treatment of psoriasis and psoriatic arthritis: a review of the literature. Skin Therapy Lett 2017;22(4):1–6.
[28] Deodhar A, Mease PJ, McInnes IB, et al. Long-term safety of secukinumab in patients with moderate-to-severe plaque psoriasis, psoriatic arthritis, and ankylosing spondylitis: integrated pooled clinical trial and post-marketing surveillance data. Arthritis Res Ther 2019;21(1):111.
[29] Deodhar A, Helliwell PS, Boehncke WH, et al. Guselkumab in patients with active psoriatic arthritis who were biologic-naive or had previously received TNFα inhibitor treatment (DISCOVER-1): a double-blind, randomised, placebo-controlled phase 3 trial. Lancet April 4, 2020;395(10230):1115–25.
[30] Coates LC, Merola JF, Mease PJ, et al. Performance of composite measures used in a trial of etanercept and methotrexate as monotherapy or in combination in psoriatic arthritis. Rheumatology (Oxford) 2021;60(3):1137–47.
[31] Berekmeri A, Mahmood F, Wittmann M, Helliwell P. Tofacitinib for the treatment of psoriasis and psoriatic arthritis. Expert Rev Clin Immunol 2018;14(9):719–30.
[32] Elmets CA, Korman NJ, Prater EF, et al. Joint AAD-NPF Guidelines of care for the management and treatment of psoriasis with topical therapy and alternative medicine modalities for psoriasis severity measures. J Am Acad Dermatol 2021;84(2):432–70.
[33] Armstrong AW, Read C. Pathophysiology, clinical presentation, and treatment of psoriasis: a review. JAMA May 19, 2020;323(19):1945–60.
[34] Rendon A, Schäkel K. Psoriasis pathogenesis and treatment. Int J Mol Sci March 23, 2019;20(6).
[35] Zhang P, Wu MX. A clinical review of phototherapy for psoriasis. Lasers Med Sci 2018;33(1):173–80.
[36] Rajitha P, Biswas R, Sabitha M, Jayakumar R. Methotrexate in the treatment of psoriasis and rheumatoid arthritis: mechanistic insights, current issues and novel delivery approaches. Curr Pharmaceut Des 2017;23(24):3550–66.
[37] Maza A, Montaudié H, Sbidian E, et al. Oral cyclosporin in psoriasis: a systematic review on treatment modalities, risk of kidney toxicity and evidence for use in non-plaque psoriasis. J Eur Acad Dermatol Venereol 2011;25(Suppl. 2):19–27.
[38] Keating GM. Apremilast: a review in psoriasis and psoriatic arthritis. Drugs 2017;77(4):459–72.
[39] Kamata M, Tada Y. Efficacy and safety of biologics for psoriasis and psoriatic arthritis and their impact on comorbidities: a literature review. Int J Mol Sci 2020;(5):21.
[40] Kim HJ, Lebwohl MG. Biologics and psoriasis: the beat goes on. Dermatol Clin 2019;37(1):29–36.

[41] Khan M, Adil SF, Alkhathlan HZ, Tahir MN, Saif S, Khan ST. COVID-19: a global challenge with old history, epidemiology and progress so far. Molecules December 23, 2020;26(1).
[42] Tu H, Tu S, Gao S, Shao A, Sheng J. Current epidemiological and clinical features of COVID-19; a global perspective from China. J Infect 2020;81(1):1–9.
[43] Chakraborty C, Sharma AR, Sharma G, Bhattacharya M, Lee SS. SARS-CoV-2 causing pneumonia-associated respiratory disorder (COVID-19): diagnostic and proposed therapeutic options. Eur Rev Med Pharmacol Sci 2020;24(7):4016–26.
[44] Wolff D, Nee S, Hickey NS, Marschollek M. Risk factors for Covid-19 severity and fatality: a structured literature review. Infection 2021;49(1):15–28.
[45] Bello-Chavolla OY, Bahena-López JP, Antonio-Villa NE, et al. Predicting mortality due to SARS-CoV-2: a mechanistic score relating obesity and diabetes to COVID-19 outcomes in Mexico. J Clin Endocrinol Metab August 1, 2020;105(8).
[46] Schiffrin EL, Flack JM, Ito S, Muntner P, Webb RC. Hypertension and COVID-19. Am J Hypertens 2020;5:373–4.
[47] Stefan N, Birkenfeld AL, Schulze MB. Global pandemics interconnected—obesity, impaired metabolic health and COVID-19. Nat Rev Endocrinol 2021;17(3):135–49.
[48] Williamson EJ, Walker AJ, Bhaskaran K, et al. Factors associated with COVID-19-related death using OpenSAFELY. Nature 2020;584(7821):430–6.
[49] Favre G, Legueult K, Pradier C, et al. Visceral fat is associated to the severity of COVID-19. Metabolism 2021;115:154440.
[50] Menter A. Psoriasis and psoriatic arthritis treatment. Am J Manag Care 2016;22(8 Suppl. l):s225–37.
[51] Yang K, Oak ASW, Elewski BE. Use of IL-23 inhibitors for the treatment of plaque psoriasis and psoriatic arthritis: a comprehensive review. Am J Clin Dermatol 2021;22(2):173–92.
[52] Ceccarelli M, Venanzi Rullo E, Berretta M, et al. New generation biologics for the treatment of psoriasis and psoriatic arthritis. State of the art and considerations about the risk of infection. Dermatol Ther 2021;34(1):e14660.
[53] Souza CS, de Castro CCS, Carneiro FRO, et al. Metabolic syndrome and psoriatic arthritis among patients with psoriasis vulgaris: quality of life and prevalence. J Dermatol 2019;46(1):3–10.
[54] Dağdelen D, Karadag AS, Kasapoğlu E, Wang JV, Erman H. Correlation of metabolic syndrome with serum omentin-1 and visfatin levels and disease severity in psoriasis and psoriatic arthritis. Dermatol Ther 2020;33(6):e14378.
[55] Perez-Chada LM, Merola JF. Comorbidities associated with psoriatic arthritis: review and update. Clin Immunol 2020;214:108397.
[56] Hussain A, Mahawar K, Xia Z, Yang W, El-Hasani S. Obesity and mortality of COVID-19. Meta-analysis Obes Res Clin Pract Jul-Aug;14(4):295–300.
[57] Dietz W, Santos-Burgoa C. Obesity and its implications for COVID-19 mortality. Obesity (Silver Spring) 2020;28(6):1005.
[58] Gisondi P, Bellinato F, Chiricozzi A, Girolomoni G. The risk of COVID-19 pandemic in patients with moderate to severe plaque psoriasis receiving systemic treatments. Vaccines (Basel) December 2, 2020;8(4).
[59] Talamonti M, Galluzzo M, Chiricozzi A, et al. Characteristic of chronic plaque psoriasis patients treated with biologics in Italy during the COVID-19 Pandemic: risk analysis from the PSO-BIO-COVID observational study. Expert Opin Biol Ther 2021;21(2):271–7.
[60] Gisondi P, Piaserico S, Naldi L, et al. Incidence rates of hospitalization and death from COVID-19 in patients with psoriasis receiving biological treatment: a Northern Italy experience. J Allergy Clin Immunol 2021;147(2):558–60.e1.
[61] Montero F, Martínez-Barrio J, Serrano-Benavente B, et al. Coronavirus disease 2019 (COVID-19) in autoimmune and inflammatory conditions: clinical characteristics of poor outcomes. Rheumatol Int 2020;40(10):1593–8.
[62] Nuño L, Novella Navarro M, Bonilla G, et al. Clinical course, severity and mortality in a cohort of patients with COVID-19 with rheumatic diseases. Ann Rheum Dis 2020;12:1659–61.
[63] Peckham H, de Gruijter NM, Raine C, et al. Male sex identified by global COVID-19 meta-analysis as a risk factor for death and ITU admission. Nat Commun December 9, 2020;11(1):6317.
[64] Zhou Y, Yang Q, Chi J, et al. Comorbidities and the risk of severe or fatal outcomes associated with coronavirus disease 2019: a systematic review and meta-analysis. Int J Infect Dis 2020;99:47–56.
[65] Rungapiromnan W, Mason KJ, Lunt M, et al. Risk of major cardiovascular events in patients with psoriasis receiving biologic therapies: a prospective cohort study. J Eur Acad Dermatol Venereol 2020;34(4):769–78.

[66] Wollina U, Fioranelli M, Goldust M, Lotti T. Psoriatic arthritis and COVID-19 pandemic: consequences in medical treatment? Dermatol Ther 2020;33(5):e13743.
[67] Akiyama S, Hamdeh S, Micic D, Sakuraba A. Prevalence and clinical outcomes of COVID-19 in patients with autoimmune diseases: a systematic review and meta-analysis. Ann Rheum Dis October 13, 2020;80:384–91.
[68] Mahil SK, Dand N, Mason KJ, et al. Factors associated with adverse COVID-19 outcomes in patients with psoriasis-insights from a global registry-based study. J Allergy Clin Immunol 2021;147(1):60–71.
[69] Yousaf A, Gayam S, Feldman S, Zinn Z, Kolodney M. Clinical outcomes of COVID-19 in patients taking tumor necrosis factor inhibitors or methotrexate: a multicenter research network study. J Am Acad Dermatol 2021;84(1):70–5.
[70] Ciurea A, Papagiannoulis E, Bürki K, et al. Impact of the COVID-19 pandemic on the disease course of patients with inflammatory rheumatic diseases: results from the Swiss Clinical Quality Management cohort. Ann Rheum Dis 2021;80(2):238–41.
[71] Gelfand JM, Armstrong AW, Bell S, et al. National Psoriasis Foundation COVID-19 Task Force guidance for management of psoriatic disease during the pandemic: version 2-Advances in psoriatic disease management, COVID-19 vaccines, and COVID-19 treatments. J Am Acad Dermatol May 2021;84(5):1254–68.
[72] Polack FP, Thomas SJ, Kitchin N, et al. Safety and efficacy of the BNT162b2 mRNA Covid-19 vaccine. N Engl J Med December 31, 2020;383(27):2603–15.
[73] Zhu FC, Guan XH, Li YH, et al. Immunogenicity and safety of a recombinant adenovirus type-5-vectored COVID-19 vaccine in healthy adults aged 18 years or older: a randomised, double-blind, placebo-controlled, phase 2 trial. Lancet August 15, 2020;396(10249):479–88.
[74] Huang Y, Yang C, Xu XF, Xu W, Liu SW. Structural and functional properties of SARS-CoV-2 spike protein: potential antivirus drug development for COVID-19. Acta Pharmacol Sin 2020;41(9):1141–9.
[75] Weinreich DM, Sivapalasingam S, Norton T, et al. REGN-COV2, a neutralizing antibody cocktail, in outpatients with Covid-19. N Engl J Med January 21, 2021;384(3):238–51.
[76] Kalil AC, Patterson TF, Mehta AK, et al. Baricitinib plus remdesivir for hospitalized adults with Covid-19. N Engl J Med 2021;384(9):795–807.
[77] Kalil AC, Stebbing J. Baricitinib: the first immunomodulatory treatment to reduce COVID-19 mortality in a placebo-controlled trial. Lancet Respir Med December 2021;9(12):1349–51.
[78] Florescu DF, Kalil AC. Janus Kinase inhibitors for the treatment of hospitalized patients with COVID-19. Curr Opin Crit Care October 1, 2021;27(5):493–6.
[79] Simonovich VA, Burgos Pratx LD, Scibona P, et al. A randomized trial of convalescent plasma in Covid-19 severe pneumonia. N Engl J Med 18 2021;384(7):619–29.
[80] Ozaras R, Berk A, Ucar DH, Duman H, Kaya F, Mutlu H. Covid-19 and exacerbation of psoriasis. Dermatol Ther 2020:e13632.
[81] Kutlu Ö, Metin A. A case of exacerbation of psoriasis after oseltamivir and hydroxychloroquine in a patient with COVID-19: will cases of psoriasis increase after COVID-19 pandemic? Dermatol Ther 2020:e13383.

CHAPTER

27

Thyroid autoimmunity and COVID-19

Ifigenia Kostoglou-Athanassiou[1], *Lambros Athanassiou*[2] and *Panagiotis Athanassiou*[3]

[1]Department of Endocrinology, Asclepeion Hospital, Athens, Greece; [2]Department of Rheumatology, Asclepeion Hospital, Athens, Greece; [3]Department of Rheumatology, St. Paul's Hospital, Thessaloniki, Greece

Introduction

Autoimmune thyroid diseases are mainly autoimmune Hashimoto's thyroiditis and Graves' disease. Autoimmune Hashimoto's thyroiditis is characterized by the presence thyroid peroxidase antibodies and thyroglobulin antibodies [1,2]. Patients may present with normal thyroid function or with hypothyroidism. Euthyroid patients may progress to subclinical hypothyroidism or hypothyroidism [3,4]. Graves' disease is characterized by the presence of TSH receptor antibodies [5–8]. Patients present with hyperthyroidism, thyroid ophthalmopathy, and pretibial myxedema [8]. Subacute thyroiditis is an inflammatory thyroid disease [9]. It presents with pain in the area of the thyroid radiating to the lower mandible and to the ears [10]. High inflammatory indices, such as CRP and ESR, characterize the disease. The disease responds to the administration of nonsteroidal antiinflammatory agents and corticosteroids [11].

Risk factors for the development of autoimmune thyroid disease are genetic, epigenetic, and environmental. Genetic factors are HLA-DR4, CD40, CTLA-4, and PTP-N22 and factors related to thyroglobulin gene and TSH receptor gene [12]. Environmental factors include the presence of iodine excess in the environment [13], infectious agents such as hepatitis C virus [14], smoking, alcohol, selenium deficiency [15], drugs such as amiodarone [16], interferon-a [17], highly active antiretroviral therapy, and immune checkpoint inhibitors [18]. Estrogens are also a risk factor for autoimmune thyroid disease [19].

The SARS-CoV-2 virus is a coronavirus. It belongs to the group of Coronaviridae related to various epidemics in the past [20]. The SARS-CoV-2 virus has caused the current pandemic [21]. It may run as a mild infection or may cause severe pneumonia, which may be lethal. The

Autoimmunity, COVID-19, Post-COVID19 syndrome and COVID-19 vaccination
https://doi.org/10.1016/B978-0-443-18566-3.00004-9

virus enters the cells via a spike which attaches to angiotensin-converting enzyme 2 (ACE2) that acts as a receptor for the virus [22]. Various cells express the ACE2, thus rendering them susceptible to invasion by the virus. Thyroid cells express the ACE2 rendering them susceptible to the SARS-CoV-2 virus [23,24].

Cases of thyroid disease have been reported in the context of infection by the SARS-CoV-2 virus. Cases of subacute thyroiditis have been reported in connection with the COVID-19 infection [25–31]. Hypothyroidism and Graves' disease have also been observed after Covid-19 infection [32].

Autoimmune thyroid diseases

Autoimmune thyroid diseases are mainly autoimmune Hashimoto's thyroiditis and Graves' disease. Autoimmune Hashimoto's thyroiditis presents with either euthyroidism, or subclinical or clinical hypothyroidism [4,33,34]. Thyroid antibodies characterizing Hashimoto's thyroiditis are thyroid peroxidase antibody and thyroglobulin antibody. In some patients other types of autoantibodies may be observed such as thyroid stimulating hormone receptor blocking (TSHR-blocking) antibodies [35]. Euthyroid patients with Hashimoto's thyroiditis may progress to subclinical or clinical hypothyroidism. In the case of subclinical or clinical hypothyroidism, the disease is treated by the administration of thyroxine [33,34]. Silent thyroiditis and postpartum thyroiditis are forms of autoimmune Hashimoto's thyroiditis [9,36].

Graves' disease is an autoimmune multisystem disorder characterized by hyperthyroidism, thyroid ophthalmopathy, pretibial myxedema, and thyroid acropathy [5,6]. The disease is characterized by the presence of TSH receptor antibodies, thyroid peroxidase, and thyroglobulin antibodies [37]. The disease usually presents with hyperthyroidism and/or thyroid ophthalmopathy. In the course of the disease, patients may become euthyroid or hypothyroid.

Subacute thyroiditis

Subacute thyroiditis is a postinflammatory or inflammatory thyroid disorder [9]. It is characterized by painful involvement of the thyroid gland, transient hyperthyroidism, elevated inflammatory indices, such as CRP and ESR and transiently elevated thyroid peroxidase and thyroglobulin antibodies. Subacute thyroiditis has been observed in association with an upper respiratory tract infection and clusters of the disease have been associated with viral infections [38,39]. The disease runs a variable course either mild or severe [40]. The patients present with hyperthyroidism, which may progress to hypothyroidism and then they become euthyroid. In some patients, hypothyroidism may be permanent [10]. The disease may recur [41,42].

The SARS-CoV-2 virus

SARS-CoV-2 is a coronavirus, a member of the Coronaviridae family [43] which is related to various epidemics which have taken place in previous years [44]. The SARS-CoV-2 virus has been related to the development of the current pandemic [45]. The virus may act as an initiating factor for the development of autoimmunity [46].

Mechanism of tissue invasion by the SARS-CoV-2 virus

The mechanism by which the SARS-CoV-2 virus invades the tissues by a spike which attaches to the angiotensin-converting enzyme 2-ACE2 that acts as a receptor for the virus [47]. The transmembrane serine protease 2 also acts as a receptor for the virus and primes the spike viral protein to facilitate viral entry into the cell [48]. Various tissues express the angiotensin-converting enzyme 2 receptor such as the adrenal, the thyroid, the testes, and perhaps the ovary [49–51].

Mechanism of autoimmunity induction

The SARS-CoV-2 virus may induce autoimmunity via various mechanisms. The virus has been shown to induce hyperstimulation of the immune system and in cases of severe disease cytokines are released in the circulation in the form of a storm called cytokine storm [52,53]. In these case, autoantibodies are produced which may induce an autoimmune disease or exacerbate an already existing autoimmune disease [54]. Mechanisms responsible for the induction of autoimmunity by the SARS-CoV-2 virus are molecular mimicry, that is, the resemblance of amino acid sequence of the virus to human proteins [55,56]. Alternatively, the induction of excessive neutrophil extracellular traps may lead to the development of autoimmunity [57]. In cases of infection by the SARS-CoV-2 virus, the development of autoantibodies, such as antiphospholipid antibodies, has been observed [58].

Autoimmune and inflammatory thyroid diseases and SARS-CoV-2

Various thyroid diseases have been observed related to the SARS-CoV-2 infection (Fig. 27.1). In particular, subacute thyroiditis or de Quervain's thyroiditis has been observed in relationship to the SARS-CoV-2 infection. Graves' disease has also been detected in relationship to the SARS-CoV-2 infection. A form of thyroiditis has also been found in relationship with the SARS-CoV-2 virus infection. Hypothyroidism has also been diagnosed immediately following a COVID-19 infection. During acute SARS-CoV-2 infection, euthyroid sick syndrome has also been found [59]. Euthyroid sick syndrome is the alteration of thyroid hormones observed during an acute disease, especially if the patient is hospitalized or admitted to an acute care unit [60]. The syndrome is characterized by low TSH levels, low FT_4, and/or low FT_3 levels.

Subacute thyroiditis

There are many case reports of patients who developed subacute thyroiditis in the context of COVID-19 infection. Mattar et al. [25] described a case of subacute thyroiditis in a patient hospitalized with COVID-19 infection. The patient presented with hyperthyroidism and ultrasonographic findings of subacute thyroiditis. They noted that subacute thyroiditis should be considered in the differential diagnosis of a patient with COVID-19 infection presenting

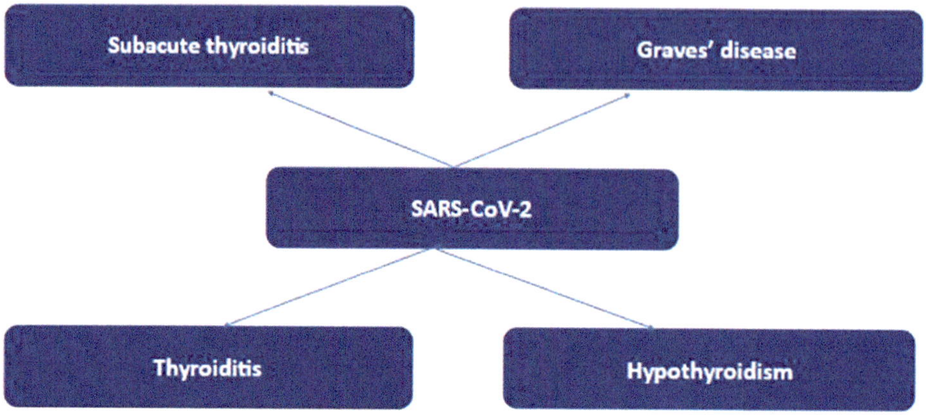

FIGURE 27.1 Thyroid diseases after SARS-CoV-2 infection.

with tachycardia without signs of progression of the Covid-19 illness. Campos-Barrera et al. [27] described a case of subacute thyroiditis in a 37-year-old female patient associated with a very mild COVID-19 infection. Similarly, Brancatella et al. [28] described a case of a female patient presenting with subacute thyroiditis following a very mild COVID-19 infection. Asfuroglu-Kalkan et al. [29] presented a female patient who developed subacute thyroiditis and was shown to have active COVID-19 infection by RT-PCR. Ruggeri et al. [31] described a case of subacute thyroiditis in a female patient 6 weeks after the onset of an upper respiratory tract infection which was diagnosed as a mild SARS-CoV-2 infection. Saad et al. [61] reviewed all articles describing an autoimmune disease related to the SARS-CoV-2 infection published in PubMed over a period of 5 months in 2020 and they found one case of subacute thyroiditis. Speer and Somogyi [26] reviewed thyroid complications after a SARS-CoV-2 infection and they found that SARS-CoV-2 infection may be complicated by subacute thyroiditis, autoimmune thyroiditis, and an atypical form of thyroiditis. They concluded that thyroid function should be monitored in patients with COVID-19 infection.

Autoimmune thyroiditis

The onset of autoimmune thyroiditis with subclinical hypothyroidism and positive TPO antibodies has been reported following a symptomatic COVID-19 infection in a Chinese 45-year-old man [62]. Lui et al. [63] studied 191 patients hospitalized for SARS-CoV-2 infection and they found that three patients had evidence of an autoimmune thyroid disease. In their cohort, they also observed patients with euthyroid sick syndrome. The development of thyroiditis leading to clinical hypothyroidism has also been reported following COVID-19 infection [32]. Clinical hypothyroidism 6 weeks after SARS-CoV-2 infection has also been observed [32].

Graves' disease

Mateu-Salat et al. [64] described two cases of Graves' disease in female middle-aged patients following a SARS-CoV-2 acute infection. Their first patient had previously diagnosed

Graves' disease in remission for more than 30 years and presented with disease recurrence following an acute COVID-19 infection. Their second patient was also a middle-aged female patient who presented with Graves' disease following an acute albeit mild Covid-19 infection. The findings of Mateu-Salat et al. are in accordance with the findings of Dotan et al. [46] who reported either onset of autoimmunity or exacerbation of previously existing autoimmune disease by the SARS-CoV-2 virus. Lanzolla et al. [65] described the onset of Graves' disease accompanied by Graves orbitopathy in a young female patient 2 months after COVID-19 infection. Feghali et al. [32] reported a case of new onset of Graves' disease 8 weeks after a COVID-19 infection in a 33-year-old patient. The onset or exacerbation of Graves' disease after SARS-CoV-2 infection in the cases so far described in the literature has been observed in female patients. This finding is in accordance with Graves' disease being more prevalent in females [14] and female sex being a risk factor for autoimmune diseases [66]. In accordance, estrogens are a risk factor for the development of autoimmune diseases [67,68].

Vaccination against SARS-CoV-2 and thyroid disease

Vaccines against SARS-CoV-2

The emergence of the SARS-CoV-2 virus caused the current pandemic and came up as a major threat for humanity. As a response to the pandemic major efforts were made to develop novel vaccines against the disease. Vaccination against the SARS-CoV-2 is a major weapon against the disease, and it has been applied successfully so far. The vaccines of Moderna and Pfizer/Biontech utilized a new mRNA strategy. Artificial mRNA is injected in the human organism which leads to the production of viral proteins by the host. Consequently, viral protein fragments are found on the cell surface of the host, are introduced to the immune system and antibodies against those proteins are produced [69]. A recombinant adenovirus vectored COVID-19 vaccine has also been developed [70]. However, there have been some reports of adverse events related to the thyroid following vaccination.

Subacute thyroiditis in the context of the SARS-CoV-2 vaccine

Several cases of subacute thyroiditis have been reported following vaccination against SARS-CoV-2. Jeevahudeen et al. [71] described a case of subacute thyroiditis in a middle-aged female patient following the second dose of the mRNA COVID-19 vaccine. Subacute thyroiditis was selflimiting and did not require any significant therapeutic modality. Siolos et al. [72] reported a case of subacute thyroiditis following the mRNA COVID-19 vaccine. Cases of subacute thyroiditis in female patients following the mRNA vaccine have also been reported by Plaza-Enriquez et al. [73] and Sotanpoor and Norouzi [74]. A case of subacute thyroiditis presenting a few hours after the second dose of the mRNA vaccine, which required corticosteroids to manage has also been studied [75]. Schimmel et al. also reported subacute thyroiditis following the mRNA COVID-19 vaccine [76]. Subacute thyroiditis following COVID-19 vaccination has also been observed in a male patient [77]. Subacute thyroiditis has also been found following the adeno-virus vectored COVID-19 vaccine [78].

Silent thyroiditis in the context of the SARS-CoV-2 vaccine

Silent thyroiditis is a form of autoimmune thyroiditis which is selflimiting. Silent thyroiditis has been reported following vaccination against COVID-19 [72].

Graves' disease in the context of the SARS-CoV-2 vaccine

The development of thyroid eye disease in a female patient with clinically controlled Graves' disease without preexisting eye involvement has been reported 3 days after the second vaccination against the SARS-CoV-2 virus [79]. The onset of Graves' disease has been reported following COVID-19 vaccination [80]. Vera-Lastra et al. [81] and Zettinig and Krebs [82] reported four cases of Graves' disease after the mRNA COVID-19 vaccine. A patient with aggravated hyperthyroidism due to Graves' has also been reported following the adenovirus vectored COVID-19 vaccine [83].

Mechanisms of thyroid disease in SARS-CoV-2

Thyroid cells express angiotensin converting enzyme 2 -ACE2 [23,50]. Thus, the SARS-CoV-2 virus attaches to the ACE2 via its spike and infects among other tissues the thyroid gland. In accordance, the extremely rare case of a patient who developed thyroid storm, an emergency situation of severe hyperthyroidism, during COVID-19 infection has been described [84]. Most cases of subacute thyroiditis and Graves' disease following COVID-19 infection are in female patients, as female patients have a stronger immune response, longer survival at the cost of increased risk for autoimmunity [85]. During vaccination against COVID-19, antibodies to the spike protein of the virus are produced and may also attach to the ACE2, thus causing thyroid disease.

Conclusion

Thyroid autoimmunity manifests itself in many forms, such as Hashimoto's thyroiditis and Graves' disease. Various factors predispose to the development of autoimmune thyroid disease such as infectious agents, viruses, and microbial factors. The SARS-CoV-2 virus may be related to the development of autoimmunity. Euthyroid sick syndrome may manifest itself in severe COVID-19 infection. Subacute thyroiditis, autoimmune thyroiditis, and subsequent hypothyroidism and Graves' disease have been described in relationship with the SARS-CoV-2 infection.

References

[1] Hiromatsu Y, Satoh H, Amino N. Hashimoto's thyroiditis: history and future outlook. Hormones (Basel) 2013;12(1):12–8.

[2] Hashimoto H. Zur kenntnis der lymphomatosen Veranderung der Sshilddruse (Struma lymphomatosa). Arch Klin Chir 1912;97:219–48.

[3] Caturegli P, De Remigis A, Rose NR. Hashimoto thyroiditis: clinical and diagnostic criteria. Autoimmun Rev Apr-May;13(4–5):391–7.

[4] Biondi B, Cappola AR, Cooper DS. Subclinical hypothyroidism: a review. JAMA July 9, 2019;322(2):153–60.
[5] Smith TJ, Hegedüs L. Graves' disease. N Engl J Med October 20, 2016;375(16):1552–65.
[6] Bartalena L. Diagnosis and management of Graves disease: a global overview. Nat Rev Endocrinol December 2013;9(12):724–34.
[7] Allelein S, Schott M. Update Graves' disease 2019. Dtsch Med Wochenschr February 2019;144(3):152–5. Update Morbus Basedow.
[8] Bahn R, Levy E, Wartofsky L. Graves' disease. J Clin Endocrinol Metab November 2007;92(11):2. p following 14A.
[9] Samuels MH. Subacute, silent, and postpartum thyroiditis. Med Clin March 2012;96(2):223–33.
[10] Görges J, Ulrich J, Keck C, Müller-Wieland D, Diederich S, Janssen OE. Long-term outcome of subacute thyroiditis. Exp Clin Endocrinol Diabetes November 2020;128(11):703–8.
[11] Duan L, Feng X, Zhang R, et al. Short-Term versus 6-week prednisone in the treatment of subacute thyroiditis: a randomized controlled trial. Endocr Pract August 2020;26(8):900–8.
[12] Dong YH, Fu DG. Autoimmune thyroid disease: mechanism, genetics and current knowledge. Eur Rev Med Pharmacol Sci 2014;18(23):3611–8.
[13] Wang B, He W, Li Q, et al. U-shaped relationship between iodine status and thyroid autoimmunity risk in adults. Eur J Endocrinol September 2019;181(3):255–66.
[14] Antonelli A, Ferrari SM, Ragusa F, et al. Graves' disease: epidemiology, genetic and environmental risk factors and viruses. Best Pract Res Clin Endocrinol Metabol January 2020;34(1):101387.
[15] Ventura M, Melo M, Carrilho F. Selenium and thyroid disease: from pathophysiology to treatment. Internet J Endocrinol 2017;2017:1297658.
[16] Bogazzi F, Tomisti L, Bartalena L, Aghini-Lombardi F, Martino E. Amiodarone and the thyroid: a 2012 update. J Endocrinol Invest 2012;35(3):340–8.
[17] Monzani F, Caraccio N, Dardano A, Ferrannini E. Thyroid autoimmunity and dysfunction associated with type I interferon therapy. Clin Exp Med April 2004;3(4):199–210.
[18] Percik R, Shoenfeld Y. Check point inhibitors and autoimmunity: why endocrinopathies and who is prone to? Best Pract Res Clin Endocrinol Metabol January 2020;34(1):101411.
[19] Lu Y, Li J. Estrogen and thyroid diseases: an update. Minerva Med August 2016;107(4):239–44.
[20] Umakanthan S, Sahu P, Ranade AV, et al. Origin, transmission, diagnosis and management of coronavirus disease 2019 (COVID-19). Postgrad Med December 2020;96(1142):753–8.
[21] Tsang HF, Chan LWC, Cho WCS, et al. An update on COVID-19 pandemic: the epidemiology, pathogenesis, prevention and treatment strategies. Expert Rev Anti Infect Ther July 2021;19(7):877–88.
[22] Bourgonje AR, Abdulle AE, Timens W, et al. Angiotensin-converting enzyme 2 (ACE2), SARS-CoV-2 and the pathophysiology of coronavirus disease 2019 (COVID-19). J Pathol July 2020;251(3):228–48.
[23] Narayan SS, Lorenz K, Ukkat J, Hoang-Vu C, Trojanowicz B. Angiotensin converting enzymes ACE and ACE2 in thyroid cancer progression. Neoplasma March 2020;67(2):402–9.
[24] Rotondi M, Coperchini F, Ricci G, et al. Detection of SARS-COV-2 receptor ACE-2 mRNA in thyroid cells: a clue for COVID-19-related subacute thyroiditis. J Endocrinol Invest May 2021;44(5):1085–90.
[25] Mattar SAM, Koh SJQ, Rama Chandran S, Cherng BPZ. Subacute thyroiditis associated with COVID-19. BMJ Case Rep August 25, 2020;13(8).
[26] Speer G, Somogyi P. Thyroid complications of SARS and coronavirus disease 2019 (COVID-19). Endocr J February 28, 2021;68(2):129–36.
[27] Campos-Barrera E, Alvarez-Cisneros T, Davalos-Fuentes M. Subacute thyroiditis associated with COVID-19. Case Rep Endocrinol 2020;2020. 8891539.
[28] Brancatella A, Ricci D, Viola N, Sgrò D, Santini F, Latrofa F. Subacute thyroiditis after Sars-COV-2 infection. J Clin Endocrinol Metab July 1, 2020;105(7).
[29] Asfuroglu Kalkan E, Ates I. A case of subacute thyroiditis associated with Covid-19 infection. J Endocrinol Invest 2020;8:1173–4.
[30] Aleksandrov Y, Semikov V, Shulutko A, Gogokhia T, Gorbacheva A, Mansurova G. Subacute thyroiditis and COVID-19 (review). Georgian Med News February 2021;(311):98–103.
[31] Ruggeri RM, Campennì A, Siracusa M, Frazzetto G, Gullo D. Subacute thyroiditis in a patient infected with SARS-COV-2: an endocrine complication linked to the COVID-19 pandemic. Hormones (Basel) 2021;1:219–21.
[32] Feghali K, Atallah J, Norman C. Manifestations of thyroid disease post COVID-19 illness: report of Hashimoto thyroiditis, Graves' disease, and subacute thyroiditis. J Clin Transl Endocrinol Case Rep 2021;22:100094.

[33] Ragusa F, Fallahi P, Elia G, et al. Hashimotos' thyroiditis: epidemiology, pathogenesis, clinic and therapy. Best Pract Res Clin Endocrinol Metabol December 2019;33(6):101367.
[34] Ralli M, Angeletti D, Fiore M, et al. Hashimoto's thyroiditis: an update on pathogenic mechanisms, diagnostic protocols, therapeutic strategies, and potential malignant transformation. Autoimmun Rev October 2020;19(10):102649.
[35] Weetman AP. An update on the pathogenesis of Hashimoto's thyroiditis. J Endocrinol Invest May 2021;44(5):883–90.
[36] Noh JY. Silent thyroiditis and subacute thyroiditis. Nihon Rinsho November 2012;70(11):1945–50.
[37] McIver B, Morris JC. The pathogenesis of Graves' disease. Endocrinol Metab Clin N Am March 1998;27(1):73–89.
[38] Desailloud R, Hober D. Viruses and thyroiditis: an update. Virol J January 12, 2009;6:5.
[39] Espino Montoro A, Medina Pérez M, González Martín MC, Asencio Marchante R, López Chozas JM. Subacute thyroiditis associated with positive antibodies to the Epstein-Barr virus. An Med Interna October 2000;17(10):546–8. Tiroiditis subaguda asociada a anticuerpos positivos al virus de Epstein-Barr.
[40] Benbassat CA, Olchovsky D, Tsvetov G, Shimon I. Subacute thyroiditis: clinical characteristics and treatment outcome in fifty-six consecutive patients diagnosed between 1999 and 2005. J Endocrinol Invest September 2007;30(8):631–5.
[41] Stasiak M, Tymoniuk B, Stasiak B, Lewiński A. The risk of recurrence of subacute thyroiditis is HLA-dependent. Int J Mol Sci March 3, 2019;20(5).
[42] Sencar ME, Calapkulu M, Sakiz D, et al. An evaluation of the results of the steroid and non-steroidal anti-inflammatory drug treatments in subacute thyroiditis in relation to persistent hypothyroidism and recurrence. Sci Rep November 15, 2019;9(1):16899.
[43] Bouayad A. Innate immune evasion by SARS-CoV-2: comparison with SARS-CoV. Rev Med Virol November 2020;30(6):1–9.
[44] Shah VK, Firmal P, Alam A, Ganguly D, Chattopadhyay S. Overview of immune response during SARS-CoV-2 infection: lessons from the past. Front Immunol 2020;11:1949.
[45] Yang Y, Peng F, Wang R, et al. The deadly coronaviruses: the 2003 SARS pandemic and the 2020 novel coronavirus epidemic in China. J Autoimmun May 2020;109:102434.
[46] Dotan A, Muller S, Kanduc D, David P, Halpert G, Shoenfeld Y. The SARS-CoV-2 as an instrumental trigger of autoimmunity. Autoimmun Rev April 2021;20(4):102792.
[47] Beyerstedt S, Casaro EB, Rangel BÉ. COVID-19: angiotensin-converting enzyme 2 (ACE2) expression and tissue susceptibility to SARS-CoV-2 infection. Eur J Clin Microbiol Infect Dis May 2021;40(5):905–19.
[48] Thunders M, Delahunt B. Gene of the month: TMPRSS2 (transmembrane serine protease 2). J Clin Pathol December 2020;73(12):773–6.
[49] Ashraf UM, Abokor AA, Edwards JM, et al. SARS-CoV-2, ACE2 expression, and systemic organ invasion. Physiol Genom February 1, 2021;53(2):51–60.
[50] Li MY, Li L, Zhang Y, Wang XS. Expression of the SARS-CoV-2 cell receptor gene ACE2 in a wide variety of human tissues. Infect Dis Poverty April 28, 2020;9(1):45.
[51] Scialo F, Daniele A, Amato F, et al. ACE2: the major cell entry receptor for SARS-CoV-2. Lung December 2020;198(6):867–77.
[52] Muralidar S, Ambi SV, Sekaran S, Krishnan UM. The emergence of COVID-19 as a global pandemic: understanding the epidemiology, immune response and potential therapeutic targets of SARS-CoV-2. Biochimie December 2020;179:85–100.
[53] Jung HE, Lee HK. Current understanding of the innate control of toll-like receptors in response to SARS-CoV-2 infection. Viruses October 22, 2021;13(11).
[54] Ehrenfeld M, Tincani A, Andreoli L, et al. Covid-19 and autoimmunity. Autoimmun Rev August 2020;19(8):102597.
[55] Kanduc D, Shoenfeld Y. Molecular mimicry between SARS-CoV-2 spike glycoprotein and mammalian proteomes: implications for the vaccine. Immunol Res October 2020;68(5):310–3.
[56] Lucchese G, Flöel A. SARS-CoV-2 and Guillain-Barré syndrome: molecular mimicry with human heat shock proteins as potential pathogenic mechanism. Cell Stress Chaperones September 2020;25(5):731–5.
[57] Apel F, Zychlinsky A, Kenny EF. The role of neutrophil extracellular traps in rheumatic diseases. Nat Rev Rheumatol August 2018;14(8):467–75.

[58] Gatto M, Perricone C, Tonello M, et al. Frequency and clinical correlates of antiphospholipid antibodies arising in patients with SARS-CoV-2 infection: findings from a multicentre study on 122 cases. Clin Exp Rheumatol Jul-Aug;38(4):754−9.
[59] Zou R, Wu C, Zhang S, et al. Euthyroid sick syndrome in patients with COVID-19. Front Endocrinol 2020;11. 566439.
[60] Lee S, Farwell AP. Euthyroid sick syndrome. Compr Physiol March 15, 2016;6(2):1071−80.
[61] Saad MA, Alfishawy M, Nassar M, Mohamed M, Esene IN, Elbendary A. COVID-19 and autoimmune diseases: a systematic review of reported cases. Curr Rheumatol Rev 2021;17(2):193−204.
[62] Tee LY, Harjanto S, Rosario BH. COVID-19 complicated by Hashimoto's thyroiditis. Singap Med J 2021;5:265.
[63] Lui DTW, Lee CH, Chow WS, et al. Thyroid dysfunction in relation to immune profile, disease status, and outcome in 191 patients with COVID-19. J Clin Endocrinol Metab January 23, 2021;106(2):e926−35.
[64] Mateu-Salat M, Urgell E, Chico A. SARS-COV-2 as a trigger for autoimmune disease: report of two cases of Graves' disease after COVID-19. J Endocrinol Invest 2020;10:1527−8.
[65] Lanzolla G, Marcocci C, Marinò M. Graves' disease and Graves' orbitopathy following COVID-19. J Endocrinol Invest 2021;9:2011−2.
[66] Ortona E, Pierdominici M, Maselli A, Veroni C, Aloisi F, Shoenfeld Y. Sex-based differences in autoimmune diseases. Ann Ist Super Sanita Apr-Jun;52(2):205−12.
[67] Di Florio DN, Sin J, Coronado MJ, Atwal PS, Fairweather D. Sex differences in inflammation, redox biology, mitochondria and autoimmunity. Redox Biol April 2020;31:101482.
[68] Moulton VR. Sex hormones in acquired immunity and autoimmune disease. Front Immunol 2018;9:2279.
[69] Heaton PM. The Covid-19 vaccine-development multiverse. N Engl J Med 2020;20:1986−8.
[70] Zhu FC, Guan XH, Li YH, et al. Immunogenicity and safety of a recombinant adenovirus type-5-vectored COVID-19 vaccine in healthy adults aged 18 years or older: a randomised, double-blind, placebo-controlled, phase 2 trial. Lancet August 15, 2020;396(10249):479−88.
[71] Jeeyavudeen MS, Patrick AW, Gibb FW, Dover AR. COVID-19 vaccine-associated subacute thyroiditis: an unusual suspect for de Quervain's thyroiditis. BMJ Case Rep November 9, 2021;14(11).
[72] Siolos A, Gartzonika K, Tigas S. Thyroiditis following vaccination against COVID-19: report of two cases and review of the literature. Metabol Open December 2021;12:100136.
[73] Plaza-Enriquez L, Khatiwada P, Sanchez-Valenzuela M, Sikha A. A case report of subacute thyroiditis following mRNA COVID-19 vaccine. Case Rep Endocrinol 2021;2021. 8952048.
[74] Soltanpoor P, Norouzi G. Subacute thyroiditis following COVID-19 vaccination. In: Clin Case Rep. 10; 2021. e04812.
[75] Kyriacou A, Ioakim S, Syed AA. COVID-19 vaccination and a severe pain in the neck. Eur J Intern Med October 18, 2021;94:95−6.
[76] Schimmel J, Alba EL, Chen A, Russell M, Srinath R. Letter to the editor: thyroiditis and thyrotoxicosis after the SARS-CoV-2 mRNA vaccine. Thyroid September 2021;31(9):1440.
[77] Sahin Tekin M, Saylısoy S, Yorulmaz G. Subacute thyroiditis following COVID-19 vaccination in a 67-year-old male patient: a case report. Hum Vaccines Immunother July 1, 2021:1−3.
[78] Oyibo SO. Subacute thyroiditis after receiving the adenovirus-vectored vaccine for coronavirus disease (COVID-19). Cureus June 2021;13(6):e16045.
[79] Rubinstein TJ. Thyroid eye disease following COVID-19 vaccine in a patient with a history Graves' disease: a case report. Ophthalmic Plast Reconstr Surg Nov-Dec;37(6):e221−3.
[80] Sriphrapradang C, Shantavasinkul PC. Graves' disease following SARS-CoV-2 vaccination. Endocrine 2021;3:473−4.
[81] Vera-Lastra O, Ordinola Navarro A, Cruz Domiguez MP, Medina G, Sánchez Valadez TI, Jara LJ. Two cases of Graves' disease following SARS-CoV-2 vaccination: an autoimmune/inflammatory syndrome induced by adjuvants. Thyroid September 2021;31(9):1436−9.
[82] Zettinig G, Krebs M. Two further cases of Graves' disease following SARS-Cov-2 vaccination. J Endocrinol Invest 2021:1−2.
[83] Sriphrapradang C. Aggravation of hyperthyroidism after heterologous prime-boost immunization with inactivated and adenovirus-vectored SARS-CoV-2 vaccine in a patient with Graves' disease. Endocrine 2021;2:226−7.
[84] Sullivan K, Helgeson J, McGowan A. COVID-19 associated thyroid storm: a case report. Clin Pract Cases Emerg Med November 2021;5(4):412−4.
[85] Shoenfeld Y, Tincani A, Gershwin ME. Sex gender and autoimmunity. J Autoimmun May 2012;38(2−3):J71−3.

CHAPTER

28

Variation of the COVID-19 characteristics between genders

Nicole Bechmann[1] *and Stefan R. Bornstein*[2]

[1]Institute of Clinical Chemistry and Laboratory Medicine, University Hospital Carl Gustav Carus, Technische Universität Dresden, Dresden, Germany; [2]Department of Internal Medicine III, University Hospital Carl Gustav Carus, Technische Universität Dresden, Dresden, Germany

Introduction

The onset of severe acute respiratory syndrome coronavirus 2 (SARS-CoV-2) has led to the COVID-19 pandemic with millions of infections and deaths worldwide. Biological sex plays an important role for the severity and outcomes of COVID-19 infections [1–3]. Genetic and hormonal differences between both sexes lead to significant divergences in metabolic, immune, and endocrine responses to viral infections and thus affect the course of SARS-CoV-2 infections. Sex-related comorbidities, lifestyle, and behavioral aspects such as smoking, alcohol consumption, and diet are additional factors that contribute to differences between women and men concerning COVID-19. Variations in social behavior might also contribute to differences between both sexes. Women perceive COVID-19 more as a serious health problem than men and are therefore more likely to comply with restrictive measures [4]. Mobile phone data from 1.2 million devices in Austria revealed gender differences in social behavior during different phases of the COVID-19 pandemic; for instance, men returned to normal social behavior more rapidly than women, while women avoided larger shopping malls during the lockdown [5]. Here, we summarize the current knowledge on how these sex-specific differences contribute to molecular and clinical variations between specific subgroups of COVID-19 patients.

Sex differences in severity and outcome of COVID-19

Although the COVID-19 pandemic has been ongoing for almost 2 years, events and determinants leading to COVID-19 death remain largely unknown. Similar to previous endemic

Autoimmunity, COVID-19, Post-COVID19 syndrome and COVID-19 vaccination
https://doi.org/10.1016/B978-0-443-18566-3.00022-0

infections, including MERS-CoV and SARS-CoV (2002), COVID-19 affects men more severely than women [2,6]. Already in early reports of SARS-CoV-2, men were described as being at higher risk for a severe course of COVID-19 compared with women, which was further associated with a higher mortality rate [6,7]. Epidemiological data from several governments compiled by the Global Health 50/50 research initiative and analyzed for gender differences confirm increased mortality in men, although the number of COVID-19 cases is comparable in both sexes [8]. A study based on data collected by the National Institute for Demographic Studies calculated an overall male to female mortality ratio per 100′000 people of 1.4. The ratio varied among age groups, being lowest among those 0−9 years (0.81) and highest among those people aged 60−69 years (2.6) [9]. Recent data in children under 18 years of age indicate that males are more likely to be hospitalized and die in hospital than females [10]. In addition to sex and age, comorbidities influence the severity of COVID-19.

Comorbidities vary between sexes with consequences for the severity of COVID-19 infections

Patients with comorbidities, such as hypertension, diabetes, cancer, and cardiovascular disease, are at higher risk for severe and even fatal COVID-19 courses, with a strikingly higher incidence of these comorbidities in males [11,12] (Fig. 28.1). Hormonal and genetic differences

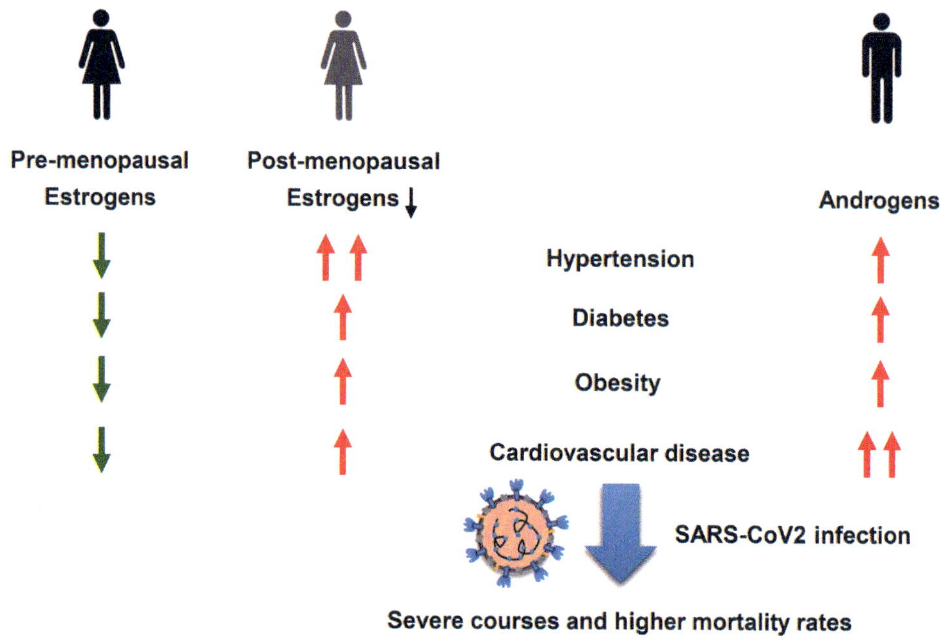

FIGURE 28.1 **Sex differences in the incidence of common comorbidities are associated with worse outcome in COVID-19 disease.** Patients with comorbidities, such as hypertension, diabetes, obesity and cardiovascular disease are at increased risk for severe courses of COVID-19 infections. In premenopausal women, the risk for such comorbidities is lowest, increasing after menopause due to estrogen deficiency. In males, the likelihood of such comorbidities is significantly increased in all age groups.

cause differential regulation of metabolic processes including insulin sensitivity, glycemic control, adipose tissue homeostasis, and lipid metabolism [13,14]. Males are more prone to impaired glucose metabolism and type 2 diabetes than females [15,16]. A recent study examined the effects of androgens on glucose homeostasis; sex-specific differences in glucose metabolism were explained in part by modulation of the gut microbiome and by circulating glutamine [17]. In a cohort study of people with diabetes, male sex and living in residential care were identified as risk factors for developing ICU-treated or even fatal COVID-19 [18]. In an observational study that included people with diabetes admitted for COVID-19, female sex was associated with a lower rate of serious outcomes; however, mortality was comparable to men [19]. After menopause, women have a tendency to accumulate visceral fat and become more insulin resistant, which leads to an increased risk for type 2 diabetes [20]. Independent of diabetes risk, people with obesity have an increased risk of mortality from COVID-19 infection; in particular visceral obesity, for which men have a predisposition, increases the risk of complications [21]. Overall, obese patients with COVID-19 are more likely to be hospitalized associated with a higher risk of in-hospital death, mechanical ventilation, and thromboembolism [22]. Sex differences in adipose tissue distribution, immune cell accumulation in adipose tissue (discussed below), and circulating levels of key adipokines might contribute to sex discrepancies in the severity of COVID-19 [23].

Sexual dimorphism in blood pressure control is well known, but the mechanisms involved remain unclear. Men have higher blood pressure and prevalence of hypertension compared with age-matched premenopausal women; however, after the fifth decade of life, the prevalence of hypertension in women begins to exceed that in men [24–26]. Differential regulation of the renin–angiotensin system, adrenergic receptors, oxidative stress, nitric oxide bioavailability, and immune cells contributes to the differences between sex [26]. Hypertension is associated with an increased risk of severe or even fatal COVID-19 courses [27]. People with hypertension and COVID-19 are at higher risk to develop severe pneumonia or organ damage and show increased inflammatory responses compared with nonhypertensive patients [28]. A linear positive causal relationship between blood pressure and cardiovascular disease underscores the need to treat hypertension early to reduce cardiovascular risk. In both sexes, cardiovascular disease is the leading cause of death. However, epidemiological observations suggest that women have a lower risk of major adverse cardiovascular events than age-matched men [29]. In women, manifestation appears to be delayed, because cardiovascular risk increases in women with age, especially after menopause, when estrogen levels decrease. Therefore, estrogens are generally considered to protect the cardiovascular system [30]. Acute cardiac injury is reported in 8%–62% of patients hospitalized with COVID-19 and is accompanied with higher COVID-19 severity [31,32]. Sex differences in the prevalence and severity of comorbidities contribute to sex disparities in COVID-19 severity and outcome and should be considered in disease stratification and treatment.

Sexual dimorphism in SARS-CoV-2 entry pathways

Two distinct SARS-CoV-2 entry pathways have been described, depending mainly on the coexpression of transmembrane protease serine subtype 2 (TMPRSS2) and angiotensin-converting enzyme 2 (ACE2) on the surface of the target cell [33] (Fig. 28.2).

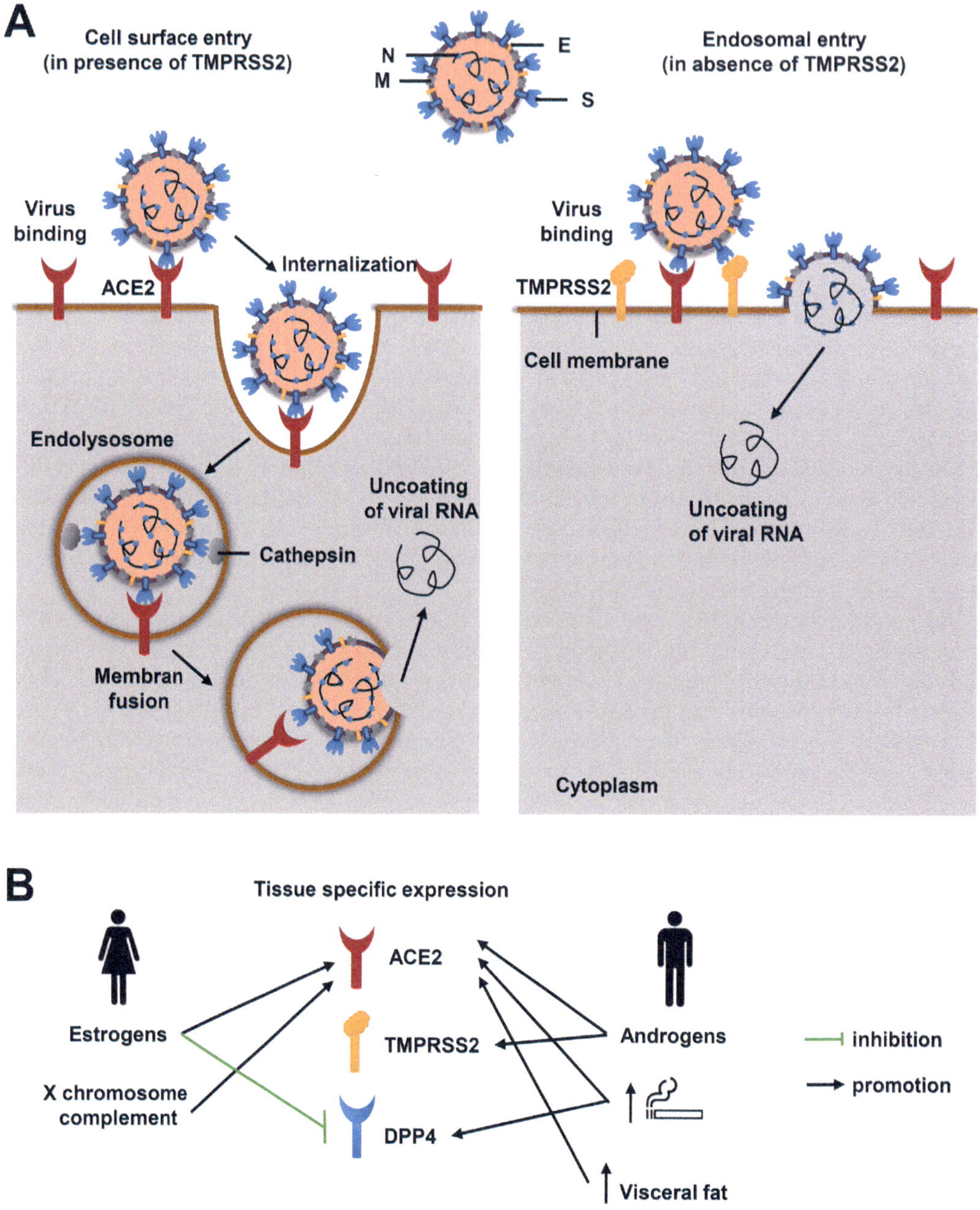

FIGURE 28.2 **SARS-CoV-2 entry pathways and sex-mediated expression of SARS-CoV-2 receptors and coreceptors.** (A) The coronavirus consists of four viral proteins—the spike (S), envelope (E), membrane (M) and nucleocapsid (N) proteins—and genomic RNA. Dependent on the presence of transmembrane protease serine subtype 2 (TMPRSS2), SARS-CoV-2 can enter target cells by two different pathway. In absence of TMPRSS2, SARS-CoV-2 binds to angiotensin-converting enzyme 2 (ACE2) and the virus-ACE2 complex internalizes via endocytosis. Within the endolysosomes, spike protein S2′ is cleaved by cathepsins allowing membrane fusion and viral RNA release in the cytoplasm of host cells for uncoating and replication. When TMPRSS2 is present, S2′clevage occurs at the cell surface, mediated by TMPRSS2, which initiates direct fusion with the membrane. (B) The expression of SARS-CoV-2 receptors and coreceptors, such as ACE2, TMPRSS2 and dipeptidyl peptidase-4 (DPP4) is dependent on the respective tissue. In addition, there are differences in expression between the sexes caused by the action of the X chromosome complement and the sex hormones, estrogen, and androgen. Moreover, smoking and visceral fat affect the expression SARS-CoV-2 receptors and coreceptors. Men accumulate more visceral fat and are more likely to smoke than women, which may contribute to differences between the two sexes in the severity of COVID-19.

For SARS-CoV-2 entry two spike (S) protein cleavage events are typically required; while the S1–S2 boundary is cleaved in the infected cell during maturation, the S2′ site is cleaved after ACE2 binding at the target cell. Cleavage of the S2′ site is mediated by different proteases, such as TMPRSS2. In absence of TMPRSS2, the SARS-CoV-2 ACE2 complex is internalized via endocytosis followed by a cathepsin-mediated S2′cleavage in the endolysosomes under acidic conditions. In the presence of TMPRSS2, S2′cleavage already occurs at the cell surface initiating fusion with the target cell membrane [33]. SARS-CoV-2 entry is thus strongly dependent on the expression of these cell surface proteins, which varies among tissues and is influenced by sex-specific factors such as sex hormones and X-chromosome complement.

Sex hormone-dependent regulation of ACE2

The membrane-bound peptidase, ACE2, is highly expressed in the lung, heard, kidney, and the gastrointestinal tract and regulates blood pressure through the renin–angiotensin–aldosterone system [34]. In addition to the tissue-specific expression pattern of ACE2, the gene encoding ACE2 is located at specific sites of the X-chromosome that generally escape inactivation of the other X-chromosome in mammalian XX cells. This silencing mechanism suppresses redundant gene expression in XX cells up to 90%, but as a consequence female cells overexpress genes located at specific sites of the X-chromosome, such as ACE2 [35]. Moreover, the female sex hormone, estrogen, upregulates the expression of ACE2, thereby contributing to differences in the ACE expression between both sexes [36]. A study in essential hypertensive patients revealed a positive correlation between the serum ACE2 activity and estrogen levels [37]. In addition, androgen-dependent mechanisms also appear to be involved in the regulation of ACE2 expression [38,39]. While some studies revealed no differences in the expression of ACE2 between the two sexes [40], others described a higher expression in aged males [38,41]. A review examining basic research studies on the influence of sex on ACE2 expression found that most studies were conducted in males (6:1 ratio) and furthermore summarized a tissue-dependent expression of ACE2 with higher levels in males [42]. The sex imbalance in studies is also widespread in clinical research, where sex-specific differences are not taken into account or are not even collected in the first place, as most studies focus on disease patterns in men [43,44]. Current discussions and recommendations will hopefully lead to rapid changes in this regard in both basic and clinical research.

Some evidence suggests a protective role of ACE2 in chronic pathologies, such as hypertension and cardiovascular disease [45]. These are also comorbidities associated with a worse COVID-19 prognosis. On the other hand, some animal models suggest that SARS-CoV infections lead to downregulation of ACE2 expression, which causes toxic accumulation of angiotensin II, resulting in an inflammatory response associated with acute lung injury [46,47]. Specific *ACE2* variants were described to be associated with an earlier penetrance, more severe hypertension, and outcomes of COVID-19 in obese smoking males [48]. Another study showed comparable ACE expression in the lungs of nonsmoking women and men; in contrast, ACE2 expression was significantly increased in the lungs of male smokers [38]. ACE2 may not only be involved in the severity of COVID-19 infections through regulation of SARS-CoV-2 virus entry, but also plays a role in comorbidities associated with poorer prognosis. Several factors, including sex hormones and X-chromosome complement, influence tissue-dependent expression of ACE2, and more comprehensive studies in both sexes are needed to fully understand the role of ACE2 and the therapeutic potential of ACE2 inhibitors.

Sex-dependent differences in the expression of transmembrane protease serine subtype 2 (TMPRSS2)

After SARS-CoV-2 binding to ACE2 on the surface of the host cell, TMPRSS2 mediates cleavage of SARS-CoV-2 spike proteins (S2′) allowing fusion with the cell membrane (Fig. 28.1A). TMPRSS2 is a widely studied gene linked to the pathogenesis of prostate cancer and is regulated by androgens [49]. Therefore, it is not surprising that single-cell RNA sequencing of lungs from healthy women and men revealed significantly increased expression of *TMPRSS2* in men, whereas mRNA levels of *ACE2* showed no sex differences [40]. In addition, *ACE2*$^{+}$ *TMPRSS2*$^{+}$ double-positive cells occurred more than three times as often in men than in women [40]. In contrast to ACE2, the expression of TMPRSS2 in the lung does not appear to be affected by smoking [38]. Unfortunately, in a double-blind, randomized, placebo-controlled multicenter trial, treatment with the TMPRSS2 inhibitor camostat mesilate failed to reduce the time to clinical recovery, nor did it reduce mortality in hospitalized COVID-19 patients [50]. In contrast, the antiandrogen enzalutamide showed potential to reduce TMPRSS2 levels in mouse lungs and human lung cells; in addition, it diminished SARS-CoV-2 entry and infection in lung cells [51]. These data suggest that addressing the virus uptake by decreasing TMPRSS2 alone is not sufficient to improve outcome of COVID-19 patients. However, systemic approaches, such as modulation of androgen receptor signaling, which would address other androgen receptor targets in addition to TMPRSS2, may offer potential therapeutic approaches for SARS-CoV-2 infections (discussed in detail below).

Sex-dependent dipeptidyl peptidase-4 (DPP4) activity

In addition, recent evidences suggested that DPP4 also known as CD26 (cluster of differentiation 26) act as a coreceptor for SARS-CoV-2 when entering host cells [52,53]. Its exopeptidase activity leads to cleavage of N-terminal dipeptides from various substrates, including cytokines, neuropeptides, and incretin [54]. The substantial dysregulation of DPP4 in inflammation, cancer, and diabetes as well as its involvement in the immune response underscore the potential of DPP4 as a druggable target. Continuous administration of DPP4 inhibitors, already widely used in diabetes, has therefore also been encouraged for patients with SARS-CoV-2 infection [55,56]. The available retrospective observational studies provide only inconsistent results for the treatment of COVID-19 patients with DPP4 inhibitors [57,58]. While some report significantly lower mortality rates among patients with diabetes receiving DPP4 inhibitors compared to those without, other studies showed no effect or even worse outcomes in patients treated with DPP4 inhibitors. However, in the absence of larger randomized controlled trials, a definitive assessment is not possible. A population-based cohort study suggests that DPP4 inhibition alter certain aspects of the innate immune response. In combination with metformin, DPP4 inhibition appears to decrease the risk of autoimmune disease, including rheumatoid arthritis, in people with diabetes compared to those treated with metformin alone [59]. This could potentially be used to modulate the higher plasma levels of innate cytokines in males that were reported in the context of COVID-19 infections [60].

Although the expression of DPP4 in the lung is comparatively low, the expression is increased in smokers and patients with chronic obstructive pulmonary disease, who are more susceptible to SARS-CoV-2 infection [61]. This might contribute to the differences between the two sexes in the severity of COVID-19, as men are much more likely to smoke than women [62]. Moreover, no differences in DPP4 expression between nonobese postmenopausal women and nonobese premenopausal women were observed, but expression was associated with body weight and body fat centralization [63]. In mice, DPP4 activity in the uterus changed during estrous cycle, with low activities during estrus and high during diestrus [64]. In ovariectomized mice, exposure to estradiol diminished DPP4 activity in the uterus compared to uteri treated with progesterone or vehicle control [64]. Treatment of mice with genistein, a phytoestrogen, also decreased DPP4 activity [65]. These results suggest a potentially estrogen-dependent mechanism in the regulation of DPP4 activity leading to lower DPP4 levels in women (Fig. 28.1B), but further studies are needed to clarify, in particular, the associated implications for COVID-19 progression.

Hypothalamic–pituitary–adrenal (HPA) axis, sex hormones, and COVID-19

It is likely that SARS-CoV-2 infection causes activation of the endocrine stress axis at multiple levels [66]. The hypothalamic–pituitary–adrenal (HPA) axis integrates and manages intrinsic and extrinsic stress stimuli within the organism leading to the secretion of glucocorticoids by the adrenal glands and showed thereby a clear sex-bias [67]. In general, females respond to acute stress with increased glucocorticoid secretion compared to men; the physiological and behavioral changes triggered by this response are essential for survival in the initial phase, but if they persist, the risk for stress-related diseases rises [68]. Due to sex differences in the HPA axis, women are at higher risk to develop such stress-related pathologies compared to men [67]. In addition, the hypothalamic–pituitary–gonadal (HPG) axis, which controls reproduction, regulates HPA axis function in a sex-dependent manner, through the production of the sex hormones, estradiol, or dihydrotestosterone [69]. Estradiol increases the activity of the HPA axis, while androgens exhibit the opposite effects [67]. In the context of the increased stress response in women, it is somewhat surprising that computer tomography studies showed that the adrenal gland is larger in men than in women [70]. In rats and mice, the opposite is the case, with female animals having larger adrenal glands than males [71]. This should be taken into account when translating preclinical results related to sex in this regard. Moreover, female mice exhibit a threefold higher turnover of adrenal tissue than males, which is due to androgens that suppress the recruitment of stem cells from the adrenal capsule and proliferation [72]. A recent study identified the adrenal gland as a prominent target for SARS-CoV-2 infections [73]. Cellular damage caused by the viral infection might lead to a predisposition to adrenal dysfunction, which is associated with hormonal imbalance and an impairment in the response to acute stress [73].

The enhanced release of stress hormones, especially of glucocorticoids, by the adrenal gland in women might contribute to the less severe course of COVID-19 and a lower mortality rate in women than in men. Moreover, treatment with potent glucocorticoids such as dexamethasone is the most effective therapy currently available to reduce inflammation and diminish progression in patients hospitalized with severe COVID-19 infections [74,75]. In a prospective, triple-blind, randomized controlled trail including 84 patients, treatment with methylprednisolone was shown to be superior to dexamethasone in reducing the length of hospitalization in patients with SARS-CoV-2 [76]. Moreover, evidence suggests that early administration of inhaled glucocorticoids in patients with COVID-19 reduces the likelihood of needing urgent medical care and time to recovery [77].

Given the emerging role of sex hormones not only in regulating the HPA axis but also in many other sex-dependent aspects associated with COVID-19 disease, it has been hypothesized that enhancing estrogen signaling or decreasing androgen signaling might be a potential strategy to improved outcomes, particularly in men infected with SARS-CoV-2. Drugs targeting these hormonal pathways have been in clinical use for many years, hence several clinical trials (e.g., NCT04475601 [78], NCT04397718 [79]) are already underway or even completed addressing this hypothesis. A randomized, controlled pilot study with 42 hospitalized men, resulted in shorter hospital stay and reduced need for oxygen supplementation for participants receiving progesterone (subcutaneous) in addition to standard treatment compared with control subjects [80]. Another prospective study of 77 hospitalized men indicated beneficial effects of antiandrogenic treatment with improved clinical outcome in severely affected COVID-19 patients [81]. In addition, a community-based study of 4532 subjects suggests that androgen-deprivation therapy, commonly used for the treatment of prostate cancer, may diminish the risk of infections with SARS-CoV-2 by reducing TMPRSS2 expression [82]. A clinical trial is currently underway to determine if treatment of men and postmenopausal women with transdermal estradiol patches may decrease severity of COVID-19 (NCT04359329). Women with COVID-19 who received hormone replacement therapy (HRT) have a lower likelihood of death compared to other women [83]. This may be due to the therapeutic benefits of HRT, including lower incidence of cardiovascular disease [84]. Postmenopausal women infected with SARS-CoV-2 present with elevated levels of proinflammatory cytokines (IL-6, IL-1), whereas HRT has the potential to diminish cytokine levels in these women to premenopausal levels [85]. Nevertheless, possible side effects associated with the administration of sex hormones, such as an increased risk of thrombosis or high dosages of glucocorticoids, should be considered.

Moreover, pregnancy is associated with persistently high estrogen levels. Studies suggest that the clinical course of COVID-19 is not severe in most of these women and that the infection does not significantly affect pregnancy and neonatal outcomes [86], but comorbidities, such as hypertension, diabetes, and asthma were risk factors for hospitalization of pregnant women [87]. Not only the sex hormones themselves, but also their precursors, dehydroepiandrosterone (DHEA) and its sulfate (DHEAS), may contribute to the observed sexual dimorphism in COVID-19. Since DHEA is a potent inhibitor of glucose-6-phosphate dehydrogenase (G6PD). Reduction in the normal G6PD activity sensitizes human cells to coronavirus 229E infections [88]. Moreover, elevated DHEA levels, which are higher in males, can cause cytotoxic effects in endothelial cells that might contribute to SARS-CoV-2-induced vascular endothelialitis [89]. These associations should be considered, especially in patients with diabetes, who already have low G6PD activity [90].

Sex discrepancies in the immune response to COVID-19

Sex has direct implications on the course of infections caused by different pathogens. Females are more likely to have a stronger immune response, which is associated with a lower susceptibility and/or vulnerability to infectious disease [91]. High levels of estradiol and progesterone in females suppress the production of proinflammatory cytokines by macrophages and instead stimulate the production of antiinflammatory cytokines in CD4+ T helper cells [92,93]. In addition, estradiol increases the production of antibodies by B cells [94]. In contrast, testosterone suppresses both adaptive and innate immune response [95]; however, low circulating testosterone levels in men hospitalized with COVID-19 were linked with enhanced disease severity, inflammation, and mortality [96,97].

Hospitalized males with severe COVID-19 showed significantly higher levels of the proinflammatory cytokines, IL-6, IL-8, and MCP-1, than females; in addition, only severely affected males present with higher levels of IL-8, GRO, sCD40L, MIP-1β, MCP-1 compared with mildly affected or control patients [98]. Females exhibit significantly higher antiinflammatory cytokine IL-10 levels compared to males [98]. In another study, male patients showed higher plasma levels of innate immune cytokines (e.g., IL-8 and IL-18) and a more robust induction of nonclassical monocytes, while female patients had a more robust T-cell activation during SARS-CoV-2 infection [99]. Only in male patients was a poor T-cell response associated with a worse disease course, whereas in female patients, higher levels of innate immune system cytokines were associated with a worse course of COVID-19 [99].

In addition to the effects of sex hormones, a number of X-linked genes (e.g., *IL-13, IL-4, IL-10, TLR7, FOXP3, XIST*) and Y-linked genes (*SOX9, SRY*) may contribute to sexual dimorphic immune responses [100]. The sex-dependent distribution and composition of adipose tissue also influences immune response in a sex-specific manner. In this context, it is not surprising that obesity has been described as a predictor of severe COVID-19 [101]. In particular, visceral fat, which accumulates predominantly in males, has been associated with more severe SARS-CoV-2 infections [102,103]. In mice, adipose tissue of males comprises more immune cells, associated with higher and longer elevated levels of cytokines than those of females [104–106]. Similar effects in human may contribute to the rapid and intense systematic inflammation in males that leads to the deleterious increase in cytokines (cytokine storm) observed in critical SARS-CoV-2 infections.

Sex-related differences in autoimmunity and COVID-19 vaccines

Another important immunologic aspect that may contribute to sex-related differences in the severity and outcome of COVID-19 disease is autoimmunity [107]. Sexual dimorphism is well known in autoimmune disease (AID), since 75%–80% of patients suffering from AID are females [108]. Nevertheless, AIDs with higher prevalence in males are characterized by acute inflammation, the presence of autoantibodies, and a proinflammatory Th1 immune response, whereas AIDs which occur more often in women have known antibody-mediated pathology (Th2 immune response) [108]. Androgens seem to foster a type 1 (Th1) cytokine profile, as in rheumatoid arthritis, while estrogens promote AID with a type 2 (Th2) cytokine profile, as in systemic lupus erythematosus [108]. Some evidence suggests that COVID-19 infections might simulate or trigger a form of organ-specific autoimmunity in predisposed patients [109–111]. Histological investigations in patients infected with SARS-CoV-2 revealed an infiltration of T lymphocytes (CD3+), most of them were CD8+ suppressors, in the lungs, adrenals, liver and intestine [112,113]. This is of particular interest since autoimmune reactions are mediated by CD8+ T cell cytotoxicity, confirming the involvement of autoimmune processes in these tissues after infection with COVID-19. Sex-dependent differences in autoimmune response, as well as higher prevalence of autoimmune disease in women, may also have implications for the course of COVID-19, but further studies are needed to make conclusive statements.

Autoimmunity is also important to consider in the context of COVID-19 vaccines, which represents the most promising, if not the only way, to contain the COVID-19 pandemic. Extremely rare cases of unusual thrombocytopenia have been described 4–28 days after immunization with ChAdOx1 nCov-19 (AstraZeneca) and Ad26.COV2.S (Johnson & Johnson/ Janssen), preferably in young women (younger than 50 years) [114,115]. Although the complete pathomechanism of this rare phenomena remains unclear, certain findings revealed high levels of antibodies to platelet factor 4 (PF4) in these patients. In contrast to heparin-induced thrombocytopenia, binding of antibodies to PF4 occurred in the absence of heparin indicating an autoimmune heparin-induced thrombocytopenia in these patients [115–117]. Unfortunately, the mortality rate in patients with cerebral sinus thrombosis after SARS-CoV-2 vaccination is high [118]. In addition, extremely rare cases of Guillain–Barré syndrome, another classical autoimmune disorder, was described after vaccination with Janssen (Johnson & Johnson) COVID-19 vaccine, which particularly occurs in males between 50 and 60 years [119,120]. Some case reports describe rare cases of myocarditis after vaccination with mRNA-based COVID-19 vaccines (24 cases/million), mainly in men (18–85 years), and some patterns of myocardial damage in these patients suggest an autoimmune myocarditis [120,121]. Sex differences appear to have an impact on the occurrence of side effects, and further research is needed to better understand the relevant connections. Despite these extremely rare potential side effects, the benefits of these vaccines clearly outweigh their risks and offer a promising way out of the pandemic.

Sexual dimorphism and long COVID syndrome

The long COVID syndrome, or also named post-COVID syndrome, is defined as a complex of nonspecific persisting symptoms, such as muscle weakness, chronic fatigue, sleep difficulties, depression or anxiety, that occur after acute COVID-19 and cannot be explained by other disease [122]. Similar to other postviral syndromes, such as chronic fatigue syndrome caused by Epstein–Barr virus, women are more likely than men to develop long COVID syndrome [123,124]. The higher probability of women to develop long COVID syndrome remains only until the age of 60, after which the risk level between women and men equalizes. In addition to female sex, older age and a high body mass index also appear to be risk factors for the development of long COVID syndrome [125]. In another study, in addition to female sex and age, active smoking was also reported as a risk factor, whereas the severity of acute COVID-19 infection did not affect the risk of developing long COVID-19 syndrome [126]. In a Swiss cohort study of 5838 people, women were more likely to report at least one persistent symptom, and decreased resilience was the most commonly reported symptom in both sexes [127]. Cardiovascular risk factors, self-reported domestic stress, and preexisting mental illness increased the risk for the development of long COVID syndrome in women [127]. Preexisting asthma has been reported to increase the risk to develop long COVID syndrome and is more common in women than men, which may further contribute to differences between sexes [128]. Persistent symptoms following acute COVID-19 infection have also been described in children [129,130]. In a small cohort of children (n = 129), 27.1% of children reported at least one symptom more than 120 days after initial diagnosis, and 20.6% of children reported three or more symptoms [130]. Most symptoms in these children were equally distributed between both sexes, with some exceptions such as headache (16.1% vs. 4.5%), altered taste (4.8% vs. 1.5%) and smell (6.5% vs. 3%), and insomnia (22.6% vs. 14.9%), which were more common in girls, but without statistical significance [131]. Results based on the collection of symptoms by physician or electronic aids (e.g., apps) might be biased by sex-specific differences in the perception and reporting of symptoms. Men with West Nile virus (WNV) infection, for example, reported significantly fewer symptoms than women, although viral loads were comparable in both sexes [132].

Currently, it is not fully understood why some people develop long COVID and others do not. In addition to multiorgan damage caused by inflammation, the involvement of autoantibodies (discussed in detail above) is also being considered as a cause [133], which may also explain the differences between the two sexes in long COVID. Since the immune response is stronger in women than in men, this leads to more severe consequences of acute COVID-19 in men on the one hand, but on the other hand, the incidence of autoimmune reactions is higher in women [131]. An improved understanding of the underlying mechanisms and risk factors, such as female sex, is critical to identify patients predisposed to the development of long COVID syndrome early, which may allow for preventive interventions and improve therapeutic outcome.

Conclusions

Variation of COVID-19 courses between sexes, with males being more severely affected than females, underscores the importance of considering biological sex regarding potential prevention and treatment strategies for COVID-19. We recently shared our personal opinion from a clinical perspective on this topic [3]. However, we are only at the beginning of defining sex-specific preventive and therapeutic approaches. Given that we are far away from sex-specific treatments in other areas of clinical practice, where gender differences have been known for decades, it becomes apparent that we still have a long way to go before we reach the goal of sex-specific recommendations for patients with COVID-19. All of the data discussed here underscore the importance of collecting and reporting sex-specific data in clinical and preclinical studies in the future, not just in COVID-19. Although the general molecular mechanisms do not differ between males and females, sex-specific differences in the expression patterns of cell surface proteins, in the levels of sex hormones, in stress and immune responses, and social behaviors are partly responsible for the observed sexual dimorphism in COVID-19. More comprehensive, prospective and mechanistic studies are needed to gain deeper insights and to understand the relationships among the various contributing factors.

References

[1] Scully EP, Haverfield J, Ursin RL, Tannenbaum C, Klein SL. Considering how biological sex impacts immune responses and COVID-19 outcomes. Nat Rev Immunol 2020:1–6.

[2] Alwani M, Yassin A, Al-Zoubi RM, Aboumarzouk OM, Nettleship J, Kelly D, et al. Sex-based differences in severity and mortality in COVID-19. Rev Med Virol 2021;31. e2223.

[3] Bechmann N, Barthel A, Schedl A, Herzig S, Varga Z, Gebhard C, et al. Sexual dimorphism in COVID-19: potential clinical and public health implications. Lancet Diabetes Endocrinol 2022;10(3):221–30.

[4] Galasso V, Pons V, Profeta P, Becher M, Brouard S, Foucault M. Gender differences in COVID-19 attitudes and behavior: panel evidence from eight countries. Proc Natl Acad Sci USA 2020;117(44):27285–91.

[5] Reisch T, Heiler G, Hurt J, Klimek P, Hanbury A, Thurner S. Behavioral gender differences are reinforced during the COVID-19 crisis. Sci Rep 2021;11(1):1–12.

[6] Chen N, Zhou M, Dong X, Qu J, Gong F, Han Y, et al. Epidemiological and clinical characteristics of 99 cases of 2019 novel coronavirus pneumonia in Wuhan, China: a descriptive study. Lancet 2020;395(10223):507–13.

[7] Zhao S, Cao P, Chong MK, Gao D, Lou Y, Ran J, et al. COVID-19 and gender-specific difference: analysis of public surveillance data in Hong Kong and Shenzhen, China, from January 10 to February 15, 2020. Infect Control Hosp Epidemiol 2020;41(6):750–1.

[8] The Sex GaC-P. https://globalhealth5050.org/the-sex-gender-and-covid-19-project/dataset/ (viewed 15 December, 2021).

[9] Bhopal SS, Bhopal R. Sex differential in COVID-19 mortality varies markedly by age. Lancet 2020;396(10250):532–3.

[10] Woodruff RC, Campbell AP, Taylor CA, Chai SJ, Kawasaki B, Meek J, et al. Risk factors for severe COVID-19 in children. Pediatrics 2022;149(1).

[11] Berenguer J, Ryan P, Rodríguez-Baño J, Jarrín I, Carratalà J, Pachón J, et al. Characteristics and predictors of death among 4035 consecutively hospitalized patients with COVID-19 in Spain. Clin Microbiol Infect 2020;26(11):1525–36.

[12] Chakravarty D, Nair SS, Hammouda N, Ratnani P, Gharib Y, Wagaskar V, et al. Sex differences in SARS-CoV-2 infection rates and the potential link to prostate cancer. Commun Biol 2020;3(1):1–12.

[13] Morris A. Sex differences for fasting levels of glucose and insulin: expanding our understanding. Nat Rev Endocrinol 2021;17(3):131.

[14] Link JC, Reue K. Genetic basis for sex differences in obesity and lipid metabolism. Annu Rev Nutr 2017;37:225–45.

[15] Menke A, Casagrande S, Geiss L, Cowie CC. Prevalence of and trends in diabetes among adults in the United States, 1988–2012. JAMA 2015;314(10):1021–9.

[16] Kautzky-Willer A, Harreiter J, Pacini G. Sex and gender differences in risk, pathophysiology and complications of type 2 diabetes mellitus. Endocr Rev 2016;37(3):278–316.

[17] Gao A, Su J, Liu R, Zhao S, Li W, Xu X, et al. Sexual dimorphism in glucose metabolism is shaped by androgen-driven gut microbiome. Nat Commun 2021;12(1):7080.

[18] McGurnaghan SJ, Weir A, Bishop J, Kennedy S, Blackbourn LA, McAllister DA, et al. Risks of and risk factors for COVID-19 disease in people with diabetes: a cohort study of the total population of Scotland. Lancet Diabetes Endocrinol 2021;9(2):82–93.

[19] Tramunt B, Smati S, Coudol S, Wargny M, Pichelin M, Guyomarch B, et al. Sex disparities in COVID-19 outcomes of inpatients with diabetes: insights from the CORONADO study. Eur J Endocrinol 2021;1(aop).

[20] Carr MC. The emergence of the metabolic syndrome with menopause. J Clin Endocrinol Metab 2003;88(6):2404–11.

[21] Stefan N, Birkenfeld AL, Schulze MB. Global pandemics interconnected—obesity, impaired metabolic health and COVID-19. Nat Rev Endocrinol 2021;17(3):135–49.

[22] Hendren NS, de Lemos JA, Ayers C, Das SR, Rao A, Carter S, et al. Association of body mass index and age with morbidity and mortality in patients hospitalized with COVID-19: results from the American Heart Association COVID-19 Cardiovascular Disease Registry. Circulation 2021;143(2):135–44.

[23] Mauvais-Jarvis F. Sex differences in metabolic homeostasis, diabetes, and obesity. Biol Sex Differ 2015;6(1):1–9.

[24] Maranon R, Reckelhoff JF. Sex and gender differences in control of blood pressure. Clin Sci 2013;125(7):311–8.

[25] Sandberg K, Ji H. Sex differences in primary hypertension. Biol Sex Differ 2012;3(1):1–21.

[26] Elmarakby AA, Sullivan JC. Sex differences in hypertension: lessons from spontaneously hypertensive rats (SHR). Clin Sci 2021;135(15):1791–804.
[27] Lippi G, Wong J, Henry BM. Hypertension and its severity or mortality in Coronavirus Disease 2019 (COVID-19): a pooled analysis. Pol Arch Intern Med 2020;130(4):304–9.
[28] Trump S, Lukassen S, Anker MS, Chua RL, Liebig J, Thürmann L, et al. Hypertension delays viral clearance and exacerbates airway hyperinflammation in patients with COVID-19. Nat Biotechnol 2021;39(6):705–16.
[29] Akyea RK, Kontopantelis E, Kai J, Weng SF, Patel RS, Asselbergs FW, et al. Sex disparity in subsequent outcomes in survivors of coronary heart disease. Heart 2022;108(1):37–45.
[30] Iorga A, Cunningham CM, Moazeni S, Ruffenach G, Umar S, Eghbali M. The protective role of estrogen and estrogen receptors in cardiovascular disease and the controversial use of estrogen therapy. Biol Sex Differ 2017;8(1):1–16.
[31] Guo T, Fan Y, Chen M, Wu X, Zhang L, He T, et al. Cardiovascular implications of fatal outcomes of patients with coronavirus disease 2019 (COVID-19). JAMA cardiology 2020;5(7):811–8.
[32] Chung MK, Zidar DA, Bristow MR, Cameron SJ, Chan T, Harding III CV, et al. COVID-19 and cardiovascular disease: from bench to bedside. Circ Res 2021;128(8):1214–36.
[33] Jackson CB, Farzan M, Chen B, Choe H. Mechanisms of SARS-CoV-2 entry into cells. Nat Rev Mol Cell Biol 2021:1–18.
[34] Turner AJ, Hiscox JA, Hooper NM. ACE2: from vasopeptidase to SARS virus receptor. Trends Pharmacol Sci 2004;25(6):291–4.
[35] Gagliardi MC, Tieri P, Ortona E, Ruggieri A. ACE2 expression and sex disparity in COVID-19. Cell Death Discov 2020;6(1):1–2.
[36] Bukowska A, Spiller L, Wolke C, Lendeckel U, Weinert S, Hoffmann J, et al. Protective regulation of the ACE2/ACE gene expression by estrogen in human atrial tissue from elderly men. Exp Biol Med 2017;242(14):1412–23.
[37] Zhang Q, Cong M, Wang N, Li X, Zhang H, Zhang K, et al. Association of angiotensin-converting enzyme 2 gene polymorphism and enzymatic activity with essential hypertension in different gender: a case–control study. Medicine 2018;97(42).
[38] Baratchian M, McManus JM, Berk MP, Nakamura F, Mukhopadhyay S, Xu W, et al. Androgen regulation of pulmonary AR, TMPRSS2 and ACE2 with implications for sex-discordant COVID-19 outcomes. Sci Rep 2021;11(1):1–11.
[39] Deng Q, ur Rasool R, Russell RM, Natesan R, Asangani IA. Targeting androgen regulation of TMPRSS2 and ACE2 as a therapeutic strategy to combat COVID-19. IScience 2021;24(3):102254.
[40] Okwan-Duodu D, Lim E-C, You S, Engman DM. TMPRSS2 activity may mediate sex differences in COVID-19 severity. Signal Transduct Target Ther 2021;6(1):1–3.
[41] Viveiros A, Gheblawi M, Aujla PK, Sosnowski DK, Seubert JM, Kassiri Z, et al. Sex-and age-specific regulation of ACE2: insights into severe COVID-19 susceptibility. J Mol Cell Cardiol 2022;164:13–6.
[42] Miličić Stanić B, Maddox S, de Souza AM, Wu X, Mehranfard D, Ji H, et al. Male bias in ACE2 basic science research: missed opportunity for discovery in the time of COVID-19. Am J Physiol Regul Integr Comp Physiol 2021;320(6):R925–37.
[43] Winham SJ, Mielke MM. What about sex? Nat Metab 2021:1–3.
[44] Mielke MM, Miller VM. Improving clinical outcomes through attention to sex and hormones in research. Nat Rev Endocrinol 2021;17(10):625–35.
[45] Hanff TC, Harhay MO, Brown TS, Cohen JB, Mohareb AM. Is there an association between COVID-19 mortality and the renin-angiotensin system? A call for epidemiologic investigations. Clin Infect Dis 2020;71(15):870–4.
[46] Imai Y, Kuba K, Rao S, Huan Y, Guo F, Guan B, et al. Angiotensin-converting enzyme 2 protects from severe acute lung failure. Nature 2005;436(7047):112–6.
[47] Zhang H, Penninger JM, Li Y, Zhong N, Slutsky AS. Angiotensin-converting enzyme 2 (ACE2) as a SARS-CoV-2 receptor: molecular mechanisms and potential therapeutic target. Intensive Care Med 2020;46(4):586–90.
[48] Hamet P, Pausova Z, Attaoua R, Hishmih C, Haloui M, Shin J, et al. SARS–CoV-2 receptor ACE2 gene is associated with hypertension and severity of COVID 19: interaction with sex, obesity, and smoking. Am J Hypertens 2021;34(4):367–76.
[49] Lin B, Ferguson C, White JT, Wang S, Vessella R, True LD, et al. Prostate-localized and androgen-regulated expression of the membrane-bound serine protease TMPRSS2. Cancer Res 1999;59(17):4180–4.

[50] Gunst JD, Staerke NB, Pahus MH, Kristensen LH, Bodilsen J, Lohse N, et al. Efficacy of the TMPRSS2 inhibitor camostat mesilate in patients hospitalized with Covid-19-a double-blind randomized controlled trial. EClinicalMedicine 2021:100849.
[51] Leach D, Mohr A, Giotis E, Cil E, Isac A, Yates L, et al. The antiandrogen enzalutamide downregulates TMPRSS2 and reduces cellular entry of SARS-CoV-2 in human lung cells. Nat Commun 2021;12(1):1–12.
[52] Qi F, Qian S, Zhang S, Zhang Z. Single cell RNA sequencing of 13 human tissues identify cell types and receptors of human coronaviruses. Biochem Biophys Res Commun 2020;526(1):135–40.
[53] Solerte SB, Di Sabatino A, Galli M, Fiorina P. Dipeptidyl peptidase-4 (DPP4) inhibition in COVID-19. Acta Diabetol 2020;57:779–83.
[54] Röhrborn D, Wronkowitz N, Eckel J. DPP4 in diabetes. Front Immunol 2015;6:386.
[55] Seliger B, Subbarayan K, Ulagappan K, Wickenhauser C, Bachmann M. Immune interaction map of human SARS-CoV-2 target genes: implications for therapeutic avenues. Front Immunol 2021;12:647.
[56] Hariyanto TI, Kurniawan A. Dipeptidyl peptidase 4 (DPP4) inhibitor and outcome from coronavirus disease 2019 (COVID-19) in diabetic patients: a systematic review, meta-analysis, and meta-regression. J Diabetes Metab Disord 2021:1–8.
[57] Bonora B, Avogaro A, Fadini G. Disentangling conflicting evidence on DPP-4 inhibitors and outcomes of COVID-19: narrative review and meta-analysis. J Endocrinol Invest 2021:1–8.
[58] Yang Y, Cai Z, Zhang J. DPP-4 inhibitors may improve the mortality of coronavirus disease 2019: a meta-analysis. PLoS One 2021;16(5):e0251916.
[59] Kim SC, Schneeweiss S, Glynn RJ, Doherty M, Goldfine AB, Solomon DH. Dipeptidyl peptidase-4 inhibitors in type 2 diabetes may reduce the risk of autoimmune diseases: a population-based cohort study. Ann Rheum Dis 2015;74(11):1968–75.
[60] Yazbeck R, Jaenisch S, Abbott C. Dipeptidyl peptidase 4 inhibitors: applications in innate immunity? Biochem Pharmacol 2021:114517.
[61] Seys LJ, Widagdo W, Verhamme FM, Kleinjan A, Janssens W, Joos GF, et al. DPP4, the Middle East respiratory syndrome coronavirus receptor, is upregulated in lungs of smokers and chronic obstructive pulmonary disease patients. Clin Infect Dis 2018;66(1):45–53.
[62] Cai H. Sex difference and smoking predisposition in patients with COVID-19. Lancet Respir Med 2020;8(4):e20.
[63] de Oliveira Siciliano P, Godoy-Matos AF, a Braga LD, Carvalho JDP, do Amaral Corrêa JO. DPP4 activity is related to body weight and central fat in postmenopausal women. Diabetes Metabol Syndr Clin Res Rev 2019;13(5):3031–4.
[64] Ohta N, Takahashi T, Mori T, Park MK, Kawashima S, Takahashi K, et al. Hormonal modulation of prolyl endopeptidase and dipeptidyl peptidase IV activities in the mouse uterus and ovary. Eur J Endocrinol 1992;127(3):262–6.
[65] Rajput MS, Sarkar PD, Nirmal NP. Inhibition of DPP-4 activity and neuronal atrophy with genistein attenuates neurological deficits induced by transient global cerebral ischemia and reperfusion in streptozotocin-induced diabetic mice. Inflammation 2017;40(2):623–35.
[66] Steenblock C, Todorov V, Kanczkowski W, Eisenhofer G, Schedl A, Wong M-L, et al. Severe acute respiratory syndrome coronavirus 2 (SARS-CoV-2) and the neuroendocrine stress axis. Mol Psychiatr 2020;25(8):1611–7.
[67] Heck AL, Handa RJ. Sex differences in the hypothalamic–pituitary–adrenal axis' response to stress: an important role for gonadal hormones. Neuropsychopharmacology 2019;44(1):45–58.
[68] Sapolsky RM, Romero LM, Munck AU. How do glucocorticoids influence stress responses? Integrating permissive, suppressive, stimulatory, and preparative actions. Endocr Rev 2000;21(1):55–89.
[69] Viau V. Functional cross-talk between the hypothalamic-pituitary-gonadal and-adrenal axes. J Neuroendocrinol 2002;14(6):506–13.
[70] John R, Putta T, Simon B, Eapen A, Jebasingh F, Thomas N, et al. Normal adrenal gland thickness on computerized tomography in an Asian Indian adult population. Indian J Radiol Imag 2018;28(4):465.
[71] Bechmann N, Berger I, Bornstein SR, Steenblock C. Adrenal medulla development and medullary-cortical interactions. Mol Cell Endocrinol 2021;528:111258.
[72] Grabek A, Dolfi B, Klein B, Jian-Motamedi F, Chaboissier M-C, Schedl A. The adult adrenal cortex undergoes rapid tissue renewal in a sex-specific manner. Cell Stem Cell 2019;25(2):290–6. e2.
[73] Kanczkowski W, Evert K, Stadtmüller M, Haberecker M, Laks L, Chen L-S, et al. COVID-19 targets human adrenal glands. Lancet Diabetes Endocrinol 2022;10(1):13–6.

[74] Group RC. Dexamethasone in hospitalized patients with Covid-19. N Engl J Med 2021;384(8):693–704.

[75] Águas R, Mahdi A, Shretta R, Horby P, Landray M, White L. Potential health and economic impacts of dexamethasone treatment for patients with COVID-19. Nat Commun 2021;12(1):1–8.

[76] Ranjbar K, Moghadami M, Mirahmadizadeh A, Fallahi MJ, Khaloo V, Shahriarirad R, et al. Methylprednisolone or dexamethasone, which one is superior corticosteroid in the treatment of hospitalized COVID-19 patients: a triple-blinded randomized controlled trial. BMC Infect Dis 2021;21(1):1–8.

[77] Ramakrishnan S, Nicolau Jr DV, Langford B, Mahdi M, Jeffers H, Mwasuku C, et al. Inhaled budesonide in the treatment of early COVID-19 (STOIC): a phase 2, open-label, randomised controlled trial. Lancet Respir Med 2021;9(7):763–72.

[78] Welén K, Överby AK, Ahlm C, Freyhult E, Robinsson D, Henningsson AJ, et al. COVIDENZA-A prospective, multicenter, randomized PHASE II clinical trial of enzalutamide treatment to decrease the morbidity in patients with Corona virus disease 2019 (COVID-19): a structured summary of a study protocol for a randomised controlled trial. Trials 2021;22(1):1–3.

[79] Nickols NG, Goetz MB, Graber CJ, Bhattacharya D, Hoo GS, Might M, et al. Hormonal intervention for the treatment of veterans with COVID-19 requiring hospitalization (HITCH): a multicenter, phase 2 randomized controlled trial of best supportive care vs best supportive care plus degarelix: study protocol for a randomized controlled trial. Trials 2021;22(1):1–8.

[80] Ghandehari S, Matusov Y, Pepkowitz S, Stein D, Kaderi T, Narayanan D, et al. Progesterone in addition to standard of care vs standard of care alone in the treatment of men hospitalized with moderate to severe Covid-19: a randomized, controlled pilot trial. Chest 2021;160:74–84.

[81] Goren A, Wambier CG, Herrera S, McCoy J, Vaño-Galván S, Gioia F, et al. Anti-androgens may protect against severe COVID-19 outcomes: results from a prospective cohort study of 77 hospitalized men. J Eur Acad Dermatol Venereol 2021;35:e13–5.

[82] Montopoli M, Zumerle S, Vettor R, Rugge M, Zorzi M, Catapano CV, et al. Androgen-deprivation therapies for prostate cancer and risk of infection by SARS-CoV-2: a population-based study (N=4532). Ann Oncol 2020;31(8):1040–5.

[83] Dambha-Miller H, Hinton W, Joy M, Feher M, de Lusignan S. Mortality in COVID-19 amongst women on hormone replacement therapy or combined oral contraception: a cohort study. medRxiv 2021. https://doi.org/10.1093/fampra/cmac041.

[84] Nappi RE, Simoncini T. Menopause transition: a golden age to prevent cardiovascular disease. Lancet Diabetes Endocrinol 2021;9(3):135–7.

[85] Okpechi SC, Fong JT, Gill SS, Harman JC, Nguyen TH, Chukwurah QC, et al. Global sex disparity of COVID-19: a descriptive review of sex hormones and consideration for the potential therapeutic use of hormone replacement therapy in older adults. Aging Dis 2021;12(2):671.

[86] Di Toro F, Gjoka M, Di Lorenzo G, De Santo D, De Seta F, Maso G, et al. Impact of COVID-19 on maternal and neonatal outcomes: a systematic review and meta-analysis. Clin Microbiol Infect 2021;27(1):36–46.

[87] Knight M, Bunch K, Vousden N, Morris E, Simpson N, Gale C, et al. Characteristics and outcomes of pregnant women admitted to hospital with confirmed SARS-CoV-2 infection in UK: national population based cohort study. Bmj 2020:369.

[88] Wu Y-H, Tseng C-P, Cheng M-L, Ho H-Y, Shih S-R, Chiu DT-Y. Glucose-6-phosphate dehydrogenase deficiency enhances human coronavirus 229E infection. J Infect Dis 2008;197(6):812–6.

[89] Ackermann M, Verleden SE, Kuehnel M, Haverich A, Welte T, Laenger F, et al. Pulmonary vascular endothelialitis, thrombosis, and angiogenesis in Covid-19. N Engl J Med 2020;383(2):120–8.

[90] Heymann AD, Cohen Y, Chodick G. Glucose-6-phosphate dehydrogenase deficiency and type 2 diabetes. Diabetes Care 2012;35(8). e58-e.

[91] Klein SL, Flanagan KL. Sex differences in immune responses. Nat Rev Immunol 2016;16(10):626–38.

[92] Wray S, Arrowsmith S. The physiological mechanisms of the sex-based difference in outcomes of COVID19 infection. Front Physiol 2021;12:71.

[93] Mauvais-Jarvis F, Klein SL, Levin ER. Estradiol, progesterone, immunomodulation, and COVID-19 outcomes. Endocrinology 2020;161(9). bqaa127.

[94] Myers MJ, Petersen BH. Estradiol induced alterations of the immune system—I. Enhancement of IgM production. Int J Immunopharm 1985;7(2):207–13.

[95] Trigunaite A, Dimo J, Jørgensen TN. Suppressive effects of androgens on the immune system. Cell Immunol 2015;294(2):87–94.
[96] Rastrelli G, Di Stasi V, Inglese F, Beccaria M, Garuti M, Di Costanzo D, et al. Low testosterone levels predict clinical adverse outcomes in SARS-CoV-2 pneumonia patients. Andrology 2021;9(1):88–98.
[97] Dhindsa S, Zhang N, McPhaul MJ, Wu Z, Ghoshal AK, Erlich EC, et al. Association of circulating sex hormones with inflammation and disease severity in patients with COVID-19. JAMA Netw Open 2021;4(5). e2111398-e.
[98] Qi S, Ngwa C, Morales Scheihing DA, Al Mamun A, Ahnstedt HW, Finger CE, et al. Sex differences in the immune response to acute COVID-19 respiratory tract infection. Biol Sex Differ 2021;12(1):1–10.
[99] Takahashi T, Ellingson MK, Wong P, Israelow B, Lucas C, Klein J, et al. Sex differences in immune responses that underlie COVID-19 disease outcomes. Nature 2020;588(7837):315–20.
[100] Ghosh S, Klein RS. Sex drives dimorphic immune responses to viral infections. J Immunol 2017;198(5):1782–90.
[101] Tamara A, Tahapary DL. Obesity as a predictor for a poor prognosis of COVID-19: a systematic review. Diabetes Metabol Syndr Clin Res Rev 2020;14(4):655–9.
[102] Petersen A, Bressem K, Albrecht J, Thieß H-M, Vahldiek J, Hamm B, et al. The role of visceral adiposity in the severity of COVID-19: highlights from a unicenter cross-sectional pilot study in Germany. Metabolism 2020;110:154317.
[103] Földi M, Farkas N, Kiss S, Dembrovszky F, Szakács Z, Balaskó M, et al. Visceral adiposity elevates the risk of critical condition in COVID-19: a systematic review and meta-analysis. Obesity 2021;29(3):521–8.
[104] Ishikawa A, Wada T, Nishimura S, Ito T, Okekawa A, Onogi Y, et al. Estrogen regulates sex-specific localization of regulatory T cells in adipose tissue of obese female mice. PLoS One 2020;15(4). e0230885.
[105] Varghese M, Griffin C, McKernan K, Eter L, Lanzetta N, Agarwal D, et al. Sex differences in inflammatory responses to adipose tissue lipolysis in diet-induced obesity. Endocrinology 2019;160(2):293–312.
[106] Camporez JP, Lyu K, Goldberg EL, Zhang D, Cline GW, Jurczak MJ, et al. Anti-inflammatory effects of oestrogen mediate the sexual dimorphic response to lipid-induced insulin resistance. J Physiol 2019;597(15):3885–903.
[107] Dotan A, Muller S, Kanduc D, David P, Halpert G, Shoenfeld Y. The SARS-CoV-2 as an instrumental trigger of autoimmunity. Autoimmun Rev 2021:102792.
[108] Amur S, Parekh A, Mummaneni P. Sex differences and genomics in autoimmune diseases. J Autoimmun 2012;38(2–3):J254–65.
[109] Gagiannis D, Steinestel J, Hackenbroch C, Hannemann M, Umathum VG, Gebauer N, et al. COVID-19-induced acute respiratory failure: an exacerbation of organ-specific autoimmunity? medRxiv 2020. https://doi.org/10.1101/2020.04.27.20077180. published online May 01, 2020 (preprint).
[110] Zhou Y, Han T, Chen J, Hou C, Hua L, He S, et al. Clinical and autoimmune characteristics of severe and critical cases of COVID-19. Clin Transl Sci 2020;13(6):1077–86.
[111] Caso F, Costa L, Ruscitti P, Navarini L, Del Puente A, Giacomelli R, et al. Could Sars-coronavirus-2 trigger autoimmune and/or autoinflammatory mechanisms in genetically predisposed subjects? Autoimmun Rev 2020;19(5):102524.
[112] Zinserling V, Vashukova M, Vasilyeva M, Isakov A, Lugovskaya N, Narkevich T, et al. Issues of pathology of a new coronavirus infection COVID-19. J Infektol 2020:5–11.
[113] Ehrenfeld M, Tincani A, Andreoli L, Cattalini M, Greenbaum A, Kanduc D, et al. Covid-19 and autoimmunity. Autoimmun Rev 2020;19(8):102597.
[114] Muir K-L, Kallam A, Koepsell SA, Gundabolu K. Thrombotic thrombocytopenia after Ad26. COV2. S vaccination. N Engl J Med 2021;384(20):1964–5.
[115] Greinacher A, Thiele T, Warkentin TE, Weisser K, Kyrle PA, Eichinger S. Thrombotic thrombocytopenia after ChAdOx1 nCov-19 vaccination. N Engl J Med 2021;384(22):2092–101.
[116] Cines DB, Bussel JB. SARS-CoV-2 vaccine–induced immune thrombotic thrombocytopenia. N Engl J Med 2021:2254–6.
[117] McGonagle D, De Marco G, Bridgewood C. Mechanisms of immunothrombosis in vaccine-induced thrombotic thrombocytopenia (VITT) compared to natural SARS-CoV-2 infection. J Autoimmun 2021;121:102662.
[118] Van Kammen MS, De Sousa DA, Poli S, Cordonnier C, Heldner MR, Van De Munckhof A, et al. Characteristics and outcomes of patients with cerebral venous sinus thrombosis in SARS-CoV-2 vaccine–induced immune thrombotic thrombocytopenia. JAMA Neurol 2021;78(11):1314–23.

[119] Dalakas MC. Guillain-Barré syndrome: the first documented COVID-19–triggered autoimmune neurologic disease: more to come with myositis in the offing. Neurol Neuroimmunol Neuroinflamm 2020;7(5).

[120] Rosenblum HG, Hadler SC, Moulia D, Shimabukuro TT, Su JR, Tepper NK, et al. Use of COVID-19 vaccines after reports of adverse events among adult recipients of Janssen (Johnson & Johnson) and mRNA COVID-19 vaccines (Pfizer-BioNTech and moderna): update from the advisory committee on immunization practices—United States, july 2021. Morb Mortal Wkly Rep 2021;70(32):1094.

[121] Shay DK, Shimabukuro TT, DeStefano F. Myocarditis occurring after immunization with mRNA-based COVID-19 vaccines. JAMA Cardiol 2021;6:1115–7.

[122] Huang C, Huang L, Wang Y, Li X, Ren L, Gu X, et al. 6-month consequences of COVID-19 in patients discharged from hospital: a cohort study. Lancet 2021;397(10270):220–32.

[123] Appel S, Chapman J, Shoenfeld Y. Infection and vaccination in chronic fatigue syndrome: myth or reality? Autoimmunity 2007;40(1):48–53.

[124] Taquet M, Dercon Q, Luciano S, Geddes JR, Husain M, Harrison PJ. Incidence, co-occurrence, and evolution of long-COVID features: a 6-month retrospective cohort study of 273,618 survivors of COVID-19. PLoS Med 2021;18(9):e1003773.

[125] Sudre CH, Murray B, Varsavsky T, Graham MS, Penfold RS, Bowyer RC, et al. Attributes and predictors of long COVID. Nat Med 2021;27(4):626–31.

[126] Bai F, Tomasoni D, Falcinella C, Barbanotti D, Castoldi R, Mulè G, et al. Female gender is associated with long COVID syndrome: a prospective cohort study. Clin Microbiol Infect 2021;28.

[127] Gebhard CE, Suetsch C, Bengs S, Deforth M, Buehler KP, Hamouda NN, et al. Sex-and gender-specific risk factors of post-COVID-19 syndrome: a population-based cohort study in Switzerland. medRxiv 2021. https://doi.org/10.1101/2021.06.30.21259757. published online July 06, 2021 (preprint).

[128] Leynaert B, Sunyer J, Garcia-Esteban R, Svanes C, Jarvis D, Cerveri I, et al. Gender differences in prevalence, diagnosis and incidence of allergic and non-allergic asthma: a population-based cohort. Thorax 2012;67(7):625–31.

[129] Ludvigsson JF. Case report and systematic review suggest that children may experience similar long-term effects to adults after clinical COVID-19. Acta Paediatr 2021;110(3):914–21.

[130] Buonsenso D, Munblit D, De Rose C, Sinatti D, Ricchiuto A, Carfi A, et al. Preliminary evidence on long COVID in children. medRxiv 2021. https://doi.org/10.1101/2021.01.23.21250375.

[131] Ortona E, Buonsenso D, Carfi A, Malorni W. Long COVID: an estrogen-associated autoimmune disease? Cell Death Discov 2021;7(1):1–3.

[132] Hoffman KW, Lee JJ, Foster GA, Krysztof D, Stramer SL, Lim JK. Sex differences in cytokine production following West Nile virus infection: implications for symptom manifestation. Pathog Dis 2019;77(2). ftz016.

[133] Bornstein SR, Voit-Bak K, Donate T, Rodionov RN, Gainetdinov RR, Tselmin S, et al. Chronic post-COVID-19 syndrome and chronic fatigue syndrome: is there a role for extracorporeal apheresis? Mol Psychiatr 2021:1–4.

CHAPTER

29

SARS-CoV-2, fertility-related autoantibodies and reproductive injury

Arad Dotan[1,2], *Darja Kanduc*[3], *Sylviane Muller*[4,5,6] *and Yehuda Shoenfeld*[1,7]

[1]Zabludowicz Center for Autoimmune Diseases, Sheba Medical Center, Ramat Gan, Israel; [2]Sackler Faculty of Medicine, Tel Aviv University, Tel Aviv, Israel; [3]Department of Biosciences, University of Bari, Bari, Italy; [4]Centre National de la Recherche Scientifique-Université de Strasbourg, Unit Biotechnology and Cell Signalling, Team Neuroimmunology and Peptide Therapeutics - Strasbourg Drug Discovery and Development Institute, Strasbourg, France; [5]Fédération Hospitalo-Universitaire OMICARE, Fédération de Médecine Translationnelle de Strasbourg, University of Strasbourg, Strasbourg, France; [6]University of Strasbourg Institute for Advanced Study, Strasbourg, France; [7]Tel Aviv University, Tel Aviv, Israel

Introduction

Since the outbreak of severe acute respiratory syndrome coronavirus 2 (SARS-CoV-2), responsible for the coronavirus disease 2019 (COVID-19) pandemic, millions of mortality cases have been confirmed due to the virus, and hundreds of millions of individuals worldwide have been infected [1]. Although a significant period of time has passed since the World Health Organization declared a global health emergency, the virus is still a primary global health concern. In some patients, SARS-CoV-2 infection may lead to severe lung inflammation with a hypercoagulative state that could escalate to multiorgan failure [2–5]. This severe clinical presentation was the primary concern up until recently. Nevertheless, many chronic manifestations are widely described in COVID-19 recovered patients, weeks after the viral infection confirmation [6]. It is estimated that approximately 80% of infected individuals develop at least one long-term symptom 2 weeks after the primary

Autoimmunity, COVID-19, Post-COVID19 syndrome and COVID-19 vaccination
https://doi.org/10.1016/B978-0-443-18566-3.00024-4

infection by SARS-CoV-2 [6]. Many health experts have raised the concern of fertility dysfunction in both men and women. Fertility preservation is of high clinical and public health importance. Hence, this chapter will examine the possibility that SARS-CoV-2 may contribute to infertility as another long-term postviral manifestation.

SARS-CoV-2 and male fertility

Spermatogenesis is the genesis of spermatozoa that occur in the male reproductive system, specifically in the seminiferous tubules of the testis. There are numerous possible causes of male infertility, including exposure to gonadotoxins, trauma, tumors, obstructive factors, iatrogenic, viral infections, and many more [7]. Viral-induced male infertility has been studied widely and in much detail in the past. Numerous viruses that belong to an extensive range of families have been found in the semen of infected men. Moreover, some of these are known to induce orchitis, resulting in impaired testicular functions and male infertility [8]. Influenza virus, MuV, HIV, Coxsackieviruses, dengue virus, rubella, and echovirus are some of the viruses associated with these pathophysiological effects. Notably, like SARS-CoV-2, all these pathogens are RNA viruses [8].

On postmortem examination of severely ill COVID-19 patients, injury to Sertoli cells and seminiferous tubules with a reduction of Leydig cells had all been identified [9]. In order to evaluate the contribution of the SARS-CoV-2 infection, in contrast to the prolonged severe disease course alone, findings were found to be statistically significant compared to severely ill non-COVID-19 patients who died following a disease course longer than 7 days ($P \leq .001$) [9]. Nevertheless, sperm impairment resulting from the SARS-CoV-2 infection is unclear as unambiguous evidence exists; sperm disorders had been identified following COVID-19, yet might result from the acute disease, which is frequently accompanied by fever, medication, and prolonged sexual abstinence [9,10].

A significant decrease in testosterone, luteinizing hormone (LH), follicle-stimulating hormone (FSH) levels, and testosterone to luteinizing hormone ratio (TLR) were found compared to non-SARS-CoV-2 infected men controls [10]. Additionally, abnormal levels of LH and testosterone had been identified in SARS-CoV-2 infected men (all $P \leq .0001$) [11]. TLR of SARS-CoV-2 infected men was found to be with a negative association with severity ($P \leq .0001$ and $P = .0236$) [10,12]. This evidence may indicate a COVID-19-induced testosterone deficiency. This effect may be due to direct injury of SARS-CoV-2 to the Leydig cells population or an indirect impact of viral-induced orchitis [9]. Nevertheless, it is well established that testosterone levels might decrease in ill men due to hypothalamic–pituitary–testicular axis suppression [13]. Thus, additional investigation is needed in order to evaluate the SARS-CoV-2 effects on gonadotropins levels in the short term, as well as in the long term.

Pathological findings of patients who died of COVID-19 exhibit injury to Sertoli cells and seminiferous tubules with a reduction of Leydig cells. These findings were significant compared to severely ill non-COVID-19 patients who died following a disease course longer than 7 days (P 0.001) [9]. Nevertheless, in the majority of cases, no SARS-CoV-2 particles were identified in electron microscopy nor in a reverse transcription-polymerase chain reaction (RT-PCR) [9], which might suggest an immune-mediated injury rather than a direct viral injury. Similarly, the absence of the virus was confirmed in many studies that investigated semen of SARS-CoV-2 infected patients. However, impairment of sperm quality may exist in

COVID-19-ill patients, depending on the severity of the illness. Significant impairment of sperm quality was found in patients with a moderate disease compared to mild disease [14]. Furthermore, another study found that 11 out of 43 (25.5%) of patients who recovered from COVID-19 infection Oligo-teratozoospermia (OTA syndrome) was detected, which represents a significantly high portion as compared to its rate in the general population (1%–3%) [10].

SARS-CoV-2 and female fertility

According to the currently available literature, there is very little evidence of long-term effects of SARS-CoV-2 infection on female fertility. Compared to COVID-19 mediated injury to male reproductive organs and male hormonal dysfunctions, sufficient female reproductive dysfunction was not shown in high-quality research. Nevertheless, multiple suspected mechanisms might contribute to female infertility (which will be described broadly in the text).

Mechanisms in which SARS-COV-2 may lead to infertility

SARS-CoV-2 may lead to infertility for several reasons: [1] strong affinity of SARS-CoV-2 for the human ACE2 receptor, [2] SARS-CoV-2 induced sex steroid hormonal abnormalities [3] increased levels of oxidative stress in COVID-19, [4] molecular mimicry between humans and components of SARS-CoV-2 leading to antigenic cross-reactivity phenomena and [5] viral-induces production of autoantibodies which are associate with infertility.

ACE2 as a port of entry of SARS-CoV-2 into cells

Angiotensin-converting enzyme II (ACE2), one of the receptors of SARS-CoV-2, is a critical enzyme in the renin–angiotensin–aldosterone system, which acts as a cellular entry portal for the virus. Systematic studies based on three independent RNA expression data banks (Human Protein Atlas, FAMTOM5, and GETx) have identified ACE2 in numerous tissues in the human body, including the small intestine, kidneys, ovaries, uterus, vagina and placenta, lungs, heart, thyroid, adipose tissue, and especially in testis [15,16]. It has therefore been postulated that SARS-CoV-2 may cause direct injury in such tissues, including reproductive organs in both genders, through cell entry via ACE2 [17–19].

Single-cell RNA sequencing analysis illustrates that ACE2 is highly expressed in seminiferous tubule cells, spermatogonia, adult Leydig, and Sertoli cells of the human testis, in a much more significant amount than most ACE2-expressing tissues [10]. Immunostaining indicates that ACE2 is diffusely expressed in Sertoli and strongly expressed in Leydig cells [9]. Thus, it was hypothesized that the testis might be a target of SARS-CoV-2, resulting in a direct injury to this cell population and a possible spermatogenic failure. Furthermore, it was shown that ACE2 expression in the testis is age-dependent, higher in 30 years old individuals than men aged 60 years [21]. Thus, younger SARS-CoV-2 infected patients might be more likely to experience COVID-19 induced orchitis and spermatogenesis disruption.

ACE2 has a critical contribution to the regulation of follicular development and ovulation, modulates luteal angiogenesis and degeneration, and affects the regular changes of endometrial tissue and embryo development [17]. Yet it is still unclear whether SARS-CoV-2 has a significant effect on female fertility.

Sex steroid hormonal abnormalities of SARS-CoV-2 infected patients

An additional clinical feature that deserves attention when interpreting the potential association between male fertility and COVID-19 is sex steroid hormone abnormalities in SARS-CoV-2 infected men. LH is a hormone produced by gonadotropic cells in the anterior pituitary gland and stimulates testosterone secretion by Leydig cells in the testis. Sertoli cells are a primary cellular target of testosterone, and their proper function is necessary for the maturation, survival of germ cells, and normal spermiogenesis. A large study that conducted measurements of circulating sex steroid levels in 286 COVID-19-ill men at hospital admission found significantly lower levels of LH and testosterone in patients with COVID-19 compared to 281 healthy men (all $P \leq .0001$) [11]. Likewise, the results were still significant after accounting for age, body mass index, Charlson Comorbidity Index, and IL-6 values ($P \leq .0001$). Testosterone levels suggest that 243 (85%) of the COVID-19-ill men had secondary hypogonadism (defined as testosterone ≤9. 2 mmol/L) with a higher risk of intensive care unit admission and death (all $P \leq .05$) [11].

On the contrary, testosterone levels might decrease in ill men following the suppression of the hypothalamic–pituitary–testicular axis [13]. Nonetheless, two different studies found a decrease in the *ratio* of testosterone to LH in SARS-CoV-2 infected men with a negative association with the severity ($P = .0236$) [12,22]. Hence, hormonal abnormalities are not likely to occur merely due to the hypothalamic-pituitary-testicular axis suppression as pathological findings show significant damage to Leydig cells (responsible for testosterone secretion). This alternative mechanism also contributes to hypogonadism and the disruption of spermatogenesis.

Oxidative stress induced by SARS-CoV-2

The body produces free radicals during normal metabolic processes, for example, inhaling and exhaling. Oxidative stress is a state that occurs when, however, there is an excess of free radicals in cells; it refers to the accumulation of oxygen reactive species (ROS) as a consequence of an imbalance between pro-oxidants and antioxidants. It is well established that oxidative stress is linked to sperm damage and male infertility, even though a certain amount of ROS is necessary for normal spermatogenesis and oocyte fertilization [23]. There are numerous sources of oxidative stress, including tobacco usage, alcohol, obesity/poor nutrition, metabolic syndrome, overexercise, cold, toxins, and infections, most of which are associated with inflammation [23]. Hence, it is not surprising that oxidative stress exists in COVID-19-ill patients due to the hyper-stimulation of the immune system and increased levels of circulating neutrophil extracellular traps (NETs) induced by the SARS-CoV-2 [24–26]. A recent study including a cohort of 32 hospitalized patients with a confirmed diagnosis of COVID-19 and healthy controls showed that the concentration of NETs that are potent triggers of autoimmunity was augmented in plasma, tracheal aspirate, and lung autopsies tissues from COVID-19 patients, and their neutrophils released higher levels of NETs [27]. Recurrent evidence has accumulated that most reaction cascades leading to NET release involve ROS. It is also documented that a close link exists between NETosis, autophagy processes, inflammasome engagement, and pyroptosis in SARS-CoV-2 patients [28,29]. It should also be mentioned here that for many individuals, the COVID-19 pandemic causes extensive psychological stress, which is an additional major cause of systemic oxidative stress production [30]. Oxidative stress can immensely harm semen quality, disrupt sperm functions, and morphology by damaging sperm DNA and inducing apoptotic pathways of spermatozoa, these effects of oxidative stress may contribute significantly to male infertility [30].

Molecular mimicry between SARS-CoV-2 and humans

Much the same as other viruses, SARS-CoV-2 may cross the blood–testis barrier, triggering a secondary autoimmune response in the testis tissue [20]. Conversely, large quantities of inflammatory cells were not found within the seminiferous tubules, nor does evidence of SARS-CoV-2 particles in most pathological investigations [9]. The absents of many inflammatory cells make the impression that the mechanism causing testis damage in SARS-CoV-2 infected patients is not through a cell-mediated immune response nor a direct injury by the virus. Possible alternatives might involve autoantibodies and the complement system that possess the capacity to contribute to testis injury and spermatogenesis disruption. It has been shown that homology of a primary sequence exists between humans and components of SARS-CoV-2 [24,31]. The mechanism in molecular mimicry disrupts the physiological function of the immune system by identifying amino acid sequence similarities between the pathogens and the human host, which may lead to autoimmune pathologies through cross-reactivity phenomena occurring after pathogen infection. Molecular mimicry is a common mechanism of autoantibodies development that may play a significant part in the pathophysiology of a secondary autoimmune reaction to pathogens and the new onset of autoimmune diseases (AIDs) [24,32]. A SARS-CoV-2 infection was previously shown to be associated with many autoantibodies and AIDs, more commonly in severely ill COVID-19 patients [3,24,33]. Our group found 41 pentapeptides of the SARS-CoV-2 spike glycoprotein, with 27 human proteins related to oogenesis, uterine receptivity, decidualization, and placentation. All the shared pentapeptides that we identified, with the exception of four, are also present in SARS-CoV-2 spike glycoprotein–derived epitopes that have been experimentally validated as immunoreactive. Our findings effectively documented the possibility that COVID-19 might lead to an immune reaction toward numerous female fertility-linked proteins and disrupt physiological reproductive functions.

It should be emphasized that our findings do not indicate female reproductive dysfunction in COVID-19 patients. Nevertheless, there is a potential cross-reactivity between the homologous peptides that could lead to the development of autoantibodies and new-onset of autoimmune-mediated manifestations.

Autoantibodies associated with infertility

Infertility resulting from the effect of autoantibodies has been extensively debated [34–36]. Specific autoantibodies such as lupus anticoagulant, anticardiolipin, anti-beta-2-glycoprotein, antithyroid peroxidase (anti-TPO), antinuclear, antiannexin V, antiprothrombin, antilaminin, antifollicle stimulating hormone autoantibodies have been associated with infertility, primarily due to premature ovarian insufficiency, in addition to pregnancy loss [35,36].

Notably, various autoantibodies are present in COVID-19 patients, including some associated with infertility, such as anticardiolipin, antinuclear, antiannexin V, and anti-TPO [24]. Development of various autoantibodies seems to acquire in acute COVID-19, yet some of the autoimmune manifestations presented by patients were developed weeks or months after the recovery from COVID-19 [24,37]. For instance, among 159 acute COVID-19 patients, antithyroid peroxidase (anti-TPO) and antithyroglobulin were present in 20% and 11%, respectively. The follow-up (after approximately 3 months) was done for 127 patients and found 7 (5.5%) who were initially negative for anti-TPO were found positive; intriguingly, only one patient initially positive for anti-TPO was found negative in the follow-up [37]. The same group also found 20.1% (41/204) with "long COVID-19," defined as the presence or persistence of symptoms upon follow-up (after approximately 3 months) [37]. These results are worrisome because they may indicate the development of autoimmunity in COVID-19 patients in the long term.

Since the SARS-CoV-2 has infected an enormous and unmeasurable number of individuals worldwide, it is hard to estimate the long test effects on global health in terms of autoimmunity. It is essential to note that the development of autoantibodies could act as the preclinical stage of autoimmune diseases. It is of great importance to recognize those autoimmune manifestations of COVID-19 in order to properly cope with their outcomes in the ongoing pandemic and the long-term postpandemic period.

References

[1] Coronavirus disease (COVID-19) – World Health Organization. Available from: https://www.who.int/emergencies/diseases/novel-coronavirus-2019.

[2] Cavalli E, Bramanti A, Ciurleo R, Tchorbanov AI, Giordano A, Fagone P, et al. Entangling COVID-19 associated thrombosis into a secondary antiphospholipid antibody syndrome: diagnostic and therapeutic perspectives (Review). Int J Mol Med September 1, 2020;46(3):903–12.

[3] Ehrenfeld M, Tincani A, Andreoli L, Cattalini M, Greenbaum A, Kanduc D, et al. Covid-19 and autoimmunity. Autoimmun Rev August 1, 2020;19(8):102597.

[4] Ryabkova VA, Churilov LP, Shoenfeld Y. Influenza infection, SARS, MERS and COVID-19: cytokine storm—the common denominator and the lessons to be learned. Clin Immunol Orlando Fla February 2021;223:108652.

[5] Shoenfeld Y. Corona (COVID-19) time musings: our involvement in COVID-19 pathogenesis, diagnosis, treatment and vaccine planning. Autoimmun Rev June 2020;19(6):102538.

[6] Lopez-Leon S, Wegman-Ostrosky T, Perelman C, Sepulveda R, Rebolledo PA, Cuapio A, et al. More than 50 long-term effects of COVID-19: a systematic review and meta-analysis. Sci Rep August 9, 2021;11(1):16144.

[7] Raheem AA, Ralph D. Male infertility: causes and investigations. Trends Urol Mens Health 2011;2(5):8–11.

[8] Liu W, Han R, Wu H, Han D. Viral threat to male fertility. Andrologia 2018;50(11). e13140.

[9] Yang M, Chen S, Huang B, Zhong J-M, Su H, Chen Y-J, et al. Pathological findings in the testes of COVID-19 patients: clinical implications. Eur Urol Focus September 15, 2020;6(5):1124–9.

[10] Cinislioglu AE, Cinislioglu N, Demirdogen SO, Sam E, Akkas F, Altay MS, Utlu M, Sen IA, Yildirim F, Kartal S, Aydin HR. The relationship of serum testosterone levels with the clinical course and prognosis of COVID-19 disease in male patients: a prospective study. Andrology January 2022;10(1):24–33.

[11] Salonia A, Pontillo M, Capogrosso P, Gregori S, Tassara M, Boeri L, et al. Severely low testosterone in males with COVID-19: a case-control study. Andrology March 9, 2021;9:1043–52.

[12] Ma L, Xie W, Li D, Shi L, Ye G, Mao Y, et al. Evaluation of sex-related hormones and semen characteristics in reproductive-aged male COVID-19 patients. J Med Virol 2021;93(1):456–62.

[13] Turner HE, Wass JAH. Gonadal function in men with chronic illness. Clin Endocrinol 1997;47(4):379–403.

[14] Holtmann N, Edimiris P, Andree M, Doehmen C, Baston-Buest D, Adams O, et al. Assessment of SARS-CoV-2 in human semen—a cohort study. Fertil Steril August 2020;114(2):233–8.

[15] Shastri A, Wheat J, Agrawal S, Chaterjee N, Pradhan K, Goldfinger M, et al. Delayed clearance of SARS-CoV2 in male compared to female patients: high ACE2 expression in testes suggests possible existence of gender-specific viral reservoirs. medRxiv April 2020;17. 2020.04.16.20060566.
[16] Hikmet F, Méar L, Edvinsson Å, Micke P, Uhlén M, Lindskog C. The protein expression profile of ACE2 in human tissues. Mol Syst Biol July 1, 2020;16(7):e9610.
[17] Shao M, Li X, Liu F, Tian T, Luo J, Yang Y. Acute kidney injury is associated with severe infection and fatality in patients with COVID-19: a systematic review and meta-analysis of 40 studies and 24,527 patients. Pharmacol Res November 1, 2020;161:105107.
[18] Peters AE, Mihalas BP, Bromfield EG, Roman SD, Nixon B, Sutherland JM. Autophagy in female fertility: a role in oxidative stress and aging. Antioxidants Redox Signal March 10, 2020;32(8):550–68.
[19] Dotan A, Kanduc D, Muller S, Makatsariya A, Shoenfeld Y. Molecular mimicry between SARS-CoV-2 and the female reproductive system. Am J Reprod Immunol 2021;86:e13494.
[20] He W, Liu X, Feng L, Xiong S, Li Y, Chen L, et al. Impact of SARS-CoV-2 on male reproductive health: a review of the literature on male reproductive involvement in COVID-19. Front Med November 19, 2020;7. 594364.
[21] Shen Q, Xiao X, Aierken A, Yue W, Wu X, Liao M, Hua J. The ACE2 expression in Sertoli cells and germ cells may cause male reproductive disorder after SARS-CoV-2 infection. J Cell Mol Med August 2020;24(16):9472–7.
[22] Ma L, Xie W, Li D, Shi L, Mao Y, Xiong Y, et al. Effect of SARS-CoV-2 infection upon male gonadal function: a single center-based study. medRxiv January 1, 2020. https://doi.org/10.1101/2020.03.21.20037267.
[23] Agarwal A, Rana M, Qiu E, AlBunni H, Bui AD, Henkel R. Role of oxidative stress, infection and inflammation in male infertility. Andrologia December 2018;50(11). e13126.
[24] Dotan A, Muller S, Kanduc D, David P, Halpert G, Shoenfeld Y. The SARS-CoV-2 as an instrumental trigger of autoimmunity. Autoimmun Rev April 1, 2021;20(4):102792.
[25] Laforge M, Elbim C, Frère C, Hémadi M, Massaad C, Nuss P, et al. Tissue damage from neutrophil-induced oxidative stress in COVID-19. Nat Rev Immunol September 2020;20(9):515–6.
[26] Narasaraju T, Tang BM, Herrmann M, Muller S, Chow VTK, Radic M. Neutrophilia and NETopathy as key pathologic drivers of progressive lung impairment in patients with COVID-19. Front Pharmacol 2020;11:870.
[27] Veras FP, Pontelli MC, Silva CM, Toller-Kawahisa JE, de Lima M, Nascimento DC, Schneider AH, Caetité D, Tavares LA, Paiva IM, Rosales R. SARS-CoV-2–triggered neutrophil extracellular traps mediate COVID-19 pathology. J Exp Med December 7, 2020;(12):217.
[28] Bonam SR, Muller S, Bayry J, Klionsky DJ. Autophagy as an emerging target for COVID-19: lessons from an old friend, chloroquine. Autophagy December 1, 2020;16(12):2260–6.
[29] Ferreira AC, Soares VC, de Azevedo-Quintanilha IG, Dias S da SG, Fintelman-Rodrigues N, Sacramento CQ, et al. SARS-CoV-2 engages inflammasome and pyroptosis in human primary monocytes. Cell Death Dis March 1, 2021;7(1):43.
[30] Dutta S, Sengupta P. SARS-CoV-2 and male infertility: possible multifaceted pathology. Reprod Sci January 1, 2021;28(1):23–6.
[31] Kanduc D, Shoenfeld Y. Molecular mimicry between SARS-CoV-2 spike glycoprotein and mammalian proteomes: implications for the vaccine. Immunol Res October 2020;68(5):310–3.
[32] Oldstone MB. Molecular mimicry and immune-mediated diseases. FASEB J Off Publ Fed Am Soc Exp Biol October 1998;12(13):1255–65.
[33] Halpert G, Shoenfeld Y. SARS-CoV-2, the autoimmune virus. Autoimmun Rev December 2020;19(12):102695.
[34] Carp HJ, Selmi C, Shoenfeld Y. The autoimmune bases of infertility and pregnancy loss. J Autoimmun May 1, 2012;38(2–3):J266–74.
[35] Deroux A, Dumestre-Perard C, Dunand-Faure C, Bouillet L, Hoffmann P. Female infertility and serum autoantibodies: a systematic review. Clin Rev Allergy Immunol August 1, 2017;53(1):78–86.
[36] Van Voorhis BJ, Stovall DW. Autoantibodies and infertility: a review of the literature. J Reprod Immunol July 1, 1997;33(3):239–56.
[37] Lui DTW, Lee CH, Chow WS, Lee ACH, Tam AR, Pang P, et al. Long COVID in patients with mild to moderate disease: do thyroid function and autoimmunity play a role? Endocr Pract September 1, 2021;27(9):894–902.

Further reading

Ace2 gene (protein coding). Available: https://www.genecards.org/cgi-bin/carddisp.pl?gene=ACE2&keywords=ACE2#protein_expression.

CHAPTER

30

Maternal and fetal issues in COVID-19-mediated thromboinflammation

Victoria Bitsadze[1], *Jamilya Khizroeva*[1], *Alexander Makatsariya*[1,2], *Ismail Elalamy*[1,3] and *Jean-Christophe Gris*[1,4]

[1]Department of Obstetrics and Gynecology, Institute of Children's Health, I.M. Sechenov First Moscow State Medical University (Sechenov University), Moscow, Russia; [2]Russian Academy of Sciences, Moscow, Russia; [3]Medicine Sorbonne University, Hematology Department of Thrombosis Center, Tenon University Hospital, Paris, France; [4]Hematology Department, University of Montpellier, Nimes, France

Introduction

A new virus called SARS-CoV-2 has literally turned the world upside down and became a spectacular example of devastating alliance of cytokine storm, thromboinflammation, and immunothrombosis (Fig. 30.1). At the same time, COVID-19 has become an excellent model for studying these important biological processes. Within a few months after the start of the pandemic, it became clear that the hemostasis disorders due to hyperinflammation play the role of the first violin in orchestrating the severe course and adverse outcomes of the disease. In critically ill COVID-19 patients, hemostatic disorders are presented in 100% of cases and their severity has a prognostic value.

Endothelial dysfunction and immunothrombosis are currently considered as the key mechanisms in COVID-19 [1].

The term immunothrombosis was first proposed by Bernd Engelmann and Steffen Massberg in 2012 to denote the pathogens- and damaged cells-induced internal effector pathway of innate immunity. In immunothrombosis, activated neutrophils and monocytes release tissue factor and extracellular nucleosomes and destroy endogenous anticoagulants, thereby contributing to the activation of coagulation caused by inflammation (hence the concept of thromboinflammation) [2].

Autoimmunity, COVID-19, Post-COVID19 syndrome and COVID-19 vaccination
https://doi.org/10.1016/B978-0-443-18566-3.00039-6

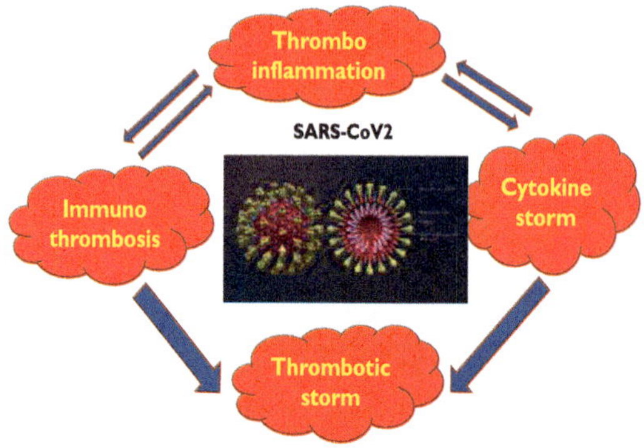

FIGURE 30.1 COVID-19—the model of devastating alliance of inflammation and coagulation.

Possible etiopathogenetic mechanisms of thromboinflammation in COVID-19

From an evolutionary point of view, immunothrombosis can be considered as a favorable mechanism of intravascular immunity. However, when immunothrombosis is not controlled, it causes unregulated activation of the blood clotting cascade, leading to the formation of microthrombosis and uncontrolled inflammation, which eventually develop into thrombosis, disseminated intravascular coagulation (DIC), and systemic inflammatory response syndrome (SIRS)—SIRS-shock.

The mechanisms of hemostasis disorders in severe COVID-19 are diverse, and there is often simultaneous activation of many pathways, including activation of platelets, external and internal pathways of coagulation cascade, suppression of fibrinolysis, etc. with the development of DIC, thrombotic microangiopathy (TMA), and even local intravascular coagulation in the lungs (Fig. 30.2). Clinical manifestations include acute respiratory distress-syndrome, venous and arterial thrombosis, also with atypical localization and multiple organ failure which may resemble a picture of catastrophic antiphospholipid syndrome (CAPS) or heparin-induced thrombocytopenia due to systemic widespread thrombosis, which, by analogy with a cytokine storm, was called thrombotic storm. Thrombotic storm is a phenomenon that, by analogy with CAPS, is characterized by multiple thrombosis developing over a short period of time, but without the circulation of high levels of antiphospholipid antibodies (APLA).

The cause of microcirculatory disorders resulting from cytokine and thrombotic storms is often TMA, which combines heterogeneous clinical conditions characterized by arteriolar and capillary thromboses with the development of hemolytic anemia thrombocytopenia, and ischemic damage.

A typical clinical manifestation of TMA is a multiple organ dysfunction. In some cases, atypical manifestations are observed, such as malignant arterial hypertension, neurological disorders, and HELLP syndrome during pregnancy.

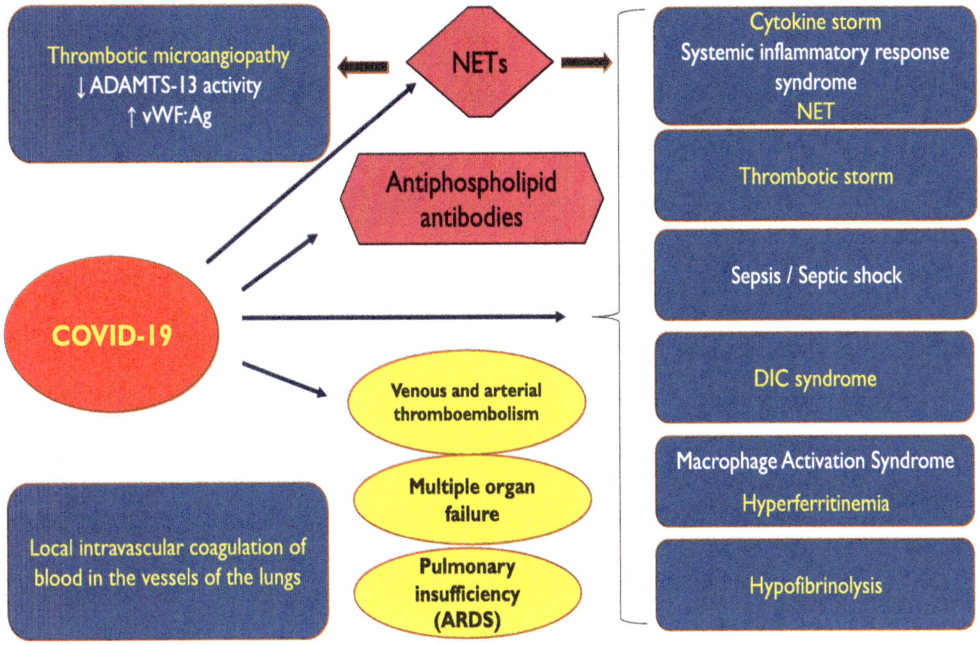

FIGURE 30.2 Multidimensional mechanisms of hemostasis disorders in severe COVID-19.

The origin of TMA may be different, but one of the most important causes is the deficiency of ADAMTS-13 (a Distntegrin and Metalloproteinase with a Thrombospondin Type 1 motif, member 13)—a zinc-containing metallo-protease that cleaves von Willebrand factor (vWF), a large protein involved in blood clotting. ADAMTS-13 degrades large vWF multimers and decreases their activity. Von Willebrand factor multimers have a high ability to activate platelets. Under conditions of SARS-CoV-2-mediated endothelial damage, ADAMTS-13 is consumed by excessive amounts of high-molecular-weight von Willebrand factor. Accumulation of an ultra-high-molecular-weight multimers in combination with adherent and aggregated platelets causes microcirculation thrombosis with the development of organ failure.

There are limited data of the role of TMA and ADAMTS-13 deficiency in severe and critically ill COVID-19 patients, but it's known that hyperinflammation is a principal cause of endothelial damage and hypercoagulation via neutrophil extracellular traps (NETs) formation. **NETs**—extracellular structures like networks of chromatin filaments lined with highly active proteases and proteins of nuclear, cytosolic, and granular origin. NETs are able to induce endothelial activation leading to excessive expression of ultra-high-molecular-weight multimers von Willebrand Factor and ADAMTS-13 depletion due the cleavage of large amount vWF. This leads to ADAMTS-13 consumption and as a result of TMA. The worst clinical picture and outcome are associated with severe ADAMTS-13 deficiency.

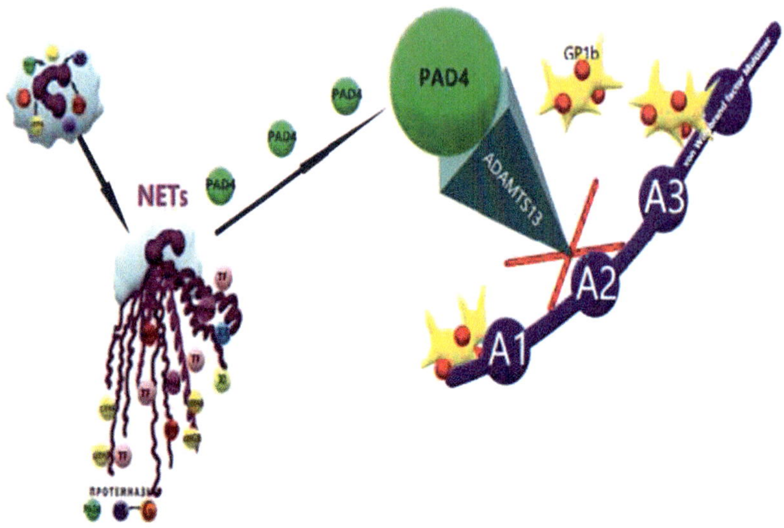

FIGURE 30.3 NETs effects on ADAMTS-13.

A direct suppression of the natural anticoagulant properties of ADAMTS-13 by neutrophil traps—NETs can also be the cause of TMA in conditions of a systemic inflammatory response and netosis (Fig. 30.3).

NETs—neutrophil extracellular traps.
PAD4—peptidyl arginine deiminase.
MPO—myeloperoxidase.
DNA—deoxyribonucleic acid.
CitH—citrullinated histone.
TF—tissue factor.
CE, UL—coagulation factors.
NE—neutrophil.
ADAMTS-13—(*a disintegrin and metalloproteinase with a thrombospondin type 1 motif, member 13*).

Neutrophils play a crucial role in the immediate response to infection using phagocytosis, release of granular contents and reactive oxygen species (ROS), and synthesis and release of NETs to kill pathogens [3]. NETs are a unique tool of innate immunity formed by the extrusion of nuclear DNA into the extracellular environment, where they capture a wide range of microorganisms, from bacteria and fungi to parasites [4]. Pathological formation of NETs—NETosis—can cause damage or cell death of neighboring tissues. It occurs in rheumatoid arthritis (RA), SLE, vasculitis, etc. [4]. The main signaling pathway initiating NETosis includes calcium mobilization, generation of ROS by NAPDH oxidase, cytoplasmic-to-nucleus transfer of neutrophil elastase (NE), myeloperoxidase (MPO), peptidyl arginine deiminase 4 (PAD4), and histone citrullination [5]. These events contribute to chromatin unfolding, a prerequisite for efficient DNA extrusion.

Massive activation of neutrophils during a cytokine storm with the release of many NETs and uncontrolled thrombo-inflammation processes underlie the development of endothelial damage in COVID-19.

Neutrophils are attracted to the site of inflammation in several stages: activation, adhesion, and extravasation. All this happens with the participation of selectins chemokines, including P-selectin, P-selectin glycoprotein ligand-1 (P-selectin glycoprotein ligand 1, PSGL-1). P-selectin is expressed on the surface of activated endothelial cells and platelets. Integrin αLβ2 and intercellular adhesion molecule 1 (intercellular adhesion molecule 1, ICAM-1) are also involved in neutrophil adhesion [6]. Intracellular material is released during the activation of neutrophils. Previously, NETosis was thought to be a terminal event for neutrophils; however, it has been shown that some neutrophils survive in this process, becoming nonnuclear and continue to have a damaging effect on tissues. NETosis is not a single process but a multitude of processes resulting in the expulsion of the contents of the nucleus [7]. Suicidal, vital, and mitochondrial types of netosis have already been described in the literature [8].

NETs overproduced in COVID-19 promote alveolitis endothelial damage and trigger intravascular coagulation [9]. Excessive activation of neutrophils with the production of extracellular traps of neutrophils contributes to acute damage to lung tissue, microthrombosis, hemorrhages, and pulmonary insufficiency. Histones are the protein components of NETs and have a cytotoxic effect. The chromatin networks in NET disrupt the alveolar-capillary barrier, leading to endothelial injury, vessel disruption, and hemorrhage [10]. Hyperproduction or an impaired utilization of NETs leads to pathological microclotting in sepsis [11]. Under the influence of endogenous and exogenous DNases, NETs are degraded, and histones are massively released from DNA binding, manifested by thrombosis [12]. Studies have shown that both arterial and venous thrombi contain neutrophils and NETs [13]; NETs are always present in thrombi, especially at the organization stage.

NETs activate the procoagulant link in various ways, disrupting fibrinolysis and anticoagulants' functioning [11]. DNA NETs triggers the coagulation cascade through an intrinsic pathway, as negatively charged surfaces increase the activation of factor XII (FXII), the initiator of this pathway [14]. NETs DNA acts as a cofactor for thrombin-dependent activation of factor XI [15] and contributes to the success of extrinsic pathway reactions associated with tissue factor [16]. The endothelium's activation and even its death [17], caused by the cytotoxic effect of histones, H2O2 is released, which further stimulates NETosis [7]. Weibel-Palade bodies located in the endothelium undergo exocytosis together with von Willebrand factor, which supports thrombosis by binding to platelets. Histones activate platelets via toll-like receptors TLR2 and TLR4 [18] and enhance thrombin-dependent platelet activation [19]. Histone H4, binding to prothrombin, promotes its autoactivation [20]. Histones disrupt the antithrombin-dependent inactivation of thrombin [21] and prevent thrombin-thrombomodulin interaction [22]. NETs histones trigger pathways to inactivate activated protein C (APC), an anticoagulant that can inhibit NETosis via PAR receptors on neutrophils [23]. Namely, both neutrophil oxidase and elastase can inactivate APC. Histones are able not only to activate hemostasis but also to increase the stability of the thrombus. They enhance structural changes in fibrin, making it more resistant to fibrinolysis. By activating plasminogen in solution, histones inhibit plasmin, acting as competitive substrates. Protection of fibrin from the action of plasminogen is also enhanced by covalent binding of histones to fibrin, catalyzed by activated transglutaminase, coagulation factor XIIIa. Using noncovalent interactions, histone-associated lateral aggregation of fibrin protofibrils occurs, leading to thickening of fibrin filaments, which, as a result, leads to difficulty in fibrinolysis processes. Plasmin is a serine protease with broad specificity that binds to arginine and lysine, making histones a candidate target for plasmin. Histones compete with fibrin for plasmin-binding sites interfere with plasmin activity and fibrinolysis triggered by tPA. DNA increases the formation of complexes of tissue plasminogen activator with an inhibitor of plasminogen activator-1 [24], reduces the intensity of plasmin synthesis from plasminogen under the action of tPA on the thrombus surface [21], binds proteins responsible for fibrin degradation, and reduces their release by fibrin clots [25], and also penetrates fibrin strands and blocks plasmin-mediated thrombus lysis.

As stated above, NETs lead to a decrease in ADAMTS13 activity. Both extracellular DNA and histone NETs can bind to vWF, leading to even greater recruitment of new neutrophils to the lesion, enhancing the pro-inflammatory effect. Plasma glycoprotein von Willebrand factor (vWF) typically ensures the delivery of platelets to the sites of damage to the vascular wall and promotes their subsequent activation and aggregation [26]. Extra-large vWF multimers (UL-vWF) released from endothelial cells can spontaneously activate circulating platelets and other blood cells, promoting thrombosis [27]. ADAMTS13 metalloproteinase specifically cleaves the multimer at Tyr1605-Met1606 regions in the A2 domain, thereby regulating the size and activity of vWF multimers and preventing thrombus formation [28].

A few publications are currently available in the world literature regarding the role of ADAMTS-13 and vWF in COVID-19 with a limited number of study patients. The results of our study in 140 intensive care unit (ICU) patients with severe COVID-19 indicate a significant correlation between ADAMTS-13 activity and adverse outcomes.

As for pregnant women, even in normal pregnancy, the activity of ADAMTS-13 is also decreased, especially in the third trimester [29,30].

Moreover, there is a so-called physiological hypercoagulation, a decrease in blood flow rate, an increase in systemic inflammation in the third trimester (it should be noted that a normal pregnancy is a model of a compensated systemic inflammatory response). It may be one of the reasons why the risk of severe illness remains more common in later pregnancy.

Circulating granulocyte colony-stimulating factor, which arises during pregnancy, promotes the formation of extracellular traps (NETs) of neutrophils. In early pregnancy, NETosis is enhanced by human chorionic gonadotropin (hCG) and then by estrogen. A complex interaction occurs between estrogen and progesterone, in which progesterone inhibits the activity of NETosis.

Much knowledge has been accumulated about the role of T-lymphocytes, regulatory T-cells, or natural killer cells in immunological tolerance during pregnancy. However, the role of the innate immune response and, in particular, the involvement of neutrophils is not completely clear. Several factors indicate that neutrophil activity is associated with severe pregnancy complications such as preeclampsia (PE), recurrent fetal loss, or poor pregnancy outcome due to autoimmune conditions [31]. The same neutrophil activity contributes to an increase in the concentration of NETs in the placenta in PE [32].

Neutrophils in healthy pregnant women show a characteristic pro-NETotic phenotype that increases with gestational age. Not only has granulocyte colony-stimulating factor (G-CSF) been shown to increase neutrophil count during pregnancy, but it also progressively increases NETosis [33]. Studies have shown that plasma nucleosome and extracellular DNA concentrations increase during pregnancy. If a pregnant woman has placenta-associated complications, such as PE, fetal growth restriction (FGR), stillbirth, placental abruption, and preterm birth, their concentration is higher than usual, especially with PE. Other nonhistone nuclear proteins, such as high-mobility group protein B1 (HMGB1), may also be secreted by activated immune cells or released passively from damaged or dying cells, playing an essential role in acute and chronic inflammatory processes. In addition, HMGB1 is released from hypoxic trophoblast, predetermining hemostasis disorders in PE [34]. In early pregnancy, NETosis is enhanced by the action of hCG, while the steroid sex hormones estradiol (E2) and progesterone (P4) complexly modulate the activity of neutrophils. While E2 promotes NET formation, P4 acts as an antagonist to inhibit the progression of NETosis. The regulatory mechanism of progesterone's influence includes preventing the transfer of NE from the cytoplasm to the nucleus [35].

As already mentioned, human pregnancy is associated with a pro-inflammatory status characterized by increased neutrophil activation, which is most pronounced in PE [36]. The involvement of activated neutrophils in the etiology of PE was confirmed by detecting a large number of NETs in the intervillous space of the affected placenta [32]. In addition, data in animal models have shown that tissue-resident pro-angiogenic decidual neutrophils [37] and activation of circulatory neutrophils via the complement cascade may contribute to the development of PE-like conditions or conditions associated with fetal loss [38]. The latter is supported by recent reports that APLA, which are frequently found in cases of recurrent fetal loss, cause NETosis [31].

In early pregnancy, increased NETosis is mainly due to the influence of hCG. Interestingly, in vitro hCG administration results in a significant increase in peptidyl arginine deiminase, type IV (PAD4) expression without a significant increase in citH3 levels. As pregnancy progresses, the interaction between granulocyte colony-stimulating factor (G-CSF) and steroid sex hormones modulates pro-NETotic activity. In this regard, elevated G-CSF concentrations during pregnancy increase the pool of circulatory neutrophils and stimulation of the pro-NETotic phenotype through increased expression of PAD4 concomitant H3 histone citrullination, essential steps in the NETosis signaling cascade [39].

Using data on maternal and fetal extracellular DNA levels in PE, preliminary conclusions can be drawn regarding the time point of NET induction [31]. In this context, it is suggested that the increase in fetal extracellular DNA is the result of placental damage, while the increase in maternal extracellular DNA may be the result of the generation of NETs [40]. Several studies have shown that elevated fetal extracellular DNA occurs early in pregnancy before symptoms of PE appear [41,42].

On the contrary, the concentration of extracellular maternal DNA is increased only after the onset of symptoms [42]. These data suggest two phases of PE; a preclinical phase associated with placental involvement; and a second clinical phase with symptoms including a maternal systemic inflammatory response [43]. The etiopathogenesis of such a multifactorial syndrome as PE is based on various mechanisms [44,45], which include an imbalance of angiogenic factors produced by the placenta [46] and dysregulation of pro-inflammatory cytokines [47], etc.

The mother's immune system is transformed during pregnancy, adapting to the semi-allogeneic fetus. During pregnancy, there is a regular shift in the CD4+ T-cell population toward T-helper-2 (Th)-2 phenotypes rather than Th1 phenotypes, which enhances the humoral immune response compared to the cellular one [48]. In addition, there is a balance between regulatory T cells (Treg) and Th17 cells with a shift toward Treg to ensure immune tolerance [49].

Changes in the immune system during pregnancy are also associated with Toll-like receptors (TLRs), particularly TLR4 [50]. There are three different levels of TLR4 activation during pregnancy. First, TLR4 activation and the inflammatory response increase during the first trimester, promoting blastocyst implantation. In TLR4 activation in the second trimester, a decrease follows to activate the antiinflammatory response to fetal growth. Eventually, TLR4 activation and the inflammatory response increase again in the third trimester to support delivery [51]. COVID-19 leads to host cell pyroptosis and release of damage-associated molecular fragments (DAMPs), which can act as ligands for TLR molecules and induce a more robust inflammatory response.

In patients with COVID-19, especially severe cases are associated with profound immune dysregulation [52]. Some studies have revealed leukocytosis, lymphopenia, and an increase in the ratio of neutrophils to lymphocytes [53]. Using immunophenotyping, natural killers' (NK) number and functional activity have been shown CD3+, CD4+, and CD8+ T cells are reduced in severe COVID-19 [54]. NK cells play a crucial role in the innate immune response and are significant sources of pro-inflammatory cytokines, granulocyte-macrophage colony-stimulating factor (GM-CSF), and interferon-gamma (IFN-γ) [55]. Compared with patients with moderate COVID-19, those with severe COVID-19 have reduced cytotoxic T-lymphocyte (CTL) counts [56]. Studies have shown that this decrease is the result of T-cell hyperactivation and/or activation of pro-apoptotic factors, including the first apoptosis signaling receptor (FAS), tumor necrosis factor (TNF)-dependent apoptosis-inducing ligand (TRAIL), and caspase 3 [57].

In severe COVID-19, monocyte/macrophage changes are similar to the condition known as familial hemophagocytic lymphohistiocytosis (HLH), a systemic inflammatory disorder involving cytokine production and cytopenia [58]. HLH can be caused either by abnormalities in genes that regulate NK degranulation and cytotoxic CD8+ T cells or by autoimmune disease, neoplasm, and viral infection [59].

Maternal–fetal–neonatal issues in COVID-19

The main concerns of the novel coronavirus disease relating to the impact on pregnancy and fetuses can be summarized in several issues:

- maternal and fetal morbidity and mortality in COVID-19: epidemiology;
- mother-to-child transmission of SARS-CoV-2 and anti-SARS-CoV-2 antibodies and their potential role;
- mother-to-child transmission of vaccine-mediated anti-SARS-CoV-2 antibodies. Are they different from the COVID-19 mediated antibodies?
- COVID-19 mediated placental damage and placenta-mediated complications (pre-eclampsia/HELLP, placental abruption, intrauterine growth restriction, etc;

- COVID-19, thromboinflammation and hidden thrombophilia (genetic and/or acquired) as a cause of endothelial damage, maternal and placental thrombosis, and placenta-mediated complications;
- should be changed the management of pregnancy and neonatal care in the light of new data of the effects of SARS-CoV-2 on maternal/placental/fetal compartment (diagnostic and therapeutic aspects)?

The RCOG (Royal College of Obstetricians and Gynecologists) in 2020 published one of the earliest summary's findings on maternal morbidity and mortality in this pandemic, mainly based on the national study by UK Obstetric Surveillance System (UCOSS) [60].

The main conclusions of this document were

- in the UK, the maternal mortality rate from COVID-19 was 2.2 per 100,000 maternities;
- symptomatic pregnant women with COVID-19 requiring hospital treatment had overall worse maternal outcomes, including an increased risk of death, although that risk remains very low;
- risk of severe illness remained more common in later pregnancy with premature birth more than twice in pregnant women with symptoms;
- pregnant women with COVID-19 have higher rates of ICU admission.

Mortality in COVID-19 is associated with two major elements—deteriorating of lung function and thrombosis (Fig. 30.4) (although it must be said that pulmonary insufficiency is mainly associated with local pulmonary thrombosis at the capillary level) [61]. The risk of hemostatic and thromboembolic complications in pregnant women with COVID-19 is also 10 and 3 times higher, respectively [62].

A later multinational cohort study (**The INTERCOVID Multinational Cohort Study)** that included 43 institutions in 18 countries demonstrates similar but not so reassuring data as UCOSS. The risk of maternal mortality is exceptionally high—more than 22 times! [63].

There are also higher risks of pregnancy-induced hypertension, PE/eclampsia/HELLP, infections requiring antibiotics, greater risk of admission to ICU/high-dependency unit, and

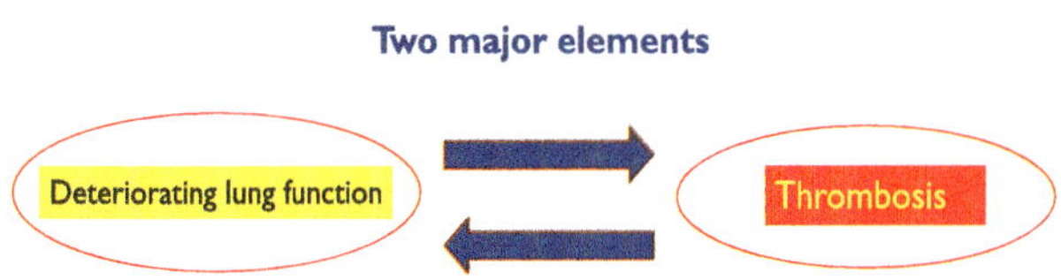

FIGURE 30.4 Mortality in COVID-19.

referral to a higher level of care (RR:1.46, 1.76, 3.38, 5.04 and 6.07, respectively; CI 95%) [63]. The relative risk of fetal distress (1.70), preterm birth (<37 gestational weeks) (1.59), low birth weight (<2500 g) (1.58) as well as maternal morbidity and mortality index (RR = 1.54), severe neonatal and perinatal morbidity and mortality index (RR = 1.58 and 1.59, respectively) are almost one and a half times higher.

Thus, based on data from multicenter cohort studies, it can be concluded that COVID-19 during pregnancy is associated with a persistent and significant increase in maternal morbidity and mortality, and neonatal complications.

Currently, in clinical practice, there are already relatively straightforward recommendations for preventing thrombosis in pregnant women with COVID-19 (RCOG, etc.). However, there are still no clear recommendations for preventing placenta-associated complications and complications in the fetus/newborn. Local immune responses at the mother–placenta–fetus border and impairments to the protective function of the placenta under conditions of SARS-CoV-2 infection remain not fully understood [64].

The pathological effects of Sars-CoV-2 on the mother–fetus dyad may be caused by placental injury and placenta-mediated complications, as well as direct exposure to the virus and/or anti-SARS-CoV-2 antibodies (Fig. 30.5).

The deleterious association of hypercoagulation, inflammation, and thrombosis in women infected with the coronavirus may also increase the risk of placental thrombosis. A case series of pregnant women with COVID-19 reported fetal vascular malperfusion or fetal vascular thrombosis mainly because of focal avascular villi and thrombi in larger fetal vessels with complement deposition [65].

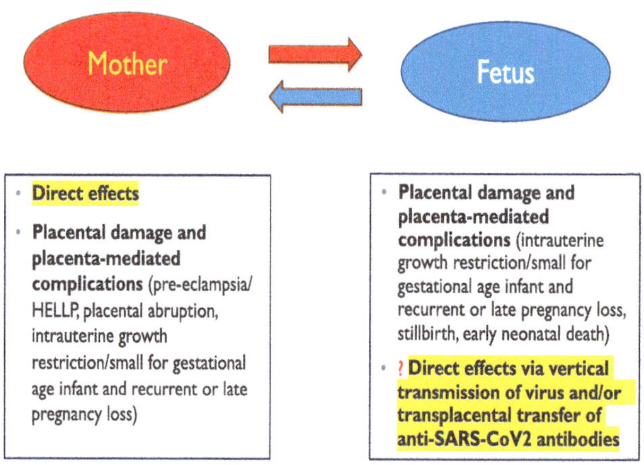

FIGURE 30.5 SARS-CoV-2 effects on the mother–fetus dyad.

Placenta

Although the SARS-CoV-2 virus primarily infects the lungs, where it can cause respiratory distress of varying severity, there is growing evidence of its adverse effects on other organs in which the angiotensin-converting enzyme 2 (ACE2) receptor is present, including the placenta.

SARS-CoV-2 enters the body and infects cells by binding to the ACE2 receptor (Fig. 30.6) [66]. ACE2 has been found to be expressed in cells of the respiratory tract and intestines, placenta, ovaries, vagina, and uterus [67]. Access to the cell is further facilitated by transmembrane serine protease 2 (TMPRSS2)-induced priming of the viral spike (S) protein. Cells that simultaneously express ACE2 and TMPRSS2 have a higher susceptibility to SARS-CoV-2 [68]. In addition, furin, trypsin, and cathepsins B and L can cleave the spike glycoprotein binding to the S1/S2 site, which facilitates virus entry [69]. ACE2 is expressed in fetal cells of the kidney, ilium, rectum, and lungs as early as 15 weeks [70]. Only a subset of cells located in the fetal adrenal gland and kidneys coexpress ACE2 and TMPRSS2. Placental cytotrophoblasts and syncytiotrophoblasts (STBs) express ACE2 starting at 7 weeks, suggesting that SARS-CoV-2 can cross the placenta at any stage of pregnancy (9). A study of the coexpression of ACE2 and TMPRSS2 in the developing embryo up to day 14 revealed the colocalization of these genes, which may indicate the possibility of increased susceptibility to SARS-CoV-2 fetal infection in early embryonic development [71].

The placenta is a protective barrier that usually prevents infection from the mother. There are three main types of placental trophoblasts: differentiated multinucleated syncytiotrophoblasts, which are in direct contact with maternal blood and line the villous tree, villous cytotrophoblast progenitors, which underlie the syncytiotrophoblast, and invasive extravillous trophoblast (EVT) cells [66].

Vertical transmission of the virus from mother to fetus can occur by:

- direct damage to the villous tree with a rupture of the protective layer of syncytiotrophoblast, which can be caused by virus-induced apoptosis and damage to blood vessels in the placenta;
- through virus-infected maternal endothelium to EVT;

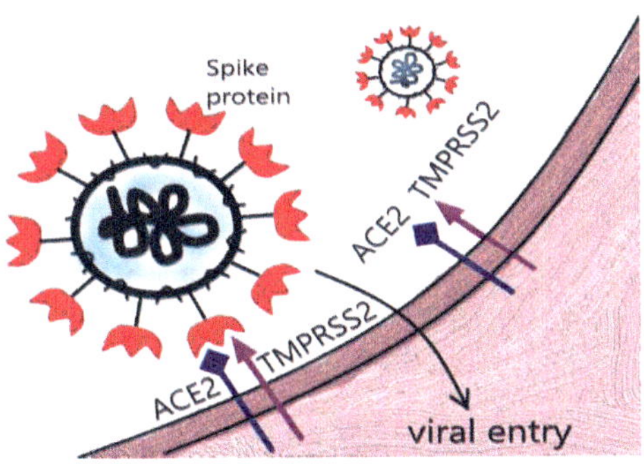

FIGURE 30.6 Entry of SARS-CoV-2.

- through the penetration of infected maternal immune cells through the syncytiotrophoblast;
- paracellular or transcellular transport (e.g., immunoglobulin-mediated transcytosis) into fetal capillaries [72];
- transmission through the aspirated amniotic fluid;
- Ascending infection from the vagina.

Fetus

Interestingly, systematic reviews and meta-analyses do not show us conclusive evidence of intrauterine transmission. Most newborns born to mothers who test positive for SARS-CoV-2 do not have the virus after delivery, indicating the presence of protective mechanisms in the placenta. However, anecdotal reports support the possibility of vertical transmission, with recent reports of newborns being infected and even showing early symptoms of the disease [73].

Whether this is due to the transplacental transmission of SARS-CoV-2 or postpartum infection, recent studies have identified the presence of SARS-CoV-2 mRNA and virions in syncytiotrophoblasts, strongly suggesting a possible transplacental transmission of the virus [74].

A study on the transplacental transfer of antibodies to SARS-CoV-2 showed effective transplacental transfer of IgG antibodies in 87% of seropositive mothers [75,76]. Studies in China have shown that the presence of IgG in the fetus may indicate transmission of this immunoglobulin from mother to fetus during pregnancy [77], but the presence of IgM in the neonatal circulation indicates that the fetus may be able to produce and secrete these immunoglobulins in response to a viral infection. So, five out of six newborns were found to have IgG antibodies and 2 (surprisingly) IgM! It is known that IgM cannot penetrate the placental barrier, then what is the reason? Destroying of the barrier function of the placenta in conditions of severe inflammatory response? Independent synthesis (self-synthesis) by the fetus? Interestingly, all newborns had elevated levels of the pro-inflammatory cytokine IL-6, although all six mothers had mild clinical manifestations of COVID-19 [78].

Of particular interest is the placental transfer of vaccine-induced antibodies [79]. As is known, after vaccination against tetanus, diphtheria, whooping cough, and influenza, vaccine-induced IgG is often detected in the blood plasma of the fetus due to its passage through the placenta [80]. Vaccination of pregnant women to protect mothers, fetuses, and infants from infection has increased over the past decade. This ensures that immunologically immature infants are protected before receiving their vaccinations. The placental transport system is highly selective for IgG antibodies and essentially excludes the transport of other major immunoglobulin classes, including Ig E, Ig M, and Ig A. Transplacental transport is regulated by the neonatal Fc receptor, which is a very complex process. The most studied factors that may modulate placental transfer are IgG subclass, antibody glycosylation, total maternal IgG concentration, maternal disease, infant gestational age, and birth weight. The intensity of antibody transmission is minimal until 16 weeks and increases during the second trimester, peaking in the third trimester, especially in the last 4 weeks of pregnancy, which can give higher antibody titers in the child than in the mother [81]. This may be due to increased cytotrophic expression in the early stages and the fact that the neonatal Fc receptor is more expressed with gestational age, and preterm infants may experience insufficient transfer of antibodies across the placenta [82].

In one published study, a pregnant woman received the BNT162b2 vaccine at 22 and 26 weeks of pregnancy. A baby born at 33 weeks' gestation still maintained positive anti-SARS-CoV-2 S antibody titers at six months of age [83].

New studies have proven transplacental transmission of antibodies against SARS-CoV-2 following vaccination with maternal COVID-19 mRNA [84–86]. A recent study showed the neutralizing effect of these antibodies; however, it is currently unclear how long these protective antibodies will be present in the child's body [87]. The mRNA containing the COVID-19 vaccine generates specific antibodies to the spike protein and induces the formation of neutralizing anti-S IgG antibodies [88]. A prospective cohort study published in March 2021 found that vaccine-derived antibodies were detected in 10 vaccinated pregnant women [85]. Neutralizing antibody titers were lower in the umbilical cord compared to maternal blood without a statistically significant difference. Even after the first dose of the vaccine, IgG was detected in the umbilical cord [85]. The optimal gestational age for vaccination has not yet been determined for effective placental immune transfer. The duration of antibodies in newborns has not yet been determined.

The latest data comes from an unprecedented vaccination campaign for pregnant women in Israel between April 2020 and March 2021 [89]. The cohort consisted of 1094 participants from eight hospitals in Israel. Result: The Pfizer-BioNTech mRNA vaccine induces a rapid rise in IgG titers and efficient placental crossover that exceeds the immune response seen in pregnant women with SARS-CoV-2 infection in the third trimester. Researchers have noted a significant and potentially reliable protective titer of anti-SARS-CoV-2 in neonatal circulation as early as two weeks after the first vaccine dose. However, robust safety evidence is still needed and should be considered in future studies to determine the role of maternal vaccination in preventing COVID-19 and its complications in infants.

Analysis of maternal and perinatal outcomes according to the severity of COVID-19 symptoms shows almost the same increased relative risk of severe neonatal and perinatal morbidity and mortality in pregnant women with any symptoms or more severe symptoms. However, pregnant women with severe COVID-19 have poorer outcomes [63]. This means that even pregnant women with mild/moderate COVID-19 are at higher risk of adverse fetal/neonatal outcomes than those without COVID-19. Perhaps this is due to the dissociation of clinical and laboratory data during pregnancy, when, despite the patient's clinical stability, laboratory tests reveal pro-inflammatory and procoagulant syndromes (even after two weeks and later, when the PCR swabs are negative), characterized mainly by an increase in the level interleukins, ferritin, and exceptionally high levels of D-dimer.

Pregnant women with mild COVID-19 and stable general condition of the mother and fetus in first days, usually get a recommendation of self-isolation at home. Therefore, placenta-mediated complications such as fetal death or placental abruption often come as a surprise to obstetricians. As a rule, such patients have additional unaccounted for and/or undiagnosed risk factors that predispose them to increased blood clotting and thrombosis (genetic thrombophilia) (FVLeiden, etc.), APLA, and comorbidity (diabetes mellitus, obesity, etc.). There are descriptions of such cases in publications [90]. We also have our own experience of placenta-mediated complications of fetal death [90] and placental abruption (our case) in pregnant women with mild COVID-19 and occult thrombophilia (FVLeiden mutation). In addition to maternal genetic thrombophilia FVLeiden, at the time of the fetal death (in first case) and placental abruption (in own case) diagnosis (despite the patients being clinically stable and PCR-were negative), laboratory tests revealed a pro-inflammatory and pro-coagulant syndrome, characterized mainly by an increase in interleukins, ferritin, and exceptionally very high level of D-dimer—more than 30 times higher (!) than the normal upper reference, which may have contributed to impaired placental perfusion and serious morphological abnormalities in the placenta. Histopathological examination of the placenta revealed inflammatory and thrombotic lesions—acute and chronic intervillusitis, villusitis and acute deciduitis, as well as signs of reduced perfusion of the maternal part of the placenta, extensive damage to the syncytiotrophoblast. In the first case upon further examination of the dead fetus, SARS-CoV-2 RNA was found in large quantities in the placenta and fetal tissues. This can indicate a transplacental passage of the virus from mother to fetus, which, possibly combined with placental thrombosis, caused fetal death. It can be assumed that the placenta becomes more permeable to the virus in conditions of an excessive inflammatory response and placental insufficiency.

In our case, a patient with placental abruption at 27 weeks of gestation had a live baby in serious clinical condition. Further examination revealed a high titer of anti-SARS-CoV-2 antibodies.

Histopathological findings in the placenta mainly demonstrated focal basal deciduitis, signs of virus-induced transformation of the amniotic epithelium, and atherosis of stem villi arteries (Fig. 30.7) for PE. Both COVID-19 and PE are characterized by endotheliopathy and systemic inflammation, which may explain similar histopathological findings in the placenta.

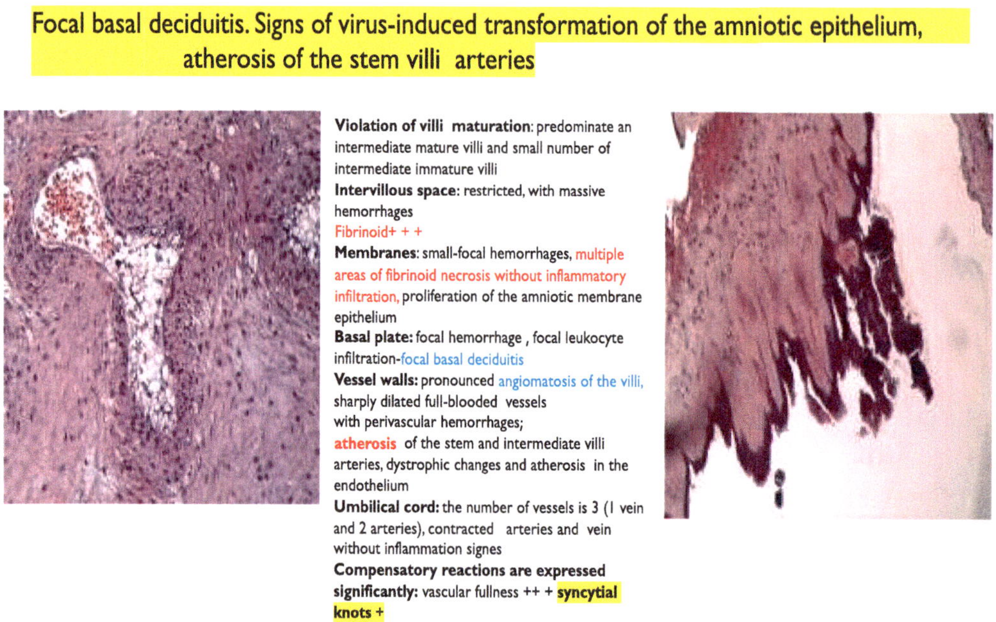

FIGURE 30.7 Placental injury and COVID-19 (histopathological findings).

Conclusion

COVID-19 during pregnancy is associated with a persistent and significant increase in the risks of maternal morbidity mortality and neonatal complications. There is a clear relationship between maternal SARS-CoV-2 infection and fetal and neonatal complications, both from placental disorders and from mother-to-child transmission of the virus and/or antibodies. Thromboinflammation and endotheliopathy caused by COVID-19 is exacerbated by latent (or known) genetic and/or acquired thrombophilia and leads to the development of placenta-mediated complications and thrombosis in both the mother and the placenta. Several described clinical cases indicate the need for a more in-depth study of the impact of COVID-19 on the mother-placenta-fetus system. Careful monitoring of pregnant women with COVID-19 (even a mild form) is required, with scheduled visits to the doctor at shorter intervals for clinical, laboratory, and dynamic visual assessment of the mother's state, placenta, and fetus. Consideration should be given to the use of additional methods for assessing fetal-placental function and laboratory testing of coagulation and inflammatory biomarkers to effectively monitor pregnant women with COVID-19 and high-risk factors to avoid adverse maternal and fetal outcomes.

Management of patients with COVID-19 is impossible without the prevention of thrombosis. Thrombogenesis in patients with severe and critical forms of COVID-19 should be suppressed at various pathogenetic levels; anticoagulant therapy alone may not be sufficient. Patients with extremely high level of D-dimer in blood serum (ISTH recommendations) and high concentrations of inflammatory markers should be hospitalized even in the absence of other signs, including clinical ones, since these signs mean excessive thrombin formation and a high risk of adverse outcomes. High D-dimer concentrations should be considered a predictive biomarker for worsening disease and/or placental-mediated complications in pregnant women with COVID-19. All pregnant women with COVID-19 (even mild to moderate cases) and no contraindications to anticoagulants should receive at least prophylactic doses of low molecular weight heparin (LMWH). LMWH is the drug of choice (of all anticoagulants) in pregnant women with COVID-19, not only because they do not pass through the placenta, but also have antiinflammatory and even possible antiviral effects [91,92] (Fig. 30.8).

Due to anticoagulant and multiple nonanticoagulant effects of LMWH, it is advisable to use LMWH as early as possible in patients with COVID-19 in order to early interruption of the most critical pathogenetic pathways, including the formation of extracellular neutrophil traps (NETs) and, accordingly, thromboinflammation and immunothrombosis.

In cases of severe COVID-19, when LMWH only therapy may not be sufficient, it is necessary to influence other mechanisms of hemostasis disorders, restore the balance between vWF and ADAMTS-13 (infusion of fresh frozen plasma or recombinant ADAMTS-13 in the future), as well as suppression of the interaction of vWF with platelets (infusion of caplacizumab).

It is also necessary to consider the possibility of influencing other targets that play an essential role in thromboinflammation in COVID-19 (immunotherapy, anticytokine drugs, complement inhibitors, etc.).

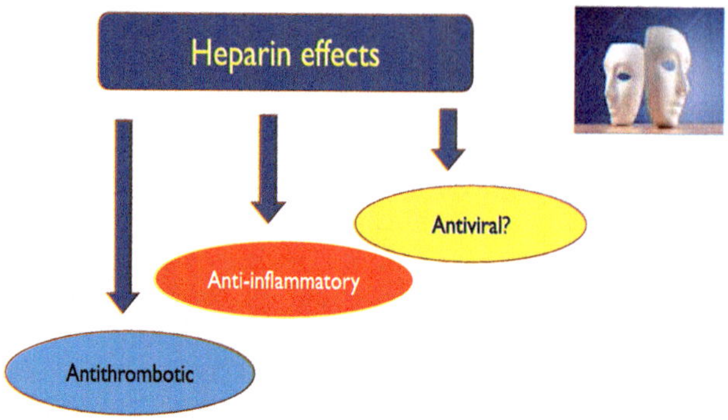

FIGURE 30.8 Different faces of heparin: not only anticoagulant effects!.

References

[1] Bonaventura A, Vecchié A, Dagna L, Martinod K, Dixon DL, Van Tassell BW, et al. Endothelial dysfunction and immunothrombosis as key pathogenic mechanisms in COVID-19. Nat Rev Immunol 2021;21(5):319–29.

[2] Engelmann B, Massberg S. Thrombosis as an intravascular effector of innate immunity. Nat Rev Immunol 2013;13(1):34–45.

[3] Borregaard N. Neutrophils, from marrow to microbes. Immunity 2010;33(5):657–70.

[4] Hahn S, Giaglis S, Chowdury CS, Hösli I, Hasler P, editors. Modulation of neutrophil NETosis: interplay between infectious agents and underlying host physiology. Seminars in immunopathology. Springer; 2013.

[5] Gupta AK, Giaglis S, Hasler P, Hahn S. Efficient neutrophil extracellular trap induction requires mobilization of both intracellular and extracellular calcium pools and is modulated by cyclosporine A. PLoS One 2014;9(5):e97088.

[6] Ley K, Laudanna C, Cybulsky MI, Nourshargh S. Getting to the site of inflammation: the leukocyte adhesion cascade updated. Nat Rev Immunol 2007;7(9):678–89.

[7] Fuchs TA, Abed U, Goosmann C, Hurwitz R, Schulze I, Wahn V, et al. Novel cell death program leads to neutrophil extracellular traps. J Cell Biol 2007;176(2):231–41.

[8] Kenny EF, Herzig A, Krüger R, Muth A, Mondal S, Thompson PR, et al. Diverse stimuli engage different neutrophil extracellular trap pathways. Elife 2017;6:e24437.

[9] Ivan FX, Rajapakse JC, Welsch RE, Rozen SG, Narasaraju T, Xiong GM, et al. Differential pulmonary transcriptomic profiles in murine lungs infected with low and highly virulent influenza H3N2 viruses reveal dysregulation of TREM1 signaling, cytokines, and chemokines. Funct Integr Genom 2012;12(1):105–17.

[10] Kobasa D, Jones SM, Shinya K, Kash JC, Copps J, Ebihara H, et al. Aberrant innate immune response in lethal infection of macaques with the 1918 influenza virus. Nature 2007;445(7125):319–23.

[11] Gould T, Lysov Z, Liaw P. Extracellular DNA and histones: double-edged swords in immunothrombosis. J Thromb Haemostasis 2015;13:S82–91.

[12] Jimenez-Alcazar M, Napirei M, Panda R, Köhler E, Kremer Hovinga JA, Mannherz H, et al. Impaired DN ase1-mediated degradation of neutrophil extracellular traps is associated with acute thrombotic microangiopathies. J Thromb Haemostasis 2015;13(5):732–42.

[13] Martinod K, Wagner DD. Thrombosis: tangled up in NETs. Blood 2014;123(18):2768–76.

[14] Factor XII contact activation. In: Naudin C, Burillo E, Blankenberg S, Butler L, Renné T, editors. Seminars in thrombosis and hemostasis. Thieme Medical Publishers; 2017.

[15] Vu TT, Leslie BA, Stafford AR, Zhou J, Fredenburgh JC, Weitz JI. Histidine-rich glycoprotein binds DNA and RNA and attenuates their capacity to activate the intrinsic coagulation pathway. Thromb Haemostasis 2016;115(1):89–98.

[16] Noubouossie DF, Whelihan MF, Yu Y-B, Sparkenbaugh E, Pawlinski R, Monroe DM, et al. In vitro activation of coagulation by human neutrophil DNA and histone proteins but not neutrophil extracellular traps. Blood 2017;129(8):1021–9.

[17] Saffarzadeh M, Juenemann C, Queisser MA, Lochnit G, Barreto G, Galuska SP, et al. Neutrophil extracellular traps directly induce epithelial and endothelial cell death: a predominant role of histones. PLoS One 2012;7(2):e32366.

[18] Semeraro F, Ammollo CT, Morrissey JH, Dale GL, Friese P, Esmon NL, et al. Extracellular histones promote thrombin generation through platelet-dependent mechanisms: involvement of platelet TLR2 and TLR4. Blood J Am Soc Hematol 2011;118(7):1952–61.

[19] Carestia A, Rivadeneyra L, Romaniuk MA, Fondevila C, Negrotto S, Schattner M. Functional responses and molecular mechanisms involved in histone-mediated platelet activation. Thromb Haemostasis 2013;110(5):1035–45.

[20] Barranco-Medina S, Pozzi N, Vogt AD, Di Cera E. Histone H4 promotes prothrombin autoactivation. J Biol Chem 2013;288(50):35749–57.

[21] Varjú I, Longstaff C, Szabó L, Farkas ÁZ, Farkas VJ, Tanka-Salamon A, et al. DNA, histones and neutrophil extracellular traps exert anti-fibrinolytic effects in a plasma environment. Thromb Haemostasis 2015;113(6):1289–98.

[22] Ammollo CT, Semeraro F, Xu J, Esmon N, Esmon C. Extracellular histones increase plasma thrombin generation by impairing thrombomodulin-dependent protein C activation. J Thromb Haemostasis 2011;9(9):1795–803.

[23] Healy LD, Puy C, Fernández JA, Mitrugno A, Keshari RS, Taku NA, et al. Activated protein C inhibits neutrophil extracellular trap formation in vitro and activation in vivo. J Biol Chem 2017;292(21):8616–29.

[24] Komissarov AA, Florova G, Idell S. Effects of extracellular DNA on plasminogen activation and fibrinolysis. J Biol Chem 2011;286(49):41949–62.

[25] Longstaff C, Varjú I, Sótonyi P, Szabó L, Krumrey M, Hoell A, et al. Mechanical stability and fibrinolytic resistance of clots containing fibrin, DNA, and histones. J Biol Chem 2013;288(10):6946–56.

[26] Löf A, Müller JP, Brehm MA. A biophysical view on von Willebrand factor activation. J Cell Physiol 2018;233(2):799–810.

[27] Zhang C, Kelkar A, Neelamegham S. von Willebrand factor self-association is regulated by the shear-dependent unfolding of the A2 domain. Blood Adv 2019;3(7):957–68.

[28] South K, Lane DA. ADAMTS-13 and von Willebrand factor: a dynamic duo. J Thromb Haemostasis 2018;16(1):6–18.

[29] Fakhouri F, Roumenina L, Provot F, Sallée M, Caillard S, Couzi L, et al. Pregnancy-associated hemolytic uremic syndrome revisited in the era of complement gene mutations. J Am Soc Nephrol 2010;21(5):859–67.

[30] Bitsadze V, Bouvier S, Khizroeva J, Cochery-Nouvellon É, Mercier É, Perez-Martin A, et al. Early ADAMTS13 testing associates with pre-eclampsia occurrence in antiphospholipid syndrome. Thromb Res 2021;203:101–9.

[31] Giaglis S, Stoikou M, Grimolizzi F, Subramanian BY, van Breda SV, Hoesli I, et al. Neutrophil migration into the placenta: good, bad or deadly? Cell Adhes Migrat 2016;10(1–2):208–25.

[32] Marder W, Knight JS, Kaplan MJ, Somers EC, Zhang X, O'Dell AA, et al. Placental histology and neutrophil extracellular traps in lupus and pre-eclampsia pregnancies. Lupus Sci Med 2016;3(1):e000134.

[33] Bouvier S, Fortier M, Vincent L, Demattei C, Mousty E, Herzog M, et al. NETosis markers in pregnancy: effects differ according to histone subtypes. Thromb Haemostasis 2021;121:877–90.

[34] Hu Y, Li H, Yan R, Wang C, Wang Y, Zhang C, et al. Increased neutrophil activation and plasma DNA levels in patients with pre-eclampsia. Thromb Haemostasis 2018;118(12):2064–73.

[35] Papayannopoulos V, Metzler KD, Hakkim A, Zychlinsky A. Neutrophil elastase and myeloperoxidase regulate the formation of neutrophil extracellular traps. J Cell Biol 2010;191(3):677–91.

[36] Osorio Y, Bonilla DL, Peniche AG, Melby PC, Travi BL. Pregnancy enhances the innate immune response in experimental cutaneous leishmaniasis through hormone-modulated nitric oxide production. J Leukoc Biol 2008;83(6):1413–22.

[37] Rochael NC, Guimarães-Costa AB, Nascimento MT, DeSouza-Vieira TS, Oliveira MP, e Souza LFG, et al. Classical ROS-dependent and early/rapid ROS-independent release of neutrophil extracellular traps triggered by Leishmania parasites. Sci Rep 2015;5(1):1–11.

[38] Hahn S, Lapaire O, Than NG. Biomarker development for presymptomatic molecular diagnosis of preeclampsia: feasible, useful or even unnecessary? Expert Rev Mol Diagn 2015;15(5):617–29.

[39] Martinod K, Demers M, Fuchs TA, Wong SL, Brill A, Gallant M, et al. Neutrophil histone modification by peptidylarginine deiminase 4 is critical for deep vein thrombosis in mice. Proc Natl Acad Sci USA 2013;110(21):8674–9.

[40] Gupta A, Hasler P, Gebhardt S, Holzgreve W, Hahn S. Occurrence of neutrophil extracellular DNA traps (NETs) in pre-eclampsia: a link with elevated levels of cell-free DNA? Ann N Y Acad Sci 2006;1075:118–22.

[41] Leung TN, Zhang J, Lau TK, Chan LY, Lo YD. Increased maternal plasma fetal DNA concentrations in women who eventually develop preeclampsia. Clin Chem 2001;47(1):137–9.

[42] Zhong XY, Laivuori H, Livingston JC, Ylikorkala O, Sibai BM, Holzgreve W, et al. Elevation of both maternal and fetal extracellular circulating deoxyribonucleic acid concentrations in the plasma of pregnant women with preeclampsia. Am J Obstet Gynecol 2001;184(3):414–9.

[43] Roberts JM, Hubel CA. The two stage model of preeclampsia: variations on the theme. Placenta 2009;30:32–7.

[44] Redman CW, Sargent IL. Latest advances in understanding preeclampsia. Science 2005;308(5728):1592–4.

[45] Brosens I, Pijnenborg R, Vercruysse L, Romero R. The "Great Obstetrical Syndromes" are associated with disorders of deep placentation. Am J Obstet Gynecol 2011;204(3):193–201.

[46] Rana S, Powe CE, Salahuddin S, Verlohren S, Perschel FH, Levine RJ, et al. Angiogenic factors and the risk of adverse outcomes in women with suspected preeclampsia. Circulation 2012;125(7):911–9.

[47] Granne I, Southcombe JH, Snider JV, Tannetta DS, Child T, Redman CW, et al. ST2 and IL-33 in pregnancy and pre-eclampsia. PLoS One 2011;6(9):e24463.

[48] Piccinni M-P, Romagnani S. Regulation of fetal allograft survival by hormone-controlled Th1-and Th2-type cytokines. Immunol Res 1996;15(2):141–50.

[49] Muyayalo KP, Huang DH, Zhao SJ, Xie T, Mor G, Liao AH. COVID-19 and Treg/Th17 imbalance: potential relationship to pregnancy outcomes. Am J Reprod Immunol 2020;84(5):e13304.

[50] Young BC, Stanic AK, Panda B, Rueda BR, Panda A. Longitudinal expression of Toll-like receptors on dendritic cells in uncomplicated pregnancy and postpartum. Am J Obstet Gynecol 2014;210(5):445. e1-. e6.

[51] Firmal P, Shah VK, Chattopadhyay S. Insight into TLR4-mediated immunomodulation in normal pregnancy and related disorders. Front Immunol 2020;11:807.

[52] Khosroshahi LM, Rokni M, Mokhtari T, Noorbakhsh F. Immunology, immunopathogenesis and immunotherapeutics of COVID-19; an overview. Int Immunopharm 2021;93:107364.

[53] Huang C, Wang Y, Li X, Ren L, Zhao J, Hu Y, et al. Clinical features of patients infected with 2019 novel coronavirus in Wuhan, China. Lancet 2020;395(10223):497–506.

[54] Chen G, Wu D, Guo W, Cao Y, Huang D, Wang H, et al. Clinical and immunological features of severe and moderate coronavirus disease 2019. J Clin Invest 2020;130(5):2620–9.

[55] Björkström NK, Strunz B, Ljunggren H-G. Natural killer cells in antiviral immunity. Nat Rev Immunol 2021:1–12.

[56] Chua RL, Lukassen S, Trump S, Hennig BP, Wendisch D, Pott F, et al. COVID-19 severity correlates with airway epithelium–immune cell interactions identified by single-cell analysis. Nat Biotechnol 2020;38(8):970–9.

[57] Mathew D, Giles JR, Baxter AE, Oldridge DA, Greenplate AR, Wu JE, et al. Deep immune profiling of COVID-19 patients reveals distinct immunotypes with therapeutic implications. Science 2020;369(6508):eabc8511.

[58] Soy M, Atagündüz P, Atagündüz I, Sucak GT. Hemophagocytic lymphohistiocytosis: a review inspired by the COVID-19 pandemic. Rheumatol Int 2021;41(1):7–18.

[59] Henderson LA, Canna SW, Schulert GS, Volpi S, Lee PY, Kernan KF, et al. On the alert for cytokine storm: immunopathology in COVID-19. Arthritis Rheumatol 2020;72(7):1059–63.

[60] Obstetricians RCo, Gynaecologists. Coronavirus (COVID-19) infection in pregnancy. 2020. 2021.

[61] Lillicrap D, Morrissey JH. 2020-Year of COVID-19. J Thromb Haemostasis 2020;18(9):2081–2081. https://doi.org/10.1111/jth.15041.

[62] Servante J, Swallow G, Thornton JG, Myers B, Munireddy S, Malinowski AK, et al. Haemostatic and thromboembolic complications in pregnant women with COVID-19: a systematic review and critical analysis. BMC Pregnancy Childbirth 2021;21(1):1–14.

[63] Villar J, Ariff S, Gunier RB, Thiruvengadam R, Rauch S, Kholin A, et al. Maternal and neonatal morbidity and mortality among pregnant women with and without COVID-19 infection: the INTERCOVID multinational cohort study. JAMA Pediatr 2021;175(8):817–26. https://doi.org/10.1001/jamapediatrics.2021.1050.

[64] Rad HS, Röhl J, Stylianou N, Allenby MC, Bazaz SR, Warkiani ME, et al. The effects of COVID-19 on the placenta during pregnancy. Front Immunol 2021:3734.
[65] Ahmed S, Zimba O, Yuri Gasparyan A. Thrombosis in Coronavirus disease 2019 (COVID-19) through the prism of Virchow's triad. Clin Rheumatol 2020;39:2529–43. https://doi.org/10.1007/s10067-020-05275-1.
[66] Wastnedge EA, Reynolds RM, Van Boeckel SR, Stock SJ, Denison FC, Maybin JA, et al. Pregnancy and COVID-19. Physiol Rev 2021;101(1):303–18.
[67] Auriti C, De Rose DU, Tzialla C, Caforio L, Ciccia M, Manzoni P, et al. Vertical transmission of SARS-CoV-2 (COVID-19): are hypotheses more than evidences? Am J Perinatol 2020;37:S31–8.
[68] Rabi FA, Al Zoubi MS, Kasasbeh GA, Salameh DM, Al-Nasser AD. SARS-CoV-2 and coronavirus disease 2019: what we know so far. Pathogens 2020;9(3):231.
[69] Pique-Regi R, Romero R, Tarca AL, Luca F, Xu Y, Alazizi A, et al. Does the human placenta express the canonical cell entry mediators for SARS-CoV-2? Elife 2020;9:e58716.
[70] Faure-Bardon V, Isnard P, Roux N, Leruez-Ville M, Molina T, Bessieres B, et al. Protein expression of angiotensin-converting enzyme 2, a SARS-CoV-2-specific receptor, in fetal and placental tissues throughout gestation: new insight for perinatal counseling. Ultrasound Obstet Gynecol 2021;57(2):242–7.
[71] Weatherbee BA, Glover DM, Zernicka-Goetz M. Expression of SARS-CoV-2 receptor ACE2 and the protease TMPRSS2 suggests susceptibility of the human embryo in the first trimester. Open Biol 2020;10(8):200162.
[72] Blumberg DA, Underwood MA, Hedriana HL, Lakshminrusimha S. Vertical transmission of SARS-CoV-2: what is the optimal definition? Am J Perinatol 2020;37(08):769–72.
[73] Gajbhiye RK, Modi DN, Mahale SD. Pregnancy outcomes, newborn complications and maternal-fetal transmission of SARS-CoV-2 in women with COVID-19: a systematic review of 441 cases. MedRxiv 2020.
[74] Patanč L, Morotti D, Giunta M. Vertical transmission of COVID-19: SARS-CoV-2 on the fetal side of the placenta in pregnancies with COVID-19 positive mothers and neonates at birth. Am J Obstet Gynecol MFM 2020:100145.
[75] Diriba K, Awulachew E, Getu E. The effect of coronavirus infection (SARS-CoV-2, MERS-CoV, and SARS-CoV) during pregnancy and the possibility of vertical maternal–fetal transmission: a systematic review and meta-analysis. Eur J Med Res 2020;25(1):1–14.
[76] Flannery DD, Gouma S, Dhudasia MB, Mukhopadhyay S, Pfeifer MR, Woodford EC, et al. Assessment of maternal and neonatal cord blood SARS-CoV-2 antibodies and placental transfer ratios. JAMA Pediatr 2021;175(6):594–600.
[77] Zeng H, Xu C, Fan J, Tang Y, Deng Q, Zhang W, et al. Antibodies in infants born to mothers with COVID-19 pneumonia. JAMA 2020;323(18):1848–9.
[78] Dong L, Tian J, He S, Zhu C, Wang J, Liu C, et al. Possible vertical transmission of SARS-CoV-2 from an infected mother to her newborn. JAMA 2020;323(18). 1846-.
[79] Gilbert PD, Rudnick CA. Newborn antibodies to SARS-CoV-2 detected in cord blood after maternal vaccination. medRxiv 2021.
[80] Fouda GG, Martinez DR, Swamy GK, Permar SR. The Impact of IgG transplacental transfer on early life immunity. Immunohorizons 2018;2(1):14–25.
[81] Wilcox CR, Holder B, Jones CE. Factors affecting the FcRn-mediated transplacental transfer of antibodies and implications for vaccination in pregnancy. Front Immunol 2017;8:1294.
[82] Palmeira P, Quinello C, Silveira-Lessa AL, Zago CA, Carneiro-Sampaio M. IgG placental transfer in healthy and pathological pregnancies. Clin Dev Immunol 2012;2012.
[83] Mangat C, Milosavljevic N. BNT162b2 vaccination during pregnancy protects both the mother and infant: anti-SARS-CoV-2 S antibodies persistently positive in an infant at 6 Months of age. Case Rep Pediatr 2021. https://doi.org/10.1155/2021/6901131. 2021.
[84] Rottenstreich A, Zarbiv G, Oiknine-Djian E, Zigron R, Wolf DG, Porat S. Efficient maternofetal transplacental transfer of anti-SARS-CoV-2 spike antibodies after antenatal SARS-CoV-2 BNT162b2 mRNA vaccination. medRxiv 2021.
[85] Gray KJ, Bordt EA, Atyeo C, Deriso E, Akinwunmi B, Young N, et al. Coronavirus disease 2019 vaccine response in pregnant and lactating women: a cohort study. Am J Obstet Gynecol 2021;225:303.
[86] Paul G, Chad R. Newborn antibodies to SARS-CoV-2 detected in cord blood after maternal vaccination—a case report. BMC Pediatr 2021;21(1):1–2.

[87] Douxfils J, Gillot C, De Gottal É, Vandervinne S, Bayart J-L, Dogné J-M, et al. Efficient maternal to neonate transfer of neutralizing antibodies after SARS-CoV-2 vaccination with BNT162b2: a case-report and discussion of the literature. Vaccines 2021;9(8):907.

[88] Jalkanen P, Kolehmainen P, Häkkinen H, Huttunen M, Tähtinen P, Lundberg R, et al. COVID-19 mRNA vaccine induced antibody responses and neutralizing antibodies against three SARS-CoV-2 variants. Nat Commun 2021;12.

[89] Beharier O, Mayo RP, Raz T, Sacks KN, Schreiber L, Suissa-Cohen Y, et al. Efficient maternal to neonatal transfer of antibodies against SARS-CoV-2 and BNT162b2 mRNA COVID-19 vaccine. J Clin Invest 2021;131.

[90] Marinho PS, Da Cunha AJLA, Chimelli L, Avvad-Portari E, Andreiuolo FM, de Oliveira-Szejnfeld PS, et al. Case Report: SARS-CoV-2 Mother-to-child transmission and fetal death associated with severe placental thromboembolism. Front Med 2021:1315.

[91] Mycroft-West CJ, Su D, Pagani I, Rudd TR, Elli S, Gandhi NS, Guimond SE, Miller GJ, Meneghetti MCZ, Nader HB, Li Y, Nunes QM, Procter P, Mancini N, Clementi M, Bisio A, Forsyth NR, Ferro V, Turnbull JE, Guerrini M, Fernig DG, Vicenzi E, Yates EA, Lima MA, Skidmore MA. Heparin inhibits cellular invasion by SARS-CoV-2: structural dependence of the interaction of the spike S1 receptor-binding domain with heparin. Thromb Haemostasis December 2020;120(12):1700–15. https://doi.org/10.1055/s-0040-1721319. Epub 2020 Dec 23. PMID: 33368089; PMCID: PMC7869224.

[92] Bitsadze VO, Slukhanchuk EV, Khizroeva JK, Tretyakova MV, Pyatigorskaya NV, Akinshina SV, Makatsariya NA, Gotsiridze KE, Babaeva NN, Grigoreva KN, Shkoda AS, Elalamy I, Gris J, Shulman S. Anticoagulant, anti-inflammatory, antiviral and antitumor properties of heparins. Obstet Gynecol Reprod 2021;15(3):295–312. https://doi.org/10.17749/2313-7347/ob.gyn.rep.2021.216 (In Russ.).

CHAPTER

31

Animal models of COVID-19 and complications

N.V. Petrova[1,2], K.K. Ganina[2] and S.A. Tarasov[1,2]

[1]FSBI Institute of General Pathology and Pathophysiology RAMS, Moscow, Russia; [2]OOO "NPF "Materia Medica Holding", Moscow, Russia

Introduction

The prevalence rate of coronavirus infection (CI), mortality, and the total number of CI-related complications highlights the necessity of large-scale nonclinical studies in order to understand pathological and immunological aspects of this infection and find effective drugs for the treatment and prevention of complications. For this purpose, validated animal models that could most completely reproduce the pathogenesis of the disease are required. There is already a number of scientific papers that describe small rodents [1–8] and ferrets [2,9], as well as nonhuman primates [10–12] as experimental models of COVID. However, the kinetics of viral replication, disease progression, and severity of symptoms vary among different animal species and viral strains [13]. Moreover, none of the CI animal models reproduces the full range of symptoms associated with this disease in humans. In addition to that, Long COVID (post-COVID syndrome) which is a condition with a diversity of symptoms that people experience after recovering from COVID-19 is another problem which draws scientific attention.

Therefore, the aim of this review was to summarize the available literature data concerning the acute and postacute animal models of SARS-CoV-2 infection.

For writing this chapter, a standard set of review writing methods was used. The literature search was performed by N.V. Petrova from May 2020 to November 2021 in the following databases: PubMed, Medline, bioRxiv, and medRxiv.

The experimental data used for this document included: animal species, age and strain, clinical symptoms of the infection, histopathology in lungs, immunological abnormalities, antibody production data, and information on the animal-to-animal transmission of SARS-CoV-2.

Autoimmunity, COVID-19, Post-COVID19 syndrome and COVID-19 vaccination
https://doi.org/10.1016/B978-0-443-18566-3.00032-3

Animal species used for SARS-CoV-2 infection

It has been shown that some animal species are susceptible to SARS-CoV-2, both in the natural environment and in experimental settings (Table 31.1).

Modeling of COVID-19 infection, rodents

Rodents

Mice

First attempts to detect SARS-CoV-2 replication in laboratory mice have been unsuccessful [14]. Apparently, mice are resistant to the virus because their ACE2 receptor differs from the human variant. For this reason, experimental models of the SARS-CoV-2 infection utilize genetically transformed (transgenic) mice. Depending on the strain, infectious dose and route of administration, age and sex of animals, it is possible to model clinical conditions of different severity.

The analysis of experimental data has shown that the severity of infection in mice intranasally challenged with SARS-CoV-2 can vary from the absence of clinical manifestations to total (100%) animal's death. In the studies performed by Bao et al. [15] and Sun et al. [16], infection of wild-type mice ($\sim 2.8 \times 10^5$ PFU) and human ACE2 C57BL/6 mice (4×10^5 PFU) did not result in animal death and produced relatively low viral load in the lungs. Intranasal SARS-CoV-2 infection (1×10^5 PFU) of adenovirally transduced hACE2 BALB/c and C57BL/6 mice (d5hACE2) did not lead to lethality either, but caused acute disease with viral load the lungs up to 6–7 Log_{10} (PFU/mL) on day 2 postinfection. Nevertheless, infection was short-lived with total duration of 7–10 days [17].

In contrast, Winkler [5], Yinda [6], Golden [18], and Jiang [19] (2020) have demonstrated that infection of K18-human ACE2 mice (1×10^4 PFU and 2×10^4 PFU) leads to total mortality, with a clear correlation between the death rate and animal gender.

Histomorphological changes in lungs varied depending on viral load and mostly manifested as cell infiltration (neutrophils and mononuclear cells), thickening of the alveolar septum, edema, focal hemorrhages, and typical lesions of pulmonary vasculature [5,6,18,19]. Moreover, these transgenic mice produced a cytokine storm in the lung that peaked by day 2 postinfection and showed marked chemokine elevation in both lungs and brain [20].

The clinical symptoms of CI in mice were represented in all the experiments by body weight loss, which was the lowest in the study by Bao et al. [15] (10%) and reached up to 20% from baseline in the paper by Jing Sun [17]. The K18-human ACE2 transgenic mice had the highest severity of CI: their weight loss was about 20% (or up to 30% in some cases), all the animals demonstrated fatigue and dyspnea [5,6].

Sun et al. [16] have described the relationship between age and clinical signs of CI, noting the absence of symptoms for young animals (4–5 weeks). The same study has also demonstrated the sensitivity of these animals to intragastric infection with SARS-CoV-2 (4×10^6 PFU), which was manifested by moderate viral replication in lung, trachea, and brain tissue. However, the severity of CI signs was significantly lower compared to intranasal virus challenge.

The use of transgenic mice would also help to more clearly identify the pathological mechanisms of the disease. In order to elucidate the possible contribution of IFN signaling in

TABLE 31.1 Susceptibility of different animal species to Sars-Cov-2 infection.

Species	Clinical signs	Antibodies	CST	References
Rodents				
hACE2 transgenic mice	• transient weight loss, • low viral load in lungs • mild interstitial pneumonia characterized by interstitial and intraalveolar mononuclear and granulocytic inflammation	+	+	[15]
d5hACE2 transduced mice	• mild clinical symptoms • lower viral titers limited to lungs • pulmonary lesions include perivascular to interstitial inflammation, edema, vascular congestion, and hemorrhage	+	nd	[16,17,57]
K18 Promoter-hACE2 Transgenic mice	• weight loss • viral replication in the lungs, cell infiltration, focal hemorrhages, edema, alveolar, interstitial and perivascular infiltration of neutrophils and mononuclear cells • development of interstitial pneumonia. • lymphopenia (blood) • cytokine (lungs) and chemokine (brain) elevations	+	nd	[5,6,18,19,58]
hACE2 mouse established by using CRISPR/Cas9	• transient weight loss, • viral replication in the lungs • development of interstitial pneumonia. • aged species demonstrated more severe clinical symptoms and cytokine response	+	nd	[16,59]
Infection with mouse-adapted model	• weight loss, • viral replication in the lungs • development of interstitial pneumonia, inflammation and immune cells infiltration. • age tropism. • cytokine response in lungs • presence of acute respiratory distress syndrome (ARDS)	+	nd	[60–62]
Syrian hamsters	• viral replication in the upper and lower respiratory tract • weight loss and tachypnea • development of broncho-interstitial pneumonia • myocarditis. • cytokine response (lungs) and blood abnormalities	+	+	[1,4,7,8,22, 25,26,55]

(Continued)

TABLE 31.1 Susceptibility of different animal species to Sars-Cov-2 infection.—cont'd

Species	Clinical signs	Antibodies	CST	References
Carnivora				
Ferrets	• viral replication predominantly in the upper respiratory tract • moderate weight loss and fever • acute bronchitis • gastrointestinal involvement • aged species demonstrated more severe clinical symptoms	+	+	[2,9,33,63,64]
Cats	• viral replication in the upper respiratory tract • clinical symptoms of CI are either mild or absent	+	+	[65]
Dogs	• viral RNA is only detected in fecal extracts • clinical symptoms are absent	+	nd	[65]
Primates. Nonhuman monkeys				
Rhesus macaques	• viral replication in the upper and lower respiratory tract and/or in some parts of the gastrointestinal tract • fatigue, dehydration and spontaneous cough • development of interstitial pneumonia • cytokines elevation in lungs • doubled level of CRP in blood • age-dependent symptoms of infection	+	nd	[37–41]
Baboons	• viral replication in the upper and lower respiratory tract • weight loss and fatigue • development of interstitial pneumonia	+	nd	[12,66]
Common marmosets	• viral replication in the upper respiratory tract • CI-related histopathological changes are mild	+	nd	[12,67]
Green monkeys	• viral replication in the upper and lower respiratory tract • loss of appetite and fatigue • development of interstitial pneumonia	+	nd	[11,68]

+—present; – absent; **CST**—cross-species transmission; **nd**—no data available.

SARS-CoV-2 pathogenesis, ACE2 mice with deletion of *IFNAR*$^{-/-}$, *IFNγ*$^{-/-}$ and *STAT1*$^{-/-}$ genes were used for SARS-CoV-2 challenge [31]. The infected *STAT1*$^{-/-}$animals (1×10^5 PFU) had the most pronounced weight loss and extensive cell infiltration in the lungs, with delayed virus clearance. These data highlight the critical role of IFN-I and STAT1 signaling in response to CI, which indicates the therapeutic potential of recombinant IFNs or STAT1 activators in human patients.

Therefore, the use of mice for CI modeling has a number of advantages: they are affordable and easy to use, reproduce clinical states of different severity (from mild to severe). However, there are some differences in the clinical manifestations of COVID infection compared to that in humans: cough is not typical for mice and no intestinal symptoms have been described, perhaps a suitable viral strain has not yet been found. Nevertheless, all of the reported features observed in mice after the infection make it possible to examine therapy and prevention of this disease exactly at the early, functionally reversible stages.

The validity and reproducibility of the experimental data obtained using inbred strains is a benefit and a drawback at the same time. Since animals of a certain inbred strain are genetically identical, they are unlikely to represent all the possible pathogenetic mechanisms of such a complex disease.

Syrian hamsters

Syrian hamsters are an excellent object for research of antivirals or vaccines against SARS-CoV-2. First important aspect is that their ACE2 cell receptor has a high affinity to the virus, which is evidenced by similar symptoms and progression of infection. The infection in these animals is accompanied by viremia (the second-third day of infection), transient weight loss, tachypnea, abnormal alterations in the lung tissue, including alveolar infiltration and pneumonia. The latter is the major CI complication in humans [21]. Indeed, in the study by Imai M. et al. [1], intranasal challenge with both a low dose (1×10^3 PFU) and a high dose ($1 \times 10^{5-6}$ PFU) led to viral replication in the upper and lower respiratory tract (7–8 Log_{10} PFU/g). Viral reproduction in the lungs peaked on day 3 postinfection for both doses. Histopathological alterations in the lung tissue were expressed as alveolar consolidation coupled with inflammation zones, cell infiltration in the interstitial region, edema, and alveolar hemorrhage. These signs could be observed already on day 3 postinfection with the high dose and on day 6 with the low dose of virus. At the end of the study, pathological signs in the lungs were improved (on day 12 postinfection) for both doses. No clear correlation between animal age and CI signs was identified, which correlates with the results of other studies [22,23]. However, in a recent study published by Selvaraj P. et al. [24] aged hamsters exhibited a more significant weight loss (about 25%), sneezing, shortness of breath, and noticeable lethargy upon infection. Animal had severe diffuse broncho-interstitial pneumonia along with myocardial disease and died between day 5 and 8 postinfection.

As another major benefit, it has been shown that SARS-CoV-2 can be effectively transmitted from infected animals (1×10^5 PFU and $\sim 5.6 \times 10^5$ PFU) to the cohoused (contact) noninfected hamsters [4,8]. Direct virus transmission was established in both currently available studies. The infection was evidenced by body weight loss ($\sim 10\%$) and viral replication predominantly in the upper respiratory tract in the first few days postinfection. Finally, neutralizing antibody production was observed for this animal species postinfection [1,7,25].

The immunological markers of CI were examined by Francis M.E. et al. [7]. Authors found significant increase in the levels of inflammatory cytokines (IL-6, IL-1beta, and TNFa) and IFN-II in respiratory tract, whereas IFN-I were inhibited. Examination of extrapulmonary tissue indicated inflammation in the kidney, liver, and heart which also lacked type I interferon upregulation.

In another study Robbert Boudewijns et al. [26] compared wild-type and $STAT2^{-/-}$ or $IL28R\text{-}a^{-/-}$ hamsters following the intranasal SARS-CoV-2 infection with $\sim 1.4 \times 10^5$ PFU dosage. In all the animals, the infection resulted in an early peak of viral replication in the lungs and pronounced viremia characterized by extrapulmonary spread of infection. Compared to the wild-type hamsters, the $IL28R\text{-}a^{-/-}$ animals showed a higher level of viral replication combined with a moderate inflammatory response and lung tissue damage. For animals with deletion of *STAT2*, different pathological outcomes were obtained: rapid spread of infection, high viremia, viral replication in the spleen, liver, and upper and lower gastrointestinal tract. The pathomorphological signs in the lungs were limited to polymorphonuclear leukocyte infiltration and detection of some apoptotic bodies in the bronchial walls.

Therefore, the data obtained demonstrate a considerable contribution of STAT2 to the inhibition of systemic viral spread and suppression of extrapulmonary viral replication, whereas IFN-III seems to be responsible for virus elimination from the lungs. Indeed, a therapeutic potential of type III IFNs in COVID-19 has been already shown [27,28].

These findings offer important insights into the pathological mechanisms of CI and its regulation. The similarity of the impact of STAT and IFN systems on the infectious process in transgenic mice and hamsters suggests that these mechanisms may be well translated into the pathophysiology of CI in humans.

To sum it up, Syrian hamsters are a very popular and well-characterized spontaneous model of CI: infection quite closely reproduces the clinical signs and symptoms observed in patients with moderate or moderate to severe CI (aged hamsters). The experimental cycle (time from infection to complete recovery) in hamsters, like that in mice, is relatively short (not more than 2 weeks). The production of neutralizing antibodies to SARS-CoV-2 antigens is another advantage of this model, which is supported by the possibility of indirect virus transmission.

Carnivora

Ferrets

Ferrets are another model for studies of human viral respiratory diseases, as these animals are susceptible to some human viruses, including influenza [29], respiratory syncytial and SARS-CoV viruses [30,31]. A major advantage of ferrets is that the structure of their respiratory system is similar to that of humans, and, consequently, can develop similar clinical symptoms of the disease. Furthermore, considering the presence of a form of ACE2 receptor compatible to SARS-CoV [32], the use of these animals for modeling CI is certainly relevant. Kim et al. [2] and Richard et al. [9] have shown that intranasal challenge of adult ferrets with SARS-CoV-2 ($\sim 2.2 \times 10^5$ and $\sim 4.2 \times 10^5$ PFU, respectively) results in viral replication and transmission, as well as antibody production. Virus replication peaked on days 3–4, and declined by days 7–9 postinfection. An insignificant number of SARS-CoV-2 RNA copies were also detected in the intestine of all the infected ferrets. As it was demonstrated by Kim et al. [2], the level of viral replication was higher in the nasal turbinates than in the lungs

(3.83 Log10 TCID50/mL and two Log10 TCID50/mL); the symptoms of infection were represented by fever (up to 40.3°C) and cough, typical for this disease. Pulmonary pathology includes lymphoplasmacytic perivasculitis and vasculitis, type II pneumocyte hyperplasia, macrophages, neutrophils in alveolar septa and lumen, and mild peribronchitis. There was a clear correlation between severity of symptoms and the age of ferrets [33] 3-year old animals showed higher viral loads in lung, longer nasal virus shedding (up to 7–9 days postinfection) compared to juvenile (≤6 months) and young adult (1–2 years) groups. Additionally, those animals showed gastrointestinal involvement, the viral copy number in rectal swabs peaked at day 4 postinfection and was almost 4.0 Log10/mL. Transcriptome analysis of aged ferret lungs revealed amelioration of gene sets related to IFN-I, macrophage (M1) and activated T-cell responses.

Successful virus transmission is one of the significant advantages of these animals. Both studies have shown that SARS-CoV-2 can be successfully transmitted directly (cocaged animals) and indirectly (animals housed separately). With direct transmission, RNA was plated from the upper respiratory and gastrointestinal tracts, followed by serum antibody production. Indirect transmission was also revealed the presence of viral RNA in the examined organs, with a slightly delayed peak of replication and lower antibody values.

Despite the explicit advantage of ferrets in terms of analyzing virus transmission, CI modeling is limited to a mild course of infection and a relatively low viral load in the lungs of infected animals. In addition, the complexity of ferrets housing makes them less attractive compared to small rodents.

Modeling of COVID-19 infection, nonhuman primates

Nonhuman primates are a natural reservoir for many infectious diseases. These animals are particularly useful for testing the safety and efficacy of drugs in the prevention and treatment a variety of infectious disease, including Zika fever [34], Ebola [35] and the novel CI caused by SARS-CoV-2 [12]. The data obtained on these animals require minimum correction when extrapolated to humans. However, the experiments themselves are expensive, and the sample size is limited by ethical issues. Moreover, nonhuman primates are not suitable for the generation of transgenic and knockout strains [36].

Rhesus macaques

Rhesus macaques are suitable for investigating SARS-CoV-2 pathogenesis, interactions between virus and the immune system and testing drug and vaccine candidates. These animals exhibited clinical signs of CI including fatigue, weight loss, and irregular breathing patterns [37,38]. In all studies, the animals were infected via different routes (predominantly the intranasal or intratracheal route with $\sim 10^{5-6}$ PFU) and no lethal cases were reported.

Rapid SARS-CoV-2 reproduction was detected in both the upper and the lower respiratory tract, peaking on days 1–2 post-infection. However, Yu J. and Deng W. [39,40] did not observe viremia in infected animals ($\sim 10^{4-5}$ PFU), which can be possibly explained by a lower virus dose.

Pathomorphological changes in the lungs included multifocal lesions and the development of mild or moderate interstitial pneumonia. Thickening of alveolar septa, accumulation of inflammatory exudate and cell infiltration into the inflammation site (mainly macrophages and neutrophils) were also observed. Like in other animal species, SARS-CoV-2 caused more severe interstitial pneumonia in old monkeys than that in young macaques [41].

Singh et al. [12] have demonstrated that all animals developed clinical signs of infection (1.05×10^6 PFU), including an increased plasma level of CRP, accompanied with the decline of red and white blood cells count. Moreover, histomorphological analysis revealed a prompt $CD4^+$ and $CD8^+$ T cell migration in lungs coupled with abnormal expression of their markers. It showed low expression of the CD69 marker (the early T cell activation antigen), CXCR3 and CCR7 receptors, as well as HLA-DR proteins, whereas the level of T cells expressing the downregulated proteins (PD-1 and LAG-3) was significantly increased, indicating alterations in the antigen presentation process during SARS-CoV-2 infection. The identified abnormalities may prompt the development of new treatment strategies against CI. Furthermore, the involvement of IFN-I and T cells in the CI resolution is consistent with the paper published by Sun et al. [17], where *STAT1*$^{-}$/$^{-}$ mice demonstrated the most pronounced infection symptoms.

Two studies [38,42] in rhesus macaques reported a transient stress leukogram by 1 day postinfection, transient neutropenia and early-onset repression of red cell indices that did not return to original baseline by day 21 postinfection. Another study revealed transient lymphopenia in *Macaca fascicularis* and *Macaca mulatta* [43].

Neutralizing antibodies in these models appear by 10–14 days postinfection. Moreover, antibodies subsequently protected the animals from repeated infection [39].

No data suggesting direct SARS-CoV-2 transmission for these animals had been published when this chapter was being prepared, but, given the similarity of CI signs and symptoms to those occurring in humans, it can be assumed that the virus can be successfully transmitted from animal to animal.

Experiments with SARS-CoV-2 infection had also been performed on other representatives of nonhuman primates [11,12]. Woolsey et al. [11] have shown that green monkeys are sensitive to a combined viral challenge (5×10^5 PFU): the high level of virus replication was followed by tissue lesions in the lungs. The pathomorphological signs of acute interstitial pneumonia included inflammatory exudate, hemorrhage, edema, and diffuse lesion together with hyaline membranes on day 5 postinfection. Tissue hypertrophy similar to cryptogenic organizing pneumonia was detected at the ends of the respiratory tract.

Moreover, the course of CI was accompanied by a shift in leukocyte subsets, as well as mild thrombocytopenia and elevated serum inflammatory markers, indicating a systemic response to the pathogen. Although the production of antibodies started as early as on day 5 postinfection, no pronounced clinical symptoms were observed in these animals, except for loss of appetite and fatigue [44].

The CI induced in baboons with a combined challenge (1.05×10^6 PFU) was similar to its course in the green monkey (1.05×10^6 PFU): high level of viral replication in the upper and lower respiratory tract, body weight loss, interstitial pneumonia with typical cell infiltration in the alveolar septa, fibrosis, accumulation of histiocytes, and neutrophils in the alveolar lumens. The animals developed bronchitis and mild tracheitis.

Marmosets proved to be the least sensitive to the infection (8.8×10^5 PFU), demonstrating low viral replication in the upper respiratory tract. The pathomorphological changes observed in the lung tissue were described as mild.

The use of nonhuman primates, like any other species, for CI modeling has a number of advantages, the most important of which is the similarity of the animals' immune system to that of the human and, consequently, the development of similar symptoms of the infection.

However, aside from the obvious ethical and technical issues with primates studies, it should be taken into account that the molecular mimicry between the viral and host proteins in case of primates differs from that in infected humans. For example, these animals have a wider variety of MHC genes compared to humans [45]. The identity of protein sequences between the virus and the host can have a considerable impact on the extent of immune response and risk of autoimmune complications, which is especially critical in vaccine development [46,47].

Modeling postacute COVID-19 infection (long covid), rodents

According to the WHO, Long COVID is a condition that occurs in individuals with a history of probable or confirmed SARS-CoV-2 infection, usually 3 months from the onset of COVID-19 symptoms and that lasts for at least 2 months and cannot be explained by an alternative diagnosis [48].

The mechanisms contributing to the appearance and development of Long COVID are largely unknown. However, there are two main theories: (1) virus-specific pathophysiologic changes and (2) a potential auto-immune contribution, which is based on reports of a small number of patients who have developed autoimmune diseases after COVID-19 infection [49]. Interestingly, the majority of COVID-19 sequelae, such as fatigue, joint and chest pain, shortness of breath, rapid or irregular heartbeat, headaches, memory issues, anxiety, and depression, overlap with the symptoms of autoimmune diseases.

The immunological changes associated with COVID-19 and especially with postacute phase of the disease are largely unknown and require further research. Nevertheless, some articles claim significant alternations in B and T cell subsets [50], lymphopenia [51] as well as an elevated levels of cytokines (in particular, IL-6, IFN-γ, IFN-λ, MCP-1 (CCL2) and VCAM-1) in blood plasma of survived patients [52]. The interesting fact is that the alterations in B-cell subsets are largely restored upon convalescence, while alterations in T cells may be present up to 6 months. The study performed by Shuwa et al. [50] revealed an elevated proportion of T effector memory cells positive for CD45RA, a higher level of $CD8^+$ T cells with cytotoxic program and enhanced level of Th1 cytokines produced by $CD4^+$and $CD8^+$ lymphocytes [50]. In another study [53], authors also showed a specific cellular immunity to SARS-CoV-2 with the predominant cytotoxic response mediated by $CD8^+$– and weaker $CD4^+$T lymphocyte response (in 34% of Long COVID patients, $CD4^+$ cell counts were lower).

We believe that a more comprehensive understanding of post-COVID side effects is essential for developing more effective prevention, diagnosis, and treatment measures. In this respect valid animal models of Long COVID-19 (post-COVID syndrome) are strongly required. Little is known about the postacute phase of SARS-CoV-2 in animals and there are a number of questions that need to be answered/investigated: (1) Do animals develop the state similar to Long COVID? (2) What are the pathological and immunological features of Long COVID in animals? (3) How do these abnormalities change over time? And finally, what is the best time frame to evaluate these aberrations?

Now there are two approaches to the development of Long COVID animal models, which correspond to different aspects of its pathogenesis: (1) the classical infectious model and (2) the autoimmune model using autoantibodies. The first concept is already supported by some (however, rather small and controversial) experimental evidence described below.

Summarizing the clinical research data of post-COVID patients, we believe that lymphopenia, the level of inflammatory cytokines, as well as differences in immune cell phenotype can be used as immunological markers of Long COVID in animals. C-reactive protein (CRP) and D-dimer levels, which are increased in COVID-19 patients with pneumonia may be also of interest. However, in a study [54] that published the results of postacute phase of the SARS-CoV-2 infection in rhesus and cynomolgus macaques authors did not find changes in CRP level. Although, there was a significant difference in animal's activity, influencing the health status of the macaques. It should be also mentioned that authors observed an increase in IL-6 levels at the end of the study in some individuals.

The kinetic of post-COVID symptoms in animals is undetermined, anyway, we should keep in mind that mice and hamsters, for example, get sick very quickly and the peak of infection occurs (depending on the strain) on day 2–4 postinfection. In this respect, we suggest to focus on more mild infection in order to get more information about what may be happening in a postacute phase of infection. However, it is still unknown how long this recovery phase lasts. Winkler et al. (2021) showed a markedly decreased number of B cells, $CD4^+$– and $CD8^+$T cells, together with monocytes in peripheral blood at 5 days postinfection even in mice receiving a nonlethal dose of virus, which is a rather promising finding.

The multiorgan damage demonstrated in hamsters after the CI, together with the cytokine response in lungs, makes these animals also valuable for the investigation of the prolonged disease in people with complications after the infection; however, the immune response in this study was accelerated by high viral dose [7]. Nouailles G. and colleagues [55] found that the infected hamsters displayed significant leukopenia at 3 and 5 days postinfection. Increased proportion of neutrophils was found at 2 days postinfection together with the increasing proportion of T cells at day 14 postinfection. Notably, calculated neutrophil-lymphocyte ratios are matching with the observations in humans with nonsevere as opposed to severe COVID-19 [56]. By day 14 postinfection, hamsters recovered with the resolution of the majority symptoms.

Therefore, we can conclude that Syrian hamsters and ACE2 mice are the most suitable species for experimental purposes, despite the variety of the described in vivo models of the SARS-CoV-2-induced acute respiratory syndrome. The animals are affordable, and the CI model is easily reproduced, with reliable and valid results. By using different animal strains, genders and ages as well as different challenge routes doses and viral strains, it is possible to reproduce both mild and moderate infection, where the side effects of COVID infection (Lond COVID) might be investigated. The ability to reproduce cytokine storm in the lung and blood abnormalities is another advantage for both of these species. What is more important, the mechanisms underlying these pathophysiological aspects can be well extrapolated to the clinic.

The production of neutralizing antibodies also makes these animals suitable for vaccine testing. Due to the high affinity of their ACE2 receptor to SARS-CoV-2 and the possibility of direct virus transmission from animal to animal, hamsters can be used in studies of the rapid spread of the infection.

Therefore, the choice of a certain animal species should primarily be based on the study aims and objectives.

Acknowledgments

Original Russian Text Petrova N.V., Ganina K.K., Tarasov S.A. Susceptability of experimental animals to SARS-CoV-2 (Coronaviridae: Coronavirinae: Betacoronavirus; Sarbecovirus) infection. 2021, published in Voprosy Virusologii Journal (in Russian), 2021, 66(2): 103–111, https://doi.org/10.36233/0507-4088-47.

References

[1] Imai M, Iwatsuki-Horimoto K, Hatta M, et al. Syrian hamsters as a small animal model for SARS-CoV-2 infection and countermeasure development. Proc Natl Acad Sci USA 2020;117(28):16587–95. https://doi.org/10.1073/pnas.2009799117.
[2] Kim YI, Kim SG, Kim SM, et al. Infection and rapid transmission of SARS-CoV-2 in ferrets. Cell Host Microbe 2020;27(5):704–9. https://doi.org/10.1016/j.chom.2020.03.023. e2.
[3] Bao L, Deng W, Huang B, et al. The pathogenicity of SARS-CoV-2 in hACE2 transgenic mice. Nature 2020;583(7818):830–3. https://doi.org/10.1038/s41586-020-2312-y.
[4] Chan JF, Zhang AJ, Yuan S, et al. Simulation of the clinical and pathological manifestations of Coronavirus Disease 2019 (COVID-19) in golden Syrian hamster model: implications for disease pathogenesis and transmissibility. Clin Infect Dis 2020;71(9):2428–46. https://doi.org/10.1093/cid/ciaa325.
[5] Winkler ES, Bailey AL, Kafai NM, et al. SARS-CoV-2 infection of human ACE2-transgenic mice causes severe lung inflammation and impaired function. Nat Immunol 2020;21(11):1327–35. https://doi.org/10.1038/s41590-020-0778-2.
[6] Yinda CK, Port JR, Bushmaker T, et al. K18-hACE2 mice develop respiratory disease resembling severe COVID-19. PLOS One 2021;17. https://doi.org/10.1101/2020.08.11.246314.
[7] Francis ME, Goncin U, Kroeker A, et al. SARS-CoV-2 infection in the Syrian hamster model causes inflammation as well as type I interferon dysregulation in both respiratory and non-respiratory tissues including the heart and kidney. PLoS Pathog 2021;17(7):e1009705. https://doi.org/10.1371/journal.ppat.1009705.
[8] Sia SF, Yan LM, Chin AWH, et al. Pathogenesis and transmission of SARS-CoV-2 in golden hamsters. Nature 2020;583:834–8. https://doi.org/10.1038/s41586-020-2342-5.
[9] Richard M, Kok A, de Meulder D, et al. SARS-CoV-2 is transmitted via contact and via the air between ferrets. Nat Commun 2020;11(1):3496. https://doi.org/10.1038/s41467-020-17367-2.
[10] Shan C, Yao YF, Yang XL, et al. Infection with novel coronavirus (SARS-CoV-2) causes pneumonia in Rhesus macaques. Cell Res 2020;30:670–7. https://doi.org/10.1038/s41422-020-0364-z.
[11] Woolsey C, Borisevich V, Prasad AN, et al. Establishment of an African green monkey model for COVID-19. bioRxiv 2020. https://doi.org/10.1101/2020.05.17.100289.
[12] Singh DK, Shashank R. Ganatra and Bindu Singh et al. SARS-CoV-2 infection leads to acute infection with dynamic cellular and inflammatory flux in the lung that varies across nonhuman primate species. bioRxiv 2020. https://doi.org/10.1101/2020.06.05.136481. 2020.06.05.136481.
[13] Muñoz-Fontela C, Dowling WE, Funnell SGP, et al. Animal models for COVID-19. Nature 2020;586(7830):509–15. https://doi.org/10.1038/s41586-020-2787-6.
[14] Li W, Greenough TC, Moore MJ, et al. Efficient replication of severe acute respiratory syndrome coronavirus in mouse cells is limited by murine angiotensin-converting enzyme 2. J Virol 2004;78(20):11429–33. https://doi.org/10.1128/JVI.78.20.11429-11433.2004.
[15] Linlin Bao HG, Deng W, Qi L, et al. Transmission of severe acute respiratory syndrome coronavirus 2 via close contact and respiratory droplets among human angiotensin-converting enzyme 2 mice. J Infect Dis 2020;222(4):551–5. https://doi.org/10.1093/infdis/jiaa281.
[16] Sun SH, Chen Q, Gu HJ, et al. A mouse model of SARS-CoV-2 infection and pathogenesis. Cell Host Microbe 2020;28(1):124–33. https://doi.org/10.1016/j.chom.2020.05.020. e4.
[17] Sun J, Zhuang Z, Zheng J, et al. Generation of a broadly useful model for COVID-19 pathogenesis, vaccination, and treatment. Cell 2020;182(3):734–43. https://doi.org/10.1016/j.cell.2020.06.010. e5.

[18] Golden JW, Cline CR, Zeng X, et al. Human angiotensin-converting enzyme 2 transgenic mice infected with SARS-CoV-2 develop severe and fatal respiratory disease. JCI Insight 2020;5(19):e142032. https://doi.org/10.1172/jci.insight.142032.

[19] Jiang RD, Liu MQ, Chen Y, et al. Pathogenesis of SARS-CoV-2 in transgenic mice expressing human angiotensin-converting enzyme 2. Cell 2020;182(1):50–8. https://doi.org/10.1016/j.cell.2020.05.027. e8.

[20] Oladunni FS, Park JG, Pino PA, et al. Lethality of SARS-CoV-2 infection in K18 human angiotensin-converting enzyme 2 transgenic mice. Nat Commun 2020;11(1):6122. https://doi.org/10.1038/s41467-020-19891-7.

[21] Huang C, Wang Y, Li X, et al. Clinical features of patients infected with 2019 novel coronavirus in Wuhan, China. Lancet 2020;395(10223):497–506. https://doi.org/10.1016/S0140-6736(20)30183-5.

[22] Osterrieder N, Bertzbach LD, Dietert K, et al. Age-Dependent progression of SARS-CoV-2 infection in Syrian hamsters. Viruses 2020;12(7). https://doi.org/10.3390/v12070779.

[23] Rosenke K, Meade-White K, Letko M, et al. Defining the Syrian hamster as a highly susceptible preclinical model for SARS-CoV-2 infection. Emerg Microb Infect 2020;9(1):2673–84. https://doi.org/10.1080/22221751.2020.1858177.

[24] Selvaraj P, Lien CZ, Liu S, et al. SARS-CoV-2 infection induces protective immunity and limits transmission in Syrian hamsters. Life Sci Alliance 2021;4(4). https://doi.org/10.26508/lsa.202000886.

[25] Rogers TF, Zhao F, Huang D, et al. Isolation of potent SARS-CoV-2 neutralizing antibodies and protection from disease in a small animal model. Science 2020;369(6506):956–63. https://doi.org/10.1126/science.abc7520.

[26] Boudewijns RTH, Kaptein SJF. STAT2 signaling as double-edged sword restricting viral dissemination but driving severe pneumonia in SARS-CoV-2 infected hamsters. bioRxiv 2020. https://doi.org/10.1101/2020.04.23.056838. 2020.04.23.056838.

[27] Jafarzadeh A, Nemati M, Saha B, Bansode YD, Jafarzadeh S. Protective potentials of type III interferons in COVID-19 patients: lessons from differential properties of type I- and III interferons. Viral Immunol 2021;34(5):307–20. https://doi.org/10.1089/vim.2020.0076.

[28] Feld JJ, Kandel C, Biondi MJ, et al. Peginterferon lambda for the treatment of outpatients with COVID-19: a phase 2, placebo-controlled randomised trial. Lancet Respir Med 2021;9(5):498–510. https://doi.org/10.1016/S2213-2600(20)30566-X.

[29] Zitzow LA, Rowe T, Morken T, Shieh WJ, Zaki S, Katz JM. Pathogenesis of avian influenza A (H5N1) viruses in ferrets. J Virol 2002;76(9):4420–9. https://doi.org/10.1128/jvi.76.9.4420-4429.2002.

[30] Martina BE, Haagmans BL, Kuiken T, et al. SARS virus infection of cats and ferrets. Nature 2003;425(6961):915. https://doi.org/10.1038/425915a.

[31] Weingartl H, Czub M, Czub S, et al. Immunization with modified vaccinia virus Ankara-based recombinant vaccine against severe acute respiratory syndrome is associated with enhanced hepatitis in ferrets. J Virol 2004;78(22):12672–6. https://doi.org/10.1128/JVI.78.22.12672-12676.2004.

[32] Wan Y, Shang J, Graham R, Baric RS, Li F. Receptor recognition by the novel coronavirus from Wuhan: an analysis based on decade-long structural studies of SARS coronavirus. J Virol 2020;94(7). https://doi.org/10.1128/JVI.00127-20.

[33] Kim YI, Yu KM, Koh JY, et al. Age-dependent pathogenic characteristics of SARS-CoV-2 infection in ferrets. Res Sq 2021;13:1–13. https://doi.org/10.21203/rs.3.rs-131380/v2. rs.3.rs-131380.

[34] Aid M, Abbink P, Larocca RA, et al. Zika virus persistence in the central nervous system and lymph nodes of rhesus monkeys. Cell 2017;169(4):610–20. https://doi.org/10.1016/j.cell.2017.04.008. e14.

[35] Nakayama E, Saijo M. Animal models for Ebola and Marburg virus infections. Front Microbiol 2013;4:267. https://doi.org/10.3389/fmicb.2013.00267.

[36] Estes JD, Wong SW, Brenchley JM. Nonhuman primate models of human viral infections. Nat Rev Immunol 2018;18(6):390–404. https://doi.org/10.1038/s41577-018-0005-7.

[37] Williamson BN, Feldmann F, Schwarz B, et al. Clinical benefit of remdesivir in rhesus macaques infected with SARS-CoV-2. bioRxiv 2020. https://doi.org/10.1101/2020.04.15.043166. 2020.04.15.043166.

[38] Munster VJ, Feldmann F, Williamson BN, et al. Respiratory disease in rhesus macaques inoculated with SARS-CoV-2. Nature 2020;585(7824):268–72. https://doi.org/10.1038/s41586-020-2324-7.

[39] Deng W, Bao L, Liu J, et al. Primary exposure to SARS-CoV-2 protects against reinfection in rhesus macaques. Science 2020;369(6505):818–23. https://doi.org/10.1126/science.abc5343.

[40] Yu J, Tostanoski LH, Peter L, et al. DNA vaccine protection against SARS-CoV-2 in rhesus macaques. Science 2020;369(6505):806–11. https://doi.org/10.1126/science.abc6284.

[41] Yu P, Qi F, Xu Y, et al. Age-related rhesus macaque models of COVID-19. Animal Model Exp Med 2020;3(1):93–7. https://doi.org/10.1002/ame2.12108.

[42] Hasenkrug KJ, Feldmann F, Myers L, et al. Recovery from acute SARS-CoV-2 infection and development of anamnestic immune responses in T cell-depleted rhesus macaques. bioRxiv 2021. https://doi.org/10.1101/2021.04.02.438262. 2021.04.02.438262.

[43] Koo BS, Oh H, Kim G, et al. Transient lymphopenia and interstitial pneumonia with endotheliitis in SARS-CoV-2-infected macaques. J Infect Dis 2020;222(10):1596–600. https://doi.org/10.1093/infdis/jiaa486.

[44] Böszörményi KP, Stammes MA, Fagrouch ZC, et al. Comparison of SARS-CoV-2 infection in two non-human primate species: rhesus and cynomolgus macaques. bioRxiv 2020. https://doi.org/10.1101/2020.11.05.369413. 2020.11.05.369413.

[45] Heijmans CMC, de Groot NG, Bontrop RE. Comparative genetics of the major histocompatibility complex in humans and nonhuman primates. Int J Immunogenet 2020;47(3):243–60. https://doi.org/10.1111/iji.12490.

[46] Kanduc D, Shoenfeld Y. Molecular mimicry between SARS-CoV-2 spike glycoprotein and mammalian proteomes: implications for the vaccine. Immunol Res 2020;68(5):310–3. https://doi.org/10.1007/s12026-020-09152-6.

[47] Kanduc D, Shoenfeld Y. On the molecular determinants of the SARS-CoV-2 attack. Clin Immunol 2020;215:108426. https://doi.org/10.1016/j.clim.2020.108426.

[48] WHO. A clinical case definition of post COVID-19 condition by a Delphi consensus. October 6 , 2021. November 12, 2021, https://www.who.int/publications/i/item/WHO-2019-nCoV-Post_COVID-19_condition-Clinical_case_definition-2021.1.

[49] Ehrenfeld M, Tincani A, Andreoli L, et al. Covid-19 and autoimmunity. Autoimmun Rev 2020;19(8):102597. https://doi.org/10.1016/j.autrev.2020.102597.

[50] Shuwa HA, Shaw TN, Knight SB, et al. Alterations in T and B cell function persist in convalescent COVID-19 patients. Med (NY) 2021;2(6):720–35. https://doi.org/10.1016/j.medj.2021.03.013. e4.

[51] Varghese J, Sandmann S, Ochs K, et al. Persistent symptoms and lab abnormalities in patients who recovered from COVID-19. Sci Rep 2021;11(1):12775. https://doi.org/10.1038/s41598-021-91270-8.

[52] Phetsouphanh C, Darley D, Wilson DB, et al. Immunological dysfunction persists for 8 months following initial mild-moderate SARS-CoV-2 infection. medRxiv 2021. https://doi.org/10.1101/2021.06.01.21257759. 2021.06.01.257759.

[53] Montes N, Domenech È, Guerrero S, Oliván-Blázquez B, Magallón-Botaya R. Analysis of cell-mediated immunity in people with long COVID. medRxiv 2021. https://doi.org/10.1101/2021.06.09.21258553. 2021.06.09.21258553.

[54] Böszörményi KP, Stammes MA, Fagrouch ZC, et al. The post-acute phase of SARS-CoV-2 infection in two macaque species is associated with signs of ongoing virus replication and pathology in pulmonary and extrapulmonary tissues. Viruses 2021;13(8). https://doi.org/10.3390/v13081673.

[55] Nouailles G, Wyler E, Pennitz P, et al. Temporal omics analysis in Syrian hamsters unravel cellular effector responses to moderate COVID-19. Nat Commun 2021;12(1):4869. https://doi.org/10.1038/s41467-021-25030-7.

[56] Liu J, Li S, Liang B, et al. Longitudinal characteristics of lymphocyte responses and cytokine profiles in the peripheral blood of SARS-CoV-2 infected patients. EBioMedicine 2020;55:102763. https://doi.org/10.1016/j.ebiom.2020.102763.

[57] Rathnasinghe R, Strohmeier S, Amanat F, et al. Comparison of transgenic and adenovirus hACE2 mouse models for SARS-CoV-2 infection. bioRxiv 2020. https://doi.org/10.1101/2020.07.06.190066. 2020.07.06.190066.

[58] Moreau GB, Burgess SL, Sturek JM, Donlan AN, Petri WA, Mann BJ. Evaluation of K18-. Am J Trop Med Hyg 2020;103(3):1215–9. https://doi.org/10.4269/ajtmh.20-0762.

[59] Liu FL, Wu K, Sun J, et al. Rapid generation of ACE2 humanized inbred mouse model for COVID-19 with tetraploid complementation. Natl Sci Rev 2021;8(2). https://doi.org/10.1093/nsr/nwaa285. nwaa285.

[60] Leist SR, Dinnon KH, Schäfer A, et al. A mouse-adapted SARS-CoV-2 induces acute lung injury and mortality in standard laboratory mice. Cell 2020;183(4):1070–85. https://doi.org/10.1016/j.cell.2020.09.050. e12.

[61] Muruato A, Vu MN, Johnson BA, et al. Mouse adapted SARS-CoV-2 protects animals from lethal SARS-CoV challenge. bioRxiv 2021. https://doi.org/10.1101/2021.05.03.442357. 2021.05.03.442357.

[62] Montagutelli X, Prot M, Jouvion G, et al. A mouse-adapted SARS-CoV-2 strain replicating in standard laboratory mice. bioRxiv 2021. https://doi.org/10.1101/2021.07.10.451880. 2021.07.10.451880.

[63] Everett HE, Lean FZX, Byrne AMP, et al. Intranasal infection of ferrets with SARS-CoV-2 as a model for asymptomatic human infection. Viruses 2021;13(1). https://doi.org/10.3390/v13010113.

[64] Patel DR, Field CJ, Septer KM, et al. Transmission and protection against reinfection in the ferret model with the SARS-CoV-2 USA-WA1/2020 reference isolate. J Virol 2021;95(13). https://doi.org/10.1128/JVI.02232-20. e0223220.

[65] Shi J, Wen Z, Zhong G, et al. Susceptibility of ferrets, cats, dogs, and other domesticated animals to SARS–coronavirus 2. Science 2020;368(6494):1016–20. https://doi.org/10.1126/science.abb7015.

[66] Tian JH, Patel N, Haupt R, et al. SARS-CoV-2 spike glycoprotein vaccine candidate NVX-CoV2373 immunogenicity in baboons and protection in mice. Nat Commun 2021;12(1):372. https://doi.org/10.1038/s41467-020-20653-8.

[67] Kozlovskaya LI, Piniaeva AN, Ignatyev GM, et al. Long-term humoral immunogenicity, safety and protective efficacy of inactivated vaccine against COVID-19 (CoviVac) in preclinical studies. Emerg Microb Infect 2021;10(1):1790–806. https://doi.org/10.1080/22221751.2021.1971569.

[68] Johnston SC, Ricks KM, Jay A, et al. Development of a coronavirus disease 2019 nonhuman primate model using airborne exposure. PLoS One 2021;16(2). https://doi.org/10.1371/journal.pone.0246366. e0246366.

CHAPTER

32

Risk assessment for aerosol infection by SARS-CoV-2 and protection by respirators and surgical masks

Eitan Israeli

Zabludowicz Center for Autoimmune Diseases, Sheba Medical Center, Ramat Gan, Israel

Background

With the COVID 19 outbreak, different speculations were raised concerning routes of infection by the emerging SARS-CoV-2. At first the health authorities around the world declared that infection may be due to droplets emitted by coughing, talking, singing, or sneezing, which will settle upon mucus membranes of the nose, mouth, and eyes. The distance of dispersal from these routes was estimated to be up to 1.8 m, and hence the 2 m "safe" social distancing between people. In addition, public health services announced that infection may occur by touching contaminated surfaces and carrying the virus to mucus membranes. Indeed, the virus can survive on surfaces for hours to days, depending on climate conditions and the surface itself, and in theory infection can be achieved, but this route is not the main one. As for infections by inhaling microdroplet aerosols, the health authorities tended to down play its importance, and some even negated it completely for some reasons. Infection by microdroplets aerosols was proved in many infectious diseases, like influenza, measles, meningitis, brucellosis, anthrax to name a few, and most of the biological agents listed as potential bio terror agents. SARS-CoV-2 was added to this list.

What are the conditions for aerosol infection?

1. The biological agent must be carried in droplets smaller than 10 um, and preferably under 1–5 um in diameter. This size can circumvent upper respiratory barriers and reach the alveoli.

Autoimmunity, COVID-19, Post-COVID19 syndrome and COVID-19 vaccination
https://doi.org/10.1016/B978-0-443-18566-3.00030-X

2. Agent concentration in aerosol must be high enough, so that a human infectious dose will be absorbed. The higher the dose, the faster illness symptoms will develop and the sickness may be more severe.
3. The agent must retain its viability (infection capacity) in air, long enough until inhaled.
4. The host must have receptors on alveoli to enable attachment and internalization by lung cells.

If all these conditions are met, and infection will ensue, developing to disease which severity depends on the immune system of the exposed host, his physiology and general health.

How are these conditions pertain to SARS-CoV-2

1. Aerosols are generated during sneezing, coughing, singing, and even speaking. A sneeze discharges around one million droplets in a wide range of diameter, from 0.1 um to a few mm. The large ones may reach 1–1.8 m and settle quickly to the ground. By flash photography, only around 40,000 can be seen by the naked eye. The rest are around or smaller than 1 um. These microdroplets can reach a distance of 7–8 m, demonstrated and depicted by movie clips by Bourouiba [1]. The aerosol cloud velocity is between 10 and 30 m/s, and this phenomenon is called "turbulent gas cloud" which pushes the droplets as far as 8 m, and because of high concentration, the rate of evaporation slows down. In a closed room with no air movement, such aerosol stays in the air at least 20 min. Upon coughing or speaking the same mechanism of generating large range of droplets, but the common diameter and numbers are smaller.
2. **The infectious dose** in humans of this virus is still not known, but from animal experiments it is estimated to be around 100 PFU [2]. From exposure experiments of monkeys, macaque, and cynomolgus, the infection dose of 10^6–10^5 $TCID_{50}$ or PFU, respectively, was determined. In engineered mice that carry the human receptor ACE2, infection through the nose ensued at doses of 67–570 PFU, and with MERS above 100 PFU. Since SARS-CoV-2 has a higher R_0 factor, 2–4 times higher, it is logical to deduce that the human infectious dose is smaller, and to be on the safe side, a dose of 100 PFU will be used in calculations. In COVID-19 patients, the concentration of viral particles from nasal swabs or lung lavage yielded up to 10^8 RNA copies per ml. Assuming that one RNA copy is equal to 1 PFU, with multiplicity of infection of 1, and that a sneeze disperses 1 mL of fluid, than 10^8 infectious viral particles are disseminated through the air. Applying risk assessment methods, this number will occupy at the beginning 1 cubic m, with concentration of 10^5 viral particles or 1000 infectious doses per liter. A person at that space, who breathes 15 L of air per min during rest, will inhale 15,000 infectious doses. The above concentration will be diluted and lowered with distance, but at 8 m, a person will be exposed to a large number of infectious doses and of course will get sick.
3. **Virus viability in aerosols** is retained for at least 3 h, and median survival time was determined to be 2.7 h. The experiment was carried out at 22 C and 65% relative humidity [3]. The test was done with both SARS 1 and SARS-CoV-2 viruses, and viability was determined by cell culture infection.

4. **The specific receptors** for the SARS-CoV-2 were identified as ACE2, which are ubiquitous in many human tissues, including epithelial cells of the lung and alveoli [4,5]. In fact, 83% of ACE2 expressing cells are type II epithelial cells (ACEII).

Airborne transmission as the dominant route for the spread of COVID-19

According to the risk assessment elucidated above, it is logical and scientifically sound to conclude that airborne transmission is the main route of infection and spread of COVID-19. Indeed, Zhang et al. from Texas University and California Institute of Technology [6] showed that the airborne transmission route is highly virulent and dominant for the spread of COVID-19. Various mitigation measures have been implemented to fight the COVID-19 pandemic, including widely adopted social distancing and mandated face covering. By analyzing the trend and mitigation measures in Wuhan, China, Italy, and New York City, from January 23 to May 9, 2020, it was illustrated that the impacts of mitigation measures are discernible from the trends of the pandemic. The analysis revealed that the difference with and without mandated face covering represents the determinant in shaping the pandemic trends in the three epicenters. This protective measure alone significantly reduced the number of infections by over 75,000 in Italy from April 6 to May 9 and over 66,000 in New York City from April 17 to May 9. Other mitigation measures, such as social distancing implemented in the United States, are insufficient by themselves in protecting the public. The authors concluded that wearing of face masks in public corresponds to the most effective means to prevent interhuman transmission, and this inexpensive practice, in conjunction with simultaneous social distancing, quarantine, and contact tracing, represents the most likely fighting opportunity to stop the COVID-19 pandemic.

Masks and respirators for protection against airborne infection

Before the COVID-19 pandemic, masks or respiratory devices were used by medical staff or industry and laboratory employees, for protection against exposure to chemical or biological agents at the workplace. There are inherent differences between these devices in building materials, shapes and fit, and of course efficiency of stopping and retaining particles. All the respiratory protection devices used by the public and professional teams during this pandemic are designed to protect from particles (solid or fluid droplets), while gases and fumes go through them freely (unless there is an active carbon layer integrated within). N95 masks are considered the gold standard in personal protective equipment because they block at least 95% of large and small particles down to smaller than 0.1 um in diameter, utilizing physical properties of the filter material [6]. The physical mechanisms involved are impaction for large particles (above 1 um), electrostatic interception (for around 1 um), and diffusion due to Brownian motion (for under 0.1 um). The filter works by trapping particles like bacteria and viruses before they pass through the mask, protecting the wearer and those around them. The N95 mask, which costs roughly $5, also fits securely to the face, eliminating most of the leakage that may occur with a loose-fitting cloth or paper mask. Surgical masks are simpler in design, usually built from three layers of polypropylene, block only 50% of airborne particles at the most, and do not provide good seal around the face. There is a "new" product in the markets called "surgical N95 respirator," a name for FDA-approved N95 respirators for use in surgery and other medical scenarios. It includes an outer fluid repelling layer, tested against synthetic blood jet. This test simulates arterial blood spill during surgery or other invasive actions. Surgical masks are single use devices. N95 are meant for single use, but in time of shortage during the pandemic, the CDC allowed reuse, provided that the respirator is intact and clean, and was set aside safely for a few days to eliminate viable microorganisms. As an alternative method, sterilization of N95 respirators was carried out by exposure to UV light, oxygen peroxide vapors, or high temperatures, with different degrees of success. The most simple and less effective are cloth masks, manufactured from variety of woven or nonwoven fabrics, such as cotton or synthetic blends. Their efficiency is between 26% and 80% depending on fabric type and number of layers. The more the layers, the greater the blocking efficiency. These masks can be washed and reused. Another personal protective device recommended by health authorities in addition to respiratory ones are face shields. Those are transparent single or multiple use devices, warn above the respirators, instead or in addition to safety glasses, and cover the whole face, protecting all the mucus membranes from splashes. They also protect the respirators and keep them clean for reuse if necessary.

SARS-CoV-2 transmission and infection with or without masks in closed places and the home

There are many examples demonstrating infections due to lack of respiratory protection, some of them well documented and investigated. Szabelwski et al. [7] from the center of disease control and prevention (CDC) investigated mass infections in an overnight camp in Georgia. The camp administration obeyed most of CDC guidelines, including polymerase chain reaction (PCR)-negative corona test 12 days before coming to camp, but failed to enforce mask wearing among the children. After one staff member had symptoms and left, the camp was closed. Among 597 people attending the camp, 76% were found to be positive to the virus, and overall attack rate was 44%. The researchers followed the households of the infected children and studied transmission of virus to others in the home. Chu et al. [8] interviewed 224 children of whom 88% had symptoms, and 526 household members. About 76% of household members contracted the disease from the children. The investigation proved that only 34% of the sick children used masks, and the highest rate of infection was in those homes. In homes where infections occurred, half the members contracted the disease. Again, these findings prove the importance of masks and distancing in preventing infections in closed places.

The risk of SARS-CoV-2 transmission from patients to hospital roommates

Karan et al. [9] assessed SARS-CoV-2 transmission between patients in shared rooms in an academic hospital between September 2020 and April 2021. In total, 11,290 patients were admitted to shared rooms, of whom 25 tested positive. Among 31 exposed roommates, 12 (39%) tested positive within 14 days. Transmission was associated with PCR cycle thresholds ≤21. Beds in the shared rooms were separated by 1.8 m, curtains were hung between them and there were six air changes per hour. These findings point to aerosol transmission and the authors therefore recommended enforcing mask wearing until receiving a negative result.

Universal masking in a health care system and SARS-CoV-2 infection among healthcare workers (HCW)

Mass General Brigham (MGB) is the largest healthcare system in Massachusetts, with 12 hospitals and more than 75,000 employees. In March 2020, MGB implemented a multipronged infection reduction strategy involving systematic testing of symptomatic HCWs and universal masking of all HCWs and patients with surgical masks [10]. This study assessed the association of hospital masking policies with the SARS-CoV-2 infection rate among HCWs. Of 9850 tested HCWs, 1271 (12.9%) had positive results for SARS-CoV-2. During the preintervention period, the SARS-CoV-2 positivity rate increased exponentially from 0% to 21.32%, with a weighted mean increase of 1.16% per day and a case doubling time of 3.6 days (95% CI, 3.0–4.5 days). During the intervention period, the positivity rate decreased linearly from 14.65% to 11.46%, with a weighted mean decline of 0.49% per day and a net slope change of 1.65% (95% CI, 1.13%–2.15%; $P < .001$) more decline per day compared with the pre intervention period. Universal masking at MGB was associated with a significantly lower rate of SARS-CoV-2 positivity among HCWs. This association may be related to a decrease in transmission between patients and HCWs and among HCWs. The decrease in HCW infections could be confounded by other interventions inside and outside of the healthcare system, such as restrictions on elective procedures, social distancing measures, and increased masking in public spaces, which are limitations of this study. Despite these local and statewide measures, the case number continued to increase in Massachusetts throughout the study period, suggesting that the decrease in the SARS-CoV-2 positivity rate in MGB HCWs took place before the decrease in the general public. Randomized trials of universal masking of HCWs during a pandemic are likely not feasible. Nonetheless, these results support universal masking as part of a multipronged infection reduction strategy in healthcare settings.

Effectivity of face masks in limiting particle dissemination and the probability of SARS-CoV-2 transmission

The effectiveness of masks in preventing the transmission of severe acute respiratory syndrome coronavirus 2 has been debated since the beginning of the COVID-19 pandemic. One important question is whether masks are effective despite the forceful expulsion of respiratory matter during coughing and sneezing. Cheng et al. [11] convincingly show that most people live in conditions in which the airborne virus load is low. The probability of infection changes nonlinearly with the amount of respiratory matter to which a person is exposed. If most people in the wider community wear even simple surgical masks, then the probability of an encounter with a virus particle is even further limited. In indoor settings, it is impossible to avoid breathing in air that someone else has exhaled, and in hospital situations where the virus concentration is the highest, even the best-performing masks used without other protective gear such as hazmat suits will not provide adequate protection. Protection efficiency will improve by combining additional measures, including social distancing and high ventilation in closed spaces. The article includes graphs and useful calculations for risk assessment and infections in different scenarios of virus air concentrations, as well as donning of protective equipment. Of special interest are the graphs depicting substantial dissemination of microparticles from the air-ways while wearing masks, upon sneezing, coughing or speaking, while upon regular breathing the masks prevent such dissemination. It is important to stress, that surgical masks fell short not by much from N95 respirators, in preventing particles dissemination. However, from the point of view, the wearer, N95 protection efficiency is more than 95%, while for surgical masks the number is between 6% and 50%.

Masks for prevention of respiratory viral infections

Chou et al. examined multiple electronic databases in order to determine the effectiveness of N95, surgical, and cloth masks in community and healthcare settings for preventing respiratory virus infections, and effects of reuse or extended use of N95 masks [12]. Randomized trials of masks and risk for respiratory virus infection, including SARS-CoV-2, and observational studies of mask use and coronavirus infection risk were included. 39 studies (18 randomized controlled trials and 21 observational studies; 33,867 participants) were included. The data showed that:

1. No study evaluated reuse or extended use of N95 masks.
2. Evidence on SARS-CoV-2 was limited to two observational studies with serious limitations.
3. Community mask use was possibly associated with decreased risk for SARS-CoV-1 infection in observational studies.
4. In high- or moderate-risk healthcare settings, observational studies found that risk for infection with SARS-CoV-1 and middle east respiratory syndrome coronavirus probably decreased with mask use versus nonuse and possibly decreased with N95 versus surgical mask use.
5. Randomized trials in community settings found possibly no difference between N95 versus surgical masks and probably no difference between surgical versus no mask in risk for influenza or influenza-like illness, but compliance was low.
6. In healthcare settings, N95 and surgical masks were probably associated with similar risks for influenza-like illness and laboratory-confirmed viral infection; clinical respiratory illness had inconsistency. The authors concluded that evidence on mask effectiveness for respiratory infection prevention is stronger in health care than community settings and N95 respirators might reduce SARS-CoV-1 risk versus surgical masks in healthcare settings. Another study [13] found that if masks will not prevent infection completely, they can lower the inhaled viral dose leading to moderate disease or even symptomless one. A more recent study by Talic et al. [14] reviewed the evidence on the effectiveness of public health measures in reducing the incidence of COVID-19, SARS-

CoV-2 transmission, and COVID-19 mortality. Seventy-two studies met the inclusion criteria, of which 35 evaluated individual public health measures and 37 assessed multiple public health measures as a "package of interventions." Eight of 35 studies were included in the meta-analysis, which indicated a reduction in incidence of COVID-19 associated with handwashing (relative risk 0.47, 95% confidence interval 0.19 to 1.12, $I^2 = 12\%$), mask wearing (0.47, 0.29 to 0.75, $I^2 = 84\%$), and physical distancing (0.75, 0.59 to 0.95, $I^2 = 87\%$). This systematic review and meta-analysis suggests that several personal protective and social measures, including handwashing, mask wearing, and physical distancing, are associated with reductions in the incidence COVID-19. Public health efforts to implement public health measures should consider community health and sociocultural needs.

The added value of face shields in preventing infections in the community and hospital

Face shields have been proposed to prevent transmission in the community, but data are lacking. Bhaskar and Arun [15] form India described transmission in a community setting before and after the use of face shields. Before face shields, 62 workers (40 women) visited 5880 homes with 31,164 persons. From the 5880 homes visited, 222 persons tested positive for SARS-CoV-2, from May 4 to May 13. Twelve workers (19%) were infected during this period. Eight developed symptoms (fever, cough, sore throat, myalgia, and anosmia) and four were asymptomatic. The 12 infected workers were moved to care centers. Four developed desaturation and mild breathing difficulty and were treated with oral hydroxychloroquine and oxygen therapy; all four recovered. Contact tracing of the workers who tested positive identified 14 van drivers, who were monitored. All were asymptomatic and tested negative between days 7 and 10 after contact with the workers. After face shield introduction, 50 workers (previously uninfected) continued to provide counseling, visiting 18,228 homes. Among the counseled 118,428 persons, 2682 subsequently tested positive for SARS-CoV-2. No worker developed asymptomatic or symptomatic infection. This study found no SARS-CoV-2 infections among community health workers after the addition of face shields to their personal protective equipment. Because the first worker became symptomatic 13 days after beginning home visits and workers had no contact with family, co-workers, or the public, there is no known alternative source of infection for the workers except the asymptomatic contacts of SARS-CoV-2 patients. The face shields may have reduced ocular exposure or contamination of masks or hands or may have diverted movement of air around the face. Mohajer et al. [16] investigated the effect of face shields on rates of infection in a hospital which is a quaternary healthcare system with more than 500 beds and 8000 health care providers (HCP). Between April 1 and April 17, 2020, the hospital instituted several infection prevention strategies to limit transmission of SARS-CoV-2 including limiting entry to facility, screening for symptoms and temperature, universal masking for HCP, universal masking for patients, social distancing (avoid having lunch with other people), and limiting meeting size to less than 10. On July 6, 2020, the hospital implemented universal face shield requirements for all healthcare personnel upon entry to facility. They decided to add face shields in order to reduce the potential for autoinoculation by preventing the HCP from touching their face, and to protect from viral entry to the eyes, nose, and mouth. In addition, they may be used as a barrier of transmission from HCP to other HCP and patients, and they can be reused for a long time, easily cleaned and available at low cost. Of 6527 HCP tested, 246 tested positive for SARS-CoV-2 (3.8%). In the preintervention period, the weekly positivity rate among HCP increased from 0% to 12.9%. During the intervention period, the weekly positivity rate among HCP decreased to 2.3%, with segmented regression showing a change in predicted proportion positive in week 13 (22.9%–2.7%, $P < .001$) and change in the postintervention slope on the log odds scale ($P < .001$). A total of 25 hospital acquired infections (HAI) cases were identified (16 possible and nine confirmed). In the preintervention period, HAI cases increased from 0 to 7. During the intervention period, HAI cases decreased to 0.

Concluding remarks

SARS-CoV-2 is expelled from the airways of COVID-19 patients and carriers at a large range of droplets, which hover in the air for a long time, keep virus viability for a few hours, can reach the alveoli in the lungs of exposed people, attach to ACE2 receptors, and cause infection and disease. The risk for infection is higher in closed places and crowded gatherings and lower in open and high rate ventilated spaces. Wearing any kind of respiratory protective device, including multilayer cloth masks, on mouth and nose of carrier or patient, significantly reduce expulsion and dissemination of viral particles, and will keep public infection rate at a low level. Protecting healthy people by any kind of mask will serve the same purpose, while medical and laboratory staff will benefit more by wearing standard NIOSH-approved respirators. N95 respirators provide good protection from all range particles, including viruses, with at least 95% efficiency, provided they are worn correctly and have a good fit around the face. Surgical masks provide partial protection, of not more than 50% to the wearer, against large range of particles including viruses, but are very prone to errors in wearing. Both devices, without exhale valve, will protect the wearer and other people as well. N95 respirators with exhale valve do not protect other people from the wearer. Face shields in combination with masks or respirators provide additional protection from infection, by reducing ocular exposure or contamination of masks or hands, as well as by diverting movement of air around the face.

References

[1] Bourouiba L. Turbulent gas clouds and respiratory pathogen emissions: potential implications for reducing transmission of COVID-19. JAMA 2020;26. https://doi.org/10.1001/jama.2020.4756.

[2] DHS Science and Technology Master Question List for COVID-19 (caused by SARS-CoV-2) Weekly Report 18 March 2020. https://www.dhs.gov/sites/default/files/publications/2020_03_18_mql_covid-19-sars- cov-2_-_cleared_for_public_release_0.pdf.

[3] van Doremalen N, Bushmaker T, Morris DH, Holbrook MG, Gamble A, Williamson BN, et al. Aerosol and surface stability of HCoV-19 (SARS-CoV-2) compared to SARS-CoV-1. N Engl J Med 2020;382:1564–7.

[4] Hamming I, Timens W, Bulthuis ML, Lely AT, Navia GJ, van Goor H. Tissue distribution of ACE2 protein, the functional receptor for SARS coronavirus. A first step in understanding SARS pathogenesis. J Pathol 2004;203:631–7.

[5] Zhang H, Penninger JM, Li Y, Zhong N, Slutsky AS. Angiotensin-converting enzyme 2 (ACE2) as a SARS-CoV-2 receptor: molecular mechanisms and potential therapeutic target. Intensive Care Med 2020;46:586–90. https://doi.org/10.1007/s00134-020-05985-9.

[6] Xinjian H, Reoponen T, McKay RT, Grinhpun SA. Effect of particle size on the performance of an N95 filtering facepiece respirator and a surgical mask at various breathing conditions. Aerosol Sci Technol 2013;47:1180–7.

[7] Szablewski CM, Chang KT, Brown MM, Chu VT, Yousaf AR, Anylachi N, et al. SARS-CoV-2 transmission and infection among attendees of an overnight camp — Georgia, June 2020. MMWR (Morb Mortal Wkly Rep) 2020;69:1023–5.

[8] Chu VT, Yousaf AR, Chang K, Schwartz NG, McDaniel CJ, Lee SH, et al. Household transmission of SARS-CoV-2 from children and adolescents. N Engl J Med 2021;385:954–6.

[9] Karan A, Klompas M, Tucker R, Baker M, Vaidya V, Rhee C. The risk of severe acute respiratory syndrome coronavirus 2 (SARS-CoV-2) transmission from patients with undiagnosed coronavirus disease 2019 (COVID-19) to roommates in a large academic medical center. Clin Infect Dis 2022;74:1097–100. https://doi.org/10.1093/cid/ciab564.

[10] Wang X, Ferro EG, Zhou G, Hashimoto D, Bhatt DL. Association between universal masking in a health care system and SARS-CoV-2 positivity among health care workers. JAMA 2020;324:703–4. https://doi.org/10.1001/jama.2020.12897.

[11] Cheng GY, Ma N, Witt C, Rapp S, Wild PS, Andreae MO, et al. Face masks effectively limit the probability of SARS-CoV-2 transmission. Science 2021;372:1439–43.

[12] Chou R, Dana T, Jungbauer R, Weeks C, McDonagh MS. Masks for prevention of respiratory virus infections, including SARS-CoV-2, in health care and community settings. Ann Intern Med 2020;173:542–55. https://doi.org/10.7326/M20-3213 [e-pub].

[13] Gandhi M, Rutherford GW. Facial masking for COVID-19 — potential for "variolation" as we await a vaccine. N Engl J Med 2020;383:e101.

[14] Talic S Shah S, Wild H, Gasevic D, Maharaj A, Ademi Z, et al. Effectiveness of public health measures in reducing the incidence of COVID-19, SARS-CoV-2 transmission, and COVID-19 mortality: systematic review and meta-analysis. BMJ 2021;375:e068302. https://doi.org/10.1136/bmj-2021-068302.

[15] Bhaskar ME, Arun S. SARS-CoV-2 infection among community health workers in India before and after use of face shields. JAMA 2020;324:1348–9. https://doi.org/10.1001/jama.2020.15586.

[16] Mohajer MA, Panthagani KM, Lasco T, Lembcke B, Hemmige V. Association between universal face shield in a quaternary care center and reduction of SARS-CoV-2 infections among healthcare personnel and hospitalized patients. Int J Infect Dis 2021;105:252–5. https://doi.org/10.1016/j.ijid.2021.02.060.

Further reading

Zhang R, Li Y, Zhang AL, Wang Y, Molina MJ. Identifying airborne transmission as the dominant route for the spread of COVID-19. Proc Natl Acad Sci USA 2020;117:14857–63. https://doi.org/10.1073/pnas.2009637117.

CHAPTER

33

Therapeutic options in COVID-19

Ehud Horwitz[1], *Ofer Perzon*[2] *and Dror Mevorach*[3]

[1]Pharmacy Division and Department of Infectious Diseases and Clinical Microbiology, Hadassah Medical Center and the Faculty of Medicine, Hebrew University, Jerusalem, Israel; [2]Department of Medicine B, Hadassah Medical Center and the Faculty of Medicine, Hebrew University, Jerusalem, Israel; [3]Department of Medicine B, and Division of Rheumatology-Immunology-Allergology and the Wohl Institute for Translational Medicine, Department of Medicine, Hadassah Medical Center and the Faculty of Medicine, Hebrew University, Jerusalem, Israel

Overview

As illustrated in Table 33.1, COVID-19 treatment can be categorized into prophylactic treatment, early-stage treatment, and late-stage treatment, for inpatients and outpatients. In early treatment, antiviral agents are used (including nirmatrelvir/ritonavir, which may also be used as a prophylactic agent against severe disease) and passive immunization

TABLE 33.1 Treatment approach in infection with SARS-CoV-2.

Vaccines	Neutralizing antibodies	Anti-virals	Neutralizing antibodies	Anticoagulants	Immune modulators
mRNA vaccines	Bamlanivimab/ etesevimab	Nirmatrelvir-ritonavir	Bamlanivimab/ etesevimab	Low molecular weight heparin for mild to severe patients	Dexamethasone/ corticosteroids
Adenovirus-vectored vaccines	Casirivimab/ imdevimab	Molnupiravir	Casirivimab/ imdevimab		Tocilizumab
	Tixagevimab/ cilgavimab? (Prophylaxis)	Remdesivir	Sotrovimab		Baricitinib
			Convalescent plasma?		
					Antivirals: Remdesivir

Autoimmunity, COVID-19, Post-COVID19 syndrome and COVID-19 vaccination
https://doi.org/10.1016/B978-0-443-18566-3.00034-7

with monoclonal antibodies. Additional prophylactic treatment for hospitalized patients includes anticoagulation. Late-stage treatment in progressive disease characterized by a cytokine storm and lung involvement is largely immunomodulatory, and includes corticosteroids, interluekin-6 inhibitors, and JAK inhibitors. Additional medications that have not been yet approved for treatment are beyond the scope of this discussion.

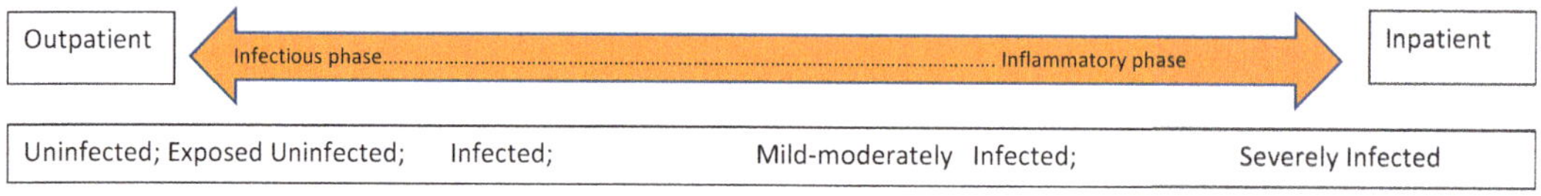

Antiviral medications

By early 2022, three main antiviral agents were incorporated into standard of care (SOC) therapy against SARS-CoV-2.

Remdesivir (formerly GS-5734), an RNA-dependent RNA polymerase inhibitor, was the first antiviral medication introduced for treating COVID-19. In *in-vitro* studies, remdesivir demonstrated activity against several pathogenic viruses. It was originally developed for hepatitis-C and Ebola virus infections, where animal studies have shown promise; however, a randomized clinical trial in Ebola patients was halted due to inferior interim results [1]. *In-vitro* activity against coronaviruses ignited renewed interest in clinical use of the drug shortly after emergence of the SARS-CoV-2 pandemic in early 2020. The availability of human safety data gathered during the development phases and clinical trials for Ebola virus infections allowed for expedited regulatory evaluation of remdesivir for treating COVID-19. Indeed, Emergency Use Authorization (EUA) was granted by the U.S. Food and Drug Administration (FDA) as early as May 2020, less than 6 months after the first reports concerning COVID-19, and European Medicines Agency (EMA) authorization followed in July 2020. These approvals were mainly based on results of the international, multicenter Adaptive COVID-19 Treatment Trial (ACTT-1), which enrolled over 1000 hospitalized patients. The study found accelerated recovery among remdesivir patients compared to patients managed with standard of care (SOC) (10 vs. 15 days, respectively, RR = 1.29, 95% CI 1.12–1.49) [2]. This effect appeared more pronounced when remdesivir was initiated within 10 days of symptom onset. Conversely, remdesivir was not significantly better than SOC in patients with severe/critical disease and in those on mechanical ventilation.

The Simple-Moderate study enrolled nearly 600 hospitalized patients not requiring supplemental oxygen, who were randomized in an open-label design to either five or 10 days of remdesivir [3]. Patients in the 5-day arm were more likely to achieve improved clinical status on day 11 compared with the 10-day arm patients (OR = 1.65, 95% CI 1.09–2.84). A second open-label, randomized clinical study in approximately 400 hospitalized adult patients with severe COVID-19, found no significant difference in efficacy or safety between a five- and a 10-day course of remdesivir [4].

The multinational, WHO-sponsored, ongoing Solidarity trial, assessing parallel COVID-19 treatment arms, published interim results in October 2020 [5]. Of 11,330 hospitalized adult patients in over 400 medical centers across 30 countries, 2750 received a 10-day course of remdesivir. None of the four trial drug arms (remdesivir, hydroxychloroquine, lopinavir/ritonavir, or interferon) showed significantly reduced mortality, the primary outcome, as compared to the SOC/no trial drug arm. Similarly, oxygen requirement and length of hospital stay were not affected by any of the trial drugs.

Following the initial EUA, remdesivir was granted formal FDA authorization in October 2020 (as Veklury®), for treating COVID-19 in patients aged 12 and above, weighing at least 40 kg, who require hospitalization. It is administered intravenously as a single 200 mg loading dose followed by 100 mg once daily, for 5 days. If no clinical improvement is observed, treatment may be extended to a total of 10 days. A 10-day course is recommended for patients requiring invasive mechanical ventilation and/or ECMO. Remdesivir is currently not recommended in patients with impaired renal function (eGFR < 30 mL/min), as such patients were excluded from the major remdesivir trials. Of note, preliminary data suggests that remdesivir use may be safe in patients with severe renal failure [6]. The most common adverse effects associated with remdesivir are nausea and impaired liver function tests.

Several systemic reviews and meta-analyses have assessed the clinical utility of remdesivir. A recent Cochrane Database review examined five randomized controlled trials collectively including approximately 7500 adult patients, a majority of whom required supplemental oxygen as either low-flow oxygen or mechanical ventilation. The review concluded that "remdesivir probably has little or no effect on all-cause mortality up to 28 days in hospitalized adults with SARS-CoV-2 infection." No conclusion could be drawn regarding remdesivir's effect on clinical status [7]. Other reviews suggest that while remdesivir did not reduce mortality, if initiated early after symptom onset in patients with nonsevere disease, it may offer other potential clinical benefits such as reduced recovery time and increased chances for clinical improvement [8].

A Canadian multi-center open-label study randomized 1267 hospitalized patients to either a 10-day remdesivir course with SOC or SOC alone [9]. The primary outcome, in-hospital death by day 28, occurred in 18.7% of remdesivir patients, compared to 22.7% of the SOC-only patients, not reaching statistical significance. However, several secondary outcomes were significantly improved in the remdesivir arm, including need for mechanical ventilation and mean oxygen-free and ventilator-free days, further suggesting a possible role for remdesivir in hospitalized patients.

Remdesivir may also be used as a three-day course in high-risk non-hospitalized patients with mild-moderate disease. This is based on findings of the randomized, double-blind placebo-controlled PINETREE study, which evaluated a 3-day remdesivir course initiated within 7 days of symptom onset in 562 unvaccinated outpatients [10]. Overall, 47%–62% of participants had at least one of the following: diabetes, hypertension, obesity. The primary endpoint, COVID-19-related hospitalization or death from any cause within 28 days, occurred in 0.7% of patients in the remdesivir arm versus 5.3% in the placebo arm (HR = 0.13, 95% CI 0.03–0.59). Adverse events were reported in approximately 45% of patients in both arms; most were mild, and few were serious or led to discontinuation (more among placebo patients compared to active treatment). This study suggests a potential for ambulatory use of remdesivir in early stages of COVID-19, provided that complex logistic barriers related to daily intravenous administration to infected individuals for 3 days can be overcome. Of note, the change in SARS-CoV-2 viral load from baseline to day 7 was similar in both groups, questioning the prospect of reduced transmissibility with this intervention.

Current IDSA COVID-19 treatment guidelines [11] suggest the use of remdesivir for both ambulatory patients at high risk for progression to severe disease as a 3-day outpatient course, and for hospitalized patients with severe disease as a 5-day course, but recommend against routine remdesivir treatment in patients with invasive ventilation and/or ECMO. Current WHO COVID-19 guidelines [12] conditionally recommend remdesivir for non-severe patients at high risk for hospitalization.

The major active remdesivir metabolite, GS-441,524, is currently under investigation as a potential inhalational therapy for COVID-19 patients [13].

Molnupiravir (Lagevrio, formerly MK-4482, EIDD-2801) was granted an EUA by the FDA in late December 2021 [14], following European and UK authorizations in November 2021, for oral treatment of mild-moderate COVID-19 adult patients with a high risk of progression to severe disease. Molnupiravir is a prodrug, which is converted to a nucleoside hydroxycitidine analog (NHC) following oral administration. NHC is incorporated by the SARS-CoV-2 RNA polymerase into its RNA. This results in erroneous, malfunctioning viral RNA, rendering the viral genome nonreplicable.

The EUA [15] was granted based on the results of the MOVe-OUT study, a randomized, double-blind clinical trial involving 1433 nonhospitalized, unvaccinated adult patients with mild-moderate COVID-19 and with at least one risk factor for progressing to severe disease requiring hospitalization [16]. Predefined risk factors were age >60 yr, obesity (BMI $\geq$ 30), diabetes, chronic kidney disease, serious heart conditions, chronic obstructive lung disease (COPD), or active cancer. Treatment had to be initiated within 5 days of symptom onset. Patients were randomized to either molnupiravir 800 mg (administered as four 200 mg tablets) or a matching placebo, twice daily for 5 days. The primary endpoint, defined as hospitalization or death of any cause through day 29, occurred in 6.8% of molnupiravir patients, versus 9.7% of placebo patients, representing an absolute risk reduction of 3% and a modest relative risk reduction of approximately 30% (95% CI 0.49–0.99). A single death was reported in the molnupiravir arm, compared to nine in the placebo arm (89% relative risk reduction, 95% CI 14–99). The main reported adverse effects were diarrhea, nausea, and dizziness, occurring in 1%–2% of patients in both the molnupiravir and placebo arms. Serious adverse events and adverse drug effect-related discontinuations occurred more frequently in the placebo arm (10% and 3%, respectively) compared with the molnupiravir arm (7% and 1%, respectively).

In contrast, the MOVe-IN study, assessing molnupiravir efficacy in adult hospitalized COVID-19 patients was suspended prematurely after interim results suggested futility [17]. A postexposure prophylaxis study, MOVe-AHEAD is ongoing.

In contrast to nirmatrelvir/ritonavir, molnupiravir and NHC are not substrates nor effectors of CYP enzymes, p-glycoprotein, or BCRP transporters. There are currently no known or expected drug-drug interactions associated with molnupiravir use; however, molnupiravir is currently contraindicated for use in children and in pregnant women due to animal evidence of bone and cartilage toxicity. No dose adjustments are necessary for patients with renal or hepatic impairment or in elderly patients.

NIH COVID-19 Treatment guidelines [18] list molnupiravir as an alternative for treating nonhospitalized patients at high risk for disease progression when the preferred options (nirmatrelvir/ritonavir or remdesivir) can be used. Similarly, Molnupiravir use is endorsed by IDSA COVID-19 treatment guidelines [12] for indications authorized under the EUA.

Nirmatrelvir is an oral antiviral protease inhibitor, specifically designed to target the SARS CoV2 main protease (Mpro). Being a substrate of human CYP-3A4, nirmatrelvir is coadministered with low-dose ritonavir, serving as a potent CYP-3A4 inhibitor, and thus boosting nirmatrelvir exposure without providing any significant antiviral activity. Copackaged nirmatrelvir and ritonavir, manufactured by Pfizer under the brand name Paxlovid®, was granted an EUA by the FDA in late December 2021 following the announcement of the final results of the phase 2/3 randomized double-blind placebo controlled EPIC-HR (Evaluation of Protease Inhibition for COVID-19 in High-Risk Patients) clinical study [19]. It was approved by the FDA for the treatment of mild-to-moderate coronavirus disease (COVID-19) in adults and pediatric patients (12 years of age and older weighing at least 40 kg or about 88 pounds) with positive results of direct SARS-CoV-2 testing who are at high risk for progression to severe COVID-19, including hospitalization or death. The EPIC-HR study enrolled 2246 unvaccinated patients randomized to either 300 mg/100 mg nirmatrelvir/ritonavir or placebo, twice daily for 5 days. For inclusion, treatment was to be started within 5 days of initial symptom onset. The primary endpoint was COVID-19-related hospitalization or death from any cause by day 28. In the nirmatrelvir/ritonavir arm, there was an 89% reduction for COVID-19-related hospitalization, occurring in 0.7% of the active treatment arm compared with 6.5% of the placebo arm, when treatment was initiated within 3 days of symptom onset, a highly significant finding ($P < .0001$). A similar 88% reduction in the primary endpoint was observed when treatment was initiated within 5 days of symptom onset. Twelve patients in the placebo arm died by day 28, while no deaths occurred in the treatment arm. A relative risk reduction of 95% was demonstrated for those aged 65 years and above. In addition, viral load was measured on day 5 for a subset of 499 participants, and was found to be 10-fold lower for those receiving active treatment versus the placebo arm.

Adverse effects were generally mild, mainly dysgeusia (6% vs. 1% with placebo), diarrhea (3% vs. 2%), hypertension, and myalgia (both 1% vs. <1%). Serious adverse effects were reported in 1.6% of active treatment versus 6.6% with placebo, and adverse effect related discontinuations also occurred less frequently with active treatment compared with placebo (2.1% vs. 4.2%). Potential drug-drug interactions pose a significant challenge when combining nirmatrelvir/ritonavir with background medications, as nirmatrelvir is a CYP-3A4 substrate and ritonavir is a potent CYP-3A4 inhibitor. The use of CYP-3A4 inducers (e.g., rifampin, carbamazepine, phenytoin, phenobarbital, St. John's wart) is a contraindication for nirmatrelvir/ritonavir use. For CYP-3A4 substrates, it is recommended to consult the FDA-approved prescribing information [20] for specific guidance, as some substrates may be continued unchanged or at a reduced dose (e.g., quetiapine, calcium-channel blockers), some need to be held (atorvastatin, salmeterol), and others are a contraindication to nirmatrelvir/ritonavir use (e.g., alfuzosin, midazolam, sirolimus, amiodarone).

Nirmatrelvir/ritonavir dose is reduced in patients with moderate renal dysfunction (eGFR = 30–60 mL/min) and is not recommended in those with eGFR lower than 30 mL/min, in severe hepatic impairment, in children under 12 years of age, or in pregnant or lactating women.

To date, nirmatrelvir/ritonavir appears to be the most effective antiviral treatment available for COVID-19 in high-risk ambulatory patients. A significant reduction in mortality and

COVID-19-related hospitalization were recently reported among high-risk, mostly immune (vaccinated, previusoly infected or both) nirmatrelvir/ritonavir recipients aged 65 years and above during the Omicron-subvariant surge [21], although this effect was not demonstrated in patients aged 40-64 years. However, the EPIC-SR study,in standard-risk patients, was prematurely discontinued due to futility [22]. Third nirmatrelvir study, EPIC-PEP, assessing use as postexposure prophylaxis, also failed to demonstrate benefit in this clinical situation [23].

Current NIH COVID-19 treatment guidelines [18] recommend nirmatrelvir/ritonavir as the preferred treatment for nonhospitalized patients at high risk for disease progression, provided that administration is initiated within 5 days of symptom onset. IDSA COVID-19 guidelines [12] also recommend nirmatrelvir/ritonavir for these patients. A detailed review with additional updated information regarding molnupiravir and nirmatrelvir/ritonavir has recently been published [24].

Passive immunization

Convalescent Plasma. The concept of utilizing passive immunization in the form of convalescent plasma (CP) for treating infectious diseases was first presented and practiced more than 100 years ago, just prior to the Spanish Flu pandemic in 1918. Since then, it has been studied against SARS, avian influenza-A (H5Na), influenza-A (H1N1), Middle-East Respiratory Syndrome (MERS), and Ebola viral infections, with variable success [25]. As the SARS-CoV2 pandemic spread globally in early 2020, it became evident that vaccines for COVID-19 prevention and medications for specific COVID-19 treatment, were unlikely to become available in the short-term. In contrast, recovering patients are readily available in pandemics, forming a potential large and accessible source for CP. Therefore, it is not surprising that CP transfusion was suggested and practiced in the very early stages of the COVID-19 pandemic [26].

CP can be obtained from donating patients who were recently recovered from COVID-19 and be used to provide antibodies to SARS-CoV2 for newly-infected COVID-19 patients. The donated plasma is handled and screened according to strict procedures and regulations to assure patient safety, and administered intravenously similarly to other plasma products, as a single dose.

CP use was initially complicated by numerous confounders, such as heterogeneity in antibody content (titer), patient characteristics, and varying concomitant treatments. Following initial case reports, case series, observational studies, and nonrandomized trials, several trials were conducted. In the United States, an open-label multicenter study assessed CP transfusion to more than 35,000 patients with severe COVID-19 (52% in ICU, 27.5% on mechanical ventilation) [27]. In patients receiving CP within 3 days of diagnosis, 7-day mortality was 8.7%; however, transfusions given later than 3 days from diagnosis resulted in a significantly higher 7-day mortality rate of 11.9% ($P < .001$), with similar findings for 30-day mortality (21.6% vs. 26.7%, respectively, $P < .0001$). A significant inverse correlation was identified between CP IgG antibody levels and mortality (relative risk 0.65 and 0.7 for 7 and 30-day mortality, respectively, for high and medium IgG antibody level vs. low-level).

Several randomized clinical trials failed to prove CP's benefit in hospitalized patients. The large RECOVERY trial randomized approximately 11,500 patients to either high-titer CP or placebo, and found similar day 28 mortality, time-to-hospital discharge, and need for mechanical ventilation in both arms [28]. Based on this study and additional studies with similar findings, CP transfusion is currently not recommended by the NIH for use in hospitalized patients without impaired humoral immunity [29].

CP's role in nonhospitalized patients without impaired humoral immunity and in hospitalized and nonhospitalized patients with impaired humoral immunity remains unclear. The SIREN-C3PO single-blind study randomly assigned 511 nonhospitalized mild-to-moderate COVID-19 patients with symptoms for up to 1 week of and at least one risk factor for progression to severe disease to either high-titer CP or placebo [30]. The trial was terminated prematurely due to futility, as CP failed to demonstrate superiority over placebo in composite primary endpoints of disease progression or in any of several predefined secondary endpoints. Five deaths occurred in the CP arm and one in the placebo arm. Infusion-related adverse reactions were also more frequent in the CP arm.

In contrast, a recent study suggests that early administration (within 8 days of symptom onset) of high-titer CP to nonhospitalized adults (regardless of risk factors) may be beneficial in terms of disease progression requiring hospitalization [31]. This multi-center, double-blind randomized study enrolled approximately 1200 such patients to either high-titer CP or placebo. The primary outcome, 28-day hospitalization, occurred in 2.9% of CP patients versus 6.3% of placebo patients, representing a statistically-significant 54% risk reduction for hospitalization.

It is noteworthy that the above-mentioned trials were carried out prior to the emergence and spread of the delta and omicron variants. It remains to be determined whether CP derived from patients infected by an early variant might be less active against other variants, or on the contrary, the polyclonal antibody content of CP is advantageous by offering activity against a wide range of mutant variants.

Immunosuppressed COVID-19 patients are at high risk for severe COVID-19, hospitalization, and death. It is biologically-plausible that CP may be of significant benefit for these patients, who cannot be vaccinated or are not expected to produce an adequate immune response to viral exposure or to vaccination [32]. Indeed, a reanalysis of RECOVERY trial data comparing mortality in seronegative and seropositive patients suggests that COVID-19 patients who are seronegative at presentation are more likely to benefit from CP transfusion [33].

As this and other evidence of potential CP benefit in immunocompromised COVID patients were obtained retrospectively and not in specific randomized clinical trials, it is yet to be established whether patients with impaired humoral immunity form a targeted subset population for CP transfusion. Accordingly, NIH COVID-19 Treatment Guidelines [29] do not make a recommendation for or against CP use in immunocompromised patients, hospitalized or nonhospitalized.

Furthermore, CP transfusion in COVID-19 is not currently endorsed by either the NIH [29] or WHO [12] guidelines. IDSA guidelines [11] currently limit high-titer-CP use to non-hospitalized patients with mild-to-moderate COVID-19 at high risk for progression to severe disease who have no other treatment options.

The original CP EUA granted by the FDA in August 2020 authorized CP use in hospitalized COVID-19 patients regardless of immune status. However, the most recent (December 2021) FDA-EUA regarding CP [34] restricted its use to immunocompromised COVID-19 patients only, either hospitalized or nonhospitalized.

Adverse effects associated with CP transfusion are generally similar to those typical of other plasma infusions, consisting of infusion-related events, transfusion-transmitted infections, and transfusion-related lung injury and volume overload. Among approximately 100,000 CP transfusion recipients in the United States, serious adverse transfusion reactions were reported in 597 cases, of which 107, 267, and 223 were considered definitely-, probably-, and possibly-transfusion-related, respectively [35].

Another SARS-CoV-2-related risk associated with CP administration is disease deterioration, as noted in specific subsets of some of the clinical trials, such as transfusion being given more than 7 days after hospitalization [36], and administration of CP containing high levels of IgG antibodies against the full transmembrane spike protein [37].

Monoclonal Antibodies. Monoclonal antibodies (MAb) for treating and preventing, COVID-19 have been recently become available. Several monoclonal antibodies were designed to specifically bind to various targets on the SARS-CoV-2 spike protein, thereby neutralizing viral attachment to human cells. This inhibits viral reproduction, reduces viral load, and disease progression is consequently averted.

To date, four MAb products have been granted an EUA for treating mild-moderate COVID-19 patients at high risk for disease progression to severe disease: bamlanivimab/etesevimab (B/E), sotrovimab, bebtelovimab and casirivimab/imdevimab (C/I). C/I and B/E were also approved for postexposure prophylaxis (PEP) in patients who are not fully vaccinated, and those who are vaccinated but are expected to have inadequate immune response due to immunosuppression after close exposure to an infected COVID-19 patient. A fifth MAb, copackaged tixagevimab/cilgavimab (T/C) received an EUA for pre-exposure prophylaxis (PrEP) for uninfected individuals aged 12 and above, who have not been recently exposed to an infected person, but are moderate to severely immune-compromised and might therefore not mount an adequate immune response to a COVID-19 vaccination, or cannot be vaccinated due to a history of severe adverse reaction to a vaccine. All four MAbs approved for treatment are given as single-dose intravenous infusions within 10 days of symptom onset. C/I can also be administered subcutaneously, and C/T is administered intramuscularly, both conferring a significant logistic advantage for outpatient use.

Initially, bamlanivimab (formerly LY-CoV555), a neutralizing human IgG1k MAb, was the first MAb to receive EUA (November 2020) [38], based on the results of the pahse-2 BLAZE-1 clinical trial [39]. This study randomized 452 outpatients with mild or moderate COVID-19, to receive single-dose intravenous bamlanivimab in one of three doses (700 mg, 2,800 mg, 7,000 mg) or placebo. Day 11 viral load versus baseline, the primary study endpoint, was found to be significantly decreased in the 2,800 mg subgroup as compared to the placebo group. In addition, bamlanivimab patients had a slightly lower symptom severity on days 2–6 and lower rates of COVID-19-related hospitalization or emergency room visits (1.6%) versus placebo (6.3%).

However, subsequent findings of the rapid emergence of bamlanivimab-resistant SARS-CoV-2 variants led to revocation of the EUA in April 2021 [40]. In order to preserve and amplify bamlanivimab efficacy, it was coformulated with etesevimab, a second MAb targeting the SARS-CoV-2 spike protein. The B/E combination was shown to be efficacious against SARS-CoV-2 variants circulating in the USA in early 2021. This was demonstrated in the phase-3 BLAZE-1 study, encompassing 1035 ambulatory mild or moderate COVID-19 patients with high risk to progression to severe disease, randomized to single dose intravenous B/E or placebo within 3 days of laboratory COVID-19 confirmation [41]. The primary endpoint, defined as COVID-19-related hospitalization or death by day 29, occurred in 2.1% of B/E patients, significantly less than that in the placebo arm (7%, relative risk reduction 70%, $P < .001$). Ten patients in the placebo arm died, while no deaths occurred in the B/E arm. In addition, day-7 viral load reduction from baseline was significantly larger in the B/E arm compared to the placebo arm.

A revised EUA for the combined MAb B/E was granted in February 2021 [42]. Its use was later halted (June 2021) following the spread of more resistant variants (Beta, Gamma), and then released in September 2021, after activity against the Delta variant was demonstrated. The B/E EUA was further revised in January 2022 [43], expanding authorization to all age groups (including neonates) for both treatment and PEP, based on reviewing data from BLAZE-1, BLAZE-2 and the yet-unpublished BLAZE-4 studies. Shortly afterward, with the emergence and rapid global spread of the dominant Omicron variant, it appeared that it's highly-mutated spike protein presents significantly reduced susceptibility to B/E (as well as to C/I). Consequently, The American Department of Health and Human Services has paused distribution of both combination MAbs in December 2021.

Casirivimab and imdevimab (C/I), both SARS-CoV-2 spike-targeting MAbs coformulated and distributed as Regen-Cov®, were granted an EUA in November 2020 for COVID-19 treatment in nonhospitalized patients aged 12 and above with mild-to-moderate disease. A Phase-3 clinical trial randomized 1355 outpatients with risk factors for severe disease to either C/I at 1200 mg or 2400 mg, or placebo [44]. COVID-19-related hospitalization or death by day 29 occurred in 1.3% of 2400 mg C/I patients versus 4.6% of placebo patients, representing a significant 71% risk reduction (a similar reduction was observed in the 1200 mg group vs. placebo). Time to symptom resolution was shorter with C/I (10 days for both doses) versus placebo (14 days), and viral load reduction on day 7 versus baseline was significantly greater in C/I patients.

Additional authorization for PEP was issued in July 2021, for exposed individuals with a high risk of progression to severe COVID-19, hospitalization, and death. This was based on a significant 81% relative risk reduction in COVID-19 infection on day 28, following a single SC 1200 mg C/I injection (600 mg of each MAb) versus placebo, in 752 high-risk individuals recently (up to 96 h) exposed to a COVID-19 positive household contact [45]. Among symptomatic participants, symptom resolution and high-viral load duration were significantly shorter among C/I patients (1.2 and 0.4 weeks, respectively) than among placebo patients (3.2 and 1.3 weeks, respectively).

C/I has also shown to be beneficial in preventing progression to symptomatic COVID-19 when administered subcutaneously to recently exposed, asymptomatic diagnosed patients. In a multinational double-blind, placebo-controlled randomized clinical trial, patients were allocated to a single subcutaneous 1200 mg C/I dose or placebo within 96 h of index case positive test collection [46]. Among 100 C/I patients, 29% progressed to symptomatic disease, compared to 42% of 104 placebo patients (OR = 0.54, 95% CI 0.3–0.97, $P = .04$). Among symptomatic patients, symptom duration was 5.6 days shorter with C/I compared to placebo, as were other secondary outcomes, the number of symptomatic weeks and number of high viral load weeks, both per 1000 participants. Treatment-emergent adverse events were reported more frequently in the placebo arm (48.1%) than in the C/I arm (33.5%), most of which were COVID-19-related, and few of which were serious.

A third approved MAb, sotrovimab (Xevudi®), strongly binds to the N343 residue on the SARS-CoV-2 spike protein, with chemically designed to allow for enhanced binding, thus exhibiting an extended half-life of approximately 50 days and boosted lung distribution. The EUA has been issued based on results of the COMET-ICE trial [47]. This double-blind, placebo-controlled clinical study enrolled 1057 patients randomized to either an intravenous single 500 mg sotrovimab dose or matching placebo, within 5 days of symptom onset. Disease progression (defined as hospitalization for >24 hr for any acute illness or death from any cause) by day 29 was found to be reduced by 79% in the active arm versus the placebo arm. In addition, viral load reduction from baseline to day 8 was significantly larger with active treatment. As part of the COMET-ICE trial, it has also been shown that intramuscular administration of sotrovimab is noninferior to intravenous administration. While sotrovimab retains activity against Omicron subvariants BA.1 and BA.1.1, it is significantly less active in neutralizing the BA.2. BA.4 and BA.5 subvariants, and is therefore currently witheld from clinical use [48].

Bebtelovimab is currently the only MAb retainig activity against all commonly circulating Omicron subvaraints [48], An FDA EUA was issued in February 2022 [49], based on results of the BLAZE-4 study (published as preprint [50]). The study primary end point - persistently high viral load on day 7 - was significantly lower in patrient groups administered 175 mg bebtelovimab. T/C (Evusheld®) was recently granted an EUA for pre-exposure prophylaxis based on a phase-3 clinical study (PROVENT), which enrolled more than 5000 uninfected participants carrying a high risk of severe disease in case of infection but with no recent exposure to an infected individual. Participants were randomized (2:1) to either C/T (each given as a separate single intramuscular injection) and followed for up to 6 months. Symptomatic COVID-19 infection w diagnosed in 0.2% of T/C recipients versus 1% in the placebo arm, a significant 77% relative risk reduction (95% CI 46–90%, $P < .001$). However, in second clinical trial, (STROM-CHASER), a statistically-insignificant 33% relative risk reduction in COVID-19 infection among postexposure high-risk individuals as compared with placebo was seen, and T/C has therefore not been authorized for PEP. In June 2022, the FDA revised T/C EUA in order to achieve better protection against emerging Omicron subvariants - T/C doses were increased to 300mg of each component, whic may be repeated every 6 months [51].

In general, adverse effects related to MAb administration were infrequent, similar to that of placebo recipients, and mild, mainly injection site reactions, headache, fatigue, cough, rash, and gastrointestinal disturbances. Few cases of anaphylactic reaction were reported. No drug-drug interactions are expected.

Current WHO guidelines conditionally recommend sotrovimab for COVID-19 patients at the highest risk for hospitalization, but this recommendation fails to address the weak activity against newer Omicron subvariants. A similar conditional recommendation for C/I is accompanied by a note concerning its predicted lack of efficacy against the omicron variant. IDSA guidelines refer to bebtelovimab as the only optional MAb active against Omicron subvariants for outpatients with mild-to-moderate disease at high risk for progression to severe disease. However, due to sparsity of clinical efficacy and safety data, it is suggested as ana alternative where first-line options (nirmatrelvir/r and remdesivir) can not be used [11]. T/C is recommended for pre-exposure prophylaxis in immunocompromised individuals at increased risk for inadequate response to vaccination or those who cannot be vaccinated, and C/I is recommended for postexposure prophylaxis in exposed individuals with a high risk for progression to severe disease. However, these are limited by activity against the Omicron variant, which, effective September 2022, is retained only by bebtelovimab (as treatment) and T/C (as pre-exposure prophylaxis).

Anticoagulation

Anticoagulation became an essential component of COVID-19 treatment in hospitalized patients after it became apparent that the hyper-inflammatory process provoked by the viral infection commonly manifests as a prothrombotic state. In general, infection-induced endothelial cell dysfunction often disrupts the balance between thrombin generation and fibrinolytic activity, thereby prompting a hyper-coagulable state. This shift toward hypercoagulability is further driven by hypoxia and other underlying processes. In COVID-19 patients, the hypercoagulable state may present as microthrombi generation within the lung microcirculation, further impeding respiratory function, in addition to macrovascular events. Reported prevalence of venous thromboembolism (VTE) among COVID-19 patients varies over a wide range, assumingly due to varying patient populations, differing VTE screening techniques, and other factors. A recent meta-analysis reported pulmonary embolism (PE) and deep vein thrombosis (DVT) prevalences of 32% and 27%, respectively, in hospitalized COVID-19 patients [52]. Consequently, prophylactic anticoagulation therapy has been suggested in COVID-19 patients in the very early stages of the pandemic, for prevention of thrombotic complications [53].

It is generally well accepted that the majority of hospitalized COVID-19 patients are likely to benefit from anticoagulation. However, several important aspects remain controversial, mainly the intensity and duration of anticoagulation. In general, hospitalized non-COVID-19 patients requiring preventive anticoagulation are administered a prophylactic anticoagulant dose. Due to the potentially-fulminant nature of COVID-19, others have suggested that moderate- or therapeutic-intensity coagulation should be given to hospitalized COVID-19 patients.

A multiplatform randomized clinical trial collecting data from three separate studies, ACTIVE-4a, ATTACC, and REMAP-CP, was launched in a joint effort to assess the value of therapeutic dose versus prophylactic-dose anticoagulation in various COVID-19 severity categories. While therapeutic dose anticoagulation did not improve outcomes compared to prophylactic dose in critically-ill patients [54], it appeared to be superior in non-critical disease, as reflected in significantly fewer days on organ support [55]. This benefit was accompanied by a doubling of major bleeding events (1.9% vs. 0.9% with therapeutic-dose and prophylactic-dose anticoagulation, respectively). These findings imply that therapeutic AC may be most beneficial when started early in the course of COVID-19, prior to deterioration to critical disease. Several explanations have been suggested for these findings, including early effect of therapeutic dose AC prior to deterioration to a largely irreversible disease pathology, and additional AC effects, which may further prevent clinical deterioration, such as prevention of microthrombi formation and antiinflammatory and antiviral activity of heparin. This and other studies [56,57] led to a revision in the NIH Treatment Guidelines, which currently recommend a therapeutic dose of AC for non-ICU hospitalized patients with a high D-dimer level who require low-flow oxygen, while maintaining the recommendation for a prophylactic-dose of AC for hospitalized ICU patients, including those requiring high-flow oxygen [58]. The American Society of Hematology also recently revised its guidelines concerning anticoagulation in acutely-ill COVID-19 patients [59], which now suggest using therapeutic-intensity over prophylactic-intensity anticoagulation. However, prophylactic-dose AC is suggested for critically-ill patients [60]. IDSA guidelines currently maintain a recommendation for prophylactic-dose AC for hospitalized patients [61].

More recently, the ACTION trial failed to demonstrate the benefit of therapeutic-dose AC to hospitalized COVID-19 patients with an elevated baseline D-dimer level, (given as either low-molecular-weight heparin to unstable patients or a direct oral anticoagulant for stable patients) [62]. Similarly, the INSPIRATION trial found no significant difference in the primary composite outcome of 30-day VTE, arterial thrombosis, need for ECMO, or death between intermediate-dose and prophylactic-dose AC in 562 ICU COVID-19 patients, with more frequent major bleeding and thrombocytopenia occurring in the intermediate-dose group [63].

It is also yet to be determined whether anticoagulation is to be given only during hospitalization, or continued after discharge for a yet-to-be-defined additional period. Current NIH treatment guidelines, as well as other guidelines, do not recommend the continuation of ambulatory anticoagulation for most COVID-19 patients [58]. However, a recent multicenter open-label randomized study including 320 patients at increased risk for VTE (as defined by as an IMPROVE-VTE score $\geq$4 or 2–3 with a D-dimer value above 500 ng/mL) found that a postdischarge 35-day course of rivaroxaban 10 mg/day, significantly reduced the efficacy primary outcome (a composite of symptomatic or fatal VTE, asymptomatic VTE on bilateral lower-limb venous ultrasound and CT pulmonary angiogram, symptomatic arterial thromboembolism, and cardiovascular death at day 35, RR = 0.33,95% CI 0.12–0.90, $P = .0293$) with no major bleeding events [64].

It is emphasized that COVID-19 patients with an underlying indication for therapeutic-dose anticoagulation (such as atrial fibrillation) should continue their chronic full-dose anticoagulation.

Immunomodulation

As the COVID-19 pandemic progressed, it became evident that the pathogenesis of severe disease involves a rapid, intense inflammatory response to the viral infection, typical of several other viral respiratory diseases. Indeed, inflammatory lung insult was reflected in an increase in inflammatory markers such as CRP, ferritin, and interleukins–1 and interleukin–6 in severe COVID-19 cases. Hence, antiinflammatory therapeutic options were suggested, studied and used for acute, severe illness. As part of this therapeutic paradigm, corticosteroids appeared to be an attractive option, due to their low cost and the extensive experience in using them in various disease states and consequent familiarity with both potential benefits and risks.

Corticosteroids were used for treating severe COVID-19 in China during the early stages of the pandemic; however, lacking sufficient clinical evidence, such use was considered controversial [65,66]. The NIH-funded RECOVERY trial was the first large trial to assess the value of corticosteroids in COVID-19 disease [67]. This open-label trial assigned 2104 hospitalized patients to receive intravenous or oral dexamethasone 6 mg once daily for up to 10 days, and 4321 patients to receive SOC, consisting of several treatment arms. The primary outcome, death by day 28, occurred in 22.9% of the dexamethasone arm versus 25.7% in the placebo arm (age-adjusted risk ratio 0.83, 95% CI 0.75–0.93, $P < .001$). This effect was most pronounced in patients on mechanical ventilation with 29.3% versus 41.4%; (rate ratio, 0.64; 95% CI 0.51–0.81), and to a lesser extent in patients requiring oxygen without ventilator support (23.3% vs. 26.2%; rate ratio, 0.82; 95% CI 0.72–0.94). In contrast, dexamethasone did not appear to benefit those not requiring respiratory support at randomization (17.8% vs. 14.0%; rate ratio 1.19; 95% CI 0.92–1.55). Recognized corticosteroid-related serious adverse effects reported were hyperglycemia (2 cases), gastrointestinal hemorrhage, and psychosis (1 case each). These findings were later supported by those of the CoDEX study in ICU-COVID-19 patients with moderate-severe acute respiratory distress syndrome [68]. This study randomized 299 patients to either SOC with daily IV dexamethasone 20 mg for 5 days followed by 10 mg/d for 5 days or until ICU discharge, or SOC alone. Dexamethasone use was associated with a significant decrease in need for mechanical ventilation and in mortality. Of note, the CoDEX trial was prematurely terminated following publication of the RECOVERY trial results, as the data and safety monitoring board found it no longer ethical to continue the trial considering the positive RECOVERY trial findings. Several additional corticosteroid studies, such as the hydrocortisone arm of the REMAP-CAP study assessing intravenous hydrocortisone in severe ICU COVID-19 patients [69], were also halted upon publication of the RECOVERY trial result. Therefore, the body of evidence concerning efficacy and safety of corticosteroids other than dexamethasone is relatively small, making dexamethasone the preferred corticosteroid for treating COVID-19.

However, it is generally accepted that glucocorticosteroids other than dexamethasone may be as effective. NIH guidelines suggest that where dexamethasone is unavailable, it may be substituted by an equivalent dose of an alternative corticosteroid [70]. However, one study reported that a 3-day course of high-dose (250–500 mg/d) IV methylprednisolone followed by 50 mg oral prednisone for 14 days significantly decreased recovery time, transfer to ICU, and inflammatory markers as compared to 6 mg/d IV dexamethasone for 7–10 days in 216 non-ICU severe COVID-19 patients [71]. Additionally, doubling the dexamethasone daily dose to 12 mg was not found to increase survival without life support measures in the randomized COVID-STEROID-2 study in 1000 adult COVID-19 patients with severe hypoxemia [72]. Similarly, the COVIDICUS multi-center, placebo-controlled, randomized clinical trial found similar 60-day mortality rates in hospitalized COVID-19 patients with severe acute hypoxemic respiratory failure administered either low-dose (6 mg/d) or high-dose dexamethasone (20 mg/d for 5 days followed by 10mg/d for 5 days) [73]. Of note, a preplanned secondary Bayesian analysis of COVID-STEROID-2 results recently concluded that the 12 mg daily dexamethasone dose is associated with a high probability of benefit and low probability of clinically-important harm compared to the 6 mg daily dose [74].

It appears that the optimal selection of a specific corticosteroid and of an optimal dosing regimen in different patient populations is yet to be determined [75].

A Cochrane Database review examined clinical data published until April 2021, and concluded that systemic corticosteroids probably slightly reduce all-cause mortality in hospitalized COVID-19 patients (moderate-certainty evidence) and may also increase ventilator-free days (low-certainty evidence) [76].

The adverse effect profile of short-term systemic corticosteroids is well recognized and includes hyperglycemia, hypertension, sleep disturbances, behavioral/cognitive changes, secondary infections, and gastrointestinal effects. As corticosteroid use in COVID-19 is generally short-termed, tapering down following the completion of the treatment course is not necessary. Being a moderate CYP-3A4 inducer, dexamethasone use may interact with coadministered medications that are substrates of this enzyme; therefore, patient medication records should be reviewed for potential drug-drug interactions prior to dexamethasone initiation.

Current NIH guidance support using corticosteroids in hospitalized COVID-19 patients requiring supplemental oxygen (as monotherapy or combined with remdesivir in patients with minimal or high-flow noninvasive ventilation, and in combination with tocilizumab or sarilumab in patients on mechanical ventilation or ECMO) [77]. These guidelines recommend against corticosteroid use in nonhospitalized patients [18]. Similarly, current IDSA treatment guidelines recommend corticosteroids for treating hospitalized patients with severe or critical disease, suggest coricosteroids for severe non-critical disease, and recommend agains corticosteroid use n mild-moderate disease in hosputalized patients without hypoxemia requiring supllemental oxygen [11].

Inhaled budesonide was evaluated I the phase-2 open-label STOIC randomized controlled study [78]. 146 nonhospitalized COVID-19 patients within 7 days of mild symptom onset were allocated to either inhaled budesonide twice daily in addition to SOC or SOC alone, until symptom resolution. The primary endpoint, COVID-19-related urgent care visit, occurred in 3% of budesonide patients versus 15% of SOC patients (difference in proportions 0·123, 95% CI 0.033−0.213, $P = .009$). Several additional secondary outcomes were also suggestive of budesonide benefit. This and other studies evaluating inhaled corticosteroids were generally small, open-label and largely subjective endpoints. Accordingly, NIH guidelines state that there is currently insufficient data for recommendations regarding use of inhaled corticosteroids.

IL-6 Inhibitors. Interleukin-6 (IL-6) is a proinflammatory cytokine, produced in response to tissue damage by various cell types such as macrophages, mast cells, fibroblasts, B- and T-lymphocytes, and others. The binding of IL-6 to IL-6 receptors propagates a cascade of downstream signaling events related to the JAK/STAT pathway, resulting in further activation of various immune system components [79]. IL-6 plasma levels were found to be elevated in severe COVID-19 disease and associated with higher mortality [80]. Based on these findings, IL-6 inhibitors were suggested as potential therapies for COVID-19 disease, targeted to impede the hyper-inflammatory process characteristic of severe disease. With characteristic long elimination half-lives (generally 5−17 days), single-dose therapies are an additional attractive feature of IL-6 inhibitors for treating COVID-19 disease.

The most-studied IL-6 inhibitor to date is the humanized recombinant IL-6 monoclonal antibody tocilizumab (Actemra®), originally approved for several rheumatologic indications and for chimeric-antigen receptor T-cell (CART therapy) related cytokine release syndrome. Following early small COVID-19 studies presenting mixed results, tocilizumab was evaluated in several larger studies. A second IL-6 inhibitor, sarilumab (Kevzara®), was less extensively studied.

The open-label adaptive-platform REMAP-CAP trial evaluated intravenous weight-based tocilizumab (given as a single dose with an optional second dose 12–24 later) and single-dose intravenous sarilumab [81]. Each was given with SOC and compared to SOC alone. The study population consisted of approximately 800 ICU patients on either noninvasive ventilation, mechanical ventilation, or cardiovascular support. The primary outcome was an ordinal composite of in-hospital mortality and organ support-free days by day 21. In the hospital, survival was defined as a secondary outcome. Both IL-6 inhibitors demonstrated a significant benefit in in-hospital survival and organ support-free days compared to SOC. The benefit appeared to be most pronounced in patients with higher baseline CRP levels. The combined IL-6 data also demonstrated a significantly improved 90-day survival rate compared to SOC. Nine serious adverse events were reported in the tocilizumab arm: five bleeding events, two cardiac events, secondary infection, and visual impairment (one case each). There were no serious adverse events reported in the sarilumab arm and 11 in the SOC arm (seven thromboses, four bleeding events).

Another open-label study, the RECOVERY trial, randomized approximately 2000 hospitalized patients with hypoxia and elevated CRP to either tocilizumab + SOC or SOC alone [82]. Tocilizumab was administered intravenously as a single weight-based tocilizumab dose with the option of a second dose 12–24 hr later if no improvement was noted. The primary outcome, 28-day mortality, occurred in 31% of tocilizumab + SOC patients versus 35% of SOC-only patients (rate ratio 0.85, 95% CI 0.76–0.94, $P = .0028$). Patients in the tocilizumab arm also had significantly earlier discharge and, if not on mechanical ventilation at baseline, a lower likelihood of deterioration to mechanical ventilation or death. Moreover, the clinical benefits conferred by tocilizumab appeared to be additive to those of systemic corticosteroids. Serious adverse events in the tocilizumab arm were otitis externa, *Staphylococcus aureus* bacteremia, and lung abscess (one case each), which resolved uneventfully. A meta-analysis conducted by the RECOVERY Trial investigators found a significant mortality benefit with tocilizumab versus SOC in hospitalized COVID-19 patients. Similarly, a recent systemic review and network meta-analysis of 36 IL-6 inhibitors trials (tocilizumab and sarilumab), combining nearly 20,000 patients, concluded that they appear to reduce mortality, but only if co-administered with a corticosteroid [83].

In contrast, the double-blind, placebo-controlled clinical REMDACTA trial failed to demonstrate the clinical benefit of tocilizumab in hospitalized severe COVID-19 pneumonia patients requiring at least 6 L/min supplemental oxygen [84]. The study randomly assigned 434 patients to receive tocilizumab with remdesivir and 215 patients to placebo with remdesivir. Tocilizumab treatment was not found to shorten the time from randomization to discharge (or to being "ready for discharge"). Mortality was also not significantly altered; death occurred in 18.2% of tocilizumab patients versus 19.7 of placebo patients. Serious adverse events were reported in approximately 30% of patients in both arms; 10.7% of tocilizumab patients discontinued treatment due to an adverse event, as did 13.1% of placebo patients. Similar rates of infections and serious infections were reported in both arms (12% and 7.8% vs. 13.4% and 10% in the tocilizumab and placebo arms, respectively).

Similarly, a multinational double-blind placebo-controlled clinical study failed to demonstrate the clinical benefit of sarilumab in hospitalized, adult COVID-19 pneumonia patients requiring oxygen supplementation or intensive care at baseline [85]. Time to clinical improvement (defined as an improvement ≥2 points on a seven-point ordinal scale) and day-29 survival did not significantly differ between sarilumab and placebo arms. In both arms, treatment-emergent adverse events occurred in 65%–70% of participants, of which approximately 12% were considered serious.

In general, recognized serious adverse effects associated with IL-6 inhibitors include liver function test abnormalities, hematological disorders (neutropenia, thrombocytopenia), secondary infections, and bowel perforations. Hence, Il-6 inhibitors are not to be administered to patients with an active bacterial infection, tuberculosis, or a history of intestinal ulceration or liver disease. Common, less serious adverse effects, include mouth ulcers, headaches, and hypertension.

As cytokines, including IL-6, may down-regulate the expression of CYP450 enzymes, IL-6 inhibition may negate this effect, resulting in induced CYP activity, which may affect multiple medications (such as certain glucocorticosteroids, calcium channel blockers, benzodiazepines, atorvastatin, phenytoin, warfarin and others). This effect may persist for weeks after termination of tocilizumab, owing to its long elimination half-life.

Despite these inconsistent findings, the FDA has granted tocilizumab a EUA for treating COVID-19 disease in June 2021, and current NIH Treatment Guidelines for Therapeutic Management of Hospitalized Adults with COVID-19 [77] list tocilizumab as an option for treating patients requiring supplemental oxygen through the high-flow device or noninvasive ventilation, mechanical ventilation, or ECMO (or any form of supplemental oxygen with rapidly increasing oxygen demand and systemic inflammation). Tocilizumab is used in combination with a corticosteoird with or without remdesivir. Sarilumab is listed as an alternative to IL-6 inhibitor where tocilizumab is not available or not feasible (to date, sarilumab has not been granted a EUA for treating COVID-19 disease). Current WHO Guidelines [86] strongly recommend IL-6 receptor blockers for the treatment of severe or critical COVID-19. Current IDSA guidelines [11] suggest using tocilizumab, in addition to SOC (such as a corticosteroid), for treating progressive severe or critical disease with elevated inflammation markers.

JAK inhibition reduces inflammation by blocking phosphorylation and activation of signal transducers and activators of transcription (STAT) involved in cytokine-mediated inflammatory processes and immune function. Baricitinib (Olumiant®) is an oral reversible Janus-Kinase (JAK) inhibitor that selectively inhibits JAK-1 and JAK-2, originally indicated for the treatment of rheumatoid arthritis (RA) and atopic dermatitis. Another JAK-inhibitor, tofacitinib (Xeljanz®), which predominantly inhibits JAK-1 and JAK-3, is indicated for juvenile idiopathic arthritis and ulcerative colitis. Owing to their immunosuppressive effects, both JAK-inhibitors have been evaluated for treating COVID-19 disease.

In the early stage of the COVID-19 pandemic, it was proposed that baricitinib may reduce the hyperinflammatory process initiated by the viral infection, topped with an antiviral effect elicited by its capability to inhibit viral entry into human cells [87]. As baricitinib has been used for treating rheumatoid arthritis prior to the COVID-19 pandemic, its safety profile has been examined in both clinical trials and post-marketing surveillance. It is noteworthy that baricitinib use in RA is long-term, as opposed to short-term use in COVID-19 disease; hence, safety issues recognized in RA may be related to chronic use and overestimate those to be expected in treating COVID-19 patients. However, as acutely-infected patients were excluded from baricitinib trials for traditional indications, generalizability of safety issues to COVID-19 patients is limited, and their significance for short-term use in COVID-19 patients is yet to be determined.

Baricitinib was used off-label in Italy for COVID-19 patients as early as March 2020 [88]. This small, non-randomized study was later followed by larger trials (detailed below). Adverse effects most commonly reported in those trials were upper respiratory tract infections (14%–24%), headache (11%–24%) and nasopharyngitis (11%–18%). In addition, similar to other JAK inhibitors, baricitinib use was associated with various laboratory findings such as decreased hemoglobin, neutrophil and lymphocyte counts, liver function test abnormalities, increased platelet count, bilirubin and CPK, and lipid parameters. Most of these effects are typical of JAK inhibitors. Clinically, serious adverse effects related to baricitinib use included thrombosis, opportunistic infections, GI perforations, malignancies, and major cardiovascular events [87].

Baricitinib dosing in COVID-19 disease is 4 mg taken orally once daily, regardless of food, for 7–14 days. The daily dose is halved in patients with moderate renal failure (eGFR 30–60 mL/min), and reduced to 1 mg with more significant impairment (eGFR 15–30 mL/min); use is contraindicated with eGFR<15 mL/min. Being an organic anionic transporter-3 (OAT3) substrate, baricitinib exposure might be increased by OAT3 inhibitors such as probenecid.

Baricitinib is currently NIH-recommended for use in hospitalized adult patients with increasing oxygen supplementation requiring a high-flow device or noninvasive ventilation, and with systemic inflammation, in combination with a corticosteroid, with or without remdesivir [77]. Current IDSA guidelines [12] recommend baricitinib for severely-ill hospitalized patients on high-flow oxygen or noninvasive ventilation, while citing limited data for mortality benefit in mechanically-ventilated patients. Similarly, baricitinib is also recommended by WHO guidelines for treating severe and critical COVID-19 patients, while recommending against use of tofacitinib due to insufficient data, unless baricitinib or IL-6 inhibitors is not available [12]. All three guidelines recommend against combining JAK inhibitors with IL-6 inhibitors.

The first large randomized clinical study to evaluate baricitinib in COVID-19 was the double-blind, placebo-controlled, multinational NIH-sponsored ACTT-2 trial, which assigned 1,033 COVID-19 hospitalized patients to either baricitinib or placebo for up to 14 days or until hospital discharge, both in addition to standard remdesivir treatment. The median time to recovery was slightly shorter in the baricitinib arm (7 days) compared to the placebo arm (8 days, recovery rate ratio 1.16, 95% CI 1.01–1.32, $P = .03$). The effect was greatest in patients on high-flow oxygen or noninvasive ventilation (recovery rate ratio 1.51, 95% CI 1.1–2.08). 28-day mortality was 5.1% versus 7.8% in the baricitinib and placebo arms, respectively (hazard ratio 0.65, 95% CI 0.39–1.09). Adverse effects, including new infections, were more frequent in the placebo arm; those most commonly reported were hyperglycemia, anemia, decreased lymphocyte count, and acute kidney injury. These results suggest that combined baricitinib + remdesivir is marginally superior to remdesivir alone, and that this effect is most pronounced in patients on high-flow oxygen or non-invasive ventilation.

Based on the ACTT-2 findings, an initial EUA for using baricitinib with remdesivir for treating hospitalized adult COVID-19 patients requiring any supplemental oxygen was granted by the FDA in November 2020.

A second NIH-sponsored, multinational, randomized, double-blind, placebo-controlled clinical study, COV-BARRIEIR, assigned 1,525 hospitalized adult COVID-19 patients to 4 mg baricitinib or placebo orally, once daily for up to 14 days in addition to SOC, which included systemic corticosteroids (approximately 79% of patients) and/or antivirals (approximately 19% remdesivir) [89]. Progression to high-flow oxygen, noninvasive ventilation, invasive mechanical ventilation (including ECMO), or death by day 28, the composite primary outcome, was slightly, yet statistically significantly reduced in the baricitinib arm (27.8%) compared to the placebo arm (30.5%; odds ratio 0.85, 95% CI 0.67–1.08, $P = 0.18$). However, day-28 all-cause mortality, a pre-defined secondary outcome, was significantly lower in the baricitinib arm (8%) versus the placebo arm (13%, hazard ratio 0.57, 95% CI 0.41–0.78, $P = .0018$), representing an NNT of 20. An additional analysis found that day-60 all-cause mortality was also significantly lower in baricitinib patients compared to placebo (10% vs. 15%, respectively, HR = 0.62, 95% CI 0.47–0.83, $P = .005$). The mortality benefit was even larger in a subset of patients requiring oxygen at baseline and not receiving concomitant corticosteroids. Serious adverse events were more frequent in the placebo arm (18%) compared to the baricitinib arm (15%), as were treatment discontinuations related to adverse effects (9% vs. 7%, respectively). Treatment-emergent infections were reported in 16% of patients in both arms, venous thromboembolic events occurring in approximately 3% of participants in both arms, and major cardiovascular events occurred in 1% in both arms. As the primary endpoint did not differ between baricitinib and placebo, despite a considerable reduction in both 28-day and 60-day mortality (defined as secondary and exploratory endpoints, respectively), COV-BARRIER findings justify further studies for better defining subgroups of patients, which may gain maximal benefit from this drug (perhaps patients with more severe disease at baseline). Following the COV-BARRIER study, the FDA reissued the baricitinib EUA in July 2021, to longer mandate the combination with remdesivir. In addition, the EUA was further expanded to include pediatric patients aged 2 years and above in May 2022.

The combined safety data of ACTT-2 and COV-BARRIER trials demonstrate that infections, venous thromboembolic events, overall treatment-emergent adverse events, serious adverse events, discontinuations due to adverse events, and any-cause death occurred more frequently in the placebo arms compared with baricitinib arms [90], thereby further assuring the safe use of baricitinib in hospitalized COVID-19 patients. The open-label RECOVERY trial platform reported that addition of baricitinib to SOC in hospitalized COVID-19 patients significantly reduced 28-day mortality rate by 13% as compared with SOC only, with no additional safety issues (although the clinical benefit was somewhat smaller than the combined 43% mortality rate reduction reported in a meta-analysis of eight previous JAK-inhibition trials [91]

The randomised, double-blind, double placebo-controlled, multi-center ACTT-4 trial, enrolled hospitalised adults COVID-19 patients who required supplemental oxygen administered by low- or , high-flow or non-invasive mechanical ventilation modalities, to receive remdesivir with either baricitinib or dexamethasone [92]. The primary outcome, day-29 mechanical ventilation free survival, was similar in both groups, but dexamethasone was associated with significantly more adverse effects, including severe and life-threatening events.

The STOP-COVID clinical trial randomized 289 hospitalized adult COVID-19 patients to either tofacitinib 10 mg or placebo, orally for 14 days or until hospital discharge [93]. The primary outcome, respiratory failure or death by day 29, occurred in 18.1% of tofacitinib patients compared to 29% of placebo patients (risk ratio 0.63, 95% CI 0.41–0.97, $P = .04$). Death from any cause by day 28 was lower in the tofacitinib arm compared to the placebo arm (2.8% vs. 5.5%, respectively, hazard ratio 0.49, 95% CI 0.15–1.63), as were odds of a worse clinical score on day 14 and day 28 (hazard ratio 0.6 and 0.54, respectively). Adverse events were reported in 26.1% of tofacitinib patients versus 22.5% of placebo patients. Elevated liver function tests, hepatic failure, acute kidney injury, and lymphopenia occurred more frequently in the tofacitinib arm; however, infection rates were similar. Acute myocardial infarction, aspiration, deep vein thrombosis, pulmonary hypertension, seizure, and ventricular tachycardia each occurred in one patient in the tofacitinib arm, while anemia, cardiogenic shock, multiple organ dysfunction syndrome, and shock each occurred in one patient in the placebo arm.

Being a CYP-3A4 substrate, the tofacitinib dose is reduced when combined with drugs moderately inhibiting this enzyme, and tofacitinib is not recommended with strong inhibitors.

Due to multiple potential drug-drug interactions, twice-daily administration, and a relatively small-sample clinical trial, it appears that tofactinib may be suitable as an alternative JAK inhibitor for treating COVID-19 disease where baricitinib is not available. This is reflected in the section regarding kinase inhibitors in NIH COVID-19 treatment guidelines [94].

To date, limited data is available regarding the use of several other JAK-inhibitors (such as ruxolitinib) and tyrosine-kinase inhibitors for treating COVID-19 disease.

Respiratory support

A detailed treatment strategy for the respiratory support of COVID-19 patients is beyond the scope of this discussion, but a general approach will be outlined in the text below, in accordance with the WHO, CDC, and NIH guidelines.

In general, oxygen should be supplemented to achieve a target peripheral oxygen saturation of ≥90%, with either a low- or a high-flow oxygen delivery system, as well as non-invasive ventilation (NIV), in accordance with patient respiratory distress, comorbidities, and hypoxemia severity.

Awake proning, when feasible, was thought to reduce the need for intubation [95] [93,96], but later studies did not find a difference in intubation rates, length of stay, or mortality with awake pronation versus standard of care [96]. Data regarding the efficacy of high flow nasal cannulae (HFNC) and NIV in COVID-19 is limited, although there are signs of benefit [97,98] [115]. HFNC is usually preferred due to better patient comfort, but NIV can be used in patients with proven indications, including obstructive sleep apnea, pulmonary edema, or chronic obstructive pulmonary disease (COPD) exacerbation. While some patients will fail these conservative approaches to oxygen support, the "right timing" for intubation remains elusive. Although practice varies and decisions should be individualized, patients should be probably intubated if they suffer from rapid and progressive deterioration, including worsening mental status, hemodynamic compromise, hypercapnia, or refractory hypoxemia, despite conservative treatment. Patients with COVID-19-related acute respiratory distress syndrome (ARDS) often require prolonged mechanical ventilation ($\geq$2 weeks) and some will require tracheostomy to facilitate weaning. In general, the treatment of mechanically ventilated COVID-related ARDS patients should follow the evidence-based ARDS guidelines, including lung-protective ventilation (tidal volume $\leq$6 mL/kg, plateau pressure $\leq$30 cm), relatively high positive end-expiratory pressure (PEEP) adjusted to the fraction of inspired oxygen [FiO_2], and lowest FiO_2 possible (preferably <0.6) to achieve the saturation target of 90%–96% [100].

In patients with moderate to severe ARDS and refractory hypoxemia (partial pressure of oxygen [PaO_2] to FiO_2 ratio of <150 mmHg), rescue procedures might include pronation, alveolar recruitment maneuvers (e.g., higher PEEP), neuromuscular blockage, pulmonary vasodilators (inhaled nitric oxide or epoprostenol) and extracorporeal membrane oxygenation (ECMO). Among these interventions, only the use of pronation and ECMO were found to lower mortality among non-COVID severe ARDS patients. Data regarding these modalities in COVID-19 patients is limited but there are signals of benefit [101–104].

While awaiting more evidence, ECMO can be used in COVID-19 patients in accordance with its general indications for other causes [105], either as a salvage treatment for patients who fail to improve despite all the above strategies or upfront in severe ARDS (PaO_2/FiO_2 < 100 mmHg). Lung transplantation may be an acceptable treatment for selected patients with irreversible respiratory failure due to Covid-19 [106].

References

[1] Mulangu S, Dodd LE, Davey Jr RT, Tshiani Mbaya O, et al. A randomized, controlled trial of Ebola virus disease therapeutics. N Engl J Med 2019;381(24):2293–303. https://doi.org/10.1056/NEJMoa1910993. pmid:31774950.

[2] Beigel JH, Tomashek KM, Dodd LE, Mehta AK, et al. Remdesivir for the treatment of Covid-19–final report. N Engl J Med 2020;383(19):1813–26. https://doi.org/10.1056/NEJMoa2007764. pmid:32445440.

[3] Spinner CD, Gottlieb RL, Criner GJ, Arribas Lopez JR, et al. Effect of remdesivir vs standard care on clinical status at 11 days in patients with moderate COVID-19: a randomized clinical trial. JAMA 2020;324(11):1048–57. https://doi.org/10.1001/jama.2020.16349. pmid:32821939.

[4] Goldman JD, Lye DCB, Hui DS, Marks KM, et al. Remdesivir for 5 or 10 days in patients with severe Covid-19. N Engl J Med 2020;383(19):1827–37. https://doi.org/10.1056/NEJMoa2015301. pmid:32459919.

[5] WHO Solidarity Trial Consortium. Repurposed antiviral drugs for Covid-19–interim WHO solidarity trial results. N Engl J Med 2021;384(6):497–511. https://doi.org/10.1056/NEJMoa2023184. pmid:33264556.

[6] Pettit NN, Pisano J, Nguyen CT, Lew AK, et al. Remdesivir use in the setting of severe renal impairment: a theoretical concern or real risk? Clin Infect Dis 2020;i73(11):e3990–5. https://doi.org/10.1093/cid/ciaa1851.

[7] Ansems K, Grundeis F, Dahms K, Mikolajewska A, et al. Remdesivir for the treatment of COVID-19. Cochrane Database Syst Rev 2021;8:CD014962. https://doi.org/10.1002/14651858.CD014962. pmid:34350582.

[8] Mechineni A, Kassab H, Manickam R. Remdesivir for the treatment of COVID 19: review of the pharmacological properties, safety and clinical effectiveness. Expert Opin Drug Saf 2021;20(11):1299–307. https://doi.org/10.1080/14740338.2021.1962284. pmid:34338121.

[9] Ali K, Azher T, Baqi M, Binnie A, et al. Remdesivir for the treatment of patients in hospital with COVID-19 in Canada: a randomized controlled trial. CMAJ (Can Med Assoc J) 2022. https://doi.org/10.1503/cmaj.211698. pmid:35045989.

[10] Gottlieb RL, Vaca CE, Paredes R, Mera J, et al. Early remdesivir to prevent progression to severe Covid-19 in outpatients. N Engl J Med 2021;386(4):305–15. https://doi.org/10.1056/NEJMoa2116846.

[11] ISDA COVID-19 real-time learning network: antivirals (updated August 30th 2022). Centers for disease control (CDC) and infectious diseases society of America (IDSA). IDSA; 2022. Available from: https://www.idsociety.org/practice-guideline/covid-19-guideline-treatment-and-management/. [Accessed 31 August 2022].

[12] Therapeutics and COVID-19: [WHO] living guideline (updated July 14th, 2022). World Health Organization (WHO); 2022. Available from: https://app.magicapp.org/#/guideline/6290. [Accessed 31 August 2022].

[13] Tempestilli M, Caputi P, Avataneo V, Notari S, et al. Pharmacokinetics of remdesivir and GS-441524 in two critically ill patients who recovered from COVID-19. J Antimicrob Chemother 2020;75(10):2977–80. https://doi.org/10.1093/jac/dkaa239. pmid:32607555.

[14] FDA. Fact sheet for healthcare providers: emergency Use Authorization for molnupiravir. Kenilworth, NJ, USA: Merck & Co, Inc; 2021. Available from, https://www.fda.gov/media/155054/download. [Accessed 30 January 2022].

[15] FDA. FDA Emergency Use Authorization for the treatment of high-risk adults with mild to moderate COVID-19. Kenilworth, NJ, USA: Merck & Co, Inc; 2021. Available from: https://www.merck.com/news/merck-and-ridgebacks-molnupiravir-receives-u-s-fda-emergency-use-authorization-for-the-treatment-of-high-risk-adults-with-mild-to-moderate-covid-19/. [Accessed 30 January 2022].

[16] Jayk Bernal A, Gomes da Silva MM, Musungaie DB, Kovalchuk E, et al. Molnupiravir for oral treatment of Covid-19 in nonhospitalized patients. N Engl J Med 2021. https://doi.org/10.1056/NEJMoa2116044.

[17] Arribas JR, Bhagani S, Lobo SM, Khaertynova I, et al. Randomized trial of molnupiravir or placebo in patients hospitalized with Covid-19. NEJM Evidence 2022;1(2). https://doi.org/10.1056/EVIDoa2100044.

[18] NIH. Therapeutic Management of Nonhospitalized Adults With COVID-19 (updated August 8th, 2022). Washington, DC, USA: U.S. National Institutes of Health (NIH); 2022. Available from: https://www.covid19treatmentguidelines.nih.gov/management/clinical-management-of-adults/nonhospitalized-adults–therapeutic-management/. [Accessed 31 August 2022].

[19] Hammond J, Leister-Tebbe H, Gardner A, et al., EPIC-HR investigators. Oral Nirmatrelvir for High-Risk, Nonhospitalized Adults with Covid-19. N Engl J Med 2022;386:1397–408. https://doi.org/10.1056/NEJMoa2118542.

[20] FDA. Fact sheet for healthcare providers: emergency use authorization for Paxlovid. New York, NY, USA: Pfizer, Inc.; 2021. Available from, www.fda.gov/media/155050/download#:~:text=The%20dosage%20for%20PAXLOVID%20is,each%20active%20ingredient%20within%20PAXLOVID./. [Accessed 30 January 2022].

[21] Arbel R, Wolff-Sagy Y, Hoshen M, et al. Nirmatrelvir Use and Severe Covid-19 Outcomes during the Omicron Surge. N Engl J Med 2022;387:790–8. https://doi.org/10.1056/NEJMoa2204919.

[22] Pfizer. Pfizer Reports Additional Data on PAXLOVIDTM Supporting Upcoming New Drug Application Submission to U.S. FDA. https://www.pfizer.com/news/press-release/press-release-detail/pfizer-reports-additional-data-paxlovidtm-supporting. [Accessed 31 August 2022].

[23] Pfizer. Pfizer Shares Top-Line Results from Phase 2/3 EPIC-PEP Study of PAXLOVIDTM for Post-Exposure Prophylactic Use. https://www.pfizer.com/news/press-release/press-release-detail/pfizer-shares-top-line-results-phase-23-epic-pep-study. [Accessed 31 August 2022].

[24] Atmar RL, Finch N/. New perspectives on antimicrobial agents: molnupiravir and nirmatrelvir/ritonavir for treatment of COVID-19. Antimicrob Agents Chemother 2022;66(8). https://doi.org/10.1128/aac.02404-21.

[25] Cao H, Shi Y. Convalescent plasma: possible therapy for novel coronavirus disease 2019. Transfusion 2020;60(5):1078–83. https://doi.org/10.1111/trf.15797. pmid:32359090.

[26] Duan K, Liu B, Li C, Zhang H, et al. Effectiveness of convalescent plasma therapy in severe COVID-19 patients. Proc Natl Acad Sci U S A 2020;117(17):9490–6. https://doi.org/10.1073/pnas.2004168117.

[27] Joyner MJ, Senefeld JW, Klassen SA, Mills JR, et al. Effect of convalescent plasma on mortality among hospitalized patients with COVID-19: initial 3-month experience. medRxiv 2020. https://doi.org/10.1101/2020.08.12.20169359. pmid:32817978.

[28] Abani O, Abbas A, Abbas F, Abbas M, et al. Convalescent plasma in patients admitted to hospital with COVID-19 (RECOVERY): a randomised controlled, open-label, platform trial. Lancet 2021;397(10289):2049–59. https://doi.org/10.1016/S0140-6736(21)00897-7.

[29] NIH. COVID-19 treatment guidelines: convalescent plasma (updated April 29th, 2022). Washington, DC, USA: U.S. National Institutes of Health (NIH); 2022. Available from: https://www.covid19treatmentguidelines.nih.gov/therapies/anti-sars-cov-2-antibody-products/covid-19-convalescent-plasma/. [Accessed 31 August 2022].

[30] Korley FK, Durkalski-Mauldin V, Yeatts SD, Schulman K, et al. Early convalescent plasma for high-risk outpatients with Covid-19. N Engl J Med 2021;385(21):1951–60. https://doi.org/10.1056/NEJMoa2103784.

[31] Sullivan DJ, Gebo KA, Shoham S, et al. Randomized controlled trial of early outpatient COVID-19 treatment with high-titer convalescent plasma. New England Journal of Medicine 2022;386:1700–11. https://doi.org/10.1056/NEJMoa2119657.

[32] Herishanu Y, Avivi I, Aharon A, Shefer G, et al. Efficacy of the BNT162b2 mRNA COVID-19 vaccine in patients with chronic lymphocytic leukemia. Blood 2021;137(23):3165–73. https://doi.org/10.1182/blood.2021011568.

[33] Hamilton FW, Lee T, Arnold DT, Lilford R, et al. Is convalescent plasma futile in COVID-19? A Bayesian re-analysis of the RECOVERY randomized controlled trial. Int J Infect Dis 2021;109:114–7. https://doi.org/10.1016/j.ijid.2021.06.034.

[34] FDA. Revised indications for the emergency use authorization of convalescent plasma for the treatment of COVID-19 (December 28, 2021). Washington, DC, USA: Food and Drug Administration (FDA), U.S. Department of Health and Human Services (HHS); 2021. Available from: https://www.fda.gov/media/141477/download/. [Accessed 30 January 2022].

[35] Senefeld JW, Johnson PW, Kunze KL, Bloch EM, et al. Access to and safety of COVID-19 convalescent plasma in the United States Expanded Access Program: a national registry study. PLoS Med 2021;18(12). https://doi.org/10.1371/journal.pmed.1003872. e1003872.

[36] Writing Committee for the REMAP-CAP Investigators. Effect of convalescent plasma on organ support–free days in critically ill patients with COVID-19: a randomized clinical trial. JAMA 2021;326(17):1690–702. https://doi.org/10.1001/jama.2021.18178.

[37] Bégin P, Callum J, Jamula E, Cook R, et al. Convalescent plasma for hospitalized patients with COVID-19: an open-label, randomized controlled trial. Nat Med (N Y, NY, U S) 2021;27(11):2012–24. https://doi.org/10.1038/s41591-021-01488-2.

[38] FDA. Fact sheet for healthcare providers: emergency Use Authorization (EUA) of bamlanivimab. Indianapolis. FDA; 2021. Available from: https://www.fda.gov/media/143603/download/. [Accessed 31 January 2022].

[39] Chen P, Nirula A, Heller B, Gottlieb RL, et al. SARS-CoV-2 neutralizing antibody LY-CoV555 in outpatients with Covid-19. N Engl J Med 2021;384(3):229–37. https://doi.org/10.1056/NEJMoa2029849. pmid:33113295.

[40] FDA. Coronavirus (COVID-19) update: FDA revokes Emergency Use Authorization for monoclonal antibody bamlanivimab. Washington DC, USA: US Food and Drug Administration (FDA), Department of Health and Human Services; 2021. Available from: https://www.fda.gov/news-events/press-announcements/coronavirus-covid-19-update-fda-revokes-emergency-use-authorization-monoclonal-antibody-bamlanivimab/. [Accessed 31 January 2022].

[41] Dougan M, Nirula A, Azizad M, Mocherla B, et al. Bamlanivimab plus etesevimab in mild or moderate Covid-19. N Engl J Med 2021;385(15):1382–92. https://doi.org/10.1056/NEJMoa2102685. pmid:34260849.

[42] Fact sheet for health care providers: emergency Use Authorization (EUA) of bamlanivimab and etesevimab. Indianapolis, IN, USA: Eli Lilly and Co; 2021. Available from: https://www.fda.gov/media/145802/download/. [Accessed 31 January 2022].

[43] FDA. Revised indications for the Emergency Use Authorization of bamlanivimab and etesevimab administered together (January 24, 2022). Washington, DC, USA: Food and Drug Administration (FDA), Department of Health and Human Services (HHS); 2022. Available from: https://www.fda.gov/media/145801/download/. [Accessed 31 January 2022].

[44] Weinreich DM, Sivapalasingam S, Norton T, Ali S, et al. REGEN-COV antibody combination and outcomes in outpatients with Covid-19. N Engl J Med 2021;385(23):e81. https://doi.org/10.1056/NEJMoa2108163. pmid:34587383.

[45] O'Brien MP, Forleo-Neto E, Musser BJ, Isa F, et al. Subcutaneous REGEN-COV antibody combination to prevent Covid-19. N Engl J Med 2021;385(13):1184–95. https://doi.org/10.1056/NEJMoa2109682. pmid:34347950.

[46] O'Brien MP, Forleo-Neto E, Sarkar N, Isa F, et al. Effect of subcutaneous casirivimab and imdevimab antibody combination vs placebo on development of symptomatic COVID-19 in early asymptomatic SARS-CoV-2 infection: a randomized clinical trial. JAMA 2022;327:432–41. https://doi.org/10.1001/jama.2021.24939. pmid:35029629.

[47] Gupta A, Gonzalez-Rojas Y, Juarez E, et al. Early Treatment for Covid-19 with SARS-CoV-2 Neutralizing Antibody Sotrovimab. N Engl J Med 2021;385:1941–50. https://doi.org/10.1056/NEJMoa2107934.

[48] IDSA COVID-19 Real-Time Learning Network. Anti-SARS-CoV-2 Monoclonal Antibodies. https://www.idsociety.org/covid-19-real-time-learning-network/therapeutics-and-interventions/monoclonal-antibodies/#Bebtelovimab. [Accessed 31 August 2022].

[49] FDA. Fact Sheet for Healthcare Providers: Emregency Use Authorization for Bebtelovimab (updated August 2022). https://www.fda.gov/media/156152/download. [Accessed 31 August 2022].

[50] Dougan M, Azizad M, Chen P, et al., MedRxiv. Bebtelovimab, alone or together with bamlanivimab and etesevimab, as a broadly neutralizing monoclonal antibody treatment for mild to moderate, ambulatory COVID-19. https://www.medrxiv.org/content/10.1101/2022.03.10.22272100v1. [Accessed 31 August 2022].

[51] FDA. FDA authorizes revisions to Evusheld dosing. https://www.fda.gov/drugs/drug-safety-and-availability/fda-authorizes-revisions-evusheld-dosing. [Accessed 1 September 2022].
[52] Kollias A, Kyriakoulis KG, Lagou S, Kontopantelis E, et al. Venous thromboembolism in COVID-19: a systematic review and meta-analysis. Vasc Med 2021;26(4):415–25. https://doi.org/10.1177/1358863X21995566. pmid:33818197.
[53] Tang N, Bai H, Chen X, Gong J, et al. Anticoagulant treatment is associated with decreased mortality in severe coronavirus disease 2019 patients with coagulopathy. J Thromb Haemostasis 2020;18(5):1094–9. https://doi.org/10.1111/jth.14817. pmid:32220112.
[54] REMAP-CAP, ACTIV-4a, and ATTACC Investigators. Therapeutic Anticoagulation with Heparin in Critically Ill Patients with Covid-19. N Engl J Med 2021;385:777–89. https://doi.org/10.1056/NEJMoa2103417.
[55] ATTACC I, ACTIV-4a A, REMAP-CAP I, Lawler PR, et al. Therapeutic anticoagulation with heparin in noncritically ill patients with Covid-19. N Engl J Med 2021;385(9):790–802. https://doi.org/10.1056/NEJMoa2105911. pmid:34351721.
[56] Sholzberg M, Tang GH, Rahhal H, AlHamzah M, et al. Effectiveness of therapeutic heparin versus prophylactic heparin on death, mechanical ventilation, or intensive care unit admission in moderately ill patients with covid-19 admitted to hospital: RAPID randomised clinical trial. BMJ 2021;375. https://doi.org/10.1136/bmj.n2400. n2400.
[57] Spyropoulos AC, Goldin M, Giannis D, Diab W, et al. Efficacy and safety of therapeutic-dose heparin vs standard prophylactic or intermediate-dose heparins for thromboprophylaxis in high-risk hospitalized patients with COVID-19: the HEP-COVID randomized clinical trial. JAMA Intern Med 2021;181(12):1612–20. https://doi.org/10.1001/jamainternmed.2021.6203. pmid:34617959.
[58] NIH: the COVID-19 Treatment Guidelines Panel's Statement on anticoagulation in hospitalized patients with COVID-19 (updated May 31st, 2022). Washington, DC, USA: National Institutes of Health (NIH), Department of Health and Human Services (HSS); 2022. Available from: https://www.covid19treatmentguidelines.nih.gov/therapies/antithrombotic-therapy/. [Accessed 31 August 2022].
[59] Cuker A, Tseng EK, Nieuwlaat R, Angchaisuksiri P, et al. American Society of Hematology living guidelines on the use of anticoagulation for thromboprophylaxis in patients with COVID-19: July 2021 update on postdischarge thromboprophylaxis. Blood Advances 2022;6(2):664–71. https://doi.org/10.1182/bloodadvances.2021005945.
[60] Cuker A, Tseng EK, Nieuwlaat R, et al. American Society of Hematology living guidelines on the use of anticoagulation for thromboprophylaxis for patients with COVID-19: March 2022 update on the use of anticoagulation in critically ill patients. Blood Adv 2022;6(17):4975–82. https://doi.org/10.1182/bloodadvances.2022007940.
[61] IDSA COVID-19 real-time learning network: thrombosis (updated January 20th, 2022).
[62] Lopes RD, de Barros ESPGM, Furtado RHM, Macedo AVS, et al. Therapeutic versus prophylactic anticoagulation for patients admitted to hospital with COVID-19 and elevated D-dimer concentration (ACTION): an open-label, multicentre, randomised, controlled trial. Lancet 2021;397(10291):2253–63. https://doi.org/10.1016/S0140-6736(21)01203-4. pmid:34097856.
[63] INSPIRATION Investigators. Effect of intermediate-dose vs standard-dose prophylactic anticoagulation on thrombotic events, extracorporeal membrane oxygenation treatment, or mortality among patients with COVID-19 admitted to the intensive care unit: the INSPIRATION randomized clinical trial. JAMA 2021;325(16):1620–30. https://doi.org/10.1001/jama.2021.4152. pmid:33734299.
[64] Ramacciotti E, Barile Agati L, Calderaro D, Aguiar VCR, et al. Rivaroxaban versus no anticoagulation for post-discharge thromboprophylaxis after hospitalisation for COVID-19 (MICHELLE): an open-label, multicentre, randomised, controlled trial. Lancet 2022;399(10319):50–9. https://doi.org/10.1016/S0140-6736(21)02392-8. pmid:34921756.
[65] Russell CD, Millar JE, Baillie JK. Clinical evidence does not support corticosteroid treatment for 2019-nCoV lung injury. Lancet 2020;395(10223):473–5. https://doi.org/10.1016/S0140-6736(20)30317-2. pmid:32043983.
[66] Shang L, Zhao J, Hu Y, Du R, et al. On the use of corticosteroids for 2019-nCoV pneumonia. Lancet 2020;395(10225):683–4. https://doi.org/10.1016/S0140-6736(20)30361-5. pmid:32122468.
[67] Recovery Collaborative Group. Dexamethasone in hospitalized patients with Covid-19. N Engl J Med 2021;384(8):693–704. https://doi.org/10.1056/NEJMoa2021436. pmid:32678530.
[68] Tomazini BM, Maia IS, Cavalcanti AB, Berwanger O, et al. Effect of dexamethasone on days alive and ventilator-free in patients with moderate or severe acute respiratory distress syndrome and COVID-19: the CoDEX randomized clinical trial. JAMA 2020;324(13):1307–16. https://doi.org/10.1001/jama.2020.17021. pmid:32876695.

[69] Angus DC, Derde L, Al-Beidh F, Annane D, et al. Effect of hydrocortisone on mortality and organ support in patients with severe COVID-19: the REMAP-CAP COVID-19 corticosteroid domain randomized clinical trial. JAMA 2020;324(13):1317–29. https://doi.org/10.1001/jama.2020.17022. pmid:32876697.

[70] NIH. COVID-19 Treatment Guidelines: Corticosteroids. Washington, DC, USA: National Institutes of Health (NIH), Department of Health and Human Services (HHS); 2022. Available from: https://www.covid19treatmentguidelines.nih.gov/therapies/immunomodulators/corticosteroids/. [Accessed 31 August 2022].

[71] Pinzón MA, Ortiz S, Holguín H, Betancur JF, et al. Dexamethasone vs methylprednisolone high dose for Covid-19 pneumonia. PLoS One 2021;16(5). https://doi.org/10.1371/journal.pone.0252057. e0252057.

[72] The COVID STEROID 2 Trial Group. Effect of 12 mg vs 6 mg of dexamethasone on the number of days alive without life support in adults with COVID-19 and severe hypoxemia: the COVID STEROID 2 randomized trial. JAMA 2021;326(18):1807–17. https://doi.org/10.1001/jama.2021.18295.

[73] Bouadma L, Mekontso-Dessap A, Burdet C, et al. High-dose dexamethasone and oxygen support strategies in intensive care unit patients with severe COVID-19 acute hypoxemic respiratory failure the COVIDICUS randomized clinical trial. JAMA Inter Med 2022. https://doi.org/10.1001/jamainternmed.2022.2168.

[74] Granholm A, Munch MW, Myatra SN, Vijayaraghavan BKT, et al. Dexamethasone 12 mg versus 6 mg for patients with COVID-19 and severe hypoxaemia: a pre-planned, secondary Bayesian analysis of the COVID STEROID 2 trial. Intensive Care Med 2022;48(1):45–55. https://doi.org/10.1007/s00134-021-06573-1. pmid:34757439.

[75] Khiali S, Entezari-Maleki T. Therapeutic application of corticosteroids in COVID-19: a focus on optimum dose and duration of therapy. J Clin Pharmacol 2021;61(9):1145–8. https://doi.org/10.1002/jcph.1929.

[76] Wagner C, Griesel M, Mikolajewska A, Mueller A, et al. Systemic corticosteroids for the treatment of COVID-19. Cochrane Database Syst Rev 2021;(8). https://doi.org/10.1002/14651858.CD014963. pmid:CD014963.

[77] NIH. Therapeutic management of hospitalized adults with COVID-19 (updated August 8th 2022). Washington, DC: National Institutes of Health (NIH), Department of Health and Human Services (HHS); 2021. 2021 Available from: https://www.covid19treatmentguidelines.nih.gov/management/clinical-management/hospitalized-adults–therapeutic-management/. [Accessed 31 August 2022].

[78] Ramakrishnan S, Nicolau Jr DV, Langford B, Mahdi M, et al. Inhaled budesonide in the treatment of early COVID-19 (STOIC): a phase 2, open-label, randomised controlled trial. Lancet Respir Med 2021;9(7):763–72. https://doi.org/10.1016/S2213-2600(21)00160-0.

[79] Velazquez-Salinas L, Verdugo-Rodriguez A, Rodriguez LL, Borca MV. The role of interleukin 6 during viral infections. Front Microbiol 2019;10:1057. https://doi.org/10.3389/fmicb.2019.01057. pmid:31134045.

[80] Zhou F, Yu T, Du R, Fan G, et al. Clinical course and risk factors for mortality of adult inpatients with COVID-19 in Wuhan, China: a retrospective cohort study. Lancet (London, England) 2020;395(10229):1054–62. https://doi.org/10.1016/S0140-6736(20)30566-3. pmid:32171076.

[81] REMAP-CAP Investigators. Interleukin-6 receptor antagonists in critically ill patients with Covid-19. N Engl J Med 2021;384(16):1491–502. https://doi.org/10.1056/NEJMoa2100433. pmid:33631065.

[82] Abani O, Abbas A, Abbas F, Abbas M, et al. Tocilizumab in patients admitted to hospital with COVID-19 (RECOVERY): a randomised, controlled, open-label, platform trial. Lancet 2021;397(10285):1637–45. https://doi.org/10.1016/S0140-6736(21)00676-0.

[83] Zeraatkar D, Cusano E, Díaz Martínez JP, et al. Use of tocilizumab and sarilumab alone or in combination with corticosteroids for covid-19: systematic review and network meta-analysis. BMJ Med 2022;1:1–14. https://doi.org/10.1136/bmjmed-2021-000036.

[84] Rosas IO, Diaz G, Gottlieb RL, Lobo SM, et al. Tocilizumab and remdesivir in hospitalized patients with severe COVID-19 pneumonia: a randomized clinical trial. Intensive Care Med 2021;47(11):1258–70. https://doi.org/10.1007/s00134-021-06507-x.

[85] Lescure F-X, Honda H, Fowler RA, Lazar JS, et al. Sarilumab in patients admitted to hospital with severe or critical COVID-19: a randomised, double-blind, placebo-controlled, phase 3 trial. Lancet Respir Med 2021;9(5):522–32. https://doi.org/10.1016/S2213-2600(21)00099-0.

[86] WHO. WHO recommends life-saving interleukin-6 receptor blockers for COVID-19 and urges producers to join efforts to rapidly increase access (Updated July 6, 2021). Geneva, Switzerland: World Health Organization (WHO); 2021. Available from: https://www.who.int/news/item/06-07-2021-who-recommends-life-saving-interleukin-6-receptor-blockers-for-covid-19-and-urges-producers-to-join-efforts-to-rapidly-increase-access/. [Accessed 10 February 2022].

[87] Jorgensen SCJ, Tse CLY, Burry L, Dresser LD. Baricitinib: a review of pharmacology, safety, and emerging clinical experience in COVID-19. Pharmacotherapy 2020;40(8):843–56. https://doi.org/10.1002/phar.2438.

[88] Cantini F, Niccoli L, Matarrese D, Nicastri E, et al. Baricitinib therapy in COVID-19: a pilot study on safety and clinical impact. J Infect 2020;81(2):318–56. https://doi.org/10.1016/j.jinf.2020.04.017.

[89] Marconi VC, Ramanan AV, de Bono S, Kartman CE, et al. Efficacy and safety of baricitinib for the treatment of hospitalised adults with COVID-19 (COV-BARRIER): a randomised, double-blind, parallel-group, placebo-controlled phase 3 trial. Lancet Respir Med 2021;9(12):1407–18. https://doi.org/10.1016/s2213-2600(21)00331-3. pmid:34480861.

[90] Fact sheet for healthcare providers: emergency Use Authorization (EUA) of baricitinib (revised December 2021). Indianapolis, IN, USA: Eli Lilly & Co; 2021. Available from: https://www.fda.gov/media/143823/download/. [Accessed 1 February 2022].

[91] RECOVERY Collaborative Group. Baricitinib in patients admitted to hospital with COVID-19 (RECOVERY): A randomised, controlled, open-label, platform trial and updated meta-analysis. Lancet 2022;400(10349):359–68. https://doi.org/10.1016/S0140-6736(22)01109-6).

[92] Wolfe CR, Tomashek KM, Patterson TF, et al. Baricitinib versus dexamethasone for adults hospitalised with COVID-19 (ACTT-4): a randomised, double-blind, double placebo-controlled trial. Lancet 2022;10(9):888–99. https://doi.org/10.1016/S2213-2600(22)00088-1.

[93] Guimarães PO, Quirk D, Furtado RH, Maia LN, et al. Tofacitinib in patients hospitalized with Covid-19 pneumonia. N Engl J Med 2021;385(5):406–15. https://doi.org/10.1056/NEJMoa2101643. pmid:34133856.

[94] NIH. Kinase Inhibitors: Janus Kinase Inhibitors and Bruton's Tyrosine Kinase Inhibitors (August 8th 2022 update). https://www.covid19treatmentguidelines.nih.gov/therapies/immunomodulators/kinase-inhibitors/. [Accessed 2 September 2022].

[95] Alhazzani W, Prahar KKS, Weatherald J, et al. Effect of awake prone positioning on endotracheal intubation in patients with COVID-19 and acute respiratory failure: a randomized clinical trial. J Am Med Assoc 2022;327(21):2104–13. https://doi.org/10.1001/jama.2022.7993.

[96] Ehrmann S, Li J, Ibarra-Estrada M, Perez Y, et al. Awake prone positioning for COVID-19 acute hypoxaemic respiratory failure: a randomised, controlled, multinational, open-label meta-trial. Lancet Respir Med 2021;9(12):1387–95. https://doi.org/10.1016/S2213-2600(21)00356-8.

[97] Grieco DL, Menga LS, Cesarano M, Rosa T, et al. Effect of helmet noninvasive ventilation vs high-flow nasal oxygen on days free of respiratory support in patients with COVID-19 and moderate to severe hypoxemic respiratory failure: the HENIVOT randomized clinical trial. JAMA 2021;325(17):1731–43. https://doi.org/10.1001/jama.2021.4682. pmid:33764378.

[98] Perkins GD, Ji C, Connolly BA, Couper K, et al. Effect of noninvasive respiratory strategies on intubation or mortality among patients with acute hypoxemic respiratory failure and COVID-19: the RECOVERY-RS Randomized Clinical Trial. JAMA 2022;327(6):546–58. https://doi.org/10.1001/jama.2022.0028. pmid:35072713.

[99] Ospina-Tascón GA, Calderón-Tapia LE, García AF, et al. Effect of high-flow oxygen therapy vs conventional oxygen therapy on invasive mechanical ventilation and clinical recovery in patients with severe COVID-19: a randomized clinical trial [published correction appears in JAMA. 2022 Mar 15;327(11):1093]. JAMA 2021;326(21):2161–71. https://doi.org/10.1001/jama.2021.20714.

[100] Fan E, Del Sorbo L, Goligher EC, Hodgson CL, et al. An official American thoracic society/European society of intensive care medicine/society of critical care medicine clinical practice guideline: mechanical ventilation in adult patients with acute respiratory distress syndrome. Am J Respir Crit Care Med 2017;195(9):1253–63. https://doi.org/10.1164/rccm.201703-0548ST. pmid:28459336.

[101] Diaz RA, Graf J, Zambrano JM, Ruiz C, et al. Extracorporeal membrane oxygenation for COVID-19-associated severe acute respiratory distress syndrome in Chile: a nationwide incidence and cohort study. Am J Respir Crit Care Med 2021;204(1):34–43. https://doi.org/10.1164/rccm.202011-4166OC. pmid:33823118.

[102] Shelhamer MC, Wesson PD, Solari IL, Jensen DL, et al. Prone positioning in moderate to severe acute respiratory distress syndrome due to COVID-19: a cohort study and analysis of physiology. J Intensive Care Med 2021;36(2):241–52. https://doi.org/10.1177/0885066620980399. pmid:33380236.

[103] Weiss TT, Cerda F, Scott JB, Kaur R, et al. Prone positioning for patients intubated for severe acute respiratory distress syndrome (ARDS) secondary to COVID-19: a retrospective observational cohort study. Br J Anaesth 2021;126(1):48–55. https://doi.org/10.1016/j.bja.2020.09.042. pmid:33158500.

[104] Aoyama H, Uchida K, Aoyama K, Pechlivanoglou P, et al. Assessment of therapeutic interventions and lung protective ventilation in patients with moderate to severe acute respiratory distress syndrome: a systematic review and network meta-analysis. JAMA Netw Open 2019;2(7):e198116. https://doi.org/10.1001/jamanetworkopen.2019.8116. pmid:31365111.

[105] Shekar K, Badulak J, Peek G, Boeken U, et al. Extracorporeal Life Support Organization Coronavirus Disease 2019 Interim Guidelines: a consensus document from an international group of interdisciplinary extracorporeal membrane oxygenation providers. Am Soc Artif Intern Organs J 2020;66(7):707–21. https://doi.org/10.1097/MAT.0000000000001193.

[106] Roach A, Chikwe J, Catarino P, et al. Lung transplantation for Covid-19-related respiratory failure in the United States. N Engl J Med 2022;386(12):1187–8. https://doi.org/10.1056/NEJMc2117024.

CHAPTER

34

Intravenous immunoglobulin and convalescent plasma treatment in the COVID-19 patient

MariaGiovanna Danieli[1], *Alberto Paladini*[2] *and Eleonora Antonelli*[2]

[1]Clinica Medica, Dipartimento di Scienze Cliniche e Molecolari and Postgraduate School in Allergology and Clinical Immunology, Università Politecnica delle Marche, Ancona, Italy; [2]Postgraduate School in Internal Medicine, Dipartimento di Medicina Interna, Ospedali Riuniti di Ancona and Dipartimento di Scienze Cliniche e Molecolari, Università Politecnica delle Marche, Ancona, Italy

Introduction

The severe acute respiratory coronavirus 2 (SARS-CoV-2) is a highly pathogenic virus emerged in late 2019 responsible of the so-called coronavirus disease 2019 (COVID-19) [1]. Most of the infected subjects are either asymptomatic carriers or present mild influenza-like symptoms. A small percentage can require hospitalization as well as intensive therapy mainly due to the severe involvement of lung, heart, and vascular system [2]. The severity of the infection is closely related to the activation of innate and adaptive immune system which results in massive inflammatory responses with consequent local and systemic damage. Seeing as how a huge release of cytokines is observed, immunomodulators represent one of the most appropriate therapeutic options, thanks to their ability to smother the immune system and preventing both the cytokines storm and the tissue damage [3]. In this regard, intravenous immunoglobulin (IVIg) play an essential role for their antiinflammatory and immunomodulatory properties through which they can control the cytokine storm, counteract the virus, and restore the immune dysregulation [4].

Autoimmunity, COVID-19, Post-COVID19 syndrome and COVID-19 vaccination
https://doi.org/10.1016/B978-0-443-18566-3.00029-3

Immunological effect of IVIg in COVID-19

As previously described, the rich presence of cytokines (e.g., IL-6 and IL-17) characterizes SARS-CoV-2 infection. Multiple studies have reported that IVIg treatment restores the balance between CD4+ T lymphocytes subpopulations, reducing the frequency of Th1 and Th17 and favoring the expansion of both Th2 and Tregs [5–7]. In addition, activated CD8+ release cytokines and cytotoxic granules as well, exacerbating the cytokines storm. Experimental models showed that IVIg interferes with the generation, the activation and the cytotoxicity of CD8+ T lymphocytes by blocking important cell surface molecules [8]. High-dose of IVIg promotes B-cell apoptosis [9] and down streams their production of cytokines by interfering Toll-like receptor 9 (TLR-9) pathway [10]. Even though data from literature evidence that IVIg can skew monocytes/macrophages to an antiinflammatory state, Saha et al. proved that under specific in vitro conditions, IVIg suppresses the polarization of both inflammatory (M1) and antiinflammatory (M2) macrophages, ensuring a global inhibition of macrophage-mediated inflammatory responses [11]. High-dose of IVIg inhibits inflammatory responsiveness of myeloid dendritic cells [12] and it can regulate granulocyte survival due to specific antibodies present in polyclonal IVIg (e.g., anti-Siglec-8/9 and anti-FAS) [13]. This latter point deserves attention because neutrophils are involved in a process called "immunothrombosis" characterized by thrombus formation in venous and arterial districts as observed in COVID-19 patients [14]. If IVIg has an impact on Natural Killer cells (NK) in SARS-CoV-2 is still an open question. NK cells have an immunoregulatory role and they considerably contribute to control viral infection. In patients with severe SARS-CoV-2 infection, recent studies demonstrate a reduction in NK cells number and function and therefore, a decreased clearance of infected cells and uncontrolled levels of inflammation markers [15].

IVIg as possible therapeutical approach for COVID-19

Experts hypothesized that IVIg may be protective in view of its nonspecific antiviral and immunomodulatory effects.

Commercially available IVIg preparations contain antibodies against several antigens of human common betacoronavirus that cross-react with SARS-CoV-2 virus [16]. The usage of high-dose IVIg therapy (25 g/day for 5 days), combined with antivirals (lopinavir/ritonavir) and methylprednisolone in severe COVID-19, resulted in elevation of lymphocyte counts, decrease in inflammatory markers, partial/complete resolution of lung lesions, and negative nasal/oropharyngeal swab tests within a few days of therapy [17]. Different schedules of IVIg therapy in adult COVID-19 disease are available in the literature, but the heterogeneity in dose, duration, other concomitant treatments, and in different clinical condition does not allow a direct comparison [4]. Cao et al. were among the first to report a case series of three patients with COVID-19 all of them successfully recovered through high-dose of IVIg (0.3–0.5 g/kg/day for 5 days) administered at the early stage of clinical deterioration [18]. In a large multicentre retrospective investigation, Shao et al. compared the use of IVIg in 174 cases versus 151 controls. Both groups were at critical or severe stage of disease, and both received standard treatment based on glucocorticoids, antivirals, and antibiotics. It was observed that 0.1–0.5 g/kg/day of IVIg for 5–15 days lead to a significant decrease of

28-day mortality in patients with critical conditions. No major benefit on survival was noted in severe-type patients treated with IVIg when compared to those who received only standard therapy [19]. A recent meta-analysis found out a relationship between the severity of COVID-19 disease and the efficacy of IVIg. Indeed, in critical subgroups IVIg could reduce the rate of mortality compared with control group. A recent randomized controlled trial (RCT) evaluated IVIg treatment in 84 severely ill patients with COVID-19 (32 in the control group and 52 in the IVIg group). All subjects received lopinavir/ritonavir, hydroxychloroquine, and supportive care. The intervention group received IVIg at a dose of 400 mg/kg/day for 3 days. The results showed no significance difference between the two groups in terms of mortality rate and need for mechanical ventilation (MV). However, the study found a positive relationship between the time from hospital admission to IVIg introduction and the length of stay in the hospital and in the intensive care unit among the survivors [20].

Overall, even if the evidence regarding the use of IVIg in patients with COVID-19 is not conclusive, the benefit of high-dose IVIg is documented in almost all studies with a rapid response, a reduction in mortality and improved pulmonary function in critically ill COVID-19 patients. COVID-19 patients with mild-moderate disease do not seem to positively react to IVIg treatment. A better outcome in severe cases seems to be linked to early administration of IVIg at a higher dosage. In most studies, IVIg treatment can decrease the length of stay in intensive care unit and the necessity for MV. Even if more well-designed trials are required to identify the clinical and biochemical characteristics of COVID-19 patients' population that could benefit from IVIg, this treatment could help in reducing the burden of the disease.

Convalescent plasm: lights and shadows

Despite its worldwide diffusion and its aggressiveness, the only effective drug approved for confirmed SARS-CoV-2 infected subjects is dexamethasone. Prestigious organization, such as the Food and Drug Administration (FDA), and the World Health Organization (WHO), strongly recommend corticosteroids as a first line treatment for critical and severe COVID-19 patients. Given the lack of evidence for treatment of COVID-19, classical approaches have remerged as options to control the novel disease and convalescent plasma (CP) is one of them. It represents a strategy of passive immunization that has been used in historical viral infections such as the Spanish flu, the severe acute respiratory syndrome (SARS), the H1N1 influenza, and the Ebola virus disease [21]. Convalescent plasma is rapidly obtained through apheresis from survived infected patients in whom antibodies against the pathogen are developed. During apheresis not only neutralizing antibodies are acquired but also antiinflammatory cytokines, clotting factors, natural antibodies, defensins, pentraxins, and other undefined proteins. In this prospective, transfusion of convalescent plasma may provide an immunomodulatory effect reducing the cytokine storm [22]. On August 23, 2020, the FDA emanated an Emergency Use Authorization (EUA) for convalescent plasma as a possible therapeutical approach for COVID-19. An EUA does not represent a drug approval by the FDA rather, it allows the organization to facilitate the availability and unapproved uses of medical products during public health emergency [21]. To assess its efficacy and effectiveness more and more RCTs have been performed without a relevant survival benefit when compared to the control group. Indeed, a meta-analysis of 16 RCTs by Cao et al. did not observe a significant reduction in the risk for death in patients with COVID-19 who received convalescent plasma. However, a subanalysis showed a reduction of 28-day mortality in severe or critical patients treated versus controls, whereas no significant differences were noted in patients with mild-moderate disease. Compared with the control group, a nonsignificant reduction in length of hospital stays rate of MV, days in intensive care unit, and in rate of ICU admissions was reported. On the other hand, the meta-analysis described a decreased duration of MV after convalescent plasma treatment [23]. Nonetheless, another meta-analysis performed by Vegivinti et al. reported significantly higher clinical improvement (despite a nonsignificant reduction in hospital length of stay) and lower mortality in the convalescent plasma group compared to the controls, although two key RCTs did not support the latter result. Overall, the study does not present a clear consensus on the efficacy of the therapy in providing a mortality benefit [24]. Additionally, in literature are described adverse effects associated with convalescent plasma transfusions such as an increased risk of pulmonary embolism due to the presence of procoagulant factors [25], antibody-dependent enhancement, and the HIV epidemic in low- and middle-income nations [26,27].

A recent multicenter randomized double-blind controlled study evaluated the efficacy of convalescent plasma versus control plasma in outpatients with symptoms of COVID-19 within 8 days. A total of 1181 patients were enrolled with good results, resulting in a relative risk reduction of hospitalization at 28 days of 54%. Convalescent plasma could therefore play a role in the prevention of severe disease in outpatients with few COVID-19 symptoms [28].

The use of hyperimmune IVIg, concentrated anti-SARS-CoV-2 immunoglobulins from convalescent plasma of immunized patients, was also investigated with controversial results. In a recent study, hyper-immune immunoglobulins from patients immunized against ancestral SARS-CoV-2 appear to have a higher neutralization capacity against SARS-CoV-2 delta and omicron variants in a pseudovirus neutralization assay. It therefore suggests a possible use of hyperimmune IVIg for the treatment and prevention of SARS-CoV-2 delta and omicron variants [29].

In a randomized, double-blind, placebo-controlled phase 3 trial, hospitalized patients with COVID-19 who presented symptoms for less than 12 days without organ failure, underwent treatment with a single hyperimmune IVIg infusion in addition to standard care. After 7 days of treatment with hyperimmune IVIg, it did not demonstrate any improvement in clinical outcome [30].

In conclusion, up to now the efficacy of convalescent plasma transfusions and hyperimmune IVIg in COVID-19 disease is controversial. Hence, accurate systematic reviews and meta-analysis based on high-quality evidence are needed to evaluate convalescent plasma and hIVIg as a possible therapeutical approach.

IVIg in autoimmune disorders induced by SARS-CoV-2

The spread of COVID-19 disease around the world led to an increase in cases of autoimmune diseases related to SARS-CoV-2 infection. Molecular mimicry between Coronavirus transcriptome and numerous molecules of our organism is just one of the mechanisms that could explain the complex interaction between the virus and our immune system. The use of intravenous immunoglobulin (IVIg) appears to show efficacy in the management of many autoimmune diseases following COVID-19 infection or vaccination, confirming the immune imbalance induced by the virus [31–36]. Moreover, in some cases, the immunomodulatory effect of IVIg has been preferred over first-line immunosuppressive therapies in order not to increase the infectious risk.

Neurological disorders after SARS-CoV-2 infection

Guillain-Barré Syndrome (GBS)

Among autoimmune disorders developing after COVID-19 disease, Guillain-Barré Syndrome (GBS) is one of the most described. A review by Zuberbühler P. et al. collected data from 48 patients with polyradiculoneuropathy diagnosed as GBS and its different subtypes. All patients had a diagnosis of COVID-19 based on RT-PCR on nasopharyngeal swab or IgG/IgM antibody positivity. Six patients had mild/asymptomatic forms of the disease without respiratory symptoms, in the other patients the characteristics and incidence of symptoms were similar to general population (cough, fever, anosmia, diarrhea, and dyspnoea). The mean latency between the onset of COVID-19 symptoms and polyradiculoneuropathy was 12 days, except for nine patients who developed neurological symptoms in the first week. In some cases, the diagnosis of GBS occurred before SARS-CoV-2 swab test. Concerning neurological manifestations, 11 (22.9%) patients presented exclusively with cranial nerve involvement, three patients (6.3%) had bilateral peripheral facial paralysis (PFP) and distal paraesthesia, 6 (12.5%) patients presented with Miller—Fisher Syndrome (MFS), one had overlapping MFS-GBS and another one was defined as Miller Fisher like syndrome, two patients (4.2%) were defined as cranial polyneuritis, one presented with bilateral ptosis, dysphagia, and dysphonia with hyporeflexia, one had bilateral PFP, dysphagia, and areflexia. Forty-two patients (87.5%) received as first-line therapy IVIg 2 g/kg; two needed a second course of IVIg and two initiated plasma exchange after the first infusion. Two patients were treated with plasmapheresis alone. Four patients were not treated in order not to increase the prothrombotic risk. However, no complications due to thrombosis or embolism were found in the other patients who received IVIg. Thirty-one patients recovered completely. Fourteen patients (29.2%) experienced respiratory failure, 11 of them needed MV, one required noninvasive ventilation, and two (4.2%) patients died after hospitalization. Respiratory failure in these patients is most likely the combined effect of muscle weakness due to GBS and lung infection due to SARS-CoV-2. Antiganglioside antibodies were evaluated in 25 patients, only two patients with Miller Fisher syndrome (MFS) tested positive, one for anti-GD1b and a second had an anti-GM1 with questionable range [37]. The low incidence of antigangliosides and the presence of a single anti-GD1b, different from the more typical GQ1b usually associated with MFS, could be explained by a different pathogenic mechanism. Viral proteins, in particular the spike protein, binding different glycoproteic epitopes, could induce a cross-reactivity against surface sugars of glycolipids on the peripheral nerves [38].

Acute disseminated encephalomyelitis (ADEM)

Another neurological disease described in association with SARS-CoV-2 infection, is acute disseminated encephalomyelitis (ADEM). ADEM is a rare autoimmune disease, causing demyelination in the brain and spinal cord. Often, the disease follows viral or bacterial infections, or rarely, after vaccination. Usually, ADEM has an acute onset, starting with neurological symptoms encephalitis-like. Mahapure et al. collected a review of ADEM cases related to COVID-

19 disease. Neurological symptoms arose between 3 and 25 days after COVID-19 manifestations, only in two cases they occurred before. They presented altered consciousness, anosmia, paraplegia, brain stem involvement, sphincter involvement, and quadriplegia. Analysis of cerebrospinal fluid (CSF) was performed in 17 patients, detecting alterations in nine cases (increased protein or lymphocytes). To exclude other infections, cultural and viral PCR panel on CSF was performed and only in one patient SARS-CoV-2 was found. Antibodies to myelin oligodendrocyte glycoprotein (MOG) and to aquaporin-4 were negative in nine patients. Radiological examinations showed ADEM-compatible picture in 13 patients, seven were acute hemorrhagic encephalomyelitis (AHEM), while one was acute necrotizing hemorrhagic leukoencephalopathy (ANHLE). Almost all patients were treated with combination therapy (steroids, IVIg, antivirals, plasmapheresis), 12 patients were treated with immunomodulatory dose IVIg and among them eight also received combination therapy with intravenous methylprednisolone. Among 21 patients examined, three died due to complications. None of the patients treated with IVIg and steroid combination died but all partially recovered. One patient showed complete recovery after IVIg treatment [39].

Myasthenia gravis

IVIg also plays a role in the treatment of exacerbations of some diseases in course of SARS-CoV-2 infection. Rein et al. described the management of COVID-19 in three patients with myasthenia gravis (MG). The first case concerns a young woman (38 years old) suffering from MG for about 10 years and treated with maintenance dose of IVIg (1 g/kg every 3–4 weeks), prednisone, and pyridostigmine. SARS-CoV-2 infection (RT-PCR positive swab test) caused fever, myalgia, and syncope. After few days also ptosis and weakness of respiratory and proximal limbs muscles arose. Respiratory failure had an independent course compared to COVID-19 disease activity and required noninvasive ventilatory support. In view of the exacerbation of the disease, treatment with immunomodulating dose IVIg (2 g/kg over 5 days) and high-dose steroid (1 mg/kg) was required, with benefit and almost complete recovery. In the other two cases, no MG exacerbations occurred. One patient receiving maintenance IVIg, prednisone, and pyridostigmine presented with ageusia, anosmia, fever, myalgia, headache, cough, rash without muscle symptoms. Neither hospitalization nor therapeutic changes were required for MG. The third patient, recently diagnosed with MG, was treated with maintenance plasmapheresis, prednisone (60 mg/day), pyridostigmine, and azathioprine (150 mg/day). COVID-19 onset was characterized by fever and cough, and he required hospitalization to replace plasmapheresis with IVIg. He did not develop severe symptoms of COVID-19 disease and he did not experience exacerbations of MG [40].

Hematological autoimmune disorders after COVID-19 infection

Immune thrombocytopenic purpura (ITP) and autoimmune hemolytic anemia (AIHA)

IVIg was useful in autoimmune hematological diseases after SARS-CoV-2 infection such as immune thrombocytopenic purpura (ITP), autoimmune hemolytic anemia (AIHA), and Fisher–Evans syndrome. A review by Taherifard et al. reported data from 55 patients who developed ITP, 22 AIHA and 3 Fisher–Evans syndrome. Among patients with ITP, 15 patients received IVIg, 13 patients were treated with steroids, 13 received a combination of IVIg and steroids, six received IVIG plus thrombopoietin receptor agonist (TPO-RA), and four patients only supportive care. Among patients treated with IVIg as first line, two did not respond (86% remission rate) and additional steroids was successfully added. Similarly, among those on steroids, no response was observed in two patients (84% remission rate) and IVIg was initiated. All patients with ITP recovered, except for two who died, one from cerebral hemorrhage in the first 24 h of hospitalization, the second from causes not related to ITP [41].

In another review, Bhattacharjee & Banerjee analyzed data from 45 ITP patients with SARS-CoV-2 infection. Mild symptoms were reported in 18% of patients, while 75% developed moderate-to-severe COVID-19 disease, and three (7%) were asymptomatic. Moreover, in six patients ITP arose during the phase of infectious resolution. Skin manifestations of ITP were purpura, ecchymosis, and petechiae in 22 cases, 31% showed no signs of bleeding. Thirteen patients were treated with variable dose of IVIg (400 mg/kg/day for 5 days or 1 g/kg for 1–3 days), while 10 patients only with prednisone (1 mg/kg/day), 11 patients received IVIg + prednisone, 5 IVIg + thrombopoietin receptor agonist (TP-RA), 3 IVIg + prednisone + TP-RA, one with TP-RA, two needed only supportive therapy. Three patients died (one from cerebral hemorrhage, two from complications due to COVID-19), 30 had complete remission, and eight had a good response to therapy [42]. A practical guideline by Pavord et al. on ITP management during COVDI-19 pandemic, recommends steroids as the first therapeutic approach with minimum dose and duration (20 mg/die as starting dose up to 1 mg/kg). They suggest IVIg (1 g/kg) as a first line when the risk for severe bleeding is high and as second line in those with absent or poor respond to steroids [43].

The review by Taherifard collected 22 patients affected by AIHA during COVID-19 disease. All patients developed AIHA between 2 and 20 days after the onset of COVID-19 symptoms and most of them (59%, almost all patients with cold agglutinin syndrome) benefited from supportive therapies, 10 patients received steroid therapy, two had previously received IVIg with poor response, two were also treated with rituximab. All patients recovered except four patients who died after hospitalization [41].

Fisher Evans syndrome

Fisher–Evans syndrome is described in three patients. In the first case, autoimmune hemolytic anemia was associated with thrombocytopenia and gastrointestinal bleeding. The patient was treated with immunomodulating dose of IVIg with normal platelets final level and no more bleeding. Ten days after remission, there was a relapse of the disease, treated again with IVIg which led to a complete recovery. In the second patient, the anemia arose on a chronic history of ITP and was treated only with steroids. The third case concerns a pregnant woman (38 weeks) who developed bruising, minor bleeding, and spontaneous membranes rupture. After the delivery, she received IVIg, rituximab, and steroid therapy with complete recovery [41].

Pemphigus

A further COVID-19-related autoimmune manifestation is pemphigus vulgaris. Some case reports of pemphigus during COVID-19 disease, treated with classic immunosuppressive therapy, are reported. Treatment with rituximab [44], high-dose of steroids, or combined steroid-methotrexate [45] is described in patients with excellent response. However, it is interesting that in some cases the use of immunomodulating dose of IVIg was preferred to conventional therapy, in order not to increase the infectious risk. Ghalamkarpour et al. described a COVID-19-related relapse of pemphigus vulgaris unresponsive to prednisone therapy (40 mg/day), treated with IVIg 25 g/day for 5 days [46]. Recommendations for the management of pemphigus vulgaris during the COVID pandemic also point to IVIg as the only immunomodulatory therapy (together with dapsone) that could be useful in the management of pemphigus, including prevention of complications and relapse of the disease [47].

Autoimmune diseases related to COVID-19 vaccine

Neurological disorders

The global COVID-19 pandemic has exerted a serious pressure to public health, bringing to the development and disposition of vaccines at an unprecedented speed. ChAdOx1nCoV-19 and BNT162b2 vaccine have proved to reduce COVID-19 infections, transmissions, hospitalizations, and deaths. Rare adverse events are difficult to detect but they are of great importance for ongoing risk-benefit evaluations and for postvaccination clinical practice. Patone et al. performed a large population-based study on more than 32 million people to analyze the neurological side effects associated with and BNT162b2 vaccines as well as SARS-CoV-2 infection. In those who received the Oxford-AstraZeneca vaccine (ChAdOx1n-CoV-19), a greater incidence of Guillain-Barré syndrome (GBS) was found (38 excess case per 10 million exposed). One possible explanation is that antibodies against adenovirus vector-based vaccine can cross-react with components of the peripheral nerves. Another finding was the co-occurrence of Guillain-Barré syndrome and Bell's palsy in this group of vaccinated subjects. Tozinameran (BNT162b2) vaccine did not prove to be associated with Guillain-Barré syndrome; instead, the authors estimated about 60 excess cases of hemorrhagic strokes per 10 million. No increased risk of hemorrhagic stroke was observed in the vaccinated with Oxford-AstraZeneca. This difference seems to be related to the increased risk of immune thrombocytopenic purpura in individuals receiving mRNA vaccines, which in turn could contribute to major bleeding events. The neurological complications after COVID-19 vaccination are rare but they can cause lifelong disabilities requiring long-term care and the need of a proper healthcare resource allocation, hence social and economic impacts. However, neurological events following vaccination are fewer than those occurring in SARS-CoV-2 infection, underlining the benefits of ongoing vaccination programs [48]. Similarly, Kaulen et al. noticed cases of GBS only after ChAdOx1nCoV-19 vaccination, whereas cases of optic neuritis and myositis were found only following BNT162b2 vaccination. However, this study was not powered to investigate incidences of neurological autoimmune manifestations following SARS-CoV-2 vaccination (due to the single-center design and the small main catchment area). Patients were treated with immunosuppressants including intravenous methylprednisolone, oral prednisolone, and IVIg. Plasma exchange was chosen in the setting of severe autoimmunity or cases unresponsive to prior immunosuppressive therapy. Overall, no patient presented progressive disease after treatment started. In conclusion, if autoimmune disorders are suspected after vaccination, early administration of immunosuppressive therapy is essential, but this might limit the production of the protective antibodies. A second vaccination dose may be considered in selected patients with autoimmune reactions under continuous immunosuppressive treatment and vigilant clinical monitoring [49].

Hematological disorders

As neurological disorders, also hematological autoimmune manifestations related to COVID-19 vaccination are described with the growth of immunization campaigns.

Rare cases of thrombocytopenia and bleeding have been reported following vaccination with RNA vaccine (BNT162b2 and Moderna). In almost all patient, thrombocytopenia recovered after conventional immunosuppressive (steroids, IVIg, rituximab) and supportive therapies. Clinical presentation like ITP and the response to treatment suggest a possible autoimmune mechanism with antibody-mediated platelet clearance typical of ITP [50].

Other case series reported the development of thrombosis and thrombocytopenia following vaccination with viral vector vaccines (Oxford-AstraZeneca and Janssen). The new syndrome, defined vaccine-induced immune thrombotic thrombocytopenia (VITT), is characterized by thrombocytopenia, high levels of D-dimers and low fibrinogen (signs of coagulation activity), thrombotic events (often in atypical sites such as cerebral venous sinus and splanchnic vein), presence of antibodies to platelet factor 4 (PF4) detected by enzyme-linked immunosorbent assay (ELISA) [51]. All these features remind heparin induced thrombocytopenia (HIT), but none of patients with VITT had previous heparin exposure. Furthermore, other laboratory assay usually tested to search anti-PF4 antibodies in HIT patients was negative in VITT [52]. The immune mechanisms could therefore be different, although the clinical course is similar. In VITT syndrome, antibodies may recognize some amino acids on PF4 surface, in a different site from the binding one recognized by anti-PF4/H antibodies in patients with HIT. The different immune mechanism may still lead to platelet activation and aggregation and would explain independence from heparin exposure and different responses to laboratory tests [53].

However, the incidence of VITT remains very low (14.9 per million after the first dose and 1.8 per million after the second dose) [54] and the safety and benefits of the vaccine are not questioned.

A practical guideline of Pavord et al. summarizes the consensus diagnostic criteria and therapeutic management by the UK Hematology Expert Group. Symptoms of thromboembolism (including headache) and bleeding on 5–30 days post-COVID-19 vaccine, thrombocytopenia (PLT <150 × 109/L), elevated D-dimer (>4000 μg/mL), thrombosis and anti-PF4 by ELISA assay are the diagnostic criteria and the presence of all allows a definitive diagnosis. Therapy is based on immediate infusion of IVIg 1 g/kg to reduce platelet activation and remove anti-PF4 antibodies and, in case of ascertained thrombosis, nonheparin anticoagulants, after assessing the risk of bleeding [43].

References

[1] Hu B, Guo H, Zhou P, Shi Z-L. Characteristics of SARS-CoV-2 and COVID-19. Nat Rev Microbiol 2021;19(3):141–54.

[2] Parasher A. COVID-19: current understanding of its pathophysiology, clinical presentation and treatment. Postgrad Med 2021;97(1147):312–20.

[3] Anka AU, Tahir MI, Abubakar SD, Alsabbagh M, Zian Z, Hamedifar H, et al. Coronavirus disease 2019 (COVID-19): an overview of the immunopathology, serological diagnosis and management. Scand J Immunol 2021;93(4):e12998.

[4] Danieli MG, Piga MA, Paladini A, Longhi E, Mezzanotte C, Moroncini G, et al. Intravenous immunoglobulin as an important adjunct in the prevention and therapy of coronavirus 2019 disease. Scand J Immunol 2021:e13101.

[5] Maddur MS, Vani J, Hegde P, Lacroix-Desmazes S, Kaveri SV, Bayry J. Inhibition of differentiation, amplification, and function of human TH17 cells by intravenous immunoglobulin. J Allergy Clin Immunol 2011;127(3). 823–30.e1-7.

[6] Maddur MS, Rabin M, Hegde P, Bolgert F, Guy M, Vallat J-M, et al. Intravenous immunoglobulin exerts reciprocal regulation of Th1/Th17 cells and regulatory T cells in Guillain-Barré syndrome patients. Immunol Res 2014;60(2–3):320–9.

[7] Maddur MS, Kaveri SV, Bayry J. Circulating normal IgG as stimulator of regulatory T cells: lessons from intravenous immunoglobulin. Trends Immunol 2017;38(11):789–92.

[8] Trépanier P, Chabot D, Bazin R. Intravenous immunoglobulin modulates the expansion and cytotoxicity of CD8+ T cells. Immunology 2014;141(2):233–41.

[9] Blank M, Shoenfeld Y. Sialic acid-IVIg targeting CD22. Blood 2010;116(10):1630–2.

[10] Kessel A, Peri R, Haj T, Snir A, Slobodin G, Sabo E, et al. IVIg attenuates TLR-9 activation in B cells from SLE patients. J Clin Immunol 2011;31(1):30–8.

[11] Saha C, Kothapalli P, Patil V, ManjunathaReddy GB, Kaveri SV, Bayry J. Intravenous immunoglobulin suppresses the polarization of both classically and alternatively activated macrophages. Hum Vaccines Immunother 2019;16(2):233–9.

[12] Tjon ASW, Gent R van, Jaadar H, Hagen PM van, Mancham S, Laan LJW van der, et al. Intravenous immunoglobulin treatment in humans suppresses dendritic cell function via stimulation of IL-4 and IL-13 production. J Immunol 2014;192(12):5625–34.

[13] Graeter S, Simon H-U, von Gunten S. Granulocyte death mediated by specific antibodies in intravenous immunoglobulin (IVIG). Pharmacol Res 2020;154:104168.

[14] Spijkerman R, Jorritsma NKN, Bongers SH, Bindels BJJ, Jukema BN, Hesselink L, et al. An increase in CD62Ldim neutrophils precedes the development of pulmonary embolisms in COVID-19 patients. Scand J Immunol 2021;93(6):e13023.

[15] van Eeden C, Khan L, Osman MS, Cohen Tervaert JW. Natural killer cell dysfunction and its role in COVID-19. Int J Mol Sci 2020;21(17):E6351.

[16] Díez J-M, Romero C, Gajardo R. Currently available intravenous immunoglobulin contains antibodies reacting against severe acute respiratory syndrome coronavirus 2 antigens. Immunotherapy 2020;12(8):571–6.

[17] Gasparyan AY, Misra DP, Yessirkepov M, Zimba O. Perspectives of immune therapy in coronavirus disease 2019. J Kor Med Sci 2020;35(18):e176.

[18] Cao W, Liu X, Bai T, Fan H, Hong K, Song H, et al. High-dose intravenous immunoglobulin as a therapeutic option for deteriorating patients with coronavirus disease 2019. Open Forum Infect Dis 2020;7(3):ofaa102.

[19] Shao Z, Feng Y, Zhong L, Xie Q, Lei M, Liu Z, et al. Clinical efficacy of intravenous immunoglobulin therapy in critical ill patients with COVID-19: a multicenter retrospective cohort study. Clin Transl Immunol 2020;9(10):e1192.

[20] Tabarsi P, Barati S, Jamaati H, Haseli S, Marjani M, Moniri A, et al. Evaluating the effects of Intravenous Immunoglobulin (IVIg) on the management of severe COVID-19 cases: a randomized controlled trial. Int Immunopharm 2021;90:107205.

[21] Pau AK, Aberg J, Baker J, Belperio PS, Coopersmith C, Crew P, et al. Convalescent plasma for the treatment of COVID-19: perspectives of the national institutes of health COVID-19 treatment guidelines panel. Ann Intern Med 2021;174(1):93–5.

[22] Rojas M, Rodríguez Y, Monsalve DM, Acosta-Ampudia Y, Camacho B, Gallo JE, et al. Convalescent plasma in Covid-19: possible mechanisms of action. Autoimmun Rev 2020;19(7):102554.

[23] Cao H, Ming L, Chen L, Zhu X, Shi Y. The effectiveness of convalescent plasma for the treatment of novel corona virus disease 2019: a systematic review and meta-analysis. Front Med 2021;8:641429.

[24] Vegivinti CTR, Pederson JM, Saravu K, Gupta N, Evanson KW, Kamrowski S, et al. Efficacy of convalescent plasma therapy for COVID-19: a systematic review and meta-analysis. J Clin Apher 2021;36(3):470–82.

[25] Sanfilippo F, La Rosa V, Oliveri F, Astuto M. COVID-19, hypercoagulability, and cautiousness with convalescent plasma. Am J Respir Crit Care Med 2021;203(2):257–8.

[26] Fleming AB, Raabe V. Current studies of convalescent plasma therapy for COVID-19 may underestimate risk of antibody-dependent enhancement. J Clin Virol 2020;127:104388.

[27] Ferreira LMR, Mostajo-Radji MA. Plasma-based COVID-19 treatments in low- and middle-income nations pose a high risk of an HIV epidemic. NPJ Vaccines 2020;5:58.

[28] Sullivan DJ, Gebo KA, Shoham S, Bloch EM, Lau B, Shenoy AG, et al. Early outpatient treatment for covid-19 with convalescent plasma. N Engl J Med 2022. https://doi.org/10.1056/NEJMoa2119657.

[29] Zahra FT, Bellusci L, Grubbs G, Golding H, Khurana S. Neutralisation of circulating SARS-CoV-2 delta and omicron variants by convalescent plasma and SARS-CoV-2 hyperimmune intravenous human immunoglobulins for treatment of COVID-19. Ann Rheum Dis 2022;81:1044–5. annrheumdis-2022-222115.

[30] ITAC (INSIGHT 013) Study Group. Hyperimmune immunoglobulin for hospitalised patients with COVID-19 (ITAC): a double-blind, placebo-controlled, phase 3, randomised trial. Lancet 2022;399(10324):530–40.

[31] Dotan A, Muller S, Kanduc D, David P, Halpert G, Shoenfeld Y. The SARS-CoV-2 as an instrumental trigger of autoimmunity. Autoimmun Rev 2021;20(4):102792.

[32] Ehrenfeld M, Tincani A, Andreoli L, Cattalini M, Greenbaum A, Kanduc D, et al. Covid-19 and autoimmunity. Autoimmun Rev 2020;19(8):102597.

[33] Halpert G, Shoenfeld Y. SARS-CoV-2, the autoimmune virus. Autoimmun Rev 2020;19(12):102695.

[34] Kanduc D, Shoenfeld Y. On the molecular determinants of the SARS-CoV-2 attack. Clin Immunol 2020;215:108426.

[35] Sachinidis A, Garyfallos A. COVID-19 vaccination can occasionally trigger autoimmune phenomena, probably via inducing age-associated B cells. Int J Rheum Dis 2022;25(1):83–5.

[36] Dotan A, Shoenfeld Y. Post-COVID syndrome: the aftershock of SARS-CoV-2. Int J Infect Dis 2022;114:233–5.

[37] Zuberbühler P, Conti ME, León-Cejas L, Maximiliano-González F, Bonardo P, Miquelini A, et al. Guillain-Barre syndrome associated to COVID-19 infection: a review of published case reports. Rev Neurol 2021;72(6):203–12.

[38] Dalakas MC. Guillain-Barré syndrome: the first documented COVID-19-triggered autoimmune neurologic disease: more to come with myositis in the offing. Neurol Neuroimmunol Neuroinflamm 2020;7(5):e781.

[39] Mahapure KS, Prabhune AS, Chouvhan AV. COVID-19-Associated acute disseminated encephalomyelitis: a systematic review. Asian J Neurosurg 2021;16(3):457–69.

[40] Rein N, Haham N, Orenbuch-Harroch E, Romain M, Argov Z, Vaknin-Dembinsky A, et al. Description of 3 patients with myasthenia gravis and COVID-19. J Neurol Sci 2020;417:117053.

[41] Taherifard E, Taherifard E, Movahed H, Mousavi MR. Hematologic autoimmune disorders in the course of COVID-19: a systematic review of reported cases. Hematology 2021;26(1):225–39.

[42] Bhattacharjee S, Banerjee M. Immune thrombocytopenia secondary to COVID-19: a systematic review. SN Compr Clin Med 2020:1–11.

[43] Pavord S, Hunt BJ, Horner D, Bewley S, Karpusheff J, Guideline Committee. Vaccine induced immune thrombocytopenia and thrombosis: summary of NICE guidance. BMJ 2021;375:n2195.

[44] Sinagra JL, Vedovelli C, Binazzi R, Salemme A, Moro F, Mazzanti C, et al. Case report: complete and fast recovery from severe COVID-19 in a pemphigus patient treated with rituximab. Front Immunol 2021;12:665522.

[45] De Medeiros VLS, Monteiro-Neto AU, França DDT, Castelo Branco R, de Miranda Coelho ÉO, Takano DM. Pemphigus vulgaris after COVID-19: a case of induced autoimmunity. SN Compr Clin Med 2021:1–5.

[46] Ghalamkarpour F, Pourani MR. Aggressive course of pemphigus vulgaris following COVID-19 infection. Dermatol Ther 2020;33(6):e14398.

[47] Kasperkiewicz M, Schmidt E, Fairley JA, Joly P, Payne AS, Yale ML, et al. Expert recommendations for the management of autoimmune bullous diseases during the COVID-19 pandemic. J Eur Acad Dermatol Venereol 2020;34(7):e302–3.

[48] Patone M, Handunnetthi L, Saatci D, Pan J, Katikireddi SV, Razvi S, et al. Neurological complications after first dose of COVID-19 vaccines and SARS-CoV-2 infection. Nat Med 2021. https://doi.org/10.1038/s41591-021-01556-7.

[49] Kaulen LD, Doubrovinskaia S, Mooshage C, Jordan B, Purrucker J, Haubner C, et al. Neurological autoimmune diseases following vaccinations against SARS-CoV-2: a case series. Eur J Neurol 2021. https://doi.org/10.1111/ene.15147.

[50] Lee E-J, Cines DB, Gernsheimer T, Kessler C, Michel M, Tarantino MD, et al. Thrombocytopenia following pfizer and moderna SARS-CoV-2 vaccination. Am J Hematol 2021;96(5):534–7.
[51] Cines DB, Bussel JB. SARS-CoV-2 vaccine-induced immune thrombotic thrombocytopenia. N Engl J Med 2021;384(23):2254–6.
[52] Favaloro EJ, Pasalic L, Lippi G. Review and evolution of guidelines for diagnosis of COVID-19 vaccine induced thrombotic thrombocytopenia (VITT). Clin Chem Lab Med 2021. https://doi.org/10.1515/cclm-2021-1039.
[53] Huynh A, Kelton JG, Arnold DM, Daka M, Nazy I. Antibody epitopes in vaccine-induced immune thrombotic thrombocytopaenia. Nature 2021;596(7873):565–9.
[54] Medicines and Healthcare products regulatory agency [Internet]. GOV.UK.

CHAPTER

35

Interaction between vitamin D deficiency and COVID-19

Vânia Borba[1,2] and Pedro Carrera-Bastos[3,4,5]

[1]Zabludowicz Center for Autoimmune Diseases, Sheba Medical Center, Ramat Gan, Israel; [2]Ariel University, Ariel, Israel; [3]Centre for Primary Health Care Research, Lund University/ Region Skane, Skane University Hospital, Malmö, Sweden; [4]Faculty of Biomedical and Health Sciences, Universidad Europea de Madrid, Madrid, Spain; [5]Centro de Estudios Avanzados en Nutrición (CEAN), Córdoba, Spain

Introduction to vitamin D

Vitamin D_3 can be synthesized in the epidermis by the action of ultraviolet B (UVB) radiation on 7-dehydrocholesterol, or, it can be obtained exogenously, via food or supplements, in the form of cholecalciferol (Vitamin D_3) or ergocalciferol (Vitamin D_2) [1]. In the blood, most vitamin D is carried by vitamin D-binding protein (DBP), and when it reaches the liver it will undergo a hydroxylation at carbon 25, thanks to 25-hydroxylase, which may be one of various cytochrome P-450 enzymes, namely, the mitochondrial enzyme CYP27A1 and the microsomal enzymes CYP2J3, CYP2D25, and CYP2R1, the latter apparently being the most important [2–4]. The resulting compound is calcifediol or calcidiol—25-hydroxyvitamin D ($25OHD_3$ or $25OHD_2$, depending on the parent molecule) [4]. After being discharged into the circulation, 25OHD will travel, mostly bound to DBP, to the kidney, where it will be converted, by the action of the enzyme 25-hydroxyvitamin D 1-α-hydroxylase (CYP27B1), located in the mitochondria of proximal convoluted tubule cells, into calcitriol—1α,25-dihydroxyvitamin D ($1\alpha,25(OH)_2D_3$ or $1\alpha,25(OH)_2D_2$, again depending on the parent compound) [4]. And both 25OHD and $1\alpha,25(OH)_2D$ can be subject to degradation, thanks to CYP24A1 (24,25-hydroxylase or 24-hydroxylase) Fig. 35.1 [5].

Autoimmunity, COVID-19, Post-COVID19 syndrome and COVID-19 vaccination
https://doi.org/10.1016/B978-0-443-18566-3.00025-6

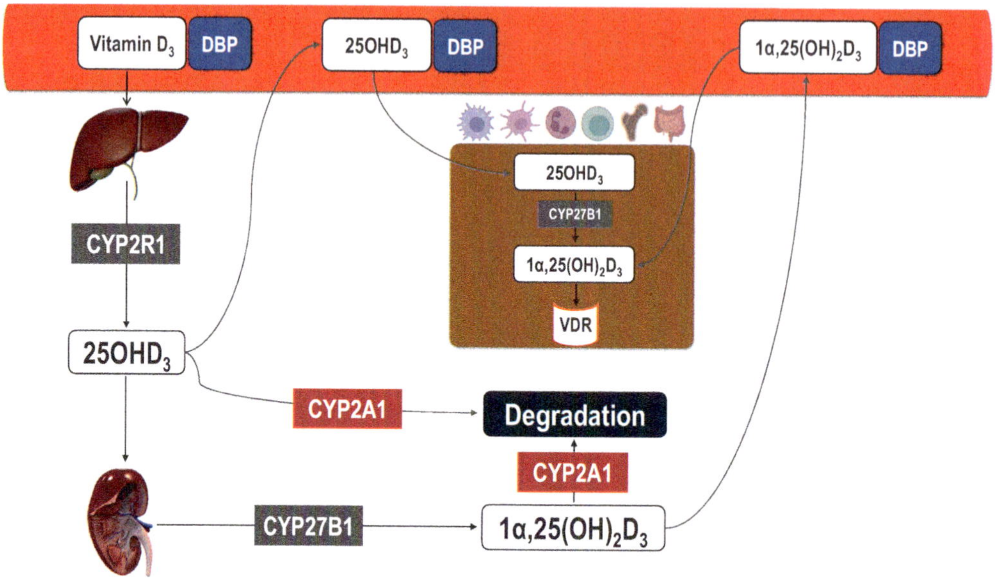

FIGURE 35.1 Vitamin D_3 bound to vitamin D binding protein (DBP) is transported to the liver, where it is hydroxylated in the C25 position by enzymes displaying 25-hydroxylase activity, especially CYP2R1. The resulting metabolite, 25-hydroxyvitamin D_3 (25OHD_3), is then transported to the kidney, where it is metabolized to 1α,25-dihydroxyvitamin D_3 (1α,25$(OH)_2D_3$) by CYP27B1, which has 1α- hydroxylase activity. Because several cells, including immune cells, express the vitamin D receptor (VDR), 1α,25$(OH)_2D_3$ can affect those cells by interacting with this receptor. Noticeably, immune cells also express CYP27B1, thus being able to locally convert 25OHD_3 to 1α,25$(OH)_2D_3$. CYP24A1, which has 24-hydroxylase activity induces the degradation of both 25OHD_3 and 1α,25$(OH)_2D_3$.

Coming back to calcitriol, this molecule, which is considered the active form of vitamin D, will serve as a ligand for the Vitamin D receptor (VDR) expressed in several extrarenal tissues [6]. Intriguingly, the VDR exerts genomic—by acting as transcription factor—and nongenomic actions, since it affects intracellular signaling [7]. Therefore, kidney-derived 1α,25$(OH)_2$D is expected to exert numerous endocrine actions in cells of different tissues, but for a long time it was only recognized for its role in the regulation of calcium, phosphate, and bone metabolism [6]. This perspective radically changed with the discovery of the VDR on a vast array of human cells, including immune cells, especially monocytes, macrophages, neutrophils, dendritic cells (DCs), eosinophils, mast cells, and T and B lymphocytes [4,8–11]. This, coupled with the evidence that several cells—for example, mast cells, monocytes, macrophages, DCs, and, to a lower extent, $CD4^+$ T lymphocytes—express CYP27B1 [8,11,12], and that some cells also contain one of the 25-hydroxylase isoforms [13], led to the acknowledgment that Vitamin D has not only several endocrine, but also paracrine and autocrine effects (Fig. 35.1), thus regulating a wide variety of physiological functions, including innate and adaptive immune responses [4,8,11], as summarized below.

Vitamin D and the immune system

Brief overview of the immune system

The immune system includes a complex set of different cell types that produce a large number of responses in order to protect the host from foreign agents, such as bacteria, fungi, viruses, and toxins, as well as mutant cells and abnormal molecules, while also contributing to tissue repair and recovery [14–16].

Concerning the different types of immune responses to microbes, these typically fall into two categories: innate and adaptive immune responses. One of the main differences between these two types of response is that the adaptive one—which is carried out by T and B lymphocytes—is highly specific for a particular pathogen and becomes more efficient after each subsequent encounter with the same aggressor [14]. As for innate immunity, although it is normally labeled as nonspecific, it has, in fact, specificity for molecules shared by groups of related microbes—that is, pathogen-associated molecular patterns (PAMPs)—and molecules produced by damaged host cells—so called danger-associated molecular patterns (DAMPs) [14]. Moreover, it is responsible for an early and rapid response to a pathogen, thus being crucial for survival. Its main components include physical and chemical barriers—for example, the epithelium and microbicidal substances produced by the epithelial surface—blood proteins—including the complement system and other mediators of the inflammatory process—and various leukocytes, such as phagocytic cells—primarily neutrophils, and monocytes/macrophages—mast cells, DCs, eosinophils, basophils, natural killer (NK) cells, and innate lymphoid cells [14,17,18].

The immunological effects of vitamin D

As mentioned, the VDR is constitutively expressed in innate immune cells, especially neutrophils, monocytes/macrophages, and DCs, and its expression is induced in lymphocytes after specific stimuli [8,10,11]. This indicates vitamin D to have an important role of in the modulation of immune and inflammatory responses. Moreover, and as discussed above, $1\alpha,25(OH)_2D$—the active form of vitamin D—can be synthesized by mast cells, monocytes, and antigen-presenting cells (APCs), such as macrophages and DCs, as well as $CD4^+$ T lymphocytes, since these cells express the enzyme 1α-hydroxylase (CYP27B1) [10]. Accordingly, toll-like receptor (TLR) activation by PAMPs in macrophages upregulates VDR and CYP27B1 gene expression, resulting in increased calcitriol synthesis and signaling, which, in turn, promotes the production of antimicrobial peptides, such as cathelicidin and β-defensin 2 [8,19]. Furthermore, $1\alpha,25(OH)_2D$ enhances autophagy in macrophages [8]. This represents an important defense mechanism characterized by the targeting of intracellular pathogens into autophagosomes which subsequently fuse with the lysosome, leading to its degradation [20]. Moreover, exposing monocytes to $1\alpha,25(OH)_2D$ increase its proliferation, as well as its phagocytic and chemotactic capacity [21].

Notwithstanding its pivotal role in maintaining adequate innate antibacterial and antiviral responses, vitamin D appears to actually downregulate the proinflammatory activity of macrophages, which are cells with a high capacity to synthesize cytokines, in particular tumor necrosis factor (TNF)-α. The TNF-α gene promoter region contains a complex set of potential regulatory elements. The transcriptional activation of the TNF-α gene in macrophages is predominantly dependent on the transcription factor designated nuclear factor binding near the k light-chain gene in the B cells (NF-κB) [22]. With the exception of mature B lymphocytes, in which NF-κB is constitutively nuclear, in virtually all other cell types, including macrophages, NF-κB is maintained in the cytoplasm through its association with inhibitor κB (IκB). When cells are activated by proinflammatory cytokines, or PAMPs, IkB is rapidly phosphorylated and polyubiquitinated, being further degraded in the proteasome. Thus, NF-κB translocates to the cell nucleus, where it induces the expression of several genes related to the inflammatory response [22,23]. Noticeably, in macrophages incubated with calcitriol and, subsequently, stimulated with LPS, vitamin D was found to increase the stability of the IkB mRNA, and decreased the phosphorylation of IkB. This reduced the translocation of NF-kB to the cell nucleus, which indicates that vitamin D plays an antiinflammatory role in macrophages [24]. In addition, calcitriol reduces gene and protein expression of TLR2 and TLR4 receptors in monocytes [11].

Similar to what has been shown in monocytes and macrophages, there is evidence that 1α,25$(OH)_2$D can increase the production of the antimicrobial peptides cathelicidin and α-defensins by neutrophils, while also increasing the synthesis of the antiinflammatory cytokine interleukin (IL)-4, and lowering the proinflammatory cytokines IL-6, IL-8, and IL-12p70, by suppressing NF-kB nuclear translocation [25]. Interestingly, calcitriol can also downregulate neutrophil apoptosis [25].

In addition, calcitriol influences epithelial integrity [11,18], as well as the synthesis of the aforementioned antimicrobial peptides (cathelicidin and β-defensin 2) by epithelial cells [8]. Moreover, it affects the activity of NK cells, whose main functions include not only the killing of infected cells but also the modulation of adaptive immune responses [8]. DCs, as well as macrophages, by acting as APCs, also affect adaptive immune responses. More specifically, when these cells, particularly DCs, present an antigen to naïve CD4+ T lymphocytes, it can elicit its differentiation into one of several lineages of effector T helper (Th) cells, namely, Th1, Th2, and Th17, depending on the cytokine milieu induced by DCs—IL-12 and IL-4, leads to Th1 and Th2 subsets, respectively, while IL-6, IL-1, and IL-23 induce Th17 differentiation. Each of these Th lymphocytes expresses distinctive types of cytokines (Th1: IL-2, interferon gamma (IFN-γ), TNF-α; Th2: IL-4, IL-5, IL-9, IL-13; Th17: IL-17, IL-21, IL-22) and performs different functions [14]. Of relevance, Th1 and Th17 cells, albeit having important roles in the protection against different types of microbes, are central players in inflammation and autoimmunity [11]. Noticeably, one of the mechanisms by which vitamin D prevents autoimmunity and aberrant inflammatory reactions is by modulating Th1 and Th17 cell differentiation and activity.

As mentioned, T lymphocytes and APCs (DCs and macrophages) express the VDR and the 1α-hydroxylase enzyme, which means they can respond to both renal-derived and locally produced 1α,25$(OH)_2$D [8]. Regarding the effect of calcitriol on DCs, which are the most important APCs in Th cell differentiation, multiple studies have shown that it can partially inhibit the differentiation of DC precursors into DCs [26], as well as their maturation and their immunostimulatory capacity, by decreasing their expression of class II Human Leukocyte Antigen (HLA) molecules—involved in the presentation of antigens by DCs—and of the costimulatory molecules CD40, CD80, and CD86 [27,28]. Furthermore, 1α,25$(OH)_2$D leads to a suppression of IL-12 synthesis by DCs, thus decreasing Th1 differentiation [11]. Moreover, it increases IL-10 production by DCs, which together with the aforementioned lower expression of costimulatory molecules, promotes induced T regulatory (iTreg) cell differentiation, which play a central role in the peripheral tolerance to autoantigens and suppress the effector activity of autoreactive Th1 and Th17 cells [8,11]. These effects of calcitriol in DCs have led to the notion that vitamin D can cause immune suppression. Nevertheless, during the process of maturation and differentiation of DCs, there is a decrease in VDR expression in these cells, which is balanced by an increase in the expression and activity of CYP27B1 as these DCs acquire a mature phenotype [29]. In this way, the calcitriol produced by mature DCs will not act autocrinally, but rather in a paracrine way in immature DCs with high VDR expression [30]. This allows for the maturation of some DCs and the activation of normal immune responses, while preventing an exaggerated response with pathological consequences [30]. Likewise, although $1\alpha,25(OH)_2D_3$ increases monocyte differentiation into macrophages and increases their antimicrobial capacity, it inhibits TLR expression in monocytes. This can be seen as a protective mechanism, by preventing an exacerbated and unregulated damaging inflammatory response [29].

Calcitriol can also act directly on Th cells. For instance, it decreases the expression of IL-2, IFN-γ, and TNF-α, while also promoting IL-4, IL-5, IL-9, and IL-13 synthesis, thereby skewing the Th1/Th2 balance in favor of a Th2 phenotype [11]. And, by inhibiting the production of IL-6, IL-21, and IL-22, $1\alpha,25(OH)_2D$ can also reduce the responses mediated by Th17 lymphocytes [8,11]. Additionally, calcitriol upregulates the expression of the Treg marker FoxP3 in naïve CD4+ T cells, which can promote Treg differentiation and suppress Th17 differentiation [8].

Vitamin D can also inhibit CD8+ T lymphocyte-mediated cytotoxicity [28] and affect B lymphocytes. Accordingly, $1\alpha,25(OH)_2D$ has been shown to reduce B-cell proliferation and differentiation into plasma cells, as well as IgG secretion, either by direct interaction with the VDR expressed in these cells, or indirectly through their effects on APCs and Th lymphocytes [29]. One of the mechanisms by which calcitriol leads to a reduction in the synthesis of proinflammatory cytokines in macrophages, and neutrophils is, as seen previously, by the suppression of the NF-κB signaling pathway in these cells. It should be noted that in B lymphocytes, $1\alpha,25(OH)_2D$ does not suppress NF-κB, but rather the expression of another transcription factor, specifically the X-box binding protein 1 (XBP1), which may explain its inhibitory role in the secretion of immunoglobulins by plasma cells [29].

Causes of vitamin D deficiency

Vitamin D deficiency is determined by measuring serum or plasma levels of 25OHD [31,32]. Although this biomarker is the most widely accepted and used to assess vitamin D status, controversy exists regarding its interpretation. This is demonstrated by many definitions of adequacy, which vary significantly. For example, in the United States, the Institute of Medicine has set the cut-off for sufficiency at 20 ng/mL (50 nmol/L) [33], whereas in England, it is merely 10 ng/mL (25 nmol/L) [34]. On the other hand, the Endocrine Society (with members from several countries) has set it at 30 ng/mL (75 nmol/L) [35]. More recently, Kimball and Holick have reviewed various lines of evidence and suggested that the optimal levels of 25OHD for multiple health outcomes should lie between 40 and

60 ng/mL (100 and 150 nmol/L, respectively) [36]. Unfortunately, vitamin insufficiency is widespread, as multiple studies demonstrate [37]. This can be explained by a wide range of factors affecting either vitamin D synthesis, intake or metabolism, as described below.

Factors that compromise the cutaneous synthesis of vitamin D

UVB radiation (wavelengths of 290–315 nm) is absorbed in the epidermis by 7-dehydrocholesterol, giving rise to previtamin D_3. This seco-steroid is then converted into Vitamin D_3, which exits the skin and enters the systemic circulation [38]. Several factors can compromise this process, specifically:

- *Solar zenith angle*

This is the angle between the local vertical—zenith—and the position of the sun in the sky at any given moment. As it increases, the amount of UVB radiation reaching the earth's surface is reduced. Consequently, any factor that increases this angle will decrease the cutaneous synthesis of previtamin D_3 and should therefore be taken into consideration when discussing vitamin D deficiency. Among the main variables affecting the solar zenith angle are latitude and season [38]. Accordingly, whereas at lower latitudes, it is possible to synthesize previtamin D_3 all year, sun exposure during the winter above and below approximately 33 degrees latitude will elicit little if any previtamin D_3 synthesis [38]. The solar zenith angle is also increased at early morning and late afternoon when the sun is not directly overhead [38].

- *Meteorological conditions*

Fully overcast clouds can cause an up to 99% reduction in UVB radiation, even when the solar zenith angle is optimal [39].

- *Air pollution*

Nitrogen dioxide, sulfur dioxide, and ozone, by absorbing UVB radiation, can reduce the cutaneous production of previtamin D_3 [38].

- *Skin pigmentation*

Melanin by being an efficient natural sunscreen with an absorption spectrum of 290–700 nm is very effective at absorbing solar UVB radiation [40]. This explains why individuals with skin types 5 and 6 (on the Fitzpatrick scale [41]), in order to synthesize the same amount of previtamin D_3 as their counterparts with skin types 1 and 2 do, require either a larger body surface area exposed to UVB radiation or more exposure time [38].

- *Aging*

By decreasing the concentration of 7-dehydrocholesterol in human epidermis, the aging process significantly reduces the synthesis of previtamin D_3. Nevertheless, and similar to what occurs in individuals with more darkly pigmented skin, older adults can effectively raise their circulating 25OHD levels by simply exposing a larger body surface area to the sun [38].

- *Sunscreen use*

As expected, the use of sunscreens that either absorb or block UVB radiation has been shown to drastically decrease previtamin D_3 synthesis, this effect being greater at higher sun protection factors [38].

Factors that decrease the intake and absorption of vitamin D

Vitamin D can be found in multiple animal foods in the form of cholecalciferol (vitamin D_3), although very few actually contain meaningful amounts (Table 35.1) [42,43]. Certain foods, such as mushrooms, also contain ergocalciferol (vitamin D_2). Nevertheless, its concentrations vary significantly [44], and there is evidence that vitamin D_2 is less stable and effective than is vitamin D_3 [1,45,46]. Therefore, in the absence of sufficient cutaneous synthesis of vitamin D, supplementation with cholecalciferol may be necessary [1]. Although there are differences in the bioavailability of the various oral vitamin D formulations, there are more important variables affecting intestinal absorption to consider. One such factor is its interaction with other nutrients, such as liposoluble vitamins A, E, and K that compete with vitamin D for intestinal absorption [47]. Certain antiobesity drugs that interfere with lipid absorption, such as orlistat, can also reduce vitamin D bioavailability [47]. Likewise, Roux-en-Y gastric bypass surgery performed in obese individuals significantly decreases vitamin D absorption [47]. There are also diseases and conditions, such as obstructive jaun-

TABLE 35.1 Dietary sources of Vitamin D [42,43].

Food	Vitamin D (IU)
Cod liver oil (10 g)	1360
Wild salmon—raw (100 g)	998
Sardine—raw (100 g)	476
Farmed trout—raw (100 g)	388
Tuna—raw (100 g)	383
Farmed salmon—raw (100 g)	245
Wild salmon—baked (100 g)	240
Wild salmon—fried (100 g)	123
Cod—raw (100 g)	104
Mackerel—raw (100 g)	24
Egg (1 unit)	20
Bovine liver—cooked (100 g)	14

dice, cystic fibrosis, celiac disease, and Crohn's disease, that impair the absorption of vitamin D [47–49]. Finally, genetic variants affecting lipid digestive enzyme may also compromise vitamin D absorption [47].

Factors that alter the metabolism of vitamin D

As illustrated in Fig. 35.1, any factor affecting the transport, metabolism, and catabolism of vitamin D can influence its status. Accordingly, genetic variants in genes that code for DBP (the main vitamin D transport protein), CYP2R1 (the major 25-hydroxylase), CYP27B1 (1-α-hydroxylase), and CYP24A1 (24-hydroxylase) have been shown to contribute to vitamin D deficiency or reduce its activity [50–56]. Certain disorders, such as liver and kidney disease, have also been shown to negatively impact vitamin D status, by perturbing its transport and metabolism [4,57]. Importantly, these diseases are characterized by inflammation [16], which can decrease the circulating levels of 25OHD [58,59]. In fact, this biomarker is considered a negative acute phase reactant [59,60], which explains, to some extent, why 25OHD concentrations may be low in patients with infectious diseases [58], especially in those in critical condition [61]. Obesity is another condition that has been shown to reduce 25OHD levels [62,63], with overweight and obese individuals having to ingest, respectively, 1.5 and 3 times more vitamin D than their lean counterparts in order to achieve the same vitamin D status [63,64]. Other factors to consider are low micronutrient status, particularly magnesium deficiency, which negatively affects DBP, CYP2R1, and CYP27B1 [65], as well as medications that upregulate CYP24A1, specifically phenytoin, carbamazepin, cyclophophamide, taxol, tamoxifen, clotrimazole, rifampicin, dexamethasone, nifedipine, spironolactone, ritononavir, saquinavir, cyproterone acetate, and herbal medicines (Kava kava, and St. John's wort) [66].

COVID-19 and vitamin D deficiency

The pandemic of Coronavirus Disease-2019 (COVID-19) caused by Severe Acute Respiratory Syndrome Coronavirus (SARS-CoV)-2 has been raising many questions around the scientific community. Starting on the individual disease susceptibility, followed by the peculiar way the virus interacts with the host immune system, as well as its capability to leave debilitating sequelae behind [67]. In that manner, it has triggered great interest in the search for the pathophysiological mechanisms of COVID-19 and its associated hyperinflammatory state [68]. SARS-CoV-2 infection causes cellular and tissue damage and triggers innate and adaptive immune responses [69]. Therefore, disease severity is due to not only to the virus itself but also to the host response [70,71]. To date, assorted investigations have elucidated plausible biological hypothesis supporting a role for vitamin D in COVID-19 disease susceptibility, severity, and recovery [72]. For example, across Europe, ecological studies have indicated an inverse correlation between estimates of vitamin D status and COVID-19 incidence and mortality [73]. And, there is a considerable overlap between risk factors for vitamin D deficiency and COVID-19 severity, including living in northerly latitudes, older age, obesity, dark skin type, and risk-predicting genetic variants [74]. Indeed, those factors have been significantly associated with increased morbidity and mortality in patients with COVID-19 [75,76].

Susceptibility for SARS-CoV-2 infection and vitamin D status

Solid evidence suggests that vitamin D deficiency contributes to the seasonal increase in respiratory viral infections, from the common cold viruses to influenza, and now possibly also to SARS-CoV-2. A large meta-analysis published in 2017 analyzed over 11,300 patients from 25 randomized studies and demonstrated the protective effect of vitamin D supplementation on respiratory tract infections in all participants ($P < .001$) [77]. More recently, an updated meta-analysis enrolling 75,541 participants emphasized the influence of vitamin D supplementation for the prevention of acute respiratory tract infections [78]. As a matter of fact and as previously mentioned, vitamin D can reduce the risk of infection by improving the antimicrobial actions of innate immune cells, as well as contributing to the integrity of physical barriers, particularly at mucosal surfaces.

As discussed above, most immune cells express the VDR, as well as enzymes that enable them to convert vitamin D into its more active form, thus enhancing the locally available concentrations to those required for immunomodulatory effects [79]. For example, calcitriol has been shown to upregulate cathelicidin in macrophages, neutrophils, and respiratory epithelial cells [25,80]. Cathelicidin has direct antiviral actions against respiratory viruses since it disrupts viral envelopes and decreases the viability of the host target cells [80]. Strikingly, there are experimental data suggesting that cathelicidin can inhibit the binding of SARS-CoV-2 to the receptor it uses to infect target cells—that is, angiotensin-converting enzyme 2 (ACE2) [80]. It has also been demonstrated that vitamin D is capable of inducing autophagy and apoptosis in infected cells, through several mechanisms [81]. Remarkably, the vitamin D binding protein (DBP), which is the major transport protein of cholecalciferol, calcifediol and calcitriol, may play an underestimated role in the development of acute respiratory syndrome, since it can significantly enhance the chemotactic activity of macrophages and neutrophils, and also participate in the resolution of tissue injury by binding to and removing extracellular actin released from dead or damaged cells [82,83].

Merzon et al. (2020) provided one of the first studies raising the association between low serum vitamin D and SARS-CoV-2 infection. The study analyzed 7807 individuals, of whom 782 (10.1%) were SARS-CoV-2-positive and 7025 (89.9%) SARS-CoV-2-negative. Univariate analysis demonstrated a significative association between low plasma 25OHD levels and an increased likelihood of infection ($P < .001$), and of hospitalization due to COVID-19 ($P < .05$) [75]. Similar results were recently presented in a large retrospective case–control study by *Israel* et al. (2022) [84]. Even more compelling are the results of an extensive meta-analysis of 72 observational studies including 1.976.099 patients, which concluded that vitamin D deficiency/insufficiency increased the odds of developing COVID-19, and was associated with disease severity ($P = .0001$) [85]. On the other hand, other studies failed to find such associations. For instance, a retrospective study using data from the UK Biobank showed that both circulating 25OHD concentrations and vitamin D deficiency were not associated with the risk of COVID-19, even after adjusting for potential confounders [86]. In any case, many of those studies are seeded in baseline measurements, including 25OHD concentration and health status, obtained a long time before the onset of COVID-19.

COVID-19 disease severity and vitamin D status

In addition to its role in modulating antiviral responses, vitamin D might contribute to the prevention or even suppression of the hyperinflammatory state—cytokine storm—observed in severe COVID-19 patients, by inhibiting or decreasing the production of proinflammatory cytokines, such as IL-6, IL-8, IL-12, TNF-α, IFN-γ, and IL-17 [8,80,87,88]. Vitamin D may offer additional protection against severe disease due to the local action of the active vitamin D metabolite, calcitriol, on the renin-angiotensin system (RAS) [89]. Accordingly, it increases the bioavailability and expression of soluble ACE2 [90,91], inhibits renin expression, and acts as a negative RAS regulator [92]. Conversely, vitamin D deficiency appears to be associated with severe COVID-19 outcomes [93]. This was especially so during the first phase of the pandemic, when SARS-CoV-2 infection was more aggressive, particularly in Southern European countries (e.g., Italy and Spain), where mortality rates were high and hypovitaminosis D is most common [94]. These correlations were also found in other epidemiological studies. For instance, retrospective meta-analyses from American and European cohorts have indicated low vitamin D status to be associated with higher rates of Intensive Care Unit (ICU) admission in patients with COVID-19 [95,96]. And an observational study from Italy that performed a survival analysis of patients with COVID-19 admitted to a respiratory intermediate care unit found severe vitamin D deficiency to be a predictor of mortality. Those with vitamin D levels <10 ng/mL (25 nmol/L) had a 50% probability of mortality, compared with a 5% risk in those with levels ≥10 ng/mL (25 nmol/L) [97]. *Chiodini* et al. (2021) published the largest meta-analysis so far, involving more than a million individuals and including up to 27 and 35 studies investigating the association between vitamin D status and ICU admission due to severe COVID-19 disease or related mortality, respectively. This found that, whatever the considered threshold (severe vitamin D deficiency, vitamin D deficiency, or vitamin D insufficiency), low 25OHD levels, assessed at the time of hospitalization, were associated with greater COVID-19 severity, and impacted on the degree of respiratory distress (e.g., requiring ICU admission) and COVID-19-related mortality [98]. More recently, *Seal* et al. (2022) were able to find concordant results in a large retrospective cohort study, enrolling 4599 US veterans with a positive SARS-CoV-2 test. After adjusting for all covariates, including race/ethnicity and poverty, the authors found a significant independent inverse dose-response relationship between increasing continuous 25OHD concentrations (from 15 to 60 ng/mL) and decreasing probability of COVID-19-related hospitalization (from 24.1% to 18.7%, $P = .009$) and mortality (from 10.4% to 5.7%, $P = .001$) [99]. Given the evidence that hypovitaminosis D impairs innate cellular immunity and may contribute to the cytokine storm [80], which is involved in COVID-19-related acute respiratory distress syndrome (ARDS) and multiorgan failure [70], those results were expected. Remarkably, the association between low vitamin D status, airways inflammation, and increased risk of respiratory infections was already known before the COVID-19 era when a large body of studies evaluated the efficacy of vitamin D supplementation as adjunctive treatment in patients with respiratory diseases [97,100].

Another important aspect relating vitamin D and COVID-19 disease is polymorphisms in the VDR and the DBP. As a matter of fact, VDR gene polymorphisms were recently found to be independently associated with the severity of COVID-19 and the survival of patients [101]. Hence, a study from Portugal, with 491 patients who tested positive for SARS-CoV-2, concluded that DBP gene polymorphisms are related to COVID-19 severity [53].

In conclusion, multiple observational studies involving nearly two million adults suggest that vitamin D deficiency/insufficiency increases susceptibility to COVID-19 infection and severity, although with a high risk of bias and heterogeneity. Association with mortality was less robust [85]. However, these data must be interpreted with caution based on a lack of statistical significance when adjusted for confounding factors, such as age, sex, and the presence of comorbidities. Such variables are determinants of COVID-19 prognosis, so it is necessary to consider these aspects in future studies.

Long COVID and vitamin D status

Post-COVID-19 syndrome (PCS) is defined by chronic clinical signs and symptoms that appear while or after suffering COVID-19 infection, persist for more than 12 weeks and cannot be explained by an alternative diagnosis [102]. This new disorder has led to the understanding that the absence of SARS-CoV-2 viral particles following COVID-19 does not necessarily mean full recovery [103]. Clinical manifestations are diverse, fluctuating, and variable [104]. The most prevalent ongoing complaints are fatigue, dyspnea, arthralgia, anosmia and dysgeusia, hair loss, cognitive symptoms, and psychosocial distress [105]. Furthermore, the persistence of symptoms is a primary determinant of mental health outcome, with anxiety, depression, sleep disturbances, and posttraumatic stress symptoms being commonly reported in COVID-19 survivors [106]. Symptom burden appears to be independent from the severity of initial infection and humoral response, with no clear predictors of who will develop long-lasting symptoms [107−109]. However, a wide variety of complaints have been reported within the PCS involving multiple organs and systems demanding long-term follow-up, and even rehospitalization due to their severity [108,110]. *Huang* et al. (2021) performed an ambidirectional cohort study enrolling 1733 patients with confirmed COVID-19 who had been discharged from *Jin Yin-tan Hospital* (Wuhan, China) between Jan 7, 2020, and May 29, 2020. The aim of this study was to describe the long-term health consequences of patients with COVID-19. Interestingly, it had been found that 76% of patients reported at least one symptom at 6 months after disease diagnosis, and the proportion was higher among women. The most prevalent complaints were fatigue or muscle weakness, sleep difficulties, anxiety, and depression. Patients with a more severe illness during their hospitalization had increasingly impaired pulmonary diffusion capacities and abnormal chest imaging manifestations [111].

The underlying biological mechanisms of PCS are unknown, although an autoimmune or chronic inflammatory response may play an important role. Some studies suggest that long COVID-19 symptoms may be due to persistent endothelial dysfunction [112], as well as various immune alterations which has led to new-onset of autoimmune-related disorders [67,69,113]. Nevertheless, due to the recentness of the COVID-19 pandemic, and the initial focus of research being on the acute phase of the disease, an accurate characterization of PCS symptomatology, evolution, and treatment has remained elusive [114,115]. In contrast to the large number of studies investigating the role of vitamin D in acute COVID-19, there is an important gap in the literature examining the relationship between vitamin D and long COVID [116]. Although we could hypothesize that vitamin D deficiency might represent a risk factor for PCS and its supplementation could provide some benefits, we could not find any study to date that confirmed this perception.

Vitamin D supplementation in COVID/long COVID patients

As mentioned, various studies have demonstrated an association between vitamin D deficiency and the severity and increased mortality of COVID-19 [117–119]. Thus, it seems likely that raising serum 25OHD concentrations after SARS-CoV-2 infection or development of COVID-19 could decrease the susceptibility, progression, and severity of COVID-19. Accordingly, several studies have investigated whether vitamin D supplementation could reduce COVID-19 susceptibility or severity. In this manner, and to allow us a better overview and comprehension of the role of vitamin D supplementation in COVID-19 patients, a summary of the clinical trials published to date was delineated on Table 35.2. A total 2104 patients in 13 clinical trials were included, six of them randomized, double-blinded, and placebo-controlled.

Irrespective of the modality and dosage, vitamin D supplementation was generally well tolerated. Only two participants out of 420 patients referred nausea/vomiting [120,121]. *Murai* et al. (2021) aimed to investigate the benefit of a single cholecalciferol dose of 200,000 IU administrated on the admission day of 120 COVID patients, matched with 120 controls, who took placebo. The baseline 25OHD level was 20.9 ng/mL. Regardless, no significant differences were observed in the range of length of hospitalization, despite that serum 25-hydroxyvitamin D levels significantly increased in the intervention group ($P < .001$) [120]. Moreover, a post hoc, ancillary, and exploratory analysis of this RCT showed no significant changes in cytokines, chemokines, and vascular endothelial growth factor (VEGF) [121]. On the other hand, a study from Turkey found that vitamin D led to a shorter hospital length of stay and decreased mortality in COVID-19 patients, even in those with comorbidities. In this study, a total of 162 patients were supplemented with different doses of cholecalciferol (total amount between 224.000 and 500.000 IU), in accordance with the baseline serum 25OHD level for 14 days [132]. In another pilot randomized open label, double-masked clinical trial from Spain, including 76 patients hospitalized for COVID-19, oral administration of high-dose calcifediol (0.532 mg on the day of admission and 0.266 mg on days 3 and 7 and weekly thereafter) significantly reduced the need for ICU admission ($P > .001$) [123]. On the same line, other clinical trials succeed to find a significant association between vitamin D supplementation and reduced risk of mortality in patients hospitalized due to COVID-19 [124,126,131]. Further, a study of SARS-CoV-2 RNA-positive patients in India, has found that 10 (63%) participants in the intervention group and 5 (21%) in the control group became SARS-CoV-2 RNA-negative after 60,000 IU of cholecalciferol supplementation for 14 days ($P < .018$). Interestingly, a significant decrease in fibrinogen levels was also noticed ($P = .007$) [122]. *Sabico* et al. (2021) compared the effect of two different doses of daily oral supplementation of vitamin D_3 in COVID-19 patients, specifically 5000 IU (high-dose group) versus 1000 IU (low-dose group). After 2 weeks of treatment, a reduced time to recovery of COVID-19 symptoms, such as cough and gustatory sensory loss was seen among the high-dose group ($P = .039$) [129]. And other favorable clinical and immunological outcomes, such as decreased biomarkers of muscle damage [125], an improvement in oxygenation level [130] and increased

TABLE 35.2 Clinical trials investigating vitamin D supplementation in COVID-19 patients, published until January 15th, 2022.

Author, country, year, CT Register	Study Design	Sample size (I/C)	Mean age & Gender	Baseline 25OHD level	Intervention	Follow-Up	Side effects	Outcomes	*P* VALUE	Ref
Murai, Brazil, 2021, NCT04449718	Randomized, DB, PC	240 I: 120 C: 120	56.2 years 43.9% female	20.9 ng/mL	I: 200,000 IU VD3 on admission + conventional care C: placebo + conventional care	During hospitalization	Vomit (1x)	No significant reduction in hospital length of stay	.62	[120]
Fernandes, Brazil, 2022, -	Randomized, DB, PC	200 I: 101 C: 99)	55.5 Years 45.5% female	–	I: single dose of 200,000 IU of VD3 C: placebo	During hospitalization	Vomit (1x)	No improvement of cytokines, chemokines, and growth factor	>0.05	[121]
Rastogi, India, 2020, NCT04459247	Randomized, DB, PC	40 I: 16 C: 24	50 years 62% female	I: 8.6 ng/mL C: 9.54 ng/mL	I: 60,000 IU of VD3 for 7 days C: placebo	21 days	–	Greater proportion of vitamin D-deficient individuals with SARS-CoV-2 infection turned SARS-CoV-2 RNA negative. Significant decrease in fibrinogen levels	<.018 0.007	[122]
Entrenas Castillo, Spain, 2020, NCT04366908	Parallel, randomized open label, double-masked	76 I: 50 C: 26	53 years 41% female	–	I: oral calcifediol (0.532 mg) at admission + 0.266 mg on day 3 and 7, and then weekly until discharge or ICU admission	Until discharge or ICU admission	–	Significantly reduced the need for ICU treatment of patients requiring hospitalization	<.001	[123]
Ling, UK, 2020, NCT04386044	Observational	444	74 years 44.9% female	31.2 ng/mL	I: approximately ≥280,000 IU VD3 in a period of up to 7 weeks	Until 7 weeks	–	High-dose cholecalciferol, regardless of baseline serum 25(OH)D levels, appears to be associated with a	.012	[124]

(Continued)

TABLE 35.2 Clinical trials investigating vitamin D supplementation in COVID-19 patients, published until January 15th, 2022.—cont'd

Author, country, year, CT Register	Study Design	Sample size (I/C)	Mean age & Gender	Baseline 25OHD level	Intervention	Follow-Up	Side effects	Outcomes	*P* VALUE	Ref
								reduced risk of mortality		
Caballero-García, Spain, 2021, –	Randomized, DB, PC	30 I: 15 C: 15	60.6 years –	21 ng/mL	I: 2000 IU VD3/day C: placebo	6 weeks	–	Decreased muscle damage indicators	<.05	[125]
Annweiler, France, 2021, NCT04560608	Observational	95 I: 67 C: 28	88 years 48.4% female	–	I: participants who had received VD3 supplements either prior to hospitalization and/or at hospital discharge C: participants who had not received any VD	3 months	–	3-month mortality was HR = 0.23 in I group compared to C group I Group had longer survival time	.002 0.008	[126]
Murai, Brazil, 2021, NCT04449718	Randomized, DB, PC	32 I: 16 C: 16	58.5 years 43.8% female	7.8 ng/mL	I: single dose of 200.000 IU of VD3 C: placebo	During hospitalization	–	No significant difference was observed in the range of length of hospital stay Serum 25-hydroxyvitamin D levels significantly increased in the I group	.74 <0.001	[127]
Maghbooli, Iran, 2021, NCT04386850	Randomized, DB, PC	106 I: 53 C: 53	50 years 41% female	19 ng/mL	I: 25 µg of $25(OH)D_3$ daily C: placebo	60 days	None	Improved immune function by increasing blood lymphocyte percentage Lower neutrophil-to-lymphocyte ratio was significantly associated with reduced ICU admission days and mortality.	<.05 0.04	[128]

Sabico, Saudi Arabia, 2021, SCTR no. 20061006	Randomized	69 I: 36 C: 33	49,8 years 35% female	53.4 nmol/L	I: 5000 IU oral vitamin D3 daily C: 1000 IU oral vitamin D3 daily	2 weeks	–	Reduced time to recovery for cough and gustatory sensory loss in I group among patients with sub-optimal VD status	.039	[129]
Elamir, USA, 2022. -	Randomized, open label	50 I: 25 C: 25	69 years 52% female	–	I: calcitriol 0.5 μg daily C: none	14 days or hospital discharge	–	Improvement in oxygenation among I group	.0305	[130]
Alcala-Diaz, Spain, 2020, -	Retrospective, open, non-randomized cohort	537 I: 79 C: 458	70 years 41% female	–	I: calcifediol (0.266 mg/capsule, 2 capsules on entry and then one capsule on day 3, 7, 14, 21, and 28 C: none	30 days	–	Calcifediol was significantly associated with lower in-hospital mortality	<.01	[131]
Gönen, Turkey, 2021, TSG-2020-34998	Open, nonrandomized cohort	185 I: 162 C: 23	50 years 31%	16.62 ng/mL	I: between 224.000 and 500.000 IU cholecalciferol (total doses for 14 days, depending on baseline serum level) C: none	14 days	–	Shorter hospital length of stay and decreased mortality in COVID-19 cases, even in the existence of comorbidities	<.05	[132]

Abbreviations: *C*, Controls; *CT*, Clinical Trial; *DB*, Double-blind; *I*, Intervention; *ICU*, Intensive Care Unit; *PC*, Placebo-controlled; *SCTR*, Saudi Clinical Trial Register; *VD*, Vitamin D.

blood lymphocyte percentage [128], were noticed in other studies with hospitalized patients who were treated with cholecalciferol, calcitriol, and calcifediol, respectively.

It should be mentioned that the heterogenicity of the various clinical trials protocols, coupled with the potential differences in both treatment programs and criteria for SARS-CoV-2 infection diagnosis and COVID-19 hospitalization adopted by the different countries during the pandemic waves, precludes a definitive conclusion. Nevertheless, we believe the overall evidence suggests that vitamin D deficiency might represent an easily modifiable risk factor for COVID-19, particularly considering the limited cost and the safety of its treatment. However, and considering the chronic consequences of COVID-19, it is necessary to examine the long-term effects of vitamin D supplementation on the enduring effects of the disease, including full recovery duration and organ damage.

COVID vaccine and vitamin D—is there a relationship?

The COVID-19 vaccines include three broad categories: protein-based vaccines, gene-based vaccines (mRNA vaccines and DNA vaccines), and a combination of gene and protein-based vaccines [133]. The immune response to vaccination with SARS-CoV-2 vaccines varies greatly between individuals. The evaluation of the efficacy and effectiveness of SARS-CoV-2 vaccines is complex, due to the lack of complete knowledge about the pathophysiology of the disease, and the diversity of vaccine formulations and strategies. However, due to the continuous emergence of new viral mutations, there is a need to enhance vaccine performance. This could be achieved not only by adapting the different vaccine formulations to new variants, but perhaps by also focusing on improving the nutritional status and baseline health and immunity of the host, in order to mitigate COVID-19 severity and increase the effectiveness of vaccination [134–137]. And given the results from the aforementioned clinical trials testing vitamin D supplementation in COVID-19 patients together with the numerous observational studies showing an inverse association between serum 25OHD levels and the incidence and severity of SARS-CoV-2 infection [138,139], vitamin D emerges as a likely candidate to be used as an adjuvant measure in COVID-19 vaccination protocols. This is further supported by the multiple interactions of vitamin D with cells of the innate and adaptive immune system [140]. Accordingly, vitamin D has been shown to:

(a). Improve THαβ CD4+ T lymphocytes, while inhibiting T helper 17 lymphocytes, and raising the production of virus-specific IgG1 antibodies and IL-10, through the activation of T-dependent B cells [141].

(b). Decrease the release of proinflammatory cytokines by macrophages, neutrophils, and CD4+ T cells, by suppressing NF-kB signaling [24,25,142], which might be relevant since baseline chronic inflammation has been associated with decreased vaccination responsiveness, as reviewed elsewhere [16,134].

A recent study by *Chillon* et al. (2021) analyzed the titers of SARS-CoV-2 IgG and its neutralization potency along with 25OHD concentrations in a cohort of healthy German adults from the time of vaccination over 24 weeks. Contrary to all expectations, no significant differences in the induced SARS-CoV-2 IgG concentrations were observed, neither with respect to baseline vitamin D status nor in relation to selfreported vitamin D supplementation. Notwithstanding, the study presents several limitations. First, it assumed that serum SARS-CoV-2 IgG concentrations represents a surrogate marker of vaccination success and did not took into consideration parameters of cellular immune response. In addition, conclusions were deduced from an analysis of healthy subjects only, not allowing extrapolations to pediatric, geriatric, or other populations [143]. Regretfully, and to the best of our knowledge, no other clinical studies have been published to date enrolling this topic. Future studies are therefore mandatory to elucidate the role of vitamin D in COVID-19 vaccination efficacy and effectiveness.

Recommendations

Vitamin D deficiency is a major public health problem worldwide in all age groups [37,144]. Thus, an important first step would be to ensure that everyone receives at least the recommended daily amount (RDA) for this nutrient [145]. Still, this is a public health measure and not a clinical-based decision. In that regard, and based on the evidence so far, and particularly under the current pandemic context, vitamin D supplementation should be mandatory in individuals with a 25OHD serum concentration lower than 20 ng/mL (50 nmol/L) [146]. Nevertheless, this should be seen as the minimum and shouldn't preclude the goal of achieving an optimal vitamin D status in individual patients, which, in order to reduce the risk of COVID-19 and its severe outcomes, including mortality, would consist in a serum concentration of 25OHD of at least 30 ng/mL (75 nmol/L)—and preferably in the range of 40–60 ng/mL (100–150 nmol/L) [31]. This is not easily achieved by the RDA, and higher doses may be needed [35], particularly, as previously mentioned, in patients with obesity, kidney, or liver disease, gene polymorphisms that negatively affect vitamin D transport or metabolism, inflammatory diseases (which obviously includes COVID-19), or taking certain medications.

On the other hand, caution is advised in individuals with certain disorders or gene polymorphisms where even moderate doses of vitamin D could cause hypercalciuria and/or hypercalcemia. Granulomatous disorders are a classic example. As previously mentioned, there are important differences between renal and macrophage vitamin D metabolism. Whereas increasing the concentration of calcium and calcitriol downregulates the expression of the 1α-hydroxylase in the kidney, macrophages do not appear to respond to this type of stimulus. This means that in conditions characterized by granulomas, such as sarcoidosis, and tuberculosis, an increased and uncontrolled synthesis of 1α,25(OH)$_2$D by macrophages with an ensuing hypercalciuria and hypercalcemia is a possibility that cannot be ignored [35,147]. According to the Endocrine Society clinical practice guideline, these patients should avoid circulating 25OHD levels above 30 ng/mL (75 nmol/L) [35]. Ideally, these patients should have their vitamin D dose individually adjusted by routine monitoring of serum 25OHD, and 1α,25(OH)$_2$D, as well as calcemia, calciuria, and parathormone [148].

Given the above, and the potential effect of the VDR in gene expression activation on the responsiveness to vitamin D supplementation [149], generic "one-size fits all" vitamin D recommendations and treatment lengths are difficult to suggest. Furthermore, the term "vitamin D supplementation" is often ambiguous and includes cholecalciferol, ergocalciferol, calcidiol, and calcitriol [1]. When comparing cholecalciferol to ergocalciferol, the preferred form should be cholecalciferol [1,45,46]. Regarding cholecalciferol versus calcifediol, the latter presents some advantages over the former. More specifically, calcifediol has a higher bioavailability and raises serum 25OHD faster than cholecalciferol and does so in a linear fashion [150]. Moreover, calcifediol, by being more potent than cholecalciferol, can be administrated in lower doses. Finally, by bypassing the first hydroxylation step catalyzed by 25-hydroxylase, calcifediol is the most suited candidate for patients with intestinal malabsorption, or disorders affecting the expression and/or activity of this enzyme, such as liver disease [150]. Despite the apparent superiority of calcifediol, cholecalciferol is less likely to elicit excessively high values of circulating 25OHD, thus having a lower risk of toxicity [151]. This makes oral cholecalciferol the preferred choice for supplementation in the general population and in most clinical conditions [1]. However, there are situations, such as hypoparathyroidism, and severe kidney insufficiency, in which calcitriol or its analogs may be more indicated than either cholecalciferol or calcifediol [31,150]. But it should only be used under strict medical supervision, because of the hypercalcemia risk [31].

In conclusion, preventing or treating vitamin D deficiency should be conducted in a personalized manner, where the dosage and form of vitamin D are adapted to the individual patient.

References

[1] Vieth R. Vitamin D supplementation: cholecalciferol, calcifediol, and calcitriol. Eur J Clin Nutr 2020;74:1493–7. https://doi.org/10.1038/s41430-020-0697-1.

[2] Tuckey RC, Cheng CYS, Slominski AT. The serum vitamin D metabolome: what we know and what is still to discover. J Steroid Biochem Mol Biol 2019;186:4–21. https://doi.org/10.1016/j.jsbmb.2018.09.003.

[3] Makris K, Bhattoa HP, Cavalier E, Phinney K, Sempos CT, Ulmer CZ, et al. Recommendations on the measurement and the clinical use of vitamin D metabolites and vitamin D binding protein - a position paper from the IFCC Committee on bone metabolism. Clin Chim Acta 2021;517:171–97. https://doi.org/10.1016/j.cca.2021.03.002.

[4] Christakos S, Dhawan P, Verstuyf A, Verlinden L, Carmeliet G. Vitamin D: metabolism, molecular mechanism of action, and pleiotropic effects. Physiol Rev 2016;96:365–408. https://doi.org/10.1152/physrev.00014.2015.

[5] Jones G, Prosser DE, Kaufmann M. 25-Hydroxyvitamin D-24-hydroxylase (CYP24A1): its important role in the degradation of vitamin D. Arch Biochem Biophys 2012;523:9–18. https://doi.org/10.1016/j.abb.2011.11.003.

[6] Charoenngam N, Shirvani A, Holick MF. Vitamin D for skeletal and non-skeletal health: what we should know. J Clin Orthop Trauma 2019;10:1082–93. https://doi.org/10.1016/j.jcot.2019.07.004.

[7] Hii CS, Ferrante A. The non-genomic actions of vitamin D. Nutrients 2016;8:135. https://doi.org/10.3390/nu8030135.

[8] Bishop E, Ismailova A, Dimeloe SK, Hewison M, White JH. Vitamin D and immune regulation: antibacterial, antiviral, anti-inflammatory. JBMR Plus 2020. https://doi.org/10.1002/jbm4.10405.

[9] Hiraguchi Y, Tanida H, Sugimoto M, Hosoki K, Nagao M, Tokuda R, et al. 1,25-Dihydroxyvitamin D3 upregulates functional C-x-C chemokine receptor type 4 expression in human eosinophils. Int Arch Allergy Immunol 2012;158(Suppl. 1):51–7. https://doi.org/10.1159/000337767.

[10] Immune cell - VDR - The Human Protein Atlas. n.d. https://www.proteinatlas.org/ENSG00000111424-VDR/immune+cell. Accessed January 16, 2022.

[11] Charoenngam N, Holick MF. Immunologic effects of vitamin D on human health and disease. Nutrients 2020;12:E2097. https://doi.org/10.3390/nu12072097.

[12] Kongsbak M, von Essen MR, Levring TB, Schjerling P, Woetmann A, Ødum N, et al. Vitamin D-binding protein controls T cell responses to vitamin D. BMC Immunol 2014;15:35. https://doi.org/10.1186/s12865-014-0035-2.

[13] Hollis BW, Wagner CL. Clinical review: the role of the parent compound vitamin D with respect to metabolism and function: why clinical dose intervals can affect clinical outcomes. J Clin Endocrinol Metab 2013;98:4619–28. https://doi.org/10.1210/jc.2013-2653.

[14] Abbas AK, Lichtman AH, Pillai S, Baker DL. Cellular and molecular immunology. 10th ed. Philadelphia, Pennsylvania: Elsevier; 2022.

[15] Paludan SR, Pradeu T, Masters SL, Mogensen TH. Constitutive immune mechanisms: mediators of host defence and immune regulation. Nat Rev Immunol 2021;21:137–50. https://doi.org/10.1038/s41577-020-0391-5.
[16] Furman D, Campisi J, Verdin E, Carrera-Bastos P, Targ S, Franceschi C, et al. Chronic inflammation in the etiology of disease across the life span. Nat Med 2019;25:1822–32. https://doi.org/10.1038/s41591-019-0675-0.
[17] Childs CE, Calder PC, Miles EA. Diet and immune function. Nutrients 2019;11:E1933. https://doi.org/10.3390/nu11081933.
[18] Gombart AF, Pierre A, Maggini S. A review of micronutrients and the immune system-working in harmony to reduce the risk of infection. Nutrients 2020;12:E236. https://doi.org/10.3390/nu12010236.
[19] Borella E, Nesher G, Israeli E, Shoenfeld Y. Vitamin D: a new anti-infective agent? Ann N Y Acad Sci 2014;1317:76–83. https://doi.org/10.1111/nyas.12321.
[20] Germic N, Frangez Z, Yousefi S, Simon H-U. Regulation of the innate immune system by autophagy: monocytes, macrophages, dendritic cells and antigen presentation. Cell Death Differ 2019;26:715–27. https://doi.org/10.1038/s41418-019-0297-6.
[21] Xu H, Soruri A, Gieseler RK, Peters JH. 1,25-Dihydroxyvitamin D3 exerts opposing effects to IL-4 on MHC class-II antigen expression, accessory activity, and phagocytosis of human monocytes. Scand J Immunol 1993;38:535–40. https://doi.org/10.1111/j.1365-3083.1993.tb03237.x.
[22] Liu T, Zhang L, Joo D, Sun S-C. NF-κB signaling in inflammation. Signal Transduct Targeted Ther 2017;2:17023. https://doi.org/10.1038/sigtrans.2017.23.
[23] Ernst O, Vayttaden SJ, Fraser IDC. Measurement of NF-κB activation in TLR-activated macrophages. Methods Mol Biol 2018;1714:67–78. https://doi.org/10.1007/978-1-4939-7519-8_5.
[24] Cohen-Lahav M, Shany S, Tobvin D, Chaimovitz C, Douvdevani A. Vitamin D decreases NFkappaB activity by increasing IkappaBalpha levels. Nephrol Dial Transplant 2006;21:889–97. https://doi.org/10.1093/ndt/gfi254.
[25] Subramanian K, Bergman P, Henriques-Normark B. Vitamin D promotes pneumococcal killing and modulates inflammatory responses in primary human neutrophils. J Innate Immun 2017;9:375–86. https://doi.org/10.1159/000455969.
[26] Hart PH, Gorman S, Finlay-Jones JJ. Modulation of the immune system by UV radiation: more than just the effects of vitamin D? Nat Rev Immunol 2011;11:584–96. https://doi.org/10.1038/nri3045.
[27] Chun RF, Liu PT, Modlin RL, Adams JS, Hewison M. Impact of vitamin D on immune function: lessons learned from genome-wide analysis. Front Physiol 2014;5:151. https://doi.org/10.3389/fphys.2014.00151.
[28] Mora JR, Iwata M, von Andrian UH. Vitamin effects on the immune system: vitamins A and D take centre stage. Nat Rev Immunol 2008;8:685–98. https://doi.org/10.1038/nri2378.
[29] Di Rosa M, Malaguarnera M, Nicoletti F, Malaguarnera L. Vitamin D3: a helpful immuno-modulator. Immunology 2011;134:123–39. https://doi.org/10.1111/j.1365-2567.2011.03482.x.
[30] Hewison M. Vitamin D and immune function: an overview. Proc Nutr Soc 2012;71:50–61. https://doi.org/10.1017/S0029665111001650.
[31] Bilezikian JP, Formenti AM, Adler RA, Binkley N, Bouillon R, Lazaretti-Castro M, et al. Vitamin D: dosing, levels, form, and route of administration: does one approach fit all? Rev Endocr Metab Disord 2021;22:1201–18. https://doi.org/10.1007/s11154-021-09693-7.
[32] Sempos CT, Heijboer AC, Bikle DD, Bollerslev J, Bouillon R, Brannon PM, et al. Vitamin D assays and the definition of hypovitaminosis D: results from the first international conference on controversies in vitamin D. Br J Clin Pharmacol 2018;84:2194–207. https://doi.org/10.1111/bcp.13652.
[33] Ross AC, Manson JE, Abrams SA, Aloia JF, Brannon PM, Clinton SK, et al. The 2011 report on dietary reference intakes for calcium and vitamin D from the Institute of Medicine: what clinicians need to know. J Clin Endocrinol Metab 2011;96:53–8. https://doi.org/10.1210/jc.2010-2704.
[34] Mayor S. Public Health England recommends vitamin D supplements in autumn and winter. BMJ 2016;354:i4061. https://doi.org/10.1136/bmj.i4061.
[35] Holick MF, Binkley NC, Bischoff-Ferrari HA, Gordon CM, Hanley DA, Heaney RP, et al. Evaluation, treatment, and prevention of vitamin D deficiency: an Endocrine Society clinical practice guideline. J Clin Endocrinol Metab 2011;96:1911–30. https://doi.org/10.1210/jc.2011-0385.
[36] Kimball SM, Holick MF. Official recommendations for vitamin D through the life stages in developed countries. Eur J Clin Nutr 2020;74:1514–8. https://doi.org/10.1038/s41430-020-00706-3.

[37] Amrein K, Scherkl M, Hoffmann M, Neuwersch-Sommeregger S, Köstenberger M, Tmava Berisha A, et al. Vitamin D deficiency 2.0: an update on the current status worldwide. Eur J Clin Nutr 2020;74:1498–513. https://doi.org/10.1038/s41430-020-0558-y.

[38] Wacker M, Holick MF. Sunlight and Vitamin D: a global perspective for health. Dermatoendocrinol 2013;5:51–108. https://doi.org/10.4161/derm.24494.

[39] Engelsen O. The relationship between ultraviolet radiation exposure and vitamin D status. Nutrients 2010;2:482–95. https://doi.org/10.3390/nu2050482.

[40] Jablonski NG, Chaplin G. Epidermal pigmentation in the human lineage is an adaptation to ultraviolet radiation. J Hum Evol 2013;65:671–5. https://doi.org/10.1016/j.jhevol.2013.06.004.

[41] Fitzpatrick TB. The validity and practicality of sun-reactive skin types I through VI. Arch Dermatol 1988;124:869–71. https://doi.org/10.1001/archderm.124.6.869.

[42] Ozkan B. Nutritional rickets. J Clin Res Pediatr Endocrinol 2010;2:137–43. https://doi.org/10.4274/jcrpe.v2i4.137.

[43] Lu Z, Chen TC, Zhang A, Persons KS, Kohn N, Berkowitz R, et al. An evaluation of the vitamin D3 content in fish: is the vitamin D content adequate to satisfy the dietary requirement for vitamin D? J Steroid Biochem Mol Biol 2007;103:642–4. https://doi.org/10.1016/j.jsbmb.2006.12.010.

[44] Phillips KM, Ruggio DM, Horst RL, Minor B, Simon RR, Feeney MJ, et al. Vitamin D and sterol composition of 10 types of mushrooms from retail suppliers in the United States. J Agric Food Chem 2011;59:7841–53. https://doi.org/10.1021/jf104246z.

[45] Houghton LA, Vieth R. The case against ergocalciferol (vitamin D2) as a vitamin supplement. Am J Clin Nutr 2006;84:694–7. https://doi.org/10.1093/ajcn/84.4.694.

[46] Balachandar R, Pullakhandam R, Kulkarni B, Sachdev HS. Relative efficacy of vitamin D2 and vitamin D3 in improving vitamin D status: systematic review and meta-analysis. Nutrients 2021;13:3328. https://doi.org/10.3390/nu13103328.

[47] Maurya VK, Aggarwal M. Factors influencing the absorption of vitamin D in GIT: an overview. J Food Sci Technol 2017;54:3753–65. https://doi.org/10.1007/s13197-017-2840-0.

[48] Margulies SL, Kurian D, Elliott MS, Han Z. Vitamin D deficiency in patients with intestinal malabsorption syndromes–think in and outside the gut. J Dig Dis 2015;16:617–33. https://doi.org/10.1111/1751-2980.12283.

[49] Lu C, Zhou W, He X, Zhou X, Yu C. Vitamin D status and vitamin D receptor genotypes in celiac disease: a meta-analysis. Crit Rev Food Sci Nutr 2021;61:2098–106. https://doi.org/10.1080/10408398.2020.1772716.

[50] Bahrami A, Sadeghnia HR, Tabatabaeizadeh S-A, Bahrami-Taghanaki H, Behboodi N, Esmaeili H, et al. Genetic and epigenetic factors influencing vitamin D status. J Cell Physiol 2018;233:4033–43. https://doi.org/10.1002/jcp.26216.

[51] Jiang X, Kiel DP, Kraft P. The genetics of vitamin D. Bone 2019;126:59–77. https://doi.org/10.1016/j.bone.2018.10.006.

[52] Duan L, Xue Z, Ji H, Zhang D, Wang Y. Effects of CYP2R1 gene variants on vitamin D levels and status: a systematic review and meta-analysis. Gene 2018;678:361–9. https://doi.org/10.1016/j.gene.2018.08.056.

[53] Freitas AT, Calhau C, Antunes G, Araújo B, Bandeira M, Barreira S, et al. Vitamin D-related polymorphisms and vitamin D levels as risk biomarkers of COVID-19 disease severity. Sci Rep 2021;11:20837. https://doi.org/10.1038/s41598-021-99952-z.

[54] Desmarchelier C, Borel P, Goncalves A, Kopec R, Nowicki M, Morange S, et al. A combination of single-nucleotide polymorphisms is associated with interindividual variability in cholecalciferol bioavailability in healthy men. J Nutr 2016;146:2421–8. https://doi.org/10.3945/jn.116.237115.

[55] Fu L, Yun F, Oczak M, Wong BYL, Vieth R, Cole DEC. Common genetic variants of the vitamin D binding protein (DBP) predict differences in response of serum 25-hydroxyvitamin D [25(OH)D] to vitamin D supplementation. Clin Biochem 2009;42:1174–7. https://doi.org/10.1016/j.clinbiochem.2009.03.008.

[56] Jones KS, Assar S, Harnpanich D, Bouillon R, Lambrechts D, Prentice A, et al. 25(OH)D2 half-life is shorter than 25(OH)D3 half-life and is influenced by DBP concentration and genotype. J Clin Endocrinol Metab 2014;99:3373–81. https://doi.org/10.1210/jc.2014-1714.

[57] Iruzubieta P, Terán Á, Crespo J, Fábrega E. Vitamin D deficiency in chronic liver disease. World J Hepatol 2014;6:901–15. https://doi.org/10.4254/wjh.v6.i12.901.

[58] Mangin M, Sinha R, Fincher K. Inflammation and vitamin D: the infection connection. Inflamm Res 2014;63:803–19. https://doi.org/10.1007/s00011-014-0755-z.

[59] Waldron JL, Ashby HL, Cornes MP, Bechervaise J, Razavi C, Thomas OL, et al. Vitamin D: a negative acute phase reactant. J Clin Pathol 2013;66:620–2. https://doi.org/10.1136/jclinpath-2012-201301.

[60] Louw JA, Werbeck A, Louw ME, Kotze TJ, Cooper R, Labadarios D. Blood vitamin concentrations during the acute-phase response. Crit Care Med 1992;20:934–41. https://doi.org/10.1097/00003246-199207000-00007.

[61] Jeng L, Yamshchikov AV, Judd SE, Blumberg HM, Martin GS, Ziegler TR, et al. Alterations in vitamin D status and anti-microbial peptide levels in patients in the intensive care unit with sepsis. J Transl Med 2009;7:28. https://doi.org/10.1186/1479-5876-7-28.

[62] Vranić L, Mikolašević I, Milić S. Vitamin D deficiency: consequence or cause of obesity? Medicina (Kaunas) 2019;55:E541. https://doi.org/10.3390/medicina55090541.

[63] Hyppönen E, Boucher BJ. Adiposity, vitamin D requirements, and clinical implications for obesity-related metabolic abnormalities. Nutr Rev 2018;76:678–92. https://doi.org/10.1093/nutrit/nuy034.

[64] Drincic A, Fuller E, Heaney RP, Armas LAG. 25-Hydroxyvitamin D response to graded vitamin D_3 supplementation among obese adults. J Clin Endocrinol Metab 2013;98:4845–51. https://doi.org/10.1210/jc.2012-4103.

[65] Dai Q, Zhu X, Manson JE, Song Y, Li X, Franke AA, et al. Magnesium status and supplementation influence vitamin D status and metabolism: results from a randomized trial. Am J Clin Nutr 2018;108:1249–58. https://doi.org/10.1093/ajcn/nqy274.

[66] Gröber U, Kisters K. Influence of drugs on vitamin D and calcium metabolism. Dermatoendocrinol 2012;4:158–66. https://doi.org/10.4161/derm.20731.

[67] Dotan A, Mahroum N, Bogdanos DP, Shoenfeld Y. COVID-19 as an infectome paradigm of autoimmunity. J Allergy Clin Immunol 2022;149:63–4. https://doi.org/10.1016/j.jaci.2021.11.009.

[68] Contreras-Bolívar V, García-Fontana B, García-Fontana C, Muñoz-Torres M. Vitamin D and COVID-19: where are we now? Postgrad Med 2021:1–13. https://doi.org/10.1080/00325481.2021.2017647.

[69] Dotan A, Muller S, Kanduc D, David P, Halpert G, Shoenfeld Y. The SARS-CoV-2 as an instrumental trigger of autoimmunity. Autoimmun Rev 2021;20:102792. https://doi.org/10.1016/j.autrev.2021.102792.

[70] Tay MZ, Poh CM, Rénia L, MacAry PA, Ng LFP. The trinity of COVID-19: immunity, inflammation and intervention. Nat Rev Immunol 2020;20:363–74. https://doi.org/10.1038/s41577-020-0311-8.

[71] Halpert G, Shoenfeld Y. SARS-CoV-2, the autoimmune virus. Autoimmun Rev 2020;19:102695. https://doi.org/10.1016/j.autrev.2020.102695.

[72] Laird E, Rhodes J, Kenny RA. Vitamin D and inflammation: potential implications for severity of covid-19. Ir Med J 2020;113:81.

[73] Pugach IZ, Pugach S. Strong correlation between prevalence of severe vitamin D deficiency and population mortality rate from COVID-19 in Europe. Wien Klin Wochenschr 2021;133:403–5. https://doi.org/10.1007/s00508-021-01833-y.

[74] Kohlmeier M. Avoidance of vitamin D deficiency to slow the COVID-19 pandemic. BMJ Nutr Prev Health 2020;3:67–73. https://doi.org/10.1136/bmjnph-2020-000096.

[75] Merzon E, Tworowski D, Gorohovski A, Vinker S, Golan Cohen A, Green I, et al. Low plasma 25(OH) vitamin D level is associated with increased risk of COVID-19 infection: an Israeli population-based study. FEBS J 2020. https://doi.org/10.1111/febs.15495.

[76] De Smet D, De Smet K, Herroelen P, Gryspeerdt S, Martens GA. Serum 25(OH)D level on hospital admission associated with COVID-19 stage and mortality. Am J Clin Pathol 2020. https://doi.org/10.1093/ajcp/aqaa252. aqaa252.

[77] Martineau AR, Jolliffe DA, Hooper RL, Greenberg L, Aloia JF, Bergman P, et al. Vitamin D supplementation to prevent acute respiratory tract infections: systematic review and meta-analysis of individual participant data. BMJ 2017;356:i6583. https://doi.org/10.1136/bmj.i6583.

[78] Jolliffe DA, Camargo CA, Sluyter JD, Aglipay M, Aloia JF, Ganmaa D, et al. Vitamin D supplementation to prevent acute respiratory infections: a systematic review and meta-analysis of aggregate data from randomised controlled trials. Lancet Diabetes Endocrinol 2021;9:276–92. https://doi.org/10.1016/S2213-8587(21)00051-6.

[79] Van Belle TL, Gysemans C, Mathieu C. Vitamin D in autoimmune, infectious and allergic diseases: a vital player? Best Pract Res Clin Endocrinol Metabol 2011;25:617–32. https://doi.org/10.1016/j.beem.2011.04.009.

[80] Charoenngam N, Shirvani A, Holick MF. Vitamin D and its potential benefit for the COVID-19 pandemic. Endocr Pract 2021;27:484–93. https://doi.org/10.1016/j.eprac.2021.03.006.

[81] Teymoori-Rad M, Shokri F, Salimi V, Marashi SM. The interplay between vitamin D and viral infections. Rev Med Virol 2019;29:e2032. https://doi.org/10.1002/rmv.2032.

[82] Speeckaert MM, Delanghe JR. Association between low vitamin D and COVID-19: don't forget the vitamin D binding protein. Aging Clin Exp Res 2020;32:1207–8. https://doi.org/10.1007/s40520-020-01607-y.

[83] Speeckaert MM, Speeckaert R, Delanghe JR. Vitamin D sufficiency and COVID-19: is vitamin D binding protein (and its polymorphism) the missing link? Endocr Pract 2021;27:645. https://doi.org/10.1016/j.eprac.2021.03.011.

[84] Israel A, Cicurel A, Feldhamer I, Stern F, Dror Y, Giveon SM, et al. Vitamin D deficiency is associated with higher risks for SARS-CoV-2 infection and COVID-19 severity: a retrospective case–control study. Intern Emerg Med 2022:1–11. https://doi.org/10.1007/s11739-021-02902-w.

[85] Dissanayake HA, de Silva NL, Sumanatilleke M, de Silva SDN, Gamage KKK, Dematapitiya C, et al. Prognostic and therapeutic role of vitamin D in COVID-19: systematic review and meta-analysis. J Clin Endocrinol Metab 2021. https://doi.org/10.1210/clinem/dgab892. dgab892.

[86] Hastie CE, Mackay DF, Ho F, Celis-Morales CA, Katikireddi SV, Niedzwiedz CL, et al. Vitamin D concentrations and COVID-19 infection in UK Biobank. Diabetes Metabol Syndr 2020;14:561–5. https://doi.org/10.1016/j.dsx.2020.04.050.

[87] Hernández JL, Nan D, Fernandez-Ayala M, García-Unzueta M, Hernández-Hernández MA, López-Hoyos M, et al. Vitamin D status in hospitalized patients with SARS-CoV-2 infection. J Clin Endocrinol Metab 2020. https://doi.org/10.1210/clinem/dgaa733. dgaa733.

[88] Diaz-Curiel M, Cabello A, Arboiro-Pinel R, Mansur JL, Heili-Frades S, Mahillo-Fernandez I, et al. The relationship between 25(OH) vitamin D levels and COVID-19 onset and disease course in Spanish patients. J Steroid Biochem Mol Biol 2021;212:105928. https://doi.org/10.1016/j.jsbmb.2021.105928.

[89] Xu J, Yang J, Chen J, Luo Q, Zhang Q, Zhang H. Vitamin D alleviates lipopolysaccharide-induced acute lung injury via regulation of the renin-angiotensin system. Mol Med Rep 2017;16:7432–8. https://doi.org/10.3892/mmr.2017.7546.

[90] Bouillon R, Quesada-Gomez JM. Vitamin D endocrine system and COVID-19. JBMR Plus 2021;5:e10576. https://doi.org/10.1002/jbm4.10576.

[91] Malkova A, Kudlay D, Kudryavtsev I, Starshinova A, Yablonskiy P, Shoenfeld Y. Immunogenetic predictors of severe COVID-19. Vaccines (Basel) 2021;9:211. https://doi.org/10.3390/vaccines9030211.

[92] Butler AE, Moin ASM, Sathyapalan T, Atkin SL. Vitamin D association with the renin angiotensin system in polycystic ovary syndrome. J Steroid Biochem Mol Biol 2021;214:105965. https://doi.org/10.1016/j.jsbmb.2021.105965.

[93] Ilie PC, Stefanescu S, Smith L. The role of vitamin D in the prevention of coronavirus disease 2019 infection and mortality. Aging Clin Exp Res 2020;32:1195–8. https://doi.org/10.1007/s40520-020-01570-8.

[94] Manios Y, Moschonis G, Lambrinou C-P, Tsoutsoulopoulou K, Binou P, Karachaliou A, et al. A systematic review of vitamin D status in southern European countries. Eur J Nutr 2018;57:2001–36. https://doi.org/10.1007/s00394-017-1564-2.

[95] Munshi R, Hussein MH, Toraih EA, Elshazli RM, Jardak C, Sultana N, et al. Vitamin D insufficiency as a potential culprit in critical COVID-19 patients. J Med Virol 2021;93:733–40. https://doi.org/10.1002/jmv.26360.

[96] Eden T, McAuliffe S, Crocombe D, Neville J, Ray S. Nutritional parameters and outcomes in patients admitted to intensive care with COVID-19: a retrospective single-centre service evaluation. BMJ Nutr Prev Health 2021;4:416–24. https://doi.org/10.1136/bmjnph-2021-000270.

[97] Carpagnano GE, Di Lecce V, Quaranta VN, Zito A, Buonamico E, Capozza E, et al. Vitamin D deficiency as a predictor of poor prognosis in patients with acute respiratory failure due to COVID-19. J Endocrinol Invest 2021;44:765–71. https://doi.org/10.1007/s40618-020-01370-x.

[98] Chiodini I, Gatti D, Soranna D, Merlotti D, Mingiano C, Fassio A, et al. Vitamin D status and SARS-CoV-2 infection and COVID-19 clinical outcomes. Front Public Health 2021;9:736665. https://doi.org/10.3389/fpubh.2021.736665.

[99] Seal KH, Bertenthal D, Carey E, Grunfeld C, Bikle DD, Lu CM. Association of vitamin D status and COVID-19-related hospitalization and mortality. J Gen Intern Med 2022. https://doi.org/10.1007/s11606-021-07170-0.

[100] Lips P, Cashman KD, Lamberg-Allardt C, Bischoff-Ferrari HA, Obermayer-Pietsch B, Bianchi ML, et al. Current vitamin D status in European and Middle East countries and strategies to prevent vitamin D deficiency: a position statement of the European Calcified Tissue Society. Eur J Endocrinol 2019;180:P23–54. https://doi.org/10.1530/EJE-18-0736.
[101] Apaydin T, Polat H, Dincer Yazan C, Ilgin C, Elbasan O, Dashdamirova S, et al. Effects of vitamin D receptor gene polymorphisms on the prognosis of COVID-19. Clin Endocrinol (Oxf) 2021. https://doi.org/10.1111/cen.14664.
[102] Carod-Artal FJ. [Post-COVID-19 syndrome: epidemiology, diagnostic criteria and pathogenic mechanisms involved]. Rev Neurol 2021;72:384–96. https://doi.org/10.33588/rn.7211.2021230.
[103] Alwan NA. Track COVID-19 sickness, not just positive tests and deaths. Nature 2020;584:170. https://doi.org/10.1038/d41586-020-02335-z.
[104] Hayes LD, Ingram J, Sculthorpe NF. More than 100 persistent symptoms of SARS-CoV-2 (long COVID): a scoping review. Front Med (Lausanne) 2021;8:750378. https://doi.org/10.3389/fmed.2021.750378.
[105] Sapkota HR, Nune A. Long COVID from rheumatology perspective — a narrative review. Clin Rheumatol 2021:1–12. https://doi.org/10.1007/s10067-021-06001-1.
[106] Patrucco F, Zeppegno P, Baricich A, Gramaglia CM, Balbo PE, Falaschi Z, et al. Long-lasting consequences of Coronavirus disease 19 pneumonia: a systematic review. Minerva Med 2021. https://doi.org/10.23736/S0026-4806.21.07594-7.
[107] Townsend L, Dyer AH, Jones K, Dunne J, Mooney A, Gaffney F, et al. Persistent fatigue following SARS-CoV-2 infection is common and independent of severity of initial infection. PLoS One 2020;15:e0240784. https://doi.org/10.1371/journal.pone.0240784.
[108] Anaya J-M, Rojas M, Salinas ML, Rodríguez Y, Roa G, Lozano M, et al. Post-COVID syndrome. A case series and comprehensive review. Autoimmun Rev 2021;20:102947. https://doi.org/10.1016/j.autrev.2021.102947.
[109] Malkova A, Kudryavtsev I, Starshinova A, Kudlay D, Zinchenko Y, Glushkova A, et al. Post COVID-19 syndrome in patients with asymptomatic/mild form. Pathogens 2021;10:1408. https://doi.org/10.3390/pathogens10111408.
[110] Ayoubkhani D, Khunti K, Nafilyan V, Maddox T, Humberstone B, Diamond I, et al. Post-covid syndrome in individuals admitted to hospital with covid-19: retrospective cohort study. BMJ 2021;372:n693. https://doi.org/10.1136/bmj.n693.
[111] Huang C, Huang L, Wang Y, Li X, Ren L, Gu X, et al. 6-month consequences of COVID-19 in patients discharged from hospital: a cohort study. Lancet 2021;397:220–32. https://doi.org/10.1016/S0140-6736(20)32656-8.
[112] Charfeddine S, Ibn Hadj Amor H, Jdidi J, Torjmen S, Kraiem S, Hammami R, et al. Long COVID 19 syndrome: is it related to microcirculation and endothelial dysfunction? Insights from TUN-EndCOV study. Front Cardiovasc Med 2021;8:745758. https://doi.org/10.3389/fcvm.2021.745758.
[113] Dotan A, Shoenfeld Y. Post-COVID syndrome: the aftershock of SARS-CoV-2. Int J Infect Dis 2022;114:233–5. https://doi.org/10.1016/j.ijid.2021.11.020.
[114] Amin-Chowdhury Z, Ladhani SN. Causation or confounding: why controls are critical for characterizing long COVID. Nat Med 2021;27:1129–30. https://doi.org/10.1038/s41591-021-01402-w.
[115] Jennings G, Monaghan A, Xue F, Mockler D, Romero-Ortuño R. A systematic review of persistent symptoms and residual abnormal functioning following acute COVID-19: ongoing symptomatic phase vs. Post-COVID-19 syndrome. J Clin Med 2021;10:5913. https://doi.org/10.3390/jcm10245913.
[116] Kerget B, Çelik E, Kerget F, Aksakal A, Uçar EY, Araz Ö, et al. Evaluation of 3-month follow-up of patients with post-acute COVID-19 syndrome. J Med Virol 2022. https://doi.org/10.1002/jmv.27579.
[117] Kazemi A, Mohammadi V, Aghababaee SK, Golzarand M, Clark CCT, Babajafari S. Association of vitamin D status with SARS-CoV-2 infection or COVID-19 severity: a systematic review and meta-analysis. Adv Nutr 2021;12:1636–58. https://doi.org/10.1093/advances/nmab012.
[118] AlSafar H, Grant WB, Hijazi R, Uddin M, Alkaabi N, Tay G, et al. COVID-19 disease severity and death in relation to vitamin D status among SARS-CoV-2-positive UAE residents. Nutrients 2021;13:1714. https://doi.org/10.3390/nu13051714.
[119] Radujkovic A, Hippchen T, Tiwari-Heckler S, Dreher S, Boxberger M, Merle U. Vitamin D deficiency and outcome of COVID-19 patients. Nutrients 2020;12:2757. https://doi.org/10.3390/nu12092757.

[120] Murai IH, Fernandes AL, Sales LP, Pinto AJ, Goessler KF, Duran CSC, et al. Effect of a single high dose of vitamin D3 on hospital length of stay in patients with moderate to severe COVID-19. JAMA 2021;325:1–9. https://doi.org/10.1001/jama.2020.26848.

[121] Fernandes AL, Murai IH, Reis BZ, Sales LP, Santos MD, Pinto AJ, et al. Effect of a single high dose of Vitamin D3 on cytokines, chemokines and growth factor in patients with moderate to severe COVID-19. Am J Clin Nutr 2022:nqab426. https://doi.org/10.1093/ajcn/nqab426.

[122] Rastogi A, Bhansali A, Khare N, Suri V, Yaddanapudi N, Sachdeva N, et al. Short term, high-dose vitamin D supplementation for COVID-19 disease: a randomised, placebo-controlled, study (SHADE study). Postgrad Med J 2020. https://doi.org/10.1136/postgradmedj-2020-139065. postgradmedj-2020-139065.

[123] Entrenas Castillo M, Entrenas Costa LM, Vaquero Barrios JM, Alcalá Díaz JF, López Miranda J, Bouillon R, et al. Effect of calcifediol treatment and best available therapy versus best available therapy on intensive care unit admission and mortality among patients hospitalized for COVID-19: a pilot randomized clinical study. J Steroid Biochem Mol Biol 2020;203:105751. https://doi.org/10.1016/j.jsbmb.2020.105751.

[124] Ling SF, Broad E, Murphy R, Pappachan JM, Pardesi-Newton S, Kong M-F, et al. High-dose cholecalciferol booster therapy is associated with a reduced risk of mortality in patients with COVID-19: a cross-sectional multi-centre observational study. Nutrients 2020;12:3799. https://doi.org/10.3390/nu12123799.

[125] Caballero-García A, Pérez-Valdecantos D, Guallar P, Caballero-Castillo A, Roche E, Noriega DC, et al. Effect of vitamin D supplementation on muscle status in old patients recovering from COVID-19 infection. Medicina (Kaunas) 2021;57:1079. https://doi.org/10.3390/medicina57101079.

[126] Annweiler C, Beaudenon M, Simon R, Guenet M, Otekpo M, Célarier T, et al. Vitamin D supplementation prior to or during COVID-19 associated with better 3-month survival in geriatric patients: extension phase of the GERIA-COVID study. J Steroid Biochem Mol Biol 2021;213:105958. https://doi.org/10.1016/j.jsbmb.2021.105958.

[127] Murai IH, Fernandes AL, Antonangelo L, Gualano B, Pereira RMR. Effect of a single high-dose vitamin D3 on the length of hospital stay of severely 25-hydroxyvitamin D-deficient patients with COVID-19. Clinics (Sao Paulo) 2021;76:e3549. https://doi.org/10.6061/clinics/2021/e3549.

[128] Maghbooli Z, Sahraian MA, Jamalimoghadamsiahkali S, Asadi A, Zarei A, Zendehdel A, et al. Treatment with 25-hydroxyvitamin D3 (calcifediol) is associated with a reduction in the blood neutrophil-to-lymphocyte ratio marker of disease severity in hospitalized patients with COVID-19: a pilot multicenter, randomized, placebo-controlled, double-blinded clinical trial. Endocr Pract 2021;27:1242–51. https://doi.org/10.1016/j.eprac.2021.09.016.

[129] Sabico S, Enani MA, Sheshah E, Aljohani NJ, Aldisi DA, Alotaibi NH, et al. Effects of a 2-week 5000 IU versus 1000 IU vitamin D3 supplementation on recovery of symptoms in patients with mild to moderate covid-19: a randomized clinical trial. Nutrients 2021;13:2170. https://doi.org/10.3390/nu13072170.

[130] Elamir YM, Amir H, Lim S, Rana YP, Lopez CG, Feliciano NV, et al. A randomized pilot study using calcitriol in hospitalized COVID-19 patients. Bone 2022;154:116175. https://doi.org/10.1016/j.bone.2021.116175.

[131] Alcala-Diaz JF, Limia-Perez L, Gomez-Huelgas R, Martin-Escalante MD, Cortes-Rodriguez B, Zambrana-Garcia JL, et al. Calcifediol treatment and hospital mortality due to COVID-19: a cohort study. Nutrients 2021;13:1760. https://doi.org/10.3390/nu13061760.

[132] Gönen MS, Alaylıoğlu M, Durcan E, Özdemir Y, Sahin S, Konukoğlu D, et al. Rapid and effective vitamin D supplementation may present better clinical outcomes in COVID-19 (SARS-CoV-2) patients by altering serum INOS1, IL1B, IFNg, cathelicidin-LL37, and ICAM1. Nutrients 2021;13:4047. https://doi.org/10.3390/nu13114047.

[133] Lai Y-J, Chang H-S, Yang Y-P, Lin T-W, Lai W-Y, Lin Y-Y, et al. The role of micronutrient and immunomodulation effect in the vaccine era of COVID-19. J Chin Med Assoc 2021;84:821–6. https://doi.org/10.1097/JCMA.0000000000000587.

[134] Morales JS, Valenzuela PL, Castillo-García A, Butragueño J, Jiménez-Pavón D, Carrera-Bastos P, et al. The exposome and immune health in times of the COVID-19 pandemic. Nutrients 2021;14:24. https://doi.org/10.3390/nu14010024.

[135] The role of vitamin D as a potential adjuvant for COVID-19 vaccines. Eur Rev. 2021. https://www.europeanreview.org/article/26637. Accessed January 9, 2022.

[136] Calder PC. Nutrition and immunity: lessons for COVID-19. Eur J Clin Nutr 2021;75:1309–18. https://doi.org/10.1038/s41430-021-00949-8.

[137] Rayman MP, Calder PC. Optimising COVID-19 vaccine efficacy by ensuring nutritional adequacy. Br J Nutr 2021;126:1919–20. https://doi.org/10.1017/S0007114521000386.

[138] Mercola J, Grant WB, Wagner CL. Evidence regarding vitamin D and risk of COVID-19 and its severity. Nutrients 2020;12:3361. https://doi.org/10.3390/nu12113361.

[139] Mardani R, Alamdary A, Mousavi Nasab SD, Gholami R, Ahmadi N, Gholami A. Association of vitamin D with the modulation of the disease severity in COVID-19. Virus Res 2020;289:198148. https://doi.org/10.1016/j.virusres.2020.198148.

[140] Chiu S-K, Tsai K-W, Wu C-C, Zheng C-M, Yang C-H, Hu W-C, et al. Putative role of vitamin D for COVID-19 vaccination. Int J Mol Sci 2021;22:8988. https://doi.org/10.3390/ijms22168988.

[141] Minton K. Vitamin D shuts down T cell-mediated inflammation. Nat Rev Immunol 2022;22:1. https://doi.org/10.1038/s41577-021-00663-3.

[142] Kolls JK, Garry RF. Role of the T cell vitamin D receptor in severe COVID-19. Nat Immunol 2022;23:5–6. https://doi.org/10.1038/s41590-021-01098-7.

[143] Chillon TS, Demircan K, Heller RA, Hirschbil-Bremer IM, Diegmann J, Bachmann M, et al. Relationship between vitamin D status and antibody response to COVID-19 mRNA vaccination in healthy adults. Biomedicines 2021;9:1714. https://doi.org/10.3390/biomedicines9111714.

[144] Palacios C, Gonzalez L. Is vitamin D deficiency a major global public health problem? J Steroid Biochem Mol Biol 2014;144 Pt A:138–45. https://doi.org/10.1016/j.jsbmb.2013.11.003.

[145] Kara M, Ekiz T, Ricci V, Kara Ö, Chang K-V, Özçakar L. "Scientific Strabismus" or two related pandemics: coronavirus disease and vitamin D deficiency. Br J Nutr 2020;124:736–41. https://doi.org/10.1017/S0007114520001749.

[146] Ulivieri FM, Banfi G, Camozzi V, Colao A, Formenti AM, Frara S, et al. Vitamin D in the Covid-19 era: a review with recommendations from a G.I.O.S.E.G. expert panel. Endocrine 2021;72:597–603. https://doi.org/10.1007/s12020-021-02749-3.

[147] Tebben PJ, Singh RJ, Kumar R. Vitamin D-mediated hypercalcemia: mechanisms, diagnosis, and treatment. Endocr Rev 2016;37:521–47. https://doi.org/10.1210/er.2016-1070.

[148] Rusińska A, Płudowski P, Walczak M, Borszewska-Kornacka MK, Bossowski A, Chlebna-Sokół D, et al. Vitamin D supplementation guidelines for general population and groups at risk of vitamin D deficiency in Poland-recommendations of the polish society of pediatric endocrinology and diabetes and the expert panel with participation of national specialist consultants and representatives of scientific societies-2018 update. Front Endocrinol (Lausanne) 2018;9:246. https://doi.org/10.3389/fendo.2018.00246.

[149] Vaughan M, Trott M, Sapkota R, Premi G, Roberts J, Ubhi J, et al. Changes in 25-hydroxyvitamin D levels post-vitamin D supplementation in people of Black and Asian ethnicities and its implications during COVID-19 pandemic: a systematic review. J Hum Nutr Diet 2021. https://doi.org/10.1111/jhn.12949.

[150] Quesada-Gomez JM, Bouillon R. Is calcifediol better than cholecalciferol for vitamin D supplementation? Osteoporos Int 2018;29:1697–711. https://doi.org/10.1007/s00198-018-4520-y.

[151] Sosa Henríquez M, Gómez de Tejada Romero MJ. Cholecalciferol or calcifediol in the management of vitamin D deficiency. Nutrients 2020;12:E1617. https://doi.org/10.3390/nu12061617.

CHAPTER

36

Side effects of the COVID-19 vaccines

Olga Vera-Lastra[1,2], Abihai Lucas Hernández[1], Alberto Ordinola Navarro[1,2,3] and Luis J. Jara[4]

[1]Internal Medicine Department, Hospital de Especialidades "Dr. Antonio Fraga Mouret" Centro Médico Nacional La Raza, Instituto Mexicano del Seguro Social, México City, México; [2]Division of Postgraduate Studies, Faculty of Medicine, Universidad Nacional Autónoma de México, México City, México; [3]Infectious Disease Department, Instituto Nacional de Ciencias Médicas y Nutrición Salvador Zubirán, México City, México; [4]Rheumatology Division, Instituto Nacional de Rehabilitación "Luis Guillermo Ibarra Ibarra", México City, México

Introduction

The ability to eradicate deadly diseases and decrease the mortality of others makes vaccines one of the most important discoveries of the last century [1]. Despite already having effective vaccines, scientific advances continue developing new antigens capable of producing more significant immune responses to achieve stronger immunity [2].

The COVID-19 pandemic has been the biggest catastrophe in recent years; its mortality has prompted researchers to accelerate an established development of vaccines in order to reduce the high mortality; without a doubt, the knowledge of previous SARS coronavirus has helped the speed of vaccine development for prompt distribution [3,4].

There have always been different varieties of vectors used in the vaccines; however, new genetically engineered RNA or DNA technology makes it possible to avoid adjuvants (part of the vaccine capable of making a stronger immune response). However, substances to maintain the stability of the vaccine have been related to adverse reactions from local to systemic affection, with favorable results in most cases [5,6].

Vaccination is the only strategy that can help us reduce the catastrophic pandemic [7]. Therefore, it is strongly suggested to be vaccinated on the appropriate dates and follow the government indications for applications and booster doses. This chapter will analyze the primary anti-COVID vaccines and their systemic adverse effects after administration.

Autoimmunity, COVID-19, Post-COVID19 syndrome and COVID-19 vaccination
https://doi.org/10.1016/B978-0-443-18566-3.00008-6

Vaccines

Vaccines have been one of the most significant advances of modern medicine and represent the most cost-effective life-saving strategy; the application has meant that diseases with high mortality have been eradicated. In addition to that, severe diseases have significantly reduced mortality [8].

Edward Jenner was among the first physician to use cowpox material to create immunity to smallpox. Jenner's work represented the first scientific attempt to control an infectious disease by deliberate vaccination. However, before Jenner, some people worked for variolation, such as Benjamin Jesty (1737–1816). The discovery and promotion of vaccination enabled the eradication of smallpox as one of the most important advances in the modern era [9].

In general, exposing some virus particles such as a DNA vector, live attenuated vaccines, or inactivated vaccines makes the subject an early exposure to create an autoimmune response. However, to increase this, adjuvants' use can help trigger a more powerful immune reaction [10].

Although this practice seems safe, The Food and Drug Administration (FDA) has an extensive review process to be realized before applications go to the community [11,12]. First, preclinical studies are performed. Subsequently, the company that wishes to develop a vaccine needs to register the investigation to the FDA, to the called Investigational New Drug Application (IND) describing the vaccine, manufactured and quality control tests. Mice are animals that have been studied the must due to the heterogeneity in terms of age and genetic diversity with humans. Subsequently, the clinical trials in general form, works like this (Fig. 36.1).

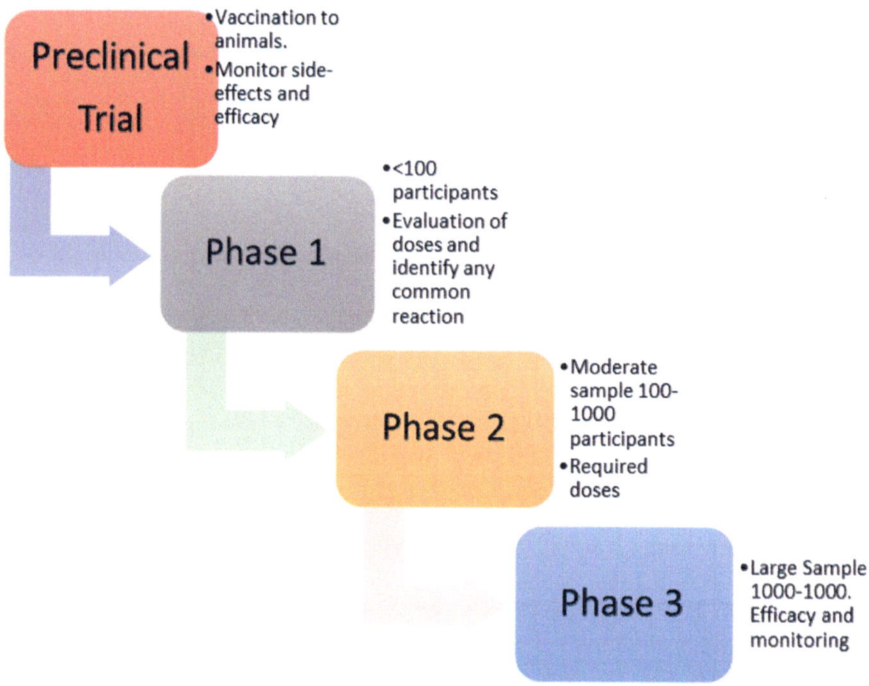

FIGURE 36.1 Showing the phases of the vaccination process.

Phase 1: 20–100 volunteers and just for a few months. It evaluates basic safety and identifies any common reactions.

Phase 2: And extensive trial with 100 participants that last for months to 2 years. Evaluating safety, efficacy, and required doses for the objectives.

Phase 3: Involve thousands of volunteers 1000–10,000, and finalize evaluating effectiveness and safety for the following years [11,12].

At the end of the trials, FDA reviews the safety and effectiveness, and after obtaining a Biologic License Application (BLA), the application could continue to the general population. Nevertheless, in addition to that, the Advisory Committee on Immunization Practices (ACIP) (A group of medical experts), develops recommendations to the Centers for Disease Control and Prevention (CDC) continues the following of the distribution [13].

Remarkably, due to the COVID-19 pandemic, this practice had to be carried out in an accelerated manner to obtain available vaccines and slow down a bit what has been the largest pandemic in recent years. The conclusion of the phases was realized by the Conditional Marketing Authorization and gave early authorization due to the pandemic [13,14].

Vaccines: mechanism of the immune response

On the first exposure to antigen, the immune system generates a primary response (innate response); besides, the first antibodies' production has been detected by the fourth and fifth days [15].

The response is as follows: The subject creates IgM antibodies with low affinity for antigen, but within several days, some B cells help to create IgG, IgA, or IgE antibodies. This change of antibodies production is possible due to helper T cells.

When further exposure to the antigen, the B cells are available to create an antibody response within 1–2 days. IgG responses are higher, stronger and substantial than IgM. Therefore, applying a vaccine would create an IgM response that activates Helpers T cells to create IgG with long substantial antibodies; after a booster, there is an activation of IgM, but since it has been previous exposure to the antigen in the first 2 days, there is an IgG response [16].

There are different pattern recognition receptors (PRR) essential in this process;

Toll-like receptors (TLRs) can regulate the persistence of germinal memory cells' differentiations pathway when triggered. TLRs play an essential role in these activations, such as activating dendritic cells (DC) and plasmacytoid and myeloid DC. Besides the activation of multiples TLRs, seems redundant, there is a synergistic activation with the multiple of these [1,9]. There is also a production of mixed TH1, Th2, and multiple MyD 88-dependent signaling pathways [8,17]. Thus, immunity's magnitude quality and persistence are hallmark issues to address.

Vaccines: molecular structure

The vaccines are mainly divided into two groups: first, a group of live attenuated vaccines that, in summary, is the weakened version of the pathogens, mimicking the protective immunity of people with the previous infection. The immunity of these vaccines would last for decades. Moreover, the latter group is the inactivated vaccines with a part of the virus that stimulates the exposure to create an immune response. However, most of these needs adjuvants to create a stronger immune response [8,11,12] (Table 36.1).

As mentioned, some vaccines include an adjuvant to make a more substantial and lasting immune response; the main adjuvants are alum, ASO4 (A substance composed of monophosphoryl Lipid A, adsorbed to alum), and Oil-in-water emulsions (MF59, AS03) [8,14].

With the adjuvant, the composition of the vaccine would look as follows: an active ingredient (the small amount of a harmless form of bacteria or virus), the adjuvant, water, preservatives, and stabilizers that maintain the vaccine quality, safe storage, and prevent contamination; for example, sorbitol and residual traces, and substances used during vaccine manufacture, measured as parts per million or billion in the final vaccine, for example, formaldehyde.

The use of an adjuvant, such as alum, can realize a gel-like substance and induce a TH2 biased response independently of TLRs with activations of the NLRP3, inflammasome, and direct activation on IL-4- producing Gr-1+ cells, essential for clonal expansion and production of B cells antibodies.

MF59 (squalane-based) and AS03 can trigger CD11b + blood cells and induce genes encoding cytokines, cytokine receptors, and adhesion molecules [10]. AS04 can induce TH1, responses and MyD88 and TRIF, enhancing proinflammatory cytokines [8,11,12]. Besides the main objective of creating neutralizing antibodies, the innate immune response is enhanced by those mechanisms, mainly by the T cell. Even though the titers of antibodies may diminish over time, the persistence of plasma cell responses may last over the years, and there would be an early activation due to all previous mechanisms.

Types of vaccines anti-COVID-19

SARS CoV-2 has been the greatest pandemic in the last years; because of that, the development of vaccines was realized in record time. Previous vaccines took 8–10 years before their use in humans. However, COVID vaccines follow-up and validation steps were developed in 8–10 months. The development of the vaccines was based on the spike glycoprotein

TABLE 36.1 Types of vaccines.

Type of vaccine	Examples
Attenuated vaccines	Smallpox, yellow fever, measles, mumps, rubella, chickenpox.
Inactive virus	Rabia, Hepatitis A
Subunit vaccines	Hepatitis B
Toxoid inactivated toxins	Diphtheria and tetanus
Carbohydrate vaccines	Pneumococcus
Conjugated vaccines	Meningococcus, hempophilus influenzae type B

as an antigen. It was readily accessible by antibodies and immunological cells [11]. The SARS CoV-2 comprises 25–28 proteins, but the spike protein shows three copies of the same protein [19,20]. There are many vaccinations platforms, but in this chapter, we will center on the most common: 1. mRNA vaccines; were developed by Pfizer-BioNTech and Moderna, utilize genetically engineered RNA or DNA to generate a protein that creates an immune response. Based on spike glycoprotein, 2. Viral Vector: Theses were developed by Astra-Zeneca, Johnson and Johnson, Reithera, and Sputnik. Viral vectors use a genetically engineered virus that creates an immune response that cannot cause the disease. 3. Inactivate vaccines. SINOVAC developed vaccines with the inactivated virus via Vero cells. 4. Protein subunits vaccines. Novavax developed these. Based on fragments of protein shells that mimic de SARS CoV-2 and create an immune response [13,14].

Besides, the mRNA vaccines do not use one of the common adjuvants; the vaccines include a lipid particle that may be responsible for an autoimmune response.

Table 36.2 shows the main characteristic of COVID-19 vaccines.

Adjuvants

Vaccines applied to the general population contain the necessary products to initiate immunogenic activity and produce antibodies that protect against diseases in the future. In order to create a more efficient immune response, certain elements have been added to vaccines; these are called "adjuvants," which comes from the Latin word "*adjuvare*," which means help. Most of these adjuvants are empirically added to vaccines without knowing the exact mechanisms that lead to the cellular immune response and the creation of

TABLE 36.2 Characteristics of the most common vaccines in COVID-19.

Vaccines	Method	Antigen	Doses	Efficacy for disease
Pfizer/BioNTech	mRNA	Spike glycoprotein	Two doses 21 days apart	95%
Moderna	mRNA	Spyke glycoprotein	Two doses 28 days apart	94%
Astra Zeneca	Adenovirus	Spyke glycoprotein	Two doses 12 weeks apart	70%
Johnson and Johnson	Adenovirus	Spyke glycoprotein	One dose	72%
NOVAVAX	Protein subunit	Prefusion 5 protein	Two doses 4–12 weeks apart	89.70%
CARAVAN	Modified mRNA	Length 5 protein	Two doses 28 days apart	47%
SINOVAC	Inactivated virus	Inactivated from vero-cells	Two doses, 14 days apart	65%
SPUTNIK	Two adenovirus	Gene spike glycoprotein	Two doses, 21 days apart	91.60%

antibodies. It should be clarified that each time a new vaccine is released on the market, both are considered one, so there is no regulation on adjuvants [21].

The adjuvants increase the duration of contact between the antigen and the immune system after applying the vaccine; therefore, the immunogenic activity is more significant [22]. One of the promising mechanisms that explain how adjuvants initiate and enhance the post-vaccine immune response is through the innate immune system, specifically the Pathogen-Associated Molecular Pattern (PAMP). These PAMPs are only found in pathogens such as viruses and bacteria, and when PAMP binds to a Pathogen Recognition Receptor (PRR) such as the Toll-like-receptor (TLR), the activation of specific immune response mechanisms initiates. TLRs are expressed in the structure of DCs and other hematolymphoid cells; therefore, by being directly related to a specific cell type, then the immune response can be activated in a specific way by initiating the immunological cascade with TLRs, which is one the interests nowadays for the manufacturing of new vaccines [21].

Multiple compounds have been used as adjuvants for the different vaccines currently available worldwide. However, some of the main adjuvants that have been used are aluminum salts such as aluminum potassium sulfate (AlK (SO4) 2) and (aluminum potassium phosphate (KAl (HPO4) 2), acting as a depot for antigens (adsorbs the antigens) and activating the immune response by the production of antibodies, on the other hand, it acts as an irritant so that the immune response increases locally recruiting leukocytes. Other adjuvants that have been used are liposomes, immune-stimulating complexes, emulsions, cytokines, and recently toll-receptor agonists have been investigated [21,22].

Since a foreign body is being introduced into the host, there is always a risk of initiating an adverse reaction. According to the World Health Organization (WHO) manual, the main adverse reactions that adjuvants have described are subcutaneous nodules, sterile abscesses, granulomatous inflammation, and contact hypersensitivity. These reactions occur mainly in those patients whose technique was not adequate when applying the vaccine since it must be intramuscular to minimize the risk of reactions [22].

Autoimmune/inflammatory syndrome (ASIA) induced by vaccines

Autoimmune/inflammatory syndrome was described in 2011 by Yehuda Shoenfeld et al. it composed a new syndrome in which four conditions were included and had the same trigger, an adjuvant. Nowadays, the Autoimmune/auto-inflammatory Syndrome (ASIA) encompasses the postvaccination phenomena, macrophagic myofasciitis syndrome (MMF), Gulf War syndrome (GWS), siliconosis, later other entities were added such as mineral oil fillers, and the sick building syndrome. In the case of postvaccination phenomena, the pathophysiology has been explained due to the vaccine's components such as aluminum (adjuvant), in which large amounts of uric acid are released in the form of monosodium urate crystals, altering the function of lysosomes after being phagocytosed by cells, cathepsin B is released and activates the system of intracellular inflammasome Nalp3 and caspase-1, secreting interleukins (1b) [18,33]. Other mechanisms related to vaccination that have been described are mediation by antigens that trigger an immunological cascade such as polyclonal activation of B cells, molecular mimicry, epitope spread, HLA expression, Toll-like receptors (TLR): as well as the release of inflammatory cytokines, modification of surface antigens, induction of new antigens, translocation of antigens, effects on virus-induced antibodies, effects on regulatory immune cells, among others [23,24]. These effects occur in very few cases of patients that receive an immunization; therefore, relating the two events is difficult since symptoms may be present from the first days until weeks or months. For vaccines, these effects have been described to begin from day two to 5 years after exposure. The postvaccination phenomena have been explained by one of the components of vaccines, aluminum, however, but it may also be secondary to other components of vaccines as bovine serum, bacteria, or stabilizers found in the vaccine (egg protein). It is possible to find different connective tissue diseases associated with the application of vaccines.

Among the vaccines associated with autoimmune disease are those against Hepatitis A and B, meningococcus, influenza, among others. Vasculitis after influenza vaccination has been described, such as microscopic polyangiitis, leukocytoclastic vasculitis, giant cell arteritis, Henoch-Scholein purpura, and polyarteritis nodosa. The vaccine against the human papillomavirus has been related to the onset of autoimmune diseases, including systemic lupus erythematosus (SLE), systemic sclerosis, Sjogren's syndrome, among others. The presentation of rheumatoid arthritis after applying vaccines such as hepatitis B and HPV has also been described. The most common diseases reported in the greatest quantity are neurological, mainly, Guillain–Barré Syndrome (during the AH1N1 pandemic in 2009), narcolepsy, acute disseminated encephalomyelitis, and transverse myelitis. Other vaccines such as polio and pertussis have been associated with Crohn's disease and ulcerative colitis [25,26]. Postvaccination autoimmune diseases are rare, but it should not be underestimated, and therefore the production of better biotechnology compounds that act as adjuvants with a better efficacy and safety profile should be promoted. It is essential to mention that the benefits of vaccines outweigh the risk of adverse effects.

These examples show that the effects of vaccination could be in different organs and with different vaccines; however, in all patients, a predisposing genetic factor should be suspected.

Covid-19 vaccination

As of November 16' 2021, 7.54 billion doses of COVID-19 vaccines have been administered, representing 52.2% of the world population [27]. With the advent of the vaccine, deaths from COVID-19 have decreased dramatically as vaccination progresses, so it is undeniable that the benefit of vaccines has been evident during this pandemic. However, as we mentioned before, the side effects of vaccines have always been present, and the COVID-19 vaccine is no exception.

Watad et al. carried out a study from December 2020 to February 2021 where 27 subjects were found with an autoimmune or auto-inflammatory disease after the COVID-19 vaccine. The average onset of symptoms was 4 days after vaccination with a range of one- to 25 days. Of the 27 cases studied, 23 could not explain the underlying disease or some other comorbidity. Therefore, the outcome is explained by the postvaccination phenomenon. Although these events do not necessarily show causality, the fact that they have occurred after vaccination forces us to be attentive to these phenomena in the general population [28].

The main clinical manifestations of autoimmunity associated with adverse effects or criteria for ASIA are described below.

Rheumatologic adverse effects

In the Watad study, 11 patients were described as having arthritis, of which 3 were anticitrullinated protein antibody-positive and rheumatoid factor positive. He also reported 3 cases of SLE, one case of dermatomyositis, three vasculitides, and one case of polymyalgia rheumatic. These cases were reported in the first months of vaccination in three different countries (USA, Israel, and the UK); however, more cases related to rheumatological diseases have been found [28].

Urban et al. described one case of a 31-year-old woman who had no previous personal or family history of rheumatologic diseases. He presented with Raynaud's phenomenon (RP) 2 weeks after her first injection of the COVID-19 vaccine containing ChAdOx1-SARS-COV-2. The clinical characteristics were compatible with a typical RP; affecting the middle fingers of both hands and the right finger of the right hand; it was accompanied by a notable temperature difference of up to 10.9°C between the individual fingers. RP has a previous association with the administration of vaccines, diphtheria-tetanus, hepatitis B, and HPV, but this is the first case reported after the COVID-19 vaccine [29].

Different vaccines and components have been linked to the presentation of autoimmune rheumatological diseases after the COVID-19 vaccination. In Italy, a 76-year-old-female presented with Henoch-Schönlein purpura (HSP) 7 days after receiving the first dose of the ChAdOx1 nCOV-19 AZD1222 vaccine. The criteria used to diagnose were from EULAR/PRINTO/PRES, on which the main symptom was palpable purpura in the absence of thrombocytopenia accompanied by other symptoms. This patient was treated with paracetamol and deflazacort as in any other HSP with a good response; a second dose was given with no new symptoms [30]. These adverse events (AE) are resumed in Table 36.3. In this table, we can observe the characteristic of autoimmune rheumatic disease postvaccines associated. According to the main results of AE secondary to vaccines, it was found more frequent in women (mean age were 44.6 years) versus men (57.7% years), 36 (76.6%) versus 11 (23.4%), respectively. The main autoimmune rheumatic disease reported was the exacerbation of SLE 49%, followed by vasculitis 42% (leukocytoclastic vasculitis, vasculitis associated with ANCA, HSP and less frequently granulomatous vasculitis), new-onset SLE (7%) and RP (2%). Vaccines with higher AE were: BNT162b2, followed by ChAdOx1-S. Fortunately, no deaths were attributed to AE from vaccines [30–55].

Cardiovascular adverse effects

Since the beginning of the COVID-19 pandemic, there have been reported cases on which SARS-COV-2 affects the cardiovascular system. These events have been explained by the entry of SARS-COV-2 into myocardial cells facilitated by the presence of angiotensin-converting enzyme 2 (ACE2), which causes activation of monocytes, T cells, and cytokines leading to activation of a hyperinflammatory response causing hypoxemia and microthrombogenesis [56]. In the case of COVID-19 vaccines, these effects are not well explained; nevertheless, cases of myopericarditis, pericarditis, Takotsubo cardiomyopathy, and other cardiovascular effects have been reported. The different cardiovascular events associated with COVID-19 are resumed in Table 36.4 [57–69]. Concerning cardiac-type adverse events, a more frequent

TABLE 36.3 Rheumatologic events after COVID-19 vaccination.

Author	Sex Age	Previous history	Vaccine type	Symptoms/Disease	Dose	Time to presentation	Time to resolution	Country
Sirufo et al. [30]	Female 76	None	ChAdOx1 nCOV-19 AZD1222	Henoch-Schönlein purpura	First dose	Seven days	Two weeks	Italy
Urban N et al. [29]	Female 31	None	ChAdOx1-SARS-COV-2	Raynaud phenomenon	First dose	Two weeks	Four weeks	Austria
Bostan et al. [31]	Female 57	Epilepsy Bipolar disorder Depression	mRNA COVID-19	Small vessel vasculitis	First and second dose	One week	One week	Turkey
Mücke et al. [32]	Male 76	Heart failure NYHA ll Alcoholic liver cirrhosis	BNT162b2	Cutaneous and gastrointestinal Immune complex vasculitis	First dose	Twelve days	Five days	Germany
Conticini et al. [33]	Male 77	Microscopic polyangiitis	BNT162b2	Relapse of microscopic polyangiitis	First dose	"Few days"	Seven days	Italy
Hakroush and Tampe [34]	Female 79	Hypertension Degenerative disc disease	BNT162b2	ANCA-associated vasculitis	Second dose	Two weeks	On follow up	Germany
Cohen et al. [35]	Female 46	Psoriasis Psoriatic arthritis Irritable bowel syndrome Leukocytoclastic vasculitis.	BNT162b2	Leukocytoclastic vasculitis flare	First and second dose	Two days	On follow up	USA
Takeyama et al. [36]	Female 48	None	BNT162b2	Intracerebral hemorrhage due to vasculitis	First dose	Two days	Four weeks	Japan
Shakoor et al. [37]	Female 78	Type 2 Diabetes Hypertension, paroxysmal atrial Fibrillation	BNT162b2	ANCA-associated vasculitis	First and second dose	Sixteen days	On follow up	USA

(Continued)

TABLE 36.3 Rheumatologic events after COVID-19 vaccination.—cont'd

Author	Sex Age	Previous history	Vaccine type	Symptoms/Disease	Dose	Time to presentation	Time to resolution	Country
Zavala-Flores et al. [38]	20 cases Female: 18 Male: 2 Age: 38.65 ± 14.13	Lupus	BNT162b2	Lupus flares	First and second	2.3 ± 0.8 days	On follow up	Peru
Kreuter et al. [39]	Female 62	Cutaneous lupus	ChAdOx1-S	Transition of cutaneous into systemic lupus erythematosus	First dose	Ten days	On follow up	Germany
Kreuter et al. [40]	Male 79	Not mentioned	BNT162b2	Subacute cutaneous lupus erythematosus	First dose	Ten days	Four weeks	Germany
Joseph and Chong [41]	Female 54	Subacute cutaneous lupus erythematosus	mRNA-1273	Subacute cutaneous lupus erythematosus flare	First dose	Four days	Two weeks	USA
Patil and Patil [42]	Female 22	Family history for autoimmune thyroiditis, allergic rhinitis, and asthma	ChAdOx1-S (Covishield)	Systemic lupus erythematosus	First and second dose	Two weeks	On follow up	India
Niebel et al. [43]	Female 73	Subacute cutaneous lupus erythematosus	BNT162b2	Exacerbation of subacute cutaneous lupus erythematosus	First dose	Ten days	On follow up	Germany
Maye et al. [44]	Male 23	IgA vasculitis	BNT162b2	Reactivation of IgA vasculitis	Second dose	24 h	Two weeks	United Kingdom
Fritzen et al. [45]	Female 60	Chronic liver disease, portal hypertension, polycythemia vera, hypothyroidism, and type 2 diabetes	ChAdOx1-S	Leukocytoclastic vasculitis	Second dose	Eleven days	Seven days	Brazil

Kondo and Yamanaka [46]	Female 45	Henoch-Schönlein purpura	BNT162b2	Henoch-Schönlein purpura reactivation	First and second dose	24 h	On follow up	Japan
Dicks and Gray [47]	Male 65	Diabetes and hypertension	BNT162b2	Leukocytoclastic vasculitis	Third dose	Two days	On follow up	USA
Bencharattanaphakhi and Rerknimitr [48]	Two cases Female 1st: 23 2nd: 26	None	CoronaVac	Leukocytoclastic vasculitis	First dose	1st: 36 h 2nd: 4 h	1st: Five days 2nd: Four weeks	Thailand
Kar et al. [49]	Female 46	None	BBV152 (Covaxin)	Cutaneous small-vessel vasculitis	First dose	Five days	Fifteen days	India
Naitlho et al. [50]	Male 62	Osteosarcoma Tonsillectomy	ChAdOx1-S	Henoch-Schönlein purpura	First dose	Eight days	Seven days	Morocco
Badier et al. [51]	Male 72	Hypertension, myocardial infarction, type 2 diabetes mellitus, obesity and asthma	ChAdOx1-S	IgA vasculitis	First dose	Fifteen days	On follow up	Not mentioned
Okuda et al. [52]	Female 37	Graves disease	BNT162b2	ANCA-associated vasculitis	First dose	Twelve days	38 days	Japan
Dash et al. [53]	Male 27	None	Not mentioned	Urticarial vasculitis	Second dose	One day	One week	India
Vassallo et al. [54]	Female 51	None	BNT162b2	Cutaneous lymphocytic vasculitis	First dose	Six hours	One week	Italy
Gillion et al. [55]	Male 77	None	ChAdOx1-S	Granulomatous vasculitis	First dose	Four weeks	Four weeks	Belgium

TABLE 36.4 Cardiovascular events after COVID-19 vaccination.

Author	Sex/Age	Previous history	Vaccine type	Symptoms/Disease	Vaccine dose	Time to presentation	Time to resolution	Country
Ashaari et al. [57]	Male/66	Type 2 diabetes Depression Previous transient ischemic attack	BNT162b2	Pericarditis	First dose	Seven days	Seven days	Ireland
Alon Nevet [58]	Three cases: Male/20, 29, 24	None	BNT162b2	Acute myocarditis	Second dose	Two days	"Rapid resolution"	Israel
Patrignani et al. [59]	Male/56	Mild COVID-19 infection 4 months earlier	BNT162b2	Acute myocarditis	First dose	Four days	Seven days	Italy
Lania-Torres et al. [60]	Male/28	Arrhythmogenic left ventricular cardiomyopathy	BNT162b2	Acute myocarditis	Second dose	Two weeks	Ten days	Spain
Singh et al. [61]	Male/24	None	BNT162b2	Acute myocarditis	Second dose	Three days	Seven days	USA
Tate et al. [62]	Female/29	None	BNT162b2	Isolated tachycardia	Second dose	Eight hours	One day	USA
Perez et al. [63]	Case series: 7 patients 6 males 1 female Age: 22–71/ Median: 44	Hypertension 5/7 Obesity 4/7 OSA (4/7) Tobacco use (3/7) Dyslipidemia (3/7) History of myocarditis (1/7) History of pericarditis (1/7)	3 patients: BNT162b 4 patients: mRNA-1273	Acute myocarditis	One case: First dose 6 cases: Second dose	Three days (range 1–13 days)	Two days (range: 2–4 days)	USA
McLean et al. [64]	Male/16	None	BNT162b2	Myopericarditis	Second dose	60 h	6 days	USA
Marshall et al. [65]	Case series: 7 patients Male: 7/ Median: 16 (range: 14–19)	None	BNT162b2	Acute myocarditis: 5 cases Myopericarditis: 2 cases	Second dose	Three days (range: 2–4 days)	Three days (range: 2–6 days)	USA

Toida et al. [66]	Female/80	Hypertension Renal sclerosis in hemodialysis Hyperparathyroidism	BNT162b2	Takotsubo cardiomyopathy	First dose	Four days	Five days	Japan
Khogali et al. [67]	Female/29	Allergy to tree nuts and peanuts Partial right nephrectomy with stable mild chronic kidney disease (CKD) since birth	mRNA-1273	Myopericarditis	Second dose	Ten days	Three weeks	Qatar
Ammirati et al. [68]	Male/56	None	BNT162b2	Acute myocarditis	Second dose	Three days	Seven days	Italy
Bautista Garcia et al. [69]	Male/39	Asthma Hypothyroidism, Chronic atrophic gastritis An isolated episode of atrial fibrillation Recurrent spontaneous pneumothorax with left apical lobectomy.	BNT162b2	Acute myocarditis	Second dose	Six hours	Six days	Spain

condition was observed in males 22 (84.6%) with an average age of 32.6 years and females 4 (15.4%) 45.5 years. The EA more frequent was acute myocarditis. The vaccine applied most frequently was Pfizer in 54% of these reviewed cases.

Endocrine adverse effects

The relationship between ASIA and endocrine diseases has been known since some years ago. There have been reports of Addison's disease after exposure to adjuvants as in vaccines; there also reported cases of subacute thyroiditis following HPV vaccination, influenza, and other adjuvants. Some other cases that have been reported are type 1 diabetes, primary ovarian failure, and Hashimoto's Thyroiditis [70]. In the case of COVID-19, there have been many cases of endocrine reactions during infection; but since the vaccination began, there have also been many reports of endocrine affections; the same principle has explained this as in the cardiovascular system, endocrine organs have been found to have angiotensin-converting enzyme two receptors which can facilitate the entry of SARS-CoV-2 into the cells causing different reactions. This is mainly seen in the thyroid gland, explained by the abundant receptors expressed on the gland [71]. Table 36.5 resumes some of the cases reported worldwide on endocrine reactions. There were 21 patients: male 4 (19%) with a mean age of 51 years old and female 17 (81%) with an average of 42 years old. The most frequent autoimmune thyroid disease was subacute thyroiditis in 14 patients (66%), followed by Graves'Disease (14%). The most frequently applied vaccine was Pfizer 33%, Chadox 24 and Modern 19% [71–84].

Dermatologic adverse effects

In the case of cutaneous AE, Grieco et al. studied 2740 subjects where the most common reaction was urticaria followed by angioedema. Nevertheless, other kinds of reactions can appear on the skin in some cases, even severe cases such as Steven-Johnson syndrome [85].

Bellinato et al. [86] studied 74 patients with cutaneous adverse reactions associated with SARS-CoV-2 Vaccines. Among the dermatological manifestations, postvaccines were injection site reactions, affecting 30%–70% and generally mild or moderate. Small case series or single case reports included filler reactions, exanthemas, vascular lesions, urticaria, eczematous dermatitis, autoimmune bullous reactions, and severe cutaneous adverse reactions. In addition, the exacerbation of chronic immune-mediated dermatoses (mainly psoriasis and atopic dermatitis) and reactivations of herpes infection were reported. The cutaneous reactions were generally mild, self-limiting, and resembled common cutaneous drug eruptions and/or COVID-19 skin manifestations [86].

In Table 36.6, some of the typical manifestations on the skin appear, regarding dermatological AE, there was 60% female (53 years) and 40% male (41 years). The pityriasis rosea was the most frequent dermatologic disease [87–105]. Pfizer was the leading vaccine with AE, followed by Astra- Zeneca ChAdOx1-S and Modern.

Hematological adverse effects

Since the first months of the pandemic, adverse hematologic reactions have been seen after COVID-19 infections, such as thrombosis. Nowadays, some of the treatments that have been

TABLE 36.5 Endocrine reactions after COVID-19 vaccination.

Author	Sex Age	Previous history	Vaccine type	Symptoms/ Disease	Dose	Time to presentation	Time to resolution	Country
Siolos et al. [72]	Two cases Females 1st: 51 2nd: 39	1st: None 2nd: Mother with hypothyroidism	1st: BNT162b2 2nd: ChAdOx1-S	1st: Subacute Thyroiditis 2nd: Silent Thyroiditis	First dose	1st: 11 days 2nd: Three weeks	1st and 2nd: Two months	Greece
Yamamoto et al. [73]	Female/ 64	Colorectal cancer Diabetes Obesity	BNT162b2	Hyperthyroidism	First dose	Six days	28 days	Japan
Murvelashvili et al. [74]	Male/51	None	mRNA-1273	Hypophysitis	Second dose	Two days	1 month	USA
Ratnayake et al. [75]	Male/75	None	ChAdOx1-S	Subacute Thyroiditis	First dose	Fourteen days	4 months	United Kingdom
Bornemann et al. [76]	Two cases Females 1st: 26 2nd: 49	None	1st: ChAdOx1-S 2nd: mRNA-1273	Subacute Thyroiditis	First dose	Two weeks	2 weeks	Germany
Vera-Lastra et al. [77]	Two cases Females 1st: 40 2nd: 28	1st: Hypertension 2nd: None	BNT162b2	Graves' disease	First dose	1st: Two days 2nd: Three days	On follow up	Mexico
Patel et al. [78]	Male/48	None	Not mentioned	Subacute Thyroiditis	Second dose	One week	Not mentioned	USA
Franquemont et al. [79]	Female/42	None	BNT162b2	Subacute Thyroiditis	First dose	Five days	Not mentioned	USA
Oyibo [80]	Female/55	Asthma	ChAdOx1-S	Subacute Thyroiditis	First dose	One week	Sequelae hypothyroidism	United Kingdom
Sahin et al. [81]	Male/67	Hypertension Atrial extra beats	CoronaVac	Subacute Thyroiditis	Second dose	Two weeks	Six weeks	Turkey

(Continued)

TABLE 36.5 Endocrine reactions after COVID-19 vaccination.—cont'd

Author	Sex Age	Previous history	Vaccine type	Symptoms/ Disease	Dose	Time to presentation	Time to resolution	Country
İremli et al. [82]	Three cases Females 1st: 35 2nd: 34 3rd: 37	1st: None 2nd: Previous COVID-19 infection 3rd: None	CoronaVac	Subacute Thyroiditis	1st: Second dose 2nd: First dose 3rd: Second dose	1st and 2nd: Four days 3rd: Seven days	1st and 2nd: On follow up 3rd: Eight weeks	Turkey
Pujol et al. [71]	Three cases 1st: Female/38 2nd: Male/32 3rd: Female/38	1st: Not mentioned 2nd: Type 1 diabetes 3rd: Schizophrenia	1st: mRNA-1273 2nd: BNT162b2 3rd: BNT162b2	1st: Subacute Thyroiditis 2nd: Silent Thyroiditis 3rd: Graves' disease	1st: First dose 2nd: First dose 3rd: First dose	1st: Eight days 2nd: 10 days 3rd: 12 days	1st: Two weeks 2nd: On follow up 3rd: On follow up	Spain
Plaza-Enriquez et al. [83]	Female/42	Colon cancer Paroxysmal supraventricular tachycardia Iron deficiency anemia Neuropathy Lumbar radiculopathy	mRNA-1273	Subacute Thyroiditis	Second dose	5–6 days	Two months	USA
Sigstad et al. [84]	Female/fourth decade	Papillary carcinoma Hashimoto's thyroiditis	BNT162b2	Subacute Thyroiditis	First dose	6 days	Not mentioned	Norway

TABLE 36.6 Dermatologic reactions after COVID-19 vaccination.

Author	Sex/ Age (years)	Previous history	Vaccine type	Symptoms/Disease	Dose	Time to presentation	Time to resolution	Country
Pérez-López et al. [87]	Female/78	Diabetes Alzheimer	BNT162b2	Bullous pemphigoid	First and second dose (reactivation)	Three days	Two weeks	Spain
Thomas et al. [88]	Male/third decade	Allergy to sulfa drugs	BNT162b2	Chronic spontaneous maculopapular urticaria	Second dose	One week	On follow up	USA
Dash et al. [89]	Male/60	Diabetes Hypertension	ChAdOx1-S	Stevens-Johnson Syndrome	First dose	Three days	Two weeks	India
Cinotti et al. [90]	Male/70	Hypertension	ChAdOx1-S	Eosinophilic dermatitis	First dose	Five days	Three weeks	Italy
Saibene et al. [91]	Female/58	Treatment with oral sertraline, lorazepam, and atorvastatin	mRNA-1273	Erythema multiforme	First and second dose (reactivation)	Five days	Two weeks	Italy
Onn et al. [92]	Female/53	None	BNT162b2	Lichenoid skin Eruption	First dose	Twelve days	Two weeks	New Zealand
Elboraey et al. [93]	Female/ "middle-aged"	None	BNT162b2	Stevens-Johnson Syndrome	Second dose	Five days	Not mentioned	Kingdom of Saudi Arabia
Majid et al. [94]	Female/65	Hypertension	ChAdOx1-S	Sweet syndrome	First	One week	Two weeks	India
Lehmann et al. [95]	Female 79	Type 2 diabetes and hypertension	BNT162b2	Guttate Psoriasis	First	Ten days	On follow up	Switzerland
Marcantonio-Santa Cruz et al. [96]	Two cases Female 1st: 22 2nd: 54	Not mentioned	BNT162b2	Pityriasis rosea	1st: Second dose 2nd: First and second dose	1st: Seven days 2nd: One week	1st: Not mentioned 2nd: Three weeks	Spain

(Continued)

TABLE 36.6 Dermatologic reactions after COVID-19 vaccination.—cont'd

Author	Sex/ Age (years)	Previous history	Vaccine type	Symptoms/Disease	Dose	Time to presentation	Time to resolution	Country
Elbæk et al. [97]	Female 47	Darier's disease	ChAdOx1-S	Darier's disease flare	First dose	Two days	On follow up	Denmark
Kong et al. [98]	Male/66	Hypertension, hyperlipidemia, diabetes, renal failure, hypotiroidism, coronary heart disease	mRNA-1273	Erupción ampollosa fija extensa a fármacos	Second dose	12 days	No	
Cazzato et al. [99]	Male/43	None	Pfizer-BioNTech	Purpuric rash	Second dose	14 days	No	Italy
Guenin et al. [100]	Female/61	None	mRNA-1273	Reaction of hipersensibilidad	Third dose	2 days	3 days	USA
Bianchi et al. [101]	6 female male/	Allergic rhinitis	Pfizer-BioNTech	Mucous-cutaneous adverse reactions: Acute urticaria	First dose	Less 24 hs		Italy
Burlando et al. [102].	Female/48 años	None	ChAdOx1-S	Acute urticaria	First dose	4 days	3 h	Italy
Adya et al [103].	Male/29	None	mRNA-1273	Pityriasis rosea	First dose	Immediate	No	India
Cyrenne et al. [104]	Female/20	Alopecia areata	Pfizer-BioNTech	Pityriasis rosea	First dose	2 days	2 weeks	Canada
Cyrenne et al. [104]	Male/40	None	Pfizer-BioNTech	Pityriasis rosea-like	Second dose	3 weeks	3 weeks	Canada
Leerunyakul et al. [105]	Female/52	Recurrent glioblastoma	ChAdOx1-S	Pityriasis rosea -like eruption	First dose	2 weeks	–	Thailand

proven to improve the chances of healing are corticosteroids and anticoagulants. In the case of vaccines for COVID-19, there have also been some reported cases of a new entity called thrombosis with thrombocytopenia syndrome or vaccine-induced (immune) thrombotic thrombocytopenia (VITT). Findings in VITT are thrombocytopenia, elevated D-dimer, reduced fibrinogen, and antibodies against platelet factor 4 (anti-PF4) that have been found in most patients with this entity [106]. The main symptom presented during this disease is thrombosis of atypical sites in classic sites such as deep vein thrombosis and pulmonary embolism [107].

Among the components of the vaccine that have been mentioned to be responsible for causing the production of anti-PF4 antibodies are adenovirus itself, the protein cassette, or other components such as polysorbate 80 [108]. Although the pathogenesis is unclear, it has been proposed that vaccination can trigger the production of PF4 autoantibodies through molecular mimicry phenomena, while vaccination compounds lead to rigorous activation of immune cells [109].

Table 36.7 [110–123] resumes some examples of VITT, including a case of Acquired hemophilia A. The main hematological complication observed was thrombosis with the presence of antibodies against platelet factor 4 (anti-PF4) induced by the ChAdOx1 nCoV-19 vaccine, followed by thrombotic thrombocytopenia and autoimmune thrombocytopenia, with a predominance of women in 72% and 28% were men.

Nephrological adverse effects

Some cases of renal involvement after the COVID-19 vaccine have been reported, especially Nephrotic Syndrome. Table 36.8 resumes some of these cases [124–135].

The most frequent nephrological complication was glomerulonephritis, predominantly in women in 57% with a mean age of 46 years and the rest in men.

Neurological adverse effects

Neurologic reactions after vaccination have been described since many years ago; of note, during the beginning of Influenza vaccination, some cases of Guillain-Barré syndrome were reported. Reactions that may appear are acute disseminated encephalomyelitis, acute ischemic stroke, transverse myelitis, headache, etc. There is no clear explanation for the apparition of these symptoms; some have explained it as molecular mimicry, neurotoxicity, or other mechanisms. Garg et al. [136] described the spectrum of neurological cases after COVID-19 vaccination; the main symptom was a headache in 62.2%, weakness in 1%, and severe cases as transverse myelitis [99]. Table 36.9 resumes some of the cases reported worldwide [137–146]. The main neurological complication observed was Guillain-Barré syndrome.

Other adverse effects

In Table 36.10 are described some other reactions after COVID-19 vaccination that could be explained due to the presence of angiotensin-converting enzyme two receptors that have been found in every organ [147–150].

TABLE 36.7 Hematological reactions after COVID-19 vaccination.

Author	Sex Age	Previous history	Vaccine type	Symptoms/Disease	Dose	Time to presentation	Time to resolution	Country
Lemoine et al. [110]	Male/70	Polymyalgia rheumatic hepatitis C	mRNA-1273	Acquired hemophilia A	First	Two days	On follow up	USA
Costello et al. [111]	Female/40	Migraine Obesity	Ad26.COV2.S	Thrombotic thrombocytopenia	First (single dose)	Six days	Not mentioned	USA
Karabulut et al. [112]	Male/48	Type 2 diabetes refractory thrombotic thrombocytopenic purpura (TTP), Idiopathic thrombocytopenic purpura (ITP)	mRNA-1273	Recurrence of thrombotic thrombocytopenic purpura	First	Five days	Ten days	USA
Appelbaum et al. [113]	Female/25	Not mentioned	mRNA-1273	Immune thrombocytopenic purpura	First	Ten days	Two weeks	USA
Greainacher et al. [114]	Eleven cases: 9 female 2: Male Range: 22 −49 years	One patient: Von Willebrand disease, anticardiolipin antibodies, and factor V Leiden.	ChAdOx1 nCov-19	1: Fatal intracranial hemorrhage. 9: Cerebral venous thrombosis 3: Splanchnic-vein thrombosis, 3: Pulmonary embolism 5: Disseminated intravascular coagulation	First	Five-sixteen days	Six patients: Died Five patients: On follow up	Germany and Austria
Schultz et al. [115]	1: Female/ 37 2: Female/ 42 3: Male/32 4: Female/ 49 5: Female/ 54	1: Pollen allergy 2: Pollen allergy 3: Asma 4: None 5: Hypertension	ChAdOx1 nCoV-19	1: Severe thrombocytopenia, thrombosis in the left transverse and sigmoid sinuses 2: Venous thrombosis with occlusion of the transverse and sigmoid sinuses and hemorrhagic infarction in the left hemisphere 3: Thrombosis of several branches of the portal vein with occlusion of the left intrahepatic portal vein and left hepatic vein.	First	1: Eight days 2: 10 days 3: Seven 4: 10 days 5: Seven	1: Died 2: Died 3: 12 days 4:10 days 5:Died	Norway

				4: Massive thrombosis in the deep and superficial cerebral veins and right cerebellar hemorrhagic infarction 5: Massive cerebral vein thrombosis				
Scully et al. [116]	23 cases. 14: Female 9: Male Range age: 21–77	One patient: Deep venous thrombosis One patient: Combined oral contraceptive pill	ChAdOx1 nCoV-19	22 patients with thrombosis. 13: Cerebral venous thrombosis 4 pulmonary embolism 1 deep venous thrombosis and bilateral adrenal hemorrhage. 2 ischemic stroke 2 portal vein thrombosis 1 patient with isolated thrombocytopenia and hemorrhagic phenotype	First	6–24 days	7 patients died	United Kingdom
Mehta et al. [117]	Two 1: Male/32 2: Male/25	1: None 2: Primary sclerosing cholangitis, migraines	ChAdOx1 nCoV-19	1:Thrombocytopenia/ 2:Thrombocytopenia/ Superior sagittal sinus thrombosis with extension into the cortical veins, and hemorrhage in lobar and subarachnoid locations	First	1: Nine days 2: Six says	1: Died 2: Died	United Kingdom
Tiede et al. [118]	Five/ Female Range age 41–67	Not mentioned	ChAdOx1 nCoV-19	Five cases of prothrombotic immune thrombocytopenia 1: CVST 2: Multiple cortical emboli and aortic arch thrombi 3: Headache, diplopia 4: Extensive splanchnic vein thrombosis 5: Cerebral artery thrombosis	First	5–11 days	Recovering	Germany
See et al. [119]	12 cases/ Female Age range: 18–60 years	Seven patients: Obesity hypothyroidism and oral contraceptive use	Ad26.COV2.S	CVST and thrombocytopenia	First (single dose)	6–15	3 died	US

(*Continued*)

TABLE 36.7 Hematological reactions after COVID-19 vaccination.—cont'd

Author	Sex Age	Previous history	Vaccine type	Symptoms/Disease	Dose	Time to presentation	Time to resolution	Country
Vayne et al. [120]	Nine cases 7 female 2 male 24–73 years	Not mentioned	ChAdOx1 nCoV-19	Severe thrombocytopenia 1: CVST splanchnic vein thrombosis	Not mentioned	9–12	Not mentioned	France
Althaus et al. [121]	Eight cases 5 female 3 male Range: 24–53	One patient: Heterozygous FVL mutation One patient: Contraception	ChAdOx1 nCoV-19	4 patients: CVST 2 patients: CVST + PE 1: PE 1: Bleeding, multiple thrombosis	Not mentioned	6–20	3 died 5 recovering	Germany
Castelli et al. [122]	One case 50/Males	None	ChAdOx1 nCoV-19	CVST (Cerebral VENOUS SINUS THROMBOSIS)	First	7	Died	Italy
Muir et al. [123]	One case Female/60	None	Ad26.COV2.S	Thrombotic thrombocytopenia CVST	First (single dose)	14	Remained critically	USA

TABLE 36.8 Nephrological reactions after COVID-19 vaccination.

Author	Sex Age	Previous history	Vaccine type	Symptoms/Disease	Dose	Time to presentation	Time to resolution	Country
Fernández et al. [124]	Four cases 1st: Female/38 2nd: Male/53 3rd: Female/59 4th: Female/67	1st: Obesity 2nd: Hypertension 3rd: Hypertension, obesity, mesangial Proliferative glomerulonephritis 4th: Sjögren Minimal change disease	1st: BBIBP-CorV 2nd: ChAdOx1-S 3rd: Gam-COVID-Vac 4th: Gam-COVID-Vac	Glomerulonephritis	First dose	1st: Seven 2nd: 10 3rd: 14 4th: Six	On follow up	Argentina
Da et al. [125]	Male/70	None	BNT162b2	Membranous Nephropathy	First and second dose	One week	On follow up	Singapore
Haji et al. [126]	Male/63	*Cannabis* use	Ad26.COV2.S	Pheochromocytoma multisystem crisis	First (single dose)	One day	On follow up	USA
Anupama et al. [127]	Female/19	Not mentioned	ChAdOx1-S (Covishield)	Nephrotic syndrome (mesangial proliferative variant of minimal change disease)	First	Eight days	Not mentioned	India
Lim et al. [128]	Male/51	None	Ad26.COV.2	Nephrotic syndrome secondary to minimal change disease	First	Seven days	42 days	Korea
Lebedev et al. [129]	Male/50	None	BNT162b2	Minimal change disease with nephrotic syndrome and acute kidney injury	First	Four days	17 days	Israel
Maas et al. 131)	Male/80	Venous thromboembolisms several years earlier	BNT162b2	Minimal change disease	First	Seven days	Ten days	Netherlands
D' Agate et al. [131]	Male/77	Type 2 diabetes mellitus	BNT162b2	Minimal change disease and acute kidney injury	First	Seven days	On follow up	USA

(Continued)

TABLE 36.8 Nephrological reactions after COVID-19 vaccination.—cont'd

Author	Sex Age	Previous history	Vaccine type	Symptoms/Disease	Dose	Time to presentation	Time to resolution	Country
Holzworth et al. [132]	Female/63	Hypertension and tobacco dependence	mRNA-1273	Minimal change disease	Only	< Seven days	Not mentioned	USA
Weijers et al. [133]	Female/61	Autoimmune hepatitis and hypothyroidism	BNT162b2	Minimal change disease	First	Ten days	21 Days	Netherlands
Thappy et al. [134]	Male/43	None	mRNA-1273	Minimal change disease	Only	Seven days	On follow up	Etiopia
Leclerc et al. [135]	Male/71	Dyslipidemia	ChAdOx1 nCoV-19	Minimal change disease with severe acute kidney injury	First	13 days	68 days	Canada

TABLE 36.9 Neurological reactions after COVID-19 vaccination.

Author	Sex Age	Previous history	Vaccine type	Symptoms/Disease	Dose	Time to presentation	Time to resolution	Country
Chavez et al. [137]	Male/82	Laryngeal cancer Barrett's Esophagus Chronic kidney disease	BNT162b2	Myasthenia gravis	First	Four weeks	On follow up	USA
Morehouse et al. [138]	Female/49	Neurofibromatosis type I Hypothyroidism Multiple vitamin deficiencies	Ad26.COV2.S	Guillain–Barré syndrome type acute, motor, and sensory axonal neuropathy	First (single dose)	Five days	On follow up	USA
Permezel et al. [139]	Male/63	Type 2 diabetes Ischemic heart disease Atrial fibrillation	ChAdOx1-S	Acute disseminated encephalomyelitis	First	Twelve days	Died on day 20th	Australia
Torrealba-Acosta et al. [140]	Male/77	Coronary artery Disease hyperlipidemia hypothyroidism	mRNA-1273	Acute aseptic meningoencephalitis with sweet syndrome	First	Two days	One week	USA
Gao et al. [141]	Female/76	Hypertension	mRNA-1273	Acute transverse myelitis Subtype: Longitudinally Extensive transverse myelitis	First	Three days	Two weeks	Taiwan
Dalwadi et al. [142]	Female/86	Atrial fibrillation Type 2 diabetes Aortic stenosis Previous ischemic stroke	mRNA-1273	Guillain–Barre syndrome	Second	Two days	On follow up	USA
Finstere [143]	Male/32	Amphetamine's consumer Guillain–Barré syndrome 14 years previous Family history of bipolar disorder and brain tumor	Vector-based	Exacerbating Guillain–Barre syndrome	First	Eight days	On follow up	Austria
Malamud et al. [144]	Male/14	Not mentioned	BNT162b2	Guillain–Barre syndrome	Second	One month	Two months	USA
Fujimori et al. [145]	Female/40	Peripheral facial nerve palsy (4 years previous)	BNT162b2	Multiple sclerosis	Second	Two weeks	Three weeks	Japan
Manea et al. [146]	Male/29	None	BNT162b2	Multiple cranial nerve palsies	First	Six days	One month	Romania

TABLE 36.10 Other types of reactions after COVID-19 vaccination.

Author	Sex Age	Previous history	Vaccine type	Symptoms/ Disease	Dose	Time to presentation	Time to resolution	Country
Rela et al. [147]	Two cases: 1st: Female/ 38 2nd: Male/62	1st: Hypothyroidism 2nd: Diabetes	ChAdOx1-S (Covishield)	Autoimmune hepatitis	Not mentioned	1st: 20 days 2nd: 16 days	1st: One month 2nd: Died 3 weeks later	India
Pan et al. [148]	Female/ 50	None	Inactivated COVID-19 vaccine	Bilateral uveitis	Not mentioned	Five days	Five weeks	China
Ganga et al. [149]	Male/58	Hypertension	mRNA-1273	Massive cervical lymphadenopathy	Not mentioned	Two days	Two weeks	USA
Parrino et al. [150]	Three cases: 1st: Female/ 37 2nd: Male/63 3rd: Male/30	1st: Glaucoma, undifferentiated connective tissue disease 2nd: Sensorineural hearing loss, asthma Depression 3rd: Hashimoto thyroiditis	BNT162b2	Tinnitus	1st and 2nd: First dose 3rd: Second	1st: Seven hours 2nd: 20 hours 3rd: One week	On follow up	Italy

Discussion

The AE associated with the application of the vaccine against COVID-19 are varied and affects different organs and systems, based on the observation of cause and effect between the appearance of clinical manifestation after application of the vaccine. Table 36.11 shows the main characteristics of the reported cases.

The suspicion of AE associated with immunization is high due to the reported cases and the time that the adverse reaction was presented. The vaccines that have been authorized so far by the WHO are all being constantly evaluated for the probable side effects, so the case reports are extremely important to find a better way of immunization without the risk of complications. As mentioned, many factors contribute to the development of adverse reactions, from the genetic factors of the recipient itself to each of the ingredients present in the vaccine, so we cannot predict in whom one or another reaction will occur. The symptoms presented did not prefer geographical area since the reports have been from different countries worldwide. We briefly reviewed the reported cases and found 232 cases in different articles. All the COVID-19 vaccines accepted by the World Health Organization have shown

TABLE 36.11 Adverse events postvaccination anti–COVID-19.

Variable	Rheumatology	Cardiovascular	Endocrine	Dermatology	Hematology	Nephrology	Neurology	Other	Total
Female	36	4	16	12	59	6	4	3	140
Male	11	23	5	8	22	9	6	4	88
Age (average)	47	26	45	51	45	58	55	50	47.125
Astra-Zeneca	8	0	4	5	64	3	1	2	87
Pfizer	33	22	8	11	0	5	4	3	86
Moderna	2	5	4	4	3	2	3	1	24
Sinofarm	0	0	0	0	0	1	0	0	1
Johnson and Johnson	0	0	0	0	14	2	1	0	17
Corona-Vac	2	0	4	0	0	0	0	0	6
Covaxin	1	0	0	0	0	0	0	0	1
Sputnik	0	0	0	0	0	2	0	0	2
Not mentioned	1	0	1	0	0	0	1	1	4
First dose	17	4	15	9	64	14	7	2	132
Second dose	4	23	6	7	0	0	3	1	44
First and second	25	0	0	3	0	1	0	0	29
Third dose	1	0	0	1	0	0	0	0	2
Not mentioned	0	0	0	0	17	0	0	4	21
Time to presentation (average days)	5	4	8	9	11	8	11	7	7.875
Time to resolution (average days)	12	4	34	14	12	32	26	26	20
On follow up	29	0	10	7	0	5	4	1	83
Died	0	0	0	0	25	0	1	1	27

AE. In this way, the adverse events that occurred most frequently were attributed to the Oxford/Astra Zeneca and BNT162b2 (Pfizer—BioNTech) vaccines.

Most cases were present in patients in whom the Astra-Zeneca vaccine was applied, which has a mechanism of action based on a viral vector and no known adjuvant. The most affected sex was female in all the evaluated areas, except in the cardiovascular system, in which men occupied 85% of the cases presented. The average age of patients with side effects was 47 years; however, vaccination has not yet begun in the child population, so the age ranges are shifted. Among the important background of those who had adverse reactions to the vaccine, the most important were hypertension and diabetes with 19 and 17 cases each, most likely because they are among the main pathologies worldwide, on the other hand, the patients with no chronic disease were 39 which corresponds to 16% of the total.

In patients in whom symptoms appeared, the average onset was 8 days, ranging from 1 to 11 days, which is consistent with previous cases reports of the postvaccine phenomena due to ASIA. Recovery in most cases occurred after 20 days (range 4–34 days). The cases with total recovery after the adverse reaction occupied 52%; on the other hand, there are still patients in follow-up (35%). Unfortunately, 27 fatal cases were reported, 25 of them secondary to thrombotic events. Regarding the percentage of postvaccine phenomena per system, the following were reported: 47 cases of rheumatology, 27 cases of cardiovascular disease, 21 endocrinological, 20 dermatological, 81 hematological, 15 nephrological, 10 neurological, and seven cases of other systems.

We observed that ASIA not only appears as a postvaccine phenomenon in those that contain any of the known adjuvants but also in vaccines such as Astra-Zeneca that has not been reported to contain any adjuvants for its mechanism of action. AstraZeneca (ChAdOx1 nCoV-19 Covid-19) vaccine favors the production of antiplatelet factor 4 (anti-PF4) antibodies, blood clots, and thrombocytopenia [151], i.e., paradoxical thrombocytopenia. Regarding, the Pfizer-BioNTech Covid-19 mRNA vaccine has also produced autoimmune diseases and ASIA effects. It has been considered that the conjugated polyethylene glycol lipids stabilize the nanoparticles of the vaccine, induce the autoimmune reaction, and not only anaphylaxis as already described [77].

Conclusion

The anti–COVID-19 vaccine has been an outstanding achievement of biotechnology; however, they are not exempt from mild to severe and local and systemic adverse events that meet ASIA criteria.

The AE application of different types of vaccines may occur due to the interaction between the susceptibility of the host and some components of vaccines. It has been proposed that molecular mimicry is one of the most important mechanisms implicated in the EA.

Adverse events have been observed in the following systems: hematologic (thrombosis, immune thrombotic thrombocytopenia), rheumatologic (vasculitis or exacerbation of the autoimmune rheumatic disease, such as systemic lupus erythematosus or the novo diseases), neurologic (Guillain Barré Syndrome, neuropathy), dermatologic (acute urticaria, pityriasis rosae), cardiac (myocarditis), endocrine (subacute thyroiditis, Graves' disease), among others.

References

[1] Killeen RM. Vaccines—one of the greatest medical advances of modern times. Can Pharm J 2007;140(2_Suppl. 1). https://doi.org/10.3821/1913-701X-140-Sp2.S2. Revue des Pharmaciens du Canada.

[2] Pardi N, Hogan MJ, Porter FW, Weissman D. mRNA vaccines—a new era in vaccinology. Nat Rev Drug Discov 2018;17(4):261–79. https://doi.org/10.1038/nrd.2017.243.

[3] De León-Rodríguez SG, Hernández-Rico B, Olmo-Vázquez GD, Cruz-Dávalos I, Bonifaz LC. SARS-CoV-2: previous coronaviruses, immune response, and development of vaccines. SARS-CoV-2: coronavirus previos, respuesta inmune y desarrollo de vacunas. Bol Med Hosp Infant Mex 2020;77(5):252–61. https://doi.org/10.24875/BMHIM.20000191.

[4] Moore JP, Klasse PJ. COVID-19 vaccines: "warp speed" needs mind melds, not warped minds. J Virol 2020;94(17). https://doi.org/10.1128/JVI.01083-20. 20. Published 2020 August 17.

[5] Gee J, Marquez P, Su J, et al. First month of COVID-19 vaccine safety monitoring - United States, December 14, 2020-January 13, 2021. MMWR Morb Mortal Wkly Rep 2021;70(8):283–8. https://doi.org/10.15585/mmwr.mm7008e3. Published 2021 February 26.

[6] Rosenblum HG, Hadler SC, Moulia D, et al. Use of COVID-19 vaccines after reports of adverse events among adult recipients of Janssen (Johnson & Johnson) and mRNA COVID-19 vaccines (Pfizer-BioNTech and Moderna): update from the Advisory Committee on immunization practices—United States, July 2021. MMWR Morb Mortal Wkly Rep 2021;70(32):1094–9. https://doi.org/10.15585/mmwr.mm7032e4. Published 2021 August 13.

[7] Gavriatopoulou M, Ntanasis-Stathopoulos I, Korompoki E, et al. Emerging treatment strategies for COVID-19 infection. Clin Exp Med 2021;21(2):167–79. https://doi.org/10.1007/s10238-020-00671.

[8] Pulendran B, Ahmed R. Immunological mechanisms of vaccination. Nat Immunol 2011;12(6):509–17. https://doi.org/10.1038/ni.2039.

[9] Riedel S. Edward Jenner and the history of smallpox and vaccination. Proc (Bayl Univ Med Cent) 2005;18(1):21–5. https://doi.org/10.1080/08998280.2005.11928028.

[10] Guimarães LE, Baker B, Perricone C, Shoenfeld Y. Vaccines, adjuvants and autoimmunity. Pharmacol Res 2015;100:190–209. https://doi.org/10.1016/j.phrs.2015.08.003.

[11] US Food and Drug Administration. Guidance for industry: content and format of chemistry, manufacturing and controls information and establishment description information for a vaccine or related product. http://www.fda.gov/downloads/BiologicsBloodVaccines/GuidanceComplianceRegulatoryInformation/Guidances/Vaccines/ucm092272.pdf.

[12] Baylor NW. The regulatory evaluation of vaccines for human use. Methods Mol Biol 2016;1404:773–87. https://doi.org/10.1007/978-1-4939-3389-1_51.

[13] Marcellino MT, Di Timoteo F, De Angelis M, Oliva A. Overview of the main anti-SARS-CoV-2 vaccines: mechanism of action, efficacy and safety. Infect Drug Resist 2021;14:3459–76. https://doi.org/10.2147/IDR.S315727. Published 2021 August 31.

[14] World Health Organization. mRNA vaccines against COVID-19: Pfizer-BioNTech COVID-19 vaccine BNT162b2: prepared by the Strategic Advisory Group of Experts (SAGE) on immunization working group on COVID-19 vaccines, December 22 2020. World Health Organization; 2020. https://apps.who.int/iris/handle/10665/338096.

[15] Dotan A, Muller S, Kanduc D, David P, Halpert G, Shoenfeld Y. The SARS-CoV-2 as an instrumental trigger of autoimmunity. Autoimmun Rev 2021;20(4). https://doi.org/10.1016/j.autrev.2021.102792.

[16] Bennett JE, Dolin R, Blaser MJ. Mandell, Douglas, and Bennett's principles and practice of infectious diseases. Philadelphia, PA: Elsevier/Saunders; 2015.

[17] Quebec T, Bennouna S, Alkan S, et al. Yellow fever vaccine YF-17D activates multiple dendritic cell subsets via TLR2, 7, 8, and 9 to stimulate polyvalent immunity. J Exp Med 2006;203(2):413–24. https://doi.org/10.1084/jem.20051720.

[18] Ravichandran S, Coyle E, Klenow L, et al. Antibody signature induced by SARS-CoV-2 spike protein immunogens in rabbits. Sci Transl Med 2020;12(550). https://doi.org/10.1126/scitranslmed.abc3539.

[19] Duan L, Zheng Q, Zhang H, Niu Y, Lou Y, Wang H. The SARS-CoV-2 spike glycoprotein biosynthesis, structure, function, and antigenicity: implications for the design of spike-based vaccine immunogens. Front Immunol 2020;11. https://doi.org/10.3389/fimmu.2020.576622. Published 2020 Oct 7.

[20] Dan JM, Mateus J, Yu K, et al. Immunological memory to SARS-CoV-2 assessed for greater than six months after infection. bioRxiv 2021;371:6529. https://doi.org/10.1101/2020.11.15.383323.
[21] Shaw AR, Feinberg MB. 92—vaccines. In: Clinical immunology. 3rd ed. Edinburgh: Mosby; 2008. p. 1353—82. Weyand RRRAFTSWSJFM, editor.
[22] World Health Organization. . Global manual on surveillance of adverse events following immunization, 2016 update. World Health Organization; 2014. https://apps.who.int/iris/handle/10665/206144.
[23] Shoenfeld Y, Agmon-Levin N. ASIA—autoimmune/inflammatory syndrome induced by adjuvants. J Autoimmun 2011;36(1):4—8. https://doi.org/10.1016/j.jaut.2010.07.003.
[24] Watad A, Quaresma M, Brown S, et al. Autoimmune/inflammatory syndrome induced by adjuvants (Shoenfeld's syndrome)—an update. Lupus 2017;26(7):675—81. https://doi.org/10.1177/0961203316686406.
[25] Vera-Lastra O, Medina G, Cruz-Dominguez Mdel P, Jara LJ, Shoenfeld Y. Autoimmune/inflammatory syndrome induced by adjuvants (Shoenfeld's syndrome): clinical and immunological spectrum. Expet Rev Clin Immunol 2013;9(4):361—73. https://doi.org/10.1586/eci.13.2.
[26] Watad A, Bragazzi NL, McGonagle D, et al. Autoimmune/inflammatory syndrome induced by adjuvants (ASIA) demonstrates distinct autoimmune and autoinflammatory disease associations according to the adjuvant subtype: insights from an analysis of 500 cases. Clin Immunol 2019;203:1—8. https://doi.org/10.1016/j.clim.2019.03.007.
[27] Ritchie H, Mathieu E, Rodés-Guirao L, Appel C, Giattino C, Ortiz-Ospina E, Joe H, Macdonald B, Beltekian D, Roser M. Coronavirus pandemic (COVID-19). Published online at OurWorldInData.org; 2020. Retrieved from, https://ourworldindata.org/coronavirus [Online Resource].
[28] Watad A, De Marco G, Mahajna H, et al. Immune-mediated disease flares or new-onset disease in 27 subjects following mRNA/DNA SARS-CoV-2 vaccination. Vaccines 2021;9(5):435. https://doi.org/10.3390/vaccines9050435. Published 2021 April 29.
[29] Urban N, Weber B, Deinsberger J, Gschwandtner M, Bauer W, Handisurya A. Raynaud's phenomenon after COVID-19 vaccination: causative association, temporal connection, or mere bystander? Case Rep Dermatol 2021;13(3):450—6. https://doi.org/10.1159/000519147. Published 2021 September 15.
[30] Sirufo MM, Raggiunti M, Magnanimi LM, Ginaldi L, De Martinis M. Henoch-schönlein purpura following the first dose of COVID-19 viral vector vaccine: a case report. Vaccines 2021;9(10):1078. https://doi.org/10.3390/vaccines9101078. Published 2021 September 25.
[31] Bostan E, Zaid F, Akdogan N, Gokoz O. Possible case of mRNA COVID-19 vaccine-induced small-vessel vasculitis [published online ahead of print, 2021 October 27]. J Cosmet Dermatol 2021. https://doi.org/10.1111/jocd.14568. 10.1111/jocd.14568.
[32] Mücke VT, Knop V, Mücke MM, et al. First description of immune complex vasculitis after COVID-19 vaccination with BNT162b2: a case report. BMC Infect Dis 2021;21(1):958. https://doi.org/10.1186/s12879-021-06655-x. Published 2021 September 16.
[33] Conticini E, d'Alessandro M, Bergantini L, et al. Relapse of microscopic polyangiitis after vaccination against COVID-19: a case report. J Med Virol 2021;93(12):6439—41. https://doi.org/10.1002/jmv.27192.
[34] Hakroush S, Tampe B. Case report: ANCA-associated vasculitis presenting with rhabdomyolysis and pauci-immune crescentic glomerulonephritis after Pfizer-BioNTech COVID-19 mRNA vaccination. Front Immunol 2021;12:762006. https://doi.org/10.3389/fimmu.2021.762006. Published 2021 September 30.
[35] Cohen SR, Prussick L, Kahn JS, et al. Leukocytoclastic vasculitis flare following the COVID-19 vaccine. Int J Dermatol 2021;60(8):1032—3. https://doi.org/10.1111/ijd.15623.
[36] Takeyama R, Fukuda K, Kouzaki Y, et al. Intracerebral hemorrhage due to vasculitis following COVID-19 vaccination: a case report [published online ahead of print, 2021 November 16]. Acta Neurochir 2021:1—5. https://doi.org/10.1007/s00701-021-05038-0.
[37] Shakoor MT, Birkenbach MP, Lynch M. ANCA-associated vasculitis following Pfizer-BioNTech COVID-19 vaccine. Am J Kidney Dis 2021;78(4):611—3. https://doi.org/10.1053/j.ajkd.2021.06.016.
[38] Zavala-Flores E, Salcedo-Matienzo J, Quiroz-Alva A, Berrocal-Kasay A. Side effects and flares risk after SARS-CoV-2 vaccination in patients with systemic lupus erythematosus [published online ahead of print, 2021 November 16]. Clin Rheumatol 2021:1—9. https://doi.org/10.1007/s10067-021-05980-5.
[39] Kreuter A, Burmann SN, Burkert B, Oellig F, Michalowitz AL. Transition of cutaneous into systemic lupus erythematosus following adenoviral vector-based SARS-CoV-2 vaccination. J Eur Acad Dermatol Venereol 2021;35(11):e733—5. https://doi.org/10.1111/jdv.17514.

[40] Kreuter A, Licciardi-Fernandez MJ, Burmann SN, et al. Induction and exacerbation of subacute cutaneous lupus erythematosus following mRNA-based or adenoviral vector-based SARS-CoV-2 vaccination [published online ahead of print, 2021 July 22]. Clin Exp Dermatol 2021. https://doi.org/10.1111/ced.14858. 10.1111/ced.14858.
[41] Joseph AK, Chong BF. Subacute cutaneous lupus erythematosus flare triggered by COVID-19 vaccine [published online ahead of print, 2021 August 29]. Dermatol Ther 2021:e15114. https://doi.org/10.1111/dth.15114.
[42] Patil S, Patil A. Systemic lupus erythematosus after COVID-19 vaccination: a case report. J Cosmet Dermatol 2021;20(10):3103–4. https://doi.org/10.1111/jocd.14386.
[43] Niebel D, Ralser-Isselstein V, Jaschke K, Braegelmann C, Bieber T, Wenzel J. Exacerbation of subacute cutaneous lupus erythematosus following vaccination with BNT162b2 mRNA vaccine. Dermatol Ther 2021;34(4). https://doi.org/10.1111/dth.15017.
[44] Maye JA, Chong HP, Rajagopal V, Petchey W. Reactivation of IgA vasculitis following COVID-19 vaccination. BMJ Case Rep 2021;14(11). https://doi.org/10.1136/bcr-2021-247188. Published 2021 November 30.
[45] Fritzen M, Funchal GDG, Luiz MO, Durigon GS. Leukocytoclastic vasculitis after exposure to COVID-19 vaccine [published online ahead of print, 2021 November 10]. An Bras Dermatol 2021;S0365–0596(21):00274–9. https://doi.org/10.1016/j.abd.2021.09.003.
[46] Kondo M, Yamanaka K. Possible HSP reactivation post-COVID-19 vaccination and booster. Clin Case Rep 2021;9(10). https://doi.org/10.1002/ccr3.5032. Published 2021 October 28.
[47] Dicks AB, Gray BH. Images in Vascular Medicine: leukocytoclastic vasculitis after COVID-19 vaccine booster [published online ahead of print, 2021 November 1]. Vasc Med 2021. https://doi.org/10.1177/1358863X211055507. 1358863X211055507.
[48] Bencharattanaphakhi R, Rerknimitr P. Sinovac COVID-19 vaccine-induced cutaneous leukocytoclastic vasculitis. JAAD Case Rep 2021;18:1–3. https://doi.org/10.1016/j.jdcr.2021.10.002.
[49] Kar BR, Singh BS, Mohapatra L, Agrawal I. Cutaneous small-vessel vasculitis following COVID-19 vaccine. J Cosmet Dermatol 2021;20(11):3382–3. https://doi.org/10.1111/jocd.14452.
[50] Naitlho A, Lahlou W, Bourial A, et al. A rare case of Henoch-Schönlein purpura following a COVID-19 vaccine-case report [published online ahead of print, 2021 September 8]. SN Compr Clin Med 2021:1–4. https://doi.org/10.1007/s42399-021-01025-9.
[51] Badier L, Toledano A, Porel T, et al. IgA vasculitis in adult patient following vaccination by ChadOx1 nCoV-19. Autoimmun Rev 2021;20(11):102951. https://doi.org/10.1016/j.autrev.2021.102951.
[52] Okuda S, Hirooka Y, Sugiyama M. Propylthiouracil-induced antineutrophil cytoplasmic antibody-associated vasculitis after COVID-19 vaccination. Vaccines 2021;9(8):842. https://doi.org/10.3390/vaccines9080842. Published 2021 July 31.
[53] Dash S, Behera B, Sethy M, Mishra J, Garg S. COVID-19 vaccine-induced urticarial vasculitis. Dermatol Ther 2021;34(5). https://doi.org/10.1111/dth.15093. e15093.
[54] Vassallo C, Boveri E, Brazzelli V, et al. Cutaneous lymphocytic vasculitis after administration of COVID-19 mRNA vaccine. Dermatol Ther 2021;34(5). https://doi.org/10.1111/dth.15076. e15076.
[55] Gillion V, Jadoul M, Demoulin N, Aydin S, Devresse A. Granulomatous vasculitis after the AstraZeneca anti-SARS-CoV-2 vaccine. Kidney Int 2021;100(3):706–7. https://doi.org/10.1016/j.kint.2021.06.033.
[56] Vera-Lastra O, Lucas-Hernández A, Ruiz-Montiel JE, et al. Myopericarditis as a manifestation of long COVID syndrome. Cureus November 10, 2021;13(11). https://doi.org/10.7759/cureus.19449. e19449.
[57] Ashaari S, Sohaib HA, Bolger K. A case report: symptomatic pericarditis post-COVID-19 vaccination. Eur Heart J Case Rep 2021;5(10). https://doi.org/10.1093/ehjcr/ytab375. Published 2021 September 24.
[58] Nevet A. Acute myocarditis associated with anti-COVID-19 vaccination. Clin Exp Vaccine Res 2021;10(2):196–7. https://doi.org/10.7774/cevr.2021.10.2.196.
[59] 59-Patrignani A, Schicchi N, Calcagnoli F, et al. Acute myocarditis following Comirnaty vaccination in a healthy man with previous SARS-CoV-2 infection. Radiol Case Rep 2021;16(11):3321–5. https://doi.org/10.1016/j.radcr.2021.07.082.
[60] Alania-Torres E, Morillas-Climent H, García-Escrivá A, et al. Case report: probable myocarditis after covid-19 mRNA vaccine in a patient with arrhythmogenic left ventricular cardiomyopathy. Front Cardiovasc Med 2021;8:759119. https://doi.org/10.3389/fcvm.2021.759119. Published 2021 October 12.
[61] Singh B, Kaur P, Cedeno L, et al. COVID-19 mRNA vaccine and myocarditis. Eur J Case Rep Intern Med 2021;8(7):002681. https://doi.org/10.12890/2021_002681. Published 2021 June 14.

[62] Tate C, Demashkieh L, Hakmeh W. Isolated tachycardia presenting after Pfizer-BioNTech COVID-19 vaccination. Cureus 2021;13(7). https://doi.org/10.7759/cureus.16706. e16706.
[63] Perez Y, Levy ER, Joshi AY, et al. Myocarditis following COVID-19 mRNA vaccine: a case series and incidence rate determination [published online ahead of print, 2021 November 3]. Clin Infect Dis 2021. https://doi.org/10.1093/cid/ciab926.
[64] McLean K, Johnson TJ. Myopericarditis in a previously healthy adolescent male following COVID-19 vaccination: a case report. Acad Emerg Med 2021;28(8):918–21. https://doi.org/10.1111/acem.14322.
[65] Marshall M, Ferguson ID, Lewis P, et al. Symptomatic acute myocarditis in 7 adolescents after Pfizer-BioNTech COVID-19 vaccination. Pediatrics 2021;148(3). https://doi.org/10.1542/peds.2021-052478.
[66] Toida R, Uezono S, Komatsu H, et al. Takotsubo cardiomyopathy after vaccination for coronavirus disease 2019 in a patient on maintenance hemodialysis [published online ahead of print, 2021 November 3]. CEN Case Rep 2021:1–5. https://doi.org/10.1007/s13730-021-00657-z.
[67] Khogali F, Abdelrahman R. Unusual presentation of acute perimyocarditis following SARS-COV-2 mRNA-1237 Moderna vaccination. Cureus 2021;13(7). https://doi.org/10.7759/cureus.16590. Published 2021 July 23.
[68] Ammirati E, Cavalotti C, Milazzo A, et al. Temporal relation between second dose BNT162b2 mRNA Covid-19 vaccine and cardiac involvement in a patient with previous SARS-COV-2 infection. Int J Cardiol Heart Vasc 2021;34:100774. https://doi.org/10.1016/j.ijcha.2021.100774.
[69] Bautista García J, Peña Ortega P, Bonilla Fernández JA, Cárdenes León A, Ramírez Burgos L, Caballero Dorta E. Acute myocarditis after administration of the BNT162b2 vaccine against COVID-19. Rev Esp Cardiol 2021;74(9):812–4. https://doi.org/10.1016/j.rec.2021.04.005.
[70] Bragazzi NL, Hejly A, Watad A, Adawi M, Amital H, Shoenfeld Y. ASIA syndrome and endocrine autoimmune disorders. Best Pract Res Clin Endocrinol Metabol 2020;34(1):101412. https://doi.org/10.1016/j.beem.2020.101412.
[71] Pujol A, Gómez LA, Gallegos C, et al. Thyroid as a target of adjuvant autoimmunity/inflammatory syndrome due to mRNA-based SARS-CoV2 vaccination: from Graves' disease to silent thyroiditis [published online ahead of print, 2021 November 18]. J Endocrinol Invest 2021:1–8. https://doi.org/10.1007/s40618-021-01707-0.
[72] Siolos A, Gartzonika K, Tigas S. Thyroiditis following vaccination against COVID-19: report of two cases and review of the literature. Metabol Open 2021;12:100136. https://doi.org/10.1016/j.metop.2021.100136.
[73] Yamamoto K, Mashiba T, Takano K, et al. A case of exacerbation of subclinical Hyperthyroidism after first administration of BNT162b2 mRNA COVID-19 vaccine. Vaccines 2021;9(10):1108. https://doi.org/10.3390/vaccines9101108. Published 2021 September 29.
[74] Murvelashvili N, Tessnow A. A case of Hypophysitis following immunization with the mRNA-1273 SARS-CoV-2 vaccine. J Investig Med High Impact Case Rep 2021;9. https://doi.org/10.1177/23247096211043386. 23247096211043386.
[75] Ratnayake GM, Dworakowska D, Grossman AB. Can COVID-19 immunisation cause subacute thyroiditis? [published online ahead of print, 2021 July 17]. Clin Endocrinol 2021. https://doi.org/10.1111/cen.14555.
[76] Bornemann C, Woyk K, Bouter C. Case report: two cases of subacute thyroiditis following SARS-CoV-2 vaccination. Front Med 2021;8:737142. https://doi.org/10.3389/fmed.2021.737142. Published 2021 August 24.
[77] Vera-Lastra O, Ordinola Navarro A, Cruz Domiguez MP, Medina G, Sánchez Valadez TI, Jara LJ. Two cases of Graves' disease following SARS-CoV-2 vaccination: an autoimmune/inflammatory syndrome induced by adjuvants. Thyroid 2021;31(9):1436–9. https://doi.org/10.1089/thy.2021.0142.
[78] Patel KR, Cunnane ME, Deschler DG. SARS-CoV-2 vaccine-induced subacute thyroiditis [published online ahead of print, 2021 September 9]. Am J Otolaryngol 2021;43(1):103211. https://doi.org/10.1016/j.amjoto.2021.103211.
[79] Franquemont S, Galvez J. Subacute thyroiditis after mRNA vaccine for Covid-19. J Endocr Soc April-May;5(-Suppl. ment_1):A956–7. https://doi.org/10.1210/jendso/bvab048.1954.
[80] Oyibo SO. Subacute thyroiditis after receiving the adenovirus-vectored vaccine for coronavirus disease (COVID-19). Cureus 2021;13(6). https://doi.org/10.7759/cureus.16045. Published 2021 June 29.
[81] Sahin Tekin M, Saylısoy S, Yorulmaz G. Subacute thyroiditis following COVID-19 vaccination in a 67-year-old male patient: a case report [published online ahead of print, 2021 July 1]. Hum Vaccines Immunother 2021:1–3. https://doi.org/10.1080/21645515.2021.1947102.

[82] İremli BG, Sendur SN, Ünlütürk U. Three cases of subacute thyroiditis following SARS-CoV-2 vaccine: postvaccination ASIA syndrome. J Clin Endocrinol Metab 2021;106(9):2600–5. https://doi.org/10.1210/clinem/dgab373.

[83] Plaza-Enriquez L, Khatiwada P, Sanchez-Valenzuela M, Sikha A. A case report of subacute thyroiditis following mRNA COVID-19 vaccine. Case Rep Endocrinol 2021;2021. https://doi.org/10.1155/2021/8952048. 8952048.

[84] Sigstad E, Grøholt KK, Westerheim O. Subacute thyroiditis after vaccination against SARS-CoV-2. Subakutt tyreoiditt etter vaksinering mot SARS-CoV-2. Tidsskr Nor Laegeforen 2021;141(2021–14). https://doi.org/10.4045/tidsskr.21.0554. 10.4045/tidsskr.21.0554. Published 2021 Oct 11.

[85] Grieco T, Maddalena P, Sernicola A, et al. Cutaneous adverse reactions after COVID-19 vaccines in a cohort of 2740 Italian subjects: an observational study [published online ahead of print, 2021 October 7]. Dermatol Ther 2021. https://doi.org/10.1111/dth.15153.

[86] Bellinato F, Maurelli M, Gisondi P, Girolomoni G. Cutaneous adverse reactions associated with SARS-CoV-2 vaccines. J Clin Med November 2021;10(22):5344. https://doi.org/10.3390/jcm10225344. Published online 2021 November 16.

[87] Pérez-López I, Moyano-Bueno D, Ruiz-Villaverde R. Bullous pemphigoid and COVID-19 vaccine [published online ahead of print, 2021 Oct 21]. Med Clin 2021;157(10):e333–4. https://doi.org/10.1016/j.medcle.2021.05.004.

[88] Thomas J, Thomas G, Chatim A, et al. Chronic spontaneous urticaria after COVID-19 vaccine. Cureus 2021;13(9). https://doi.org/10.7759/cureus.18102. Published 2021 September 19.

[89] Dash S, Sirka CS, Mishra S, Viswan P. COVID-19 vaccine-induced Stevens-Johnson syndrome [published online ahead of print, 2021 June 3]. Clin Exp Dermatol 2021;46:1615–7. https://doi.org/10.1111/ced.14784. 10.1111/ced.14784.

[90] Cinotti E, Perrot JL, Bruzziches F, et al. Eosinophilic dermatosis after AstraZeneca COVID-19 vaccination [published online ahead of print, 2021 November 9]. J Eur Acad Dermatol Venereol 2021;36:e171–2. https://doi.org/10.1111/jdv.17806.

[91] Saibene AM, Alliata A, Cozzi AT, et al. Erythema multiforme major following SARS-CoV-2 vaccine. Clin Case Rep 2021;9(10). https://doi.org/10.1002/ccr3.4947. Published 2021 October 13.

[92] Onn PY, Chang CL. Lichenoid cutaneous skin eruption and associated systemic inflammatory response following Pfizer-BioNTech mRNA COVID-19 vaccine administration. Respirol Case Rep 2021;9(11). https://doi.org/10.1002/rcr2.860. Published 2021 October 4.

[93] Elboraey MO, Essa EESF. Stevens-Johnson syndrome post second dose of Pfizer COVID-19 vaccine: a case report. Oral Surg Oral Med Oral Pathol Oral Radiol 2021;132(4):e139–42. https://doi.org/10.1016/j.oooo.2021.06.019.

[94] Majid I, Mearaj S. Sweet syndrome after Oxford-AstraZeneca COVID-19 vaccine (AZD1222) in an elderly female [published online ahead of print, 2021 September 29]. Dermatol Ther 2021. https://doi.org/10.1111/dth.15146.

[95] Lehmann M, Schorno P, Hunger RE, et al. New onset of mainly guttate psoriasis after COVID-19 vaccination: a case report. J Eur Acad Dermatol Venereol 2021;35(11):e752–5. https://doi.org/10.1111/jdv.17561.

[96] Marcantonio-Santa Cruz OY, Vidal-Navarro A, Pesqué D, et al. Pityriasis rosea developing after COVID-19 vaccination. J Eur Acad Dermatol Venereol 2021;35(11):e721–2. https://doi.org/10.1111/jdv.17498.

[97] Elbæk MV, Vinding GR, Jemec GBE. Darier's disease flare following COVID-19 vaccine. Case Rep Dermatol 2021;13(2):432–6. https://doi.org/10.1159/000517256. Published 2021 August 18.

[98] Kong J, Cuevas-Castillo F, Nassar M, et al. Bullous drug eruption after second dose of mRNA-1273 (Moderna) COVID-19 vaccine: case report. J Infect Public Health October 2021;14(10):1392–4. https://doi.org/10.1016/j.jiph.2021.06.021.

[99] Cazzato G, Paolo Romita P, Foti C, et al. Purpuric skin rash in a patient undergoing Pfizer-BioNTech COVID-19 vaccination: histological evaluation and perspectives. Vaccines July 8, 2021;9(7):760. https://doi.org/10.3390/vaccines9070760.

[100] Guénin SH, Kresch M, Elbogen E, Lebwohl MG. Cutaneous reaction reported after third Moderna COVID-19 vaccine. JAAD Case Rep December 2021;18:49–50. https://doi.org/10.1016/j.jdcr.2021.10.017.

[101] Bianchi L, Biondi F, Hansel K, et al. Skin tests in urticaria/angioedema and flushing to Pfizer-BioNTech SARS-CoV-2 vaccine: limits of intradermal testing. Allergy April 22, 2021. https://doi.org/10.1111/all.14839.

[102] Burlando M, Herzum A, Cozzani E, Parodi A. Acute urticarial rash after COVID-19 vaccination containing Polysorbate 80. Clin Exp Vaccine Res September 2021;10(3):298–300. https://doi.org/10.7774/cevr.2021.10.3.298.

[103] Adya KA, Inamadar AC, Albadri W. Post Covid-19 vaccination papulovesicular pityriasis rosea-like eruption in a young male. Dermatol Ther September 2021;34(5). https://doi.org/10.1111/dth.15040.

[104] Cyrenne BM, Al-Mohammedi F, DeKoven JG, et al. Pityriasis rosea-like eruptions following vaccination with BNT162b2 mRNA COVID-19 Vaccine. J Eur Acad Dermatol Venereol May 29, 2021. https://doi.org/10.1111/jdv.17342. 10.1111/jdv.17342.

[105] Leerunyakul K, Pakornphadungsit K, Suchonwanit P. Case report: pityriasis rosea-like eruption following COVID-19 vaccination. Front Med September 7, 2021;8:752443. https://doi.org/10.3389/fmed.2021.752443.

[106] Favaloro EJ. Laboratory testing for suspected COVID-19 vaccine-induced (immune) thrombotic thrombocytopenia. Int J Lab Hematol 2021;43(4):559–70. https://doi.org/10.1111/ijlh.13629.

[107] Favaloro EJ, Pasalic L, Lippi G. Review and evolution of guidelines for diagnosis of COVID-19 vaccine induced thrombotic thrombocytopenia (VITT) [published online ahead of print, 2021 October 29]. Clin Chem Lab Med 2021;60. https://doi.org/10.1515/cclm-2021-1039.

[108] Makris M, Pavord S, Lester W, Scully M, Hunt B. Vaccine-induced Immune Thrombocytopenia and Thrombosis (VITT) [published correction appears in Res Pract Thromb Haemost. 2021 Aug 10;5(5):e12585]. Res Pract Thromb Haemost 2021;5(5). https://doi.org/10.1002/rth2.12529. Published 2021 June 1.

[109] Dotan A, Shoenfeld Y. Perspectives on vaccine induced thrombotic thrombocytopenia. J Autoimmun 2021;121:102663. https://doi.org/10.1016/j.jaut.2021.102663.

[110] Lemoine C, Giacobbe AG, Bonifacino E, et al. A case of acquired haemophilia A in a 70-year-old post COVID-19 vaccine [published online ahead of print, 2021 October 28]. Haemophilia 2021. https://doi.org/10.1111/hae.14442.

[111] Costello A, Pandita A, Devitt J. Case report: thrombotic thrombocytopenia after COVID-19 Janssen vaccination. Am Fam Physician 2021;103(11):646–7.

[112] Karabulut K, Andronikashvili A, Kapici AH. Recurrence of thrombotic thrombocytopenic purpura after mRNA-1273 COVID-19 vaccine administered shortly after COVID-19. Case Rep Hematol 2021. https://doi.org/10.1155/2021/4130138. Published 2021 September 13.

[113] Appelbaum J, Arnold DM, Kelton JG, et al. SARS-CoV-2 spike-dependent platelet activation in COVID-19 vaccine-induced thrombocytopenia [published online ahead of print, 2021 November 1]. Blood Adv 2021. https://doi.org/10.1182/bloodadvances.2021005050. bloodadvances.2021005050.

[114] Greinacher A, Thiele T, Warkentin TE, et al. Thrombotic thrombocytopenia after ChAdOx1 nCov-19 vaccination. N Engl J Med 2021;384(22):2092–101. https://doi.org/10.1056/NEJMoa2104840.

[115] Schultz NH, Sørvoll IH, Michelsen AE, et al. Thrombosis and thrombocytopenia after ChAdOx1 nCoV-19 vaccination. N Engl J Med 2021;384(22):2124–30. https://doi.org/10.1056/NEJMoa2104882. Epub ahead of print. PMID: 33835768.

[116] Scully M, Singh D, Lown R, et al. Pathologic antibodies to platelet factor 4 after ChAdOx1 nCoV-19 vaccination. N Engl J Med 2021;384(23):2202–11. https://doi.org/10.1056/NEJMoa2105385.

[117] Mehta PR, Apap Mangion S, Benger M, et al. Cerebral venous sinus thrombosis and thrombocytopenia after COVID-19 vaccination - A report of two UK cases. Brain Behav Immun 2021;1591(21):514–7. https://doi.org/10.1016/j.bbi.2021.04.006.

[118] Tiede A, Sachs UJ, Czwalinna A, et al. Prothrombotic immune thrombocytopenia after COVID-19 vaccine. Blood 2021;138:350–3. https://doi.org/10.1182/blood.2021011958.

[119] See I, Su JR, Lale A, et al. US case reports of cerebral venous sinus thrombosis with thrombocytopenia after Ad26.COV2.S Vaccination, March 2 to April 21, 2021. JAMA 2021. https://doi.org/10.1001/jama.2021.7517.

[120] Vayne C, Rollin J, Gruel Y, et al. PF4 immunoassays in vaccine-induced thrombotic thrombocytopenia. N Engl J Med 2021;385:376–8. https://doi.org/10.1056/NEJMc2106383.

[121] Althaus K, Möller P, Uzun G, et al. Antibody-mediated procoagulant platelets in SARS-CoV-2- vaccination associated immune thrombotic thrombocytopenia. Haematologica 2021;106:2170–9. https://doi.org/10.3324/haematol.2021.279000.

[122] Castelli GP, Pognani C, Sozzi C, et al. Cerebral venous sinus thrombosis associated with thrombocytopenia post-vaccination for COVID-19. Crit Care 2021;25(1):137. https://doi.org/10.1186/s13054-021-03572-y.

[123] Muir KL, Kallam A, Koepsell SA, Gundabolu K. Thrombotic thrombocytopenia after Ad26.COV2.S vaccination. N Engl J Med 2021;384(20):1964–5. https://doi.org/10.1056/NEJMc2105869.

[124] Fernández P, Alaye ML, Chiple MEG, et al. Glomerulopathies after vaccination against COVID-19. Four cases with three different vaccines in Argentina [published online ahead of print, 2021 September 25]. Nefrologia 2021. https://doi.org/10.1016/j.nefro.2021.09.003.

[125] Da Y, Goh GH, Khatri P. A case of membranous nephropathy following Pfizer-BioNTech mRNA vaccination against COVID-19. Kidney Int 2021;100(4):938–9. https://doi.org/10.1016/j.kint.2021.07.016.

[126] Haji Jr N, Ali S, Wahashi EA, et al. Johnson and Johnson COVID-19 vaccination triggering pheochromocytoma multisystem crisis. Cureus 2021;13(9). https://doi.org/10.7759/cureus.18196.

[127] Anupama YJ, Patel RGN, Vankalakunti M. Nephrotic syndrome following ChAdOx1 nCoV-19 vaccine against SARScoV-2. Kidney Int Rep 2021;6(8):2248. https://doi.org/10.1016/j.ekir.2021.06.024.

[128] Lim JH, Han MH, Kim YJ, et al. New-onset nephrotic syndrome after Janssen COVID-19 vaccination: a case report and literature review. J Kor Med Sci 2021;36(30). https://doi.org/10.3346/jkms.2021.36.e218. Published 2021 August 2.

[129] Lebedev L, Sapojnikov M, Wechsler A, et al. Minimal change disease following the Pfizer-BioNTech COVID-19 vaccine. Am J Kidney Dis 2021;78(1):142–5. https://doi.org/10.1053/j.ajkd.2021.03.010.

[130] Maas RJ, Gianotten S, van der Meijden WAG. An additional case of minimal change disease following the Pfizer-BioNTech COVID-19 vaccine. Am J Kidney Dis 2021;78(2):312. https://doi.org/10.1053/j.ajkd.2021.05.003.

[131] D'Agati VD, Kudose S, Bomback AS, et al. Minimal change disease and acute kidney injury following the Pfizer-BioNTech COVID-19 vaccine. Kidney Int 2021;100(2):461–3. https://doi.org/10.1016/j.kint.2021.04.035.

[132] Holzworth A, Couchot P, Cruz-Knight W, Brucculeri M. Minimal change disease following the Moderna mRNA-1273 SARS-CoV-2 vaccine. Kidney Int 2021;100(2):463–4. https://doi.org/10.1016/j.kint.2021.05.007.

[133] Weijers J, Alvarez C, Hermans MMH. Post-vaccinal minimal change disease. Kidney Int 2021;100(2):459–61. https://doi.org/10.1016/j.kint.2021.06.004.

[134] Thappy S, Thalappil SR, Abbarh S, et al. Minimal change disease following the Moderna COVID-19 vaccine: first case report. BMC Nephrol 2021;22(1):376. https://doi.org/10.1186/s12882-021-02583-9.

[135] Leclerc S, Royal V, Lamarche C, Laurin LP. Minimal change disease with severe acute kidney injury following the Oxford-AstraZeneca COVID-19 vaccine: a case report. Am J Kidney Dis 2021;78(4):607–10. https://doi.org/10.1053/j.ajkd.2021.06.008.

[136] Garg RK, Paliwal VK. Spectrum of neurological complications following COVID-19 vaccination [published online ahead of print, 2021 October 31]. Neurol Sci 2021:1–38. https://doi.org/10.1007/s10072-021-05662-9.

[137] Chavez A, Pougnier C. A case of COVID-19 vaccine associated new diagnosis myasthenia gravis. J Prim Care Community Health 2021;12. https://doi.org/10.1177/21501327211051933.

[138] Morehouse ZP, Paulus A, Jasti SA, Bing X. A rare variant of Guillain-Barre syndrome following Ad26.COV2.S vaccination. Cureus 2021;13(9). https://doi.org/10.7759/cureus.18153. Published 2021 September 21.

[139] Permezel F, Borojevic B, Lau S, de Boer HH. Acute disseminated encephalomyelitis (ADEM) following recent Oxford/AstraZeneca COVID-19 vaccination [published online ahead of print, 2021 November 4]. Forensic Sci Med Pathol 2021:1–6. https://doi.org/10.1007/s12024-021-00440-7.

[140] Torrealba-Acosta G, Martin JC, Huttenbach Y, et al. Acute encephalitis, myoclonus and Sweet syndrome after mRNA-1273 vaccine. BMJ Case Rep 2021;14(7). https://doi.org/10.1136/bcr-2021-243173. Published 2021 July 26.

[141] Gao JJ, Tseng HP, Lin CL, et al. Acute transverse myelitis following COVID-19 vaccination. Vaccines 2021;9(9):1008. https://doi.org/10.3390/vaccines9091008. Published 2021 September 10.

[142] Dalwadi V, Hancock D, Ballout AA, Geraci A. Axonal-variant Guillian-Barre syndrome temporally associated with mRNA-based Moderna SARS-CoV-2 vaccine. Cureus 2021;13(9). https://doi.org/10.7759/cureus.18291. Published 2021 September 26.

[143] Finsterer J. Exacerbating Guillain-Barré syndrome eight days after vector-based COVID-19 vaccination. Case Rep Infect Dis 2021. https://doi.org/10.1155/2021/3619131.

[144] Malamud E, Otallah SI, Caress JB, Lapid DJ. Guillain-barré syndrome after COVID-19 vaccination in an adolescent [published online ahead of print, 2021 October 8]. Pediatr Neurol 2021;126:9–10. https://doi.org/10.1016/j.pediatrneurol.2021.10.003.

[145] Fujimori J, Miyazawa K, Nakashima I. Initial clinical manifestation of multiple sclerosis after immunization with the Pfizer-BioNTech COVID-19 vaccine [published online ahead of print, 2021 October 20]. J Neuroimmunol 2021;361:577755. https://doi.org/10.1016/j.jneuroim.2021.577755.

[146] Manea MM, Dragoş D, Enache I, Sirbu AG, Tuta S. Multiple cranial nerve palsies following COVID-19 vaccination-Case report [published online ahead of print, 2021 November 2]. Acta Neurol Scand 2021. https://doi.org/10.1111/ane.13548.

[147] Rela M, Jothimani D, Vij M, Rajakumar A, Rammohan A. Auto-immune hepatitis following COVID vaccination. J Autoimmun 2021;123:102688. https://doi.org/10.1016/j.jaut.2021.102688.

[148] Pan L, Zhang Y, Cui Y, Wu X. Bilateral uveitis after inoculation with COVID-19 vaccine: a case report [published online ahead of print, 2021 September 30]. Int J Infect Dis 2021;113:116–8. https://doi.org/10.1016/j.ijid.2021.09.075.

[149] Ganga K, Solyar AY, Ganga R. Massive cervical lymphadenopathy post-COVID-19 vaccination [published online ahead of print, 2021 October 2]. Ear Nose Throat J 2021. https://doi.org/10.1177/01455613211048984.

[150] Parrino D, Frosolini A, Gallo C, et al. Tinnitus following COVID-19 vaccination: report of three cases [published online ahead of print, 2021 June 13]. Int J Audiol 2021:1–4. https://doi.org/10.1080/14992027.2021.1931969.

[151] Cari L, Fiore P, Naghavi Alhosseini M, et al. Blood clots and bleeding events following BNT162b2 and ChAdOx1 nCoV-19 vaccine: an analysis of European data. J Autoimmun August 2021;122. https://doi.org/10.1016/j.jaut.2021.102685.

CHAPTER

37

The post-COVID syndrome

Soprun Lidiia[1,2], *Natalia Gavrilova*[2,3,4], *Varvara A. Ryabkova*[1,5,6], *Lukashenko Maria*[1] and *Kamaeva Evelina*[1]

[1]Laboratory of the Mosaic of Autoimmunity, Saint Petersburg State University, Saint Petersburg, Russia; [2]Saint Petersburg State University Hospital, Saint Petersburg, Russia; [3]Department of Faculty Therapy, Saint Petersburg State University, Saint Petersburg, Russia; [4]Department of Pulmonology, Scientific Research Institute of Phthisiopulmonology, Saint Petersburg, Russia; [5]Department of Pathology, Saint Petersburg State University, Saint Petersburg, Russia; [6]Pavlov First Saint Petersburg State Medical University, Saint Petersburg, Russia

Long COVID or post-COVID-19 syndrome: background and current case definition

Tracing the history of post-COVID syndrome one could find that as early as in April 2020, newspapers started publishing first-person accounts documenting how challenging recovery from COVID-19 could be (e.g., [1]). On 5 May, the *British Medical Journal* (*BMJ*) published the account of Paul Garner—an infectious diseases professor, who reported suffering seven weeks through a "roller coaster of ill health, extreme emotions and utter exhaustion" [2]. Garner termed it "the Covid 'long tail'" The term "long-haulers" came from Amy Watson, patient convener of "Long haul Covid fighters," and this name has become very popular in mass media. In May 2020, results of the first surveys of COVID-19 prolonged symptoms performed by the team of patients were published [3]. On 9 July, Anthony Fauci, the Director of the US's National Institute of Allergy and Infectious Diseases, and an internationally prominent pandemic advisor, stated "if you look anecdotally, there is no question that there are a considerable number of individuals who have a post-viral syndrome." Fauci mentioned as evidence "chat groups that you just click on and see people who recovered that really do not get back to normal" [4]. Ultimately, in July 2020, peer-reviewed studies started reporting sequelae (cardiological, neurological) even in "mild" COVID-19 [5–7]. By August 2020,

Autoimmunity, COVID-19, Post-COVID19 syndrome and COVID-19 vaccination
https://doi.org/10.1016/B978-0-443-18566-3.00027-X

TABLE 37.1 Case definition proposed for post-COVID-19 syndrome in the scientific literature or by healthcare providers.

Symptoms persisting beyond four weeks after symptom onset suggestive of COVID-19 [8]
Signs and symptoms that develop during or after an infection consistent with COVID-19, continue for more than 12 weeks and are not explained by an alternative diagnosis (NICE guidelines)
Continuing signs/symptoms beyond 4 weeks that can be attributed to COVID-19 infection
Persistent symptoms and/or delayed or long-term complications of SARS-CoV-2 infection beyond 4 weeks from the onset of symptoms [10]
The onset of persistent or recurrent episodes of one or more of the following symptoms, within x* weeks of infection with SARS-CoV-2 and continuing for y* weeks or more (The Royal society)
Post-viral fatigue or chronic fatigue syndrome, systemic exertion intolerance disease (SEID), also known as myalgic encephalomyelitis

WHO met with patients from the LongCovidSOS group and affirmed the need for recognition, research, and rehabilitation. By September 2020, WHO had established the ICD-10 code for the post-COVID-19 condition [8].

WHO reported several definitions, proposed in the literature for post-COVID-19 condition [9]. However, WHO admitted that at this stage, they are unable to come up with a consensus definition of post-COVID-19 condition to be used in all settings and in all patients. Different case definitions for post-COVID-19 syndrome proposed in the scientific literature or by healthcare providers are summarized in Table 37.1. Temporal criteria used to define long COVID-19 varied substantially from 3 to 24 weeks after the acute phase and/or hospital discharge but the most common time point is 12 weeks [11].

Epidemiology

A new coronavirus infection is a zooanthroponous respiratory infection caused by the SARS-CoV-2 coronavirus. The natural reservoir of the SARS-CoV-2 virus, as well as other coronaviruses, are bats. They are the ones that cause human infections after circulation in host animals: civets, camels, and lizards [12,13]. Genetic evolutionary analysis of SARS-CoV-2 has shown that this virus is genetically related to bat coronaviruses [14]. Mammals that eat bats can serve as an additional reservoir, with further distribution among humans. Phylogenetic studies of the isolated strains have shown that the genomic sequences of viruses found in bats are 99% identical to those isolated from patients with COVID-19. The genetic sequence of SARS-CoV-2 is similar to the sequence of SARS-CoV by at least 79% [15].

There are conflicting data on the incidence of post-COVID-19 complications. It seems rational to consider the early clinical symptoms (4—12 weeks after acute COVID-19) as a manifestation of the subacute course of the disease and only beyond that time consider existing symptoms as a manifestation of post-COVID syndrome [10]. Different studies give different numbers of patients who have at least one symptom after recovering from COVID-19: more than 80% in the Italian study [16], 63% in Spain and China [17,18], 32% in the United States [19]. Although the persisting symptoms and complications are mostly seen in survivors of severe illness, long-term effects are not infrequently described in people with mild infections that do not require hospitalization [20]. However, it has not yet been established how gender, age, ethnicity, underlying health conditions, viral dose, or progression of COVID-19 significantly affect the risk of developing long-term effects of COVID-19.

Susceptibility to the causative agent of the virus is high among all population groups, there are no gender differences. The distribution of COVID-19 among the population of different countries has common patterns and is higher among older people, among people with impaired immunity and the presence of chronic diseases, in which the frequency of deaths also increases [21].

Sick children are one of the significant sources of the spread of COVID-19 [22]. Despite the fact that the incidence in the age group from 0 to 19 years is low in comparison with other age groups, children are more often infected from adults than adults from children and are most often carriers and asymptomatic carriers of the disease.

COVID-19 disease risk groups include

- people aged 65 and older;
- patients with chronic diseases (diseases of the respiratory system, cardiovascular system, oncological diseases, diabetes mellitus);
- employees of medical organizations.

The mortality rate for this infection varies from 0.8% to 4%.

Clinical symptoms of the post-COVID patients

Clinical symptoms of the post-COVID patients can be divided into several groups. Up to date, there are a number of studies, describing follow-up of the patients after the discharge from the hospital and coronavirus treatment. The most common complaints, that patients are describing are pulmonological (dyspnea, pain), cardiovascular (tachycardia), neuropsychological (chronic fatigue, memory loss, attention deficit, sleep disturbance), musculoskeletal (arthralgia, myalgia, diffuse pain), as well as immunological (pyrexia, swollen lymph nodes, flu-like symptoms) [23].

Tomar et al. in their study described patients after 14 days (15–50 days) of discharge, where 82% of patients had at least one persistent symptom of the post-COVID. Fatigue (74%) was the highest overall symptom at follow-up, followed by shortness of breath (44%) and muscle weakness (36%) [24].

Lopez et al. performed a meta-analysis of 18,251 publications, of which 15 met the inclusion criteria. They assessed the prevalence of 55 long-term effects, conducted 21 meta-analyzes, and included 47,910 patients (age 17–87 years). It has been estimated that 80% of infected patients with SARS-CoV-2 have developed one or more long-term symptoms. The five most common symptoms were fatigue (58%), headache (44%), impaired attention (27%), hair loss (25%), and shortness of breath (24%) [20].

In another systematic review, Fu et al. examined the key clinical characteristics of COVID-19 patients. The report summarized a total of 43 studies and included 3600 patients. The most common clinical signs associated with COVID-19 included fever (83.3%), cough (60.3%), fatigue (38.0%), sputum hyperproduction (30%), shortness of breath (30%), myalgia (30%), sore throat (16.7% and 11.2% in critical and noncritical cases, respectively), and headache (11.3% and 11.9% in critical and noncritical cases, respectively). However, research has shown that the majority of COVID-19 patients are asymptomatic [12,25,26].

Fatigue is the most common symptom of long-term and acute COVID-19, which can persist several months after the illness. The causes of prolonged fatigue can be varied. In addition to the dysfunction of cerebral blood flow autoregulation discussed below, the possibility of persistence of a COVID infection with the development of low-grade inflammation can be possible. An increase in the concentration of pro-inflammatory cytokines can lead to multiple organ dysfunction, including chronic fatigue and cognitive dysfunction [24].

Symptoms seen in COVID-19 survivors are somewhat similar to chronic fatigue syndrome (CFS), which includes severe disabling fatigue, pain, neurocognitive disability, sleep disturbances, autonomic dysfunction. Myalgic encephalomyelitis (ME) or CFS is a complex and controversial clinical condition with no established causative factors, and 90% of ME/CFS have not been diagnosed. Possible causes of CFS include viruses, immune dysfunction, endocrine metabolic dysfunction, and neuropsychiatric factors. Infectious agents associated with CFS were Epstein–Barr virus, cytomegalovirus, enterovirus, and herpes virus. It is tempting to speculate that SARS-CoV-2 could be added to the list of viral agents that cause ME/CFS [20].

The damage to the striated muscles and myocardial tissues is widespread in these patients and is also one of the leading symptoms of post-COVID. Myalgia and myositis often debut in combination with other immunological syndromes such as arthralgia, headache, subfebrile fever. The heart muscle dysfunction is mainly described as a functional disorder, without signs of ischemia and an increase in cardiomarkers due to the immunological inflammation [24]; however, some authors note the presence of the SARS-CoV-2 virus in the myocardial tissue, without signs of myocarditis [6].

Several neuropsychiatric symptoms, like headache, brain fog, attention deficit, and anosmia, are also quite common. The etiology of neuropsychiatric symptoms in patients with COVID-19 is complex and multifactorial. It may be due to a direct consequence of infection, cerebrovascular disease (including hypercoagulability), physiological compromise (hypoxia), drug side effects, and social aspects of the potentially fatal illness. Adults following COVID-19 are at double risk of receiving a new mental health diagnosis. The most common psychiatric conditions were anxiety disorders, insomnia, and dementia. Sleep disturbances can also contribute to the manifestation of mental disorders [20].

Shortness of breath and cough is one of the most common complaints that are described in up to 20% of patients with the post-COVID syndrome. Abnormalities in CT scans of the lungs persisted in patients even for 60–100 days after the initial visit. In a follow-up study in China of noncritical cases of hospitalized COVID-19 patients, radiographic changes persisted in nearly two-thirds of patients 90 days after discharge [15]. Although most of the available studies do not include baseline pulmonary dysfunction or radiographic abnormalities, results indicate improvement or resolution of abnormal CT findings. However, residual radiological findings or impaired pulmonary function require additional study of their clinical significance and long-term consequences [20].

Pathophysiological hypotheses of the post-COVID syndrome

Novel coronavirus infection and autoimmunity

The SARS-CoV-2 virus is a single-stranded RNA coronavirus that is widespread in nature [13]. Infection occurs mainly by airborne droplets and the incubation period is, on average,

3–7 days. The virus enters the human cells through binding to angiotensin-converting enzyme 2 (ACE2) receptors. Depending on the mode of transmission of the virus and entry, SARS-CoV-2 mainly affects the respiratory system, causing lung pathology, such as alveolar damage, interstitial fibrosis, and lung tissue infiltration [27]. ACE2 receptors are represented in various human tissues and, therefore, the spectrum of complications can also be quite diverse [28,29]. Besides, the ACE2 enzyme exists in the soluble form, which would potentially bind to SARS-CoV-2 spike proteins with antigen formation [30]. If formed antibodies target the ACE2 cellular enzyme, all organs and tissues that have ACE2 receptors would be affected.

The immune response to SARS-CoV-2 can be hypertrophied, leading to the development of a cytokine storm and various autoimmune complications, as well as immunothrombosis [24,27]. One of the possible explanations for this hyperactive immune response can also be a molecular mimicry, where a foreign antigen can induce immune cells against the autoantigen caused by the similarity of the sequences of foreign and auto-peptides. It is known that molecular mimicry is implicated in many diseases such as multiple sclerosis and Guillain-Barré syndrome. The first study called attention to the possibility of the cross-reactivity in the case of COVID-19 infection reported a vast sharing of SARS-CoV-2 spike glycoprotein—which is a major antigen of the virus with human surfactant-related proteins. It is assumed that this mechanism might explain the immunopathology associated with the coronavirus infection that leads to severe SARS-CoV2-associated lung diseases [31]. Further analysis of peptide sharing between SARS-CoV-2 and mammalian species revealed massive overlap between spike glycoprotein and, substantially, humans and mice proteomes. Remarkable that such organisms can develop pathologic consequences of SARS-CoV-2 infection [31]. In support of this hypothesis, Kanduc in her research described 460 specific human peptides matching with immunoreactive viral epitopes [31]. These peptides are involved in metabolic, developmental, and regulatory functions and may be possible targets of autoimmunity in SARS-CoV-2 infection, implied in pregnancy dysfunctions, pulmonary, neurological, cardiac, and vascular disorders [14,32]. The author suggests that patients' sera can be tested for antibodies against these proteins for surveillance of patients in the post-COVID period, which might be useful for future scientific and clinical investigations.

Various autoantibodies have been described in COVID-19 patients that possibly contribute to the severity and complications of COVID-19. The first complications were associated with the occurrence of Guillain-Barré syndrome in patients with COVID-19. Lucchese et al. in their study looked for the presence of similarities between SARS-CoV-2 peptide sequences and human autoantigens associated with Guillain-Barré syndrome. They found a common immunogenic sequence between SARS-CoV-2 and heat shock proteins HSP90B, HSP90B2, and HSP60 [33]. These autoantibodies are implicated in many autoimmune neurological diseases that support this hypothesis [27]. Mohheadkar et al. have used computational techniques to identify proteins that may act as autoantigens in COVID-19 patients. Searching for sequence homology between human proteins and SARS-CoV-2 they identified four candidate proteins. These are heat shock protein A5 (HSPA5), titin, ryanodine receptor 2 (RYR2), which have sequence homology with spike and heat shock proteins alpha family class B member 1 (HSP90AB1) [34]. Further investigation of potential trigger proteins could provide useful information in the diagnosis and treatment of these patients.

"Traditional" autoantibodies are common in post-COVID patients. The most widespread are antinuclear antibodies (33%−50%), antiphospholipid antibodies (24%−57%), antibodies to TNF-alpha (10.2%) [35]. The antibodies against antigens of the autonomic nervous system may also play an important role. The most promising candidates are antibodies against adrenergic (α1, α2, β1, β2) receptors, muscarinic (M1−M5) acetylcholine receptors, endothelin A receptor, and angiotensin II receptor type 1. It should be noted that besides to the isolation of these autoantibodies, it is also necessary to establish their functional activity. Wallukat et al. examined occurrence of functionally active autoantibodies targeting G-protein coupled receptors in 31 patients with persisted post-COVID-19 symptoms [36]. The study showed an unexpectedly high amount of these autoantibodies, between two and seven different functional autoantibodies were identified in all 31 investigated patients. Moreover, β2-adrenoceptor and the muscarinic M2-receptor were found in almost all examined patients, it is remarkable that such a combination has already been reported before in sera of patients suffering from coronavirus-independent fatigue syndrome [37], PoTS and dysautonomia [38]. Autoantibodies against the angiotensin II AT1 receptor and the angiotensin 1-7 MAS receptor were present in 90% cases which can explain vasoactive processes involved in pathogenesis of post-COVID-19. The study of both the presence of autoantibodies and their activity can provide an understanding of associated neurological, cardiovascular disorders, microvascular, and endothelial complications.

In a small study of nine COVID-19 patients, five had autoantibodies for at least seven months. Interestingly, that autoantibodies were detected in 5/5 patients with reported persistent symptoms and 2/4 without continued symptoms [39].

Autoantibodies that targeted immune-relevant proteins such as cytokines (e.g., type I interferons), chemokines or their receptors, as well as particular leukocyte subsets (B cells, T cells, natural killer cells, and monocytes) have been found in acute COVID-19 in another study. These antibodies were functional, not just innocent bystanders: they had immunomodulatory effects in vitro and were associated with virological and immune parameters in vivo. Immune-targeting autoantibodies exacerbate disease severity in a mouse model of SARS-CoV-2 infection. If such autoantibodies persist, they can be partly responsible for the development of post-COVID-19 syndrome [40].

The role of small fiber neuropathy in the development of post-COVID syndrome

There is a hypothesis that a combination of autoimmune, hemodynamic, and neurological complications leads to the development of post-COVID syndrome. There are studies that describe the dysfunction of both central and peripheral nervous systems in this kind of patients [41]. Single cases of encephalitis or encephalomyelitis are evaluated in the setting of a new coronavirus infection [42]. However, data on the detection of SARS-CoV-2 in CSF are not very reliable [43]. Many authors believe that the virus did not persist in the central nervous system, if the blood−brain barrier was not permeable [5,44,45].

Autoimmune lesions of the peripheral nervous system, on the other hand, can play a very important role in the further development of post-COVID syndrome. There are single cases of Guillain-Barré syndrome and necrotizing autoimmune myositis associated with SARS-CoV-2 infection [41]. However, there might be a more serious and complicated lesion of the peripheral nervous system, that can lead to a large number of complications. This disease is called small fiber neuropathy (SFN). As a result of immunological inflammation, the nerve fibers of the smallest diameter (A-delta and C-types), which innervate the skin, mucous membranes and internal organs, may develop a dysfunction. These unmyelinated and low myelinated fibers are among the most sensitive to damaging factors and, apparently, suffer from the development of a wide range of metabolic, immunological, toxic. and infectious conditions. Given that these changes cannot be evaluated during standard electroneuromyography, SFN may remain unrecognized by both doctors and patients [27,46].

The ubiquitous prevalence of this type of nerve in the body leads to a wide and varied spectrum of symptoms. The main clinical manifestations include common pain syndromes and dysautonomia. Since small nerve fibers transmit pain impulses, pain, paresthesia, and allodynia are very typical for these patients. It is worth noting that numbness should not be observed with isolated SFN. Autonomic dysfunction includes diverse symptoms from the cardiovascular, urinary system, gastrointestinal tract, skin, and mucous membranes. Due to the wide range of varied symptoms, the diagnosis of SFN can be difficult to establish.

The role of macro- and microcirculation disorders in the pathogenesis of post-COVID syndrome

Various disorders of macro- and microcirculation are often observed in patients with post-COVID syndrome and can significantly worsen the quality of life of patients. Microcirculation disorders can manifest in the form of thrombosis and endotheliitis, which are probably associated with both the activation of neutrophils and platelets, and with the impaired innervation of the microvessels due to the SFN development. These complications can lead to the development of ground glass opacities in lungs and prolonged hypoxia, as well as Kawasaki disease in children [24]. There are also hypotheses that it may be associated with cognitive impairment and multisystemic inflammatory syndrome. One of the methods for diagnosing such conditions is laser Doppler flowmetry. During this study, an expansion of the microvascular bed may be revealed, which can be interpreted as manifestations of acute inflammation or as paretic vasodilation due to the denervation [47]. The role of the microcirculatory disorders is significantly understudied and may be underestimated in the post-COVID patients.

The most significant cardiovascular dysfunction at the macrolevel is the development of orthostatic disorders. Orthostatic hypotension and postural orthostatic tachycardia are common complications in the post-COVID patients and may be evaluated during the active or passive orthostatic tests. In his paper, Novak described a COVID-19 patient who developed chronic fatigue, orthostatic dysfunction and brain fog, corresponding to the Orthostatic Hypoperfusion Syndrome (OCHOS), a form of orthostatic intolerance, as well as painful SFN with a good response to immunotherapy [41]. The development of such macro and microcirculatory disorders can be important in the development of the post-COVID patients and may contribute to the development of such common complaints as chronic fatigue, tachycardia, and cognitive deficit (Fig. 37.1).

1. ACE2 receptors are widely distributed in various human tissues that might be affected by anti-ACE2 antibodies.

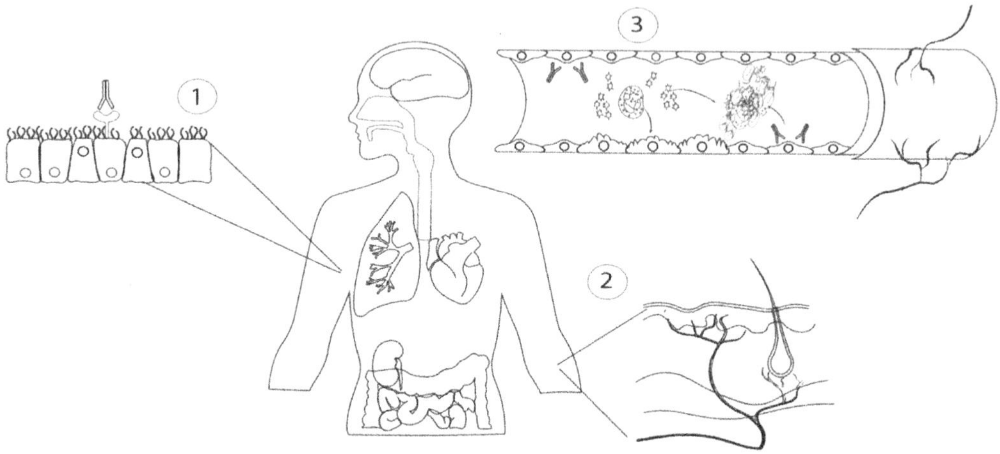

FIGURE 37.1 Pathophysiological hypotheses of the clinical symptoms in post COVID syndrome.

2. SFN due to ubiquitous prevalence of this type of nerve may lead to pain syndromes and dysautonomia.
3. Macro- and microcirculation disorders include thrombosis and endotheliitis due to activation of neutrophils and platelets and presence of antiphospholipid antibodies, impaired innervation of the microvessels due to the SFN and antiautonomic nervous system antibodies what might contribute to the development of chronic fatigue, tachycardia, and cognitive deficit.

Differential diagnosis

As mentioned earlier, the manifestations of post-COVID syndrome can be divided into several groups, and, depending on the symptom, differential diagnosis of various manifestations of long COVID can be carried out. For example, chest pain and coughing are common. These symptoms do not have a broad differential meaning, since diseases that cause similar symptoms (bronchitis, bacterial pneumonia) do not fundamentally differ in drug therapy.

According to Tomar et al., fatigue is the most frequent manifestation of this condition, which allows us to simultaneously identify the similarities between it and various autoimmune diseases and at the same time draw a number of differences with such diseases as fibromyalgia, Guillain-Barré syndrome, and others. Also, the differential diagnosis of post-COVID syndrome and chronic fatigue syndrome (as well as myalgia, arthralgia) in the future may provide a new understanding of the common pathophysiology of these conditions [48].

The presence of headaches in patients undergoing COVID can also be a starting point in the differential diagnosis of post-COVID and other neurological conditions. The putative pathophysiological basis of pain in this case is glymphatic dysfunction arising from the accumulation of toxins in the central nervous system [49]. It is not completely clear whether the effectiveness of this procedure in some patients can be associated with an increase in the flow of glymphatic fluid and clearance of interstitial fluid, and how significant a differential value may be of headache.

One of the most important differential decisions must be made between post-COVID and various pathological conditions of the cardiovascular system, since one of the most common cardiac manifestations is orthostatic hypotension and postural orthostatic tachycardia [41]. For example, a symptom of orthostatic hypotension can often be a manifestation of such diseases as atherosclerosis, anemia of various origins, Addison's disease, etc [50]. Postural tachycardia is extremely rare in diseases of the cardiovascular system; however, if the diagnosis is inaccurate, it can be easily confused with the usual tachycardia that occurs in dangerous conditions such as heart attack and heart failure. As for microcirculation disorders, in this aspect, post-COVID resembles various vascular autoimmune diseases. In the review by Leif Østergaard, the issues of damage to the endothelium and vascular pericytes as a result of the effect of the virus on the body are deeply covered. The author also notes that the pathophysiology of these processes is similar to the development of immunocomplex vasculitis of small vessels, such as Schönlein-Henoch purpura and anti-C1q vasculitis [51].

Differential diagnostics of cognitive impairments of the brain stands a bit apart. Brain fog is also common in various depressive disorders, bipolar disorder, and schizophrenia. L Sher notes that persistent psychiatric symptoms in COVID-19 survivors, such as depression, anxiety, posttraumatic symptoms, and cognitive impairment, can confuse the picture of independent psychiatric illness [52]. The author also notes that these conditions enhance the development of suicidal thoughts and behavior in this cohort of patients. This fact requires an accurate differential diagnosis of post-COVID from other psychiatric diseases, since the approaches of therapy will differ in each case [12,27,28].

Conclusion

Post-COVID syndrome is a multifactorial condition characterized by a combination of neurological, autoimmune, cardiovascular factors as well as psychological stress and neuro-endocrine dysfunction. The most common complaints include shortness of breath, pain syndrome, tachycardia, flu-like syndrome, chronic fatigue, impaired attention, memory, and sleep. These symptoms can develop within 2–4 weeks after acute novel coronavirus infection and persist for many months. The principles of therapy include, first of all, a multidisciplinary approach and treatment of autoimmune disorders, which can play a key role in the pathogenesis of post-COVID syndrome. Intravenous immunoglobulins in combination with other immunomodulatory techniques can enable millions of patients around the world to improve their quality of life and return to normal activities.

References

[1] Lowenstein F. We need to talk about what coronavirus recoveries look like. The New York Times. 2020. 13 April. Available from: https://www.nytimes.com/2020/04/13/opinion/coronavirus-recovery.html.

[2] Garner P. For 7 weeks i have been through a roller coaster of ill health, extreme emotions, and utter exhaustion. The BMJ. 2020. Available from:https://blogs.bmj.com/bmj/2020/05/05/paul-garner-people-who-have-a-more-protracted-illness-need-help-to-understand-and-cope-with-the-constantly-shifting-bizarre-symptoms/.

[3] Assaf G. COVID-19 prolonged symptoms survey—analysis report. 2020. https://patientresearchcovid19.com/research/report-1/.

[4] Fox M. Coronavirus may cause fatigue syndrome, Fauci says. 2020. CNN. 9 July. Available from: HYPERLINK, https://www.cnn.com/world/live-news/coronavirus-pandemic-07-09-20-intl/index.html.

[5] Paterson RW, Brown RL, Benjamin L, Nortley R, Wiethoff S, Bharucha T, Jayaseelan DL, Kumar G, Raftopoulos RE, Zambreanu L, et al. The emerging spectrum of COVID-19 neurology: clinical, radiological and laboratory findings. Brain 2020;143:3104–20.

[6] Puntmann VO, Carerj ML, Wieters I, et al. Outcomes of cardiovascular magnetic resonance imaging in patients recently recovered from coronavirus disease 2019 (COVID-19). JAMA Cardiol 2020;5(11):1265–73. https://doi.org/10.1001/jamacardio.2020.3557.

[7] Tenforde MW. Symptom duration and risk factors for delayed return to usual health among outpatients with COVID-19 in a multistate health care systems network — United States, March–June 2020. Morb Mortal Wkly Rep 2020;69:993–8. https://doi.org/10.15585/mmwr.mm6930e1.

[8] Callard F. Very, very mild: Covid-19 symptoms and illness classification. Somatosphere. 2020. http://somatosphere.net/2020/mild-covid.html/.

[9] World Health Organization. Annual report WHO's response to Covid-19. Geneva: World Health Organization; 2021. 2022. Licence: CC BY-NC-SA 3.0 IGO. HYPERLINK C:/Users/gavrn/Downloads/WHO-SPRP-2021-annual-report.pdf WHO-SPRP-2021-annual-report.pdf.

[10] Nalbandian A, Sehgal K, Gupta A, Madhavan MV, McGroder C, Stevens JS, Cook JR, Nordvig AS, Shalev D, Sehrawat TS, Ahluwalia N, Bikdeli B, Dietz D, Der-Nigoghossian C, Liyanage-Don N, Rosner GF, Bernstein EJ, Mohan S, Beckley AA, Seres DS, Choueiri TK, Uriel N, Ausiello JC, Accili D, Freedberg DE, Baldwin M, Schwartz A, Brodie D, Garcia CK, Elkind MSV, Connors JM, Bilezikian JP, Landry DW, Wan EY. Post-acute COVID-19 syndrome. Nat Med April 2021;27(4):601–15. https://doi.org/10.1038/s41591-021-01283-z.

[11] Yong SJ. Long COVID or post-COVID-19 syndrome: putative pathophysiology, risk factors, and treatments. Infect Dis (Lond) October 2021;53(10):737–54. https://doi.org/10.1080/23744235.2021.1924397. Epub 2021 May 22. PMID: 34024217;.

[12] Zhao D, et al. A comparative study on the clinical features of coronavirus 2019 (COVID-19) pneumonia with other pneumonias. Clin Infect Dis 2020;71(15):756–61. https://doi.org/10.1093/cid/ciaa247.

[13] Hu B, et al. Discovery of a rich gene pool of bat SARS-related coronaviruses provides new insights into the origin of SARS coronavirus. PLoS Pathog 2017;13(11).

[14] Liu PP, Blet A, Smyth D, Li H. The science underlying COVID-19: implications for the cardiovascular system. Circulation 2020.

[15] Rizzo P, et al. COVID-19 in the heart and the lungs: could we 'Notch' the inflammatory storm? Basic Res Cardiol 2020;115:31.

[16] Carfì A, Bernabei R, Landi F. Gemelli against COVID-19 post-acute care study group. Persistent symptoms in patients after acute COVID-19. JAMA 2020;324(6):603–5. https://doi.org/10.1001/jama.2020.12603.

[17] Huang C, et al. 6-month consequences of COVID-19 in patients discharged from hospital: a cohort study. Lancet 2021;397:220–32. https://doi.org/10.1016/S0140-6736(20)32656-8.

[18] Moreno-Pérez O, et al. Post-acute COVID-19 syndrome. Incidence and risk factors: a Mediterranean cohort study. J Infect 2021. https://doi.org/10.1016/j.jinf.2021.01.004.

[19] Chopra V, Flanders SA, O'Malley M. Sixty-day outcomes among patients hospitalized with COVID-19. Ann Intern Med 2020:576–8. https://doi.org/10.7326/M20-5661.

[20] Lopez-Leon S, Wegman-Ostrosky T, Perelman C, et al. More than 50 long-term effects of COVID-19: a systematic review and meta-analysis. Sci Rep 2021;11:16144. https://doi.org/10.1038/s41598-021-95565-8.

[21] Beating coronavirus: flatten the curve, raise the line—COVID-19: what you need to know (CME eligible). Coursera 2020. In press.

[22] Xu Y, et al. Characteristics of pediatric SARS-CoV-2 infection and potential evidence for persistent fecal viral shedding. Nat Med 2020;26(4):502–5. https://doi.org/10.1038/s41591-020-0817-4.

[23] Santhosh L et al. "How I Do It: Rapid Design & Implementation of Post-COVID Clinics". Chest 4158. https://doi.org/10.1016/j.chest.2021.03.044.

[24] Tomar BS, Singh M, Nathiya D, Sharma A, Sharma E, Bareth H, Suman S, Ruparelia DP, Patel JB, Gajera VK, NIMS COVID 19 Investigator Group. Prevalence of symptoms in patients discharged from COVID care facility

of NIMS hospital: is RT PCR negativity truly reflecting recovery? a single-centre observational study. Int J Gen Med March 2021;25(14):1069–78. https://doi.org/10.2147/IJGM.S295499. PMID: 33790636; PMCID: PMC8006813.

[25] Fu L, Wang B, Yuan T, Chen X, Ao Y, Fitzpatrick T, Li P, Zhou Y, Lin Y, Duan Q, et al. Clinical characteristics of coronavirus disease 2019 (COVID-19) in China: a systematic review and meta-analysis. J Infect 2020;80:656–65.

[26] Oran DP, Topol EJ. Prevalence of asymptomatic SARS-CoV-2 infection : a narrative review. Ann Intern Med 2020;173(5):362–7. https://doi.org/10.7326/M20-3012.

[27] Al-Ramadan A, Rabab'h O, Shah J, Gharaibeh A. Acute and post-acute neurological complications of COVID-19. Neurol Int 2021;13(1):102–19. https://doi.org/10.3390/neurolint13010010. Published 2021 Mar 9.

[28] Rojas M, Rodríguez Y, Monsalve DM, Acosta-Ampudia Y, Camacho B, Gallo JE, Rojas-Villarraga A, Ramírez-Santana C, Díaz-Coronado JC, Manrique R, Mantilla RD, Shoenfeld Y, Anaya JM. Convalescent plasma in Covid-19: possible mechanisms of action. Autoimmun Rev July 2020;19(7):102554. https://doi.org/10.1016/j.autrev.2020.102554. Epub 2020 May 5. PMID: 32380316; PMCID: PMC7198427.

[29] Wirth K, Scheibenbogen C. A unifying hypothesis of the pathophysiology of myalgic encephalomyelitis/chronic fatigue syndrome (ME/CFS): recognitions from the finding of autoantibodies against ß2-adrenergic receptors. Autoimmun Rev June 2020;19(6):102527. https://doi.org/10.1016/j.autrev.2020.102527. Epub 2020 Apr 1. PMID: 32247028.

[30] Halpert G, Shoenfeld Y. SARS-CoV-2, the autoimmune virus. Autoimmun Rev December 2020;19(12):102695. https://doi.org/10.1016/j.autrev.2020.102695. Epub 2020 Oct 28. PMID: 33130000; PMCID: PMC7598743.

[31] Kanduc D, Shoenfeld Y. On the molecular determinants the SARS-CoV-2 attack. Clin Immunol 2020;215:108426. https://doi.org/10.1016/j.clim.2020.108426.

[32] Bansal M. Cardiovascular disease and COVID-19. Diabetes Metabol Syndr 2020;14:247–50.

[33] Lucchese G, Flöel A. SARS-CoV-2 and Guillain-Barré syndrome: molecular mimicry with human heat shock proteins as potential pathogenic mechanism. Cell Stress Chaperones 2020. https://doi.org/10.1007/s12192-020-01145-6.

[34] Mohkhedkar M, Venigalla SSK, Janakiraman V. Autoantigens that may explain postinfection autoimmune manifestations in patients with coronavirus disease 2019 displaying neurological conditions. J Infect Dis 2021;223:536–7.

[35] Gao ZW, Zhang HZ, Liu C, Dong K. Autoantibodies in COVID-19: frequency and function. Autoimmun Rev 2021;20(3):102754. https://doi.org/10.1016/j.autrev.2021.102754.

[36] Wallukat G, Hohberger B, Wenzel K, Fürst J, Schulze-Rothe S, Wallukat A, Hönicke AS, Müller J. Functional autoantibodies against G-protein coupled receptors in patients with persistent Long-COVID-19 symptoms. J Transl Autoimmun 2021;4:100100. https://doi.org/10.1016/j.jtauto.2021.100100. Epub 2021 Apr 16. PMID: 33880442;.

[37] Löbel M, Mooslechner AA, Bauer S, Günther S, Letsch A, Hanitsch LG, Grabowski P, Meisel C, Volk HD, Scheibenbogen C. Polymorphism in COMT is associated with IgG3 subclass level and susceptibility to infection in patients with chronic fatigue syndrome. J Transl Med 2015;13:264. https://doi.org/10.1186/s12967-015-0628-4.

[38] Kharraziha I, Axelsson J, Ricci F, Di Martino G, Persson M, Sutton R, Fedorowski A, Hamrefors V. Serum activity against G protein-coupled receptors and severity of orthostatic symptoms in postural orthostatic tachycardia syndrome. J Am Heart Assoc 2020;9(15):e015989. https://doi.org/10.1161/JAHA.120.015989.

[39] Bhadelia N, et al. Distinct autoimmune antibody signatures between hospitalized acute COVID-19 patients, SARS-CoV2 convalescent individuals, and unexposed pre-pandemic controls medRxiv [preprint]. Medicine, Biology; 2021 Jan 25. Submitted for publication.

[40] Wang E, et al. Diverse functional autoantibodies in patients with COVID-19. medRxiv [preprint]vol. 12; December 2020. p. 2020. 12.10.20247205.

[41] Novak P. Post COVID-19 syndrome associated with orthostatic cerebral hypoperfusion syndrome, small fiber neuropathy and benefit of immunotherapy: a case report. eNeurologicalSci December 2020;21:100276. https://doi.org/10.1016/j.ensci.2020.100276. Epub 2020 Sep 20. PMID: 32984564; PMCID: PMC7502253.

[42] Koralnik IJ, Tyler KL. COVID-19: a global threat to the nervous system. Ann Neurol July 2020;88(1):1–11. https://doi.org/10.1002/ana.25807 Epub.

[43] Lewis A, Frontera J, Placantonakis DG, Lighter J, Galetta S, Balcer L, Melmed KR. Cerebrospinal fluid in COVID-19: a systematic review of the literature. J Neurol Sci 2021:421.

[44] Neumann B, Schmidbauer ML, Dimitriadis K, Otto S, Knier B, Niesen W-D, Hosp JA, Günther A, Lindemann S, Nagy G, et al. Cerebrospinal fluid findings in COVID-19 patients with neurological symptoms. J Neurol Sci 2020;418:117090.

[45] Solomon IH, Normandin E, Bhattacharyya S, Mukerji SS, Keller K, Ali AS, Adams G, Hornick JL, Padera RF, Sabeti P. Neuropathological features of covid-19. N Engl J Med 2020;383:989–92.

[46] Ehrenfeld M, Tincani A, Andreoli L, Cattalini M, Greenbaum A, Kanduc D, Alijotas-Reig J, Zinserling V, Semenova N, Amital H, Shoenfeld Y. Covid-19 and autoimmunity. Autoimmun Rev August 2020;19(8):102597. https://doi.org/10.1016/j.autrev.2020.102597. Epub 2020 Jun 11. PMID: 32535093; PMCID: PMC7289100.

[47] Ryabkova VA, Churilov LP, Shoenfeld Y. COVID-19 and ABO blood groups. Isr Med Assoc J March 2021;23(3):140–2. PMID: 33734622.

[48] Wostyn P. COVID-19 and chronic fatigue syndrome: is the worst yet to come? Med Hypotheses Jan 2021;146:110469. https://doi.org/10.1016/j.mehy.2020.110469. Epub 2021 Jan 2. PMID: 33401106; PMCID: PMC7836544.

[49] Wostyn P, De Deyn PP. The putative glymphatic signature of chronic fatigue syndrome: A new view on the disease pathogenesis and therapy. Med Hypotheses Sep 2018;118:142–5. https://doi.org/10.1016/j.mehy.2018.07.007. Epub 2018 Jul 6. PMID: 30037603.

[50] Joseph A, Wanono R, Flamant M, Vidal-Petiot E. Orthostatic hypotension: A review. Nephrol Ther Apr 2017;13(Suppl 1):S55–67. https://doi.org/10.1016/j.nephro.2017.01.003. PMID: 28577744.

[51] Østergaard L. SARS CoV-2 related microvascular damage and symptoms during and after COVID-19: consequences of capillary transit-time changes, tissue hypoxia and inflammation. Physiol Rep February 2021;9(3):e14726. https://doi.org/10.14814/phy2.14726.

[52] Sher L. Post-COVID syndrome and suicide risk. QJM April 27, 2021;114(2):95–8. https://doi.org/10.1093/qjmed/hcab007. PMID: 33486531; PMCID: PMC7928695.

CHAPTER

38

Disease course and pathogenesis of post-COVID-19 condition

Varvara A. Ryabkova[1,2,3] *and Leonid P. Churilov*[1,2,4]

[1]Laboratory of the Mosaic of Autoimmunity, Saint Petersburg State University, Saint Petersburg, Russia; [2]Department of Pathology, Saint Petersburg State University, Saint Petersburg, Russia; [3]Pavlov First Saint Petersburg State Medical University, Saint Petersburg, Russia; [4]Saint Petersburg Research Institute of Phthisiopulmonology, Saint Petersburg, Russia

Post-COVID-19 condition: disease course

According to the official clinical case definition released by World Health Organization (WHO) on October 6, 2021, "post COVID-19 condition occurs in individuals with a history of probable or confirmed SARS-CoV-2 infection, usually 3 months from the onset of COVID-19 with symptoms that last for at least 2 months and cannot be explained by an alternative diagnosis. Common symptoms include fatigue, shortness of breath, cognitive dysfunction but also others which generally have an impact on everyday functioning. Symptoms may be new onset, following initial recovery from an acute COVID-19 episode, or persist from the initial illness. Symptoms may also fluctuate or relapse over time" [1]. The precise incidence of long-term sequelae after acute COVID-19 remains unknown, but published reports indicate that approximately 10%–20% of COVID-19 patients experience lingering symptoms for weeks to months following acute SARS-CoV-2 infection [1]. The definition of post-COVID-19 condition highlights three important aspects of its timeline: minimum time period from the onset of symptoms, minimum duration of symptoms, and disease course. Acute COVID-19 episode lasts till negative PCR test for viral RNA is obtained. Symptoms and abnormalities present 4–12 weeks beyond acute COVID-19 are regarded as "subacute" or "ongoing symptomatic" COVID-19 [2]. Although post-COVID-19 condition is generally considered as the prolongation of the acute COVID-19 symptoms, it could manifest some time (usually 1–2 months) after the virological recovery. One should also keep in mind that activation of the innate immune system, such as that instigated by SARS-CoV-2, is an early event in the pathogenesis of a number of autoimmune diseases, occurring possibly several years prior to the first symptoms. Thus, the full spectrum of post-COVID-19

Autoimmunity, COVID-19, Post-COVID19 syndrome and COVID-19 vaccination
https://doi.org/10.1016/B978-0-443-18566-3.00006-2

manifestations is to be studied. However, to date it is widely assumed that progressive course of symptoms is not typical for the post-COVID-19 condition. At the same time, some patients describe relapsing-remitting course of the disease. A recent meta-analysis showed that 63.2%, 71.9%, and 45.9% of patients (both hospitalized and not-hospitalized) exhibited ≥1 post-COVID-19 symptom at 30, 60, or ≥90 days after disease onset/hospitalization [3]. These data clearly illustrated both the possibility of the delayed onset of post-COVID-19 condition and the trend of improving of the symptoms over time in more than a half of cases.

Post-COVID-19 condition: disease course probable links of pathogenesis

The pathogenesis of post-COVID syndrome is multifaceted, and some clinical manifestations may result from more than one mechanism. All proposed mechanisms of the post-COVID-19 health problems could be divided into several groups, according to the results of the webinar held on this issue by WHO on June 15, 2021: (1) Inflammatory/hyperinflammatory state; (2) Immune dysregulation/autoimmune; (3) Coagulation/vasculopathy; (4) Direct viral toxicity/viral persistence; (5) Autonomic dysfunction; (6) Endocrine/metabolic; (7) Inadaptation of the ACE-2 pathway [4].

Neuroinvasion of SARS-CoV-2

The first step on the road to the understanding of post-COVID-19 condition is to answer the question: Is the post-COVID-19 condition unique? Can one draw parallels between this entity and any previously known diseases? Or if it is unique, what are the causes of this uniqueness?

Similar observations of long-term sequelae (persistent shortness of breath, fatigue, mental health problems, and reduced quality of life) have been reported following the SARS-CoV-1 outbreak in 2003 and Middle East Respiratory Syndrome outbreak in 2012 as well [5]. Mental health reduction, persistent fatigue, diffuse myalgia, weakness, depression, and nonrestorative sleep at least in some individuals were stable, persisted for more than 1 year [5]. The post-COVID-19 condition has also a similarity to the postviral syndromes that followed the Spanish Flu of 1918, caused by the A(H1N1) influenza virus [6], the outbreaks of Ebola [7], West Nile fever [8], and Dengue fever [9]. Among nonepidemic viruses, the Epstein–Barr virus (EBV) is a well-known source of postviral fatigue syndrome [10]. Some bacterial pathogens have been also described as the causative agents of postinfectious fatigue syndromes, for example, Coxiella burnetii (Q fever) and Borrelia burgdorferi (Lyme disease) [10]. What do these pathogens have in common? The epidemic viruses mentioned above are able to invade central nervous system, presumably through olfactory bulb [11], or cause blood–brain barrier disruption and neuroinflammation [12–14]. EBV was detected in postmortem human brain samples in 91/101 (90%) of multiple sclerosis cases compared to 5/21 (24%) of control samples with other neurologic diseases [15]. Peripheral EBV infection in a rabbit model induced infiltration of brain parenchyma and spinal cord by blood-derived macrophages, T- and B-lymphocytes, which formed aggregates together with microglial cells, suggesting ongoing neuroinflammatory process [16]. Involvement of the central nervous system during Q fever and Lyme disease is not rare due to the penetration of the blood–brain barrier by these pathogens [17,18].

A number of reports showed brain alterations in patients who died from COVID-19 [19]. However, most of the findings do not seem to be specific to SARS-CoV-2 infection—they are more likely because of systemic inflammation and coagulopathy caused by COVID-19. Thus, according to a recent systematic review, hypoxic changes were the most frequently reported alteration of brain tissue, followed by ischemic and hemorrhagic lesions and reactive astrogliosis and microgliosis [19]. There was no clear evidence of the classical neuropathology of viral CNS infections in most cases—with no lymphocytic leptomeningitis or encephalitis, microglial nodules, pronounced or frequent perivascular lymphocytic cuffing, focal demyelination, or viral inclusions. At the same time, SARS-CoV-2 RNA and proteins were detected in brain tissues (including microvasculature, cortical neurons, astrocytes, choroid plexus and meninges) in human autopsy studies. The neuroinvasive capacity of SARS-CoV-2 has been also recently demonstrated both in vitro in such models as stem cell-derived neural cells and cerebral organoids [20] and in vivo in animal models (including mouse, hamster, ferret, and nonhuman primates) [21]. One of the main arguments against SARS-CoV-2 neuroinvasion is that the mRNA levels of ACE2 appear to be very low in the human CNS. However, several recent studies report some new SARS-CoV-2-binding receptors, including neuroreceptors (e.g., NRP1, BSG, and TMPRSS2) suggesting that SARS-CoV-2 may use other gates for neurotropism in addition to ACE2 [21]. SARS-CoV-2 infectivity in animal models varies due to different distributions and density of the proteins which mediated the propagation of SARS-CoV-2 to the CNS between these models and the human brain and due to the different capacity of the virus to interact with various ACE2 species [21]. There is evidence for all three possible routes of the neuroinvasion of SARS-COV-2 (via olfactory nerves, via direct infection of vascular endothelial cells, and via the blood–brain barrier disrupted by the inflammatory response). Thus, on the one hand, the productive infection within the olfactory bulb was reported in K18-hACE2 transgenic mice following intranasal inoculation in the absence of viremia at any time after infection [22]; the presence of SARS-CoV-2 or inflammatory features of olfactory bulb was observed in 57 cases (28.9%) among published reports of brain autopsy in fatal COVID-19 [19]; a systematic literature review of the neuroimaging abnormalities in SARS-CoV-2 revealed predominant involvement of the olfactory system with disruptions across four olfactory structures, and abnormalities also extended to the corpus callosum, cingulate cortex, and insula, jointly implicating the olfactory brain network [23]. On the other hand, SARS-CoV-2 RNA was also detected in human brain samples in the CNS regions that have no direct connection to the olfactory mucosa (e.g., cerebellum) [19], that predominantly composed of blood vessels (e.g., choroid plexus) or that contain regions with lack of blood–brain barrier (e.g., dorsal medulla) [24]. However, it requires further investigation, whether the described brain abnormalities are relevant for the post-COVID-19 condition which could develop also after mild disease. The neuroimaging studies of post-COVID-19 are scarce and inconsistent. Early studies reported a profile of brain PET hypometabolism in patients with persistent symptoms following COVID-19 (although the pattern varied from predominant frontoparietal hypometabolism [25] to the hypometabolism particularly of the right parahippocampal gyrus and thalamus [26] or the involvement of limbic/paralimbic regions extending to the brainstem and cerebellum) [27]. At the same time Dressing et al. [28] have recently shown the lack of significant findings on 18F-FDG PET, and only mild impairments on neuropsychological testing in patients with long-COVID syndrome in contrast to the severe and lasting disability reported by the patients (e.g., cognitive symptoms, inability to work). The authors speculated that the pathophysiological background of self-reported cognitive symptoms, disability, and even mild impairments in the neuropsychological test battery in these patients was primarily caused by fatigue, and suggested that fatigue itself resulted from the immune dysregulation processes. At the same time, the first longitudinal imaging study comparing brain scans acquired from individuals before and after SARS-CoV-2 infection (401 patients) to the scans from a well-matched control group (384 individuals) identified significant effects of COVID-19 in the brain with a loss of gray matter in the left parahippocampal gyrus, the left lateral orbitofrontal cortex, anterior cingulate cortex, insula, supramarginal gyrus, and temporal pole [29]. These findings thus consistently relate to the loss of gray matter in limbic cortical areas directly linked to the primary olfactory and gustatory system. The hospitalized patients showed greater reduction in gray matter thickness in limbic regions. Finally, significantly greater cognitive decline between the two timepoints was seen even in the nonhospitalized SARS-CoV-2 positive group compared to the controls, and this decline was associated with greater atrophy of crus II, a cognitive lobule of the cerebellum. To sum up, extensive investigation is required to answer: what is the main mechanism of the CNS involvement in COVID-19 and post-COVID-19 condition; what is the main route of CNS SARS-CoV-2 infection; and whether the CNS morphological or functional abnormalities revealed in the acute of chronic phase of COVID-19 correlate with the persistent symptoms in post-COVID-19 condition.

Immune-related mechanisms

Thus, it is not certain that chronic fatigue and the other long-term complications in some COVID-19 patients are related to the invasion of SARS-COV-2 into the brain. To date, most researchers and clinicians agree that the long-term COVID-19 symptoms are associated with the SARS-CoV-2 ability to disturb the immune system function. It is well-known that systemic inflammatory response (SIRS) is present in severe COVID-19. Presumably, the perturbation or overactivation of the immune system can continue after the clearance of the virus or result from the persistence of the fragments of viral genes and underlie the prolonged symptoms of COVID-19. Several studies have reported the persistence of viral proteins and RNA in intestinal biopsies [30]. Discovery of SARS-CoV-2 S1 protein in the nonclassical monocytes in patients with post-COVID-19 condition 15 months postinfection represents further evidence for the theory of the viral latency which provides triggers for the immune system, fueling chronic inflammation [31]. One should remember that in response to SIRS of different etiology long-lasting counterbalancing compensatory antiinflammatory response syndrome (CARS) occurs that leads to postinfectious/posttraumatic immunosuppression [32]. This concept was initially developed in sepsis, entirely confirmed in posttraumatic shock and traumatic disease of postshock patients [33] and, in line with this concept, patients with prolonged sepsis (or those rescued from traumatic shock and entered into next stage of traumatic disease) are prone to latent virus reactivation [34]. A recent study has shown that it can be also true for the post-COVID-19 condition: 66.7% (20/30) of patients with post-COVID-19 condition versus 10% (2/20) of control subjects were positive for EBV reactivation based on positive titers for EBV early antigen-diffuse (EA-D) IgG or EBV viral capsid antigen (VCA) IgM [35]. A similar level of EBV reactivation was reported among patients with prolonged symptoms who were 21–90 days (short-term) postdiagnosis of COVID-19, indicating that reactivation may occur soon after or concurrently with COVID-19 infection. Notably, that myalgic encephalomyelitis/chronic fatigue syndrome (ME/CFS) was first described in reference to a post-EBV infection fatigue and EBV is the most researched source of postviral fatigue syndrome [10]. It is interesting that reports of individuals with post-COVID-19 condition whose symptoms resolved within days of receiving COVID-19 vaccinations are emerging [30]. While these reports are primarily anecdotal and formal clinical studies are needed to evaluate this phenomenon, given these responses are brisk (occurring within days of vaccination), this supports the hypothesis of latent chronic infection of SARS-COV-2 due to the postinfectious immunosuppression; vaccination might serve to simply boost the existing, suboptimal adaptive immune response, clear residual infections, and in turn eliminate the symptoms of post-COVID-19 condition. At the same time, it is possible that post-COVID-19 condition is heterogenous by its nature and vaccination-induced resolution is only seen in those individuals with chronic latent infection, but not in SARS-CoV-2-induced autoimmunity [30]. It has been shown that latent polyautoimmunity characterized by increased levels of different autoantibodies and proinflammatory cytokines and observed during the acute phase of COVID-19 persisted in patients with post-COVID-19 condition [36]. Meanwhile, transient immunosuppressive state, which is a characteristic of acute COVID-19, could be closely linked with chronic inflammatory process even after successful clearance of the virus. It was observed in clinical practice before the COVID pandemic that transient immunosuppression or immunodeficiency which occurs before a sudden reactivation of the immune components was associated with the triggering of autoimmunity or autoinflammation phenomena [37]. This hypothesis of inappropriate immune reconstitution in genetically susceptible individuals with the loss of self-tolerance was proposed [37] and could explain the occurrence of post-COVID-19 condition in immunocompetent patients who is not appeared to suffer from the prolonged immunosuppression after acute COVID-19.

Vascular mechanisms

Besides virus-related mechanisms and immune dysfunction, it could be persistent vasculopathy that takes part in the pathogenesis of post-COVID-19 condition. COVID-19 is associated with severe vascular inflammation, both in the pulmonary and extrapulmonary vasculature, both on the macro- and microvascular level [38]. This involves diffuse endothelial damage with pyroptosis and apoptosis as well as a procoagulant change of the vascular endothelium. A preliminary study of vascular changes in patients with persistent symptoms after COVID-19 with [18F]FDG-PET/CT suggested that SARS-CoV-2 induces inflammation of large vessels (thoracic aorta, right iliac artery, and femoral arteries) [39]. Notably, that [18F]FDG vascular uptake in post-COVID-19 condition in this study demonstrated smooth linear pattern, similar to that observed in large vessel vasculitis as opposed to atherosclerosis with focal and nonlinear pattern. At the same time, it is not clear how large vessels vasculitis can result in cognitive dysfunction, for example, which is very common in post-COVID-19 condition and appear to be related to the dysfunction of small vessels. At the same time, endothelial dysfunction, which was revealed by Ambrosine et al. [40] with flow-mediated dilation method in convalescent COVID-19 patients 2 months from swab test negativization, directly correlated with the severity of pulmonary impairment in this group of patients. In addition, a recent study of microvascular circulation in post-COVID-19 condition highlighted the role of the endothelial dysfunction in the pathogenesis of persistent nonrespiratory symptoms [41]. The authors focused on the evaluation of endothelial quality index (EQI) by finger thermal monitoring with E4 diagnosis Polymath and showed that 49.7% of patients had impaired EQI. Furthermore, persistent symptoms especially chest pain, fatigue, and neurocognitive symptoms (nonrespiratory symptoms) after COVID-19 were mainly associated with endothelial dysfunction, even after adjustment for age, sex, diabetes, hypertension, dyslipidemia, coronary heart disease, and severe clinical status of COVID-19 infection with the need for oxygen. In multivariate analysis, endothelial dysfunction was an independent risk factor of post-COVID-19 condition. Although it is well-known that acute COVID-19 is associated with hemostatic changes, which can persist up to 8 months after hospital discharge [42], hemostatic markers were not associated with functional impairment in post-COVID-19 condition at eight or 12 months after initial disease [42] or 68 days after symptom resolution or hospital discharge following adjustment for age, sex, and severity of initial infection [43]. These findings suggest that other mechanisms apart from hypercoagulability could contribute to the persistent symptoms after COVID-19. However, further research is needed on the interactions between coagulation, inflammation, autoimmunity, and symptoms in post-COVID-19 condition.

Autonomic dysfunction

Some of the most common symptoms of post-COVID-19 condition (orthostatic intolerance, palpitations/tachycardia, temperature intolerance, labile blood pressure, new-onset hypertension, gastrointestinal symptoms such as abdominal pain, bloating, nausea, xerostomia) could be explained by autonomic instability. Notably, that one of the most prevalent primary autonomic disorders, postural tachycardia syndrome (POTS), is commonly associated with antecedent or concomitant bacterial, viral, and parasitic infection [44]. The studies reporting the results of autonomic nervous testing, which can objectively assess autonomic nervous system function in post-COVID-19, are scarce. According to Hinduja et al. [45], sudomotor dysfunction was revealed in 26% of patients with post-COVID-19 syndrome in India by assessing electrochemical skin conductance of the hands and feet. Barizien et al. [46] described a significant dissociation of the NOL index (a multiparameter artificial intelligence-driven index which is based on heart rate variability and reflects parasympathetic/sympathetic balance) between post-COVID-19 participants with fatigue and control participants without a history of COVID-19. At the same time, Townsend et al. [47] reported no signs of cardiovascular autonomic dysfunction on reflex testing as measured by Ewing's autonomic battery with beat-to-beat blood pressure and heart rate measurement during deep breathing, Valsalva, cold pressor testing, and a 5-min stand test in 20 patients with fatigue and 20 nonfatigued patients at a median of 166 days following COVID-19, despite 14/20 fatigued patients (70%) reported palpitations, dizziness or lightheadedness, or chest discomfort on active stand. The proposed mechanisms of dysautonomia in post-COVID-19 condition include (1) viral invasion or disruption of baroreflex pathways in the carotid artery or the nucleus tractus solitarious of the medulla; (2) deconditioning; (3) effects of functional autoantibodies to the G-protein-coupled receptors including adrenergic and muscarinic acetylcholine receptors. Despite some indirect evidence favoring the first mechanism (detection of the SARS-CoV-2 RNA in dorsal medulla in autopsy brain samples [24], the ability of some respiratory viruses in animal models to enter the brain via sensory nerves of the vagus in respiratory organs [21] and location of the vagal nerve nuclei in the medulla), studies in animal models are required to support this hypothesis. The onset of dysautonomia is often concurrent with the acute COVID-19 which would argue against deconditioning being the main mechanism of dysautonomia in patients with post-COVID-19 condition [48]. Regarding the third proposed mechanism, autoantibodies against the β2-adrenoceptor and the muscarinic

M2 receptor has been found in the sera of 29/29 patients with different symptoms after recovery from acute COVID-19 as well as in 2/2 symptoms-free survivor of COVID-19 [49]. These autoantibodies induced a positive and a negative chronotropic response on their targeted receptors, respectively. However, the authors did not specify at what point after acute COVID-19 the assessment of autoantibodies was performed. Together with H. Heidecke we also detect these autoantibodies in patients both with and without persistent symptoms following COVID-19 (in 9/16 and 2/3 individuals with and without symptoms respectively) (unpublished data). These findings could question the role of these autoantibodies in the pathogenesis of post-COVID-19 condition suggesting their role as passive by-standers. The neurotransmitter receptors mentioned above are present not only within autonomic nervous system, but also on many other cells, like platelets, endothelium, immune cells, and endocrinocytes. In this context the term "dysautonomia" should not be interpreted as solely neural disorder, but one should keep in mind that dysfunction of adrenergic and muscarinic transmitter systems could cause a wider spectrum of pathophysiological consequences.

Endocrine mechanisms

The prolonged critical illness, which was a well-known condition also before the COVID-19 era, may appear to represent the completely distinct type of post-COVID-19 health problems, having nothing in common with post-COVID-19 condition which develops in nonhospitalized patients. The latter shares a lot of features with ME/CFS [50]. But a hypothesis of a common mechanisms of the prolonged critical illness and ME/CFS proposed in recent paper by Stanculescu et al. [51] let us suggest that despite varying degrees of severity of the acute-COVID-19 in hospitalized and nonhospitalized patients, the mechanisms of their post-COVID-19 health problems could have something in common. Independent of the nature of the critical illness, the acute phase is associated with an excessive response of proinflammatory cytokines which coexists or transits early to antiinflammatory phenotype whose downside is injury-associated immunosuppression [52]. These mechanisms of immune dysfunction in post-COVID-19 condition have been discussed above. In prolonged critical illness, the initial inflammatory surge has generally settled but a uniform dysregulation of the endocrine axes occurs, which is characterized by the suppression of the pituitary gland's pulsatile secretion of tropic hormones [53]. Although the pituitary's pulsatile secretion and its relationships to metabolic and immune functions remain largely unstudied in ME/CFS, the endocrine patterns observed in severe ME/CFS are not unlike those of *prolonged* critical illness [51]. Lessons from past experience with SARS have taught us that multiple endocrine axes can be affected by SARS-CoV, manifesting as hypothyroidism, follicular thyroid cells dysfunction, and delayed central hypocortisolism [54]. Regarding hypothalamic–pituitary–adrenal axis, Leow et al. [55] evaluated cortisol, ACTH levels, and 24-h urinary free cortisol in SARS survivors and found that 39.3% of the patients had hypocortisolism and among them 83.3% had secondary adrenal insufficiency. In 2004, Wheatland [56] suspected the existence of homologies between adrenocorticotropic hormones (ACTH) in various mammals and SARS coronavirus replicase 1AB protein, as well as between ACTH and influenza virus peptides, that may cause anti-ACTH autoimmunity in both SARS and influenza. Due to the etiopathogenetic similarity between SARS-CoV and SARS-CoV-2, endocrine involvement in COVID-19 is likely to be present. However, according to the study of 70 COVID-19 survivors

3 months after recovery, all of them had normal peak cortisol level after Synacthen test, although 62.9% of participants suffered from persistent fatigue [57]. The levels of growth hormone and IGF-1 were also similar in the same group of patients with post-COVID-19 fatigue, compared to those without it, and did not alter with number of persistent symptoms [58]. We reported that human ACTH receptor (but not ACTH itself) shares peptides with SARS-COV-2 [59]. It can be suggested that SARS-CoV-2 causes the production of functional autoantibodies against ACTH receptor, which can interrupt physiological interactions within hypothalamic–pituitary–adrenal axis. Similar antigen mimicry exists also between immunogenic epitopes of SARS-CoV-2 S-protein and key enzyme of adrenocortical steroidogenesis, 21-hydroxylase (CYP21A2), one of the main targets in autoimmune adrenalitis [60]. Meanwhile, potent adrenocortical response in cytokine storm as well as in any other variant of SIRS is the main antishock protective mechanism, so altering adrenals and geopardizing their defensive action, COVID-19 may promote distress-related organ failure with all its sequels. Thyroid gland has also gained considerable attention in both acute COVID-19 and post-COVID-19 condition. The dysfunction of hythothalamic–pituitary–thyroid axis has been clinically linked with the acute phase of COVID-19, which is characterized in severe cases by the occurrence of Low T3 Syndrome/Nonthyroidal Illness Syndrome [61]. However, abnormal thyroid function tests in acute COVID-19 generally resolved [62]. Although there are case reports of new onset autoimmune thyroid diseases following COVID-19, and a number of COVID-19 survivors have an increase in antithyroid peroxidase antibodies titers 3 months after acute COVID-19 [63], development of post-COVID-19 condition was more likely in those with negative antithyroid peroxidase antibodies upon follow-up [62]. Thyroid hormones are key regulators of mitochondrial oxidation and related metabolic processes. Interestingly, both myalgic encephalomyelitis/chronic fatigue syndrome and long COVID, as well as chronic autoimmune thyroiditis –all are characteristic for mitochondrial dysfunction, oxidative stress and hypoergosis [64,65]. Further research is required to determine persistent effects of COVID-19 on endocrine function.

References

[1] WHO. A clinical case definition of post COVID-19 condition by a Delphi consensus. 2021.

[2] Nalbandian A, Sehgal K, Gupta A, Madhavan MV, McGroder C, Stevens JS, et al. Post-acute COVID-19 syndrome. Nat Med 2021;27:601–15. https://doi.org/10.1038/s41591-021-01283-z.

[3] Fernández-de-las-Peñas C, Palacios-Ceña D, Gómez-Mayordomo V, Florencio LL, Cuadrado ML, Plaza-Manzano G, et al. Prevalence of post-COVID-19 symptoms in hospitalized and non-hospitalized COVID-19 survivors: a systematic review and meta-analysis. Eur J Intern Med 2021;92:55–70. https://doi.org/10.1016/J.EJIM.2021.06.009.

[4] Diaz JV. WHO update: post COVID-19 condition Clinical case definition and update on clinical activities. Lecture presented at: WHO webinar 2: understanding mechanisms of post COVID-19 condition. October 6, 2021.

[5] Ramakrishnan RK, Kashour T, Hamid Q, Halwani R, Tleyjeh IM. Unraveling the mystery surrounding post-acute sequelae of COVID-19. Front Immunol 2021;12:2574. https://doi.org/10.3389/FIMMU.2021.686029/BIBTEX.

[6] Honigsbaum M, Krishnan L. Taking pandemic sequelae seriously: from the Russian influenza to COVID-19 long-haulers. Lancet 2020;396:1389–91. https://doi.org/10.1016/S0140-6736(20)32134-6.

[7] Clark DV, Kibuuka H, Millard M, Wakabi S, Lukwago L, Taylor A, et al. Long-term sequelae after Ebola virus disease in Bundibugyo, Uganda: a retrospective cohort study. Lancet Infect Dis 2015;15:905–12. https://doi.org/10.1016/S1473-3099(15)70152-0.

[8] Garcia MN, Hause AM, Walker CM, Orange JS, Hasbun R, Murray KO. Evaluation of prolonged fatigue post—West Nile virus infection and association of fatigue with elevated antiviral and proinflammatory cytokines. Viral Immunol 2014;27:327. https://doi.org/10.1089/VIM.2014.0035.

[9] Sigera PC, Rajapakse S, Weeratunga P, De Silva NL, Gomes L, Malavige GN, et al. Dengue and post-infection fatigue: findings from a prospective cohort—the Colombo Dengue Study. Trans R Soc Trop Med Hyg 2021;115:669—76. https://doi.org/10.1093/TRSTMH/TRAA110.

[10] Islam MF, Cotler J, Jason LA. Post-viral fatigue and COVID-19: lessons from past epidemics. Fatigue Biomed Heal Behav 2020;8:61—9. https://doi.org/10.1080/21641846.2020.1778227.

[11] Mori I. 1918 H1N1 influenza virus infection—induced proinflammatory cytokines in the olfactory bulb could trigger lethargic disease. J Infect Dis 2018;218:1686—7. https://doi.org/10.1093/INFDIS/JIY380.

[12] Calderón-Peláez MA, Velandia-Romero ML, Bastidas-Legarda LY, Beltrán EO, Camacho-Ortega SJ, Castellanos JE. Dengue virus infection of blood-brain barrier cells: consequences of severe disease. Front Microbiol 2019;10. https://doi.org/10.3389/FMICB.2019.01435.

[13] Schreiber-Stainthorp W, Solomon J, Lee JH, Castro M, Shah S, Martinez-Orengo N, et al. Longitudinal in vivo imaging of acute neuropathology in a monkey model of Ebola virus infection. Nat Commun 2021;12:1—12. https://doi.org/10.1038/s41467-021-23088-x. 121 2021.

[14] Diamond MS, Klein RS. West Nile virus: crossing the blood-brain barrier. Nat Med 2004;10:1294—5. https://doi.org/10.1038/nm1204-1294. 1012 2004.

[15] Hassani A, Corboy JR, Al-Salam S, Khan G. Epstein-Barr virus is present in the brain of most cases of multiple sclerosis and may engage more than just B cells. PLoS One 2018;13. https://doi.org/10.1371/JOURNAL.PONE.0192109.

[16] Hassani A, Reguraman N, Philip P, Shehab S, Khan G. Epstein—Barr virus infection causes inflammation in the brain in a rabbit model. Mult Scler Relat Disord 2021;51:102997. https://doi.org/10.1016/J.MSARD.2021.102997.

[17] Ford L, Tufts DM. Lyme neuroborreliosis: mechanisms of B. Burgdorferi infection of the nervous system. Brain Sci 2021;11. https://doi.org/10.3390/BRAINSCI11060789.

[18] Bernit E, Pouget J, Janbon F, Dutronc H, Martinez P, Brouqui P, et al. Neurological involvement in acute Q fever: a report of 29 cases and review of the literature. Arch Intern Med 2002;162:693—700. https://doi.org/10.1001/ARCHINTE.162.6.693.

[19] Maiese A, Manetti AC, Bosetti C, Del Duca F, La Russa R, Frati P, et al. SARS-CoV-2 and the brain: a review of the current knowledge on neuropathology in COVID-19. Brain Pathol 2021;31:e13013. https://doi.org/10.1111/BPA.13013.

[20] Song E, Zhang C, Israelow B, Lu-Culligan A, Prado AV, Skriabine S, et al. Neuroinvasion of SARS-CoV-2 in human and mouse brain. J Exp Med 2021:218. https://doi.org/10.1084/JEM.20202135/VIDEO-1.

[21] Wan D, Du T, Hong W, Chen L, Que H, Lu S, et al. Neurological complications and infection mechanism of SARS-COV-2. Signal Transduct Targeted Ther 2021;6:1—16. https://doi.org/10.1038/s41392-021-00818-7.

[22] Kumari P, Rothan HA, Natekar JP, Stone S, Pathak H, Strate PG, et al. Neuroinvasion and encephalitis following intranasal inoculation of SARS-CoV-2 in K18-hACE2 mice. Viruses 2021;13:132. https://doi.org/10.3390/V13010132.

[23] Najt P, Richards HL, Fortune DG. Brain imaging in patients with COVID-19: a systematic review. Brain, Behav Immun Heal 2021;16:100290. https://doi.org/10.1016/J.BBIH.2021.100290.

[24] Serrano GE, Walker JE, Arce R, Glass MJ, Vargas D, Sue LI, et al. Mapping of SARS-CoV-2 brain invasion and histopathology in COVID-19 disease. MedRxiv 2021. https://doi.org/10.1101/2021.02.15.21251511. 2021.02.15.21251511.

[25] Hosp JA, Dressing A, Blazhenets G, Bormann T, Rau A, Schwabenland M, et al. Cognitive impairment and altered cerebral glucose metabolism in the subacute stage of COVID-19. Brain 2021;144:1263—76. https://doi.org/10.1093/BRAIN/AWAB009.

[26] Sollini M, Morbelli S, Ciccarelli M, Cecconi M, Aghemo A, Morelli P, et al. Long COVID hallmarks on [18F] FDG-PET/CT: a case-control study. Eur J Nucl Med Mol Imag 2021;48:1. https://doi.org/10.1007/S00259-021-05294-3.

[27] Guedj E, Campion JY, Dudouet P, Kaphan E, Bregeon F, Tissot-Dupont H, et al. 18F-FDG brain PET hypometabolism in patients with long COVID. Eur J Nucl Med Mol Imag 2021;48:2823–33. https://doi.org/10.1007/S00259-021-05215-4/FIGURES/4.

[28] Dressing A, Bormann T, Blazhenets G, Schroeter N, Walter LI, Thurow J, et al. Neuropsychological profiles and cerebral glucose metabolism in neurocognitive long COVID-syndrome. J Nucl Med 2021;121:262677. https://doi.org/10.2967/JNUMED.121.262677. jnumed.

[29] Douaud G, Lee S, Alfaro-Almagro F, Arthofer C, Wang C, McCarthy P, et al. Brain imaging before and after COVID-19 in UK biobank. MedRxiv 2021. https://doi.org/10.1101/2021.06.11.21258690.

[30] O'Donnell JS, Chappell KJ. Chronic SARS-CoV-2, a cause of post-acute COVID-19 sequelae (Long-COVID)? Front Microbiol 2021;12:2232. https://doi.org/10.3389/FMICB.2021.724654/BIBTEX.

[31] Patterson BK, Francisco EB, Yogendra R, Long E, Pise A, Rodrigues H, et al. Persistence of SARS CoV-2 S1 protein in CD16+ monocytes in post-acute sequelae of COVID-19 (PASC) up to 15 months post-infection. bioRxiv 2021. https://doi.org/10.1101/2021.06.25.449905. 2021.06.25.449905.

[32] Arlati S. Pathophysiology of acute illness and injury. Oper Tech Recent Adv Acute Care Emerg Surg 2019:11–42. https://doi.org/10.1007/978-3-319-95114-0_2.

[33] Hietbrink F, Koenderman L, Rijkers GT, Leenen LPH. Trauma: the role of the innate immune system. World J Emerg Surg 2006;1. https://doi.org/10.1186/1749-7922-1-15.

[34] Walton AH, Muenzer JT, Rasche D, Boomer JS, Sato B, Brownstein BH, et al. Reactivation of multiple viruses in patients with sepsis. PLoS One 2014;9:e98819. https://doi.org/10.1371/JOURNAL.PONE.0098819.

[35] Gold JE, Okyay RA, Licht WE, Hurley DJ. Investigation of long COVID prevalence and its relationship to epstein-barr virus reactivation. Pathogens 2021;10. https://doi.org/10.3390/PATHOGENS10060763.

[36] Acosta-Ampudia Y, Monsalve DM, Rojas M, Rodríguez Y, Zapata E, Ramírez-Santana C, et al. Persistent autoimmune activation and proinflammatory state in post-COVID syndrome. MedRxiv 2021. https://doi.org/10.1101/2021.11.17.21266457. 2021.11.17.21266457.

[37] Cañas CA. The triggering of post-COVID-19 autoimmunity phenomena could be associated with both transient immunosuppression and an inappropriate form of immune reconstitution in susceptible individuals. Med Hypotheses 2020;145:110345. https://doi.org/10.1016/J.MEHY.2020.110345.

[38] Christensen RH, Berg RMG. Vascular inflammation as a therapeutic target in COVID-19 "long haulers": HIITing the spot? Front Cardiovasc Med 2021;8:643626. https://doi.org/10.3389/FCVM.2021.643626.

[39] Sollini M, Ciccarelli M, Cecconi M, Aghemo A, Morelli P, Gelardi F, et al. Vasculitis changes in COVID-19 survivors with persistent symptoms: an [18F]FDG-PET/CT study. Eur J Nucl Med Mol Imag 2021;48:1460–6. https://doi.org/10.1007/S00259-020-05084-3/FIGURES/4.

[40] Ambrosino P, Calcaterra I, Molino A, Moretta P, Lupoli R, Spedicato GA, et al. Persistent endothelial dysfunction in post-acute COVID-19 syndrome: a case-control study. Biomedicines 2021;9. https://doi.org/10.3390/BIOMEDICINES9080957.

[41] Charfeddine S, Ibn Hadj Amor H, Jdidi J, Torjmen S, Kraiem S, Hammami R, et al. Long COVID 19 syndrome: is it related to microcirculation and endothelial dysfunction? insights from TUN-EndCOV study. Front Cardiovasc Med 2021;8:1702. https://doi.org/10.3389/FCVM.2021.745758.

[42] Meijenfeldt FA von, Havervall S, Adelmeijer J, Thalin C, Lisman T. Persistent endotheliopathy in the pathogenesis of long COVID syndrome: comment from von Meijenfeldt et al. J Thromb Haemostasis 2021. https://doi.org/10.1111/JTH.15580.

[43] Fogarty H, Townsend L, Morrin H, Ahmad A, Comerford C, Karampini E, et al. Persistent endotheliopathy in the pathogenesis of long COVID syndrome. J Thromb Haemostasis 2021;19:2546–53.

[44] Blomberg J, Gottfries C-G, Elfaitouri A, Rizwan M, Rosén A. Infection elicited autoimmunity and myalgic encephalomyelitis/chronic fatigue syndrome: an explanatory model. Front Immunol 2018;9:229–49. https://doi.org/10.3389/fimmu.2018.00229.

[45] Hinduja A, Moutairou A, Calvet JH. Sudomotor dysfunction in patients recovered from COVID-19. Neurophysiol Clin 2021;51:193–6. https://doi.org/10.1016/J.NEUCLI.2021.01.003.

[46] Barizien N, Le Guen M, Russel S, Touche P, Huang F, Vallée A. Clinical characterization of dysautonomia in long COVID-19 patients. Sci Rep 2021;11:1–7. https://doi.org/10.1038/s41598-021-93546-5.

[47] Townsend L, Moloney D, Finucane C, McCarthy K, Bergin C, Bannan C, et al. Fatigue following COVID-19 infection is not associated with autonomic dysfunction. PLoS One 2021;16:e0247280. https://doi.org/10.1371/JOURNAL.PONE.0247280.

[48] Goodman BP, Khoury JA, Blair JE, Grill MF. COVID-19 dysautonomia. Front Neurol 2021;12:543. https://doi.org/10.3389/FNEUR.2021.624968/BIBTEX.

[49] Wallukat G, Hohberger B, Wenzel K, Fürst J, Schulze-Rothe S, Wallukat A, et al. Functional autoantibodies against G-protein coupled receptors in patients with persistent long-COVID-19 symptoms. J Transl Autoimmun 2021;4:100100. https://doi.org/10.1016/J.JTAUTO.2021.100100.

[50] Wong TL, Weitzer DJ. Long COVID and myalgic encephalomyelitis/chronic fatigue syndrome (ME/CFS)-A systemic review and comparison of clinical presentation and symptomatology. Medicina (Kaunas) 2021;57:418. https://doi.org/10.3390/medicina57050418.

[51] Stanculescu D, Larsson L, Bergquist J. Hypothesis: mechanisms that prevent recovery in prolonged ICU patients also underlie myalgic encephalomyelitis/chronic fatigue syndrome (ME/CFS). Front Med 2021;8:628029. https://doi.org/10.3389/FMED.2021.628029.

[52] Pfortmueller CA, Meisel C, Fux M, Schefold JC. Assessment of immune organ dysfunction in critical illness: utility of innate immune response markers. Intensive Care Med Exp 2017;5:1–16. https://doi.org/10.1186/S40635-017-0163-0.

[53] Langouche L, Van Den Berghe G. Hypothalamic-pituitary hormones during critical illness: a dynamic neuroendocrine response. 2014. https://doi.org/10.1016/B978-0-444-59602-4.00008-3.

[54] Das L, Dutta P, Walia R, Mukherjee S, Suri V, Puri GD, et al. Spectrum of endocrine dysfunction and association with disease severity in patients with COVID-19: insights from a cross-sectional, observational study. Front Endocrinol 2021;12:824. https://doi.org/10.3389/FENDO.2021.645787/BIBTEX.

[55] Leow MKS, Kwek DSK, Ng AWK, Ong KC, Kaw GJL, Lee LSU. Hypocortisolism in survivors of severe acute respiratory syndrome (SARS). Clin Endocrinol 2005;63:197–202. https://doi.org/10.1111/J.1365-2265.2005.02325.X.

[56] W. R. Molecular mimicry of ACTH in SARS - implications for corticosteroid treatment and prophylaxis. Med Hypotheses 2004;63:855–62. https://doi.org/10.1016/J.MEHY.2004.04.009.

[57] Clarke SA, Phylactou M, Patel B, Mills EG, Muzi B, Izzi-Engbeaya C, et al. Normal adrenal and thyroid function in patients who survive COVID-19 infection. J Clin Endocrinol Metab 2021;106:2208–20. https://doi.org/10.1210/CLINEM/DGAB349.

[58] Clarke S, Phylactou M, Patel B, Mills E, Muzi B, Izzi-Engbeaya C, et al. Pituitary and gonadal axes in patients with 'Long COVID': post hoc analysis. Endocr Abstr 2021:77. https://doi.org/10.1530/ENDOABS.77.P82.

[59] Churilov L, Kanduc D, Ryabkova V. COVID-19: adrenal response and molecular mimicry. Isr Med Assoc J 2021;23:618–9.

[60] Churilov LP, Normatov MG, Utekhin VJ. Molecular mimicry between SARS-CoV-2 and human endocrinocytes: aprerequisite of post-COVID endocrine autoimmunity? Pathophysiology 2022;29(3).

[61] Llamas M, Garo ML, Giovanella L. Low free-T3 serum levels and prognosis of COVID-19: systematic review and meta-analysis. Clin Chem Lab Med 2021;59:1906–13. https://doi.org/10.1515/CCLM-2021-0805/PDF.

[62] Lui DTW, Lee CH, Chow WS, Lee ACH, Tam AR, Pang P, et al. Long COVID in patients with mild to moderate disease: do thyroid function and autoimmunity play a role? Endocr Pract 2021;27:894. https://doi.org/10.1016/J.EPRAC.2021.06.016.

[63] Lui DTW, Lee CH, Chow WS, Lee ACH, Tam AR, Fong CHY, et al. Insights from a prospective follow-up of thyroid function and autoimmunity among COVID-19 survivors. Endocrinol Metab 2021;36:582. https://doi.org/10.3803/ENM.2021.983.

[64] Wood E, Hall KH, Tate W. Role of mitochondria, oxidative stress and the response to antioxidants in myalgic encephalomyelitis/chronic fatigue syndrome: a possible approach to SARS-CoV-2 'long-haulers'? Chronic Dis Transl Med 2021;7(1):14–26. https://doi.org/10.1016/j.cdtm.2020.11.002.

[65] Zimmermann FA, Neureiter D, Feichtinger RG, et al. Deficiency of respiratory chain complex I in Hashimoto thyroiditis. Mitochondrion 2016;26:1–6. https://doi.org/10.1016/j.mito.2015.11.002.

CHAPTER

39

Long-term assessment of autoantibodies in post-COVID syndrome

Natalia Gavrilova[1,2,3], *Anna Malkova*[4,5], *Soprun Lidiia*[3,6], *Varvara A. Ryabkova*[6,7,8] *and Kamaeva Evelina*[6]

[1]Department of Faculty Therapy, Saint Petersburg State University, Saint Petersburg, Russia; [2]Department of Pulmonology, Scientific Research Institute of Phthisiopulmonology, Saint Petersburg, Russia; [3]Saint Petersburg State University Hospital, Saint Petersburg, Russia; [4]Ariel University, Ariel, Israel; [5]Saint Petersburg State University, Saint Petersburg, Russia; [6]Laboratory of the Mosaic of Autoimmunity, Saint Petersburg State University, Saint Petersburg, Russia; [7]Department of Pathology, Saint Petersburg State University, Saint Petersburg, Russia; [8]Pavlov First Saint Petersburg State Medical University, Saint Petersburg, Russia

Novel coronavirus infection is associated with both innate and acquired autoimmune reactions. The autoimmune hypothesis of the pathogenesis of post-COVID-19 syndrome is being described in various studies that evaluate autoantibodies (Aab) to human tissues, many of which have a direct correlation with the COVID-19 symptoms [1,2]. Among the most widespread Aab in the acute COVID-19 disease, rheumatoid factor (RF), and antinuclear antibodies (ANA) were described. Cluster analysis by Anaya et al. revealed that those patients with high frequency of RF, anti-β2 Glycoprotein 1 IgM (anti-β2GP1) antibodies, and ANA had a longer hospital stay required more vasopressors during hospitalization and were more likely to develop critical disease [3].

A number of studies have shown that the SARS-CoV-2 virus has homologous regions with human proteins and at least three candidate proteins have been isolated, which include heat shock protein A5 (HSPA5), titin, ryanodine receptor 2 (RYR2) [4]. Thus, there is a possibility of cross-reactivity of virus proteins with the tissues of the human body and the production of the certain Aab. This chapter describes the most studied of the identified Aab in patients suffering from a novel coronavirus infection, which may be important in clinical practice.

Autoimmunity, COVID-19, Post-COVID19 syndrome and COVID-19 vaccination
https://doi.org/10.1016/B978-0-443-18566-3.00040-2

Antibodies to the autonomic nervous system in patients with post-COVID-19 syndrome

An important role in the development of post-COVID syndrome is probably played by various autonomic Aab, the presence of which was evaluated according to the several studies [5]. Thus, Aab to β2-adrenoceptor, α1-adrenoceptor, and angiotensin II receptor type 1 receptor described in the study by Wallukat et al. [6] can be considered as one of the most promising biomarkers. The concept of an autoimmune response to the G-protein coupled receptors is based on the fact that Aab of this type can have functional activity, affecting the functioning of the cardiovascular system. Patients with post-COVID-19 syndrome often complain of orthostatic disorders (primarily postural orthostatic tachycardia, POTS), palpitations, darkening in the eyes, and chronic fatigue, which pathophysiologically could be developed due to the functionally active Aab to autonomic nervous system. There are works where blood serum of patients with various manifestations of POTS was examined to assess the concentration of Aab, where more than half of the patients showed increased titers of Aab against the adrenergic alpha 1 receptor and against the muscarinic acetylcholine M4 receptor [2,7]. Nevertheless, in such cases, the question remains about the actual degree of functional activity of these Aab and their ability to influence the autoregulation of the cardiovascular system. Wallukat et al. [6] showed that in a group of 31 patients with post-COVID syndrome, in each case, from 2 to 7 G-protein coupled receptors Aab were detected, that functioned as receptor agonists, causing both a positive chronotropic effect (antibodies to adrenoreceptors and angiotensin II receptor type 1 receptor), as well as a negative chronotropic effect (muscarinic antibodies, MAS and ETA antibodies) in a study on cardiomyocytes of neonatal rats. In another study [8], serum from patients with POTS was added to a culture of human embryonic kidney 293 cells that are overexpressing adrenergic α1 receptor, adrenergic β2 receptor, cholinergic muscarinic type 2 receptor, and opioid receptor-like 1. As a result, *in vitro* was obtained activation of all four types of receptors, which may be critical for understanding the pathogenesis of this condition and determining the treatment regimen for patients. In a number of studies, Aab to the autonomic nervous system were described even in patients in the acute period of a novel coronavirus infection and persisted for several months after it, which may also be important for choosing the treatment tactics [7–9].

Post-COVID-19 syndrome, rheumatological diseases, and antibodies to the components of the immune system

In many medical centers around the world, there has been a significant surge in rheumatic diseases in patients with post-COVID-19 syndrome. At the same time, the primary question—whether the novel coronavirus infection was the cause of these conditions or was a trigger that activates this process—still remains to be resolved. The most widespread autoimmune conditions that develop in such patients include antiphospholipid syndrome, IgA nephropathy, autoimmune liver diseases, rheumatoid arthritis and systemic lupus erythematosus, as well as some neurological autoimmune disorders [10].

One of the most common "traditional" autoantibodies described in patients with a post-COVID-19 condition include antinuclear (ANA), antiphospholipid (aPL), and anti-TNF-alpha antibodies [11]. Autoantibodies that targeted cytokines (type I interferons), chemokines or their receptors, as well as particular leukocyte subsets (B cells, T cells, natural killer cells, and monocytes) have also been identified in patients with acute COVID-19, which may correlate with the presence and severity of a cytokine storm in such patients, and, therefore, help determine the prognosis and treatment regimen in such patients [12].

Acosta-Ampudia et al. [9] monitored patients in acute phase of COVID and after 1, 7, and 11 months after the disease. They found that such patients had high level of anti-Sars-Cov2 S1 IgG, increased anti-double stranded DNA, anti-thyroglobulin, anti-β2GP1 IgM autoantibodies. Moreover, despite of the general lymphopenia, increased number of effector T cells, B naïve cells, Th9, and decreased number of naïve T cells were observed. The authors concluded that the clinical manifestations in the post-COVID-19 condition could be associated with the persistence of a proinflammatory and effector phenotype induced by SARS-CoV-2 infection. According to their data, long-term persistent immune activation could contribute to reactivity and the development of autoimmunity processes. Based on the study results, the research group proposed potential therapeutic targets for management of post-COVID syndrome, such as TNF or IL-6 blockade and immunomodulatory drugs.

Chang et al. created the bead-based antigen arrays to detect IgG autoantibodies associated with connective tissue diseases, anticytokine antibodies, and antiviral antibody responses in 147 hospitalized subjects and 41 healthy controls [13]. According to the published data, individual patients with COVID-19 had higher titers autoantibodies, including ANA, anti-dsDNA, different anti-ribosomal, thyroid autoantibodies, in comparison with healthy controls. In another study which used rapid extracellular antigen profiling 172 patients with COVID-19 and 22 healthcare workers with mild disease or asymptomatic infection were investigated for autoantibodies against 2770 extracellular and secreted proteins [12]. The researchers found that patients with COVID-19 exhibit marked increases in autoantibody reactivities as compared to uninfected individuals and show a high prevalence of autoantibodies against immunomodulatory proteins (including cytokines, chemokines, complement components, and cell-surface proteins). Moreover, specific clinical characteristics were associated with Aab against tissue-associated antigens. For example, Aab against various tissue-associated antigens were correlated with inflammatory clinical markers such as D-dimer, ferritin, C-reactive protein, and lactate in patients with COVID-19. The patients with autoantibodies against HCRTR2, which is an orexin receptor enriched in the hypothalamus, had a marked negative correlation with low Glasgow coma scale scores.

One of the most important clinical issues is the presence of aPL Aab, which are often evaluated in post-COVID-19 syndrome, especially in its severe forms. aPL antibodies typically include anticardiolipin antibodies, anti-β2-glycoprotein I (β2GPI) antibodies, and lupus anticoagulants. The question of their clinical significance and the degree of functional activity is constantly studied in the literature [14]. Cavalli et al. examined the prevalence of aPL Aab in COVID-19 patients, which showed overall higher titers, compared to the healthy population [15]. The question of the risk of thrombosis and its association with the aPS Aab in the post-COVID-19 syndrome needs to be further investigated, as well as the dynamics of the titers of these Aab in patients with acute and postacute COVID-19 disease [16]. Though the absolute levels of Aab in this type of patients may be lover in comparison with the rheumatic diseases (e.g., antiphospholipid syndrome), the presence of autoimmune complication in COVID-19 may sufficiently worsen the prognosis. As Pascolini et al. showed 40% of patients with ANA and aPS Aab died during the hospitalization due to the COVID-19 complications, when in patients without autoimmune reactions, the mortality rate was as low as 5%. The authors emphasize the small amounts of study groups (33 and 31 patients, respectively); therefore, the results of this study must be considered as preliminary [17].

One of the most severe neurological complications in the post-COVID-19 condition is Guillain-Barré syndrome (GBS) that may be developed due to the molecular similarities between SARS-CoV-2 peptide sequences and heat shock proteins HSP90B, HSP90B2, and HSP60 [18]. These autoantibodies are implicated in many other autoimmune neurological diseases that support this hypothesis [19]. It is still unclear, whether COVID-19 infection directly leads to GBS development, though at least two case studies referred to it lately [20,21].

Possible causes of autoantibodies production in the post-COVID-19 condition

The most discussed cause of autoimmune inflammation in patients with post-COVID-19 disease is molecular mimicry of Sasr-Cov2 proteins with human antigens. A row of possible human proteins which have matches with 15mer palindromic SARS-CoV-2 peptide was described lately [22]. Among them are proteins associated with neuronal functions: Neuronal acetylcholine receptor subunit alpha-2, G protein-coupled receptor 89C, Arginyl-tRNA synthetase-like, tsukushin, phospholipid phosphatase-related protein type 5, metabotropic glutamate receptor 5, plasminogen receptor. The plasminogen receptor suggested to be a risk factor for COVID-19 susceptibility [23] and is highly expressed at the proinflammatory macrophages—microglial cells, what is typical for neuroinflammatory diseases [9].

One of the explanations of the development of autoimmune complications might be also the molecular similarity of SARS-CoV-2 S-protein with surfactant proteins, which was shown in the Kanduc et al. study [24]. Also peptides shared between spike glycoproteins from HCoV-229E and SARS-CoV-2 and human surfactant-related proteins were revealed, among which there are several that can be associated with neuronal complications: alpha-2C adrenergic receptor and AGRF5, G-protein coupled receptor 116 [24]. In the next study of this group [25], it was shown that SARS-CoV-2 spike glycoproteins shares numerous pentapeptides with antiinflammatory proteins what might explain the development cytokine storms, including systemic multiorgan hyperinflammation, macrophage activation syndrome, ferritinemia, endothelial dysfunction, and acute respiratory syndrome. There are also matches with G-protein receptors: G-protein coupled receptor 176, Probable G-protein coupled receptor 25, Probable G-protein coupled receptor 83, G-protein coupled receptor 84.

According to the hypothesis of Townsend et al. [26], delayed lung damage after SARS-CoV-2 infection may be caused by an autoimmune response to ACE2, which can be explained by the forced presentation of the ACE2 protein in complex with CoV spike in Fc receptor-positive antigen-presenting cells. In the study conducted by Arthur et al. [27], 81% of the convalescent patients and 93% of patients acutely hospitalized had detectable ACE2 antibodies in comparison with patients without history of SARS-CoV-2 infection. However, the data on clinical characteristics were not provided; therefore, it's difficult to correlate the presence of autoantibodies to ACE2 with organ damage.

According to Cappello F et al., hypoxia during the infection might induce expression of anti-stress proteins, including heat shock proteins (Hsp) that have a high level of structural conservation and share various similar antigens within and across species. It might be the cause of immunological crossreactivity between Hsp/chaperones and virus proteins that leads to autoimmune reactivity [28]. Generated antibodies might damage endothelium cells with the development of thrombosis, disseminated intravascular coagulation, and multiorgan failure [29,30].

Conclusion

Novel coronavirus infection remains to be one of the most serious problems of modern health care, mainly, due to its prevalence and insufficient knowledge of the pathogenesis of this disease. Autoimmune complications can be an important link in achieving the goals of treatment, prognosis, and rehabilitation of these patients. Autoantibodies to the autonomic nervous system, antinuclear, antiphospholipid antibodies, and RF are the most frequently evaluated ones. A lot of studies have been tackling the role of the novel coronavirus infection as a trigger for classic autoimmune diseases, but the extent of the virus's influence on rheumatic diseases is still a matter of debate. The identification of autoantibodies and the development of the evidence-based knowledge about their role in the post-COVID-19 syndrome will allow the elaboration of the new recommendations for the diagnosis and treatment of these patients.

References

[1] Halpert G, Shoenfeld Y. SARS-CoV-2, the autoimmune virus. Autoimmun Rev December 2020;19(12):102695. https://doi.org/10.1016/j.autrev.2020.102695. Epub 2020 Oct 28. PMID: 33130000; PMCID: PMC7598743.

[2] Ehrenfeld M, Tincani A, Andreoli L, Cattalini M, Greenbaum A, Kanduc D, Alijotas-Reig J, Zinserling V, Semenova N, Amital H, Shoenfeld Y. Covid-19 and autoimmunity. Autoimmun Rev August 2020;19(8):102597. https://doi.org/10.1016/j.autrev.2020.102597. Epub 2020 Jun 11. PMID: 32535093; PMCID: PMC7289100.

[3] Anaya JM, Monsalve DM, Rojas M, Rodríguez Y, Montoya-García N, Mancera-Navarro LM, Villadiego-Santana AM, Rodríguez-Leguizamón G, Acosta-Ampudia Y, Ramírez-Santana C. Latent rheumatic, thyroid and phospholipid autoimmunity in hospitalized patients with COVID-19. J Transl Autoimmun 2021;4:100091. https://doi.org/10.1016/j.jtauto.2021.100091. Epub 2021 Mar 2. PMID: 33681751; PMCID: PMC7920824.

[4] Mohkhedkar M, Venigalla SSK, Janakiraman V. Autoantigens that may explain postinfection autoimmune manifestations in patients with coronavirus disease 2019 Displaying neurological conditions. J Infect Dis 2021;223:536–7.

[5] Dotan A, Shoenfeld Y. Post-COVID syndrome: the aftershock of SARS-CoV-2. Int J Infect Dis January 2022;114:233–5. https://doi.org/10.1016/j.ijid.2021.11.020. Epub 2021 Nov 14. PMID: 34785367; PMCID: PMC8590600.

[6] Wallukat G, Hohberger B, Wenzel K, et al. Functional autoantibodies against G-protein coupled receptors in patients with persistent Long-COVID-19 symptoms. J Transl Autoimmun 2021;4:100100. https://doi.org/10.1016/j.jtauto.2021.100100.

[7] La Cava A. Antiphospholipid antibodies and COVID-19. Autoimmun Rev October 2021;20(10):102910. https://doi.org/10.1016/j.autrev.2021.102910. Epub 2021 Jul 22. PMID: 34303846; PMCID: PMC8297967.

[8] Seyed Hosseini E, Riahi Kashani N, Nikzad H, Azadbakht J, Hassani Bafrani H, Haddad Kashani H. The novel coronavirus disease-2019 (COVID-19): mechanism of action, detection and recent therapeutic strategies. Virology December 2020;551:1–9. https://doi.org/10.1016/j.virol.2020.08.011. Epub 2020 Sep 24. PMID: 33010669; PMCID: PMC7513802.

[9] Acosta-Ampudia Y, Monsalve DM, Rojas M, Rodríguez Y, Zapata E, Ramírez-Santana C, Anaya J-M. Persistent autoimmune activation and proinflammatory state in post-COVID syndrome. MedRxiv; 2021. p. 2021. https://doi.org/10.1101/2021.11.17.21266457. 11.17.21266457.

[10] Chen Y, Xu Z, Wang P, Li XM, Shuai ZW, Ye DQ, Pan HF. New-onset autoimmune phenomena post-COVID-19 vaccination. Immunology December 27, 2021. https://doi.org/10.1111/imm.13443. Epub ahead of print. PMID: 34957554.

[11] Gao ZW, Zhang HZ, Liu C, Dong K. Autoantibodies in COVID-19: frequency and function. Autoimmun Rev 2021;20(3):102754. https://doi.org/10.1016/j.autrev.2021.102754.

[12] Wang E, et al. Diverse functional autoantibodies in patients with COVID-19. medRxiv [preprint]. December 12, 2020. 2020.12.10.20247205.

[13] Chang SE, Feng A, Meng W, Apostolidis SA, Mack E, Artandi M, Barman L, Bennett K, Chakraborty S, Chang I, Cheung P, Chinthrajah S, Dhingra S, Do E, Finck A, Gaano A, Geßner R, Giannini HM, Gonzalez J, Greib S, Gündisch M, Hsu AR, Kuo A, Manohar M, Mao R, Neeli I, Neubauer A, Oniyide O, Powell AE, Puri R, Renz H, Schapiro J, Weidenbacher PA, Wittman R, Ahuja N, Chung HR, Jagannathan P, James JA, Kim PS, Meyer NJ, Nadeau KC, Radic M, Robinson WH, Singh U, Wang TT, Wherry EJ, Skevaki C, Luning Prak ET, Utz PJ. New-onset IgG autoantibodies in hospitalized patients with COVID-19. Nat Commun 2021;12:1–15. https://doi.org/10.1038/s41467-021-25509-3.

[14] Taha M, Samavati L. Antiphospholipid antibodies in COVID-19: a meta-analysis and systematic review. RMD Open 2021;7. https://doi.org/10.1136/rmdopen-2021-001580.

[15] Cavalli E, Bramanti A, Ciurleo R, Tchorbanov AI, Giordano A, Fagone P, Belizna C, Bramanti P, Shoenfeld Y, Nicoletti F. Entangling COVID-19 associated thrombosis into a secondary antiphospholipid antibody syndrome: diagnostic and therapeutic perspectives (Review). Int J Mol Med 2020;46:903–12. https://doi.org/10.3892/ijmm.2020.4659.

[16] Stelzer M, Henes J, Saur S. The role of antiphospholipid antibodies in COVID-19. Curr Rheumatol Rep 2021;23(9):72. https://doi.org/10.1007/s11926-021-01041-7. Published 2021 Jul 14.

[17] Pascolini S, Vannini A, Deleonardi G, Ciordinik M, Sensoli A, Carletti I, Veronesi L, Ricci C, Pronesti A, Mazzanti L, Grondona A, Silvestri T, Zanuso S, Mazzolini M, Lalanne C, Quarneti C, Fusconi M, Giostra F, Granito A, Muratori L, Lenzi M, Muratori P. COVID-19 and immunological dysregulation: can autoantibodies be useful? Clin Transl Sci March 2021;14(2):502–8. https://doi.org/10.1111/cts.12908. Epub 2021 Jan 20. PMID: 32989903; PMCID: PMC7536986.

[18] Lucchese G, Flöel A. SARS-CoV-2 and Guillain-Barré syndrome: molecular mimicry with human heat shock proteins as potential pathogenic mechanism. Cell Stress Chaperones 2020;25(5):731–5. https://doi.org/10.1007/s12192-020-01145-6.

[19] Al-Ramadan A, Rabab'h O, Shah J, Gharaibeh A. Acute and post-acute neurological complications of COVID-19. Neurol Int 2021;13(1):102–19. https://doi.org/10.3390/neurolint13010010. Published 2021 Mar 9.

[20] Toscano G, Palmerini F, Ravaglia S. Guillain-Barrė syndrome associated with SARS-CoV-2. NEJM 2020. https://doi.org/10.1056/NEJMc2009191.

[21] Seaghat Z, Karimi N. Guillain-Barrė syndrome associated with COVID-19 infection: a case report. J Clin Neurosci 2020. https://doi.org/10.1016/j.jocn.2020.04.062.

[22] Gunning 3rd WT, Kvale H, Kramer PM, Karabin BL, Grubb BP. Postural orthostatic tachycardia syndrome is associated with elevated G-protein coupled receptor autoantibodies. J Am Heart Assoc September 17, 2019;8(18):e013602. https://doi.org/10.1161/JAHA.119.013602. Epub 2019 Sep 9. PMID: 31495251; PMCID: PMC6818019.

[23] Kharraziha I, Axelsson J, Ricci F, Di Martino G, Persson M, Sutton R, Fedorowski A, Hamrefors V. Serum activity against G protein-coupled receptors and severity of orthostatic symptoms in postural orthostatic tachycardia syndrome. J Am Heart Assoc August 4, 2020;9(15):e015989. https://doi.org/10.1161/JAHA.120.015989. Epub 2020 Jul 30. PMID: 32750291; PMCID: PMC7792263.

[24] Kanduc D, Shoenfeld Y. On the molecular determinants of the SARS-CoV-2 attack. Clin Immunol 2020;215:108426. https://doi.org/10.1016/j.clim.2020.108426.

[25] Kanduc D. From anti-SARS-CoV-2 immune response to the cytokine storm via molecular mimicry. Antibodies 2021;10:36. https://doi.org/10.3390/antib10040036.

[26] Townsend A. Autoimmunity to ACE2 as a possible cause of tissue inflammation in Covid-19. Med Hypotheses 2020;144. https://doi.org/10.1016/j.mehy.2020.110043.

[27] Arthur JM, Forrest JC, Boehme KW, Kennedy JL, Owens S, Herzog C, Liu J, Harville TO. Development of ACE2 autoantibodies after SARS-CoV-2 infection. PLoS One 2021;16:e0257016. https://doi.org/10.1371/JOURNAL.PONE.0257016.

[28] Cappello F, Gammazza AM, Dieli F, de Macario EC, Macario AJ. Does sars-cov-2 trigger stress-induced autoimmunity by molecular mimicry? A hypothesis. J Clin Med 2020;9:1–14. https://doi.org/10.3390/jcm9072038.

[29] Marino Gammazza A, Légaré S, Lo Bosco G, Fucarino A, Angileri F, Conway de Macario E, Macario AJ, Cappello F. Human molecular chaperones share with SARS-CoV-2 antigenic epitopes potentially capable of eliciting autoimmunity against endothelial cells: possible role of molecular mimicry in COVID-19. Cell Stress Chaperones 2020;25:737–41. https://doi.org/10.1007/s12192-020-01148-3.

[30] Cappello F. Is COVID-19 a proteiform disease inducing also molecular mimicry phenomena? Cell Stress Chaperones 2020;25:381–2. https://doi.org/10.1007/s12192-020-01112-1.

CHAPTER

40

Post-COVID-19 syndrome and fibromyalgia

Francesco Ursini[1,2], *Piero Ruscitti*[3] *and Roberto Giacomelli*[4]

[1]Medicine & Rheumatology Unit, IRCCS Istituto Ortopedico Rizzoli, Bologna, Italy; [2]Department of Biomedical and Neuromotor Sciences (DIBINEM), University of Bologna, Bologna, Italy; [3]Rheumatology Unit, Department of Biotechnological and Applied Clinical Sciences, Università degli Studi dell'Aquila, L'Aquila, Italy; [4]Unit of Allergology, Department of Medicine, Campus Bio-Medico University Hospital, Roma, Italy

Severe acute respiratory syndrome coronavirus 2 (SARS-CoV-2), which is responsible for the coronavirus disease 2019 (COVID-19), has caused a global medical emergency [1]. A growing body of evidence is suggesting the possible subacute and long-term effects in patients suffering from COVID-19, affecting multiple organ systems [2]. In this context, the residual effects of SARS-CoV-2 infection have been recently reported, including fatigue, dyspnoea, chest pain, cognitive disturbances, arthralgia, and a profound decline of quality of life [3–5]. Thus, the so-called long COVID has been proposed to describe these signs and symptoms which may continue or, in some cases, develop following the acute phase of COVID-19. This condition may comprise both ongoing symptomatic COVID-19 (from 4 to 12 weeks) and post-COVID-19 syndrome (12 weeks or more) [6]. In other coronavirus infections, including the SARS epidemic of 2003 and the Middle East respiratory syndrome (MERS) outbreak of 2012, a similar constellation of persistent symptoms was shown, thus reinforcing the possible concern about the clinically significant consequences of COVID-19 [7–9]. Previous studies, which assessed the long-term health problems in survivors of these two outbreaks, demonstrated a reduced lung function as well as a decreased ability to exercise in some survivors up to 6 months after discharge from hospital [7–9]. Mental health problems, such as stress, anxiety, and depression, were also observed in up to one-third of 2003 SARS and MERS survivors, after 6 months and beyond [7–9]. The quality of life was observed to be low even 12 months after discharge from the hospital in these patients [7–9]. On these bases, some works have presently suggested the postacute infectious consequences of COVID-19, with studies from the United States, Europe, and China reporting outcomes for those patients

Autoimmunity, COVID-19, Post-COVID19 syndrome and COVID-19 vaccination
https://doi.org/10.1016/B978-0-443-18566-3.00011-6

who were hospitalized and survived for this disease. A rate of occurrence between 30% and 80% was reported suggesting the relevance of this issue among patients with COVID-19 [3,10–15]. As far as the pathogenesis is concerned, potential mechanisms contributing to the pathophysiology of this post-acute COVID-19 condition may include (i) virus-specific pathophysiologic changes; (ii) immunologic aberrations and inflammatory damage in response to the acute infection; (iii) expected sequelae of postcritical illness [6]. The latter is a well-known syndrome which may include the onset or the worsening of abnormalities in physical, cognitive, and psychiatric domains after critical illness [16–19]. The pathophysiology of postintensive care syndrome is considered to be multifactorial and may involve microvascular ischemia and injury, immobility, and metabolic alterations during the critical disease [20].

During acute COVID-19, musculoskeletal pain is reported in one-third of patients [21] and it may be also part of the spectrum of post-COVID-19 syndrome, along with other manifestations [6]. Musculoskeletal pain is the cardinal symptoms of fibromyalgia, a disease characterized by chronic widespread pain, fatigue, sleep disturbances, and functional symptoms [22]. Fibromyalgia is the third most frequent musculoskeletal condition, and its prevalence increases with age [22]. However, although diagnosis has improved with the evolution of more accurate diagnostic criteria [23–25], a considerable proportion of physicians still fail to recognize the syndrome. Many factors may contribute to the development of fibromyalgia: genetic predisposition, personal experiences, emotional-cognitive factors, the mind–body relationship, and a biopsychological ability to cope with stress [22]. However, the pathogenesis of fibromyalgia is not entirely clarified yet. Pain augmentation/dysperception may be associated with exquisite neuromorphological modifications and imbalance between pronociceptive and antinociceptive pathways arising from an intricate interplay between genetic predisposition, stressful life events, psychological characteristics, and emerging peripheral mechanisms, such as small fiber neuropathy or neuroinflammation [22]. In this context, the role of viral infection as a triggering factor for the development of fibromyalgia has been postulated since many years; several viruses have been invoked, such as hepatitis C, parvovirus B19, human immunodeficiency virus (HIV), Epstein–Barr virus and human herpesvirus-6 (HHV-6), and human herpesvirus-7 (HHV-7) [26] but evidence remains still inconclusive. The first demonstration of a potential correlation between SARS-CoV-2 and subsequent development of fibromyalgia came from an online survey performed by our group and aimed at investigating the prevalence and predictors of post-COVID-19 fibromyalgia [27]. Among 616 individuals (77.4% women) recovering from COVID-19 participating in the survey, 189 (30.7%) satisfied the American College of Rheumatology survey criteria for fibromyalgia (56.6% women). Respondents with fibromyalgia exhibited features suggestive of a more serious form of COVID-19, including a higher rate of hospitalization and more frequent treatment with supplemental oxygen. Intriguingly, in multivariate logistic regression analysis male gender (OR: 9.95, 95% CI 6.02 to 16.43, $P < 0.0001$) and obesity (OR: 41.20, 95% CI 18.00 to 98.88, $P < 0.0001$) were the strongest predictors of being classified as having post-COVID-19 FM. Taken together, these data suggest a speculative mechanism in which obesity and male gender synergistically affect the severity of COVID-19 that, in turn, may rebound on the risk of developing post-COVID-19 fibromyalgia and determine its severity [27]. Similarly, Bierle et al. reported the results of a retrospective analysis of patients referred to the Mayo Clinic General Internal Medicine division for the evaluation of central sensitization syndrome from the beginning of the COVID-19 pandemic (November 2019). Of the total 465 cases reviewed, 42 (9%) met criteria for post-COVID central sensitization syndrome, with a clinical presentation mainly characterized by pain (90.2%), fatigue (73.8%), dyspnoea (42.9%), and orthostatic intolerance (38.1%) [28].

Despite the mechanism underlying post-COVID-19 fibromyalgia remains unclear, preliminary evidence from clinical and preclinical research suggests that several COVID-19-specific mechanisms may contribute to the pathophysiology of the subsequent musculoskeletal syndrome, for example, a sustained virus-induced injury to endothelium or neuromuscular structures [29,30]. Interestingly, early reports suggest an increased prevalence of small fiber neuropathy—a well-recognized determinant of fibromyalgia symptoms—and autonomic dysfunction in patients recovering from COVID-19 [31–33].

Furthermore, it is possible to hypothesize a role of immunological derangement and smouldering inflammation triggered by SARS-CoV-2. Indeed, it is interesting to note that some of the proinflammatory cytokines involved in COVID-19 and post-COVID-19 syndrome manifestations, such as interleukin (IL)-1 and IL-6 [6], may contribute to the pathogenesis of fibromyalgia [34] as well. Finally, other indirect and nonspecific processes—for example, prolonged bed rest, deconditioning, posttraumatic stress disorder—may prevail at least in some patients. For this reason, according to the current knowledge, treatment should be focused at treating both central sensitization and physical deconditioning. The possible multiple components of the pathogenesis and maintenance of this condition may necessitate a multimodal treatment approach. Common practice is to start with painkillers such as paracetamol and/or tramadol associated with pain modulators (e.g., amitriptyline, duloxetine, or pregabalin). A multimodal, individualized, rehabilitation program should be initiated as early as possible. The long-term prognosis of post-COVID-19 fibromyalgia is still unknown, although it is possible to expect a full recovery in a significant proportion of patients.

References

[1] Rothan HA, Byrareddy SN. The epidemiology and pathogenesis of coronavirus disease (COVID-19) outbreak. J Autoimmun May 2020;109:102433. https://doi.org/10.1016/j.jaut.2020.102433. Epub 2020 Feb 26. PMID: 32113704; PMCID: PMC7127067.

[2] Gupta A, Madhavan MV, Sehgal K, Nair N, Mahajan S, Sehrawat TS, Bikdeli B, Ahluwalia N, Ausiello JC, Wan EY, Freedberg DE, Kirtane AJ, Parikh SA, Maurer MS, Nordvig AS, Accili D, Bathon JM, Mohan S, Bauer KA, Leon MB, Krumholz HM, Uriel N, Mehra MR, Elkind MSV, Stone GW, Schwartz A, Ho DD, Bilezikian JP, Landry DW. Extrapulmonary manifestations of COVID-19. Nat Med July 2020;26(7):1017–32. https://doi.org/10.1038/s41591-020-0968-3. Epub 2020 Jul 10. PMID: 32651579.

[3] Carfì A, Bernabei R, Landi F. Gemelli against COVID-19 post-acute care study group. Persistent symptoms in patients after acute COVID-19. JAMA August 11, 2020;324(6):603–5. https://doi.org/10.1001/jama.2020.12603. PMID: 32644129; PMCID: PMC7349096.

[4] Tenforde MW, Kim SS, Lindsell CJ, Billig Rose E, Shapiro NI, Files DC, Gibbs KW, Erickson HL, Steingrub JS, Smithline HA, Gong MN, Aboodi MS, Exline MC, Henning DJ, Wilson JG, Khan A, Qadir N, Brown SM, Peltan ID, Rice TW, Hager DN, Ginde AA, Stubblefield WB, Patel MM, Self WH, Feldstein LR, Network Investigators IVY. CDC COVID-19 response team; IVY network investigators. Symptom duration and risk factors for delayed return to usual health among outpatients with COVID-19 in a multistate health care systems network - United States, March-June 2020. MMWR Morb Mortal Wkly Rep July 31, 2020;69(30):993–8. https://doi.org/10.15585/mmwr.mm6930e1. PMID: 32730238; PMCID: PMC7392393.

[5] Huang C, Huang L, Wang Y, Li X, Ren L, Gu X, Kang L, Guo L, Liu M, Zhou X, Luo J, Huang Z, Tu S, Zhao Y, Chen L, Xu D, Li Y, Li C, Peng L, Li Y, Xie W, Cui D, Shang L, Fan G, Xu J, Wang G, Wang Y, Zhong J, Wang C, Wang J, Zhang D, Cao B. 6-month consequences of COVID-19 in patients discharged from hospital: a cohort study. Lancet January 16, 2021;397(10270):220–32. https://doi.org/10.1016/S0140-6736(20)32656-8. Epub 2021 Jan 8. PMID: 33428867; PMCID: PMC7833295.

[6] Nalbandian A, Sehgal K, Gupta A, Madhavan MV, McGroder C, Stevens JS, Cook JR, Nordvig AS, Shalev D, Sehrawat TS, Ahluwalia N, Bikdeli B, Dietz D, Der-Nigoghossian C, Liyanage-Don N, Rosner GF, Bernstein EJ, Mohan S, Beckley AA, Seres DS, Choueiri TK, Uriel N, Ausiello JC, Accili D, Freedberg DE, Baldwin M, Schwartz A, Brodie D, Garcia CK, Elkind MSV, Connors JM, Bilezikian JP, Landry DW, Wan EY. Post-acute COVID-19 syndrome. Nat Med April 2021;27(4):601–15. https://doi.org/10.1038/s41591-021-01283-z. Epub 2021 Mar 22. PMID: 33753937.

[7] Ahmed H, Patel K, Greenwood DC, Halpin S, Lewthwaite P, Salawu A, Eyre L, Breen A, O'Connor R, Jones A, Sivan M. Long-term clinical outcomes in survivors of severe acute respiratory syndrome and Middle East respiratory syndrome coronavirus outbreaks after hospitalisation or ICU admission: a systematic review and meta-analysis. J Rehabil Med May 31, 2020;52(5):jrm00063. https://doi.org/10.2340/16501977-2694. PMID: 32449782.

[8] Lam MH, Wing YK, Yu MW, Leung CM, Ma RC, Kong AP, So WY, Fong SY, Lam SP. Mental morbidities and chronic fatigue in severe acute respiratory syndrome survivors: long-term follow-up. Arch Intern Med December 14, 2009;169(22):2142–7. https://doi.org/10.1001/archinternmed.2009.384. PMID: 20008700.

[9] Lee AM, Wong JG, McAlonan GM, Cheung V, Cheung C, Sham PC, Chu CM, Wong PC, Tsang KW, Chua SE. Stress and psychological distress among SARS survivors 1 year after the outbreak. Can J Psychiatr April 2007;52(4):233–40. https://doi.org/10.1177/070674370705200405. PMID: 17500304.

[10] Chopra V, Flanders SA, O'Malley M, Malani AN, Prescott HC. Sixty-day outcomes among patients hospitalized with COVID-19. Ann Intern Med April 2021;174(4):576–8. https://doi.org/10.7326/M20-5661. Epub 2020 Nov 11. PMID: 33175566; PMCID: PMC7707210.

[11] Arnold DT, Hamilton FW, Milne A, Morley AJ, Viner J, Attwood M, Noel A, Gunning S, Hatrick J, Hamilton S, Elvers KT, Hyams C, Bibby A, Moran E, Adamali HI, Dodd JW, Maskell NA, Barratt SL. Patient outcomes after hospitalisation with COVID-19 and implications for follow-up: results from a prospective UK cohort. Thorax April 2021;76(4):399–401. https://doi.org/10.1136/thoraxjnl-2020-216086. Epub 2020 Dec 3. PMID: 33273026; PMCID: PMC7716340.

[12] Moreno-Pérez O, Merino E, Leon-Ramirez JM, Andres M, Ramos JM, Arenas-Jiménez J, Asensio S, Sanchez R, Ruiz-Torregrosa P, Galan I, Scholz A, Amo A, González-delaAleja P, Boix V, Gil J, research group COVID19-ALC. Post-acute COVID-19 syndrome. Incidence and risk factors: a Mediterranean cohort study. J Infect March 2021;82(3):378–83. https://doi.org/10.1016/j.jinf.2021.01.004. Epub 2021 Jan 12. PMID: 33450302; PMCID: PMC7802523.

[13] Halpin SJ, McIvor C, Whyatt G, Adams A, Harvey O, McLean L, Walshaw C, Kemp S, Corrado J, Singh R, Collins T, O'Connor RJ, Sivan M. Postdischarge symptoms and rehabilitation needs in survivors of COVID-19 infection: a cross-sectional evaluation. J Med Virol February 2021;93(2):1013–22. https://doi.org/10.1002/jmv.26368. Epub 2020 Aug 17. PMID: 32729939.

[14] Jacobs LG, Gourna Paleoudis E, Lesky-Di Bari D, Nyirenda T, Friedman T, Gupta A, Rasouli L, Zetkulic M, Balani B, Ogedegbe C, Bawa H, Berrol L, Qureshi N, Aschner JL. Persistence of symptoms and quality of life at 35 days after hospitalization for COVID-19 infection. PLoS One December 11, 2020;15(12):e0243882. https://doi.org/10.1371/journal.pone.0243882. PMID: 33306721; PMCID: PMC7732078.

[15] Garrigues E, Janvier P, Kherabi Y, Le Bot A, Hamon A, Gouze H, Doucet L, Berkani S, Oliosi E, Mallart E, Corre F, Zarrouk V, Moyer JD, Galy A, Honsel V, Fantin B, Nguyen Y. Post-discharge persistent symptoms and health-related quality of life after hospitalization for COVID-19. J Infect December 2020;81(6):e4–6. https://doi.org/10.1016/j.jinf.2020.08.029. Epub 2020 Aug 25. PMID: 32853602; PMCID: PMC7445491.

[16] Needham DM, Dinglas VD, Morris PE, Jackson JC, Hough CL, Mendez-Tellez PA, Wozniak AW, Colantuoni E, Ely EW, Rice TW, Hopkins RO, NIH NHLBI ARDS Network. Physical and cognitive performance of patients with acute lung injury 1 year after initial trophic versus full enteral feeding. EDEN trial follow-up. Am J Respir Crit Care Med September 1, 2013;188(5):567–76. https://doi.org/10.1164/rccm.201304-0651OC. PMID: 23805899; PMCID: PMC3827703.

[17] Pandharipande PP, Girard TD, Jackson JC, Morandi A, Thompson JL, Pun BT, Brummel NE, Hughes CG, Vasilevskis EE, Shintani AK, Moons KG, Geevarghese SK, Canonico A, Hopkins RO, Bernard GR, Dittus RS, Ely EW. BRAIN-ICU study investigators. Long-term cognitive impairment after critical illness. N Engl J Med October 3, 2013;369(14):1306–16. https://doi.org/10.1056/NEJMoa1301372. PMID: 24088092; PMCID: PMC3922401.

[18] Kress JP, Hall JB. ICU-acquired weakness and recovery from critical illness. N Engl J Med April 24, 2014;370(17):1626–35. https://doi.org/10.1056/NEJMra1209390. PMID: 24758618.

[19] Hosey MM, Needham DM. Survivorship after COVID-19 ICU stay. Nat Rev Dis Prim July 15, 2020;6(1):60. https://doi.org/10.1038/s41572-020-0201-1. PMID: 32669623; PMCID: PMC7362322.

[20] Inoue S, Hatakeyama J, Kondo Y, Hifumi T, Sakuramoto H, Kawasaki T, Taito S, Nakamura K, Unoki T, Kawai Y, Kenmotsu Y, Saito M, Yamakawa K, Nishida O. Post-intensive care syndrome: its pathophysiology, prevention, and future directions. Acute Med Surg April 25, 2019;6(3):233–46. https://doi.org/10.1002/ams2.415. PMID: 31304024; PMCID: PMC6603316.

[21] Ciaffi J, Meliconi R, Ruscitti P, Berardicurti O, Giacomelli R, Ursini F. Rheumatic manifestations of COVID-19: a systematic review and meta-analysis. BMC Rheumatol October 28, 2020;4:65. https://doi.org/10.1186/s41927-020-00165-0. PMID: 33123675; PMCID: PMC7591274.

[22] Sarzi-Puttini P, Giorgi V, Marotto D, Atzeni F. Fibromyalgia: an update on clinical characteristics, aetiopathogenesis and treatment. Nat Rev Rheumatol November 2020;16(11):645–60. https://doi.org/10.1038/s41584-020-00506-w. Epub 2020 Oct 6. PMID: 33024295.

[23] Wolfe F, Smythe HA, Yunus MB, Bennett RM, Bombardier C, Goldenberg DL, Tugwell P, Campbell SM, Abeles M, Clark P, et al. The American college of rheumatology 1990 criteria for the classification of fibromyalgia. Report of the multicenter criteria committee. Arthritis Rheum February 1990;33(2):160–72. https://doi.org/10.1002/art.1780330203. PMID: 2306288.

[24] Wolfe F, Clauw DJ, Fitzcharles MA, Goldenberg DL, Katz RS, Mease P, Russell AS, Russell IJ, Winfield JB, Yunus MB. The American college of rheumatology preliminary diagnostic criteria for fibromyalgia and measurement of symptom severity. Arthritis Care Res May 2010;62(5):600–10. https://doi.org/10.1002/acr.20140. PMID: 20461783.

[25] Wolfe F, Clauw DJ, Fitzcharles MA, Goldenberg DL, Häuser W, Katz RL, Mease PJ, Russell AS, Russell IJ, Walitt B. 2016 revisions to the 2010/2011 fibromyalgia diagnostic criteria. Semin Arthritis Rheum December 2016;46(3):319–29. https://doi.org/10.1016/j.semarthrit.2016.08.012. Epub 2016 Aug 30. PMID: 27916278.

[26] Buskila D, Atzeni F, Sarzi-Puttini P. Etiology of fibromyalgia: the possible role of infection and vaccination. Autoimmun Rev October 2008;8(1):41–3. https://doi.org/10.1016/j.autrev.2008.07.023. Epub 2008 Aug 13. PMID: 18706528.

[27] Ursini F, Ciaffi J, Mancarella L, Lisi L, Brusi V, Cavallari C, D'Onghia M, Mari A, Borlandelli E, Faranda Cordella J, La Regina M, Viola P, Ruscitti P, Miceli M, De Giorgio R, Baldini N, Borghi C, Gasbarrini A, Iagnocco A, Giacomelli R, Faldini C, Landini MP, Meliconi R. Fibromyalgia: a new facet of the post-COVID-19 syndrome spectrum? results from a web-based survey. RMD Open August 2021;7(3):e001735. https://doi.org/10.1136/rmdopen-2021-001735. PMID: 34426540; PMCID: PMC8384499.

[28] Bierle DM, Aakre CA, Grach SL, Salonen BR, Croghan IT, Hurt RT, Ganesh R. Central sensitization phenotypes in post acute sequelae of SARS-CoV-2 infection (PASC): defining the post COVID syndrome. J Prim Care Community Health 2021 ;12. https://doi.org/10.1177/21501327211030826. PMID: 34231404; PMCID: PMC8267019.

[29] Libby P, Lüscher T. COVID-19 is, in the end, an endothelial disease. Eur Heart J September 1, 2020;41(32):3038–44. https://doi.org/10.1093/eurheartj/ehaa623. PMID: 32882706; PMCID: PMC7470753.

[30] Guerrero JI, Barragán LA, Martínez JD, Montoya JP, Peña A, Sobrino FE, Tovar-Spinoza Z, Ghotme KA. Central and peripheral nervous system involvement by COVID-19: a systematic review of the pathophysiology, clinical manifestations, neuropathology, neuroimaging, electrophysiology, and cerebrospinal fluid findings. BMC Infect Dis June 2, 2021;21(1):515. https://doi.org/10.1186/s12879-021-06185-6. PMID: 34078305; PMCID: PMC8170436.

[31] Abrams RMC, Simpson DM, Navis A, Jette N, Zhou L, Shin SC. Small fiber neuropathy associated with SARS-CoV-2 infection. Muscle Nerve; November 12, 2021. https://doi.org/10.1002/mus.27458. Epub ahead of print. PMID: 34766365; PMCID: PMC8661991.

[32] Hinduja A, Moutairou A, Calvet JH. Sudomotor dysfunction in patients recovered from COVID-19. Neurophysiol Clin March 2021;51(2):193–6. https://doi.org/10.1016/j.neucli.2021.01.003. Epub 2021 Jan 26. PMID: 33551341; PMCID: PMC7835104.

[33] Shouman K, Vanichkachorn G, Cheshire WP, Suarez MD, Shelly S, Lamotte GJ, Sandroni P, Benarroch EE, Berini SE, Cutsforth-Gregory JK, Coon EA, Mauermann ML, Low PA, Singer W. Autonomic dysfunction following COVID-19 infection: an early experience. Clin Auton Res June 2021;31(3):385–94. https://doi.org/10.1007/s10286-021-00803-8. Epub 2021 Apr 16. PMID: 33860871; PMCID: PMC8050227.

[34] Rodriguez-Pintó I, Agmon-Levin N, Howard A, Shoenfeld Y. Fibromyalgia and cytokines. Immunol Lett October 2014;161(2):200–3. https://doi.org/10.1016/j.imlet.2014.01.009. Epub 2014 Jan 23. PMID: 24462815.

CHAPTER

41

Treatment and prevention of the post-COVID syndrome

Natalia Gavrilova[1,2,3], *Soprun Lidiia*[3,4], *Varvara A. Ryabkova*[4,5,6], *Lukashenko Maria*[4] and *Kamaeva Evelina*[4]

[1]Department of Faculty Therapy, Saint Petersburg State University, Saint Petersburg, Russia; [2]Department of Pulmonology, Scientific Research Institute of Phthisiopulmonology, Saint Petersburg, Russia; [3]Saint Petersburg State University Hospital, Saint Petersburg, Russia; [4]Laboratory of the Mosaic of Autoimmunity, Saint Petersburg State University, Saint Petersburg, Russia; [5]Department of Pathology, Saint Petersburg State University, Saint Petersburg, Russia; [6]Pavlov First Saint Petersburg State Medical University, Saint Petersburg, Russia

In December 2019, one of the most severe pandemics in modern history, COVID-19 infection, originated in China, which led to the devastating consequences in the global healthcare system. In 2020, about one in five COVID-19 patients required hospitalization and 5% remained in the intensive care units, that strongly contributed to the healthcare crisis all over the world [1,2].

In 2020–21, the medical and scientific specialists demonstrated unprecedented unity in the prevention and treatment of this disease. However, more than 175 million people worldwide are still infected, and up to 3.8 million people have died from complications of the novel coronavirus infection [3]. At the beginning of the pandemic, the most pressing issue was the growing respiratory and cardiovascular failures, the prevention of bacterial complications, and providing respiratory support for the patients [4–6]. However, after a while it became clear that COVID-19 infection also leads to the long term and sometimes very serious complications, probably of an autoimmune nature, that can last for months, limiting patients' capabilities, and reducing their quality of life [7]. The pathophysiology of these coronavirus complications, their principles of diagnosis and therapy remain unclear and require active and effective clarification [8,9].

Autoimmunity, COVID-19, Post-COVID19 syndrome and COVID-19 vaccination
https://doi.org/10.1016/B978-0-443-18566-3.00012-8

Principles of treatment of the post-COVID syndrome

As mentioned previously, two types of coronavirus complications should be distinguished. Some patients, who suffered from the COVID-19, had a severe course of the disease, which required respiratory support and, sometimes, staying in the intensive care unit. Such patients may experience respiratory dysfunction for a long time during the convalescence period, intensive care unit complications, and exacerbations of chronic respiratory and cardiovascular diseases [10,11]. For such patients, appropriate recommendations for rehabilitation are being actively developed all over the world that are mostly based on the principles of rehabilitation for severe pneumonia convalescents. The questions of therapy and rehabilitation of this group of patients lie in the field of pulmonology and internal diseases and not covered in this chapter.

The second type of the post-COVID complications is much less clear and requires extensive further studies [12,13]. The following chapter will be based on the authors' clinical experience in the treatment of such patients and, therefore is limited by the authors' knowledge, population characteristics of the examined patients (North-West region of Russian Federation), and a short follow-up period, which is currently no more than 6–8 months for the earliest patients that applied to the clinic.

These patients usually did not have a severe course of the novel coronavirus infection, most of them were not hospitalized or visit the intensive care unit. The majority of them described a mild course of illness or not mentioned any clinical manifestation at all, being diagnosed with the COVID-19 infection only with raised antibody titers. Nevertheless, within a few weeks, these patients developed an autoimmune-like complication with three basic groups of symptoms, including immunological and neurological complaints, as well as the internal organ dysfunction [3,8]. The principles of patient management that the authors consider appropriate for the treatment and prevention of these symptoms will be described in this chapter.

Immunological manifestations of post-COVID-19 syndrome

Immunological manifestations include fever, myalgia, arthralgia, flu-like symptoms, and constant fatigue [3,7,8]. Therapy of these clinical manifestations is rather complicated and requires careful exclusion of other causes of this condition and the work of a multidisciplinary team of specialists, including GP, neurologist, infectious disease specialist, and rheumatologist.

Primary rehabilitation techniques include physical rehabilitation, Pilates, and yoga classes [14]. In the presence of fatigue complaints, a graduated increase in the intensity of physical activity can be recommended. Such protocols have been developed for patients with chronic fatigue syndrome and can also be applied to the post-COVID syndrome rehabilitation. The important issue of both these diseases is a condition called postexertional malaise [15]. Some patients, overworking themselves with physical exercises during the rehabilitation period, may feel severe fatigue for several days after the session, which reduces the quality of life and discontinue the rehabilitation plan. It is much more useful for such patients to prescribe programs with a gradual increase in physical activity that are described elsewhere.

The most widespread immunological complains include pyrexia, myalgia, and flu-like symptoms. The prescription of NSAIDs that remains a treatment of choice in the acute period of viral and bacterial infections, in our experience, does not show reliable results in the post-COVID-19 condition and requires further research, providing only partial relief for the patients [16]. An exception should be made for the post-COVID arthritis, where NSAIDs are still the first-line therapy [17,18]. Diet recommendations include, at first place, adequate water regime. A gluten-free diet developed for the celiac disease may show its effectiveness in the post-COVID-19 disease as well as for other autoimmune conditions [19–21]. Its beneficial role may possibly be explained due to the growth stimulation of a certain microbiota composition that is necessary to decrease the systemic inflammation.

Immunomodulatory therapy is the most promising treatment for the severe cases of the post-COVID syndrome. Intravenous immunoglobulins (IVIg) have proven beneficial in the treatment of chronic fatigue syndrome and various autoimmune pathologies, and therefore a positive effect of IVIg is possible in this group of patients. Several regimes of IVIg appointment are possible. First of all, this is the standard scheme of 0.4 g/kg of body weight per day for 3–5 days, which is widely used in the treatment of various autoimmune diseases [22–25]. Its relative disadvantages include the high cost and the possibility of thrombotic complications. It is also possible to use low-dose IVIG therapy, where the total daily dose for the patient does not exceed 5 g, and course lasts for 3–5 days. The possibility of subcutaneous IVIg administration and other therapy regimens are being studied [26]. It is also possible to combine this medication with other types of immunosuppressants—plasmapheresis, steroids, and biological therapy.

Isolated prescription of the corticosteroids needs further studies to evaluate their effectiveness in treating fatigue, immunologic, and neurologic complications of the post-COVID-19 disorder [27]. However, based on our clinical experience, it is necessary to distinguish a group of patients, who have clinical manifestations of autoimmune adrenal insufficiency. Symptoms include fatigue, loss of energy, malaise, weight loss, nausea, anorexia, postural hypotension and hypoglycemia, and increased salt requirements [28]. In such patients, it is necessary to carefully identify the manifestations of adrenal insufficiency, evaluate the autoantibodies to the adrenal gland, and prescribe appropriate hormonal therapy if necessary.

Plasmapheresis is a rather controversial method in the autoimmune disorder treatment [29,30]. It is important to note that plasmapheresis alone does not achieve beneficial effects due to the possibility of an increase in the titer of autoantibodies after the completion of the procedure and, therefore, an increase in clinical symptoms. The use of plasmapheresis in combination with other immunosuppressive methods requires further studies.

Unfortunately, there are no reliable methods to protect patients from the development of post-COVID-19 syndrome described. Most likely, genetic factors play an important role in its development, which determine the severity of the response to the pathogen and the possibility of manifestation of autoimmune disorders. A possible way to ensure the safety of patients from the development of autoimmune disorders may be the loss of contacts with the trigger factors, including such adjuvants as silicone implants, some types of dental implants, as well as harmful environmental factors and occupational hazards [31].

Neurological complications of the COVID-19

Neurological disorders remain a surprisingly large group and have very diverse manifestations in a patient with post-COVID-19 syndrome. The main complains include polyneuropathy, autonomic dysfunction, cognitive impairment, "brain fog", manifestations of anxiety and depression, impaired sense of smell, vision, and hearing [32–34]. There are also possible manifestations of more severe autoimmune neurological disorders, such as Guillain-Barré syndrome, myelopathy, cranial nerves neuropathy, and other complications [35,36].

In the early period of autoimmune disorders, the development of emotional instability, depression, anxiety, sleep disturbances, and a special type of cognitive dysfunction called "brain fog" is often described. Post-COVID patients describe all of the above complaints, which are also included in the Delphi Consensus by the World Health Organization on October 6, 2021 as a manifestation of post-COVID-19 syndrome [37].

The efforts of a psychologist and psychotherapist in the rehabilitation of such patients can hardly be overestimated [38]. In addition to helping with the stress of the disease, reduced physical activity, the presence of autonomic and pain syndromes, painkillers, anxiolytics, and antidepressants can be prescribed. An important feature of the treatment of these conditions is, first of all, to identify the degree of anxiety and depression, which also affect the cognitive state of patients. Also, cognitive decrease in this group of patients may be the result of impaired brain blood supply, microcirculation dysfunction, and postural orthostatic tachycardia, which will be mentioned in the section describing dysautonomia of the internal organs [22].

A separate group of the post-COVID-19 complications include patients with manifestations of classical clinical pattern of polyneuropathy with pain syndrome and dysautonomia. The difficulties in the establishing this diagnosis begin, when no electrophysiological pattern on electroneuromyography is evaluated. In the most cases, this is a manifestation of the small fiber neuropathy, with the destruction of the smallest nerve fibers A delta and C type [22,39]. Sjogren's disease, systemic lupus erythematosus, celiac disease are the classical examples of the autoimmune disorders that may lead to the development of such complication [40]. On the other hand, in patients with fibromyalgia, chronic fatigue syndrome, and post-COVID-19 condition may also suffer from small fiber dysfunction. Diagnostic methods include skin biopsy, corneal confocal microscopy, quantitative sensory testing, and some validated scales such as COMPASS-31, SFN-SIQ, SFN-RODS, and others [41]. Once the diagnosis is established, the standard clinical protocols for the treatment of polyneuropathy may be applied, including anticonvulsants, antidepressants, medications that improve nerve conduction, and metabolism.

Small fiber neuropathy may play an important role in pathogenesis of fibromyalgic syndrome [42] associated with a novel coronavirus infection. Such patients are characterized by a widespread pain in four or five areas of the body for more than three months after an episode of a viral infection, muscle spasms, dysautonomia, sleep disorders, cognitive impairment, brain fog, and chronic fatigue. In the treatment of such patients, an important role is played by the timely evaluation of pain and the anticonvulsants, antidepressants, and muscle relaxers prescription, along with the physical therapy and rehabilitation.

Pathogenetic therapy with intravenous immunoglobulins may be beneficial, though such conception requires further research.

Loss of smell is a classic manifestation of the novel coronavirus infection. It is important to note that many patients will recover their olfactory function within a few months, while others either do not recover their sense of smell or have perversions of olfactory sensations. Treatment of this condition is complex and requires long-term management by both medical specialists and patients: olfactory training, intranasal corticosteroid drops, oral corticosteroids, and Omega 3 supplies [43].

Internal organ dysfunction in patients with post-COVID-19 condition

This section will not cover respiratory disorders, since, according to the authors' opinion, they are a considered to be a complication of an acute novel coronavirus infection and are widely covered in the recommendations for the treatment and rehabilitation of these patients.

One of the most common internal organ dysfunctions in patients with post-COVID-19 condition is a cardiovascular dysfunction. Such patients may develop microcirculatory disorders, as well as dysregulation of blood pressure and pulse, for example, postural orthostatic tachycardia and, in rare cases, orthostatic hypotension. Microcirculation disorders are corrected with appropriate medications [22,44]. This therapy may be of great value in patients who has complains like hair loss, unsatisfying skin and nail condition, and, possibly, also in patients with cognitive impairment. A conception is described, according to which cognitive disorders may be the result of a lack of blood circulation in certain parts of the brain in the post-COVID-19 patients. Orthostatic tachycardia is characterized with the increase by 30 beats or more for at least 2 min of observations when the patient is moved from the horizontal to the vertical position. Tachycardia, fatigue, darkening in the eyes, cognitive impairment, may be described in such patients [44]. This complication can be evaluated in 24 h Holter monitoring, passive and active orthostatic tests. Treatment for such patients may include physical rehabilitation, beta-blockers prescription, and breathing exercises aimed to decrease the daytime heart rate [45].

Conclusion

The main principle of successful therapy for post-COVID syndrome is a holistic, multidisciplinary approach involving a large team of medical specialists. Damage to small nerve fibers and the development of micro-, microcirculatory, and respiratory disorders in combination with autoimmune dysfunction, the development of hypercoagulability and immunological inflammation contributes to the progression of multiple organ dysfunction in these patients. Therefore, treatment options include corrections of all of the abovementioned conditions that require further extensive research.

References

[1] Santhosh L et al. "How i do it: rapid design & implementation of post-COVID clinics". Chest 4158. https://doi.org/10.1016/j.chest.2021.03.044.

[2] Malkova A, Kudryavtsev I, Starshinova A, Kudlay D, Zinchenko Y, Glushkova A, Yablonskiy P, Shoenfeld Y. Post COVID-19 syndrome in patients with asymptomatic/mild form. Pathogens October 30, 2021;10(11):1408. https://doi.org/10.3390/pathogens10111408. PMID: 34832564; PMCID: PMC8620929.
[3] Ehrenfeld M, Tincani A, Andreoli L, Cattalini M, Greenbaum A, Kanduc D, Alijotas-Reig J, Zinserling V, Semenova N, Amital H, Shoenfeld Y. Covid-19 and autoimmunity. Autoimmun Rev August 2020;19(8):102597. https://doi.org/10.1016/j.autrev.2020.102597. Epub 2020 Jun 11. PMID: 32535093; PMCID: PMC7289100.
[4] Tomar BS, Singh M, Nathiya D, Sharma A, Sharma E, Bareth H, Suman S, Ruparelia DP, Patel JB, Gajera VK, NIMS COVID 19 Investigator Group. Prevalence of symptoms in patients discharged from COVID care facility of NIMS hospital: is RT PCR negativity truly reflecting recovery? a single-centre observational study. Int J Gen Med March 2021;25(14):1069–78. https://doi.org/10.2147/IJGM.S295499. PMID: 33790636; PMCID: PMC8006813.
[5] Oran DP, Topol EJ. Prevalence of asymptomatic SARS-CoV-2 infection: a narrative review. Ann Intern Med 2020;173(5):362–7. https://doi.org/10.7326/M20-3012.
[6] Lopez-Leon S, Wegman-Ostrosky T, Perelman C, et al. More than 50 long-term effects of COVID-19: a systematic review and meta-analysis. Sci Rep 2021;11:16144. https://doi.org/10.1038/s41598-021-95565-8.
[7] Ryabkova VA, Churilov LP, Shoenfeld Y. Influenza infection, SARS, MERS and COVID-19: cytokine storm - the common denominator and the lessons to be learned. Clin Immunol February 2021;223:108652. https://doi.org/10.1016/j.clim.2020.108652. Epub 2020 Dec 14. PMID: 33333256; PMCID: PMC7832378.
[8] Halpert G, Shoenfeld Y. SARS-CoV-2, the autoimmune virus. Autoimmun Rev December 2020;19(12):102695. https://doi.org/10.1016/j.autrev.2020.102695. Epub 2020 Oct 28. PMID: 33130000; PMCID: PMC7598743.
[9] Moreno-Pérez O, et al. Post-acute COVID-19 syndrome. Incidence and risk factors: a Mediterranean cohort study. J Infect 2021;82(3):378–83. https://doi.org/10.1016/j.jinf.2021.01.004.
[10] Chopra V, Flanders SA, O'Malley M. Sixty-day outcomes among patients hospitalized with COVID-19. Ann Intern Med 2020;174(4):576–8. https://doi.org/10.7326/M20-5661.
[11] Fu L, Wang B, Yuan T, Chen X, Ao Y, Fitzpatrick T, Li P, Zhou Y, Lin Y, Duan Q, et al. Clinical characteristics of coronavirus disease 2019 (COVID-19) in China: a systematic review and meta-analysis. J Infect 2020;80:656–65.
[12] Dotan A, Muller S, Kanduc D, David P, Halpert G, Shoenfeld Y. The SARS-CoV-2 as an instrumental trigger of autoimmunity. Autoimmun Rev April 2021;20(4):102792. https://doi.org/10.1016/j.autrev.2021.102792. Epub 2021 Feb 19. PMID: 33610751; PMCID: PMC7892316.
[13] Dotan A, Shoenfeld Y. Post-COVID syndrome: the aftershock of SARS-CoV-2. Int J Infect Dis January 2022;114:233–5. https://doi.org/10.1016/j.ijid.2021.11.020. Epub 2021 Nov 14. PMID: 34785367; PMCID: PMC8590600.
[14] Barker-Davies RM, O'Sullivan O, Senaratne KPP, Baker P, Cranley M, Dharm-Datta S, Ellis H, Goodall D, Gough M, Lewis S, Norman J, Papadopoulou T, Roscoe D, Sherwood D, Turner P, Walker T, Mistlin A, Phillip R, Nicol AM, Bennett AN, Bahadur S. The Stanford Hall consensus statement for post-COVID-19 rehabilitation. Br J Sports Med August 2020;54(16):949–59. https://doi.org/10.1136/bjsports-2020-102596. Epub 2020 May 31. PMID: 32475821; PMCID: PMC7418628.
[15] Wostyn P. COVID-19 and chronic fatigue syndrome: is the worst yet to come? Med Hypotheses January 2021;146:110469. https://doi.org/10.1016/j.mehy.2020.110469. Epub 2021 Jan 2. PMID: 33401106; PMCID: PMC7836544.
[16] Moore N, Bosco-Levy P, Thurin N, Blin P, Droz-Perroteau C. NSAIDs and COVID-19: a systematic review and meta-analysis. Drug Saf September 2021;44(9):929–38. https://doi.org/10.1007/s40264-021-01089-5. Epub 2021 Aug 2. PMID: 34339037; PMCID: PMC8327046.
[17] Kocyigit BF, Akyol A. Reactive arthritis after COVID-19: a case-based review. Rheumatol Int November 2021;41(11):2031–9. https://doi.org/10.1007/s00296-021-04998-x. Epub 2021 Sep 22. PMID: 34550429; PMCID: PMC8456072.
[18] Colatutto D, Sonaglia A, Zabotti A, Cereser L, Girometti R, Quartuccio L. Post-COVID-19 arthritis and sacroiliitis: natural history with longitudinal magnetic resonance imaging study in two cases and review of the literature. Viruses August 6, 2021;13(8):1558. https://doi.org/10.3390/v13081558. PMID: 34452422; PMCID: PMC8402767.

[19] Passali M, Josefsen K, Frederiksen JL, Antvorskov JC. Current evidence on the efficacy of gluten-free diets in multiple sclerosis, psoriasis, type 1 diabetes and autoimmune thyroid diseases. Nutrients August 1, 2020;12(8):2316. https://doi.org/10.3390/nu12082316. PMID: 32752175; PMCID: PMC7468712.

[20] Palmieri B, Vadala' M, Laurino C. Gluten-free diet in non-celiac patients: beliefs, truths, advantages and disadvantages. Minerva Gastroenterol Dietol June 2019;65(2):153–62. https://doi.org/10.23736/S1121-421X.18.02519-9. Epub 2018 Dec 14. PMID: 30545212.

[21] Krysiak R, Szkróbka W, Okopień B. The effect of gluten-free diet on thyroid autoimmunity in drug-naïve women with hashimoto's thyroiditis: a pilot study. Exp Clin Endocrinol Diabetes July 2019;127(7):417–22. https://doi.org/10.1055/a-0653-7108. Epub 2018 Jul 30. PMID: 30060266.

[22] Novak P. Post COVID-19 syndrome associated with orthostatic cerebral hypoperfusion syndrome, small fiber neuropathy and benefit of immunotherapy: a case report. eNeurologicalSci December 2020;21:100276. https://doi.org/10.1016/j.ensci.2020.100276. Epub 2020 Sep 20. PMID: 32984564; PMCID: PMC7502253.

[23] Bureau BL, Obeidat A, Dhariwal MS, Jha P. Peripheral neuropathy as a complication of SARS-cov-2. Cureus November 12, 2020;12(11):e11452. https://doi.org/10.7759/cureus.11452. PMID: 33214969; PMCID: PMC7673277.

[24] Karbiener M, Farcet MR, Schwaiger J, Powers N, Lenart J, Stewart JM, Tallman H, Kreil TR. Plasma from post-COVID-19 and COVID-19-vaccinated donors results in highly potent SARS-CoV-2 neutralization by intravenous immunoglobulins. J Infect Dis September 2021;20:jiab482. https://doi.org/10.1093/infdis/jiab482. Epub ahead of print. PMID: 34543421; PMCID: PMC8499975.

[25] Gupta S, Chandra A, Ray BK, Pandit A. Treatment related fluctuation and response to intravenous immunoglobulin therapy in post COVID-19 Guillain-Barre syndrome. Diabetes Metabol Syndr 2021 ;15(5):102246. https://doi.org/10.1016/j.dsx.2021.102246. Epub 2021 Aug 13. PMID: 34416468; PMCID: PMC8361026.

[26] Kolahchi Z, Sohrabi H, Ekrami Nasab S, et al. Potential therapeutic approach of intravenous immunoglobulin against COVID-19. Allergy Asthma Clin Immunol 2021;17:105. https://doi.org/10.1186/s13223-021-00609-3.

[27] Abdelalim AA, Mohamady AA, Elsayed RA, Elawady MA, Ghallab AF. Corticosteroid nasal spray for recovery of smell sensation in COVID-19 patients: a randomized controlled trial. Am J Otolaryngol 2021 ;42(2):102884. https://doi.org/10.1016/j.amjoto.2020.102884. Epub 2021 Jan 4. PMID: 33429174; PMCID: PMC7836546.

[28] Sánchez J, Cohen M, Zapater JL, Eisenberg Y. Primary adrenal insufficiency after COVID-19 infection. AACE Clin Case Rep November 14, 2021. https://doi.org/10.1016/j.aace.2021.11.001. Epub ahead of print. PMID: 34805497; PMCID: PMC8590605.

[29] Güler T, Yurdakul FG, Acar Sivas F, Kiliç Z, Adigüzel E, Yasar E, Bodur H. Rehabilitative management of post-acute COVID-19: clinical pictures and outcomes. Rheumatol Int December 2021;41(12):2167–75. https://doi.org/10.1007/s00296-021-05003-1. Epub 2021 Sep 27. PMID: 34580754.

[30] Truong AD, Auld SC, Barker NA, Friend S, Wynn AT, Cobb J, Sniecinski RM, Tanksley CL, Polly DM, Gaddh M, Connor M, Nakahara H, Sullivan HC, Kempton C, Guarner J, Duncan A, Josephson CD, Roback JD, Stowell SR, Maier CL. Therapeutic plasma exchange for COVID-19-associated hyperviscosity. Transfusion April 2021;61(4):1029–34. https://doi.org/10.1111/trf.16218. Epub 2020 Dec 9. PMID: 33231313; PMCID: PMC7753437.

[31] Watad A, Quaresma M, Bragazzi NL, Cervera R, Tervaert JWC, Amital H, Shoenfeld Y. The autoimmune/inflammatory syndrome induced by adjuvants (ASIA)/Shoenfeld's syndrome: descriptive analysis of 300 patients from the international ASIA syndrome registry. Clin Rheumatol February 2018;37(2):483–93. https://doi.org/10.1007/s10067-017-3748-9. Epub 2017 Jul 25. PMID: 28741088.

[32] Solomon IH, Normandin E, Bhattacharyya S, Mukerji SS, Keller K, Ali AS, Adams G, Hornick JL, Padera RF, Sabeti P. Neuropathological features of covid-19. N Engl J Med 2020;383:989–92.

[33] Paterson RW, Brown RL, Benjamin L, Nortley R, Wiethoff S, Bharucha T, Jayaseelan DL, Kumar G, Raftopoulos RE, Zambreanu L, et al. The emerging spectrum of COVID-19 neurology: clinical, radiological and laboratory findings. Brain 2020;143:3104–20.

[34] Koralnik IJ, Tyler KL. COVID-19: a global threat to the nervous system. Ann Neurol July 2020;88(1):1–11. https://doi.org/10.1002/ana.25807 Epub.

[35] Lucchese G, Flöel A. SARS-CoV-2 and Guillain-Barré syndrome: molecular mimicry with human heat shock proteins as potential pathogenic mechanism. Cell Stress Chaperones 2020;25(5):731–5.

[36] Al-Ramadan A, Rabab'h O, Shah J, Gharaibeh A. Acute and post-acute neurological complications of COVID-19. Neurol Int 2021;13(1):102–19. https://doi.org/10.3390/neurolint13010010. Published 2021 Mar 9.
[37] https://www.who.int/publications-detail-redirect/WHO-2019-nCoV-Post_COVID-19_condition-Clinical_case_definition-2021.1.
[38] Vink M, Vink-Niese A. Could cognitive Behavioural therapy Be an effective treatment for long COVID and post COVID-19 fatigue syndrome? lessons from the qure study for Q-fever fatigue syndrome. Healthcare (Basel) December 11, 2020;8(4):552. https://doi.org/10.3390/healthcare8040552. PMID: 33322316; PMCID: PMC7764131.
[39] Abrams RMC, Simpson DM, Navis A, Jette N, Zhou L, Shin SC. Small fiber neuropathy associated with SARS-CoV-2 infection. Muscle Nerve November 12, 2021. https://doi.org/10.1002/mus.27458. Epub ahead of print. PMID: 34766365; PMCID: PMC8661991.
[40] Basantsova NY, Starshinova AA, Dori A, Zinchenko YS, Yablonskiy PK, Shoenfeld Y. Small-fiber neuropathy definition, diagnosis, and treatment. Neurol Sci July 2019;40(7):1343–50. https://doi.org/10.1007/s10072-019-03871-x. Epub 2019 Apr 9. PMID: 30968230.
[41] Shouman K, Vanichkachorn G, Cheshire WP, Suarez MD, Shelly S, Lamotte GJ, Sandroni P, Benarroch EE, Berini SE, Cutsforth-Gregory JK, Coon EA, Mauermann ML, Low PA, Singer W. Autonomic dysfunction following COVID-19 infection: an early experience. Clin Auton Res June 2021;31(3):385–94. https://doi.org/10.1007/s10286-021-00803-8. Epub 2021 Apr 16. PMID: 33860871; PMCID: PMC8050227.
[42] Martínez-Lavín M. Fibromyalgia and small fiber neuropathy: the plot thickens! Clin Rheumatol December 2018;37(12):3167–71. https://doi.org/10.1007/s10067-018-4300-2. Epub 2018 Sep 20. PMID: 30238382.
[43] Hopkins C, Alanin M, Philpott C, Harries P, Whitcroft K, Qureishi A, Anari S, Ramakrishnan Y, Sama A, Davies E, Stew B, Gane S, Carrie S, Hathorn I, Bhalla R, Kelly C, Hill N, Boak D, Nirmal Kumar B. Management of new onset loss of sense of smell during the COVID-19 pandemic - BRS Consensus Guidelines. Clin Otolaryngol January 2021;46(1):16–22. https://doi.org/10.1111/coa.13636. Epub 2020 Sep 24. PMID: 32854169; PMCID: PMC7461026.
[44] Dixit NM, Churchill A, Nsair A, Hsu JJ. Post-Acute COVID-19 Syndrome and the cardiovascular system: what is known? Am Heart J May 2021;5:100025. https://doi.org/10.1016/j.ahjo.2021.100025. Epub 2021 Jun 24. PMID: 34192289; PMCID: PMC8223036.
[45] Larsen NW, Stiles LE, Miglis MG. Preparing for the long-haul: autonomic complications of COVID-19. Auton Neurosci November 2021;235:102841. https://doi.org/10.1016/j.autneu.2021.102841. Epub 2021 Jul 3. PMID: 34265539; PMCID: PMC8254396.

Index

Note: 'Page numbers followed by "f" indicate figures and "t" indicates tables'.

D

J

K

L

N

R

S

CPI Antony Rowe
Eastbourne, UK
December 10, 2022